Published by the American Medical Association

January 1989
Volume 124, Number 1

archives of Surgery

EDITORIALS

Hail and Farewell — *A. E. Baue*

A New Editor for the Archives — *M. D. Springer*

Inaugural Editorial — *C. H. Organ, Jr*

PROGRAM OF THE SOCIETY OF SURGICAL ONCOLOGY—1988—PART I

The Prognostic Significance of Lymph Node Metastases After Preoperative Chemotherapy for Locally Advanced Breast Cancer — *D. R. McCready, G. N. Hortobagyi, S. W. Kau, T. L. Smith, A. U. Buzdar, C. M. Balch*

A Comparison of Palpable and Nonpalpable Breast Cancers — *T. J. Pagana, W. J. Lubbe, S. M. Schwartz, G. D. Sprechini*

Nonpalpable In Situ Ductal Carcinoma of the Breast — *G. F. Schwartz, A. S. Patchefsky, S. D. Finklestein, S. H. Sohn, A. Prestipino, S. A. Feig, J. S. Singer*

Breast Carcinoma In Situ — *D. W. Kinne, J. A. Petrek, M. P. Osborne, A. A. Fracchia, A. A. DePalo, P. P. Rosen*

Implications of Accurate Pathologic Margins in the Treatment of Primary Breast Cancer — *T. G. Frazier, R. W. Y. Wong, D. Rose*

Lability of Steroid Hormone Receptors Following Devascularization of Breast Tumors — *L. M. Ellis, J. L. Wittliff, M. S. Bryant, H. S. Sitren, W. E. Hogancamp, W. W. Souba, K. I. Bland*

Cancer Centers—Origins and Purpose — *W. W. Shingleton*

Results of Surgical Excision of One to 13 Hepatic Metastases in 98 Consecutive Patients — *J. P. Minton, W. B. Hamilton, A. Sardi, C. Nieroda, B. Sickle-Santanello, P. J. O'Dwyer*

Experimental Liver Metastasis — *T. S. Ravikumar, J. D'Emilia, C. Cocchiaro, B. Wolf, V. King, G. Steele, Jr*

Intra-abdominal Recurrence of Colorectal Cancer Detected by Radioimmunoguided Surgery (RIGS System) — *A. Sardi, M. Workman, C. Mojzisik, G. Hinkle, C. Nieroda, E. W. Martin, Jr*

Rationale for Aggressive Colonoscopy in Patients With Colorectal Neoplasia — *K. S. Dasmahapatra, K. Lopyan*

Prospective Phase I Trial of Conservative Management of Low Rectal Lesions — *D. R. McCready, D. M. Ota, T. A. Rich, D. Thielvoldt, J. M. Jessup*

Staging Renal Carcinoma — *M. A. Benson, J. R. Haaga, M. I. Resnick*

Photodynamic Therapy for Esophageal Tumors — *J. S. McCaughan, Jr, T. A. Nims, J. T. Guy, W. J. Hicks, T. E. Williams, Jr, L. R. Laufman*

Effect of Timing of Lymphokine Presentation on Generation of Cytotoxic T Lymphocytes — *M. M. Stringfellow, R. E. Wilson, S. J. Burakoff, S. H. Herrmann*

Natural Killer Sensitivity of Colorectal Carcinoma Targets — *D. J. Bägli, G. D. Steele, Jr, T. Barlozzari*

Complete Contents p 5

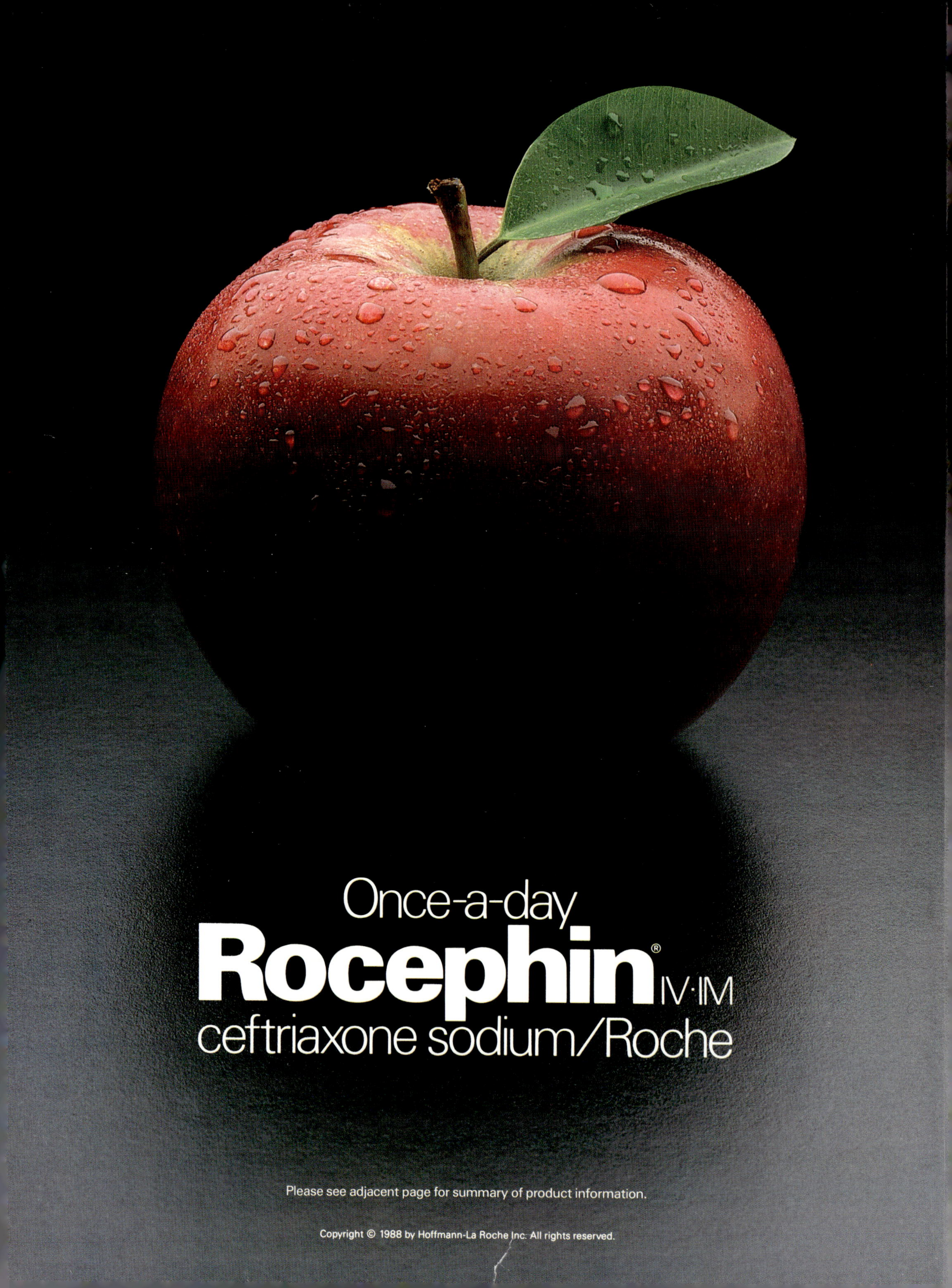
Once-a-day
Rocephin® IV·IM
ceftriaxone sodium/Roche
Please see adjacent page for summary of product information.
Copyright © 1988 by Hoffmann-La Roche Inc. All rights reserved.

Archives of Surgery

JANUARY 1989 VOLUME 124 NUMBER 1

Official Publication of the Western Surgical Association, Surgical Infection Society, New England Surgical Society, Society of Surgical Oncology, Pacific Coast Surgical Association

EDITORIALS

Hail and Farewell ... 17
Arthur E. Baue, MD, St Louis

A New Editor for the Archives ... 18
Michael D. Springer, Chicago

Inaugural Editorial ... 19
Claude H. Organ, Jr, MD, Oakland, Calif

PAPERS READ BEFORE THE ANNUAL MEETING OF THE SOCIETY OF SURGICAL ONCOLOGY, NEW ORLEANS, MAY 22 TO MAY 25, 1988—Part I

The Prognostic Significance of Lymph Node Metastases After Preoperative Chemotherapy for Locally Advanced Breast Cancer ... 21
David R. McCready, MD; Gabriel N. Hortobagyi, MD; Shu W. Kau, RN; Terry L. Smith, MS; Aman U. Buzdar, MD; Charles M. Balch, MD, Houston
- The number of lymph nodes with metastatic cancer had more prognostic value than other factors.

A Comparison of Palpable and Nonpalpable Breast Cancers ... 26
Timothy J. Pagana, MD; Willem J. Lubbe, MD; Sheldon M. Schwartz, MD; Gene D. Sprechini, PhD, Williamsport, Pa
- Obviously, nonpalpable breast cancers were smaller and more frequently noninvasive and less frequently had metastasized to lymph nodes.

Nonpalpable In Situ Ductal Carcinoma of the Breast: Predictors of Multicentricity and Microinvasion and Implications for Treatment ... 29
Gordon F. Schwartz, MD; Arthur S. Patchefsky, MD; Sidney D. Finklestein, MD; Sae H. Sohn, MD; Anthony Prestipino, MD; Stephen A. Feig, MD; Jodi S. Singer, MD, Philadelphia
- Ductal carcinoma in situ as an incidental finding may be treated by excision alone.

Breast Carcinoma In Situ ... 33
David W. Kinne, MD; Jeanne A. Petrek, MD; Michael P. Osborne, MD; Alfred A. Fracchia, MD; Angelo A. DePalo, MD; Paul Peter Rosen, MD, New York
- Axillary dissection is not indicated for in situ breast cancer.

Implications of Accurate Pathologic Margins in the Treatment of Primary Breast Cancer ... 37
Thomas G. Frazier, MD, Bryn Mawr, Pa; Randolph W. Y. Wong, MD, Philadelphia; David Rose, MD, Bryn Mawr, Pa
- Patients with clear or close margins after segmental resection of breast cancer were found to have residual tumor with subsequent reexcision.

Lability of Steroid Hormone Receptors Following Devascularization of Breast Tumors ... 39
Lee M. Ellis, MD, Gainesville, Fla; James L. Wittliff, PhD, Louisville; Michael S. Bryant, MD, Harry S. Sitren, PhD, Gainesville, Fla; William E. Hogancamp, Louisville; Wiley W. Souba, MD, ScD, Kirby I. Bland, MD, Gainesville, Fla
- Thirty minutes of tissue ischemia before processing resulted in a decrease in estrogen and androgen receptors.

Cancer Centers—Origins and Purpose: The James Ewing Lecture ... 43
William W. Shingleton, MD, Durham, NC
- Comprehensive cancer centers have been important, but continuous evaluation of their effectiveness is necessary.

Results of Surgical Excision of One to 13 Hepatic Metastases in 98 Consecutive Patients ... 46
John P. Minton, MD, PhD; Walter B. Hamilton; Armando Sardi, MD; Carol Nieroda, MD; Brenda Sickle-Santanello, MD; Patrick J. O'Dwyer, MD, Columbus, Ohio
- Resection of multiple liver metastases by local removal using electrocautery was associated with prolonged survival in a number of patients.

Experimental Liver Metastasis: Implications of Clonal Proclivity and Organ Specificity ... 49
T. S. Ravikumar, MD; John D'Emilia, MD; Celia Cocchiaro; Barbara Wolf, MD; Vincent King; Glenn Steele, Jr, MD, PhD, Boston
- Spontaneous metastases to lung and liver were established in this animal model.

The **ARCHIVES OF SURGERY** (ISSN 0004-0010) is published monthly by the American Medical Association, 535 N Dearborn St, Chicago, IL 60610, and is an official publication of the Association. Second-class postage paid at Chicago, IL 60610 and at additional mailing office.

SUBSCRIPTION RATES—The subscription rates for the ARCHIVES OF SURGERY are as follows: $50 for one year, $85 for two years in the United States and US possessions; all other countries, one year, $60; two years, $105 for surface delivery. (For expedited air delivery to most countries, add $15 surcharge for one-year subscription, $30 for two years.) Rates for subscriptions for delivery to Japan or South Korea are available through exclusive agents—contact the publisher. ***Special rates for residents and medical students in the United States and US possessions are available.*** Address inquiries to the American Medical Association, Circulation and Fulfillment Division, 535 N Dearborn St, Chicago, IL 60610. Phone: (312)280-7168.

CHANGE OF ADDRESS—POSTMASTER, send all address changes for the ARCHIVES OF SURGERY to Caryl L. Wertheimer, Director of Fulfillment, 535 N Dearborn St, Chicago, IL 60610. Notification of address change must be made at least six weeks in advance, include both old and new addresses, a recent mailing label, and your new zip code.

CONTENTS—Continued

Intra-abdominal Recurrence of Colorectal Cancer Detected by Radioimmunoguided Surgery (RIGS System) 55
Armando Sardi, MD; Mark Workman; Cathy Mojzisik, RN, MS; George Hinkle, RPh; Carol Nieroda, MD; Edward W. Martin, Jr, MD, Columbus, Ohio
- In some patients undergoing second-look operations, recurrent tumor was located only by the technique of radiolabeled monoclonal antibodies.

Rationale for Aggressive Colonoscopy in Patients With Colorectal Neoplasia 63
Kumar S. Dasmahapatra, MD, Kevin Lopyan, MD, Newark, NJ
- Metachronous colon cancers were found by colonoscopy as late as 60 months after an initial cancer resection.

Prospective Phase I Trial of Conservative Management of Low Rectal Lesions 67
David R. McCready, MD; David M. Ota, MD; Tyvin A. Rich, MD; Diva Thielvoldt, RN; J. Milburn Jessup, MD, Houston
- In selected patients with low rectal cancer, local excision and radiotherapy was done with early, good results.

Staging Renal Carcinoma: What Is Sufficient? 71
Mark A. Benson, MD; John R. Haaga, MD; Martin I. Resnick, MD, Cleveland
- Computed tomography is the principal technique for overall staging of renal cell carcinoma.

Photodynamic Therapy for Esophageal Tumors 74
James S. McCaughan, Jr, MD; Thomas A. Nims, MD; Jerry T. Guy, MD; William J. Hicks, MD; Thomas E. Williams Jr, MD; Leslie R. Laufman, MD, Columbus, Ohio
- Improvement in ability to swallow was provided in a number of patients.

Effect of Timing of Lymphokine Presentation on Generation of Cytotoxic T Lymphocytes 81
Monica M. Stringfellow, MD; Richard E. Wilson, MD; Steven J. Burakoff, MD; Steven H. Herrmann, MD, Boston
- Both interleukin 1 and interleukin 6 are required for optimal generation of cytotoxic T lymphocytes.

Natural Killer Sensitivity of Colorectal Carcinoma Targets: Correlation With Degree of Differentiation 89
Darius J. Bägli, MD, CM; Glenn D. Steele, Jr, MD, PhD; Teresa Barlozzari, PhD, Boston
- Poorly differentiated colorectal cancer cells were susceptible to natural killer cell lysis.

Cachectin Activity in the Serum of Cachectic, Tumor-Bearing Rats 94
Mark C. Stovroff, MD; Douglas L. Fraker, MD; Jeffrey A. Norton, MD, Bethesda, Md
- Serum cachectic activity correlated with tumor burden, and the levels became undetectable following tumor resection.

The Flip Side of Tumor Immunity 102
Richmond T. Prehn, MD, Liisa M. Prehn, MD, Seattle
- Immunosuppression may be as likely to have a therapeutic effect as immunoaugmentation.

Recombinant Human Tumor Necrosis Factor Alone and With Chemotherapeutic Agents: Effect on Nude Mouse–Supported Human Bladder Cancer Heterografts 107
Anurag K. Das, MD; Philip J. Walther, MD, PhD; Niall J. Buckley, MD; Susan H. M. Poulton, Durham, NC
- Synergism between recombinant human tumor necrosis factor and chemotherapeutic agents was found only with etoposide.

Squamous Cell Carcinoma Arising in Previously Burned or Irradiated Skin 115
Michael J. Edwards, MD; Rose M. Hirsch, MD; J. Ralph Broadwater, MD; David T. Netscher, MD; Frederick C. Ames, MD, Houston
- Chronic ulceration in scar tissue should suggest this diagnosis.

Is Limb-Sparing Surgery Applicable to Neurogenic Sarcomas of the Extremities? 118
John S. Bolton, MD; Jean-Nicolas Vauthey, MD; Gist H. Farr, Jr, MD; Edward I. Sauter, MD; John C. Bowen III, MD; David G. Kline, MD, New Orleans
- Patients with high-grade neurogenic sarcomas of the extremities have a high risk of local recurrence after limb-sparing operative treatment.

Patterns of Recurrence After Resection of Osteosarcoma of the Extremity: Strategies for Treatment of Metastases 122
James F. Huth, MD, Frederick R. Eilber, MD, Los Angeles
- The prognosis is particularly bad with metastases to the lung and other sites.

Clinical Experience With Regional Pancreatectomy for Adenocarcinoma of the Pancreas 127
William F. Sindelar, MD, PhD, Bethesda, Md
- Regional pancreatectomy with en bloc pancreatectomy and removal of regional nodes, duodenum, gastric antrum, and intrapancreatic portal vein produced little survival benefit for most patients.

REGULAR DEPARTMENTS

Correspondence and Brief Communications 133

Books 134

Calendar of Events 135

Instructions for Authors 10

Index to Advertisers 13

Archives of Surgery FEBRUARY 1989 VOLUME 124 NUMBER 2

Official Publication of the Western Surgical Association, Surgical Infection Society, New England Surgical Society, Society of Surgical Oncology, Pacific Coast Surgical Association

PAPERS READ BEFORE THE ANNUAL MEETING OF THE SOCIETY OF SURGICAL ONCOLOGY, NEW ORLEANS, LA, MAY 22 TO MAY 25, 1988—Part II

Conservative Surgery and Radiation Therapy for Early Breast Cancer: Long-term Cosmetic Results 153
Mary Ann Rose, MD, Boston, Mass; Ivo Olivotto, MD, Vancouver, Canada; Blake Cady, MD; Clinton Koufman, MD; Robert Osteen, MD; Barbara Silver; Abram Recht, MD; Jay R. Harris, MD, Boston, Mass
• Satisfactory cosmetic results after conservative operations and radiation therapy are maintained for at least seven years.

Local Recurrent Mammary Carcinoma Failing Multimodality Therapy: A Solution 158
Patricia M. McCormack, MD; Manjit S. Bains, MD; Michael E. Burt, MD, PhD; Nael Martini, MD; Ted Chaglassian, MD; David A. Hidalgo, MD, New York, NY
• Chest wall resection and reconstruction offer significant palliation.

Extent of Lymph Node Dissection in Melanoma of the Trunk or Lower Extremity 162
Daniel G. Coit, MD, Murray F. Brennan, MD, New York, NY
• More extensive lymphadenectomy was not associated with improved survival or decreased recurrence.

Hepatectomy Prolongs Survival of Mice With Induced Liver Metastases 167
Manuel H. Castillo, MD; Ralph J. Doerr, MD; Norman Paolini, Jr, MS; Stephen Cohen, PhD; Martin Goldrosen, PhD, Buffalo, NY
• Hepatectomy prolonged survival when performed after tumor cell injection.

Partial Hepatectomy Augments the Liver's Antitumor Response 170
Ralph Doerr, MD; Manuel Castillo, MD; Paul Evans, MS; Norman Paolini, MS; Martin Goldrosen, PhD; Stephan A. Cohen, PhD, Buffalo, NY
• Partial hepatectomy enhanced the antitumor activity of nonparenchymal liver cells.

Prolongation of Survival of Nude Mice Bearing Human Colon Cancer: Treatment With Yttrium 90–Labeled Anti–Carcinoembryonic Antigen Antibody 175
David M. Hyams, MD; Jose M. Esteban, MD; Barbara G. Beatty, PhD, Duarte, Calif; Philip M. Wanek, RPh, San Diego, Calif; J. David Beatty, MD, Duarte, Calif
• Different dosing regimens had very different results in this animal model.

Survival of Patients With Stage B2 Colon Carcinoma: The Gastrointestinal Tumor Study Group Experience 180
Russell Nauta, MD, Washington, DC; Donald M. Stablein, PhD, Potomac, Md; E. Douglas Holyoke, MD, Buffalo, NY
• Because of excellent survival, patients with stage B2 colon carcinoma are seldom candidates for adjuvant trials of toxic therapy.

Interactions of Human Colorectal Carcinoma Cells With Basement Membranes: Analysis and Correlation With Differentiation 183
George W. Daneker, Jr, MD; Andrew J. Piazza; Glenn D. Steele, Jr, MD, PhD; Arthur M. Mercurio, PhD, Boston, Mass
• Tumor cell adherence and poor differentiation correlate with invasion of basement membranes.

The **ARCHIVES OF SURGERY** (ISSN 0004-0010) is published monthly by the American Medical Association, 535 N Dearborn St, Chicago, IL 60610, and is an official publication of the Association. Second-class postage paid at Chicago, IL 60610 and at additional mailing office.

SUBSCRIPTION RATES—The subscription rates for the ARCHIVES OF SURGERY are as follows: $50 for one year, $85 for two years in the United States and US possessions; all other countries, one year, $60; two years, $105 for surface delivery. (For expedited air delivery to most countries, add $15 surcharge for one-year subscription, $30 for two years.) Rates for subscriptions for delivery to Japan or South Korea are available through exclusive agents—contact the publisher. ***Special rates for residents and medical students in the United States and US possessions are available.*** Address inquiries to the American Medical Association, Circulation and Fulfillment Division, 535 N Dearborn St, Chicago, IL 60610. Phone: (312)280-7168.

CHANGE OF ADDRESS—POSTMASTER, send all address changes for the ARCHIVES OF SURGERY to Caryl L. Wertheimer, Director of Fulfillment, 535 N Dearborn St, Chicago, IL 60610. Notification of address change must be made at least six weeks in advance, include both old and new addresses, a recent mailing label, and your new zip code.

CONTENTS—Continued

The Desmoid Tumor: Not a Benign Disease 191
Mitchell C. Posner, MD; Man H. Shiu, MD; James L. Newsome, MD; Steven I. Hajdu, MD; Jeffrey J. Gaynor, PhD; Murray F. Brennan, MD, New York, NY
- Desmoid tumors are malignant soft-tissue neoplasms that require aggressive therapy.

Scar or Recurrent Rectal Cancer: Positron Emission Tomography Is More Helpful for Diagnosis Than Immunoscintigraphy 197
Peter Schlag, MD; Burkhard Lehner, MD; Ludwig G. Strauss, MD; Peter Georgi, MD; Christian Herfarth, MD, Heidelberg, Federal Republic of Germany
- All patients with increased uptake of flu-deoxyglucose F 18 by positron emission tomography had recurrent rectal cancer.

Prognostic Significance of Cellular Immunity to Autologous Breast Carcinoma and Glycoprotein 55 202
Maurice M. Black, MD; Reinhard E. Zachrau, MD; Roy H. Ashikari, MD, Valhalla, NY; Benjamin F. Hankey, ScD, Bethesda, Md
- Cellular immunity as measured by skin window reactivity to autologous breast cancer is prognostically favorable.

Photodynamic Therapy for Cutaneous and Subcutaneous Malignant Neoplasms 211
James S. McCaughan, Jr, MD; Jerry T. Guy, MD; William Hicks, MD; Leslie Laufman, MD; Thomas A. Nims, MD; John Walker, Columbus, Ohio
- Photodynamic therapy produced a complete response with no evidence of tumor in a number of patients.

Antioxidants vs Carotenoids: Inhibitors or Promoters of Experimental Colorectal Cancers 217
Thomas A. Colacchio, MD; Vincent A. Memoli, MD; Laurie Hildebrandt, Hanover, NH
- Ascorbic acid and alpha-tocopherol demonstrated a chemopreventive effect against induced murine tumors.

Plasma Ultrafiltration as Cancer Therapy 222
Alan Wile, MD, Orange, Calif
- Serum ultrafiltration therapy in six patients reduced their serum suppressor factors.

Endoscopic Ablation of Esophageal Malignancies With the Neodymium-YAG Laser and Electrofulguration 225
Hector R. Nava, MD; Marlys E. Schuh, MD; Raman Nambisan, MD; John L. Clark, MD; Harold O. Douglass, Jr, MD, Buffalo, NY
- Both techniques improved swallowing with mean survival for these patients of 11 months.

Are Complications in Intraoperative Radiation Therapy More Frequent Than in Conventional Treatment? 229
Douglas T. Cromack, MD; Michelle M. Maher, RN; Harald Hoekstra, MD, PhD; Timothy J. Kinsella, MD; William F. Sindelar, MD, PhD, Bethesda, Md
- No, complications are not more frequent with intraoperative radiation therapy!

The Influence of Natural Killer Cells in Neuroblastoma 235
John V. Reynolds, FRCS(I); Jian Shou, MD; Hoon Choi, MD; Robert Sigal, MD; Moritz M. Ziegler, MD; John M. Daly, MD, Philadelphia, Pa
- In vivo depletion of natural killer cells enhanced tumor growth and decreased survival in this animal model.

ORIGINAL ARTICLES

Pseudocysts in Chronic Pancreatitis: Surgical Results in 102 Consecutive Patients 240
Tuula Kiviluoto, MD; Leena Kivisaari, MD; Eero Kivilaakso, MD; Matti Lempinen, MD, Helsinki, Finland
- In patients with chronic pancreatitis and pseudocysts, internal drainage or resection produced the most satisfactory results.

Single-Dose Antibiotic Prophylaxis in Contaminated Abdominal Surgery 244
John C. Hall, FRACS, Perth, Western Australia; J. McK. Watts, FRACS, Lexi Press, RN, Bedford Park, South Australia; P. O'Brien, FRACS, Melbourne, Australia; J. Turnidge, FRACP, P. McDonald, FRACP, Bedford Park, South Australia
- In patients undergoing contaminated abdominal operations, a single dose of prophylactic antibiotic was as effective as an extended course of antibiotics.

Long-term Survival in Carcinoma of the Biliary Tract: Analysis of Prognostic Factors in 146 Resections 248
Kiyoaki Ouchi, MD; Seiki Matsuno, MD; Toshio Sato, MD, Sendai, Japan
- Following resection, 41% of patients with gallbladder cancer and approximately 23% of patients with bile duct cancer lived 5 years.

Follow-up of Patients With Aspirated Breast Cysts Is Necessary 253
Hisham Hamed, MD; Andrew Coady, MS; Murid A. Chaudary; Ian S. Fentiman, MD, London, England
- Reexamination six weeks following aspiration of a breast cyst is necessary.

REGULAR DEPARTMENTS

Correspondence and Brief Communications 256

Books 258

Instructions for Authors 148

Index to Advertisers 149

Archives of Surgery

MARCH 1989 VOLUME 124 NUMBER 3

Official Publication of the Western Surgical Association, Surgical Infection Society, New England Surgical Society, Society of Surgical Oncology, Pacific Coast Surgical Association

ORIGINAL ARTICLES

Evaluation of Prostacyclin Production by Human Gallbladder 277
Donald L. Kaminski, MD; Y. G. Deshpande, MS; Scott Westfall, MD; David Herbold, MD, St Louis, Mo
- Prostacyclin formation may be an important mediator of the inflammatory changes of cholecystitis.

The Efficacy of Oral Antimicrobials in Reducing Aerobic and Anaerobic Colonic Mucosal Flora 281
Jonathan I. Groner, MD; Charles E. Edmiston, Jr, PhD; Candace J. Krepel; Gordon L. Telford, MD; Robert E. Condon, MD, MS, Milwaukee, Wis
- Oral antibiotics with mechanical cleansing, but not mechanical preparation alone, decreased mucosa-associated bacteria.

Emergency Abdominal Operations in the Patient With Acquired Immunodeficiency Syndrome 285
Joshua H. Burack, MD; Marc S. Mandel, MD; Lawrence S. Bizer, MD, Bronx, NY
- Mortality rate was high following emergency intra-abdominal operations in AIDS patients.

Errors in Estimating Energy Expenditure in Critically Ill Surgical Patients 287
Vincente Cortes, MD, Miami, Fla, Loren D. Nelson, MD, Nashville, Tenn
- Because of overestimation of the stress factor, calculated or estimated energy expenditure was greater than measured energy expenditure.

Hemostasis of Solid Viscus Trauma by Intraparenchymal Injection of Fibrin Glue 291
Carl J. Hauser, MD, Los Angeles, Calif
- Intraparenchymal hepatic fibrin glue injection was a more effective hemostatic agent than was topical fibrin glue.

Neutron Therapy for Nonresectable Radioresistant Tumors 294
Lionel Cohen, MD, Frank R. Hendrickson, MD, Batavia, Ill
- High-energy fast neutron beams are a valuable adjunct to manage some tumors that are resistant to conventional therapy.

Gallbladder Response to Enteral Lipids in Injured Patients 301
Ronald C. Merrell, MD; Priscilla Miller-Crotchett, RN; Patricia Lowry, MD, Houston, Tex
- After injury these patients had modest enlargement and diminished contractions of the gallbladder that were not improved with enteral lipids.

Gastric Adenocarcinoma: A Disease in Transition 303
Blake Cady, MD, Boston; Ricardo L. Rossi, MD, Mark L. Silverman, MD, Burlington, Mass; William Piccione, MD, Chicago, Ill; Thomas A. Heck, MD, Dayton, Ohio
- Twenty-seven (47%) of 57 patients who underwent resection for cure survived five years.

Is Extensive Lymphadenectomy Necessary for Surgical Treatment of Intramucosal Carcinoma of the Stomach? 309
Keiji Iriyama, MD; Toyomatsu Asakawa, MD; Hiroshi Koike, MD; Hiroshi Nishiwake, MD; Hiroshi Suzuki, MD, Tsu, Japan
- Lymph node metastases are unlikely in patients with protruding, intramucosal intestinal type gastric carcinomas less than 5 cm in size.

DNA Ploidy and Tumor Invasion in Human Gastric Cancer: Histopathologic Differentiation 314
Daisuke Korenaga, MD; Masaru Haraguchi, MD; Takeshi Okamura, MD; Hideo Baba, MD; Atsushi Saito, MD; Keizo Sugimachi, MD, Fukuoka, Japan
- Aneuploid DNA patterns were associated with more aggressive gastric cancer than were diploid DNA profiles.

The **ARCHIVES OF SURGERY** (ISSN 0004-0010) is published monthly by the American Medical Association, 535 N Dearborn St, Chicago, IL 60610, and is an official publication of the Association. Second-class postage paid at Chicago, IL 60610 and at additional mailing office.

SUBSCRIPTION RATES—The subscription rates for the ARCHIVES OF SURGERY are as follows: $50 for one year, $85 for two years in the United States and US possessions; all other countries, one year, $60; two years, $105 for surface delivery. (For expedited air delivery to most countries, add $15 surcharge for one-year subscription, $30 for two years.) Rates for subscriptions for delivery to Japan or South Korea are available through exclusive agents—contact the publisher. ***Special rates for residents and medical students in the United States and US possessions are available.*** Address inquiries to the American Medical Association, Circulation and Fulfillment Division, 535 N Dearborn St, Chicago, IL 60610. Phone: (312)280-7168.

CHANGE OF ADDRESS—POSTMASTER, send all address changes for the ARCHIVES OF SURGERY to Subscription Department, 535 N Dearborn St, Chicago, IL 60610. Notification of address change must be made at least six weeks in advance, include both old and new addresses, a recent mailing label, and your new zip code.

CONTENTS—Continued

Prophylactic Antibiotherapy in Abdominal Surgery: First- vs Third-Generation Cephalosporins 323
Nelly Rotman, MD, Creteil, France; Jean-Marie Hay, MD, Colombes, France; Françoise Lacaine, MD, Paris, France; Pierre-Louis Fagniez, MD, Creteil, France; Association de Recherche en Chirurgie Cooperative Group, Bois-Colombes, France
• Cephalosporin prophylaxis was helpful in clean operations, in clean contaminated operations, and in patients with general increased risk of infection.

Guidelines for Practical Utilization of Intraoperative Frozen Sections 331
Marianne U. Prey, MD, St Louis, Mo; Thomas Vitale, MD, Melbourne, Fla; Scott A. Martin, MD, St Louis, Mo
• Intraoperative frozen-section interpretation was associated with 0.15% false-positive and 2.8% false-negative diagnosis rates.

Comparison of Antibody Response With Delayed Hypersensitivity in Severely Injured Patients 339
Michael J. Hershman, FRCS; William G. Cheadle, MD; Sarah H. Appel; Christopher D. George, FRCS; Pattie F. Davidson, RN; Karen M. Cost, PhD; Hiram C. Polk, Jr, MD, Louisville, Ky
• Clinical outcome and antibody response were determined by the extent of initial bacterial contamination.

Computed Tomography and Diagnostic Peritoneal Lavage in Blunt Abdominal Trauma: Their Combined Role 344
Paul A. Kearney, Jr, MD; Thomas Vahey, MD; Richard E. Burney, MD; Gary Glazer, MD, Ann Arbor, Mich
• Peritoneal lavage was helpful in detecting injuries missed by computed tomography.

The Training and Utilization of Surgical Physician Assistants: A Retrospective Study 348
Linda Ballard Brandt; Malcolm S. Beinfield, MD; Horace A. Laffaye, MD, Norwalk, Conn; Arthur E. Baue, MD, St Louis, Mo
• A surgical postgraduate training program for physician assistants provided coverage of surgical patients in hospitals without surgical residencies.

Physiologic Effects of Steep Positioning in the Surgical Intensive Care Unit 352
Loren D. Nelson, MD, Hans B. Anderson, RRT, Miami, Fla
• Continuous rotation reversed the adverse effects on oxygenation caused by positional changes.

Nosocomial Abscess: Results of an Eight-Year Prospective Study of 32 284 Operations 356
Mary M. Olson, RN, BSN, Melody O'Connor Allen, MD, Minneapolis, Minn
• Postoperative infection surveillance was associated with a decrease in wound infection and abscess formation rates.

Determinants of Urea Nitrogen Production in Sepsis: Muscle Catabolism, Total Parenteral Nutrition, and Hepatic Clearance of Amino Acids 362
Mauro Pittiruti, MD; John H. Siegel, MD; Gabriele Sganga, MD; Bill Coleman; Charles E. Wiles III, MD; Robert Placko, Baltimore, Md
• Septic patients who survived had strikingly different metabolic alterations from septic patients with multiple organ failure.

Isolated Regional Perfusion in the Treatment of Subungual Melanoma 373
Peter C. Baas, MD; Harald J. Hoekstra, MD, PhD; Heimen Schraffordt Koops, MD, PhD; J. Wolter Oosterhuis, MD, PhD; Jan Oldhoff, MD, PhD, Groningen, the Netherlands
• Regional hyperthermic cytotoxicity drug perfusion prevented local recurrence following amputation for subungual melanoma.

CLINICAL NOTES

Influence of Estrogen Receptors on Survival and Recurrence in Patients With Breast Cancer Without Lymph Node Metastases 377
Hope S. Maki, MD, James L. Hoehn, MD, Marshfield, Wis
• Estrogen receptor status did not adversely affect outcome in lymph node-negative breast cancer patients.

A Foregut Carcinoid Tumor Causing Zollinger-Ellison Syndrome 381
Gordon B. Werbel, MD; Suzanne P. Nelson, MD; Philip G. Robinson, MD; John Anastasi, MD; Raymond J. Joehl, MD; Robert V. Rege, MD, Chicago, Ill
• A benign gastric carcinoid tumor contained gastrin and produced severe peptic ulcer disease.

TECHNIQUE

Fibrin Glue Achieves Hemostasis in Patients With Coagulation Disorders 385
Harry B. Kram, MD; Ragu C. Nathan, MD; Frederick J. Stafford, MD; Arthur W. Fleming, MD; William C. Shoemaker, MD, Los Angeles, Calif
• Fibrin glue is especially useful in patients with parenchymal organ hemorrhage and disordered coagulation.

REGULAR DEPARTMENTS

Correspondence and Brief Communications 388
Books 390
Calendar of Events 391
Index to Advertisers 270
Instructions for Authors .... **See February issue, p 148**

Archives of Surgery

APRIL 1989 VOLUME 124 NUMBER 4

Official Publication of the Western Surgical Association, Surgical Infection Society, New England Surgical Society, Society of Surgical Oncology, Pacific Coast Surgical Association

EDITORIAL

The Veterans Administration and Surgical Education in the United States 407
James M. Guernsey, MD, FACS, Martinez, Calif

PAPERS READ BEFORE THE 12TH ANNUAL SURGICAL SYMPOSIUM OF THE ASSOCIATION OF VETERANS ADMINISTRATION SURGEONS, MINNEAPOLIS, MINN, MAY 12 TO MAY 16, 1988

Common Bile Duct Healing: Do Different Absorbable Sutures Affect Stricture Formation and Tensile Strength? 408
Kenneth W. Sharp, MD; Charles B. Ross, MD; Vicki N. Tillman; John F. Dunn, MD, Nashville, Tenn
- The type of absorbable suture used had no effect on the anastomotic strictures or breaking strength of a common bile duct anastomosis.

Epidural Anesthesia in Patients Undergoing Thoracic Surgery 415
Barbara K. Temeck, MD; Paul W. Schafer, MD; Woo Y. Park, MD; John W. Harmon, MD, Washington, DC
- Epidural anesthesia with light general anesthesia was quite satisfactory in high-risk patients requiring thoracotomies.

Use of Sequential B-Mode Ultrasonography to Manage Abdominal Aortic Aneurysms 419
Fred N. Littooy, MD, Maywood, Ill; George Steffan, PA, Hines, Ill; Howard P. Greisler, MD, Maywood, Ill; Theresa L. White, RN, Hines, Ill; William H. Baker, MD, Maywood, Ill
- A threshold of 5 cm in diameter to consider elective repair remains feasible.

Pelvic Fracture Hemorrhage: Priorities in Management 422
B. Mark Evers, MD; Henry M. Cryer, MD; Frank B. Miller, MD, Louisville, Ky
- Patients continue to die of pelvic fracture hemorrhage despite angiography, embolization, MAST, and external fixation.

Anastomotic Tensile Strength Following In Situ Replacement of an Infected Abdominal Aortic Graft 425
Raymond Vetsch, MD; Dennis F. Bandyk, MD; David D. Schmitt, MD; Thomas M. Bergamini, MD; James D. Storey, MD; Jonathan B. Towne, MD, Milwaukee, Wis
- Replacement of infected canine aortic grafts resulted in satisfactory healing.

Hemodynamic Effects on Endothelial Cell Monolayer Detachment From Vascular Prostheses 429
Howard P. Greisler, MD; Eric D. Endean, MD; John J. Klosak, MD, Maywood, Ill; Joan Ellinger, Scott C. Henderson, Hines, Ill; Si M. Pham, MD; Steven J. Durham, MD; David P. Showalter, MD; Jeffery Levine, PhD; Harvey S. Borovetz, PhD, Pittsburgh, Pa
- Cultured endothelial cells remained adherent to graft surfaces during artificial flow states.

Pentoxifylline Increases Extremity Blood Flow in Diabetic Atherosclerotic Patients 434
Richard W. Schwartz, MD; Nancy M. Logan; Paul J. Johnson, MD; William E. Strodel, MD; Joseph G. Fine, MD; Andris Kazmers, MD; Gordon L. Hyde, MD, Lexington, Ky
- In eight of ten patients there was an increase in dorsalis pedis arterial flow.

Microvascular Free-Tissue Transfer: The Atlanta Veterans Administration Medical Center Experience 438
Grant W. Carlson, MD, John J. Coleman III, MD, Atlanta, Ga
- Free microvascular tissue transfer effectively solved many reconstruction and wound problems. Results improved with increased experience.

The Role of Isolated Profundaplasty for the Treatment of Rest Pain 441
David M. McCoy, MD; Alan P. Sawchuk, MD; James J. Schuler, MD; Joseph R. Durham, MD; Jens Eldrup-Jorgensen, MD; Thomas H. Schwarcz, MD; Joseph P. Meyer, MD; D. Preston Flanigan, MD, Chicago, Ill
- Isolated profundaplasty was beneficial in 57% of patients but this could have been increased if selection had been based on hemodynamic measurements.

Recombinant Human Tumor Necrosis Factor Produces Hemodynamic Changes Characteristic of Sepsis and Endotoxemia 445
William J. Schirmer, MD; James M. Schirmer; Donald E. Fry, MD, Cleveland, Ohio
- Injection of human TNF in rats produced the hyperdynamic changes of sepsis with reduced hepatic blood flow.

The **ARCHIVES OF SURGERY** (ISSN 0004-0010) is published monthly by the American Medical Association, 535 N Dearborn St, Chicago, IL 60610, and is an official publication of the Association. Second-class postage paid at Chicago, IL 60610 and at additional mailing office.

SUBSCRIPTION RATES—The subscription rates for the ARCHIVES OF SURGERY are as follows: $50 for one year, $85 for two years in the United States and US possessions; all other countries, one year, $60; two years, $105 for surface delivery. (For expedited air delivery to most countries, add $15 surcharge for one-year subscription, $30 for two years.) Rates for subscriptions for delivery to Japan or South Korea are available through exclusive agents—contact the publisher. ***Special rates for residents and medical students in the United States and US possessions are available.*** Address inquiries to the American Medical Association, Circulation and Fulfillment Division, 535 N Dearborn St, Chicago, IL 60610. Phone: (312) 280-7168.

CHANGE OF ADDRESS—POSTMASTER, send all address changes to ARCHIVES OF SURGERY. Attention: Subscription Department, 535 N Dearborn St, Chicago, IL 60610. Notification of address change must be made at least six weeks in advance, include both old and new addresses, a recent mailing label, and your new zip code.

CONTENTS—Continued

The Association of *Escherichia coli* Virulence and Pulmonary Microvascular Damage 449
Roderick A. Barke, MD; David L. Dunn, MD, PhD; Agustin P. Dalmasso, MD; Melody O'Connor-Allen, MD; Richard L. Simmons, MD; Edward W. Humphrey, MD, PhD, Minneapolis, Minn
• Increased virulence of organisms was associated with increased lung microvascular damage.

Effect of Eflorithine on Intestinal Regeneration 454
Jon S. Thompson, MD; Shailendra K. Saxena, MD, MS; John G. Sharp, PhD, Omaha, Neb
• Inhibition of polyamine synthesis impaired growth of new intestinal mucosa.

Effective Hepatic Blood Flow During Cardiopulmonary Bypass 458
William W. Hampton, MD; Michael C. Townsend, MD; William J. Schirmer, MD; David M. Haybron, MD; Donald E. Fry, MD, Cleveland, Ohio
• Effective hepatic blood flow was decreased in patients during cardiopulmonary bypass.

Concomitant Cholecystectomy for Asymptomatic Cholelithiasis 460
Larry E. Bragg, MD, Jon S. Thompson, MD, Omaha, Neb
• Incidental cholecystectomy is recommended in patients with asymptomatic gallstones who require a laparotomy for other reasons.

Reversal of Pigment Gallstone Disease in a Canine Model 463
Lillian G. Dawes, MD; David L. Nahrwold, MD; Sanford I. Roth, MD; Robert V. Rege, MD, Chicago, Ill
• Dietary-induced pigment gallstones disappeared following discontinuation of the lithogenic diet in dogs.

Terminal Loop Cutaneous Ureterostomy in Cadaveric Kidney Transplantation 467
R. Neal Garrison, MD; Frederick R. Bentley, MD; Mohammad Amin, MD, Louisville, Ky
• Terminal loop cutaneous ureterostomy is a safe, effective means of urinary drainage in kidney transplantation when the bladder cannot be used.

Pentagastrin Stimulation of Human Colon Carcinoma 470
D. Byron McGregor, MD; Laura L. Morriss, PhD; Pacita B. Manalo, MD; Richard A. Bomberger, MD; Ronald S. Pardini, PhD, Reno, Nev
• Pentagastrin exerted a stimulatory effect that varied with the type of cell line of human colon cancer.

Inhibition of the Stimulated Canine Exocrine Pancreas by Amino Acids and Fat 473
Richard S. Stubbs, MB, ChB, MD, FRCS, FRACS, Wellington, New Zealand, Bruce E. Stabile, MD, San Diego, Calif
• Intravenous amino acids and intraduodenal lipid inhibited stimulated canine pancreatic secretion but probably by different mechanisms.

Detection of the Cancer-Prone Colon, Using Transepithelial Impedance Analysis 480
Richard J. Davies, MD; Renah Joseph; Horacio Asbun, MD; Marc Sedwitz, MD, San Diego, Calif
• Cancer-susceptible mice had a greater increase in electrical conductance after receiving a chemical carcinogen.

Recent Trends in the Management of Incisional Herniation 485
Raymond C. Read, MD, PhD, Gordon Yoder, PAC, Little Rock, Ark
• Recurrence rates after primary ventral hernia repair were 25% and 40% after a second ventral hernia repair.

Biochemical Adaptation of Venous Patches Placed in the Carotid Circulation 490
Dean M. Govostis, MD; Dennis F. Bandyk, MD; Thomas M. Bergamini, MD; Jonathan B. Towne, MD, Milwaukee, Wis
• Vein patch closure of arteries resulted in enhanced prostacyclin production compared with arteries closed primarily.

ORIGINAL ARTICLE

Limitations to Donating Adequate Autologous Blood Prior to Elective Orthopedic Surgery 494
Lawrence T. Goodnough, MD; J. Wasman; Kathleen Corlucci; Ann Chernosky, Cleveland, Ohio
• Autologous blood procurement was limited by low hematocrits and limited erythropoietic response to phlebotomy.

CLINICAL NOTE

Adenocarcinoma Arising in an Ileostomy: Report of Two Cases and Review of the Literature 497
Patricia L. Roberts, MD; Malcolm C. Veidenheimer, MD; Sharon Cassidy, RN, ET; Mark L. Silverman, MD, Burlington, Mass
• Adenocarcinoma occurred in ileostomy stomas in two patients many years after construction of the ileostomy.

BRIEF CLINICAL NOTE

Successful Reconstruction of Late Portal Vein Stenosis After Hepatic Transplantation 503
Velma P. Scantlebury, MD; Albert B. Zajko, MD; Carlos O. Esquivel, MD, PhD; Ignazio R. Marino, MD; Thomas E. Starzl, MD, PhD, Pittsburgh, Pa
• Portal vein stenosis occurred following liver transplantation in three young patients and was successfully corrected by operation.

TECHNIQUE

Cardiac Contusion: The Effect on Operative Management of the Patient With Trauma Injuries 506
Patrick Ross, Jr, MD, PhD; Linda Degutis, MSN; Christopher C. Baker, MD, New Haven, Conn
• Blunt trauma patients who have sustained a cardiac contusion can undergo elective operations with a low incidence of complications.

REGULAR DEPARTMENTS

Correspondence and Brief Communications 508
Calendar of Events 510
Books 511
Index to Advertisers 394
Instructions for Authors .... **See February 1989 issue, p 148**

Archives of Surgery

MAY 1989 VOLUME 124 NUMBER 5

Official Publication of the Western Surgical Association, Surgical Infection Society, New England Surgical Society, Society of Surgical Oncology, Pacific Coast Surgical Association

EDITORIAL

The New England Surgical Society 529
Claude H. Organ, Jr, MD, Oakland, Calif

PAPERS READ BEFORE THE 69TH ANNUAL MEETING OF THE NEW ENGLAND SURGICAL SOCIETY, MONTREAL, CANADA, SEPT 15 TO SEPT 17, 1988

Seldom Come By: The Worthwhileness of a Career in Surgery 530
Clement A. Hiebert, MD, Portland, Me

Lung Transplantation: Samuel Jason Mixter Lecture 535
F. Griffith Pearson, MD, FRCSC, Toronto, Canada

Management of General Surgical Complications Following Cardiac Transplantation 539
Verdi J. DiSesa, MD; Robert L. Kirkman, MD; Nicholas L. Tilney, MD; Gilbert H. Mudge, MD; John J. Collins, Jr, MD; Lawrence H. Cohn, MD, Boston, Mass
• In 11 of 12 patients undergoing heart transplantation, an aggressive approach to abdominal complications was successful.

Ibuprofen Causes Reduced Toxic Effects of Interleukin 2 Administration in Patients With Metastatic Cancer 542
Timothy J. Eberlein, MD; Deric D. Schoof, PhD; Hamish R. Michie, FRCS; Anthony F. Massaro; Ulrike Burger; Douglas W. Wilmore, MD; Richard E. Wilson, MD, Boston, Mass
• The cyclooxygenase inhibitor ibuprofen reduced toxicity but not the rate of response to interleukin 2 therapy.

Tamoxifen as an Alternative to Surgical Resection for Selected Geriatric Patients With Primary Breast Cancer 548
Richard G. Margolese, MD, Montreal, Canada, Roger S. Foster, Jr, MD, Burlington, Vt
• Eighteen of 30 elderly patients had regression of the primary tumor with tamoxifen therapy alone.

Primary Cancer of the Liver: Evaluation, Treatment, and Prognosis 552
William V. McDermott, MD; Blake Cady, MD; Basil Georgi, MD; Glenn Steele, Jr, MD; Urmila Khettry, MD, Boston, Mass
• Median survival in patients with a tumor in a normal liver was 32 months as compared with 19 months in patients with tumors and chronic liver disease.

Management of Biliary Obstruction: A Comparison of Percutaneous, Endoscopic, and Operative Techniques 556
Janice G. Rothschild, MD; Marshall M. Kaplan, MD; Victor G. Millan, MD; Randolph B. Reinhold, MD, Boston, Mass
• Endoscopic therapy was safe and helpful with stone disease as compared with percutaneous hepatic drainage, but an abdominal operation seemed better for malignancy.

Liver Abscess: The Need for Complete Gastrointestinal Evaluation 561
Jeffrey L. Cohen, MD, Hartford, Conn; F. Maureen Martin, MD, Boston, Mass; Ricardo L. Rossi, MD, David J. Schoetz, Jr, MD, Burlington, Mass
• The pyogenic liver abscess often has a disease process in the biliary or gastrointestinal tract.

Intrahepatic Cholangiojejunostomy as a Palliative Procedure in Primary Sclerosing Cholangitis 565
James R. Goldenring, MD, PhD, C. Elton Cahow, MD, New Haven, Conn
• Effective palliation was provided by intrahepatic cholangiojejunostomy if secondary biliary cirrhosis had not developed.

The **ARCHIVES OF SURGERY** (ISSN 0004-0010) is published monthly by the American Medical Association, 535 N Dearborn St, Chicago, IL 60610, and is an official publication of the Association. Second-class postage paid at Chicago, IL 60610, and at additional mailing office.

SUBSCRIPTION RATES—The subscription rates for the ARCHIVES OF SURGERY are as follows: $50 for one year, $85 for two years in the United States and US possessions; all other countries, one year, $60; two years, $105 for surface delivery. (For expedited air delivery to most countries, add $15 surcharge for one year subscription, $30 for two years.) Rates for subscriptions for delivery to Japan or South Korea are available through exclusive agents—contact the publisher. ***Special rates for residents and medical students in the United States and US possessions are available.*** Address inquiries to the American Medical Association, Circulation and Fulfillment Division, 535 N Dearborn St, Chicago, IL 60610. Phone: (312)280-7168.

CHANGE OF ADDRESS—POSTMASTER, send all address changes to the ARCHIVES OF SURGERY, Attention: Subscription Department, 535 N Dearborn St, Chicago, IL 60610. Notification of address change must be made at least six weeks in advance, include both old and new addresses, a recent mailing label, and your new zip code.

CONTENTS—Continued

Intrapleural Regional Analgesia for Pain Management in Cholecystectomy 568
Moustafa A. El-Naggar, MD; Frank J. Schaberg, Jr, MD; Martin R. Phillips, MD, Pawtucket, RI
• Insertion of an intrapleural catheter and injection of 30 mL of bupivacaine provided prolonged pain relief after cholecystectomy.

Management of Pancreatic Fistulas 571
F. Maureen Martin, MD; Ricardo L. Rossi, MD; J. Lawrence Munson, MD; Stephen G. ReMine, MD; John W. Braasch, MD, Burlington, Mass
• Fistulas associated with pancreatitis are the most heterogeneous and difficult to manage.

Cholecystokinin Augmentation of 'Surgical' Pancreatitis: Benefits of Receptor Blockade 574
Irvin M. Modlin, MD; Anton J. Bilchik, MD; Karl A. Zucker, MD; Thomas E. Adrian, PhD, MRCPath; Jeffrey Sussman, MD; Scott M. Graham, MD, New Haven, Conn
• Cholecystokinin (CCK) potentiated and a CCK receptor blocking agent decreased the severity of experimental pancreatitis.

Selective Nonoperative Management of Blunt Splenic Trauma in Adults 581
James R. Elmore, MD; David E. Clark, MD; Robert J. Isler, MD; William R. Horner, MD, Portland, Me
• Multiple injuries, age over 64 years, and a requirement for more than 2 U of blood indicate the now frequent need for a laparotomy.

Progress in Experimental Porcine Small-Bowel Transplantation 587
Hironori Kaneko, MD; Wayne Hancock, MD, PhD; Robert T. Schweizer, MD, Hartford, Conn
• Successful small-bowel transplantation can be achieved with adequate immunosuppression in a large animal.

Use of the Triplex Scanner in Diagnosis of Deep Venous Thrombosis 593
Alfred V. Persson, MD; Catherine Jones; Russell Zide; Edward R. Jewell, MD, Burlington, Mass
• The results of triplex scanning can be safely used alone to diagnose or exclude deep venous thrombosis.

The Impact of an Ambulatory Surgical Service in a Community Hospital 601
Horace A. Laffaye, MD, New Haven, Conn
• The average savings per patient having an operation on an ambulatory basis was $2000 and 3.07 hospital days.

Routine Intraoperative Angioscopy in Lower Extremity Revascularization 604
Arnold Miller, MD, ChB; David R. Campbell, MD; Gary W. Gibbons, MD; Frank B. Pomposelli, Jr, MD; Dorothy V. Freeman, MD; Stephen J. Jepsen, MD; Robert S. Lees, MD; Jonathan L. Isaacsohn, MD; David Purcell, MD; Mark Bolduc, MD; Frank W. LoGerfo, MD, Boston, Mass
• Intraoperative angioscopy is a good alternative to the intraoperative arteriogram in monitoring the technical effectiveness of the procedure.

Limb Salvage Despite Extensive Tissue Loss 609
Jack L. Cronenwett, MD; Martha D. McDaniel, MD; Robert M. Zwolak, MD, PhD; Daniel B. Walsh, MD; Joseph R. Schneider, MD; William F. Reus, MD; Lawrence B. Colen, MD, Hanover, NH
• Ninety-three percent of limbs that would have required amputation were salvaged by combining revascularization with reconstruction.

Recent Experience With Thoracoabdominal Aneurysm Repair 620
Richard P. Cambria, MD; David C. Brewster, MD; Ashby C. Moncure, MD; Bengt Ivarsson, MD; R. Clement Darling, MD; J. Kenneth Davison, MD; William M. Abbott, MD, Boston, Mass
• The risk/benefit ratio in most patients seems to be weighted toward elective resection.

Splenectomy: The Treatment of Choice for Human Immunodeficiency Virus–Related Immune Thrombocytopenia? . . . 625
Thanjavur S. Ravikumar, MD; J. Davis Allen, MD; Albert Bothe, Jr, MD; Glenn Steele, Jr, MD, Boston, Mass
• Splenectomy provided a durable and lasting response for human immunodeficiency virus-related thrombocytopenia.

ORIGINAL ARTICLE

Gallstone Disease: The Clinical Manifestations of Infectious Stones 629
Alison L. Smith, MD; Lygia Stewart, MD; Robert Fine, MD; Carlos A. Pellegrini, MD; Lawrence W. Way, MD, San Francisco, Calif
• Gallstone disease is more virulent in patients whose gallstones contain bacteria.

REGULAR DEPARTMENTS

Correspondence and Brief Communications 636

Books 637

Index to Advertisers 580

Instructions for Authors 520

Archives of Surgery

JUNE 1989 VOLUME 124 NUMBER 6

Official Publication of the Western Surgical Association, Surgical Infection Society, New England Surgical Society, Society of Surgical Oncology, Pacific Coast Surgical Association

ORIGINAL ARTICLES

Preliminary Clinical Experience With the Titanium Greenfield Vena Caval Filter 657

Lazar J. Greenfield, MD, Kyung J. Cho, MD, Ann Arbor, Mich; S. Osher Pais, MD, Baltimore, Md; Michael Van Aman, MD, Columbus, Ohio

- A titanium model of the Greenfield filter provides ease of insertion, and the sheath technique should prevent misplacement.

Arterial Mycotic Aneurysm and Rupture: A Potentially Fatal Complication of Pancreas Transplantation in Diabetes Mellitus 660

Andreas G. Tzakis, MD; Patricia B. Carroll, MD; Robert D. Gordon, MD; Itsuo Yokoyama, MD; Leonard Makowka, MD, PhD; Thomas E. Starzl, MD, PhD, Pittsburgh, Pa

- A mycotic aneurysm must be suspected in patients with a pancreatic transplant who present with unexplained hypotension, cardiac arrest, or gastrointestinal bleeding.

Results of Operative Treatment of Gastrointestinal Tract Tumors in Patients Over 80 Years of Age 662

Ph. Morel, MD; R. A. Egeli, MD; S. Wachtl, MD; A. Rohner, MD, Geneva, Switzerland

- Operative treatment of gastrointestinal tract malignancy in patients greater than 80 years of age improved their activity level and resulted in a 48% survival rate at 3 years.

Surgical Manipulation and the Tensile Strength of Polypropylene Sutures 665

Philip B. Dobrin, MD, PhD, Maywood, Ill

- Accidental knots and grasping with forceps decreased the tensile strength of these sutures.

Thromboxane A_2-Receptor Blockade and Prostacyclin in Porcine *Escherichia coli* Shock 669

Erik Svartholm, MD, PhD; David Bergqvist, MD; Ulla Hedner, MD, PhD; June Ljungberg; Ulf Haglund, MD, PhD, Malmö, Sweden

- Although thromboxane A_2 is one of the mediators of pulmonary vascular responses, it is not important for the hemostatic changes in this model.

Inflammatory Aneurysms of the Abdominal Aorta 673

Hans H. Moosa, MD; Andrew B. Peitzman, MD; David L. Steed, MD; Thomas B. Julian, MD; Fredric Jarrett, MD; Marshall W. Webster, MD, Pittsburgh, Pa

- A CT scan with contrast for periaortic inflammation is the most reliable diagnostic test.

Strategy in Reoperative Surgery for Hyperparathyroidism 676

Polly S. Y. Cheung, MBBS, FRCS; Anders Borgstrom, MD; Norman W. Thompson, MD, Ann Arbor, Mich

- Second operations for hyperparathyroidism will be less frequent after thorough initial neck exploration, correct interpretation of the pathology, and adequate parathyroid resection.

How Accurate Is Fine-Needle Biopsy in Malignant Neoplasia of the Pancreas? 681

Livingston Parsons, Jr, MD, Charles H. Palmer, MD, Albuquerque, NM

- Aspiration biopsy of the pancreas performed percutaneously or intraoperatively was associated with a high incidence of false-negative results.

Colorectal Neodymium-YAG Photoablative Therapy: Comparing Applications and Complications on Both Sides of the Peritoneal Reflection 684

Donald E. Low, MD; Richard A. Kozarek, MD; Terrence J. Ball, MD; David J. Patterson, MD; Lucius D. Hill, MD, Seattle, Wash

- Laser photoablative therapy for colorectal carcinoma can be used with equal efficiency and safety on either side of the peritoneal reflection.

Small-Bowel Perforation Complicating the Open Treatment of Generalized Peritonitis 689

Walter J. B. Mastboom, MD; Han H. C. Kuypers, MD, PhD; Frans J. Schoots, MD; Theo Wobbes, MD, PhD, Nijmegen, the Netherlands

- Small-bowel perforations developed without apparent cause in a number of patients being treated for peritonitis by the open method.

Angiotropin Treatment Prevents Flap Necrosis and Enhances Dermal Regeneration in Rabbits 693

Michael Höckel, MD, PhD, Mainz, West Germany, John F. Burke, MD, Boston, Mass

- Angiotropin pretreatment can prevent flap necrosis and augment dermal regeneration after rounding.

The **ARCHIVES OF SURGERY** (ISSN 0004-0010) is published monthly by the American Medical Association, 535 N Dearborn St, Chicago, IL 60610, and is an official publication of the Association. Second-class postage paid at Chicago, IL 60610, and at additional mailing office.

SUBSCRIPTION RATES—The subscription rates for the ARCHIVES OF SURGERY are as follows: $50 for one year, $85 for two years in the United States and US possessions; all other countries, one year, $60; two years, $105 for surface delivery. (For expedited air delivery to most countries, add $15 surcharge for one year subscription, $30 for two years.) Rates for subscriptions for delivery to Japan or South Korea are available through exclusive agents—contact the publisher. ***Special rates for residents and medical students in the United States and US Possessions are available.*** Address inquiries to the American Medical Association, Circulation and Fulfillment Division, 535 N Dearborn St, Chicago, IL 60610. Phone: (312)280-7168.

CHANGE OF ADDRESS—POSTMASTER, send all address changes to the ARCHIVES OF SURGERY, Attention: Subscription Department, 535 N Dearborn St, Chicago, IL 60610. Notification of address change must be made at least six weeks in advance, include both old and new addresses, a recent mailing label, and your new zip code.

CONTENTS—Continued

Simple Intestinal Obstruction Causes Bacterial Translocation in Man 699
Edwin A. Deitch, MD, Shreveport, La
• Bacteria were cultured from mesenteric lymph nodes obtained from patients with simple intestinal obstruction.

Management of Severe Incisional Abscesses Following Laparotomy: Early Reclosure Under Cover of Metronidazole and Ampicillin 702
Finn Gottrup, MD, PhD, Randers, Denmark; P. Gjøde, MD, Aalborg, Denmark; F. Lundhus, MD, Randers, Denmark; H. Andrup, MD, Aalborg, Denmark; C. N. Holm, MD, Viborg, Denmark; S. Terpling, MD, Randers, Denmark
• Management of abdominal wound abscesses by incision and drainage, antibiotics, and early reclosure was safe and effective.

Oral Prophylaxis With Neomycin and Erythromycin in Colorectal Surgery: More Proof for Efficacy Than Failure 705
Per-Arne Kling, MD, Sven Dahlgren, MD, Umeå, Sweden
• Results were similar with oral neomycin-erythromycin or intravenous cephtriaxone-etronidazole preparation in colorectal surgery.

The Effect of New Monofilament Absorbable Sutures on the Healing of Musculoaponeurotic Incisions, Gastrotomies, and Colonic Anastomoses 708
Pamela A. Foresman; Richard F. Edlich, MD, PhD; George T. Rodeheaver, PhD, Charlottesville, Va
• Two new monofilament absorbable sutures, Maxon and PDS, were equally effective in experimental wounds.

Diagnosis and Treatment of Duodenoenteric Fistulas Complicating Crohn's Disease 712
Kenneth K. W. Lee, MD, Wolfgang H. Schraut, MD, Chicago, Ill
• In patients with Crohn's disease, duodenoenteric fistulas were due to enterocolonic rather than duodenal Crohn's disease.

Excision of the Burn Wound in Patients With Large Burns 718
William F. McManus, MD; Arthur D. Mason, Jr, MD; Basil A. Pruitt, Jr, MD, Fort Sam Houston, Tex
• The apparent advantages of excision of large burn wounds may only reflect patient selection.

Diagnostic Pneumoperitoneum in the Pediatric Patient With a Unilateral Inguinal Hernia 721
Gregory A. Timberlake, MD; M. Gage Ochsner, MD; Randall W. Powell, MD, San Diego, Calif
• In pediatric patients, intraoperative pneumoperitoneum during inguinal herniorrhaphy was used to diagnose a contralateral hernia.

Prostaglandin E_2 in Pyloric Stenosis 724
Gideon Goldman, MD; Elsa Tiomny, MD; Perry J. Kahn, MD; Dalia Somjen, PhD; Zamir Halpern, MD; Tuvia Gilat, MD; Theodor Wiznitzer, MD, Tel-Aviv, Israel
• Decreased PGE_2 levels were present in patients with pyloric obstruction.

The Effect of Endotoxin on Glucose Metabolism in Skeletal Muscle Requires the Presence of Plasma 727
Joseph F. Amaral, MD; Jeffry D. Shearer, MA; Balduino Mastrofrancesco, MS; Donald S. Gann, MD; Michael D. Caldwell, MD, PhD, Providence, RI
• Endotoxin does not have a direct effect on glucose uptake of skeletal muscle.

Hypertonic Saline Resuscitation in a Porcine Model of Severe Hemorrhagic Shock 733
Gregory G. Stanford, MD; C. Richard Patterson, MD; Lynda Payne, RN; Timothy C. Fabian, MD, Memphis, Tenn
• Hypertonic saline was effective in resuscitating pigs with hemorrhagic shock.

CLINICAL NOTES

Percutaneous Nephrostomy in the Management of Renal Candidiasis 739
Orlando Ortiz, MD, Won J. Lee, MD, New Hyde Park, NY
• Percutaneous nephrostomy allowed drainage, extraction of the fungus ball, and irrigation with amphotericin B.

Echinococcal Disease in an Extended Family and Review of the Literature 741
CPT Franco Musio, MC, USA, Dimitrios Linos, MD, Athens, Greece
• Echinococcal disease developed in seven of 11 members of an extended family group.

BRIEF CLINICAL NOTES

Emergent Endoscopic Retrograde Cholangiopancreatography: A Highly Specific Test for Acute Pancreatic Trauma 745
Sharon R. Hayward, MD; Charles E. Lucas, MD; Choichi Sugawa, MD; Anna M. Ledgerwood, MD, Detroit, Mich
• A normal pancreatogram ruled out pancreatic transection in this trauma patient.

Percutaneous Transhepatic Ultrasonic Cholelithotripsy 747
Anurag K. Das, MD; John L. Weinerth, MD; Steven C. Rose, MD; R. Randal Bollinger, MD, PhD, Durham, NC
• Transhepatic lithotripsy was utilized to remove gallstones in this patient.

TECHNIQUE

Argon Laser Treatment of Radiation Proctitis 749
John J. O'Connor, MD, Bethesda, Md

REGULAR DEPARTMENTS

Correspondence and Brief Communications 751
Index to Advertisers 644
Instructions for Authors 737

Hail and Farewell

I thank those who have contributed so much to the *Archives of Surgery* over the past 12 years, and I salute the new Editor, Dr Claude H. Organ, Jr. It was a great privilege for me to succeed Dr Richard Warren in 1976, and the intervening years have been joyful and challenging. Responsibility for the editorial content of a major surgical publication is of greater consequence.

I am most grateful, first of all, to those who make a publication possible: the readers and the writers. The *Archives of Surgery* now is received internationally by over 75 000 readers who have consistently demonstrated their interest and support by high readership surveys and positive responses to queries about relevance and value of our printed material. The writers—authors, investigators, clinicians, and teachers—have provided a wealth of material from which to select and publish. So much that is worthwhile cannot be accommodated. So much that is important must wait for many months before it can be printed. This weighs heavily on an editor, and I appreciate the courtesy and good humor of those who must wait or go elsewhere.

The real heroes of a peer-review publication are the reviewers and members of the Editorial Board. Careful, considerate, thoughtful, and expert reviews have become a hallmark of our Editorial Board members and the many anonymous external reviewers. How many of our manuscripts—yours, mine—have been improved, clarified, and made more accurate and succinct by their considered comments? Theirs' is a labor of love for matters surgical. A monthly listing of the Editorial Board members on the masthead and a yearly listing of the names of our many other reviewers are hardly compensation for their efforts. I greatly appreciate and salute their excellent work.

The publications staff of the American Medical Association in Chicago has been an immense help—enjoyable to work with, supportive during my occasional editorial lapses, and always ensuring a quality publication. My thanks to them.

Finally, a special thanks to the *Archives of Surgery* office staff and my associates. Dr Ben Eiseman has served as Book Review Editor for many years, and his thoughtful and always entertaining reviews have made this a popular feature of the journal. Dr Hastings K. Wright served as Associate Editor during the New Haven days and was a great help in establishing our peer-review system and in taking over for me during a sabbatical and other junkets. Dr Donald L. Kaminski has been both an immense help and a scholarly addition in St Louis as Associate Editor, serving truly in a labor of love for surgery. Mrs Nancy Nyhan served superbly as editorial assistant during the New Haven years. My business managers at Yale, Joe Podgorski and Elinor Ingenito, were an immense help. My wife Rosemary provided the transition from New Haven to St Louis and made it possible to move the editorial office and get off to a fast and excellent start at St Mary's Health Center. In recent years, Kathy Illyes and Kit Hereford have served admirably as editorial assistant and associate, and I am very grateful to them. Sister Betty Brucker, FSM, and St Mary's Health Center have been most gracious in providing a home for the editorial office.

I also welcome Dr Organ to his new task. The *Archives of Surgery* will be in excellent hands, and I am most pleased to pass the pen on to him. His capabilities as a scholar, clinician, and leader will stand him in good stead as the ARCHIVES moves into a new era of scientific publication. It is most appropriate and exciting now to have new leadership. The time has come for more creative thinking and renewed vigor. I have tremendously enjoyed and benefited from my tour and will miss many aspects of the job. I do, however, look forward to recovery from "briefcase elbow" (lateral epicondyle extensor carpi radialis brevis inflammation produced by carrying a heavy briefcase filled with manuscripts through airports and parking lots). As this recovery occurs, my tennis game should subsequently improve, although some members of the Editorial Board would challenge that possibility.

I look forward now to joining all of you as readers of the *Archives of Surgery* and thank you for the wonderful experiences I have had.

ARTHUR E. BAUE, MD
St Louis

A New Editor for the Archives

The American Medical Association is proud to announce the appointment of Claude H. Organ, Jr, MD, as Editor of the *Archives of Surgery*.

The selection of Dr Organ was the result of the most exhaustive search process in recent AMA history. As is the custom, a search committee comprising several of the leading figures in the specialty was formed, with the Editor of one of the other AMA Specialty Journals—in this case, William W. McLendon, MD, of the *Archives of Pathology & Laboratory Medicine*—serving as chairman. The initial call for nominations resulted in more than 75 letters of recommendation; the initial list of candidates read like a *Who's Who* of the surgical field. The committee assiduously pared this number down to 30 active candidates. After more than a year of deliberation, letter writing, and conference calls the committee presented a list of five finalists, in order of preference, to George D. Lundberg, MD, AMA Vice-President for Scientific Information. Dr Organ's name was at the top of the list.

Claude H. Organ, Jr, was graduated cum laude from Xavier University in New Orleans and received his medical degree from Creighton University School of Medicine in Omaha in 1952. His ties to Creighton are long and strong: he went on to perform his residency there and received an MS in surgery in 1957. After a tour of duty as a lieutenant commander in the US Navy, stationed at the US Naval Hospital at Camp Pendelton, Calif, Dr Organ returned to Creighton as an instructor of surgery. He rose quickly through the academic hierarchy and in 1971 was named Professor and Chairman of the Department of Surgery and Chief Physician in Surgery at Creighton Memorial St Joseph Hospital.

In 1982, seeking a warmer climate and more time in the teaching arena, Dr Organ accepted a professorship at the University of Oklahoma, Oklahoma City, where he served until the fall of last year.

No stranger to multiple challenges, Dr Organ is beginning another professional chapter concurrent with his new editorship of the Archives. Recently he moved to Oakland, Calif, to become Professor of Surgery and Director of Surgical Residency at the University of California Davis–East Bay. This exciting and innovative new program will combine the resources of several institutions—Highland Hospital Center, Martinez Veterans Administration Center, Kaiser Oakland, Merritt Hospital, and Oakland Children's Hospital—to establish UC Davis's academic presence in the East Bay.

In addition to his notable career in academic medicine, Dr Organ recently served with distinction as Chairman of the American Board of Surgery, the first black to achieve that high honor. He is a former President of the Southwestern Surgical Congress and maintains memberships in national and international medical societies too numerous to list here.

A speaker of international renown, Dr Organ is much in demand as a lecturer and visiting professor. In May 1986 he was awarded an honorary fellowship in the Royal College of Surgeons of South Africa. He has authored more than 100 articles and book chapters, primarily in the areas of endocrinology, oncology, and surgical gastroenterology.

Perhaps Dr Organ's most important—and, for him, enjoyable—contribution to surgery has been as an educator. His skill, humor, and larger-than-life presence in the surgical theater have instructed and inspired countless surgical residents.

His appointment as Editor of the Archives provides an extraordinary opportunity to extend this role to a larger arena. The *Archives of Surgery* has the largest circulation of any surgical publication in the world—currently 73 000. The journal is received by virtually all physicians in the

Claude H. Organ, Jr, MD. New Editor, *Archives of Surgery.*

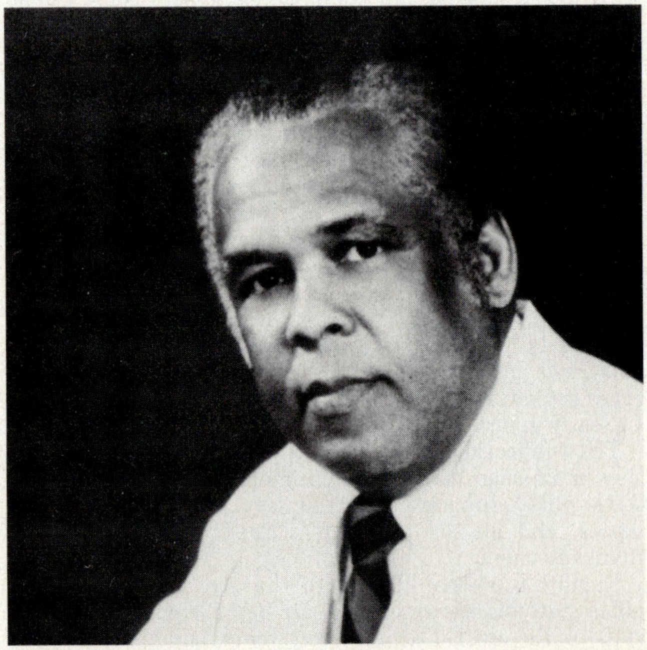

areas of general and orthopedic surgery as well as those in urology and numerous surgical subspecialties. The new Editor has an enormous task ahead of him: to address this vast, diversified audience of surgeons, to inform, to teach, and to explore all areas of interest to the specialty at large.

Dr Organ inherits a journal that ranks among the top in its field thanks to the efforts of his predecessor, Arthur E. Baue, MD. Dr Baue took the reins of the ARCHIVES in 1977 and skillfully guided the journal through some very difficult times. Over the years he has established relationships with several prominent surgical societies, watched the number of manuscript submissions steadily increase, and kept the journal on a solid foundation. Art Baue has been one of the senior statesmen of the AMA journals, and we will miss his wit and wise counsel.

In Claude Organ the ARCHIVES has found a surgeon of enormous worldwide stature to assume this important editorship. The catalogue of Dr Organ's professional achievements, although impeccable and impressive, is only part of the reason for his appointment. Meeting him confirms what his curriculum vitae only suggests: this is an extraordinary person. That fact quickly becomes apparent to colleagues, students, and staff members who work with him. It became obvious to the search committee that ultimately recommended him, based on the glowing endorsements and lavish praise from his surgical colleagues around the world, and to the AMA staff in our initial contacts with him as he sets up his base in Oakland. Claude Organ's life and career have been a model of excellence for persons of all races and nationalities to admire and emulate. The ARCHIVES is proud to welcome him to the circle of editors and looks forward to his leadership.

MICHAEL D. SPRINGER
Managing Editor and Director
AMA Specialty Journals
Chicago

Inaugural Editorial

Each successive generation of doctors stands, as it were, upon the shoulders of its predecessors.
F. M. R. Walske (1888)

The honor of becoming the seventh Editor of the American Medical Association's *Archives of Surgery* becomes immediately muted by the intensity of the task ahead. I am pleased and flattered to follow in the footsteps of previous editors Dean Lewis (1937 to 1940), Waltman Walters (1941 to 1942, 1946 to 1961), Lester Dragstedt (1943 to 1945), J. Garrett Allen (1962 to 1969), Richard Warren (1970 to 1976) and Arthur Baue (1977 to 1988). These illustrious predecessors, highly respected by their peers, have established a tradition for the ARCHIVES for almost half a century of American surgery.

During the last 12 years, Arthur E. Baue has performed a superb job of reestablishing the ARCHIVES as one of the foremost journals in this hemisphere and guided its destiny during a period of unparalleled changes in American surgery. These years have been characterized by an explosion of information, innumerable diagnostic and therapeutic additions, and geometric technical and communication advances. Art Baue has dared to publish controversial articles while applying his unique clinical and scientific research expertise to the contents of this journal. The vignettes he has added to the ARCHIVES have made it informative and readable for a wider variety of academic and community surgeons whose composition is constantly undergoing change. This is confirmed by the 62% increase in average total circulation from 44 523 in 1983 to 71 673 in 1987. Baue's editorial, "Peer and/or Peerless Review"[1] is a thoughtful classic that editors and editorial board members would be wise to read and keep in their reprint file.

We express our appreciation to Dr Baue for his seminal contributions. He has consented to remain as the senior consulting editor of the ARCHIVES. In addition, appreciation is extended to Dr D. L. Kaminski as associate editor; Mrs Katherine Illyes, editorial assistant; Katherine Hereford, secretary; Dr George D. Lundberg; Michael D. Springer; editorial board members who served under Dr Baue during his 12-year tenure; and the AMA Publications Staff.

The AMA established the *Archives of Internal Medicine* in 1910, and after considerable discussion approved the publication of the *American Archives of Surgery* in 1911. Assuming it would result in serious damage to their publications, the editors of the *Annals of Surgery* (L. S. Pilcher) and *Surgery, Gynecology and Obstetrics* (F. H. Martin) protested the publication of the ARCHIVES. The AMA Board of Trustees, however, decided to proceed with this publication.

The first issue of the *Archives of Surgery* was published in July 1920. The editorial board included Drs Dean Lewis,

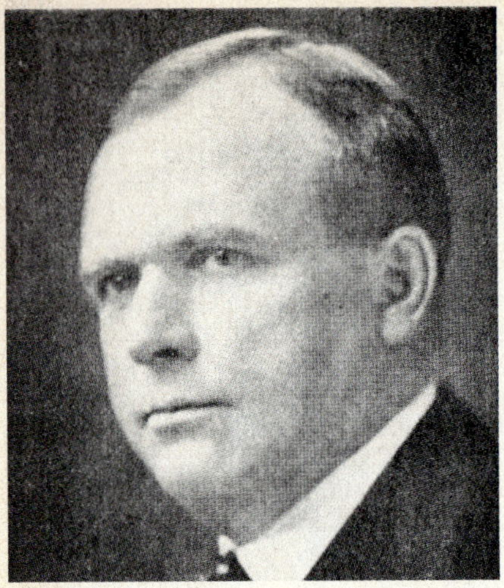

Dean Lewis

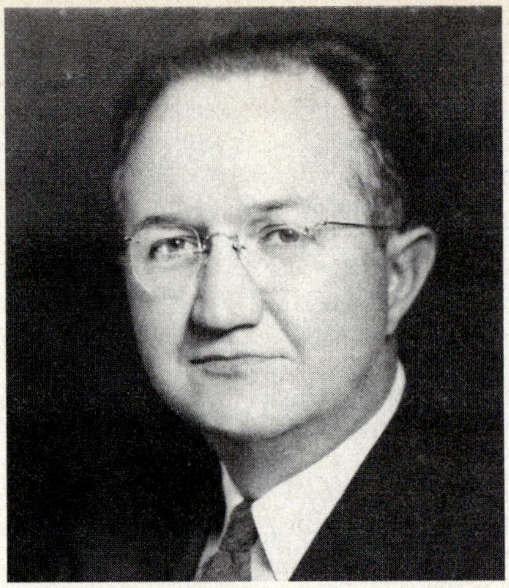

Lester Dragstedt

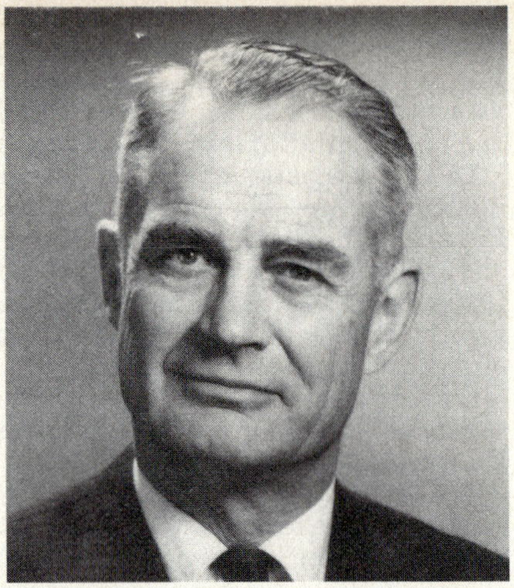

Richard Warren

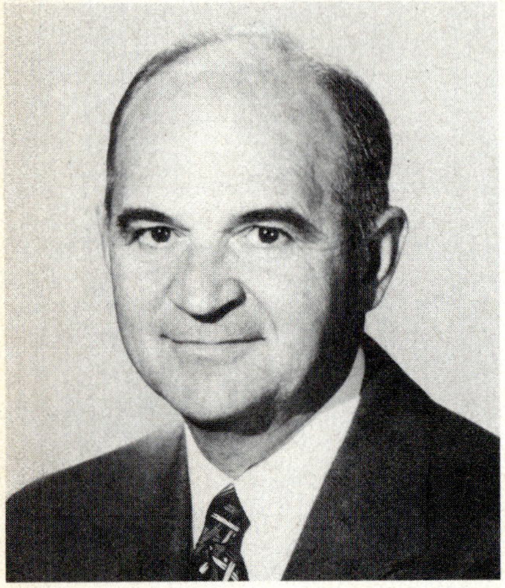

Waltman Walters

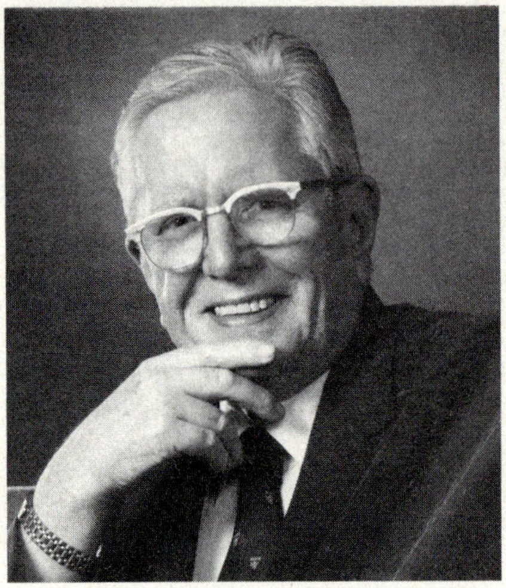

J. Garrett Allen

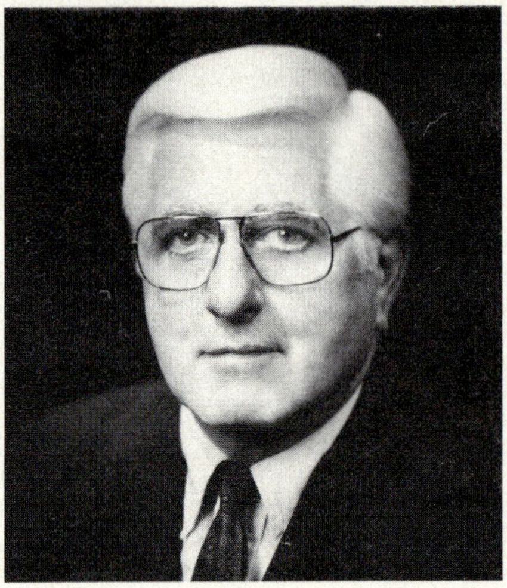

Arthur Baue

Evarts Graham, Hugh Cabot, Thomas Cullen, William Darrach, and William J. Mayo. In the inaugural editorial William J. Mayo stated,

> It is the hope of the editorial board that the *Archives of Surgery* may be one of the organs of expression in this growing field of surgical education, and that it may furnish an opportunity for the publication of original articles pertaining to research and investigation in those subjects which lay the foundation for sound surgical progress.[2]

In reviewing past editions of the ARCHIVES, this philosophy has been maintained over the years with remarkable consistency. The initial edition contained papers by Cushing, MacCallum, Bevan, Judd, Lewis, and Cutler—stellar surgeons of that era. Editors must stand in admiration and utter disbelief that Dean Lewis, the initial Editor, reviewed personally every paper considered for publication, a policy rapidly abandoned at his death. Thereafter, all editorial board members shared equally in the review process. Despite the early trend of publishing papers principally involving experimental surgical problems (intellectual elitism?), the policy of the editorial board gradually changed to encompass outstanding contributions and advancements in clinical surgery. The initial budget of the ARCHIVES was no less noteworthy: The Board of Trustees yearly set aside the sum of $600, which was given to the Editor to meet expenses. Gratefully these budgetary processes have undergone reasonable changes.

In the coming years the *Archives of Surgery* will adhere to the basic principle as outlined by William Mayo in the inaugural issue, ie, to offer surgeons a comprehensive journal constantly on the cutting edge of clinical surgery and relevant research. The ARCHIVES will be alert to and sensitive of duplicate publications, the challenge of controlled circulation journals, the increasing demands for supplements and festschrifts, as well as spiraling publication costs. We will encourage and seek original work and improve the time sequence of review and publication. Editorials from a wide range of individuals in the surgical disciplines will be published as the ARCHIVES offers a creative, analytical forum as we enter the 21st century.

CLAUDE H. ORGAN, JR, MD
Oakland, Calif

1. Baue A: Peer and/or peerless review: Some vagaries of the editorial process. *Arch Surg* 1985;120:885-888.
2. Fishbein M: *A History of the American Medical Association: 1847 to 1947*. Philadelphia, WB Saunders Co, 1947, pp 154-159.

The Prognostic Significance of Lymph Node Metastases After Preoperative Chemotherapy for Locally Advanced Breast Cancer

David R. McCready, MD; Gabriel N. Hortobagyi, MD; Shu W. Kau, RN; Terry L. Smith, MS; Aman U. Buzdar, MD; Charles M. Balch, MD

• We compared the prognostic value of surgical lymph node staging after preoperative chemotherapy relative to other patient and tumor variables in 136 patients with locally advanced breast cancer (T3-4 and/or N2-3) who received preoperative chemotherapy followed by mastectomy and axillary dissection as part of a prospective protocol. Univariate analysis revealed that the number of metastatic lymph nodes, clinical tumor stage at presentation, clinical and pathologic response, and menopause status were significant variables associated with survival and disease-free survival, but clinical node stage at presentation and estrogen receptor status were not. The number of metastatic lymph nodes had more prognostic value than the other factors, and when evaluated by multivariate regression, surgical node staging added significantly more information to the remaining variables. Surgical staging is an important component of treatment for patients with breast cancer undergoing preoperative chemotherapy because it can provide an accurate and quantitative method for subgrouping patients with different survival rates and it can be used to compare results between preoperative chemotherapy trials.

(*Arch Surg* 1989;124:21-25)

The most important prognostic variable for patients with surgically treated breast cancer is the presence and quantity of regional lymph node metastases.[1] Surgical staging of the axillary lymph nodes has traditionally been performed before chemotherapy is offered, but many centers have started to use chemotherapy as initial treatment for patients with clinically staged locally advanced breast cancer (LABC; defined as stage III[2]).[3,4] The effect of chemotherapy, given before surgical-pathologic staging, on the prognostic significance of the number of lymph node metastases is unknown.

The purpose of this study was to determine the prognostic importance of the number of axillary lymph node metastases relative to other patient and tumor variables in patients with LABC receiving preoperative chemotherapy. Univariate and multivariate analyses were used to determine which factors were associated with survival and disease-free survival (DFS) in this group of heterogeneous patients, since favorable prognoses have been previously associated with less advanced clinical subgroups (eg, T3, N0)[5,6] and the pathologic response to chemotherapy.[7] The results of this study will allow different regimens to be compared more reliably since patient selection factors vary greatly[8] and because of the inherent inaccuracy of comparisons based on clinical axillary node stage.[9]

PATIENTS AND METHODS

In 1974, chemotherapy was begun as initial treatment at M. D. Anderson Hospital, Houston, for patients with LABC. Patients who were clinically staged to have either T3-4 and/or N2-3 breast cancer (stage III) by the American Joint Committee on Cancer criteria[2] were judged to have LABC. Patients with inflammatory breast cancer, with detectable distant metastases, or who had received prior chemotherapy, were excluded. All patients provided written consent and had a core or incisional biopsy performed to establish histologic diagnosis and, if possible, to measure estrogen receptor content. Patients were initially evaluated in joint planning clinics where medical and surgical oncologists and radiotherapists were present. This protocol, which ended in 1985, accrued 191 patients, but 17 were excluded because of major protocol violations. Thirty-one patients did not have surgery, including three patients with progressive disease and 28 in whom radiation therapy was the only locoregional treatment. Of the patients who came to surgery, a further seven did not have an axillary dissection. The remaining 136 patients who completed this preoperative chemotherapy regimen and underwent a total mastectomy with axillary dissection were followed up prospectively and formed the basis of this analysis. All the patients in this analysis were rendered disease free at the time of surgery.

Accepted for publication July 8, 1988

From the Division of Surgery, Department of General Surgery (Drs McCready and Balch), the Breast Medical Oncology Service, Department of Medical Oncology (Drs Hortobagyi and Buzdar and Ms Kau), and the Department of Biomathematics (Ms Smith), University of Texas M. D. Anderson Cancer Center, Houston.

Read before the Annual Meeting of the Society of Surgical Oncology, New Orleans, May 23, 1988.

Reprint requests to Department of Medical Oncology, University of Texas M. D. Anderson Cancer Center, 1515 Holcombe Blvd, Houston, TX 77030 (Dr Hortobagyi).

Table 1.—Clinical Stage at Presentation*					
	T1	T2	T3	T4	Row Total
N0	0	0	3	4	**7**
N1	0	0	13	25	**38**
N2	1	5	11	22	**39**
N3	0	1	1	14	**16**
Column Total	**1**	**6**	**28**	**65**	**100**

*Values are percentages.

The preoperative chemotherapy has been described previously[3] and consisted of fluorouracil, 500 mg/m² intravenously on days 1 and 8, doxorubicin, 50 mg/m² on day 1, and cyclophosphamide, 500 mg/m² intravenously on day 1. After three to six 21-day cycles of chemotherapy, a total mastectomy and level I and II axillary dissection was performed. Postoperatively, the patients resumed chemotherapy for six to 18 months, and then consolidative external beam radiotherapy was scheduled; some patients received their radiation therapy immediately after surgery. Following completion of all treatment, the patients were followed up at four-month intervals for the first two years, every six months for the next two years, and yearly thereafter.

Response to chemotherapy was evaluated by physical examination. A complete response was defined as total disappearance of the primary tumor and nodal disease. A partial response consisted of a greater than 50% reduction of the product of the two largest tumor diameters measured clinically. Pathologic response was graded as negative if no tumor could be found in the mastectomy specimen; microscopic residual if no tumor could be felt or seen with the naked eye but there were some viable tumor cells seen on microscopy; and gross residual if gross tumor was present. The negative and microscopic categories were combined for survival analysis because the number in each group was small. The number of axillary lymph nodes containing histologically proved breast cancer metastases was recorded by the pathologist from the mastectomy and axillary dissection specimen.

The Kaplan-Meier[10] method was used to calculate and plot the DFS and overall survival curves and the generalized Wilcoxon test was used to test differences between them.[11] Survival and DFS were calculated from the onset of chemotherapy and date of mastectomy, respectively. Patients who died without evidence of disease were counted as dead of disease in the survival analysis but were censored from DFS analysis. Survival distributions are summarized by five-year estimates to facilitate comparisons with other studies. The Cox regression model[12] was used to determine the prognostic importance of surgical node information relative to other factors. Because interest centered on whether it was important prognostically to acquire information on node status at surgery, in addition to prognostic information otherwise available, surgical node status was initially omitted from consideration and other factors were selected for inclusion in the model, using a forward selection procedure and cutoff significance level of .05. Addition of surgical node status to the selected model allowed a test of whether this information provided significant prognostic information to the already obtained factors. Associations between factors were tested by χ^2 analysis.

RESULTS

Clinical tumor stage at presentation and the clinical and pathologic response to preoperative chemotherapy and menopausal status were all important prognostic variables of survival and DFS when examined independently, but the number of metastatic axillary lymph nodes found at the time of surgery had significantly more prognostic value than the other characteristics individually and added significant information ($P<.01$) to a model using a combination of the other variables.

The pretreatment clinical staging of the patients with LABC in this study is given in Table 1. The median age was 50 years (range, 24 to 78 years), and median follow-up of the 63 survivors was 56 months (range, seven to 145 months). The overall actuarial survival and DFS at five years were 53% and 41%, respectively.

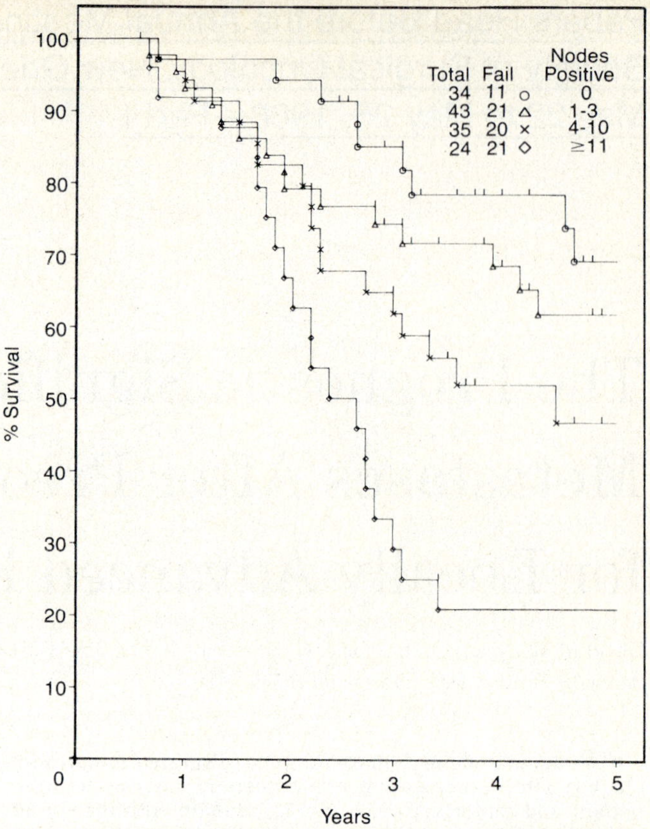

Fig 1.—Actuarial survival of patients with locally advanced breast cancer grouped according to number of metastatic axillary lymph nodes present after preoperative chemotherapy. Number of metastatic nodes was found to be significant prognostic variable of survival by univariate analysis (Wilcoxon, $P<.001$) and multivariate analysis (Cox, $P<.01$).

Univariate Analysis

Differences in survival and DFS according to the number of positive nodes were highly statistically significant, with a marked linear trend for decreased survival associated with increasing number of nodes. Survival and DFS of patients grouped by the number of positive nodes (0, 1 to 3, 4 to 10, and >10) are illustrated in Figs 1 and 2. The survival (±SE) at five years of patients with no positive axillary lymph nodes was 70%±9%, and was 62%±8% if one to three metastatic nodes were present, 47%±9% for patients with four to ten positive nodes, and 21%±8% if greater then ten nodes with metastases were found ($P<.001$). The five-year DFS was 72%±8%, 46%±8%, 35%±9%, and 6%±6%, respectively, and these differences were significant ($P<.001$). If patients with greater than or equal to four nodes were considered as one group, survival at five years was 38% and the DFS was 20%.

Two important subgroups were identified using the surgically staged node information. Patients with negative axillary nodes had an excellent prognosis, with a median survival of 91 months, but the 24 patients with more than ten positive nodes had a dismal survival rate. Only three patients in the subset are currently alive, and two of these have bone metastases. Six patients had disease recurrence within eight months of surgery.

Patients who presented with clinical stage T4 breast cancer, that is, the tumors extended into the chest wall or produced edema (including peau d'orange) or ulceration of the skin overlying the tumor, had worse prognoses (five-year survival, 42%; DFS, 30%) than those patients with less extensive primary tumors (T1-3; five-year survival, 78%, $P=.002$; DFS, 64%, $P<.001$). Clinical tumor stage at presentation was second only to the number of metastatic nodes in prognostic value when examined independently (Table 2).

Complete clinical response to the preoperative chemotherapy was associated with a significantly increased survival (94% at five years, $P=.01$) and DFS (87%, $P=.01$), but there was little difference between those patients who had a partial response and those who had no response (Table 2). Pathologic assessment of the mastectomy specimen revealed that patients with no discernible residual tumor or microscopic residual tumor (65% five-year survival, 70% DFS) after preoperative chemotherapy had significantly better survival and DFS than those patients with gross residual breast cancer remaining after preoperative chemotherapy (five-year survival, 49%, $P=.03$; DFS, 33%, $P=.001$).

Patients who were premenopausal had significantly better survival ($P=.04$) and DFS ($P=.002$) than did postmenopausal patients (Table 2), but clinical node stage at presentation was not a significant predictor of survival ($P=.08$) or DFS ($P=.06$). There were few differences in survival or DFS of the patients with tumors high in estrogen receptors compared with those with low estrogen receptor content.

Multivariate Analysis

To determine whether the number of metastatic lymph nodes added more prognostic information to other patient or tumor variables, the factors listed in Table 2 were evaluated for stepwise inclusion in Cox regression models of survival and DFS. The number of positive nodes was initially excluded from consideration. Factors selected for inclusion were clinical tumor stage at presentation, clinical response, and menopause status (Table 3). Models were then fit that included these terms plus a fourth term indicating the number of positive nodes after preoperative chemotherapy. The improvement in the fit of the model was statistically significant ($P<.01$) and suggests that surgical lymph node staging can significantly increase the prognostic information otherwise available.

Associated Factors

The number of involved lymph nodes was significantly associated with both clinical ($P<.01$) and pathologic ($P=.02$) response to chemotherapy, but pretreatment clinical tumor stage, clinical node stage at presentation, or menopausal status were not associated with the number of positive nodes (Table 4). The absence of nodal metastases tended to parallel pathologically determined chemotherapeutic response in the primary cancer. Sixteen (52%) of 31 patients who had no gross residual breast cancer had no positive lymph nodes, and none of these patients with minimal amounts of residual cancer had more than ten metastatic nodes. Similarly, ten (59%) of 17 patients who experienced a complete clinical response had no positive lymph nodes at surgery.

COMMENT

The objective of this study was to determine whether preoperative chemotherapy altered or diminished the value of surgical lymph node staging in patients with LABC. These results demonstrate that the presence and quantity of lymph node metastases remains the most important prognostic variable associated with survival and DFS after preoperative chemotherapy for patients with LABC. Menopausal status, clinical tumor stage at presentation, and response to chemotherapy are also individually important.

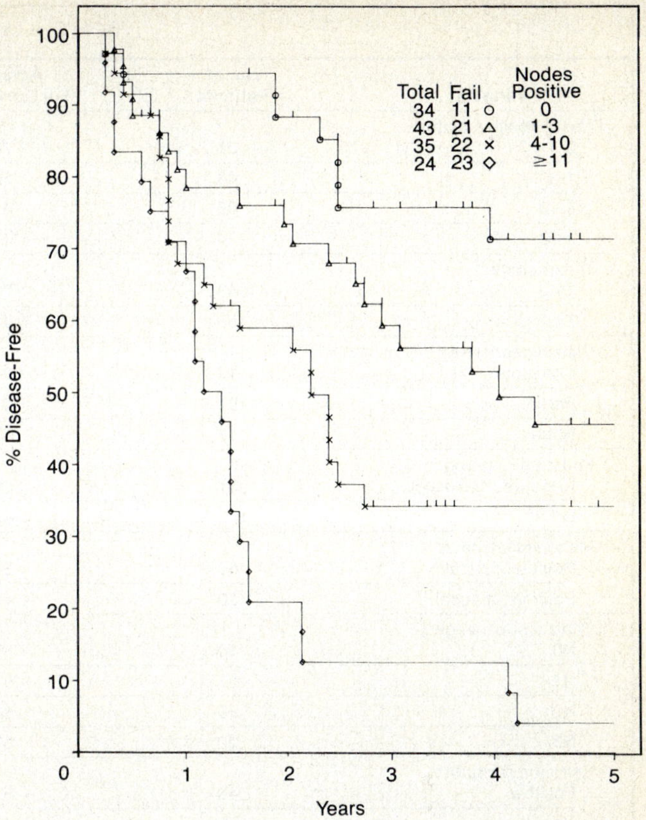

Fig 2.—Actuarial disease-free survival of patients with locally advanced breast cancer grouped according to number of axillary lymph nodes with metastases after preoperative chemotherapy. Number of positive nodes was most significant prognostic variable for disease-free survival by univariate (Wilcoxon, $P<.001$) and multivariate regression analysis (proportional hazards, Cox, $P<.01$).

Patients with LABC are heterogeneous with respect to prognosis.[6] This heterogeneity, combined with the lack of a consistent definition of LABC and the inherent inaccuracy related to clinical staging, make comparisons between treatment regimens difficult. The survival differences reported between treatment modalities may be more the result of patient selection than the effects of therapy.[8] Surgical-pathologic staging should result in more reliable treatment comparisons.

Traditionally, staging and, by definition, the measurement of prognostic variables are performed at the time of definitive surgical treatment. It is not surprising that some variables can lose their predictive value when other therapeutic modalities are initiated before surgery. Preoperative radiotherapy has been shown to obviate the prognostic value of Haagenson's grave signs, size of the primary tumor, and clinical node status.[13] Clinical node stage at presentation and estrogen receptor status were not significant after preoperative chemotherapy in this series.

There were 34 patients (25%) who had no metastatic axillary nodes after preoperative chemotherapy, which is double the number of patients with negative nodes found in stage III breast cancer treated with radical mastectomy without preoperative intervention.[14] This increased nega-

Table 2.—Univariate Analysis*					
Variable	**No. of Patients**	**Actuarial 5-y Survival, %**	***P***	**Actuarial 5-y DFS, %**	***P***
No. of positive nodes					
0	34	70	<.001	72	<.001
1-3	43	62		46	
4-10	35	47		35	
>10	24	21		5	
Tumor stage					
T1-3	48	78	.002	65	.001
T4	88	42		30	
Clinical response					
Complete	17	94	.01	87	.01
Partial	101	47		35	
None	18	43		30	
Pathologic response					
Negative, microscopic	31	65	.03	70	.001
Gross	105	49		33	
Menopausal status					
Premenopausal	66	61	.04	55	.002
Postmenopausal	70	45		29	
Clinical node stage					
N0	10	57	.08	48	.06
N1	51	67		48	
N2	53	48		37	
N3	22	37		32	
Estrogen receptor†					
Positive	46	57	.25	39	.83
Negative	59	45		40	

*By generalized Wilcoxon test.[11] DFS indicates disease-free survival.
†The receptor status was unknown in 31 patients.

Table 3.—Multivariate Analysis*				
	Survival		**DFS**	
Independent Factors	**Order of Entry**	***P***	**Order of Entry**	***P***
Surgical node staging†	. . .	<.01	. . .	<.01
Clinical tumor stage at presentation	1	<.01	1	<.01
Clinical response	2	.01	3	.02
Menopausal status	3	.04	2	.01

*DFS indicates disease-free survival. Analysis by proportional hazards model of Cox.[12] Regression equation for survival: $1n[\lambda(t)/\lambda o(t)] = +0.380(N) - 0.950(T) - 1.790(Response) - 0.396(Menopause)$; regression equation for DFS: $1n[\lambda(t)/\lambda o(t)] = +0.568(N) - 1.003(T) - 0.518(Menopause) - 1.243(Response)$. For these equations, codes for covariates are as follows: surgical nodes (N), no nodes, 0; one to three nodes, 1; four to ten nodes, 2; over ten nodes, 3; menopausal status, postmenopausal, 0; premenopausal, 1; tumor grade (T), T1-3, 1; T4, 0; response, partial or no response, 0; complete response, 1.

†The number of metastatic nodes had the highest score statistic, and the addition of this surgical staging variate resulted in significantly more prognostic information than a combination of the strongest other factors (see "Patients and Methods" section).

Table 4.—Associated Factors					
	No. of Nodes With Metastases				
Characteristic	**0**	**1-3**	**4-10**	**>10**	***P***
Pathologic response to preoperative chemotherapy					
Negative	32	2	3	0	<.01
Microscopic	15	23	8	0	
Gross	53	75	89	100	
Clinical response to preoperative chemotherapy					
Complete	29	7	11	0	.02
Partial	62	8	72	79	
None	9	9	17	21	
Menopausal status					
Premenopausal	65	49	43	33	.68
Postmenopausal	35	51	57	67	
Clinical tumor stage at presentation					
T1-3	38	37	34	29	.90
T4	62	63	66	71	
Clinical node stage at presentation					
N0	21	2	3	4	.35
N1	38	44	31	33	
N2	26	42	49	38	
N3	15	12	17	25	

*Values are percentages. *P* values are by χ^2 test.

tive node rate suggests lymph node metastases may be influenced by preoperative chemotherapy in those patients with responsive tumors. Variables that reflect response (number of lymph node metastases, clinical response, and pathologic response) and are thus measured after initial treatment may be more valuable than those measured at presentation.

The accuracy of surgical staging after preoperative chemotherapy may be the result of three factors. The number of positive lymph nodes is a quantifiable characteristic, is an index of systemic disease,[15] and is influenced by the cancer's response to chemotherapy, thus reflecting any downstaging that has occurred.

The absence of nodal metastases was significantly associated with a complete clinical and pathologic response in this series, and this suggests that downstaging of the nodal metastases paralleled the reduction of the primary cancer. The improved survival of subgroups of these downstaged patients (ie, those with complete clinical or pathologic response) also implies that prognosis depends on the amount of tumor present after chemotherapy rather than the tumor stage at presentation.

Further evidence of downstaging is provided by comparing the DFS from adjuvant postoperative chemotherapy trials for clinical stage I and II (pathologic stage T1-2, N1) breast cancer with that of our series for LABC after preoperative chemotherapy. The Milan group[16] has reported five-year survival rates for patients with one to three, four to ten, and greater than ten positive nodes of approximately 60%, 45%, and 38%, respectively, and in our series the respective survival was 62%, 47%, and 21%. However, it must be mentioned that other series have reported higher survival rates with adjuvant chemotherapy.[17]

Surgery is an integral component of the multimodality management of patients with LABC because mastectomy can improve local control,[18,19] and surgical staging provides important prognostic information. The subgroup of patients with greater than ten metastatic nodes after preoperative chemotherapy had a very poor prognosis. A more aggressive postoperative chemotherapeutic regimen is being planned for these patients with the hope that other agents will be able to prolong survival. Future protocols designed to employ only chemotherapy and radiotherapy without surgical staging will be unable to stratify and identify these subgroups of patients that may benefit from different treatments.

We wish to acknowledge the expert help of Mamie Gatlin and Janice Webb in typing the manuscript.

References

1. Fisher B, Slack NH, Bross ID, et al: Cancer of the breast: Size of neoplasm and prognosis. *Cancer* 1969;24:1071-1080.
2. American Joint Committee on Cancer: *Manual for Staging of Cancer,* ed 2. Philadelphia, JB Lippincott, 1983.
3. Hortobagyi GN, Blumenschein GR, Spanos W, et al: Multimodal treatment of locoregionally advanced breast cancer. *Cancer* 1983;51:763-768.
4. Ragaz J, Baird R, Rebbick P, et al: Neoadjuvant (preoperative) chemotherapy for breast cancer. *Cancer* 1985;56:719-724.
5. MacKay EN, Sellers AH: A prospective trial of the TNM classification of breast cancer by the regional cancer treatment centres in Ontario, 1960-1964. *Int J Cancer* 1970;6:5127-5128.
6. Hortobagyi GN, Kau SW, Buzdar AU, et al: Induction chemotherapy for stage III primary breast cancer, in Salmon SE (ed): *Adjuvant Therapy of Cancer V.* New York, Grune & Stratton, 1987, pp 419-428.
7. Feldman LD, Hortobagyi GN, Buzdar AU, et al: Pathological assessment of response to induction chemotherapy in breast cancer. *Cancer Res* 1986;46:2578-2581.
8. Davila E, Vogel CL: Management of locally advanced breast cancer (stage III): A review. *Int Adv Surg Oncol* 1984;7:297-327.
9. Fisher B, Wolmark N, Bauer M, et al: The accuracy of clinical nodal staging and of limited axillary dissection as a determinant of histologic nodal status in carcinoma of the breast. *Surg Gynecol Obstet* 1981;152:765-772.
10. Kaplan EL, Meier P: Nonparametric estimation from incomplete observations. *J Am Stat Assoc* 1958;53:457-481.
11. Gehan E: A generalized Wilcoxon test for comparing arbitrarily censored samples. *Biometrika* 1965;52:203-233.
12. Cox DR: Regression models and life tables. *J R Stat Soc* 1972;34:187-220.
13. Rao DV, Bedwinek J, Perez C, et al: Prognostic indicators in stage III and localized stage IV breast cancer. *Cancer* 1982;50:2037-2043.
14. Fracchia AA, Evans JF, Eisenberg BL: Stage III carcinoma of the breast: A detailed analysis. *Ann Surg* 1980;192:705-710.
15. Fisher B: Biological and clinical considerations regarding the use of surgery and chemotherapy in the treatment of primary breast cancer. *Cancer* 1977;40:574-587.
16. Bonadonna G, Valagussa P: Contribution of prognostic factors of adjuvant chemotherapy in breast cancer. *Recent Results Cancer Res* 1984;96:34-45.
17. Bonadonna G, Rossi A, Tancini G, et al: CMF adjuvant programs at the Milan Cancer Institute. *Recent Results Cancer Res* 1984;96:66-73.
18. Toonkel LM, Fix I, Jacobson LH, et al: Locally advanced breast carcinoma: Results with combined regional therapy. *Int J Radiat Oncol Biol Phys* 1986;12:1583-1587.
19. Balawajder I, Antich PP, Boland J: An analysis of the role of radiotherapy alone and in combination with chemotherapy and surgery in the management of advanced breast carcinoma. *Cancer* 1983;51:574-580.

Discussion

Q Would you please clarify your definition of response?

A We used two different responses: clinical response and pathologic response. The 17 patients alluded to first were clinical responders. They had complete clinical response; there was no tumor felt. Some of those had microscopic tumor in the mastectomy specimen, and some of them even could have had gross tumor that might be found once the breast was cut. But there were two separate measurements: clinical and pathologic.

Q But you said that of those 17 who had a complete clinical response, only one had a recurrence in five years.

A Only one died; that was a survival curve. I believe there were three recurrences.

Q In those patients who had a complete response, could you argue for not doing a full level I and II nodal dissection and just simply removing a few nodes, or not removing any, since 85% had no nodes involved?

A That could be an argument. There were no patients with more than ten nodes. While doing the mastectomy to show that there is no gross or residual tumor, I do not think it adds much to sample those lateral axillary nodes.

Q Would inadequate sampling contribute to apparent node negativity?

A The median number of nodes found was 13. In Dr Fortner's series of operable stage III breast cancer, there was a 12% incidence of negative nodes; there was about a 25% incidence in this series. I do not have the number of nodes actually sampled from his study to account for that. These were lateral axillary dissections, and I do not really know what our historical control would be for lateral axillary dissections, or how many nodes would be involved. I am not sure if the number of nodes is less after preoperative chemotherapy. It seems that the number of positive nodes is less, but I am not sure if the number of nodes found is less.

A Comparison of Palpable and Nonpalpable Breast Cancers

Timothy J. Pagana, MD; Willem J. Lubbe, MD; Sheldon M. Schwartz, MD; Gene D. Sprechini, PhD

• Chi-square statistics were used to compare prognostic factors of 60 patients with nonpalpable breast cancer (NPBC) and 112 patients with palpable breast cancer. Noninvasive cancers were more frequent, tumor size was smaller, and nodal metastasis was significantly less frequent in the NPBC group. However, the frequency of nodal metastasis was similar when adjusted for size and grade. There was no significant difference in the incidence of age and menopausal status of the patients, histologic types, hormone receptor status, and histologic/nuclear grade between these two groups. The findings were consistent with the hypothesis that NPBCs are potentially lethal tumors and that mammograms detect them earlier, ie, these tumors are smaller, localized, and, therefore, more curable.

(*Arch Surg* 1989;124:26-28)

The mortality for breast cancer has not changed in the last 30 to 40 years. All recent improvements in surgery, chemotherapy, and radiation therapy have not improved survival.[1,2] Unfortunately, the present knowledge of the risk factors of breast cancer does not provide a basis for reducing its incidence. In an effort to reduce the mortality, many large studies have evaluated the benefit of early detection on survival of patients with breast cancer. Recent reports[3,4] have indicated an improved survival among certain populations of mammographically screened patients. This has led to a dramatic increase in the number of women undergoing screening mammography. As a result, more nonpalpable breast cancers (NPBCs) are being detected. But, are these "tiny" nonpalpable mammographically detected cancers "real" cancers? There has been some contention that many of these small cancers are not life threatening, would not be expected to progress to the point of metastasis, and would remain unchanged indefinitely if left untreated.

In an attempt to determine whether or not NPBCs are "killer" cancers, we compared prognostic factors of NPBCs and palpable breast cancers (PBCs) detected at our institutions.

Accepted for publication July 15, 1988.

From the Divine Providence Cancer Treatment Center, Williamsport, Pa (Drs Pagana and Lubbe), The Williamsport (Pa) Hospital and Medical Center (Dr Schwartz), and the Department of Mathematics, Lycoming College, Williamsport, Pa (Dr Sprechini).

Read before the Annual Meeting of the Society of Surgical Oncology, New Orleans, May 23, 1988.

Reprint requests to 699 Rural Ave, Williamsport, PA 17701 (Dr Pagana).

PATIENTS AND METHODS

The sample consisted of 172 women whose conditions were diagnosed as breast cancer from a group of 482 patients who had undergone breast biopsies. Information was collected on the 60 women (35%) with NPBC and the 112 women (65%) with PBC. All women were consecutively treated at our institutions (Divine Providence Cancer Treatment Center, Williamsport, Pa, or The Williamsport [Pa] Hospital and Medical Center) between 1983 and 1987. These two groups of women with breast cancer were compared with respect to age, menopausal status, histologic type, histologic grade, hormone receptor status, size, and incidence of lymph node metastasis. Invasive cancers were given histologic grades according to the system described by Fisher et al.[5,6] Noninvasive cancers were given a nuclear grade by using criteria also described by Fisher and colleagues[5,6] in the same reports. Chi-square tests were used to make most comparisons that involved incidence; *t* tests were used to compare means.

RESULTS

Histology

Of the 60 NPBCs, 42 (70%) were invasive ductal, two (3%) were invasive lobular, 15 (25%) were intraductal, and one (2%) was noninvasive lobular. Of the 112 PBCs, 101 (90%) were invasive ductal, seven (6%) were invasive lobular, three (3%) were intraductal, and one (1%) was noninvasive lobular. A χ^2 test indicated that there was a significantly greater percentage of noninvasive cancer in the NPBC group ($P = .0001$). When noninvasive cancers were excluded, a χ^2 test showed no significant difference in histology between the two groups ($P = .73$).

Size

A *t* test showed that the cancers in the NPBC group were significantly smaller ($P = .0001$) than the PBC group (Table 1). The median and mean size of the NPBC group were 1.0 and 1.3 cm, respectively. The median and mean size for the PBC group were 2.0 and 2.4 cm, respectively.

Age and Menopausal Status

A *t* test yielded no significant difference between the mean age of the NPBC group (61 years) and the mean age of the PBC group (63 years) ($P = .17$). Likewise, no significant difference was found in menopausal status among the two groups (χ^2 test, $P = .33$). Fifteen patients (25%) of the

Table 1.—Size Comparison for NPBCs and PBCs*

Size, cm	No. NPBCs	No. PBCs
<1	37	28
1	12	19
2	9	31
3	2	19
4	0	3
5	0	5
6	0	2
7	0	1
8	0	3
9	0	1

*NPBCs indicates nonpalpable breast cancers; PBCs, palpable breast cancers. Significance by Student's *t* test, $P = .00001$.

Table 2.—Comparison of Hormone Receptor Assay for NPBCs and PBCs*

ER	PR	No. NPBCs	No. PBCs
Positive	Positive	17	40
Positive	Negative	12	11
Positive	ND	3	7
Negative	Positive	1	4
Negative	Negative	15	35
Negative	ND	2	3
Total Positive		**33**	**62**
Total Negative		**17**	**38**
ND		10	12

*NPBCs indicates nonpalpable breast cancers; PBCs, palpable breast cancers; ER, estrogen receptor; PR, progesterone receptor; and ND, not done. Significance by χ^2 test, $P = .64$.

NPBC group and 21 patients (19%) of the PBC group were premenopausal.

Histological/Nuclear Grade

Chi-square tests were used to compare histologic and nuclear grades. Histologic grades of invasive cancers were similar among the two groups ($P = .91$). Among the NPBC group, three (7%) were grade 1, 19 (43%) were grade 2, and 22 (50%) were grade 3. Among the PBC group, seven (6%) were grade 1, 43 (40%) were grade 2, and 58 (54%) were grade 3. The nuclear grade of noninvasive breast cancers was also similar ($P = .08$), although the percentage of noninvasive cancers was small in the PBC group. Among the NPBC group, four (25%) were grade 1, eight (50%) were grade 2, and four (25%) were grade 3. Among the PBC group, two (50%) were grade 1, two (50%) were grade 2, and none were grade 3.

Hormone Receptor Status

No significant difference in the hormone receptor status between the two groups was found with a χ^2 test. Thirty-three patients (66%) of the NPBC group were hormone receptor positive, and 62 patients (56%) of the PBC group were positive ($P = .64$). In ten of the nonpalpable cancers and 12 of the palpable cancers, no hormone receptive assay was obtained (Table 2).

Lymph Node Status

The results of a χ^2 test indicated that the NPBC group, as a whole, had a significantly lower incidence of nodal metastasis than their palpable counterparts ($P = .0001$). Six patients (10%) of the NPBC group and 46 patients (45%) of the PBC group had positive lymph nodes. This difference was still significant even when noninvasive cancers were excluded from both groups. However, the significant difference disappeared when similar size and grade tumors were compared (Table 3).

Table 3.—Comparison of Incidence of Lymph Node Metastasis With Tumor Size and Grade Kept Constant*

Grade	Size, cm	NPBCs Positive	NPBCs Negative	PBCs Positive	PBCs Negative	P†
2	<1	1	9	5	8	.14
3	<1	2	9	2	7	.63
2	1	1	6	4	6	.28
3	1	0	3	1	6	.70
2	2	0	2	6	6	.38
3	2	2	4	5	11	.65

*NPBCs indicates nonpalpable breast cancers; PBCs, palpable breast cancers.
†By Fisher's exact test.

COMMENT

Breast cancer occurs in one out of ten American women.[7] Detection after metastasis has occurred leads to immeasurable personal suffering and financial cost. Detection and treatment of breast cancer before metastasis has occurred should be associated with decreased morbidity and mortality. We have shown, as have others,[8-11] that the use of screening mammography in asymptomatic women can detect small cancers that are rarely associated with metastasis. But, are these nonpalpable neoplasms really cancer caught at an "early" stage? Or, are they a more "benign" form of breast cancer that would never develop any further during the life of the patient? There are no reliable pathohistologic criteria that can resolve these questions. Legal and ethical standards would preclude completion of a study designed to follow untreated NPBCs for a long period of time. Also, the performance of a diagnostic biopsy usually completely removes these tiny cancers and, thereby, eliminates the opportunity to study a group of patients who may refuse treatment.

Several investigators have attempted to resolve this dilemma. Moskowitz[12,13] performed mammogram screening on over 10 000 women. If he had found an exaggerated incidence of breast cancer in this screened population, he could have concluded that the use of screening mammography detected clinically significant plus clinically insignificant breast cancers. Instead, he found that the incidence of cancer in the screened population was not significantly different from the incidence of cancers otherwise expected in this population. That is to say, he did not detect an exaggerated incidence of breast cancers in the screened population. He concluded that tiny cancers detected by screening mammography would have become clinically significant if left untreated. Brinton et al[14] arrived at the same conclusion by comparing the risk factors of small and large invasive cancer groups; they showed a close similarity between the risk factors of these two groups of breast cancers, thereby supporting the notion that these two groups are biologically closely related.

We have chosen to compare reliable prognostic factors of NPBCs and PBCs to see if they may act similarly aggressive. The prognostic variables included patient age and menopausal status, tumor size, hormone receptor status, histology, histologic grading, and the incidence of lymph node metastasis. Not all of these factors, however, are a measurement of the intrinsic activity of breast cancer alone. Some of these factors are also a result of other aspects of the clinical situation. For example, while tumor size may be a measure of the intrinsic nature of breast cancer, it is also reflective of a duration of growth.[15] Likewise, while the incidence of lymph node metastasis may be the most important prognostic factor of breast cancer, it is also a result of many other prognostic variables, such as tumor size and histologic grade.[16,17] Therefore, by and of itself, tumor size and the incidence of lymph node metastasis cannot be studied as independent accurate indicators of the intrinsic nature of breast cancer. With regard to the incidence of lymph node metastasis, it is interesting to note that there was no statistically significant difference between the two groups when the size and histologic grade were kept constant. This serves to indicate comparable aggressiveness between these two groups. The numbers within these subgroups are small, however.

Histologic grading and hormone receptor status are, independently, most reflective of the intrinsic nature of breast cancer.[18-22] These are probably not related to other factors, such as duration of growth and size. In our study, we found no difference between the NPBC and PBC groups with regard to histologic grading or hormone receptor status, further supporting a biologic similarity between the two groups.

Although we have shown that NPBCs were smaller, were less frequently infiltrating, and were generally associated with a lower incidence of lymph node metastasis when compared with their palpable counterparts, there was no difference between these two groups of cancers with regard to age and menopausal status of the patient, size/grade-adjusted incidence of lymph node metastasis, histology, histologic/nuclear grade, and hormone receptor status. We conclude, therefore, that because of their similarity with PBC, tiny NPBCs are not just a benign form of breast cancer that may never kill. Rather, we suggest that NPBCs are potential killer cancers detected in their preclinical state. If left undetected or untreated, they could develop into a palpable cancer that would metastasize and kill.

This report, however, does not attempt to resolve whether or not noninvasive breast cancer represents an "earlier" stage of invasive cancer. Most investigators, however, believe that this is a natural progression, especially for ductal cancer. We agree, and in light of our data, therefore, encourage the use of screening mammography for asymptomatic women in high-risk categories. We believe this screening diminishes mortality because it detects cancers earlier and at a time when treatment can provide an excellent opportunity for cure.

We appreciate the consulting assistance of Kathleen D. Pagana, RN, PhD, in the preparation of this manuscript.

References

1. Shapiro S: Evidence on screening for breast cancer from a randomized trial. *Cancer* 1977;39:2772-2782.
2. Idem I: Imaging of the breast: A perspective. *Surg Clin North Am* 1984;64:1061-1072.
3. Seidman H, Gelb S, Silverberg E, et al: Survival experience in the breast cancer detection demonstration project. *CA* 1987;37:258-290.
4. Shapiro S, Venet W, Strax P, et al: Selection, follow-up, and analysis in the health insurance plan study: A randomized trial with breast cancer screening. *NCI Monogr* 1985;67:65-74.
5. Fisher E: Histologic grading of breast cancer. *Pathol Annu* 1980;15:239-251.
6. Fisher ER, Gresous RM, Fisher B: Pathology of invasive breast cancer: A syllabus derived from findings of the National Surgical Breast Adjuvant Project. *Cancer* 1975;36:1-85.
7. Strax P: Mass screening for control of breast cancer. *Cancer* 1984;53:665-670.
8. Bigelow R, Smith R, Goodman P, et al: Needle localization of nonpalpable breast masses. *Arch Surg* 1985;120:565-569.
9. Rodes N, Lopez M, Pearson D, et al: The impact of breast cancer screening of survival. *Cancer* 1986;57:581-585.
10. Symmonds R, Roberts J: Management of non-palpable breast abnormalities. *Ann Surg* 1987;205:520-528.
11. Meyer J, Kopans D, Stumper P, et al: Occult breast abnormalities: Percutaneous preoperative needle localization. *Radiology* 1984;150:335-337.
12. Moskowitz M: Mammographic screening: Significance of minimal breast cancers. *AJR* 1981;136:735-738.
13. Moskowitz M: Minimal breast cancer redux. *Radiol Clin North Am* 1983;21:93-113.
14. Brinton L, Hoover R, Fraumeni J: Epidemiology of minimal breast cancer. *JAMA* 1983;249:483-487.
15. Gullino P: Natural history of breast cancer. *Cancer* 1977;39:2697-2703.
16. Fisher B, Slack N, Bross I: Cancer of the breast: Size of neoplasia and prognosis. *Cancer* 1969;24:1071-1080.
17. Feig S, Schwartz G: Prognostic pathologic factors among breast cancers detected by screening mammography. *Recent Results Cancer Res* 1984;90:148-160.
18. Contesso G, Mourisse H, Friedman S, et al: Importance of histologic grade in a long-term prognosis of breast cancer: Study of 1010 patients uniformly treated at the Institut Gustave-Roussy. *J Clin Oncol* 1987;5:1378-1386.
19. Fisher E, Fisher B: The relationship of pathologic and some clinical discriminants to the spread of breast cancer. *Int J Radiat Oncol Biol Phys* 1977;2:747-750.
20. Hans-Olov A, Kilander D: Prediction of survival in breast cancer. *Acta Chir Scand*, 1984, suppl 519, pp 25-34.
21. Bishop H, Elston C, Blamey R, et al: Relationship with estrogen receptor to survival and breast cancer. *Lancet* 1979;2:283-284.
22. Knight W, Livingston R, Gregory E, et al: Estrogen receptor as an independent prognostic factor for early recurrence in breast cancer. *Cancer Res* 1977;37:4669-4671.

Discussion

Q How do you define nonpalpable, and how do you perform biopsy on NPBCs?

A Nonpalpable was described as capability of the clinician to palpate the neoplasm. All of these tumors underwent biopsy with the use of preoperative x-ray localization and all of the tumors had postoperative roentgenograms of the mammogram specimen.

Q I am still a little confused about this study. Are we to conclude that nonpalpable, noninvasive, intraductal carcinoma is potentially a killer cancer from this analysis?

A No. We do not purport to resolve the problem of noninvasive cancers becoming invasive killer cancers; that would require the study of noninvasive cancers in a longer follow-up of that group.

Q Was size a discriminating factor as to whether or not to perform biopsy?

A We do not consider size to be a discriminating factor as to whether or not we should take a biopsy specimen of a lesion. If the lesion is new or if the lesion has irregular borders or, in any way, looks suspicious or is associated with microcalcification, we will proceed with a biopsy.

Q How many of the nonpalpable cancers were, in fact, associated with microcalcifications? Was that the common presenting mammographic finding?

A Thirty percent of microcalcifications were cancerous; likewise, nearly 30% of breast nodules without calcification were cancerous, and the combination of calcification in a mass did not really increase the incidence of cancer. Therefore, around 60% of the NPBCs had microcalcification within.

Nonpalpable In Situ Ductal Carcinoma of the Breast

Predictors of Multicentricity and Microinvasion and Implications for Treatment

Gordon F. Schwartz, MD; Arthur S. Patchefsky, MD; Sidney D. Finklestein, MD; Sae H. Sohn, MD; Anthony Prestipino, MD; Stephen A. Feig, MD; Jodi S. Singer, MD

• Fifty breasts with nonpalpable ductal carcinoma in situ (DCIS) were examined for the presence of microinvasion, multicentricity, and number of involved ducts to see if the biopsy specimen could have predicted the findings in the remainder of the breast. When DCIS was an incidental finding, fewer ducts were involved and no evidence of either microinvasion or multicentricity was found. Solid and cribriform DCIS were rarely multicentric or microinvasive; micropapillary DCIS was often multicentric, rarely microinvasive; comedocarcinoma was more likely to be both microinvasive and multicentric. Ductal carcinoma in situ as an incidental finding may be treated by excision alone; papillary and micropapillary DCIS are best treated by therapy aimed at the entire breast, although axillary dissection may not be required. Therapy for comedocarcinomas should include the entire breast and the axillary nodes.

(*Arch Surg* 1989;124:29-32)

Until we solve the mystery of breast cancer prevention, how fortunate our patients would be if we could promise them the detection of this dread disease when it was nonpalpable, noninvasive, and nonthreatening. In recent years, the ubiquitous use of screening mammography in asymptomatic women has led to the earlier detection of breast cancer as clusters of microcalcifications, nonpalpable masses, and areas of parenchymal distortion, without any overt clinical evidence of disease. Many of these malignant neoplasms are not yet invasive, and the frequent diagnosis of ductal carcinoma in situ (noninvasive) (DCIS) has become a consequence of these screening mammograms. Although described rarely before this era, one third of patients in our own series of over 300 breast cancers detected by mammography had DCIS or DCIS with microinvasion.[1] Small is not a synonym for inconsequential, since 30% of clinically nonpalpable, frankly invasive cancers may have axillary metastasis, but none of this published group of patients with DCIS had a positive axillary node.

If specific identifiable characteristics of DCIS that determine the likelihood of associated multicentricity or microinvasion exist, they might be used to predict what might be occurring in the remainder of the breast or in the regional nodes. Thus, the biopsy findings might then determine what, if any, further treatment might be required in each individual patient with DCIS. If node metastasis is unlikely, then axillary dissection could be avoided in selected patients; there might be a group of patients with DCIS confirmed on biopsy for whom no further treatment might be reasonable.

This study was designed to attempt to answer these questions by comparing biopsy and subsequent mastectomy findings in women with DCIS. Mastectomy specimens in patients with nonpalpable DCIS were examined for residual tumor at the biopsy site, accompanying microinvasion, multicentricity, and axillary node metastasis, so that we could determine if the biopsy findings could predict the status of the entire breast and axilla. A strong positive correlation between biopsy findings and breast status would have significant implications for treatment, permitting therapeutic decisions on the basis of the biopsy results alone.

PATIENTS AND METHODS

Records of the pathology department and tumor registry of Thomas Jefferson University Hospital, Philadelphia, were reviewed for the years between 1970 and 1985 for patients indexed as having DCIS or DCIS with microinvasion. Patients with palpable masses that proved to be malignant, even if the biopsy demonstrated only DCIS, were excluded. If, however, a palpable mass led to biopsy, but the mass itself was benign and DCIS was an incidental finding in the biopsy specimen, the patient was

Accepted for publication Sept 2, 1988.

From the Departments of Surgery (Drs Schwartz, Sohn, and Singer), Pathology (Drs Patchefsky and Prestipino), and Radiology (Dr Feig), Jefferson Medical College; and the Department of Pathology, Hahnemann University (Dr Finklestein), Philadelphia. Dr Patchefsky is now with Hahnemann University, Philadelphia.

Read in part before the Annual Meeting of the Society of Surgical Oncology, New Orleans, May 23, 1988.

Reprint requests to 1015 Chestnut St, Suite 510, Philadelphia, PA 19107 (Dr Schwartz).

included. Women with Paget's disease, if there was no evidence of invasive cancer and no accompanying breast mass, were also included, as were patients with nipple discharge without an accompanying mass. Patients with lobular carcinoma in situ (lobular neoplasia) were excluded.

Mastectomy was an important criterion for inclusion in this study so that the entire breast would be available for microscopic examination. Thus, the study group included patients who underwent total mastectomy alone, mastectomy with axillary dissection (modified radical mastectomy), or radical mastectomy. Parenthetically, the diagnosis of DCIS has been made more frequently in recent years than before 1980. Many of our recent patients have chosen breast conservation, usually wide local excision, axillary dissection, and irradiation, and, therefore, could not be included in this study.

Biopsy and mastectomy specimens were processed in the surgical pathology department according to a standard protocol. The following details about each specimen were recorded: (1) Histologic pattern of DCIS. The patterns of papillary, micropapillary, solid, cribriform, or comedocarcinoma were used. When more than one type was present, the specimen was assigned to the diagnosis that predominated. (2) Presence of microinvasion at the biopsy site. We have previously defined microinvasion as mainly a DCIS showing focal microinvasion below the basement membrane in one or several individual ducts, but in not more than 10% of the surface of the histologic sections examined.[2] (3) Number of involved ducts, ie, the cross-sectional duct structures containing tumor in all of the tumor-bearing slides. All of the biopsy material was submitted for study; the average number of slides per biopsy specimen was eight. Total number of ducts involved was recorded by adding the numbers of ducts involved in each slide, including both the biopsy material and the site of the biopsy in the subsequent mastectomy specimen. Counting the total number of involved ducts in both specimens, biopsy and mastectomy, minimized any variations in number of involved ducts due to differences in biopsy size. Cancerization of lobules was counted as a single ductal unit. (4) Presence of multicentric ductal carcinoma in the mastectomy specimen.

Mastectomy specimens were processed according to the protocol outlined by the Pathology Working Group of the National Breast Cancer Task Force.[3] A minimum of four sections was provided from each quadrant as well as four sections from the retroareolar area. Multicentricity was defined as the presence of invasive ductal or lobular carcinoma, microinvasive ductal carcinoma, or DCIS in an area or quadrant outside the biopsy site. The presence of lobular carcinoma in situ at the biopsy site or elsewhere was ignored in the determination of multicentricity. If the lesion was centrally located, deep to the nipple-areolar complex, the cancer was considered multicentric only if additional foci of carcinoma were found outside a perimeter of 5 cm from the edge of the nipple and areola. Axillary nodes, when included, were divided into three anatomic groups using levels defined by the pectoralis minor muscle. Nodes were found by hand dissection of the fresh specimens, and each node was cut at one level unless it was large enough to warrant more sections.

RESULTS

The study group comprised 47 women, 29 to 75 years of age (mean, 56 years; median, 57 years), with 50 DCISs, three women having synchronous bilateral cancers (Table 1). Patients were followed up through June 30, 1987, with a mean follow-up of 7.7 years and a median follow-up of seven years. Mode of presentation is shown in Table 2. Thirty-two breasts altogether (64%) had undergone biopsy for suspicious mammographic findings, and in 29, DCIS was the lesion responsible for the mammographic finding. Fourteen of these lesions were comedocarcinomas. In three women with mammographic abnormalities, the DCIS was an incidental finding, with the lesion provoking the biopsy being benign. Each patient with bilateral in situ carcinoma had the same mode of presentation in each breast.

The mode of detection apparently influenced the likelihood of both multicentricity and microinvasion, as noted in Tables 3 and 4. Of the 50 breasts studied, 18 (36%) contained multicentric foci of DCIS, one patient having both multicentric DCIS and invasive ductal cancer in the same breast as well as a single positive level I axillary node. No other patient had multicentric foci of more aggressive carcinoma than that found in the biopsy specimen. The DCIS presenting as nipple discharge or as Paget's disease was accompanied by a greater incidence of multicentricity than was DCIS detected by mammography or as an incidental finding. Thirteen breasts with DCIS (26%) demonstrated microinvasion in the biopsy specimen. The cancers detected mammographically were more likely to be microinvasive than those presenting with nipple discharge or erosion. None of the patients in whom DCIS was detected incidentally had either multicentric or microinvasive cancer.

Table 1.—Age Distribution of Patients With DCIS*

Age, y	No. (% of Total)
≤30	1 (2)
31-40	2 (4)
41-50	11 (23)
51-60	15 (32)
61-70	13 (28)
>70	5 (11)
Total	**47 (100)**

*DCIS indicates ductal carcinoma in situ.

Table 2.—Detection of DCIS*

Mode of Detection	No. (% of Total)
Mammography (calcifications)	29 (58)
Incidental finding	**10 (20)**
Palpable (benign) mass	7 (14)
Mammography	3 (6)
Nipple discharge—no mass palpable	7 (14)
Paget's carcinoma—no mass palpable	4 (8)
Total	**50 (. . .)**

*DCIS indicates ductal carcinoma in situ.

Table 3.—Mode of Detection vs Microinvasion in DCIS*

Mode of Detection	Not Microinvasive No. (%)	Microinvasive No. (%)	Total
Mammography	20 (69)	9 (31)	**29**
Incidental finding	10 (100)	0 (0)	**10**
Palpable mass	7 (. . .)	. . . (. . .)	. . .
Mammogram	3 (. . .)	. . . (. . .)	. . .
Nipple discharge	5 (71)	2 (29)	**7**
Paget's carcinoma	2 (50)	2 (50)	**4**
Total	**37 (74)**	**13 (26)**	**50**

*DCIS indicates ductal carcinoma in situ.

Table 4.—Mode of Detection vs Multicentricity in DCIS*

Mode of Detection	Not Multicentric No. (%)	Multicentric No. (%)	Total
Mammography	18 (62)	11 (38)	**29**
Incidental finding	10 (100)	0 (0)	**10**
Palpable mass	7 (. . .)	. . . (. . .)	. . .
Mammogram	3 (. . .)	. . . (. . .)	. . .
Nipple discharge	2 (29)	5 (71)	**7**
Paget's carcinoma	2 (50)	2 (50)	**4**
Total	**32 (64)**	**18 (36)**	**50**

*DCIS indicates ductal carcinoma in situ.

Table 5.—Histologic Findings vs Multicentricity in DCIS*

Histologic Findings	Not Multicentric No. (%)	Multicentric No. (%)	Total
Comedocarcinoma	11 (58)	8 (42)	19
Cribriform	5 (100)	0 (0)	5
Papillary	8 (67)	4 (33)	12
Solid	7 (100)	0 (0)	7
Micropapillary	1 (14)	6 (86)	7
Total	**32 (. . .)**	**18 (. . .)**	**50**

*DCIS indicates ductal carcinoma in situ.

Table 6.—Histologic Findings vs Microinvasion in DCIS*

Histologic Findings	Not Microinvasive No. (%)	Microinvasive No. (%)	Total
Comedocarcinoma	9 (47)	10 (53)	19
Cribriform	5 (100)	0 (0)	5
Papillary	11 (92)	1 (8)	12
Solid	6 (86)	1 (14)	7
Micropapillary	6 (86)	1 (14)	7
Total	**37 (74)**	**13 (26)**	**50**

*DCIS indicates ductal carcinoma in situ.

With respect to the numbers of involved ducts in patients with DCIS, 20 (40%) of the 50 breasts examined had ten or fewer ducts involved, but ten breasts (20%) had 100 or more involved ducts. As might be expected, patients in whom DCIS was an incidental finding had the smallest number of involved ducts (mean, seven ducts), and these were mostly papillary, cribriform, and solid histologic types of DCIS. The number of ducts involved by DCIS correlated with multicentricity more than it did with microinvasion, but multicentric and microinvasive carcinomas were scattered throughout all levels of ductal involvement, even among those cases with minimal numbers of involved ducts. There was no "safe" level of duct involvement below which neither multicentricity nor microinvasion was evident. However, in every patient but one (who presented with nipple discharge), if more than 100 ducts were involved by DCIS, multicentricity was also noted. There was no significant number of involved ducts—a "breakpoint"—that implied microinvasion; the 13 breasts with microinvasive DCIS had levels of duct involvement ranging from ten to 571. Although a trend toward microinvasion was noted as the number of involved ducts increased, several patients with the greatest numbers of involved ducts did not have accompanying microinvasion.

The incidence of multicentricity and microinvasion in each histologic type of DCIS is noted in Tables 5 and 6. Although few in number, solid and cribriform DCIS were never multicentric and rarely microinvasive; papillary DCIS was rarely either multicentric or microinvasive. Micropapillary DCIS was frequently (six of seven) multicentric but rarely microinvasive. Comedocarcinomas were more likely to be either multicentric or microinvasive than the other histologic varieties of DCIS; two such lesions, with seven and 11 involved ducts, respectively, demonstrated microinvasion and multicentricity. The only patient with multicentric invasive carcinoma and an involved axillary node had a comedocarcinoma detected as mammographic calcifications, with 224 involved ducts and microinvasion detected in the biopsy specimen.

COMMENT

The diagnosis of DCIS has become more common as the use of mammography for screening asymptomatic women has become an accepted component of optimal health care. However, a variety of macroscopic and microscopic lesions are classified by this same term or synonyms, eg, DCIS, intraductal carcinoma, noninvasive duct carcinoma, and, until recently, palpable and mammographically detected tumors have not been categorized separately with respect to treatment or outcome.

None of the 50 cases of DCIS reported in this study presented as a palpable malignant mass in the breast. Eleven cases had clinical evidence of disease, ie, seven with nipple discharge and four with nipple erosion. Twenty-nine breasts underwent biopsies because of microcalcifications that proved to be malignant, and the remaining ten cases of DCIS were truly incidental findings in patients undergoing biopsy for either palpable or mammographic findings that proved benign.

Recognizing that the number of breasts examined was small, our observations concerning the number of involved ducts, microscopic tumor type, multicentricity, and microinvasion have several implications. Comedo and micropapillary forms of DCIS were more likely to be multicentric than were papillary, cribriform, and solid types, and comedocarcinomas alone were likely to be accompanied by microinvasion. In comedocarcinoma, even the small ones (involving few ducts) demonstrated this proclivity to microinvasion, implying a relatively short noninvasive growth phase. The micropapillary form of DCIS, strongly correlating with multicentricity but not with microinvasion, perhaps arises in multiple foci simultaneously but remains indolent for a longer time.

The most interesting group of patients was the group in which DCIS was an incidental finding. None of these patients had either multicentric DCIS or evidence of microinvasion. These lesions also tended to be small, all but one involving 20 ducts or less, none involving more than 35 ducts. There was only one comedocarcinoma in this group that involved only five ducts. All of the incidental in situ carcinomas discovered by mammography were adjacent to the benign lesion. The three incidental in situ carcinomas found in palpable breast disease were more difficult to localize with respect to the dominant benign lesion since these specimens were larger. Perhaps the lack of multicentricity or microinvasion in these incidental in situ carcinomas denotes a subset of DCIS with a less aggressive biologic potential.

This study also establishes that there is no safe (minimum) level of duct involvement that guarantees against multicentricity or microinvasion. As already noted, however, DCIS of the solid or cribriform types and those that are accidental discoveries are seemingly less aggressive than those that are comedocarcinomas.

The studies of DCIS that address the question of the natural history of untreated disease imply that 30% to 50% of these patients will subsequently develop an invasive carcinoma of that breast.[4,5] Current treatment recommendations are at least in part a reflection of the uncertainty of this prediction. If there were a means by which these odds could be defined more reliably in each particular situation, therapy could be tailored more precisely and individually. This concept has been recognized and already implemented to some degree by Gump et al,[6] Silverstein et al,[7] and Schnitt et al,[8] but without clear-cut guidelines for treatment based on an accurate assessment of risk of multicentricity, microinvasion, or axillary node metastasis.

If our observations in this small number of patients are confirmed so that the qualitative and quantitative characteristics of DCIS within the entire breast may be approximated by the detailed evaluation of the biopsy specimen, patients may be informed of their treatment options with greater certainty that the most suitable strategy will be suggested. If any patients, for example, are chosen for treatment by excision alone, without further attention to the remainder of the breast or to the regional nodes, it should be those women in whom the diagnosis of DCIS is an incidental finding. Women with nonpalpable solid or cribriform types of DCIS are also candidates for excision only, if the biopsy indicates a small number of involved ducts. Women with nonpalpable papillary or micropapillary subsets of DCIS apparently are still best served by treatment of the entire breast, either by mastectomy or irradiation, but axillary dissection is probably not indicated. Women with comedocarcinoma are at higher risk for microinvasion than those with other forms of DCIS. Although the risk of axillary node metastasis is small (one patient in this series), at least level I axillary dissection should be considered for those women with comedocarcinomas with large numbers of involved ducts or with documented microinvasion in the biopsy specimen.

Although not specifically addressed by this study, we concur with Gump et al[6] that macroscopic (palpable) DCIS should not be considered in the same way as nonpalpable DCIS. Patients with macroscopic disease deserve the same treatment as those with invasive carcinomas of the same size, with the recognition that axillary metastasis is less likely and the outcome more favorable.

Until the recent popularity and widespread acceptance of breast-conserving procedures, the threat of mutilation often impeded the early detection of breast cancer, since the reward for diligence was perceived as more threatening than the disease itself. As we continue to refine therapy to fit individual patient circumstances, it is a reasonable expectation that still earlier discovery will continue to be paralleled by lesser and lesser treatment.

References

1. Schwartz GF, Feig SA, Patchefsky AS: Significance and staging of nonpalpable carcinomas of the breast. *Surg Gynecol Obstet* 1988;166:6-10.
2. Schwartz GF, Patchefsky AS, Feig SA, et al: Clinically occult breast cancer: Multicentricity and implications for treatment. *Ann Surg* 1980; 191:8-12.
3. Pathology Working Group, Breast Cancer Task Force: Standardized management of breast cancer specimens. *Am J Clin Pathol* 1973;60:789-798.
4. Betsill WL, Rosen PP, Lieberman PH, et al: Intraductal carcinoma: Long term follow-up after treatment by biopsy alone. *Cancer* 1978;239: 1863-1867.
5. Page DL, Dupont WD, Rogers OW, et al: Intraductal carcinoma of the breast: Followup after biopsy only. *Cancer* 1982;49:751-758.
6. Gump FE, Jicha DL, Ozello L: Ductal carcinoma in situ (DCIS): A revised concept. *Surgery* 1987;102:790-795.
7. Silverstein MJ, Rosser RJ, Gierson ED, et al: Axillary lymph node dissection for intraductal breast carcinoma: Is it indicated? *Cancer* 1987; 59:1819-1824.
8. Schnitt SJ, Silen W, Sadowsky NL, et al: Ductal carcinoma in situ (intraductal carcinoma) of the breast. *N Engl J Med* 1988;318:898-903.

Discussion

Q May I ask you about how you quantitate the number of ducts? Since the duct is a branching structure, it seems that the frequency of your sections would determine the number of involved ducts.

A We counted the number of ducts on serial sections. This was determined by having two separate pathologists count the tubular structures that they could see to arrive at a consensus. The comments you make, in terms of serial sections, are well taken, and an attempt was made to try to avoid that in counting the ducts. To some degree this was subjective.

Q In reference to the mammographic findings, I presume the incidental finding was one in which the mammogram did not detect the lesions at that site. Please clarify this.

A Several of the patients had palpable masses and, of course, the DCIS was an incidental finding elsewhere in the specimen, not in the palpable mass. In the patients who had DCIS as an incidental finding, several had calcifications as the finding on the mammogram, but the calcifications were totally benign, such as microscopic cystic disease or another diagnosis, and the DCIS was not associated with the area of calcification.

Q Is there a relationship then in your overall study between the mammographic findings and multicentric involvement in either areas of calcifications or otherwise?

A Only in one sense. I think it is more important to determine not so much what the mammographic findings might be, but how the mammographic findings are correlated with the histologic features; those mammographic findings that proved to be calcifications within the ducts of a carcinoma were much more likely to be associated with both multicentric and microinvasive carcinoma. We can see calcifications that are extraductal in patients who have cribriform, papillary or micropapillary types of carcinoma, but when the calcifications were seen as little purple spots right in the middle of the carcinoma, this type was more likely to be associated with multicentricity and microinvasion.

Q Did I understand that one patient in your series had positive axillary nodes and that an invasive breast cancer was incidentally found at a site remote from the intraductal site?

A That's correct.

Q Then why are you advocating node dissections?

A Well, it depends whether one looks at this as mostly negative or possibly positive. The latter approach is safer. I certainly only advocated node dissections in those patients with carcinomas who had high ductal involvement and who had microinvasion at the site. Those were the only patients for whom I had advocated lymph node dissection.

Breast Carcinoma In Situ

David W. Kinne, MD; Jeanne A. Petrek, MD; Michael P. Osborne, MD;
Alfred A. Fracchia, MD; Angelo A. DePalo, MD; Paul Peter Rosen, MD

• A total of 150 patients with in situ breast cancer were treated from 1970 through 1976, with a median follow-up of 11.5 years. There were 42 patients with microinvasion and 25 with bilateral disease, analyzed separately. Eight patients who became unavailable for follow-up within five years (but who had no evidence of disease [NED]) were excluded. Eighty-five patients had ductal carcinoma in situ, 43 had lobular carcinoma in situ, and 22 had a mixed type. Modified radical mastectomy was done in 112 cases. One of 128 patients had positive axillary nodes; axillary dissection is not indicated for in situ breast cancer. Of the 150 patients, one with ductal disease died of disease. Six died of other causes, free of disease. Of 18 treated by excision alone, two underwent mastectomy for recurrence and had NED. Patients with microinvasion had involved nodes in 10%, and 94% had NED. However, all bilateral cases had NED.

(*Arch Surg* 1989;124:33-36)

Retrospective analyses of patients with in situ breast carcinoma showed that most patients were treated by mastectomy, and that survival rates, free of disease, were over 90% and approximated 100%.[1-3] Often these series did not have long-term follow-up[4-6] and/or did not include pathologic analysis of failures.[7] The latter included higher-than-expected incidences of axillary node involvement or a higher rate of distant metastases than would have been expected.[8]

Some of these problems were due to definition; before the use of mammography, patients with ductal carcinoma in situ (DCIS) presented with clinical findings. They had either a mass, Paget's disease of the nipple, or bloody nipple discharge. Haagensen[9] considered that all such patients had microinvasion and should be treated by radical mastectomy. This definition allowed up to 50% of such lesions to be invasive. It was not surprising that up to 25% of patients had positive axillary nodes in that setting, and survival after radical mastectomy was about 75%.

A more accepted definition of in situ breast cancer is that complete histologic analysis shows no areas of invasion. In this setting, involvement of axillary nodes is seen in less than 1% of cases[10] and survival with no evidence of disease (NED) after mastectomy is close to 100%.

This study attempts to answer two questions seldom addressed in the past: What is the outcome of patients with in situ breast cancer followed up for more than ten years? Also, does careful pathologic review in patients with unusual findings (positive axillary nodes) or unexpected outcome after mastectomy (local recurrence, distant metastases) reveal microinvasion? Additional subgroups for analyses were those with predominantly in situ disease but with microinvasion and patients with bilateral breast cancer whose disease on the initial side was in situ.

PATIENTS AND METHODS

All patients treated for in situ breast carcinoma at Memorial Sloan-Kettering Cancer Center, New York, between 1970 and 1976 were analyzed. Patients were divided into those with pure DCIS, lobular carcinoma in situ (LCIS), or mixed DCIS-LCIS. Patients with previous carcinoma were excluded. Two hundred twenty-five patients were analyzed, but the study was restricted to patients with unilateral in situ breast cancer. Therefore, 42 patients with predominantly in situ cancer but evidence histologically of microinvasion were analyzed separately, as were 25 patients with bilateral breast cancer.

Long-term follow-up was stressed; of the remaining 158 patients, eight were excluded because their follow-up was less than five years. All were free of disease when last seen. Thus, a median follow-up of 11.5 years was achieved (range, five to 17.4 years).

RESULTS

Patients had DCIS in 85 cases, DCIS and LCIS in 22, and LCIS in 43. The indication for biopsy was usually a mass, which most often was not caused by these diseases. A mammogram was the indication for biopsy more often in patients with DCIS than with LCIS, but DCIS also presented as Paget's disease or nipple discharge. Mammography was not done often in this earlier series, but results were more often positive in patients with DCIS than with LCIS. Mammograms were suggestive in 49 of 55 patients with DCIS and ten of 14 with DCIS and LCIS. They were positive less frequently in LCIS (13 of 22), and

Accepted for publication Sept 2, 1988.

From the Breast Service, Department of Surgery (Drs Kinne, Petrek, Osborne, Fracchia, and DePalo) and Department of Pathology (Dr Rosen), Memorial Sloan-Kettering Cancer Center, New York.

Read before the Annual Meeting of the Society of Surgical Oncology, New Orleans, May 23, 1988.

Reprint requests to 1275 York Ave, New York, NY 10021 (Dr Kinne).

Table 1.—Treatment*

	No. of Patients		
	DCIS	DCIS+LCIS	LCIS
Modified radical mastectomy	67	15	30
Radical mastectomy	13	2	0
Biopsy	3	3	12
Total mastectomy	2	2	1
Radiation	0	0	0

*DCIS indicates ductal carcinoma in situ; LCIS, lobular carcinoma in situ.

Table 2.—Patient Status*

	No. of Patients		
	DCIS	DCIS+LCIS	LCIS
No evidence of disease	79	22	42
Dead of other cause	5	0	1
Dead of disease	1	0	0
Total	**85**	**22**	**43**

Table 3.—Treatment and Outcome of Patients With Microinvasion (n=42)

	No. (%) of Patients
Radical mastectomy	13
Modified radical mastectomy	25
Positive axillary nodes	4/41 (10)
No evidence of disease	39/42 (94)
Dead of disease	3

mammograms were less often the reason for biopsy in this group.

Treatment is listed in Table 1. The majority of patients underwent modified radical mastectomy (112 cases). Fifteen patients were treated by radical mastectomy, 18 by biopsy alone, and five by total mastectomy. No patient underwent radiation therapy or received systemic treatment. Histologic confirmation of axillary node involvement was seen in only one patient of 128 who underwent node dissection (modified radical mastectomy or radical mastectomy). Of the remainder treated by total mastectomy (five) or biopsy alone (18), none developed positive nodes. This confirms the infrequency with which axillary nodes are involved by noninvasive breast cancer.

The status of the patients is shown in Table 2. A total of six patients died of other causes, free of breast cancer at their last examination.

The one patient listed as having died of disease underwent modified radical mastectomy for microscopic DCIS. Axillary lymph nodes were negative pathologically, but two years later she presented with contralateral axillary metastases and parasternal recurrence. Biopsy specimens of both showed a similar histologic pattern of poorly differentiated infiltrating breast cancer. She died a few years later with distant metastases. Although we suspect she had a contralateral invasive breast cancer, it never manifested itself, and therefore she is listed as having died of DCIS. If one accepts this judgment, of 107 patients with DCIS in this series (85 with pure DCIS and two with DCIS and LCIS), 106 were free of disease.

Considering the limits of a retrospective study, some patients were selected by their surgeons (or were self-selected) to undergo no further treatment of in situ breast cancer after excision alone. In an era before wide excision or pathologic assessment of margins, these 18 patients fared well. Two developed ipsilateral breast recurrence (both six years after biopsy), and both had NED after modified radical mastectomy, with negative axillary nodes. Thus, all 18 patients were free of disease.

Patients with microinvasion represent an interesting subgroup, given pathologic difficulties in this assessment. In 42 such patients, all treated by mastectomy with axillary node dissection (Table 3), four (10%) had positive axillary nodes. This perhaps subtle microscopic finding carries a significant risk of regional spread. Three patients died of disease (39 [94%] had NED), indicating the need for accurate diagnosis. This is increasingly important with more DCIS cases being found by mammography.

The 25 patients who developed contralateral breast cancer were analyzed separately also, and all were free of disease. In all cases, the primary side had in situ carcinoma, and in 14, due to contralateral biopsy, bilateral in situ disease was diagnosed and treated. Of interest, eight patients developed metachronous invasive cancer, two with positive nodes requiring adjuvant chemotherapy. All patients had NED at this writing.

These results reflect changes in classification after pathologic review of six questionable cases (done by P.P.R.). Assuming that all patients with in situ disease should do well after mastectomy, questionable cases that were reviewed were those DCIS cases initially thought (1) to have positive axillary nodes (two cases); (2) to have died of disease (two patients); (3) to be alive with disease (one); and (4) to have NED after local recurrence (one patient). Five of these six were changed after this review, three due to unsuspected microinvasion, one for development of invasive cancer in the contralateral breast, and one after having died of disease.

The one patient listed as having died of DCIS had undergone modified radical mastectomy. No microinvasion was noted, and all axillary nodes were negative for recurrence. Four years later she developed contralateral axillary metastases and parasternal recurrence. Biopsy specimens of both lesions showed poorly differentiated invasive breast cancer, and she died of disease four years later. In all likelihood, she had a contralateral invasive breast cancer, but because it never manifested, she was listed as having died after treatment of DCIS.

COMMENT

Due to detection by mammography, breast carcinoma in situ, especially DCIS, is being seen in greater numbers than in the past.[11] In previous years, most patients with DCIS presented with a mass, Paget's disease of the nipple, or nipple discharge, as was true for this series (1970 through 1976). Lobular carcinoma in situ, without a characteristic mammographic pattern, continues to be seen in pathologic analyses of otherwise benign breast biopsy specimens.

The definition of DCIS has changed also. Haagensen[9] considered this disease to harbor invasive elements in virtually all cases, and the diagnosis of intraductal carcinoma was made if less than half the lesion had histologically invasive elements. This explained a high incidence of positive axillary lymph nodes in his series (29%) and a ten-year survival rate of about 70% after radical mastectomy. The same definition was apparently used by the American College of Surgeons survey,[8] with a similar rate of axillary lymph node involvement and a comparable survival rate.

A more modern definition of in situ breast cancer (especially DCIS) eliminates patients whose carcinoma has any invasive components (even microinvasion); the entire histologic pattern is noninvasive.[10] When this definition is adhered to, mastectomy specimens will show unsuspected invasive carcinoma in approximately 5% of cases and pathologically involved axillary lymph nodes in less than 1% of patients.

A revised concept of DCIS has been proposed by Gump et al.[12] Gross DCIS is defined as those lesions presenting as clinical entities (mass, Paget's disease, or nipple discharge), whereas microscopic DCIS is those nonpalpable lesions detected by mammography or noted pathologically as incidental findings. When separated into these two groups, analysis of mastectomy specimens shows that gross DCIS carries a 13% incidence of multifocal microinvasion, and one of 52 patients had involved axillary nodes. Patients with microscopic DCIS had no coexistent invasive cancer and no positive nodes.

Lobular carcinoma in situ has not undergone similar changes in definition, principally because it never presented as a clinical entity and has no characteristic mammographic pattern.[13] Other important differences between DCIS and LCIS are (1) that LCIS has a more frequent bilateral expression and (2) that, when treated by excisional biopsy only, patients with LCIS develop ipsilateral breast carcinoma less frequently, and within a longer time frame, than do patients with DCIS.[14-16]

Previous series from this institution analyzing patients with in situ breast cancer have documented good results with mastectomy.[1,5,6,17] Only one patient with DCIS died of disease. Others died of other causes with NED or died of breast cancer after developing contralateral invasive cancer. However, follow-up was in the range of five years.

Sunshine et al[18] reported on 112 patients with in situ breast cancer followed up a minimum of ten years. Four patients died with metastatic disease (three with DCIS and one with LCIS). Excluding patients who died of other causes, the survival rate free of disease was 95% for patients with DCIS and 97% for those with LCIS. These authors found a high incidence of bilaterality and advocated bilateral mastectomy for patients with in situ breast cancer.

In our present series, only one of 150 patients had axillary metastases, and that a micrometastasis to one level I node. A complete axillary dissection accompanying total mastectomy is not justified if pathologic certainty of no microinvasion can be assured. Total mastectomy with removal of some lower axillary nodes near the tail of the breast is the treatment of choice. Immediate (or delayed) reconstruction can be carried out if patients wish. The avoidance of an axillary dissection in more modern series of microscopic DCIS is even more strongly recommended.[12,19]

Eighteen patients in this series did well after biopsy alone; two developed ipsilateral invasive carcinoma six years later and both underwent modified radical mastectomy, with axillary nodes negative. Both had NED more than 11 years later. The reason for selection of this management was not apparent, but apparently this approach may be successful. Whereas we have known this to be true for patients with LCIS, the outcome of patients diagnosed with DCIS treated by observation only, or excision plus radiotherapy, awaits results from trials[20] and longer follow-up.[21]

The finding that microinvasion in a predominantly in situ breast cancer carries a risk of axillary node metastases has been confirmed in other studies.[22,23] Axillary node dissection should be carried out in this setting, and also when the pathologic descriptions indicate that microinvasion cannot be ruled out. In the current series, careful pathologic review of six patients who had findings or outcomes unlikely related to pure in situ disease changed the final classification in five. Two patients said to have had DCIS and who subsequently died of disease were found to have had microinvasion in the breast. Both had negative nodes after modified radical mastectomy. Of two patients thought to have had DCIS with positive axillary nodes, one had microinvasion. One patient with DCIS, alive with metastases, developed a contralateral invasive cancer, probably the cause of the distant disease.

The last patient, the only one with DCIS to have died of disease, probably had contralateral invasive cancer, but because it was never established, she is listed as the one death. Four years after she underwent modified radical mastectomy for microscopic DCIS, with negative nodes, she presented with ipsilateral chest wall recurrence and contralateral axillary metastases. She underwent biopsy of both lesions, and poorly differentiated invasive breast carcinoma was diagnosed. Bilateral adrenalectomy led to regression, but she died of distant disease four years later. Although we suspect she had a contralateral invasive breast cancer, one never appeared clinically and she did not undergo autopsy.

References

1. Ashikari R, Hajdu SI, Robbins GF: Intraductal carcinoma of the breast (1960-1969). *Cancer* 1971;28:1182-1187.

2. Brown PW, Silverman J, Owens E, et al: Intraductal 'noninfiltrating' carcinoma of the breast. *Arch Surg* 1976;111:1063-1067.

3. Von Reuden DG, Wilson RE: Intraductal carcinoma of the breast. *Surg Gynecol Obstet* 1984;158:105-111.

4. Rosen PP, Braun DW Jr, Kinne DW: The clinical significance of pre-invasive breast carcinoma. *Cancer* 1980;46:919-925.

5. Wanebo HJ, Huvos AG, Urben JA: Treatment of minimal breast cancer. *Cancer* 1974;33:349-357.

6. Ashikari R, Huvos AG, Snyder RE: Prospective study of non-infiltrating carcinoma of the breast. *Cancer* 1977;39:435-439.

7. Carter D, Smith RRL: Carcinoma in situ of the breast. *Cancer* 1977; 40:1189-1193.

8. Rosner D, Bedwani RN, Vana J, et al: Noninvasive breast carcinoma: Results of a national survey by the American College of Surgeons. *Ann Surg* 1980;192:139-147.

9. Haagensen CD: *Disease of the Breast*, ed 2. Philadelphia, WB Saunders Co, 1971, p 586.

10. Rosen PP, Senie R, Schottenfeld D, et al: Noninvasive breast carcinoma: Frequency of unsuspected invasion and implications for treatment. *Ann Surg* 1979;189:377-382.

11. Gump FE: In situ cancers, in Harris JR, Hellman S, Henderson IC, et al (eds): *Breast Disease*. Philadelphia, JB Lippincott, 1987, pp 359-368.

12. Gump FE, Jicha DL, Ozello L: Ductal carcinoma in situ (DCIS): A revised concept. *Surgery* 1987;102:790-795.

13. Frykberg ER, Santiago F, Betsill WL Jr, et al: Lobular carcinoma in situ of the breast. *Surg Gynecol Obstet* 1987;164:285-301.

14. Betsill WL, Rosen PP, Lieberman PH, et al: Intraductal carcinoma: Long-term follow-up after treatment by biopsy alone. *JAMA* 1978;239:1863-1867.

15. Page DL, Dupont WD, Rogers LW, et al: Intraductal carcinoma of the breast: Follow-up after biopsy only. *Cancer* 1982;49:751-758.

16. Rosen PP, Lieberman PH, Braun DW Jr, et al: Lobular carcinoma in situ of the breast: Detailed analysis of 99 patients with an average follow-up of 24 years. *Am J Surg Pathol* 1978;2:225-251.

17. Farrow JH: Current concepts in the detection and treatment of the earliest of the early breast cancers. *Cancer* 1970;25:468-477.

18. Sunshine JA, Moseley HS, Fletcher WS, et al: Breast carcinoma in situ: A retrospective review of 112 cases with a minimum ten year follow-up. *Am J Surg* 1985;150:44-51.

19. Silverstein MJ, Rosser RJ, Gierson ED, et al: Axillary lymph node dissection for intraductal breast carcinoma: Is it indicated? *Cancer* 1987;59:1819-1824.

20. Fisher ER, Sass R, Fisher B, et al: Pathologic findings from the National Surgical Adjuvant Breast Project (Protocol 6): I. Intraductal

carcinoma (DCIS). *Cancer* 1986;57:197-208.
21. Schnitt SJ, Silen W, Sadowsky NL, et al: Ductal carcinoma in situ (intraductal carcinoma) of the breast. *N Engl J Med* 1988;318:898-903.
22. Schuh ME, Nemoto T, Penetrante RB, et al: Intraductal carcinoma: Analysis of presentation, pathologic findings, and outcome of disease. *Arch Surg* 1986;121:1303-1307.
23. Schwartz GF, Feig SA, Rosenberg AL, et al: Staging and treatment of clinically occult breast cancer. *Cancer* 1984;53:1379-1384.

Discussion

Q Did you separate your palpable cancers and those that were picked up by mammography?

A We do have them separated out. Most of the patients in this series had biopsy because of a mass. We do have ten with Paget's disease and 12 who presented with nipple discharge. Mammography was an infrequent indication for biopsy in the whole series.

Q Any explanation for such an excellent prognosis in the bilateral group even with metachronous invasive cancers?

A No; actually you could say our follow-up wasn't too good in that series, because the first side presented as in situ, and in eight cases they had metachronous invasive cancer, two with positive nodes. So maybe in that subset we didn't do so well, but they've all done well since.

Q What do you do for your second opinions who come to you with in situ disease in only one side?

A The common situation is that they probably have an abnormal mammogram, and we discuss the options for treatment with them. If it's DCIS I'm a little less comfortable than Dr Schwartz about a follow-up–only policy, but we would embark on that or a radiation policy in a patient interested in breast preservation. We would want a follow-up mammogram that shows no microcalcification and probably a reexcision to check for margins. The pathologist from Nimegan, Holland, has looked at a subset of patients with DCIS and mapped out how many centimeters away from the lesion multicentricity actually exists. His finding is that multicentricity is almost always within a quadrant. That, plus the Lagios data from San Francisco, leads us to believe that there probably is a subset of patients with microscopic DCIS in a small focus who want neither a mastectomy with immediate reconstruction nor radiation therapy and who are willing to accept a quadrantectomy. We will ink the margins and look very carefully for the presence of multicentric disease in that quadrant. I think this may be an in-between approach we're willing to embark upon. We're not going to have a large number of patients in a prospective study. We just can't do that. But this, to me, is a very rational approach to this disease for patients who understand why we're doing it and can't put up with the other two options.

There are lots of options in this society today. You can tell them about the National Surgical Adjuvant Breast Project trial. I haven't had too many who are interested in a computerized approach to how this disease is handled. We have a subset who understand that mastectomy is probably not necessary, but they feel that the peace of mind they gain with that, whether or not they have immediate delayed reconstruction, is worth it. They may have friends who have died of breast cancer. They may have a positive family history or other factors. That has to be offered to them as an option, obviously, and it doesn't include a node dissection in our hands for what is in situ disease. The node dissection we reserve for patients who are going to get treated by mastectomy or by radiation therapy, for those who have obvious microinvasion, or a smaller subset of patients in whom the most competent of our pathologists will say they cannot rule out microinvasion. That's a reason to do a low axillary lymph node dissection.

So we have basically two options that we offer the patients; it's a mastectomy or it's radiation therapy after all disease is out, with all the reservations that we and our radiation oncologists, frankly, have about the effects of radiation. Until studies like the National Surgical Adjuvant Breast Project reveal what happens to people who are untreated, we may be putting them at some risk. There's no doubt, in the little information we have from breast preservation approaches with radiation, that some of those recurrences both in the radiated breast or the nonirradiated breast are invasive carcinoma. So we're now taking a subset of patients who had a 100% cure rate with a mastectomy and we're allowing them to progress to invasive cancer with all that it means potentially for their prognosis, and I'm uncomfortable telling a patient that I think that.

Implications of Accurate Pathologic Margins in the Treatment of Primary Breast Cancer

Thomas G. Frazier, MD; Randolph W. Y. Wong, MD; David Rose, MD

• **Eighty-seven patients who underwent mastectomy or reexcision following a previous segmental resection with pathologic margins evaluated at that time were restudied following their definitive therapy. Of these, 40 (46.0%) had involved margins, 28 (32.2%) had close margins, and 19 (21.8%) had clear margins. Residual tumor was subsequently found in 21 (52.5%) of 40, nine (32.1%) of 28, and five (26.3%) of 19, respectively. Analysis of specimens for quadrant of residual tumor showed 27 (31.0%) of 87 patients in the same quadrant, and 11 (14.7%) of 75 present in a different quadrant. The assessment of microscopic margins may be misleading since 29.8% (14/47) of patients with clear or close margins subsequently had residual tumor, and 47.5% (19/40) of those with involved margins had no residual tumor found. Further studies are essential to define the optimum guidelines for tumor excision at the time of segmental resection.**

(*Arch Surg* 1989;124:37-38)

As primary radiation therapy has evolved to an acceptable option in the treatment of early breast cancer, the emphasis on segmental resection now focuses not only on favorable pathologic factors for primary radiation therapy but also on the optimum surgical technique to maximize survival and minimize local failure. This report seeks to evaluate the accuracy of our current methods of deciding on margins of resection and to explore further the incidence of multicentricity as it relates to the natural history of breast cancer.

PATIENTS AND METHODS

We reviewed 452 consecutive patients with breast cancer treated by the same surgeons (T.G.F. and D.R.). Two hundred sixteen (48%) had an excisional biopsy as their initial diagnostic procedure. After reviewing the clinical records and pathologic reports, 96 (44%) of these were stratified into one of two groups. Nine patients had original biopsies at other institutions and were not originally marked for margins and were therefore excluded from the study. Of the 87 remaining patients, 75 fell into group A, those patients who initially had excisional biopsy followed by modified radical mastectomy for local control. Twelve patients fell into group B, those patients who opted for segmental resection only but who underwent reexcision of their original biopsy site because of involved margins. The patients ranged in age from 33 to 85 years and had a mean age of 61.7 years.

All 87 patients had their original margin evaluation according to protocol B-06 of the National Surgical Adjuvant Breast Project.[1]

Accepted for publication Sept 2, 1988.

From the Department of Surgery, Bryn Mawr Hospital, Pa (Drs Frazier and Rose), and the Department of Surgery, Thomas Jefferson University, Philadelphia (Drs Frazier, Wong, and Rose). Dr Wong is now with the Department of Surgery, University of Arizona, Tucson.

Read before the Annual Meeting of the Society of Surgical Oncology, New Orleans, May 23, 1988.

Reprint requests to 600 Haverford Rd, Haverford, PA 19041 (Dr Frazier).

The periphery of the specimen was stained with india ink. Margins were considered uninvolved if they were clear of the inked margin. They were considered involved if the tumor cells were within the inked borders or less than one high-power field away.

At the time of mastectomy or reexcision, multiple sections were taken to check for residual carcinoma. In the mastectomy specimen, random sections were taken from other quadrants and from any other suspicious areas as well.

RESULTS

Seventy-five patients (86.2%) had mastectomy for local control and 12 patients (13.8%) had reexcision. The distribution according to histologic type of tumor and nodal status is given in Table 1. As expected, infiltrating ductal carcinoma was the most common pathologic finding, and 25 patients (28.7%) had nodal involvement. Table 2 gives the pathologic results regarding residual tumors in the second-procedure specimens. Five (26.3%) of 19 patients with clear margins, nine (32.1%) of 28 patients with close margins, and 21 (52.5%) of 40 patients with involved margins had residual tumor. In the 75 patients with mastectomy, 11 (14.7%) had tumor foci in a quadrant separate from the original biopsy quadrant. Seven (63.6%) of these 11 had residual tumor in the same biopsy quadrant as well. Subsequent subset analysis showed no difference for age, histologic type of tumor, nodal disease, or hormone receptor analysis.

Table 1.—Histologic Features and Axillary Node Status*

Histologic Feature	No. (%)	Nodal Involvement, No. (%)
Infiltrating ductal	62 (71.3)	18 (29)
Infiltrating ductal and LCIS	8 (9.2)	4 (50)
Lobular	4 (4.6)	1 (25)
Medullary	3 (3.4)	0 (0)
Infiltrating ductal and infiltrating lobular	2 (2.3)	1 (50)
Infiltrating lobular and LCIS	2 (2.3)	1 (50)
Mucinous	2 (2.3)	0 (0)
Other	4 (4.6)	0 (0)
Total	**87 (100)**	**25 (28.7)**

*LCIS indicates lobular carcinoma in situ.

Table 2.—Residual Tumor at Reexcision or Mastectomy

Margins	No. (%)
Involved	21/40 (52.5)
Close	9/28 (32.1)
Clear	5/19 (26.3)
Total	**35/87 (40.2)**

COMMENT

Logically, the complete excision of a tumor is not only desirable from a therapeutic standpoint but is also desirable from the standpoint of a lower local recurrence rate than are incomplete excisions.[2,3] The question remains, however, as to how much tissue is actually required to assure complete removal. Studies have ranged from removal of a complete quadrant and underlying fascia[4] to gross removal with only a small rim of normal tissue.[5] Since the publication of the initial results of protocol B-06 of the National Surgical Adjuvant Breast Project,[1] surgical margins that are microscopically free have become the benchmark for comparison, since this was a truly randomized prospective clinical trial. Although numerous reports have expressed the difficulties encountered in assessing margins,[6] no one heretofore has correlated the margins with residual disease. These results underscore the difficulty associated with margins that are close or involved, making the job of the pathologist extremely difficult; equally impressive is the fact that over one fourth of those patients with clear margins had residual tumor present. Of significance as well was the finding that even in patients with margins involved, residual tumor was found only half of the time. This raises a number of issues for consideration: (1) Should a much wider area of resection be an integral part of planning in the segmental resection? (2) Are gross margins as evaluated by the operative surgeon satisfactory for breast conservation surgery? (3) Should every patient receive a "boost" of x-radiation to the segmental site or the quadrant involved? (4) What tumor factors will predispose the patients to a high likelihood of residual disease, and should these factors influence initial treatment toward total mastectomy?

Obviously, these and other questions can only be answered by greater experience and further subset analysis of the various pathologic and tumor factors. Such approaches might include flow cytometry, nuclear grading, and other pathologic criteria. Until such criteria are developed, however, the present standard of microscopically free margins should continue, but serious consideration to a local boost must be given in each patient undergoing less than mastectomy for local control.

References

1. Fisher E, Sass R, Fisher B, et al: Pathologic findings from the National Surgical Adjuvant Breast Project (protocol 6). *Cancer* 1986;57:1717-1724.

2. Schnitt SJ, Connolly JL, Harris JR, et al: Pathologic predictors of early local recurrence in stage I and II breast cancer treated by primary radiation therapy. *Cancer* 1984;53:1049-1057.

3. Recht A, Silver B, Schnitt SJ, et al: Breast relapse following primary radiation therapy for early breast cancer: I. Classification frequency and salvage. *Int J Radiat Oncol Bio Phys* 1985;11:1271-1276.

4. Veronesi U, Saccozzi R, Del Vecchio M, et al: Comparing radical mastectomy with quadrantectomy, axillary dissection and radiotherapy in patients with small cancers of the breast. *N Engl J Med* 1981;305:6-11.

5. Osteen R, Connolly J, Recht A, et al: Identification of patients at high risk for local recurrence after conservative surgery and radiation therapy for stage I and II breast cancer. *Arch Surg* 1987;122:1248-1252.

6. Carter D: Margins of 'lumpectomy' for breast cancer. *Hum Pathol* 1986;17:330-333.

Discussion

Q For the future, would you consider research directed at better assessment of margins?

A I think I would. I would be interested to hear what some of the pathologists in the room have to say about that because I think this is very difficult. I think sometimes we lean too heavily on what the pathologists tell us in terms of the margins.

Q Has anybody found a foolproof method for an accurate margin assessment?

A I am not a pathologist. I do not see how you could be sure, when you are doing your reincision, that there is no residual tumor. The way we do our reexcisions is to actually take the scar and take out the whole biopsy cavity. Some people reexcise only that portion of the segmental site where the margins were close or involved. They go in through the same scar. It really varies from person to person. The way we did all of our reexcisions was to reexcise the scar and the entire biopsy cavity and ink that.

Q When these were done using local anesthesia, did you find any difference in how the biopsy was done?

A They were really done half and half. The mode of initial resection did not seem to matter. They were all prepared and sent to the pathologist in the same fashion.

Q Did not the Joint Center for Irradiation have the same problem and find that the amount of residual disease in the breast on reexcision could be predicted by the extent of intraductal carcinoma in the original biopsy specimen?

A We did not find that to be a parameter. I think that needs to be looked at. Again, this is a small series, and I would hope that some of the people at Memorial and M. D. Anderson, which have much larger series, would look at this.

A I would like to make a suggestion, since we are more interested in what we leave behind than what we take out. After we have done a so-called lumpectomy, we then take specimens from what we would be leaving behind and very carefully clip those with small clips. We send specimens from four to six places to the surgical pathologist and have him separately mark those as the margins past the lumpectomy site. The clips that we leave very clearly mark those sites for the radiation oncologist.

Q I hate to be a spoil sport, but does any of this have anything to do with outcomes?

A No. Not yet, anyway.

Q Are we becoming so preoccupied with process that we forget why we are doing what we are doing? The idea of knowing whether the margins are free really depends to some degree on fastidiousness and less on luck. Yes, we dip the whole thing in ink with a biopsy specimen if we know that the surgeon is not going to follow this immediately with a mastectomy. We do leave the whole borders and make a determination not on frozen section but on paraffin section if there is not to be a mastectomy immediately.

There are data to show that diffuse intraductal carcinoma within the tumor or intraductal carcinoma away from the tumor within the biopsy site are predictors of failure of excision with radiation therapy. So marginal involvement is information worth having. But with the business of finding that so many with tumor in the margin of the resection had no tumor in the mastectomy, a lot depends on the effort put into the reconstruction. When you get right down to it, the biology of this seems to me to be more important than the process. When we think about noninvasive cancer of the breast, we have no way of measuring at what point we have interrupted that process. The fact that there are multiple foci in some patients, and few foci in others, may reflect the fact that in the one with one or two ducts involved we have interrupted the process at an earlier phase and in the other we have interrupted it at a more advanced phase.

So to say that one or two ducts involved means that you do not have to do anything about it would be answered only with time. Even when that breast is removed for a few ducts of intraductal carcinoma and nothing is found, how do we know what would have been there six months, two years, or three years later had we left that breast? So I think that we are pushing back the frontiers of knowledge, but we still need time to answer some of these questions. I would make a plea that if there are going to be attempts to answer the questions by withholding treatment that this be done in a context of a clinical trial so that after a time, we will be able to answer the question. It is, I think, very important to embark on therapeutic programs that can be measurable so that we can adjust what we are doing by scientific information.

Lability of Steroid Hormone Receptors Following Devascularization of Breast Tumors

Lee M. Ellis, MD; James L. Wittliff, PhD; Michael S. Bryant, MD;
Harry S. Sitren, PhD; William E. Hogancamp; Wiley W. Souba, MD, ScD; Kirby I. Bland, MD

• Ischemia may invalidate hormone-receptor analyses. This study determined the effects of progressive ischemia on steroid hormone–receptor analyses. Breast cancer was induced in 50- to 60-day-old female Holtzman rats by intragastric administration of 25 mg of 7,12-dimethylbenz[a]antracene. After 90 days, rats were anesthetized and breast tumors were devascularized in vivo. At 0, 30, 60, 90, and 150 minutes, a biopsy specimen from each tumor was taken and rapidly frozen. Steroid binding capacity for estrogen (ER), progesterone (PR), and androgen (AR) receptors was determined by incubation with tracer receptor ligand. Ischemia decreased ER and AR levels by 30 minutes, whereas PR levels were unchanged through 150 minutes of ischemia. Following mastectomy, tylectomy, or breast biopsy, PR may be the most reliable of the hormone receptors for determining endocrine-responsive breast cancer. However, for accurate determination of all hormone receptors, specimens should be frozen in liquid nitrogen immediately, then preserved at −70°C, or processed immediately.

(*Arch Surg* 1989;124:39-42)

Quantification of steroid hormone–receptor levels in breast cancer now plays an integral role in selecting patients for hormonal therapy.[1-9] If both the estrogen receptor (ER) and the progesterone receptor (PR) are positive, nearly 80% of patients will demonstrate an objective response to hormonal therapy.[1,8] Conversely, if the ER is negative, fewer than 10% of patients with breast cancer will respond to endocrine manipulation.[1,8] Recently, the androgen receptor (AR) has also been found to be predictive of endocrine-responsive breast cancer.[10,11] Therefore, it is imperative that accurate steroid hormone–receptor analysis be performed to manage the patient with breast cancer properly. However, since steroid hormone receptors are labile cytoplasmic proteins, the conditions for procurement and processing of tissue for analysis may be critical for accuracy and proper interpretation. Several studies have noted a decrease in ER content in mastectomy specimens compared with biopsy tissue from the same patient.[12-14] This discrepancy may be due, in part, to surgically induced ischemia during mastectomy.

It is generally recommended that tissue be frozen within 30 to 45 minutes following surgery.[8] However, the period from devascularization of the specimen to surgical excision may further lengthen the period before proper tissue preservation. This period may allow for significant receptor autolysis, and thus may render a false-negative analysis. This study was conducted to determine the effects of progressive ischemia on sex steroid hormone–receptor analyses in an experimental breast tumor model.

MATERIALS AND METHODS

The 7,12-dimethylbenz[a]antracene (DMBA) chemically induced breast cancer in rats was chosen as the tumor-host system. The majority of these tumors are hormonally dependent and thus serve as a model of endocrine-dependent breast cancer.[15,16] Additionally, in a review of experimental breast cancers, Hilf[17] stated that DMBA-induced breast carcinoma and human mammary carcinoma are similar with regard to various metabolic processes. McGuire and DeLaGarza[18] noted a strong similarity between ERs in human breast cancer and the experimental rat mammary model. Therefore, this experimental host-tumor system serves as an appropriate model for human breast cancer.

Female Holtzman rats, 40 to 50 days old, were housed four to a cage under constant temperature (25°C to 30°C) and with a 12 hour/12 hour light-dark cycle. They were fed tap water and stock chow (Purina Rodent Chow) ad libitum.

Experimental Protocol

At 50 to 60 days of age, rats were lightly anesthetized by halothane exposure. Fifteen milligrams of DMBA dissolved in 1.5 mL of corn oil was administered by intragastric intubation. One week later, 10 mg of DMBA was given in a similar fashion. Ninety days later, rats were anesthetized with ketamine (50 mg/kg intramuscularly). Tumors were then sharply enucleated in vivo without the use of cautery or instillation of chemicals, and the skin was approximated over the tumor with clamps. The procedure was designed to simulate mastectomy. At 0, 30, 60, 90, and 150 minutes, a viable biopsy specimen was taken from each

Accepted for publication Aug 26, 1988.

From the Departments of Surgery (Drs Ellis, Bryant, Souba, and Bland) and Food Science and Human Nutrition (Dr Sitren), University of Florida, Gainesville; and the Department of Biochemistry (Dr Wittliff and Mr Hogancamp), University of Louisville School of Medicine.

Read before the Annual Meeting of the Society of Surgical Oncology, New Orleans, May 24, 1988.

Reprint requests to Department of Surgery, University of Florida College of Medicine, Box J-286, JHMHC, Gainesville, FL 32610 (Dr Bland).

tumor and rapidly frozen in liquid nitrogen. Euthermia was maintained (37°C to 37.5°C) during anesthesia. Tumors were stored at −70°C before shipping and analyses.

Analytical Methods

Tissues were packed in dry ice and forwarded to the Hormone Receptor Laboratory, James Graham Brown Cancer Center, University of Louisville, for ER, PR, and AR assays.

Sample Preparation.—At the time of tissue assay, conducted two to three weeks after tissue procurement, tissues were rapidly thawed at 4°C and homogenized in cold buffer (10 mmol/L of TRIS hydrochloride) containing 1.5 mmol/L of edetic acid, 10 mmol/L of monothioglycerol, 10% glycerol (wt/vol), and 10 mmol/L of sodium molybdate (pH, 7.4) with two to four 10-s bursts using an electronic homogenizer (Ultra-Turrac 18/10 shaft 10 N). Cytosol (supernatant) was prepared by centrifugation of the homogenate at 105 000 g for 30 minutes at 4°C. Protein level was determined by the method of Bradford[19] utilizing bovine serum albumin as a standard. All subsequent procedures were performed in an ice-water bath.

Quantification of Steroid Hormone Receptor Profiles.—To determine affinity and concentration of steroid hormone receptors in the cytosol preparations, aliquots (0.1 mL) were incubated overnight (16 to 18 hours) at 3°C with six increasing concentrations of either tritiated estradiol-17β (3 to 0.15 nmol/L) for ERs, tritiated R5020 (8 to 0.4 nmol/L) for PRs, or tritiated mibolerone (6 to 0.5 nmol/L) for ARs in 0.05 mL of TRIS buffer with or without a 200-fold excess of unlabeled inhibitor. Assays were conducted as described by Bland et al[20] using the inhibitors described for each receptor.

Statistical Analysis

Results were standardized by defining the value at baseline as 100% (control). Corresponding values at the later periods were then expressed as a percent of control. Statistical analysis was performed by two-way analysis of variance with significant differences occurring at the 95% confidence interval. Treatment means were compared with controls.

RESULTS

Of the 18 rats (approximately 80%) developing mammary tumors, 11 tumors were selected for study based on tissue integrity, size, and growth properties. Nearly 80% of these rats had multiple tumors. However, only one tumor from each rat was used for analysis.

The Table shows that ischemia significantly decreased ER levels within the first 30 minutes ($P=.05$). The ER values remained decreased throughout 150 minutes of ischemia. Similarly, AR levels were significantly lower by 30 minutes of ischemia ($P=.002$) and remained so throughout 150 minutes. The largest decrease in ER and AR levels occurred within the first 30 minutes of ischemia. In contrast, PR levels were unchanged throughout 150 minutes.

Mean (±SEM) values at baseline for ER, PR, and AR were 70±10, 149±34, and 20±2 femtomoles/mg of cytosol protein, respectively.

To determine the half-life of these hormone receptors under these experimental conditions, the receptor values were plotted logarithmically as a function of time. By this method, the half-life of the ER was approximately 175 minutes and that of the AR was approximately 50 minutes. The half-life of the PR could not be accurately calculated in this system due to its stability in regard to ischemia over this period. It is apparent that the half-life is substantially greater than that of the other hormone receptors using this tumor model.

COMMENT

Determination of tissue steroid hormone–receptor levels is now a routine and necessary procedure in the management of breast cancer. A plethora of clinical investigations have reported the use of steroid hormone–receptor analysis in predicting hormonal responsiveness as well as survival.[1-9] To effectively utilize knowledge of the tissue concentrations of these labile proteins and assure reproducibility, standardization of assay techniques must be established. Quality control was initiated in the Hormone Receptor Laboratory at the University of Louisville in 1978.[8] However, due to the lability of these cytoplasmic proteins, variation in surgical techniques and in preservation techniques may affect receptor analysis. Several comparative studies have documented a decrease in hormone-receptor levels from biopsy specimens vs mastectomy specimens.[12-14] These observations prompted this investigation on the effects of progressive ischemia on steroid hormone–receptor levels. Theoretically, a prolonged surgical procedure or a delay in proper preservation of tissue may invalidate steroid hormone–receptor analysis. Thus, an individual with breast cancer may falsely be labeled hormone-receptor negative. This patient, with a false-negative result, may not receive optimal adjuvant therapy.

The present study was designed to simulate mastectomy. Tumors were enucleated in vivo and core body temperature was maintained. Furthermore, this study was also similar to other studies examining receptor levels from biopsy specimens and from completion mastectomy. In the present study, results obtained were similar to those of several other studies[12-14] in that ER content was decreased at the termination of the procedure. Our study demonstrated a marked decrease in ER and AR content in the first 30 minutes.

It should be noted that the ERs and PRs may be occupied by endogenous hormones, since the experiment was conducted in animals with intact ovaries. It is known that in the absence of ligand, these receptors are even more labile, as would be the case in the postmenopausal patient with breast cancer. Therefore, it is possible that in postmenopausal patients with breast cancer, the hormone receptors may undergo autolysis at an even greater rate. The PR content was maintained throughout 150 minutes of ischemia. Other investigators have noted that the PR may be the more sensitive of the steroid hormone receptors in predicting hormonal responsiveness.[3,6,7] Fisher et al,[7] in a randomized prospective study of 1891 patients with breast cancer on the National Adjuvant Breast and Bowel Project, found that the PR tumor content was a stronger predictor than the ER content in predicting response to cytotoxic chemotherapy plus tamoxifen. Osborne et al,[3] in an earlier study of 65 patients, found that the presence of the PR may be a better predictor of hormonal responsiveness than the quantitative value of the ER. Clark et al[6] stated that the PR value may be of equal or greater value than the tumor ER content in predicting disease-free survival. These findings may be due, in part, to "false-negative" interpretation of ER levels secondary to surgically induced

Steroid Hormone Receptor vs Ischemic Time*

	Ischemic Time, min				
	0	30	60	90	150
ER (n=11)	100	79±10†	67±11†	54±11†	56±13†
PR (n=11)	100	101±21	101±26	94±14	84±27
AR (n=11)	100	57±12†	53±15†	28±9†	42±12†

*Values are mean±SEM, expressed as percent of control at baseline. ER indicates estrogen receptor; PR, progesterone receptor; and AR, androgen receptor.
†$P\leq.05$ compared with baseline by analysis of variance.

ischemia or improper tissue preservation, inasmuch as the ER appears more susceptible to ischemia and autolysis than the PR.

Several investigators have studied the levels of the steroid hormone receptors in biopsy specimens and from subsequent completion mastectomy specimens. However, there is no general consensus in regard to the validity of receptor analysis in the mastectomy specimen. Young et al[14] compared ER levels in biopsy and mastectomy specimens from 58 patients. They found a 44% false-negative ER determination in the mastectomy specimen. They also noted tl at 13 (42%) of 31 patients who were ER positive at mastectomy had at least a 50% drop in the ER level when compared with the level found at biopsy.

Newsome et al[13] found a 15% to 100% (mean, 70%) decrease in ER levels in completion mastectomy specimens when compared with biopsy specimens. It was concluded that the decrease in ER levels is inversely proportional to the period from devascularization to freezing. They speculate, as do we, that the ER-negative patients who respond to hormonal therapy may represent inadequate sample procurement. Hassan et al[12] in a similar study found that ER levels were 1.6 to 6.5 times greater in the biopsy specimen than in the mastectomy specimen.

In contradistinction, several authors have concluded that the mastectomy specimen *is* adequate tissue for receptor analysis. Leight et al[21] in studying biopsy and mastectomy specimens from 21 patients concluded that the biopsy specimen is preferred to the mastectomy specimen but that tissue from a properly handled mastectomy specimen is satisfactory for receptor analysis.

Meyer et al[22] studied 71 cases where biopsy and mastectomy specimens were available. They found a small significant reduction in the ER-positive assays in the mastectomy specimen compared with the biopsy tissue. They found no difference in the PR levels between tissues. Despite noting that false-negative ER interpretations may occur, they concluded that "significant losses do not occur" following completion mastectomy.

Inconsistent conclusions from these studies may be due to several factors. First, as in our study, the initiation of ischemia may affect receptor levels. However, variation in surgical technique, including the use of electrocautery, may cause variations in the degree of ischemia induced. Second, instillation of various chemicals into the wound, such as saline, water, alcohol, or betadine, may also alter receptor levels. Furthermore, there is a variable amount of tumor heterogeneity in regard to receptor concentrations. Most of the previously mentioned studies had too few patients to overcome this problem. The value of the present study is in the fact that only one variable was tested, namely, ischemia.

Bridges et al[23] studied levels of the ERs and PRs as well as their positivity in 131 women with breast cancer. Patients were divided into three groups: group 1 underwent biopsy followed by mastectomy with receptor being determined in the biopsy specimen; group 2 underwent modified radical mastectomy (MRM) in continuity with axillary dissection; and group 3 underwent en bloc mastectomy with tissue procurement within 15 to 20 minutes after the onset of surgery with axillary lymph node dissection performed separately following mastectomy. The frequency of ER and PR positivity was 72% and 40% following biopsy, 68% and 49% following MRM, and 89% and 64% following en bloc mastectomy, respectively. Although not statistically significant, the receptors showed a trend toward higher levels in the en bloc mastectomy specimens with rapid tissue procurement. Of note is the fact that the patients who underwent biopsy were younger than the other two groups. Regardless, when comparing the two mastectomy groups, these data suggest that rapid procurement of breast cancer specimens may allow for more accurate quantification of steroid hormone–receptor levels. However, these authors state that tissue from mastectomy specimens, if kept cold and rapidly frozen, may still be reliably used for quantification of the hormone receptors. Nonetheless, it is generally held that rapid and efficient procurement and processing of tissues is necessary for accurate hormone-receptor analysis.[8] To our knowledge, this is the first study elucidating the period over which ischemia affects breast tumor steroid hormone–receptor levels. Procurement within 30 minutes following devascularization is necessary to obtain accurate quantification of all three steroid hormone receptors.

At present, AR levels are not routinely analyzed or utilized in managing patients with breast cancer. However, several clinical studies suggest that knowledge of the quantitative value of AR may enhance prediction of those patients likely to respond to endocrine therapy.[10,11] If this holds true, then accurate determination of AR levels in neoplastic tissue is imperative.

In this experimental model, ischemia decreased ER and AR levels after only 30 minutes, whereas PR levels were maintained throughout 150 minutes. To obtain accurate analysis of all three steroid hormone receptors, tissue samples should be obtained before devascularization. Certainly, following breast biopsy, a portion of the specimen should be preserved for hormone-receptor analysis. It remains to be determined if biopsy of tissue just before mastectomy (and devascularization) should be obtained for hormone-receptor analysis rather than analyzing the mastectomy specimen itself. In circumstances where the PR is positive, yet the ER and/or AR are negative, consideration of the sensitivity and stability of the PR should be evaluated. In such a circumstance, false-negative values may have been obtained for the ER and/or AR, and the patient potentially may benefit from hormonal therapy.

We thank Marjorie McGarva and Cheryl Turner for preparation of the manuscript.

References

1. Bloom ND, Tobin EH, Schreibman B, et al: The role of progesterone receptors in the treatment of breast cancer. *Cancer* 1980;45:2992-2997.
2. Furmanski P, Saunders DE, Brooks SC, et al: The prognostic value of estrogen determinations in patients with primary breast cancer: An update. *Cancer* 1980;46:2794-2796.
3. Osborne CK, Yochmowitz MG, Knight WA III, et al: The value of estrogen and progesterone receptors in the treatment of breast cancer. *Cancer* 1980;46:2884-2888.
4. Skinner LG, Barnes DM, Ribeiro GG: The clinical value of multiple steroid receptor assays in breast cancer management. *Cancer* 1980;46: 2939-2945.
5. Fisher B, Redmond C, Brown A, et al: Treatment of primary breast cancer with chemotherapy and tamoxifen. *N Engl J Med* 1981;305:1-6.
6. Clark GM, McGuire WL, Hubay CA, et al: Progesterone receptors as a prognostic factor in stage II breast cancer. *N Engl J Med* 1983;309:1343-1347.
7. Fisher B, Redmond C, Brown A, et al: Influence of tumor estrogen and progesterone receptor levels on the response to tamoxifen and chemotherapy in primary breast cancer. *J Clin Oncol* 1983;1:227-241.
8. Wittliff JL: Steroid-hormone receptors in breast cancer. *Cancer* 1984;53:630-643.
9. Vollenweider-Zerargui L, Barrelet L, Wong Y, et al: The predictive value of estrogen and progesterone receptors' concentration on the clinical behavior of breast cancer in women. *Cancer* 1986;57:1171-1180.
10. Bryan RM, Mercer RJ, Bennett RC, et al: Androgen receptors in breast cancer. *Cancer* 1984;54:2436-2440.
11. Brentani MM, Franco EL, Oshima CTF, et al: Androgen, estrogen and progesterone receptor levels in malignant and benign breast tumors: A multivariate analysis approach. *Int J Cancer* 1986;38:637-642.

12. Hassan J, Luhan PA, Kohl MW: Comparison of estrogen receptor levels in breast cancer samples from mastectomy and frozen section specimens. *Cancer* 1981;47:138-139.
13. Newsome JF, Avis FP, Hammond JE, et al: Sampling procedures in estrogen receptor determinations. *Ann Surg* 1981;193:549-554.
14. Young SC, Burkett RJ, Stewart C: Discrepancy in ER levels of breast carcinoma in biopsy vs mastectomy specimens. *J Surg Oncol* 1985;29:54-56.
15. Huggins C, Briziarelli G, Sutton H Jr: Rapid induction of mammary carcinoma in the rat and the influence of hormones on the tumors. *J Exp Med* 1959;109:24-41.
16. Boylan ES, Fowler EH, Wittliff JL: Morphology, growth characteristics and oestrogen-binding capacity of DMBA-induced mammary tumours from ovariectomized rats. *Br J Cancer* 1977;35:602-609.
17. Hilf R: Will the best model of breast cancer please come forward? *Natl Cancer Inst Monogr* 1971;34:43-54.
18. McGuire WL, DeLaGarza M: Similarity of the estrogen receptor in human and rat mammary carcinoma. *J Clin Endocrinol Metab* 1973;36:548-552.
19. Bradford MM: A rapid and sensitive method for the quantification of microgram quantities of proteins utilizing the principle of protein-dye binding. *Anal Biochem* 1976;72:248-254.
20. Bland KI, Freedman BE, Harris PL, et al: The effects of ischemia on estrogen and progesterone receptor profiles in the rodent uterus. *J Surg Res* 1987;42:653-660.
21. Leight GS Jr, Wells SA Jr, McCarty KS Jr: Sex steroid receptor concentration in breast carcinoma tissue: Effect of devascularization during mastectomy. *Surgery* 1984;95:256-260.
22. Meyer JS, Schechtman K, Valdes R Jr: Estrogen and progesterone receptor assays on breast carcinoma from mastectomy specimens. *Cancer* 1983;52:2139-2143.
23. Bridges KG, Keshgegion AA, Kumar HAM, et al: Influence of surgical technique on estrogen and progesterone receptor determinations in breast cancer. *Cancer* 1985;51:2317-2320.

Discussion

Q Were you able to account in any way for possible effects due to the anesthetic?

A It is known that aberrations in the circulating hormone levels may alter receptor analysis. The ER level differs in premenopausal and postmenopausal patients and also differs according to the phase of the menstrual cycle; however, we do not have any evidence to show that ketamine or halothane, the two agents that we use, alter circulating hormone levels, but they may. However, these tumors were devascularized at time zero, so theoretically no blood flow should have been going to the tumor, affecting hormone levels.

Q Are you sure that this decrease in cytoplasmic receptor is not really a manifestation of an increased nuclear receptor? You were measuring essentially the cytoplasmic receptor. Studies done with electrocautery have shown that when you cauterize a specimen, the receptor is actually driven into the nucleus. Is it possible that the decrease you saw in your cytoplasmic determination with time is a similar event, due to ischemia or temperature or a variety of other factors that you have not controlled for?

A That may be true. We may not be measuring the true ER in that whole cell. However, the majority of laboratories do measure the cytoplasmic ERs or PRs, and if we are trying to make the study clinically applicable, I think that is where it holds true. If you measure nuclear receptors, they may be increased relative to controls; we did not do that.

Q Did you do monoclonal antibody studies?

A We did not do the study with monoclonal antibodies. I did happen to review the literature on comparison of monoclonal antibody studies vs standard methods of hormone-receptor analyses before this meeting in which there were a couple of studies looking at the effects of heat lability. The dextran-coated charcoal method and monoclonals were just as likely to find decreased levels with increasing temperature. There are no studies comparing ischemic time.

Q I think your findings are very important in view of a paper presented this morning with 1500 patients in the Scottish trial of tamoxifen. In their postmenopausal patients, ER-negative patients showed a highly significant effect of adjuvant tamoxifen. Those of us who follow these receptor studies usually quote an incidence of less than 10% for those patients who respond. However, I think this may be due to difficulty with the assay. Is this a metastasizing tumor model? If so, how do the metastases correlate with your initial receptor data?

A Over a longer period, you may have lymph node metastases. However, there were no apparent metastases at 90 days, and the amount of tissue that would be involved would not be enough to do assays.

Q Your analysis implies that there was variation between tumors. Did you also look at variation or heterogeneity within the tumor?

A We did. We took some control tumors and took five specimens from each tumor for assay. The coefficient of variation was about 30% for heterogeneity for all of the tumors. We originally had planned to use 25 tumors to try to cover for that large variation; however, due to necrosis and a tumor yield of approximately 80%, we only came up with 11 tumors for final analysis.

In Other AMA Journals

ARCHIVES OF INTERNAL MEDICINE

Age, Sex, and Race Inequality in Renal Transplantation

Carl M. Kjellstrand, MD

We calculated the chance of receiving a kidney transplant in the United States in 1983, and in the Midwest from 1979 through 1985, considering age, sex, and race. In the United States, 23 026 patients began long-term dialysis and 6112 (27%) received a kidney transplant. Transplant rates were 31% for men and 21% for women. White patients had a 30% rate and nonwhite patients a 20% rate. Patients less than 11 to 35 years old had an 85% rate vs a 3% rate for those older than 56 years. When race, age, and sex were analyzed together, nonwhite patients aged 21 to 45 years had only half the chance of receiving a transplant compared with white patients of the same age and sex. Women aged 46 to 60 years had less than half the chance of receiving a transplant when compared with men of the same age and race. These data show that there are age, sex, and race imbalances in the distribution of renal transplantation. We believe these imbalances only partially have a morally neutral biological, medical, social, and cultural explanation and that there should be a fairer distribution of kidney transplants (*Arch Intern Med* 1988;148:1305-1309).

Reprint requests to Division of Nephrology, Department of Medicine, Box 60500, Karolinska Hospital, 10401 Stockholm, Sweden (Dr Kjellstrand).

Cancer Centers—Origins and Purpose

The James Ewing Lecture

William W. Shingleton, MD

• Cancer centers in the United States date back to the beginning of this century, although there were few until the late 1950s and 1960s. The National Cancer Act of 1971 introduced a new era in serving as a major stimulus to the development of comprehensive cancer centers. Research scientists and physicians in centers have contributed significantly to the new knowledge of normal and abnormal regulation of cell growth and differentiation and to the advances in the diagnosis and treatment of cancer. The future for cancer centers is very bright. They will continue to play a major role in the advancement of knowledge about cancer. However, centers must be reevaluated at intervals to correct any deficiencies and to stimulate new and innovative approaches. Surgical oncologists should become more involved in cancer center research. Comprehensive cancer centers should develop more effective regional cancer control and prevention programs. Reevaluation of centers by the National Cancer Institute, Bethesda, Md, and its advisory body, the National Cancer Advisory Board, along with cancer center leaders, should result in a consensus concerning changes to enhance their contribution to a solution to the cancer problem.

(*Arch Surg* 1989;124:43-45)

It has now been 17 years since the passage of the National Cancer Act of 1971. One section of the act authorized the establishment of 15 new cancer centers in the United States. Three years later, at the time the act was renewed, the ceiling on the number of such centers was removed. A number of questions have arisen concerning the purpose and accomplishment of these new and previously existing cancer centers. Are there unique features about cancer centers that enhance the ability of scientists in these centers to reach a solution to the cancer problem more effectively and rapidly? What has been the pattern of their development over the years relative to goals and purpose, organizational structure, and source of funding? What has been the impact of centers on the care of patients with cancer? How well have they accomplished their mission?

Accepted for publication July 6, 1988.

Dr Shingleton is Professor Emeritus at Duke University Medical Center, Durham, NC.

Read before the Annual Meeting of the Society of Surgical Oncology, New Orleans, May 24, 1988.

Reprint requests to Duke Comprehensive Cancer Center, Box 3814, Duke University Medical Center, Durham, NC 27710 (Dr Shingleton).

In an effort to answer some of these questions, this article will present, in an abbreviated fashion, (1) a historical perspective on the development of cancer centers, (2) a description of types and organization of centers, (3) the impact of the National Cancer Act of 1971 on the development of comprehensive cancer centers, and (4) some comments on problems, accomplishments, and future outlook for centers.

HISTORICAL BACKGROUND

Several categorical institutes devoted to a study of the cancer problem were established at the turn of the century.[1(p12)] The Roswell Park Memorial Institute, Buffalo, a state-supported institution, dates from 1898. A research program in cancer was inaugurated in 1906 at Memorial Hospital for the Treatment of Cancer and Allied Diseases, New York, and expanded in 1939 to become the Memorial Sloan-Kettering Cancer Center, New York. The University of Texas M. D. Anderson Cancer Center, Houston, was established in 1941 by an act of the state legislature. The American Oncologic Hospital, Philadelphia, was founded in 1904, and the Lankanau Research Institute, Philadelphia, was founded in 1925; these institutions have evolved into the present-day Fox Chase Cancer Center in Philadelphia. The Children's Hospital Research Foundation, established in 1947, was the forerunner of the present Dana-Farber Cancer Center in Boston. It is to be noted that these early institutions were funded initially either by private funds, state funds, or a combination of both. Several other privately supported categorical cancer institutes (later referred to as centers) originated in the 1950s and 1960s. These include St Jude's Children's Research Hospital in Memphis, Fels Institute in Philadelphia, the Michigan Cancer Foundation in Detroit, and the Institute of Cancer Research of Columbia University in New York.[1(p13)]

The first federally supported cancer research laboratory began operation in 1922 in the US Public Health Service.[2(pix)] The National Cancer Institute (NCI), Bethesda, Md, was established in 1937 by an act of Congress, the first institute of the later National Institutes of Health (NIH).[2(p13)] The earliest government contract funding for biomedical research in universities originated during World War II. This was followed soon after the war by the award of Public Health Service research grants to individuals, administered by the NIH (Palmer Saunders, PhD, oral communication, April 1988). The NIH Clinical Center, Bethesda, Md, was dedicated in 1953, with each institute assigned a specific number of beds for research.[1(p1)] One of the most important features of this clinical center was the close collaboration that developed between laboratory and clinical research scientists. It has been stated that this center served as a prototype for later NIH support of clinical research in university medical centers.

The first extramural grant support program to universities for clinical research was initiated in 1960, and it was known as the Clinical Research Centers Program.[1(p2)] This policy reflected the addition of institutional research funding to the already established individual investigator-initiated research grant program. There were 19 funded university clinical research centers by the late 1960s. According to Walter et al,[1(p2)] there was a lack of sufficiently funded cancer research beds in these clinical research centers for cancer clinicians to participate effectively in NCI clinical cooperative studies. This resulted in the development and funding by the NCI of a Clinical Cancer Centers Program. The Health Research Facilities Grant Program of the NIH, which was available at that time, aided in the construction of facilities for these clinical cancer centers. The Program Project Grant (PO-1), the Cancer Clinical Research Center Grant (PO-2), and the Cancer Center Core Grant (P-30) were soon added as new mechanisms to support research in these centers. By 1963, there were 12 funded clinical cancer centers.[1(p3)]

Pertinent to these developments was the passage by Congress in 1965 of an act that established a Regional Medical Program to address the problems of heart disease, cancer, and stroke. The intent of this legislation was to organize regional community support for the earlier application of current research knowledge into medical practice related to these chronic diseases. These objectives, as related to cancer, were inadequately realized.[1(p3)] However, funds from this program helped to establish an NCI Planning Grant Program for cancer centers. These grants provided seed money for individuals at universities and not-for-profit institutions to work together in developing a cancer center. A number of institutions were successful in developing a cancer center as a result of these grants.[1(p3)]

The most important additional event that contributed to the further growth and support of cancer centers was the passage of the National Cancer Act of 1971. One section of this act authorized the director of the NCI to "provide for the establishment of fifteen new centers for clinical research training and demonstration of advanced diagnostic and treatment methods relating to cancer.[3(p103)] A conceptual basis for establishing these centers can be found in the summary statement of the Report of the National Panel of Consultants on the Conquest of Cancer that was prepared for the Committee on Labor and Public Welfare of the US Senate. Benno Schmidt, chairman of the panel, presented the summary recommendations of the report in testimony before this Senate committee in early December 1970.[3(p253)] The report called for passage of congressional legislation to establish a "National Program for the Conquest of Cancer," with provisions calling for additional funding of cancer research.[4] The pertinent section of this report, related to centers, stated the following:

> Existing cancer centers should be strengthened and additional cancer centers in different parts of the country should be created. The solution to the cancer problem lends itself to a multidisciplinary effort, where teams of highly qualified specialists are available to interact on problems of research, both clinical and non-clinical, teaching, diagnosis, prevention programs, and the development of improved methods in the delivery of medical care, including rehabilitation. Among those who work in the cancer field there is great emphasis on the advantages of a critical mass—a critical mass of scientists and physicians committed to the cooperative solution of the cancer problem, of research facilities, of patients, and of financial and other resources. This is simply another way of saying that the comprehensive cancer center offers the best organizational structure for the expanded attack on cancer.

Since passage of the National Cancer Act of 1971, 21 comprehensive cancer centers have been established; 20 currently remain. The emphasis in these centers has been to foster a multidisciplinary approach to cancer research and patient care, to provide a focal point for public awareness of the cancer problem and the need for support of research, to serve as a regional base for cancer control and prevention activities, and to develop organized support programs for patients with cancer. A majority of these centers are based in or allied to university medical schools.

TYPES OF CENTERS

Cancer centers can be classified in a variety of ways. A center may be classified according to a stated purpose or goal, organization, or source of funding. The major objective of some centers is to conduct basic biological laboratory research, and of others, primarily clinical research. Some of these "specialized" centers have both activities. Comprehensive centers, in addition to basic laboratory and clinical research, have programs in cancer epidemiology, cancer control and prevention, research training, and community outreach activities, including public and professional information and education. A center may be classified relative to organizational structure, ie, as freestanding, joint venture, departmental, matrix, or consortium. Based on the primary source of funding, they may be classified as federal, state, private, or a combination of these sources.

At the present time, there are 57 centers that have NCI-funded core support grants.[5] Two of the 20 comprehensive centers are the consortium type. A consortium center is one in which several medical schools participate. Fifteen of the comprehensive centers are associated with private universities, and five are associated with state-supported institutions. Twenty-five of the 37 specialized centers are clinical, and 12 are laboratory/basic; 30 are university associated, and seven are freestanding.

COMMENT

One of the problems related to cancer centers has been to define what constitutes a "center." This difficulty has led to some confusion on the part of both the public at large, as well as the scientific community. In my opinion, a center is best defined, in general terms, as being composed of a multidisciplinary group of research scientists and/or physicians who are bound together with a unity of purpose, who share concepts, facilities, and other resources, and who have developed an organizational structure that fosters effective management practices to achieve the desired goals of the group. Initially, there was considerable debate concerning the term *comprehensive* as applied to cancer centers. To attempt to satisfy the language related to centers present in the National Cancer Act of 1971, the NCI, with the advice and approval of the National Cancer Advisory Board, determined that there should be a group of centers that would have a broad approach to the cancer problem, including research, clinical care, prevention, and community outreach, with a precise organizational structure, and that these centers would be recognized by the

NCI as "comprehensive cancer centers."[1(p9)] A list of ten requirements was developed initially for the purpose of characterizing a comprehensive center. These were later modified and condensed to six requirements that are still in current use.[6] These requirements are, in abbreviated form, as follows: the center should (1) have an NCI-funded Cancer Center Support (Core) Grant; (2) possess a high-quality research program in laboratory, clinical, epidemiologic, and evaluative research that exists in an environment conducive to a collaborative effort among basic and clinical disciplines and epidemiologists, and with the participation by clinical scientists in regional and/or national clinical trials; (3) serve as a focal point for local and regional programs to control cancer through research activities in areas, such as prevention, detection, diagnosis, treatment, and rehabilitation; and (4) serve as a focal point for local and regional information, as well as lay and professional education programs, and possess a training program for professional and support personnel. The center should also (5) have a formal commitment of support from the parent institution indicating that the center director has (*a*) control of designated space and equipment, (*b*) necessary control over staff appointments, (*c*) control of grouped beds and ambulatory facilities, and (*d*) responsibility for planning, preparation of budgets, and development of an administrative structure that will assure sound management practices. Finally, the center should (6) have a geographic impact to assist the national capability to conduct regional trials, regional cancer control programs, and regional training, education, and information activities.

The scope of activities in comprehensive centers is somewhat variable from center to center due to the fact that some centers have emphasized certain activities and de-emphasized others. A reevaluation of comprehensive cancer centers by the NCI and the National Cancer Advisory Board is in progress at the present time.[7] The following questions are under discussion: (1) What has been the major accomplishment of cancer centers to date? (2) How many comprehensive cancer centers should there be in the United States? (3) Should these centers be geographically located? (4) How can "comprehensiveness" of a center be evaluated? (5) How should centers be funded in the future? (6) To what extent are comprehensive centers involved in cancer control and prevention research in their region? (7) How should a "partnership" be established between centers and the NCI to plan future directions of cancer research?

The question regarding the accomplishment of centers is the question that is most frequently addressed. Precise data are lacking to quantify these accomplishments, since in the matrix-type center, it is difficult to select out the relative contributions of the center from those of the parent institution. However, it is the opinion of many that cancer centers have made very significant contributions in basic and clinical cancer research, patient care, training, and education. Additionally, centers have recruited a significant number of new investigators into cancer research. Approximately 50% of all funded investigator-initiated research grants are held by scientists who are members of a cancer center (R. Morrison, oral communication, March 1988). Centers have attracted private and institutional funds that, combined with available federal funds, have made possible the addition of large amounts of new research space and equipment and have subsidized a significant amount of research activity. It is the opinion of many working in the cancer field that cancer centers have become one of the most effective, but not the only, location where new findings arising from basic laboratory research can be most rapidly and efficiently evaluated. Centers have emphasized compassionate care for patients by developing a variety of patient support programs.

An example of the matrix-type university cancer center is the Comprehensive Cancer Center at Duke University, Durham, NC, established in 1972. Fifty-five members of the medical school faculty were founding members. An organizational structure was created, with the center director reporting directly to the University Chancellor for Health Affairs; all center members originally held primary appointments in a medical school department. The growth of the center has been dramatic. There are now 200 members of the center, research space has tripled in amount, and funds for research have increased tenfold. There are, at present, 225 active clinical research protocols and approximately 1500 patients annually accessed into these studies. There were 2700 scientific publications by members of the center during the past six years. A recent reorganization of the center will permit the recruitment of 14 to 16 tenure tract investigators, with primary appointment in the cancer center and secondary appointment in a medical school department. The center is now being referred to as a "matrix-plus" type.

An enterprise as large as the NCI Cancer Centers Program has, as one might expect, encountered several problems during its evolution. Initially, there was some reluctance on the part of some faculty members and administrators of university medical schools to embrace the idea of superimposing a categorical center on an organization that operates with a discipline-oriented departmental structure. There has been a lack of full participation by surgeons in research programs in some institutions with cancer centers. Reduced federal funding of cancer support grants for centers at times has caused retrenchment of research activities in some centers. Additional problems that affect research performance in centers are (1) the issue of animals in research, (2) Federal Drug Administration constraints on new cancer drug approval, (3) inadequate ways to finance hospital costs of inpatient cancer research, (4) financing the high cost of new approved drugs, and (5) constraints arising from legal and ethical issues related to research.

A small number of "cancer centers" have been established with private funding without or with minimal peer-reviewed NCI-supported research, and without an NCI-funded core support grant. A private for-profit corporation is in the process of establishing "comprehensive cancer centers" in several locations in the country.

References

1. Walter WA, Saunders JP, Putney HD: Origins of the Cancer Center Program of the National Cancer Institute, in Miranda E (ed): *Association of American Cancer Institutes Newsletter*, June 1985. Buffalo, Roswell Park Memorial Institute, 1985.
2. Strickland SP: *Politics, Science, and Dread Disease*. Cambridge, Mass, Harvard University Press, 1972.
3. Rettig RA: *Cancer Crusade*. Princeton, NJ, Princeton University Press, 1977.
4. *National Program for Conquest of Cancer*, US Senate document 92-9, 92nd Congress, 1970.
5. *List of Existing National Cancer Institute-Supported Cancer Centers*. Silver Spring, Md, National Cancer Institute Cancer Centers Branch, Division of Prevention and Control, 1988.
6. *Guidelines for Recognition of a Cancer Center as Comprehensive*. Silver Spring, Md, National Cancer Institute, Division of Prevention and Control, June 1985.
7. Boyd J (ed): *The Cancer Letter*, April 29, 1988, vol 14, No. 18, pp 1-5.

Results of Surgical Excision of One to 13 Hepatic Metastases in 98 Consecutive Patients

John P. Minton, MD, PhD; Walter B. Hamilton; Armando Sardi, MD; Carol Nieroda, MD; Brenda Sickle-Santanello, MD; Patrick J. O'Dwyer, MD

• Metastatic carcinoma to the liver is generally considered to be associated with a poor prognosis, with five-year survival of only 20% to 30% after resection of solitary lesions. Ninety-eight consecutive patients underwent the surgical removal of one to 13 metastatic lesions from the liver. A rising carcinoembryonic antigen level was considered an indication for reexploration. All gross tumor was removed in every patient; 66 had more than one metastasis. Survival was unexpectedly high: 91 of 98 were alive at 12 months, 50 (70%) of 71 at 13 to 24 months, 23 (66%) of 36 at 25 to 36 months, 14 (74%) of 19 at 37 to 48 months, six (60%) of ten at 49 to 60 months, four (80%) of five at 61 to 72 months, and two (50%) of four 73 to 84 months after resection of multiple liver metastases. The procedure appears to be a safe and, in some patients, beneficial surgical technique for the removal of multiple hepatic metastases.

(*Arch Surg* 1989;124:46-48)

Hepatic metastases from gastrointestinal tract cancer are fatal, and multiple metastases to the liver have been considered not a surgically treatable condition. The median survival of untreated patients with hepatic metastases ranges from 3.1 to nine months.[1] Successful early detection of metastases to the liver is difficult because the anatomic location of the liver makes clinical discovery of metastases less than 3 cm in diameter difficult.[2] Resection of solitary hepatic metastasis has become the treatment of choice, with five-year survival ranging from 20% to 30%,[3-6] but multiple hepatic metastases are often ignored from a surgical standpoint. Biopsies may not even be performed in patients with more than one metastatic lesion. Patients with unresectable lesions are treated with intra-arterial or portal vein chemotherapy when appropriate.

During the past seven years, 98 patients with one or more hepatic metastases (one to 13) have been operated on and all detectable metastatic tumor was removed, with acceptably low blood loss, no mortality, and low morbidity. We present the results of these operations as well as a description of our technique, which, for lack of a better description, we call the "Swiss cheese" procedure because the liver frequently looks like a Swiss cheese when the operation is completed.

Accepted for publication Sept 21, 1988.

From the Department of Surgery, Ohio State University College of Medicine, Columbus.

Read before the Annual Meeting of the Society of Surgical Oncology, New Orleans, May 25, 1988.

Reprint requests to Department of Surgery, Ohio State University College of Medicine, 410 W Tenth Ave, Columbus, OH 43210 (Dr Minton).

PATIENTS AND METHODS

Patients

Between 1980 and 1987, 98 patients were evaluated for second-look operations because of a rising carcinoembryonic antigen (CEA) level or other objective evidence of metastasis to the liver. Primary cancer had occurred in the colon in 72, in the rectum in 12, in the breast in six, in the ovary and pancreas in two each, in the kidney and esophagus in one each, and as melanoma in two.

Serial CEA levels were measured every two months for two years and then every three months for three years after primary colon and rectal cancer resection.[7] Based on a persistent rise in the CEA level, 98 patients were readmitted to the hospital. Liver and spleen scans, abdominal echograms, and computed tomographic (CT) scans were obtained, and the presence of an elevated CEA level was confirmed. A rise in the CEA level above the baseline established after resection has proved to be a reliable indicator of recurrence.

Computed tomographic scans of the abdomen and liver were performed, along with gastrointestinal tract barium contrast roentgenographic examinations. Of the 98 patients, 19 (19%) were reoperated on with a rising CEA level as the only indication; 66 had a positive CT scan of the liver. When multiple metastases were demonstrated outside the abdominal cavity, in lungs or bone, operation was not undertaken.

Surgical Approach

Through a midline xyphoid-to-pubis incision with xyphoidectomy, the abdomen was explored and adhesions were taken down. When tumor was found elsewhere in the abdomen, it was resected (59 of 98 patients). The right lobe of the liver was dislocated from its attachments to the diaphragm and retroperitoneum by means of the elongated electrocautery tip set on 55 coagulation only. The triangular ligament of the left lobe was detached in the same fashion. The falciform ligament was detached from the diaphragm. Liver lesions were identified by bimanual examination of each lobe. With an assistant holding the dislocated liver lobe in the midline of the abdomen, the electrocautery was placed on 110 coagulation and dissection with a 1-cm margin of normal liver was carried out around each lesion. The flat cautery blade worked best, and a laser unit vacuum removed the smoke. Sodium oxychloroscene (Chlorpactin) (7 g/1000 mL H_2O) irrigation to the dissection site was used only when active bleeding occurred. Oxidized regenerated cellulose (Surgicel) was packed and held on persistent bleeding sites. Small metal clips were wedged onto vessels and bile ducts before transection when possible. A 2- to 3-mm brushlike stroke with the flat cautery tip away from the tumor provided the technical motion best for hemostasis during the dissection. One or more No. 1 Black-Braided nylon (Surgilon) sutures were placed through each lesion for the assistant to retract to expose the undersurface of the tumor during dissection. Occasionally, bending the distal one fourth of the electrocautery tip 45° facilitated the dissection. Large vessels were usually found deep, and counterpressure from the assistant's fingers on the back of the liver decreased bleeding. The Pringle maneuver was seldom used, and usually it was not even necessary to isolate the portal triad to secure vascular control.

When all detectable lesions were removed and the defects were dry, Oxidized regenerated cellulose pressure packets were removed. If the surgeon was concerned about the completeness of the tumor resection, Oxidized regenerated cellulose soaked in fluorouracil was left in the cavity. Drains were usually not used. However, when multiple lesions were removed, a closed fluted No. 19 drain was inserted. If no bile leak was seen by the third day, the drain was removed.

When four or more lesions were removed from the liver, hepatic artery Broviac and a portal vein Hickman catheters were placed in the gastroepiploic artery and vein for the delivery of chemotherapy. To check catheter placement, 3 mL of fluorescein dye was injected only into the arterial catheter to ensure that the dye evenly fluoresced in the right and left lobes of the liver, not the intestines. If the dye appeared in the intestines and the catheter position could not be improved, the hepatic artery was identified and the gastroduodenal branch isolated and catheterized with the catheter tip placed in the common hepatic artery for infusion to the left and right lobes of the liver. The catheters were inserted through the skin in the right upper quadrant of the abdomen. Before discharge, the patient was taught how to care for the catheter and self-administer chemotherapy consisting of 2 mL of fluorouracil in each catheter at 6 PM five of seven days per week, followed by heparin.

RESULTS

Of the 98 patients operated on, 59 had resection of metastases outside the liver. A total of 191 liver lesions were resected; 108 were in the right lobe and 83 in the left lobe. Metastases ranged from 0.5 to 20 cm in diameter, with the most frequent lesion size being 2.0 cm in diameter (44 metastases). Thirty-two patients had solitary hepatic metastases; 66 had more than one. Table 1 shows the number of lesions resected per person; Table 2 shows the size of the lesions resected and the lobe from which they were removed. The average intraoperative blood loss was 434 mL (range, minimal to 1200 mL). No blood transfusions were given during the last 50 operations.

The average hospital stay was ten days (range, five to 18 days), with 58% discharged on the tenth day. There were no deaths in the operating room or within 30 days postoperatively. Three patients had bile fistulas; two stopped draining in less than one month and one drained for three months. One patient suffered a postoperative myocardial infarct.

Ninety (91%) of the 98 patients were alive at the end of one year, 50 (70%) of 71 at 13 to 24 months, 23 (66%) of 35 at 25 to 36 months, 14 (74%) of 19 at 37 to 48 months, six (60%) of ten at 49 to 60 months, four (80%) of five at 61 to 72 months, and two (50%) of four 73 to 84 months after operation.

COMMENT

Acceptance of the concept that more than one metastatic liver lesion can be removed will obviously take time and a record of successful surgical experience. Our series of patients reflects our experience with the resection of multiple metastatic lesions, primarily from colon cancer. Excision of more than one lesion began innocently, when several small (1- to 3-cm) lesions were discovered during a CEA-directed second-look operation.[8] These were superficial and easily removed with the electrocautery, associated with no excessive blood loss, no residual tumor, no postoperative morbidity or mortality, and a CEA level that was normal one month after operation.

Table 1.—Hepatic Metastases Resected

No. of Hepatic Metastases	No. of Patients
1	32
2	34
3	5
4	3
5	3
6	2
7	1
8	1
9	1
13	1

Table 2.—Size and Location of Hepatic Metastases Resected

	No. of Patients	
Diameter, cm	Right Lobe	Left Lobe
0.5	1	0
1.0	18	11
1.5	12	15
2.0	24	20
2.5	10	5
3.0	6	11
3.5	12	1
4.0	9	9
5.0	3	4
5.5	2	0
6.0	0	2
7.0	2	1
7.5	1	0
8.0	5	0
9.0	0	1
9.5	0	1
10.0	1	1
15.0	2	0
20.0	0	1

The insertion of catheters for postoperative chemotherapy was suggested by Taylor and West's[9] report that after primary colon cancer resection, the injection of fluorouracil into the portal vein decreased metastatic cancer to the liver. The insertion of both a hepatic artery and portal vein catheter was thought to be better. If either catheter failed, a second catheter was available. Undetectable residual metastases would receive chemotherapy from both arterial and venous routes. Insertion of both catheters took little extra time, and the arterial perfusion pattern could be confirmed by injection of 3 mL of fluorescein dye. When there were fewer than four metastases, catheters were not placed unless the metastatic lesions were of different size, suggesting persistent tumor shedding rather than a single embolic event.

Technically, most of these lesions are easily removed without risk of excessive blood loss. However, there are three areas that deserve comment because of potential bleeding. In the right lobe, the posterior lateral and superior area, and anteriorly at the vena cava in the area of the junction of the right, left, and central hepatic veins, care must be taken to avoid bleeding, since exposure through a midline incision does not permit easy access to accomplish hemostasis in patients who are obese or those who have a high diaphragm.

Preoperative tumor detection by CT scan, magnetic

resonance image, and ultrasound is, at best, barely adequate. When more than one lesion exists, or when lesions are 2 cm in diameter or smaller, they are seldom identified. The best detector of metastases is a careful intraoperative bimanual examination. The intraoperative ultrasound is an interesting instrument that shows the location of vessels in relation to the tumor, but it has not demonstrated a metastatic lesion that could not be felt.

The shapes of the metastatic lesions resected were spherical, ovoid, and, occasionally, dumbell shaped. A true three-dimensional orientation is important in dealing with each lesion. Surface lesions tended to appear spherical on bimanual examination but only occasionally were as deep in the liver as they were wide.

When smaller lesions are removed, each margin must be checked at least by gross examination. When margins were questionable, the defects remaining after tumor removal were reexcised or laser vaporized and packed with oxidized regenerated cellulose soaked in a 6% aqueous phenol (Aqua Phenol) solution or fluorouracil in an attempt to reduce the survival of residual tumor cells. No untoward effects were observed in any patient from such packing or chemotherapy.

The self-administration of chemotherapy significantly reduces the overall cost of this management technique. Evening (6 PM) administration was selected because of reported tumor susceptibility to chemotherapy at that time and host resistance.[10] The lack of any significant toxic reactions and the unexpectedly long survival suggest that all gross tumor resection coupled with prolonged chemotherapy given directly into the hepatic circulation for extended periods of time is safe and effective in patients with hepatic metastases from colorectal tumors.

This study was supported by the American Cancer Society, National Chapter, Phi Beta Psi Sorority, and the H. L. Block Liver Metastasis Research Fund, and the Grand Chapter of the Ohio Eastern Star.

References

1. Jaffe BM, Donegan WL, Watson F, et al: Factors influencing survival in patients with untreated hepatic metastases. *Surg Gynecol Obstet* 1968; 127:1-11.

2. Kortz WJ, Meyers WC, Hanks JB, et al: Hepatic resection for metastatic cancer. *Am Surg* 1984;199:182-186.

3. Adson MA, Van Herrden JA, Adson MH, et al: Resection of hepatic metastases from colorectal cancer. *Arch Surg* 1984;119:647-651.

4. Fortner JG, Silva JS, Gorbey RB, et al: Multivariate analysis of personal series of 247 consecutive patients with liver metastasis from colorectal cancer (I). *Ann Surg* 1984;199:306-316.

5. Foster JH, Berman MM: Solid liver tumors, in *Major Problems in Clinical Surgery*. Philadelphia, WB Saunders Co, 1977, vol 22, p 214.

6. Wilson SM, Adson MA: Surgical treatment of hepatic metastases from colorectal cancers. *Arch Surg* 1976;111:330.

7. Minton JP, James KK, Hurtubise PE, et al: The use of serial carcinoembryonic antigen determinations to predict recurrence of carcinoma of the colon and the time for a second-look operation. *Surg Gynecol Obstet* 1978;147:208-210.

8. Minton JP, Hoehn JL, Gerber DM, et al: Results of a 400-patient carcinoembryonic antigen second-look colorectal cancer study. *Cancer* 1985; 55:1284-1290.

9. Taylor IR, West C: Adjuvant cytotoxic liver perfusion for colorectal cancer. *Br J Surg* 1979;66:833-837.

10. Roemeling RV, Hrushesky WJM, Kennedy BJ, et al: Programmed automatic FUDR chronotherapy improves therapeutic index. *Surg Forum* 1986;37:400-402.

Discussion

Q What are your criteria for and against embarking on this exercise?

A If there is diffuse disease in the lungs or obviously diffuse disease in the liver, then those patients are not candidates for exploration. If you have solitary or multiple solitary lesions or individually definable lesions in the liver, then they, I think, become candidates for this type of procedure. The surgeon at the operating table has to make a decision on what can be done safely and what cannot be done safely. During the operation a little pressure from the posterior aspect of the liver by the assistant and electrocautery on the highest coagulation setting really helps keep the blood loss to a minimum, and one can do these metastases safely and most of the time remove all the disease.

Q So there is no maximum above which you would say that you would not do it. Is it more a question of technical ability to get to where they are and do them?

A I have two patients with eight metastases removed surviving right now. I think the more disease you have, the less likely you are going to be able to keep these patients under control.

Q I have a question specifically about the chemotherapy regimen that you used. How long do patients continue to receive chemotherapy? I think you said you administered chemotherapy to all patients who had four or more metastases. What number of your long-term survivors are in fact in that group and what number are in the four or fewer metastases group?

A You have to take into consideration that the five-, six-, and seven-year survivors are people who had either one or two lesions. Those people did not get the lines, and I became a little more aggressive as I became more comfortable with the concept, and that is when we get into our multiple lesions. Patients with multiple lesions receive chemotherapy until their catheter is either thrombosed or broken and they refuse to have a new catheter put back in or until five years.

Q What dosage schedule are you using?

A It is very simple. I simply use 2 mL in each catheter at 6 PM until they experience diarrhea or toxic reaction, and then we just stop treatment until they recover and then reduce the dose and start them back on their home self-administration.

Q Both we and Hughes in the big national study found that margins less than 1 cm were highly correlated with poor outcome. I wondered what kind of margins you strove for. In looking at your data, it looked to me as if the median number of nodules was less than two for the whole series. So I guess the question I am actually asking is, how many had the larger numbers? In almost all the reports, the survival of patients with more than three or four separate nodules has been very poor, although not zero. I wonder about the other prognostic features too. For instance, most of the reports in the literature do not indicate a correlation between size of the nodule and the outcome, as if this were a biologic phenomenon of solitary lesions rather than a temporal phenomenon of catching them early. I wonder what your thoughts would be about that.

A To answer the question of the number of individuals with solitary lesions, I will go through those numbers: 32 had one lesion, 34 had two lesions, five had three lesions, three had four lesions, three had five lesions, two had six lesions, one had seven lesions, one had eight lesions, one had nine lesions, and one had 13 lesions.

We are still looking at flow cytometry. I do not have a good answer for that. The other factor probably related to poor survival is whether they do or do not make CEA. The patients who did not warn us early on, of course, had larger and frequently more extensive disease. The patients who had small lesions and high CEA values probably had a better clinical survival. I do not have all those data completed yet, but those are important factors, and I do agree that the biologic nature of the tumor is the answer in these people.

We always try for margins of 1 cm. I did not get these margins all the time and when margins were close or positive. What I did was take some oxidized regenerated cellulose and soak it in 6% aqueous phenol and pack it in the hole left by tumor removal. Nothing can survive local phenol. It is the same phenol that you use to inject around nerves to decrease the pain in pancreatic carcinoma. Patients tolerate it well.

Q Where did the recurrences develop in those who experienced recurrence?

A They were almost equal in the lung, liver, and abdomen. Those who died with recurrent tumors were just about equal, but I was impressed with the years of extended survival in patients with "Swiss cheese" resections that later failed.

Experimental Liver Metastasis

Implications of Clonal Proclivity and Organ Specificity

T. S. Ravikumar, MD; John D'Emilia, MD; Celia Cocchiaro; Barbara Wolf, MD;
Vincent King; Glenn Steele, Jr, MD, PhD

• "Spontaneous" lung metastases develop in over 50% of the animals bearing subcutaneous isografts of WB-2054, a rat colon carcinoma. A metastatic variant has been developed by "Fidler" type in vivo selection, yielding 100% lung metastasis. In a five-week assay to test the organ specificity of this lung metastatic variant, however, "experimental" liver and lung metastases could be induced in 100% and 60% of animals on portal venous and intravenous injections, respectively. The results demonstrate selection of a metastatic variant from heterogeneous primary tumor, and suggest at least two interacting mechanisms: (1) mechanical (the anatomy of the blood-borne metastatic pathways) and (2) biologic (factors intrinsic to primary tumor subpopulations that can be selected for metastatic proclivity). In addition, liver metastases were successfully established from colon tumors induced by cecal wall injection of tumor cells. Such a spontaneous liver metastasis model will be useful to study the specific mechanisms involved during metastasis of colon cancer to the liver.

(*Arch Surg* 1989;124:49-54)

Death from liver metastases remains a significant problem in cancer-related mortality. Colorectal carcinoma metastasizes to the liver in up to 70% of patients who develop advanced disease.[1] Other gastrointestinal tumors and extra-abdominal tumors of diverse origin metastasize to the liver frequently.[2] No effective therapy is available for nonresectable hepatic metastases.[3]

Experimental studies for understanding the mechanisms of organ-specific metastases are germane to designing proper therapeutic strategies. Such studies are limited by the lack of suitable animal models for liver metastasis.[4] A spectrum of chemically induced rodent and murine tumors and xenografts of human colon carcinoma in nude mice or rats have been described to study human colon cancer metastasis, not all of them reflecting accurately the complex steps involved in the metastatic pathway.[4-9] Few of these models display reproducible metastatic properties that are analogous to the clinical setting, and most of these systems involve induction of metastases by subcutaneous, tail vein, or intrasplenic injection. A shortcoming of the nude mice models to study the mechanisms of metastasis is that spontaneous metastases do not occur ordinarily in nude mice or occur only very rarely.[10,11] Though the in vivo studies using human tumor xenografts in immunosuppressed nude mice may be acceptable for many experimental purposes, tumor models utilizing syngeneic animal systems offer advantages of being able to study the metastatic "cascade" in immunocompetent hosts.

To this end, we have attempted to develop a model to study metastasis in a chemically induced syngeneic rat colon cancer, which has previously been shown to bear reasonable analogy to human colon carcinoma.[12,13] We have successfully established liver metastases from colon tumors induced by cecal wall injection of tumor cells, thereby providing a model that follows all the steps of the complex metastatic pathway.

Though it is generally accepted and proved in several animal tumor systems that metastasis is a nonrandom multistep process with selection of cell variants with predetermined target organ specificity,[14,15] autopsy data of patients dying of colon cancer reveal a cascade phenomenon of metastasis, conforming to a circulatory "watershed" principle.[16,17] These data are persuasive as to the interplay between the biologic characteristics of tumor cell subpopulations, host organ microenvironmental influences, and the circulation dynamics of tumor cell dissemination in the development of tumor metastasis. In this study, we have also tested the implications of organ specificity vs circulation dynamics by utilizing a metastatic variant of the rat colon cancer cell line and inducing experimental lung and liver metastases.

MATERIALS AND METHODS

Animals

Wistar-Furth–Brown Norwegian F_1 hybrid rats (WF × BN F_1) were bred in our institutional animal facility by mating female Wistar-Furth rats and male Brown Norwegian rats (Harlan Sprague-Dawley). The F_1 hybrid rats were used at 8 to 9 weeks of age. The animals were allowed free access to food and water.

Accepted for publication Sept 2, 1988.

From the Laboratory of Cancer Biology, Department of Surgery, New England Deaconess Hospital/Harvard Medical School, Boston.

Read before the Annual Meeting of the Society of Surgical Oncology, New Orleans, May 23, 1988.

Reprint requests to 110 Francis St, Suite 3A, Boston, MA 02215 (Dr Ravikumar).

Tumors

The WB-2054 tumor is a poorly differentiated mucin-producing colon adenocarcinoma, induced by 1,2-dimethylhydrazine in a WF×BN F_1 rat. This tumor is syngeneic to the F_1 hybrid rats. The tumor line is maintained both by serial in vivo passage in the subcutis and by in vitro cell culture. A metastatic variant of the WB-2054 cell line was established as described below.

Single-cell suspensions were prepared from solid tumor isografts by mechanically disaggregating small tumor pieces, suspended in RPMI 1640 medium with 1000 IU/mL of penicillin and 100 mg/mL of streptomycin. The cells were washed three times in the same medium and resuspended at appropriate concentration in phosphate-buffered saline.

Induction of Spontaneous Metastases

The term *spontaneous* metastasis is used to describe the ability of cell subpopulations from within the primary tumor isografts to progress and form metastatic foci to regional lymphatics and distant organs. Eight- to 9-week-old male WF×BN F_1 hybrid rats were injected subcutaneously in the thigh with 1×10^6 cells. Tumors thus induced were resected (under ether inhalation anesthesia) at four weeks and the rats were followed up for an additional eight weeks. At this time, all rats were killed by ether inhalation and autopsied for evaluation of lungs and livers for metastasis.

Isolation of Metastasis Variant

A cell line with enhanced metastatic ability was selected by an in vivo method similar to the description by Fidler.[18] Cells derived from spontaneous lung metastases in rats bearing primary tumor isografts were reimplanted subcutaneously, and the procedure was repeated serially in an attempt to isolate cells with enhanced metastatic ability.

Growth Kinetics of Primary Tumor and Metastatic Variant

Single-cell suspensions ($1 \times {}^{-}10^6$ live cells) of WB-2054 primary tumor and its metastatic variant were injected subcutaneously into the thigh of male WF×BN F_1 hybrid rats. Tumor isograft growth was measured twice weekly with Vernier calipers and the tumor volume determined by the method of Attia and Weiss.[19]

Metastatic Progression of Tumors

Two groups of rats were injected subcutaneously with 1×10^6 cells of either the WB-2054 primary tumor or its metastatic variant. Groups of rats were serially killed at weekly intervals, at three to eight weeks following tumor cell inoculation. Lungs and liver were dissected and examined for gross and microscopic evidence of metastasis.

Induction of Experimental Metastases

The term *experimental* metastasis signifies metastases developing after intravascular injection of neoplastic cells.[20] Single-cell suspensions (1×10^6 cells) of either primary tumor or the metastatic variant were injected intravascularly using a 26-gauge needle. For intravenous injection, the rats were subjected to light ether inhalation anesthesia, and the jugular vein was exposed in the neck by a 5-mm incision. Following the injection of tumor cells, gentle pressure was applied over the venipuncture site for about a minute and the skin closed with a metallic clip. For portal vein injections, a midline abdominal incision was made with the animal under ether anesthesia, the duodenal loop was exposed, and the tumor cells were injected into the portal vein. Sterile absorbant sponge was placed under gentle pressure over the injection site as the needle was withdrawn to prevent bleeding and peritoneal spillage of tumor cells. The abdominal wall was approximated with running 3-0 chromic catgut sutures and the skin approximated with metallic clips. Five weeks following tumor cell injections, the rats were killed for harvesting liver and lungs. Gross inspection and microscopic examination of 10% formaldehyde–fixed tissue was carried out to detect metastatic deposits.

Table 1.—Incidence of Lung Metastases Eight Weeks Following Resection of WB-2054-Primary Isografts

Experiment	No. of Rats: Isograft	No. of Rats: Lung Metastases	Percentage of Lung Metastases
1	10	5	50
2	6	4	67
3	12	7	58
Total	**28**	**16**	57

Induction of Spontaneous Liver Metastases by Cecal Injection of Tumor Cells

Male WF×BN F_1 rats were anesthetized by ether inhalation, and the cecum was exposed via a midline abdominal incision. Five million viable tumor cells (in 0.05 mL of phosphate-buffered saline) of WB-2054 or its metastatic variant were injected into the cecal wall from the serosal side using a sterile tuberculin syringe and a 27-gauge needle. The serosal surface of the injection site was dabbed with 95% alcohol swab to kill any tumor cells on the peritoneal surface. The abdominal wall was closed as described above. The rats were subjected to laparotomy every four weeks and examined for the presence of cecal tumors and liver, lymph node, or peritoneal metastases. In rats with established cecal tumors and metastases, the organs were removed and processed for histologic analysis.

Statistical Analysis

The χ^2 test with Yates' correction was used to assess the statistical significance of the incidence of parenchymal metastases.

RESULTS

Spontaneous Metastases From WB-2054 Primary Tumor Isografts

Four weeks after subcutaneous injection of 1×10^6 WB-2054 colon tumor cells into the thigh, all rats developed tumors measuring approximately 2 to 3 cm in diameter, when the tumors were resected. At eight weeks following resection of these primary tumors from the thigh, the lungs and the liver were examined grossly and microscopically. None of the rats developed liver metastasis. The incidence of lung metastases observed in three sequential experiments is summarized in Table 1. The mean incidence of lung metastases was 57% (range, 50% to 67%). We also found that at this period of eight weeks, the metastases in all animals became grossly visible, such that the lungs grossly negative for metastases were also negative on light microscopy using 10% formaldehyde–fixed tissues stained by hematoxylin-eosin.

Isolation of a Metastatic Variant

A Fidler-type selection experiment was carried out to yield a metastatic variant of the WB-2054 tumor. The third selection tumor was chosen as the metastatic variant, as it induced lung metastases in all the rats, the size of lung metastases being significantly larger than those produced by the primary tumor line. The primary tumor line will hereafter be referred to as WB-2054-P and the lung metastatic variant WB-2054-M. The histologic nature of WB-2054-M was poorly differentiated mucin-producing adenocarcinoma, identical to that of WB-2054-P.

Growth Kinetics of WB-2054-P and WB-2054-M

To ensure that the metastatic proclivity of WB-2054-M was not simply due to rapidity of proliferation, we compared the growth curves of WB-2054-P and WB-2054-M isografts induced by subcutaneous inoculation of 1×10^6 cells in two groups of rats. Figure 1 is a semilog plot of the tumor

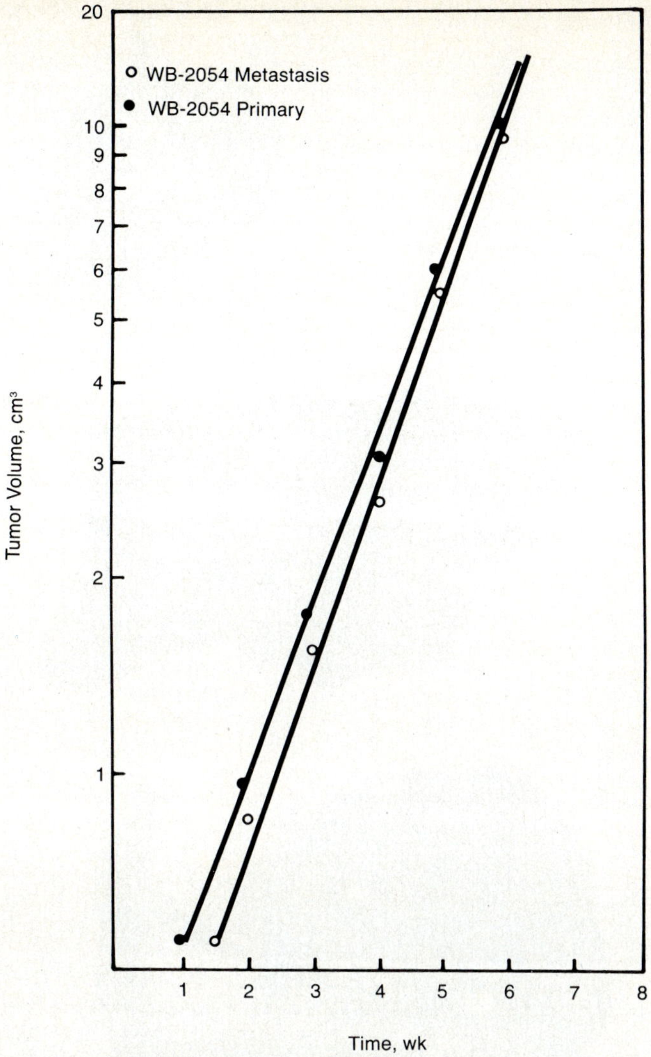

Fig 1.—Semilog plot of comparative growth kinetics of WB-2054-P and WB-2054-M isografts (n = 3, each group).

volume of exponentially growing tumors. There is no significant difference in the growth kinetics between the tumor lines. After six weeks, the tumors became necrotic, with breakdown of skin, and the volume measurements were unreliable.

Time to Spontaneous Metastasis Development

Serial killing of rats at weekly intervals to examine for lung metastases development was carried out to evaluate the rate of metastatic progression. Both WB-2054-P and WB-2054-M metastasized to lungs after a latent period five weeks following primary tumor resection.

Experimental Metastases to Liver and Lung

Groups of five rats were randomized to receive intravenous or portal venous injection of 1×10^6 cells of either WB-2054-P or WB-2054-M tumor. Five weeks after the tumor cell injection, the rats were killed and all intra-abdominal and thoracic viscera were examined for metastases. Table 2 summarizes the aggregate of two experiments. Intravenous injection of WB-2054-P did not produce parenchymal metastases in any of the rats in this five-week assay. When injected via portal vein, however, 50% of rats developed multiple gross liver metastases; none of these rats developed lung metastases. Intravenous injection of WB-2054-M resulted in 60% of rats developing pulmonary metastases. Surprisingly, all animals (100%) receiving portal venous inoculation of WB-2054-M cells, which is a lung metastasis variant, developed liver metastases. One such tumor is shown in Fig 2. Equally interesting, intravenous, WB-2054-M injection did not give rise to liver metastasis, nor did portal venous injection result in lung metastasis. These findings suggest that the arrest of tumor cells in the first capillary bed may be an important determinant of the site specificity of metastases.

Light microscopy of all the harvested organs was carried out to confirm the incidence of metastases (Figs 3 and 4).

Table 2.—Parenchymal Metastases Five Weeks Following Tumor Cell Injection*

Cells and Route	Metastases: Lung	Metastases: Liver
WB-2054-P		
IV	0/10	0/10
PV	0/10	5/10
WB-2054-M		
IV	6/10†	0/10
PV	0/10	10/10‡

*WB-2054-P and WB-2054-M indicate primary and metastatic variants, respectively; IV, intravenous; and PV, portal venous. Values are numbers of rats.

†$P<.005$, primary vs metastatic variants, χ^2 test.

‡$P<.01$, primary vs metastatic variants, χ^2 test.

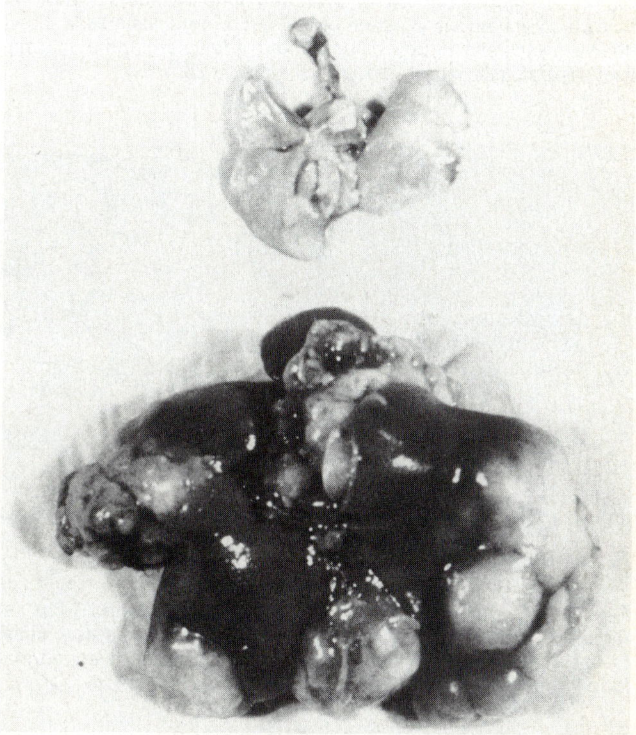

Fig 2.—Gross liver metastases in rat five weeks after portal venous injection of 1×10^6 WB-2054-metastasis cells. Note absence of lung metastases.

Induction of Spontaneous Liver Metastases by Cecal Injection

Cecal injection of WB-2054-P (n = 3) and WB-2054-M (n = 3) tumor cells resulted in development of colonic

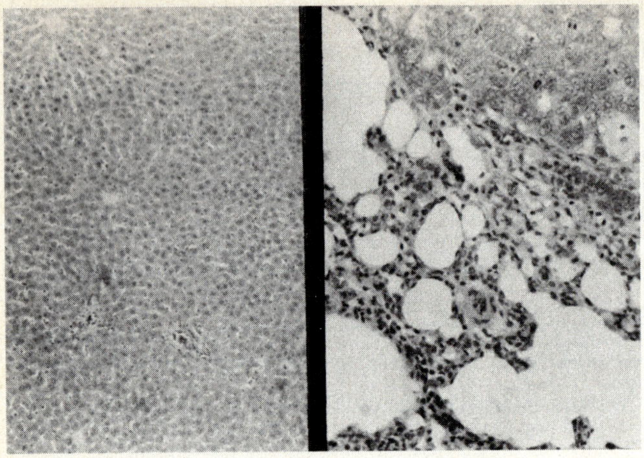

Fig 3.—Photomicrograph of liver and lung harvested from rat following intravenous injection of WB-2054-metastasis cells. Lung shows metastatic poorly differentiated adenocarcinoma; normal liver (hematoxylin-eosin, left, ×175; right, ×250).

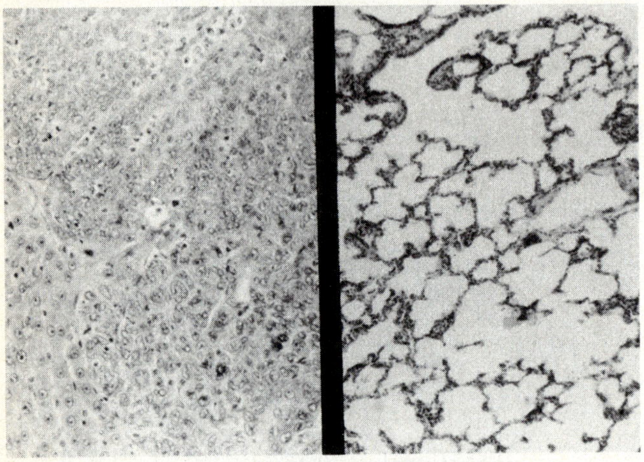

Fig 4.—Photomicrograph of liver and lung harvested from rat receiving portal venous injection of WB-2054-metastasis cells. Metastatic poorly differentiated adenocarcinoma in liver; normal lung (hematoxylin-eosin, left, ×175; right, ×250).

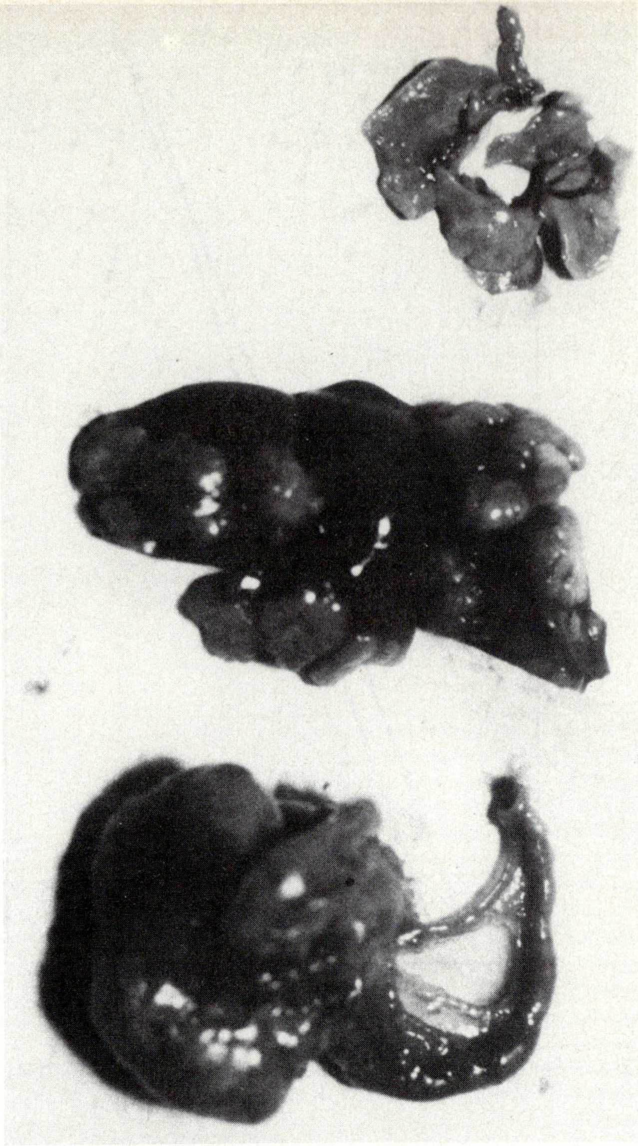

Fig 5.—Induction of cecal tumor by injection of 5×10^6 WB-2054-metastasis cells into cecal wall. Liver shows gross metastases, and lungs are free of tumor.

tumors in all rats. At eight weeks, gross liver metastases developed in two of the three rats receiving WB-2054-M cells, but no liver metastases were seen in rats inoculated with WB-2054-P cells (Fig 5). This experiment demonstrates that the variant tumor with metastatic proclivity could establish spontaneous liver metastases by progressing through all the steps of the metastatic pathway, ie, growth in the colon, progression through the basement membrane, invasion into the vascular bed, dissemination to the liver, and colonization and growth in the liver parenchyma.

COMMENT

The data lend support to the hypothesis that nonrandom selection of metastatic subpopulations from heterogeneous primary tumor is an intrinsic biologic event in the multistep metastatic pathway. Pursuant to this selection process, the metastatic variant selected for proclivity to lung targeting metastasized both to liver and lung, depending on the route of injection. Mechanical factors relating to the anatomy of the lymphatic and blood-borne metastatic pathways seem to be important in determining the target organ site rather than a "programming" of the selected metastatic clones to target-specific organs. Additionally, experimental and spontaneous organ-specific metastases could be induced in this model, which lends itself to study various factors involved in lung and liver metastases.

The development of an experimental system for organ-specific metastasis has been prompted by a paucity of suitable animal models to address the questions relating to various steps of the metastatic process in a direct fashion. Nude mice models to study the metastatic characteristics of human tumors are increasingly in use recently. Although for most purposes these models are optimal, the low incidence of metastases even with highly aggressive human tumors, the extreme rarity of spontaneous metastases, and the immunodeficient host milieu have provided the rationale to seek an alternative model with analogy to human colon cancer.[4,7,10,11] A syngeneic model may offer advantage to evaluate immunotherapeutic strategies in an immunocompetent host.[5] Furthermore, the dimethylhydrazine-induced colon cancer model has been extensively characterized in our laboratory and has been demonstrated to bear reasonable analogy to human colorectal cancer in several respects.[12,13] The ability to induce spontaneous liver and lung metastases in this study makes the analogy even closer.

It is generally accepted that metastasis is not a random process; rather, it involves selection of preexistent tumor cells with higher metastatic potential.[14,15,18,21] The establishment of a metastatic variant by Fidler-type selection in our model supports this tenet. Furthermore, this proclivity does not necessarily correlate with the growth properties of tumor per se, which is demonstrable in this and other models.[8] Heterogeneity during tumor progression and metastasis has been demonstrated with reference to expression of various membrane antigens, karyotypic abnormalities, enzyme and hormone production, and changes in cell surface glycoproteins and glycolipids.[11,22-27] Phenotypic differences between WB-2054-P and WB-2054-M will be pursued in subsequent in vitro studies.

Our finding that a lung metastatic tumor line metastasized avidly to the liver is at variance with the concept of organ specificity of metastases. The postulate of evolution of clonal cell populations that target to lung, liver, or other organs is supported by several studies.[14,18,20] Suppression of tumor metastases by specific organs, organ-specific adhesion of tumor cells, and elaboration of specific factors by target organs are some of the additional mechanisms proposed to support this postulate.[6,28-32] Clinical and experimental observations against such an organ-specific theory have also been put forward. A large autopsy study of patients dying of colon cancer revealed a cascade phenomenon of metastases: development of hepatic metastases via portal veins, metastases to lungs from liver, and finally arterial metastases to other sites from lung.[16,17] In contrast, in patients dying of gastrointestinal cancers outside the portal watershed (upper esophagus, lower rectum), the initial site of dissemination was to the lungs, with subsequent arterial dissemination to other sites. Additionally, strong evidence against organ specificity of metastatic clones has been put forward by Gorman et al.[33] Using a VX-2 carcinoma model in rabbits with portacaval shunt construction, they showed that a primary tumor metastasized according to nonorganophilic circulation dynamics. These clinical and experimental observations are in concordance with our data on experimental metastases. It thus seems likely that spontaneous tumors in humans and in animal models are influenced by an interplay between intrinsic properties of tumor cells, microenvironmental influences in the organs in which the cells arrest, and rheologic considerations.[34]

Despite the fact that organ colonization of cells after direct injection into blood vasculature is not necessarily predictive of spontaneous metastatic potential as shown in this study and by others,[35] such tumor models still are useful to study the interaction between tumor cells and host organ environment. The observation that metastatic cells frequently colonize lung and liver suggests that specific interactions occur at these sites. Specific receptors on tumor cell surface (eg, laminin), specific alterations in glycoproteins (eg, sialoglycoproteins), and elaboration of specific enzymes (eg, type IV collagenase) may be some of the contributing mechanisms.[27,31,36,37] Since it has been suggested that inhibition of sialyl transferase can prevent liver metastasis, we are now attempting to test this hypothesis in our model.[38]

Another postulate that will be addressed in this model is the role of fixed tissue macrophage–tumor cell interactions contributing to lung and liver metastases. Kupffer's cell encirclement of tumor cells injected intraportally was correlated with the metastasizing potential of certain tumor lines in vivo.[39] Stimulation of reticuloendothelial cells has been shown to inhibit metastases and the suppression of these fixed macrophages to increase metastases to liver and lung.[40,41] The establishment of spontaneous metastases to both the lung and the liver in the present study lends itself to study the mechanisms involved in organ-specific tumor cell interactions.

We thank Suzanne Jackson for expert manuscript preparation.

References

1. Kemeny N, Yagoda A, Brown D, et al: Therapy for metastatic colorectal carcinoma with a combination of methyl-CCNU, 5-fluorouracil, vincristine and strepozotocin (MOF-Strep). *Cancer* 1980;45:876-881.

2. Foster JH, Ensminger WF: Treatment of metastatic cancer to liver, in DeVita V Jr, Hellman S, Rosenberg SA (eds): *Cancer: Principles and Practice of Oncology*, ed 2. Philadelphia, JB Lippincott, 1985, pp 2117-2132.

3. Cady B: Natural history of primary and secondary tumors of the liver. *Semin Oncol* 1983;86:550-555.

4. Schirrmacher V: Cancer metastasis: Experimental approaches, theoretical concepts, and impact for treatment strategies. *Adv Cancer Res* 1985;43:1-73.

5. Dunnington DJ, Buscarino C, Gennaro D, et al: Characterization of an animal model of metastatic colon carcinoma. *Int J Cancer* 1987;39:248-254.

6. Bresalier RS, Roper SE, Hujanen ES, et al: A new model for human colon cancer metastasis. *Int J Cancer* 1987;39:625-630.

7. Goldrosen M: Murine colon adenocarcinoma: Immunobiology of metastases. *Cancer* 1980;45:1223-1228.

8. Giavazzi R, Campbell DE, Jessup JM, et al: Metastatic behavior of tumor cells isolated from primary and metastatic human colorectal carcinomas implanted into different sites in nude mice. *Cancer Res* 1986;46:1928-1933.

9. Drewinko B, Yang KY, Leibowitz A, et al: Cellular discriminants for a biological classification of human colon carcinoma. *Cancer Res* 1984;44:4241-4253.

10. Sordat BCM, Veyama Y, Fogh J: Metastasis of tumor xenografts in the nude mouse, in Fogh J, Giovanalla BC (eds): *The Nude Mouse in Experimental and Clinical Research.* Orlando, Fla, Academic Press Inc, 1982, vol 2, pp 95-147.

11. Varki NM, Roome L, Sparkes RS, et al: Microscopic metastasis of a human lung carcinoma cell line in athymic nude mice: Isolation of a metastatic variant. *Int J Cancer* 1987;40:46-52.

12. Ross DS, Steele G, Madara J, et al: Effects of specific active immunization on tumor recurrence following primary tumor resection in WF rats with 1,2-dimethylhydrazine induced bowel cancer. *JNCI* 1984;73:731-735.

13. Madara JL, Harte P, Deasy J, et al: Evidence for an adenoma-carcinoma sequence in dimethylhydrazine induced neoplasms of rat intestinal epithelium. *Am J Pathol* 1983;110:230-237.

14. Poste G, Fidler IJ: The pathogenesis of cancer metastasis. *Nature* 1980;283:139-146.

15. Nicolson GL: Generation of phenotypic diversity and progression in metastatic tumors. *Cancer Metastasis Rev* 1984;3:24-42.

16. Weiss L, Voit A, Lane WW: Metastatic patterns in patients with carcinomas of the lower esophagus and upper rectum. *Invasion Metastasis* 1984;4:47-60.

17. Weiss L, Grundmann E, Tarhorst J, et al: Hematogenous metastatic patterns in colonic carcinoma: An analysis of 1541 necropsies. *J Pathol* 1986;150:195-203.

18. Fidler IJ: Selection of successive tumor lines for metastasis. *Nature N Biol* 1973;242:148-149.

19. Attia MA, Weiss DW: Immunology of spontaneous mammary carcinomas in mice: V. Acquired tumor resistance and enhancement in strain A mice injected with mammary tumor virus. *Cancer Res* 1966;26:1787-1800.

20. Fidler IJ: Rationale and methods for the use of nude mice to study the biology and therapy of human cancer metastasis. *Cancer Metastasis Rev* 1986;5:29-49.

21. Nicolson G, Custead SE: Tumor metastasis is not due to adaptation of cells to a new organ environment. *Science* 1982;215:176-178.

22. Natali PG, Bigotti A, Nicotra MR, et al: Distribution of human class I histocompatibility antigens in normal and malignant tissues of nonlymphoid origin. *Cancer Res* 1984;44-47:4679-6687.

23. Lowe FC, Isaacs JT: Biochemical methods for predicting metastatic ability of prostatic cancer utilizing the Dunning R-3327 rat prostatic adenocarcinoma system as a model. *Cancer Res* 1984;44:744-752.

24. Spremulli EN, Scott C, Campbell D, et al: Characterization of two metastatic subpopulations originating from a single human colon carcinoma. *Cancer Res* 1983;43:3828-3835.
25. Kendal WS, Wang R, Frost P: Spontaneous mutation rates in cloned murine tumors do not correlate with metastatic potential, whereas the prevalence of karyotypic abnormalities in the parental tumor does. *Int J Cancer* 1987;40:408-413.
26. Parish CR, Coombe DR, Jakobsen KB, et al: Evidence that sulphated polysaccharides inhibit tumor metastases by blocking tumor-cell–derived heparanases. *Int J Cancer* 1987;40:511-518.
27. Irimura T, Carlson DA, Price J, et al: Differential expression of a sialoglycoprotein with an approximate molecular weight of 900 000 on metastatic human colon carcinoma cells growing in culture and in tumor tissues. *Cancer Res* 1988;48:2353-2360.
28. Horak E, Darling DL, Tarin D: Analysis of organ-specific effects on metastatic tumor formation by studies in vitro. *JNCI* 1986;76:913-922.
29. Nicolson GL, Dulski K, Basson C, et al: Preferential organ attachment and invasion in vitro by B-16 melanoma cell selected for differing metastatic colonization and invasive properties. *Invasion Metastasis* 1985;5:144-158.
30. Netland PA, Zetter BR: Organ-specific adhesion of metastatic tumor cells in vitro. *Science* 1984;224:1113-1115.
31. Terranova VP, Hujanen ES, Martin GR: Basement membrane and the invasive activity of metastatic tumor cell. *JNCI* 1986;77:311-316.
32. Hujanen ES, Terranova VP: Migration of tumor cell to organs-derived chemoattractants. *Cancer Res* 1985;45:3517-3521.
33. Gorman JR, Abrahamson J, Mordohovich D, et al: Nonorganophilic hematogenous dissemination in the presence of positive lymph nodes of a malignant tumor in rabbits. *Invasion Metastasis* 1984;4:44-59.
34. Juacaba SF, Jones LD, Tarin D: Organ preferences in metastatic colony formation by spontaneous mammary carcinomas after intra-arterial inoculation. *Invasion Metastasis* 1983;3:208-220.
35. Stackpole CW: Distinct lung-colonizing and lung-metastasizing cell populations in B15 mouse melanoma. *Nature* 1981;289:798-800.
36. Liotta LA, Rao NC, Barsky SH: Tumor invasion and the extracellular matrix. *Lab Invest* 1983;49:636-649.
37. Yogeeswaran G, Salk PL: Metastatic potential is positively correlated with cell surface sialylation of cultured murine tumor cell lines. *Science* 1981;212:1514-1516.
38. Kijima-Suda I, Miyamoto Y, Toyoshima S, et al: Inhibition of experimental pulmonary metastasis of mouse colon adenocarcinoma 26 sublines by a sialic acid: Nucleoside conjugate having sialyltransferase inhibiting activity. *Cancer Res* 1986;46:858-862.
39. Roos E, Dingemanik P: Phagocytosis of tumor cells by immune Kupffer cells in vivo and in the perfused mouse liver, in James K, McBride B, Stuart A (eds): *The Macrophage and Cancer.* Edinburgh, University of Edinburgh, 1977, pp 216-224.
40. Holmberg SB, Hafstrom L, Kjellberg G: RES function and tumor take and tumor growth in the liver and in the kidney: An experimental study in rats. *Eur J Cancer Clin Oncol* 1987;23:1883-1887.
41. Pearson HJ, Anderson J, Chamberlain J, et al: The effect of Kupffer cell stimulation or depression on the development of liver metastases in the rat. *Cancer Immunol Immunother* 1986;23:214-216.

Discussion

Q Did you look microscopically at single-cell suspensions between the primary tumor and your third variant to see if there was any gross difference of the cell membrane? Do you plan to do any biochemical studies to see if there is a difference in the composition?

A Yes, we are in the process of looking at the tumor cell heterogeneity between the primary and the metastatic variants, as well as looking at the interaction between the tumor cells and the host organ subpopulation of macrocytes.

Q What would happen if you did your intracecal injections and tried to do your selections for liver first, perhaps using either your portal vein or an intrasplenic approach, and then compared the two different metastatic variants for biologic activity by, say, titration studies?

A The lung metastasis variant was chosen because it was easy to induce subcutaneous tumor isografts in a large number of animals and, from there, big lung metastases. So far, the cecal injection of the primary tumor does not induce liver metastases, mainly because of the slower kinetics by which animals develop large cecal tumors, obstruction, and peritoneal carcinomatosis. We chose a time point—for example, four to six weeks—where the cecal tumors would be able to be resected but with primary closure and the animals followed up for later development of liver metastases. These studies are in progress.

Q With the lung tumor that you injected intraportally and that formed a metastasis in the liver, if you isolated that metastasis and gave it back intravenously, would it go to the lung again or to the liver in the next generation?

A To the lung again, unfortunately.

Q The Cleveland Clinic group made a subcutaneous pouch that seemed to work quite well. Have you tried that? Does it work?

A We have been successful in doing that, but I do not think we need to do that if we can be successful by injecting into the tip of the cecum and resecting it when the tumors are 1 cm.

Intra-abdominal Recurrence of Colorectal Cancer Detected by Radioimmunoguided Surgery (RIGS System)

Armando Sardi, MD; Mark Workman; Cathy Mojzisik, RN, MS; George Hinkle, RPh;
Carol Nieroda, MD; Edward W. Martin, Jr, MD

• Since 1986, 32 patients with metastatic colorectal cancer have undergone second-look radioimmunoguided surgery (RIGS system). The primary tumor was located in the right and transverse colon in 11 patients, left and sigmoid colon in 16, and rectum in five. The carcinoembryonic antigen level was elevated in 30 patients (94%); all patients underwent a computed tomographic scan of the abdomen and pelvis. The overall sensitivity of the computed tomographic scan was 41% (abdomen other than liver, 27%; liver, 58%; and pelvis, 22%). The RIGS system identified recurrent tumor in 81% of the patients. The most common site of metastasis was the liver (41%), independent of the primary location. Local/regional recurrences alone accounted for 40% of all recurrences. In six patients (18%), recurrent tumor was found only with the RIGS system. The RIGS system is more dependable in localizing clinically obscure metastases than other methods, and carcinoembryonic antigen testing remains the most accurate preoperative method to indicate suspected recurrences.
(*Arch Surg* 1989;124:55-59)

Knowledge of the natural history and failure patterns following the initial resection of colorectal cancer is of primary importance to physicians in choosing adjuvant regimens, as well as in carrying out an aggressive approach to recurrent colorectal cancer.

Many authors have demonstrated the benefits of hepatic resection for liver recurrences of colorectal cancer[1-4] and of the second-look approach to extrahepatic recurrences.[5-7] Many reports on the natural history of the disease are based on the results of physical examination and external scanning, which are known to be inaccurate in determining the extent and location of disease. Radioimmunoguided surgery (RIGS system) has been used at The Ohio State University College of Medicine, Columbus, to locate recurrent tumor and has altered the surgical approach in 26% of patients[8] by identifying tumor not clinically detectable. In this report, we identify the sites of recurrence in a group of patients who underwent reoperations for recurrent colorectal cancer with the assistance of the RIGS system.

PATIENTS AND METHODS

From January 1986 to November 1987, 32 patients underwent second-look surgery for recurrent colorectal carcinoma. Patients with suspected recurrent colorectal cancer who were considered possible candidates for radioimmunoguided surgery were seen in The Ohio State University Clinic.

Diagnostic evaluation of the patients included an air contrast barium enema, a computed tomographic (CT) scan of the abdomen and pelvis, a serum carcinoembryonic antigen (CEA) assay, and colonoscopy. A chest x-ray film, bone scan, and CT scan of the chest were done to exclude patients with extra-abdominal metastatic disease. The presence of either pulmonary or bone metastases excluded the patient from the study.

Patients who were accepted for the study received an injection of iodine 125–radiolabeled antibody. Before the injection, they were treated with a supersaturated solution of potassium iodide salt solution (SSKI) to block the uptake of free radiolabeled iodine by the thyroid gland.

Forearm subcutaneous hypersensitivity testing to the unlabeled antibody (0.1 mg in 0.1 mL of sodium chloride) was performed on the day of injection. If the result was positive, the patient was released from the study. If no reaction occurred, the radiolabeled antibody was given by intravenous injection over ten to 15 minutes, and the patient remained under observation for 15 minutes. Operation was scheduled when precordial counts, measured by the gamma-detecting probe (GDP), were less than 20 counts per 2 s. This usually occurred between two to three weeks after injection (range, three to 34 days).

Patients were admitted to the hospital one day before the operation. Routine bowel preparation was done.

Accepted for publication July 8, 1988.

From the Department of Surgery, Division of Surgical Oncology, The Ohio State University College of Medicine, Columbus. Drs Sardi and Nieroda are fellows of the American Cancer Society. Dr Sardi is now with the Ochsner Clinic, New Orleans.

Read before the Annual Meeting of the Society of Surgical Oncology, New Orleans, May 24, 1988.

Reprint requests to Department of Surgery, Division of Surgical Oncology, The Ohio State University College of Medicine, N-924 Doan Hall, 410 W Tenth Ave, Columbus, OH 43210 (Dr Martin).

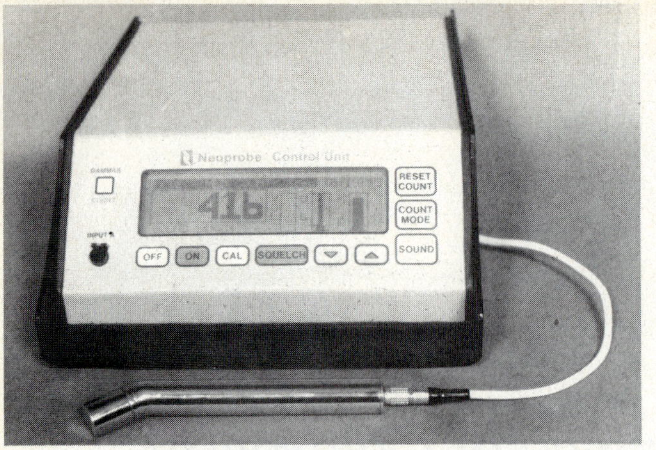

Gamma-detecting probe (Neoprobe).

GDP

The GDP (Neoprobe, Neoprobe Corp, Columbus, Ohio) is an 18-cm-long by 2-cm-diameter stainless steel tube with an angled tip (120°) for better maneuverability (Figure). Collimation can be varied by a movable stainless steel collimator. The tip of the probe contains a highly radiosensitive cadmium telluride crystal that relays through a preamplifier to emit a digital readout and an auditory signal. The intensity and the frequency of the auditory signal are directly proportional to the level of radioactivity detected. A ratio of 2:1 has been considered to be significant because it is the value at which the audible signal in tumor is clearly different from that in normal tissue.

Monoclonal Antibodies

Two monoclonal antibodies (MoAbs), prepared by hybridoma technology, were used.[9]

All antibodies were labeled with iodine 125 using the (Iodo-Gen) method that has been previously described.[8] The characteristics of MoAbs B72.3 and 17-1A have been previously described.[10-12]

SURGICAL PROCEDURE

A midline xiphopubic incision permitted a thorough exploration of the abdominal cavity with complete mobilization of the liver and small bowel, evaluation of periportal, para-aortic, and celiac nodes, and inspection of previous resection sites and the mesentery. The GDP was used to count obvious tumors and scan the abdomen for areas of increased radioactivity. Areas of obvious tumor were resected if possible, and areas with increased probe counts but without obvious tumor were obtained as biopsy specimens and were sent for frozen-section preparation and examination. Probe readings of normal tissue from which the tumor originated were taken to compare tumor-to-tissue counts. Additional counts were routinely obtained from the liver, stomach, kidney, aorta, small bowel, and colon. Each reading was repeated in triplicate.

Ex vivo probe counts were performed on the gross specimens, and routine and probe-directed samples were obtained for evaluation. Formaldehyde-fixed, paraffin-embedded samples were processed for routine hematoxylin-eosin staining.

Following resection of all recurrent tumor, the bed of resection was counted with the GDP. If increased counts were encountered, the suspicious areas were taken as biopsy specimens, frozen sections were obtained, and, if possible, further resection was carried out until normal counts were obtained. All areas of recurrent tumor were documented and correlated with the final histopathologic results.

Local failure was defined as a recurrence within the tumor bed, in adjacent organs by direct extension, or in regional nodal groups. Regional nodal groups included lymph nodes up to the takeoff of the colic vessels or lymph node–bearing areas adjacent to previous areas of resection. Diffuse disease was defined as three or more sites of noncontiguous tumor recurrence.

Table 1.—Stage of Primary According to Location (Astler-Coller Classification)

	Location, No. of Patients			
Stage	R/Transverse Colon	L/Sigmoid Colon	Rectum	Total
B1	0	4	0	**4**
B2	3	2	1	**6**
C1	1	1	0	**2**
C2	7	9	4	**20**

RESULTS

A total of 32 patients were studied. The mean age of the 18 men and 14 women was 64 years, with a range of 29 to 82 years.

The modified Dukes' classification of primary tumor was B1 in four patients, B2 in six patients, C1 in two patients, and C2 in 20 patients. The distribution according to primary tumor location is presented in Table 1. Patients were divided into three groups according to patterns of blood supply to see if there was a correlation with the pattern of recurrence: group 1, right and transverse colon (11 patients); group 2, left and sigmoid colon (16 patients); and group 3, rectum (five patients).

The mean time to recurrence was 21 months, with a range of two to 69 months: group 1, 24 months (range, five to 69 months); group 2, 20 months (range, two to 59 months); and group 3, 17 months (range, nine to 28 months).

Sites of Recurrence

Sites of recurrence and their relation to the location of primary tumor are presented in Table 2. Of the 11 patients in group 1, four (36%) had metastasis to the liver only. One patient (9%) had diffuse intra-abdominal disease, as well as liver involvement, and one patient each had recurrences in the mesocolon, mesocolon and small bowel, right paracolic gutter, celiac nodes and retroperitoneum, retroperitoneum and small-bowel mesentery. These last six recurrences could be grouped as local/regional recurrences (55%). In the 11 patients in group 1, there were no pelvic recurrences, and five patients (45%) had some form of liver involvement, either alone or in combination with other sites.

Of the 16 patients in group 2, seven (44%) had metastases to the liver only, one (6%) to the liver and pelvis, four (25%) to the pelvis only, and one (6%) to the pelvis and the anastomosis. Three patients (19%) had diffuse intra-abdominal disease, two of whom had liver involvement as well. Of these 16 patients, ten (62.5%) had liver involvement, and eight (50%) had pelvic involvement, while five (31%) had a local/regional recurrence only.

Of the five patients in group 3, two (40%) had only liver metastases, one (20%) had liver and pelvic metastases, and two (40%) had pelvic metastases. In all, three patients had liver involvement, and three had pelvic involvement.

Overall, 13 (41%) of 32 patients had only liver recurrences, six (19%) had pelvic recurrences alone, two (6%) had liver and pelvic recurrences, and four (12%) had diffuse disease. The other seven patients (22%) had some form of local/regional recurrences. When these seven patients are added to the six patients with pelvic recurrences, 40% had some form of local/regional recurrences alone (Table 3).

Table 2.—Recurrence Sites According to Primary Location in Three Patient Groups

Group*	Recurrence Site, No. (%) Liver	Liver and Pelvis	Pelvis	Diffuse	Other
1	4 (36)	0	0	1 (9)	6 (55)
2	7 (44)	1 (6)	4 (25)	3 (19)	1 (6)
3	2 (40)	1 (20)	2 (40)	0	0

*Group 1, R/transverse colon; group 2, L/sigmoid colon; and group 3, rectum.

Table 3.—Local/Regional Recurrences by Location of Primary

Group*	No. (%) Local/Regional Alone	Overall Local/Regional
1	6 (55)	7 (64)
2	5 (31)	13 (81)
3	2 (40)	3 (60)
Total	**13** (40)	**23** (72)

*Primary location: group 1, R/transverse colon; group 2, L/sigmoid colon; and group 3, rectum.

Table 4.—Preoperative CT Scan of Liver, Abdomen, and Pelvis*

CT Scan	% Accuracy	Sensitivity	Specificity
Abdomen†	71	27	100
Liver	71	58	91
Pelvis	75	22	100
Total	73	41	98

*CT indicates computed tomographic; accuracy = (true-positive[TP] + true-negative[TN])/Total No.; sensitivity = TP/(TP + false-negative); and specificity = TN/(TN + false-positive).

†Refers to CT scan in areas of abdomen other than liver.

Evaluation of Diagnostic Tests

CEA Values.—Carcinoembryonic antigen values were elevated preoperatively in 30 patients (94%). False-negative CEA values (<2.5 ng/mL) were seen in two patients with symptoms who had pelvic recurrences. The overall mean CEA value was 58 ng/mL (range, 1.9 to 298 ng/mL).

CT Scan Results.—Twenty-eight patients had a preoperative CT scan (Table 4). We evaluated the ability of the CT scan to identify tumor in the liver, abdomen (other than liver), and pelvis. Three patients with intra-abdominal disease (other than liver) had a true-positive result, 17 had a true-negative result, none had a false-positive result, and eight had a false-negative result. The sensitivity of the CT scan was 27%, specificity was 100%, and accuracy was 71%. In two of the patients in whom results were considered to be true positive, the amount of disease was underestimated by the CT scan.

Evaluation of results in patients with liver metastases showed that ten had a true-positive result, ten had a true-negative result, one had a false-positive result, and seven had a false-negative result. Sensitivity was 59%, specificity was 91%, and accuracy was 71%. In the ten patients with a true-positive result, the amount of tumor was underestimated by the CT scan in three.

Results of the CT scan of the pelvis were a true-positive in two patients, a true-negative in 19, a false-positive in none, and a false-negative in seven. Sensitivity was 22%, specificity was 100%, and accuracy was 75%. Overall, the sensitivity of the CT scan was 41%, specificity was 98%, and accuracy was 73%.

Other preoperative testing included magnetic resonance imaging of the pelvis in three patients with true-positive results and magnetic resonance imaging of the abdomen in one patient with a false-positive result. Liver/spleen scans in seven patients showed one true-positive result, four true-negative results, one false-positive result, and one false-negative result. Three hepatic arteriograms showed one true-negative result and two false-negative results. All studies combined showed an overall sensitivity of 43%, specificity of 96%, and accuracy of 71%.

Radioimmunoguided Surgery (RIGS System) Results

In 26 (81%) of the 32 patients, the RIGS system identified tumor. In six patients (18%), tumor that was not otherwise clinically evident was found only with the RIGS system. These included a celiac node metastasis in one patient, tumor in the pelvis in one, tumor in the right gutter in one, and tumor in the bed of liver resection in three. In two (6%) of these patients, it was the only tumor found. In three patients, further resection was carried out until free margins of resection were obtained. Twenty-four patients received an injection of MoAb B72.3, and in 20 instances (83%), the antibody recognized tumor. Monoclonal antibody 17-1A was injected in eight patients, and tumor was identified in six (75%). The time between the injection of the MoAb and surgery was 16 days (range, three to 34 days).

COMMENT

During the last decade, aggressive treatment of colorectal cancer metastases to the liver has come into vogue. Five-year survival rates range from 25% to 52%.[1-4] The five-year survival for patients who have undergone multiple reoperations for different patterns of intra-abdominal recurrences has ranged from 23% to 60%,[13,14] with a recent report showing a five- and ten-year actuarial survival rate of 46% and 10%, respectively, in patients with two or more recurrences.[15]

Our series excluded patients with extra-abdominal metastases and, as previously reported, we advocate an aggressive reoperative approach for recurrent colorectal cancer confined to the abdomen.[6,14,15] It has been demonstrated that 37% to 63% of all colorectal cancer recurrences will be confined to the abdomen.[16,17] All patients in our study had pathologic confirmation of sites of recurrences through exploratory laparotomy with the use of the RIGS system. Knowledge of the patterns of recurrences is of primary importance.

Analysis of the patterns of failure after primary colorectal resections showed that the most common site of recurrence regardless of the primary location is the liver, with 16 (50%) of 32 patients showing some degree of liver involvement. Thirteen (40%) of these patients had liver metastasis only. In a previous report by Willett et al,[16] colorectal cancer recurred in the liver in 88 (54%) of 163 patients, but only 31 patients (19%) had liver recurrences alone. Sugarbaker et al[17] found that 63% of recurrences were intra-abdominal, with 24% having liver involvement and 6% with only liver metastases. This difference may be due to the fact that only 60% or less of patients with abdominal failures in this series had surgical or autopsy documentation of the recurrence, and our study included

Table 5.—Local Failure Rates Reported by Different Investigators*

Source, y	No.	% Local/Regional Failure Only	% Total Local Failure
Cass et al,[19] 1976	105	60	78
Olson et al,[20] 1980	69	33	52
Russell et al,[21] 1984	186	14	29
Willett et al,[16] 1984	533	6	19
Gunderson et al,[22] 1985	91	22	48
Sugarbaker et al,[17] 1987	68	9	42
Minsky et al,[23] 1988	294	6	9

*The definition and determination of local failures differ markedly among different investigators.

only patients with confirmed intra-abdominal recurrences and no evidence of extra-abdominal disease. As pointed out by August et al,[18] the problem of the cascade phenomenon (metastases from metastases) makes autopsy studies less relevant to the design of treatment protocols. Therefore surgeons who are involved in the second-look approach to recurrent colorectal cancer should seek recurrence in the liver, regardless of the location of the primary tumor.

Local/regional recurrences alone were seen in two (40%) of five patients with primary rectal cancer, in six (55%) of 11 with right and transverse colon primaries, and in five (31%) of 16 with left and sigmoid colon primaries. The overall local/regional recurrence was 40% (Table 3). This higher incidence of local/regional recurrence, compared with that in other series (Table 5), may be due to the fact that our patients were more closely followed up with repeated CEA determinations every six to eight weeks, which does not allow enough time for the cascade phenomenon to manifest itself. Also, our results are based on the total of intra-abdominal recurrences and not on the total number of patients at risk. The definition of local failure also differs significantly between the different series, and all our patients had surgical and pathologic confirmation of the recurrence. Confirmation was not based on physical examination or laboratory test results as in other series.

Overall local failure rates have been shown to increase with the advancing stage of disease.[16] Primary tumor, staged B3, C2, and C3, have reported local failure rates in excess of 20%.[16,17] In our series, 22 patients had C lesions. The high local recurrence rate can be explained by the failure of surgeons to remove all residual microscopic disease at the time of primary operation.

Some surgeons may question the idea that only a very few patients benefit from a radical colon or rectal excision. Those patients whose tumor involves no lymph nodes constitute approximately 50% of all patients with large-bowel cancer.[24] Whether or not a segmental resection would give the same survival rate as does a radical hemicolectomy depends on the extent of lymphatic spread. If lymphatic spread is limited to epicolic and paracolic lymph nodes (one to five nodes involved), segmental resection only should be as adequate as radical hemicolectomy. However, a subset of patients with involvement of intermediate nodes may have a complete resection only if a radical hemicolectomy with extensive resection of the colonic mesentery is performed. Segmental resection would leave this group of patients with a high likelihood of having residual disease. Gabriel et al[25] proposed that the location of involved nodes influences survival. Patients with local nodes positive for disease (Dukes' C1 group) had improved survival compared with those patients with positive nodes at the point of the prominent vascular ligature (his C2 group).

The use of the RIGS system has been demonstrated in previous studies to alter the surgical approach in 26% of patients, by identifying tumor not clinically detectable.[8] The MoAbs presently used localized in 81% of patients.

In our study, additional tumor was identified in six patients (18%) by the RIGS system, allowing us to resect residual tumor not clinically evident. It may be possible that the use of this technique at the time of primary resection would decrease the incidence of recurrences, especially the high local/regional recurrence that has been reported by us, as well as by other investigators (Table 5). Using a meticulous histopathologic technique, Herrera-Ornelas et al[26] demonstrated that 64% of lymph node metastases were in nodes that measured less than 5 mm. This is one of the reasons that clinical examination alone is not adequate to determine the extent of disease and that other adjuvant techniques are needed.

Newer developments in the MoAb technique may create antibodies with higher affinity, making the RIGS system an even more reliable technique.

Carcinoembryonic antigen determination remains the most accurate preoperative method to detect recurrences; the CEA value was elevated preoperatively in 30 (94%) of the patients. The two patients whose CEA values were normal were symptomatic and were found to have pelvic recurrences. It has been previously reported that patients with pelvic recurrences tend to have lower or negative CEA values,[27] but such recurrences are also more accessible to identification by physical examination.

In contrast, the overall sensitivity of the CT scan was only 41%. For liver recurrences, it was slightly higher (58%), but its value to detect recurrences in other areas of the abdomen and pelvis decreases, especially in areas of the small-bowel mesentery.

Sugarbaker et al[17] found that following primary resection for colorectal cancer, the abdominal CT scan performed three times each year yielded little useful information. Although the sensitivity of the abdominal CT scan in the investigation of patients with suspected recurrent disease was 85%, the false-positive rate was high (45%). The two areas that most frequently showed false-positive findings were the liver and pelvis. Based on these results, the CT scan is not an accurate method to detect recurrences, and response to treatment protocols is greatly jeopardized by relying on this technique.

We conclude that the RIGS system is more dependable in localizing clinically obscure metastases than other methods and that CEA testing remains the most accurate method to detect recurrences.

The authors thank Charlie Agnone, Peter Ferrara, MD, and William Farrar, MD, for their research assistance and Susan Stamper and Helene Ayres for their secretarial-editorial assistance.

References

1. Adson MA, van Heerden JA: Major hepatic resections for metastatic colorectal cancer. *Ann Surg* 1980;191:576-582.
2. Iwatsuki S, Shaw BW Jr, Starzl TE: Experience with 150 liver resections. *Ann Surg* 1983;197:247-253.
3. Adson MA, van Heerden JA, Adson MH, et al: Resection of hepatic metastases from colorectal cancer. *Arch Surg* 1984;119:647-651.
4. Shunzaburo I, Esquivel CO, Gordon RD, et al: Liver resection for metastatic colorectal cancer. *Surgery* 1986;100:804-810.
5. Minton JP, Hoehn JL, Gerger DM, et al: Results of a 400-patient carcinoembryonic antigen second-look colorectal cancer study. *Cancer* 1985;55:1284-1290.
6. Martin EW Jr, Minton JP, Carey LC: CEA-directed second-look

surgery in the asymptomatic patient after primary resection of colorectal carcinoma. *Ann Surg* 1985;202:310-317.

7. Steele G Jr, Zamcheck N, Wilson R, et al: Results of CEA-initiated second-look surgery for recurrent colorectal cancer. *Am J Surg* 1980;139:544-548.

8. Sickle-Santanello BJ, O'Dwyer PJ, Mojzisik C, et al: Radioimmunoguided surgery using the monoclonal antibody B72.3 in colorectal tumors. *Dis Colon Rectum* 1987;30:761-765.

9. Kohler M, Milstein C: Continuous cultures of fused cells secreting antibody of predefined specificity. *Nature* 1975;256:494-497.

10. Nuti M, Teramoto YA, Costantini RM, et al: A monoclonal antibody (B72.3) defines patterns of distribution of a novel tumor-associated antigen in human mammary carcinoma cell populations. *Int J Cancer* 1982;29:539-545.

11. Thor A, Ohuchi N, Szpak CA, et al: Distribution of oncofetal antigen tumor-associated glycoprotein-72 defined by monoclonal antibody B72.3. *Cancer Res* 1986;46:3118-3124.

12. Herlyn M, Steplewski Z, Herlyn D, et al: Colorectal carcinoma-specific antigen: Detection by means of monoclonal antibodies. *Proc Natl Acad Sci USA* 1979;76:1438-1443.

13. Wanebo J, Stevens W: Surgical treatment of locally recurrent colorectal cancer. *Probl Gen Surg*, January-March 1987, vol 4, pp 115-129.

14. Sardi A, Minton JP, Nieroda C, et al: Multiple reoperations in recurrent colorectal carcinoma: An analysis of morbidity, mortality, and survival. *Cancer* 1988;61:1913-1919.

15. Minton JP, Sardi A: Carcinoembryonic antigen and second-look operation. *Probl Gen Surg*, January-March 1987, vol 4, pp 104-114.

16. Willett CG, Tepper JE, Cohen AM, et al: Failure patterns following curative resection of colonic carcinoma. *Ann Surg* 1984;200:685-690.

17. Sugarbaker PH, Gianola FJ, Dwyer A, et al: A simplified plan for follow-up of patients with colon and rectal cancer supported by prospective studies of laboratory and radiologic test results. *Surgery* 1987;102:79-87.

18. August DA, Sugarbaker PH, Schneider PD: Lymphatic dissemination of hepatic metastases: Implications for the follow up and treatment of patients with colorectal cancer. *Cancer* 1985;55:1490-1494.

19. Cass AW, Million RR, Pfaff WW: Patterns of recurrence following surgery alone for adenocarcinoma of the colon and rectum. *Cancer* 1976;37:2861-2865.

20. Olson RM, Perencevich NP, Malcolm AW, et al: Patterns of recurrence following curative resection of adenocarcinoma of the colon and rectum. *Cancer* 1980;45:2969-2974.

21. Russell AH, Tong D, Dawson LE, et al: Adenocarcinoma of the proximal colon: Sites of initial dissemination and patterns of recurrence following surgery alone. *Cancer* 1984;53:360-367.

22. Gunderson LL, Sosin H, Levit S: Adenocarcinoma of the colon: Areas of failure in a reoperation series (second or symptomatic looks). *Int J Radiat Oncol Biol Phys* 1985;11:731-741.

23. Minsky BD, Mies C, Rich TA, et al: Potentially curative surgery of colon cancer: Patterns of failure and survival. *J Clin Oncol* 1988;6:106-118.

24. Sugarbaker PH: Carcinoma of the colon—prognosis and operative choice. *Curr Probl Surg* 1981;18:754-802.

25. Gabriel WB, Dukes C, Bussey HJR: Lymphatic spread in cancer of the rectum. *Br J Surg* 1935;23:395-413.

26. Herrera-Ornelas L, Justiniano J, Castillo N, et al: Metastases in small lymph nodes from colon cancer. *Arch Surg* 1987;122:1253-1256.

27. Mavligit GM, McMurtrey MJ: Role of CEA: A challenge of a verdict. *JAMA* 1978;24:1714.

Discussion

Q This is an interesting study. I wonder if the authors might consider looking at two subgroups of patients specifically. One is a subgroup of patients in whom multiple intra-abdominal metastases are found. Is each one of these metastases surveyed individually with the authors' probe? The second is a subgroup in whom there are multiple sites that the probe indicates are hot spots and pathologic analyses are performed on these sites. If one looks at these multiple sites, do the correlation and the specificity and sensitivity of the authors' assay hold up?

A For the first question, when we find diffuse intra-abdominal metastases, we really do not make an effort to scan the whole abdomen, because we cannot offer anything more surgical to these patients. There have been some patients in whom each tumor may have different counts because of the heterogeneity of tumor cell lines. However, usually if the primary has been picked up, most of the metastases will be picked up. The studies have demonstrated that this is reliable in 94% of the patients when the primary has picked up the antibody.

Q Can the authors use this method with any kind of external camera before the operation?

A One of the problems with the system now is the type of isotope used. Iodine 125, although very good for use with the probe, cannot be used for external scanning because of its low energy level (25 to 35 meV). Iodine 123, although of an appropriate energy level for external scanning, has the problem that the half-life is only 13 hours. Since we have needed to wait approximately two to three weeks (actually we follow the precordial counts to determine the time for surgery, which has varied from three to 36 days, but mostly about 24 days) for the whole (IgG) MoAb to clear from the blood pool background, this half-life is too short. We are presently in the process of examining dual labeling of MoAbs.

Q How often did this method detect tumor that you would not have found with your laparotomy?

A Approximately 16% of the time.

Q Have you had an occasion to try this repeatedly? That is, can you use this method again on a patient or does this sensitize the patient to the protein?

A Actually, multiple times. Approximately 30 patients have received more than one injection. We do a routine skin hypersensitivity test on those patients prior to reinjection. With the first injection we found a 0.3% incidence of positive skin reactivity; in patients who received more than one injection, this rose to 4%. Any patient having a positive skin test did not receive a subsequent injection. One patient who had a negative skin hypersensitivity test did develop an allergic reaction that responded very quickly to diphenhydramine hydrochloride (Benadryl) administration. The other patients were able to receive up to four injections without any problems.

Q Did the CEA level drop postoperatively in those patients and have any of them had a subsequent recurrence that was not recognized at the first reoperation?

A In most of our patients the CEA level has dropped postoperatively when resection has been possible. It is still very early to tell much about subsequent recurrences. I know that there have been at least two patients who have had recurrences, but I can't give you any further details at this time.

DEFINING A NEW STANDA

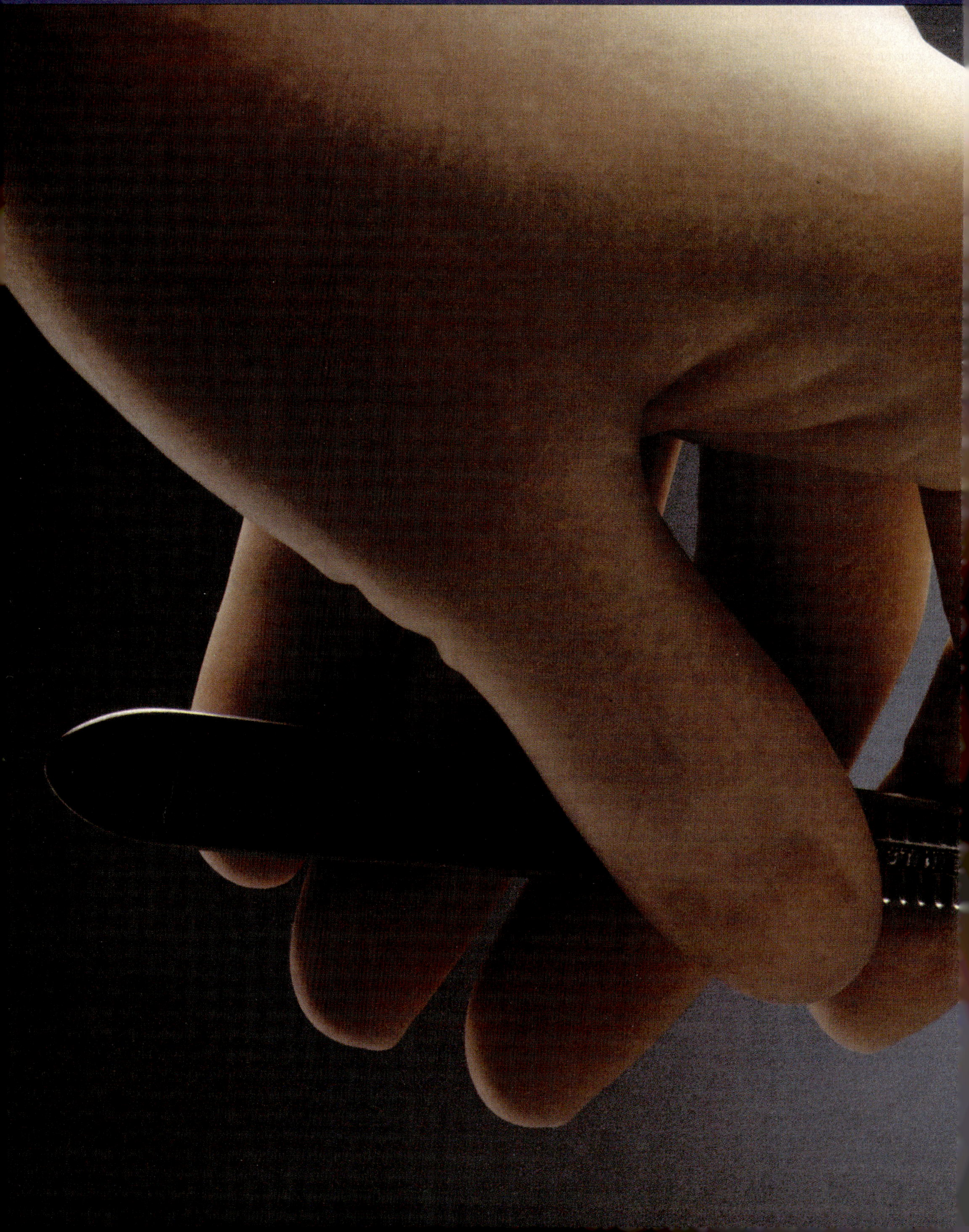

Rationale for Aggressive Colonoscopy in Patients With Colorectal Neoplasia

Kumar S. Dasmahapatra, MD, Kevin Lopyan, MD

• The role of colonoscopy in patients with colorectal neoplasia is not well established. The results of colonoscopy, from 1982 through 1987, in 42 patients with cancers who underwent preoperative colonoscopy (group 1), 64 patients with benign polyps (group 2), and 51 patients who were examined only postoperatively (group 3) were reviewed. These results indicated that (1) approximately one third of all findings would have been missed if endoscopy had been performed to only 60 cm; (2) there was a high incidence of synchronous lesions (33.3% in group 1 and 34.4% in group 2); (3) 57% of patients with synchronous cancer and 63.6% of patients with synchronous polyps developed metachronous lesions, compared with 10.7% and 11.9% of patients with a single lesion; (4) there was a higher incidence of metachronous lesions seen in group 3, compared with group 1; and (5) the median interval for noting metachronous lesions in patients who underwent colonoscopy preoperatively was approximately 18 months. These findings endorsed preoperative colonoscopy and aggressive follow-up in patients with colorectal tumors.

(*Arch Surg* 1989;124:63-66)

The last two decades have seen the emergence of colonoscopy as the dominant diagnostic modality in the management of patients with colon cancer. The incidence of synchronous cancers ranges from 1.5% to 10.7%,[1-11] and the incidence of synchronous polyps ranges from 12% to 86%.[1-11] It has also been suggested that preoperative colonoscopy may change the extent of surgery in up to 88% of patients.[1,4-6,12] Many authors have shown that postoperative surveillance colonoscopy helps to detect a significant number of patients with metachronous polyps and cancers.[9,12-15]

While many investigators believe that routine preoperative colonoscopy is a necessity,[1,4-6,8,9] others think that it is not required and that adequate intraoperative palpation and early postoperative colonoscopy will help manage synchronous lesions.[13] Much of the data regarding postoperative colonoscopy is clouded by the absence of preoperative endoscopy findings in many of the patients.[12,14,15] Furthermore, there is no consensus as to the timing and duration of postoperative follow-up.

To answer some of these questions, we have reviewed our experience with over 3500 colonoscopies from 1982 through 1987, and we evaluated the role of preresection and postresection colonoscopy in patients with cancers and benign polyps. We have also compared the results of surveillance endoscopy in patients who underwent preoperative endoscopy with those who did not.

PATIENTS AND METHODS

Eight hundred sixty-seven patients underwent a colonoscopy as the primary diagnostic modality for the evaluation of frank (n = 353) or occult (n = 514) rectal bleeding. The examination was performed up to the cecum in 95% of the patients. Fifty patients were found to have cancers, and 64 patients were found to have benign neoplastic polyps. An additional 43 patients who had not had preoperative colonoscopy, but who were placed on surveillance colonoscopy following curative resection of their cancers, were also included in this study. Patients were divided into the following three groups.

Group 1

This group consisted of 42 patients who were noted to have cancers on their initial colonoscopy and in whom the entire colon was examined. The eight remaining patients with cancers had obstructing cancers and did not have a complete colonoscopy. The mean age of this group was 58.5 years (age range, 42 to 78 years).

Group 2

This group consisted of 64 patients who were noted to have benign polyps on initial examination. Forty-one patients had one to eight (mean, 1.8) adenomatous polyps that ranged from 0.5 to 4.0 cm in diameter, and 23 patients had one to three (mean, 1.1) villous adenomas that ranged from 0.5 to 5.0 cm in diameter. Except for one patient with a large polyp in the rectum, all patients had a colonoscopic polypectomy. Patients with hyperplastic polyps and three patients with carcinoma in situ in the polyps have been excluded from these data and from further analysis. The mean age of this group of patients was 51.5 years (age range, 32 to 79 years).

Group 3

This group consisted of 51 patients, 43 of whom had undergone a colon resection for cancer, without having had a preoperative

Accepted for publication July 15, 1988.

From The Division of Surgical Oncology, University of Medicine and Dentistry of New Jersey–New Jersey Medical School, Newark, and East Orange (NJ) Veterans Administration Medical Center.

Read before the Annual Meeting of the Society of Surgical Oncology, New Orleans, May 24, 1988.

Reprint requests to Surgical Service (112), Veterans Administration Medical Center, East Orange, NJ 07019 (Dr Dasmahapatra).

colonoscopy. Eight patients with obstructive colon cancers who had not had a complete preoperative colonoscopy are also included in this group. The mean age of these patients was 56.0 years (age range, 43 to 82 years).

Since 1982, following definitive therapy, all patients have been placed on a follow-up program that required a colonoscopy every six months for one year and yearly thereafter. This was in addition to their regular clinic visits where carcinoembryonic antigen level determinations and liver function tests were performed at three-month intervals during their first year and six to 12 months thereafter. Only 12 patients (7.6%) have been unavailable for follow-up, and the remaining patients have had a minimum follow-up of 18 months. Statistical comparisons have been performed using the two-tailed Student's t test and χ^2 analysis where appropriate.

RESULTS

Figure 1 shows the approximate location of the findings in patients with cancer who had their entire colon examined preoperatively. As illustrated, 29% of abnormal findings were beyond the reach of a 60-cm scope. These lesions were at or proximal to the splenic flexure area. Synchronous lesions were noted in 33.3% (11/42) of patients. There was a 7.1% incidence of synchronous carcinomas, and 26.2% (11/42) of patients had synchronous polyps. A follow-up colonoscopy after definitive treatment revealed a 19.1% incidence of metachronous neoplasms. There was a 7.1% incidence (3/42) of a metachronous cancer and a 12% incidence of polyps. Anastomotic recurrences were seen in 7.1% (3/42). The time interval for noting metachronous lesions ranged from six to 54 months, with a median of 18.0 months. The median follow-up period in this group has been 28.0 months (range, 18 to 60 months). Of 14 patients who had synchronous lesions, eight (57%) developed metachronous lesions. In comparison, only three (10.7%) of 28 patients with solitary lesions developed metachronous lesions. This difference was statistically significant ($P<.005$, χ^2 analysis).

Figure 2 shows the approximate location of the polyps in patients in group 2. Thirty-four percent of lesions were beyond 60.0 cm, and synchronous polyps were noted in 34.4% (22/64) of patients. A follow-up colonoscopy following initial definitive treatment revealed metachronous lesions in 29.7% of patients. Twenty-five percent of patients had polyps, and 4.7% (3/64) of patients developed adenocarcinomas of the colon. The median interval for noting metachronous lesions was 19 months, with a range of six to 36 months. The median follow-up in this group was 31 months (range, 18 to 60 months). Of 22 patients who had synchronous lesions, 14 (63.6%) developed metachronous lesions. In comparison, only five (11.9%) of 42 patients with initial solitary polyps developed metachronous lesions. As was seen in group 1, this difference was also statistically significant ($P<.001$, χ^2 analysis).

Figure 3 shows the findings in group 3 patients. Metachronous lesions were noted in 49% (25/51) of patients. An anastomotic recurrence was seen in one patient. The median interval for noting metachronous neoplasms was 8.0 months (range, six to 60 months). In 43 patients, the preoperative barium enema was reviewed. Four patients (9.3%) with synchronous lesions had been identified. One patient was noted to have a synchronous cancer, and three patients had benign polyps. No other synchronous lesion was noted at the time of surgery. A retrospective review of the barium enemas did not reveal any missed lesions.

The findings in the three patient groups are compared in the Table. There was a significantly higher incidence of metachronous lesions in patients who did not undergo preoperative colonoscopy, compared with patients with cancer whose entire colon had been evaluated preoperatively (49% vs 19.1%, $P<.005$). The eight-month median time interval for noting metachronous lesions in group 3, although shorter than the interval in groups 1 and 2 (18 and 19 months, respectively), was not statistically significant. A valid comparison of the incidence of synchronous lesions in patients who were evaluated by colonoscopy (groups 1 and 2) vs barium enemas (group 3) was not possible because not all the x-ray films were available for review, and only nine of 43 patients had air contrast studies.

COMMENT

The data from our study indicate that routine preoperative colonoscopy in patients with cancer helps to detect a large number of synchronous lesions. The incidence of

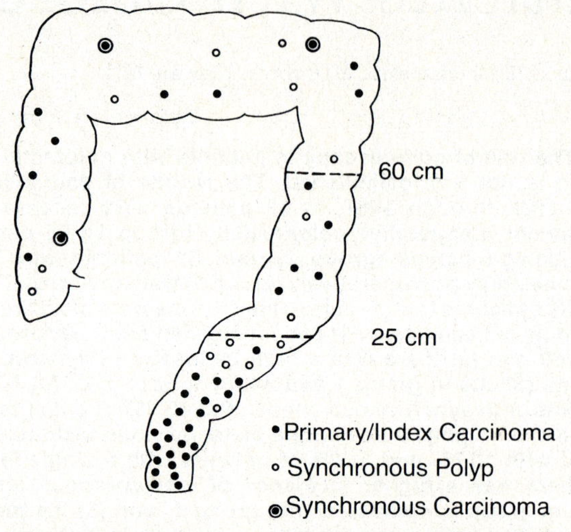

Fig 1.—Findings in patients with cancer undergoing preoperative colonoscopy (group 1).

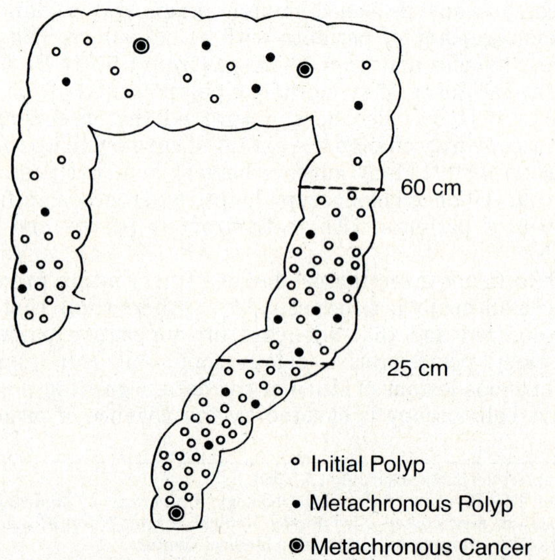

Fig 2.—Initial and follow-up findings in patients with polyps (group 2).

synchronous cancers (7.1%) and polyps (26.2% in group 1 and 34.4% in group 2) is in agreement with many previously published series.[1-11] A preoperative colonoscopy not only helps to remove small benign polyps at the time of evaluation, but proponents of this modality believe that the additional colonoscopic findings may change the extent of colon resection in up to 88% of patients.[1,4-6,12] Sollenberger et al[13] recently have challenged this concept, and they believe that adequate intraoperative palpation, together with an early postoperative colonoscopy, avoids the risk and expense of a preoperative colonoscopy. Our data revealed that in patients who had not had a preoperative colonoscopy, no new intraoperative findings were noted in any of the patients in group 3. Heald and Bussey[3] have reported that only 31% of synchronous cancers in their series were palpable. Definite answers to this question, therefore, can only be obtained from well-controlled, prospective, randomized studies. Barium enemas, although widely used preoperatively, have been shown to miss more than a third of the lesions that are detected by colonoscopy.[16] Pagana et al[4] reported that barium enemas had only a 17% reliability rate as a preoperative diagnostic tool. In our study, barium enemas were done on patients in whom a complete colonoscopy was not possible or in patients who underwent diagnostic studies on a different clinical service.

We believe that flexible sigmoidoscopy is inferior to colonoscopy in evaluating patients with rectal bleeding or in the follow-up of patients after resection. Our data, shown in Figs 1 through 3, indicate that approximately a third of the lesions would have been missed if the examination had been limited to only 60 cm or up to the splenic flexure. Data from Greene[17] and Slater et al[18] have shown that there is an apparent shift to the right in the incidence of cancers and polyps, and Dawson et al[19] have shown experimentally that mucosal changes, similar to that which occurs adjacent to cancerous areas, may occur without a pattern or regularity in the entire colon. Therefore, despite the fact that most colon tumors occur in the distal part of the colon, a complete examination is critical when evaluating patients for possible colon tumors.

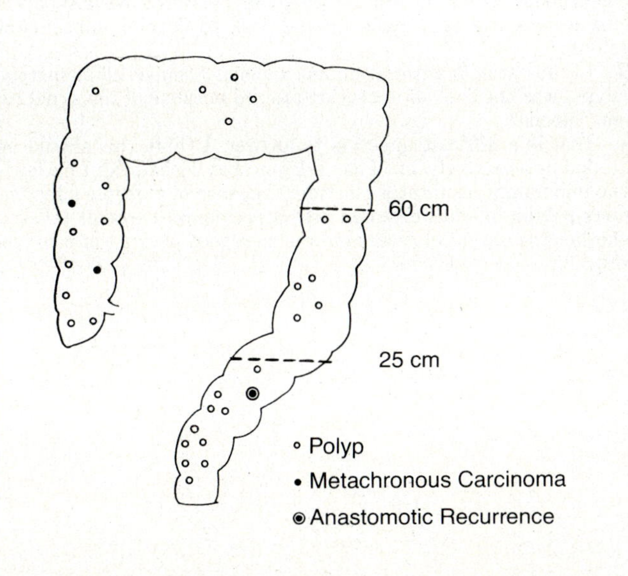

Fig 3.—Follow-up findings of patients who did not undergo colonoscopy preoperatively (group 3).

Patients with initial synchronous lesions were noted to have a higher incidence of metachronous lesions. This was true for patients with cancers, as well as for those with polyps. Eight (57%) of 14 patients with synchronous cancers and 14 (63.6%) of 22 patients with synchronous polyps developed metachronous lesions, most of which were benign polyps. This is in contrast to only three (10.7%) of 28 metachronous lesions in patients with an initial single cancer and five (11.9%) of 42 metachronous lesions in patients with a single polyp on initial examination. These findings are in agreement with those reported by Carlsson et al[9] and Kronborg et al.[15] These data suggest that patients with synchronous lesions represent a group at greater risk to develop subsequent polyps or cancers than patients with a single lesion.

The timing and duration of postoperative colonoscopy remain unresolved issues. The timing of the initial postoperative endoscopy has varied from three to 38 months.[9,14,15] In our study, excluding the patients who were unavailable for follow-up, all patients had their first postresection or postpolypectomy colonoscopy between six and eight months. Patients who underwent a complete colonoscopy initially (groups 1 and 2) had a median interval of 18 and 19 months, respectively, from the treatment of the primary lesion to the noting of metachronous lesions. These are similar to the figures reported by Carlsson et al,[9] although earlier reports from the same institution had reported much longer time intervals.[14] Patients who were examined preoperatively could therefore be examined at yearly intervals, although those patients who are at risk to develop anastomotic recurrences may undergo a colonoscopy earlier. The significantly higher incidence of noting metachronous lesions in patients who did not undergo a colonoscopy preoperatively (group 3) could simply be explained by the fact that many of these "metachronous" lesions might, in reality, have existed synchronously. The median time interval for noting metachronous lesions in group 3 was shorter than in groups 1 and 2 but not statistically significant. These data support the view that patients who do not undergo endoscopy preoperatively need to be followed up carefully and should undergo early postoperative colonoscopy.

In our study, metachronous lesions have been noted as

Comparative Results in Three Patient Groups

Group	% of Lesions >60 cm	Incidence, % Synchronous Lesions	Incidence, % Metachronous Lesions	Recurrence, %	Median Interval (Range) From Primary Lesion to Metachronous Lesion, mo
1 (n=42)	29	Cancer, 7.1; polyps, 26.2	Cancer, 7.1; polyps, 12	7	18 (6-54)
2 (n=64)	34	34.4	Cancer, 4; polyps, 25	...	19 (6-36)
3 (n=51)	...	...	Cancer, 4; polyps, 45	2	8 (6-60)

late as 60 months after treatment. Although this may justify yearly colonoscopy for at least five years, definite answers regarding how long patients need to be followed up require studies with longer follow-up data. The results from our study certainly endorse the use of preoperative colonoscopy and support aggressive follow-up endoscopy in patients with colorectal neoplasias.

References

1. Langevin JM, Nivatvongs S: The true incidence of synchronous cancer of the large bowel: A prospective study. *Am J Surg* 1984;147:330-333.
2. Moertel CG, Bargen JA, Dockerty MB: Multiple carcinomas of the large intestine: A review of the literature and a study of 261 cases. *Gastroenterology* 1958;34:85-98.
3. Heald RH, Bussey HJR: Clinical experiences at St Mark's Hospital with multiple synchronous cancers of the colon and rectum. *Dis Colon Rectum* 1975;18:6-10.
4. Pagana TJ, Ledesma EJ, Mittelman A, et al: The use of colonoscopy in the study of synchronous colorectal neoplasms. *Cancer* 1984;53:356-359.
5. Maxfield RJ: Colonoscopy as a routine preoperative procedure for carcinoma of the colon. *Am J Surg* 1984;147:477-480.
6. Isler JT, Brown PC, Lewis GF, et al: The role of preoperative colonoscopy in colorectal cancer. *Dis Colon Rectum* 1987;30:435-439.
7. Cunliffe WJ, Haselton PS, Tweedle DEF, et al: Incidence of synchronous and metachronous colorectal carcinoma. *Br J Surg* 1984;71:941-943.
8. Thorson AG, Christensen MA, Davis SJ: The role of colonoscopy in the assessment of patients with colorectal cancer. *Dis Colon Rectum* 1986;29:306-311.
9. Carlsson G, Petrelli NJ, Nava H, et al: The value of surveillance after curative resection for colorectal cancer or synchronous adenomatous polyps. *Arch Surg* 1987;122:1261-1263.
10. Reilly JC, Rusin LC, Theuerkauf FJ Jr: Colonoscopy: Its role in cancer of the colon and rectum. *Dis Colon Rectum* 1982;25:532-538.
11. Swinton NW, Parshley PF: Multiple cancers of the colon and rectum. *Dis Colon Rectum* 1962;5:378-380.
12. Unger SW, Wanebo HJ: Colonoscopy: An essential monitoring technique after resection of colorectal cancer. *Am J Surg* 1983;145:71-76.
13. Sollenberger LL, Eisenstat TE, Rubin RJ, et al: Is preoperative colonoscopy necessary in carcinoma of the colon and rectum? *Am Surg* 1988;54:113-115.
14. Nava HR, Pagana TJ: Postoperative surveillance of colorectal carcinoma. *Cancer* 1982;49:1043-1047.
15. Kronborg O, Hage E, Deichgraeber E: The remaining colon after radical surgery for colorectal cancer: The first three years of a prospective study. *Dis Colon Rectum* 1983;26:172-176.
16. Gilbertsen V: Colon cancer screening. *Gastrointest Endosc* 1980;26:31-32.
17. Greene FL: Distribution of colorectal neoplasms: A left to right shift of polyps and cancer. *Am Surg* 1983;49:63-65.
18. Slater GI, Haber RH, Aufses AH, et al: Changing distribution of carcinoma of the colon and rectum. *Surg Gynecol Obstet* 1984;158:216-218.
19. Dawson PM, Habib NA, Rees HC, et al: Mucosal field change in colorectal cancer. *Am J Surg* 1987;153:281-283.

Discussion

Q I have a question about the group of patients who had cancer and underwent a preoperative colonoscopy. In that group, there were metastatic cancers, and I am troubled by that. Were they at the suture line? Were they actually recurrences, or were they missed? If the interval was, in fact, six months between the colonoscopies, I do not understand how they were able to develop metachronous carcinomas within that time.

A The patients who had carcinomas noted at six months had not had a preoperative colonoscopy.

Q In the group of patients who had their colon cleared of all polyps and who then developed another lesion at 18 months, how big was the lesion, and what were the lesions that they developed?

A The mean size of the lesions, which was not mentioned, was 1 cm. Most of the lesions were actually small. It was difficult to measure them accurately, and we got the reports from the pathologist who measured them at the time that they sectioned them. We did point out that we excluded patients with hyperplastic polyps; these were the very tiny polyps that were not included in this analysis.

Q Was any attempt made to look at the number of polyps cleared at the initial session to determine the subsequent chances of developing other neoplastic lesions and to correlate those two?

A We did not look at the number of polyps, but we did look at synchronous vs single lesions; obviously, patients with synchronous lesions are at a much greater risk to develop subsequent lesions.

Q In the patients with carcinoma and synchronous adenomatous polyps, was the type of operation altered because of the synchronous lesions?

A That is a difficult question to answer. I think this should be studied prospectively, but I can tell you that we had eight patients who underwent a subtotal colectomy because of multiple adenomatous polyps in addition to an adenocarcinoma. I cannot tell you whether the extent of resection was increased because of colonoscopy.

Prospective Phase I Trial of Conservative Management of Low Rectal Lesions

David R. McCready, MD; David M. Ota, MD; Tyvin A. Rich, MD;
Diva Thielvoldt, RN; J. Milburn Jessup, MD

• The purpose of this study was to assess anal function and to compare the morbidity of local excision and postoperative radiotherapy for rectal adenocarcinoma with the morbidity of abdominoperineal resection. A posterior parasacral approach was used for local excision. All patients had negative margins, and all but one were continent after completion of radiotherapy. Seven patients (29%) had either a wound infection or a fistula in the local excision group. No local failures occurred, although follow-up was only 13 months. Thirteen (50%) of the 26 patients who underwent an abdominoperineal resection developed at least one complication. Combined treatment that spares the rectal sphincters may be preferable in selected patients with low rectal cancer, if long-term disease-free survival is maintained.

(*Arch Surg* 1989;124:67-70)

The standard treatment for adenocarcinoma of the distal part of the rectum is abdominoperineal resection (APR), which was described originally by Miles[1] in 1908. However, local excision of carefully selected, favorable rectal cancers can be as effective as APR in controlling local disease and providing long-term survival without the formation of a permanent colostomy.[2-4] The successful use of local excision alone, using a transanal[5] or posterior approach,[4,6] depends on the selection of this treatment for patients who have exophytic,[7] small (<3 to 4 cm),[4] and well-differentiated cancers[8] that have not penetrated the muscularis propria of the rectum. Approximately 12% to 25% of such patients will have lymph node metastases.[8,9] Yet, clinical assessment of tumor penetration is wrong in about 20% of patients,[10] and if the cancer has invaded through the bowel wall, the chance of lymph node metastases is greater than 50%,[8] and local recurrence rates increase.[8]

Accepted for publication Sept 30, 1988.

From the Division of Surgery, Department of General Surgery (Drs McCready, Ota, and Jessup and Ms Thielvoldt) and Department of Clinical Radiotherapy (Dr Rich), University of Texas M. D. Anderson Cancer Center, Houston.

Read before the Annual Meeting of the Society of Surgical Oncology, New Orleans, May 25, 1988.

Reprint requests to Department of General Surgery, University of Texas M. D. Anderson Cancer Center, 1515 Holcombe Blvd, Box 106, Houston, TX 77030 (Dr Jessup).

Although APR is usually advised for those patients who, at the time of local excision, are found to have cancers that penetrate through the muscularis propria[4] (T3) or have metastasized to regional lymph nodes,[7] recent evidence suggests that external-beam radiotherapy (XRT), with doses of at least 45 Gy, can control clinically occult local disease after conservative surgery,[11] as well as after APR.[12] Trials using preoperative XRT suggest that, in doses of 45 to 50 Gy, XRT can decrease the number of lymph node metastases found at surgery.[13]

To determine whether the combination of complete local excision of rectal cancers using the posterior parasacral (transsphincteric[14] or transsacral[6]) excision (PSE), followed by XRT, can be safely extended to patients with rectal cancers that penetrate into the muscularis propria (T2), as well through the muscle (T3), a prospective trial was initiated. In this phase I to II protocol, well- or moderately well-differentiated rectal neoplasms, up to 4 cm in diameter and within 0 to 10 cm of the anal verge, were excised with negative margins. Patients with T2 or T3 lesions received postoperative XRT, in addition to PSE, while patients with benign lesions or T1 (confined to the submucosa) cancers just underwent PSE.

The success of this protocol, aimed at preserving anal function, is predicated on the assumption that combined modality treatment (PSE and XRT) will control local disease as well as radical surgery (APR) does T2 and T3 lesions, up to 4 cm in diameter, and that the complications of this treatment program will not exceed those associated with APR. The purpose of this study was to assess the complications of the local excision of rectal cancers using a parasacral approach in combination with selective postoperative XRT and to compare the morbidity of patients who underwent these treatments with the morbidity of a concurrent group of patients with rectal cancer who were treated with APR at this institution.

PATIENTS AND METHODS

All patients had biopsy proved adenocarcinoma of the rectum or villous adenoma before surgery. Those patients who refused standard therapy (APR) or whose tumors were benign provided informed consent and were entered into this prospective protocol that was approved by the institutional review board. No other colonic lesions were present on either colonoscopy or barium enema. Along with a history and physical examination, preoperative tests included a carcinoembryonic antigen determination, liver function tests (determinations of serum bilirubin, lactate dehydrogenase, aspartate aminotransferase, and alkaline phosphatase levels), serum electrolyte determinations, complete blood cell count with platelets count, and a chest x-ray film. A computed tomographic scan of the pelvis was performed to exclude gross (>2 cm) nodal disease. Patients were excluded if the primary tumor was fixed to the sacrum or pelvis regardless of size, if the tumor was larger than 30% of the bowel wall circumference, or if lymph nodes were palpable or were visualized (>2 cm) on a pelvic computed tomographic scan. The patients' treatment could be converted to APR if there was cancer at the margins of resection or if perirectal lymph node metastases were found.

A PSE was performed at the University of Texas M. D. Anderson Cancer Center, Houston, by one of two approaches: transsphincteric[14] or transsacral.[6] Two to six weeks after surgery, when the wound was healed and bowel function was normal, XRT was begun. Patients who developed rectocutaneous fistulas began XRT after a diverting colostomy was fashioned.

Initial radiotherapy treatment fields were designed to include the entire pelvis plus the immediately draining perirectal lymph nodes and the parasacral incision. This area was given a minimum dose of 45 Gy in five weeks using 1.8 Gy per fraction, five days per week. The radiation portals were then reduced to cover the site of excision with a margin of 3 to 5 cm and treated to a minimum dose of 53 Gy. Photons with an energy of 18 meV or greater were used. Three fields (posterior plus two lateral) were used with strict avoidance of single posterior or direct perineal fields. Patients were treated in the prone position with an open tabletop device to allow mobilization of the small intestine away from the posterior part of the pelvis.

During the same time period, patients with rectal lesions who were treated with APR, but not preoperative radiotherapy, formed the comparison group. Perineal wounds were closed primarily, and the pelvic floor was reperitonealized. Wound infections were defined as drainage of pus that required dressing changes. The diagnoses of neurogenic bladder and impotence were made after consultation with the urology service. All patients whose conditions were diagnosed as neurogenic bladders required self-catheterization. A complication with the colostomy was recorded only if it required an operative revision. The diagnosis of a fistula was made clinically.

Two indexes of anal function were evaluated. The number of bowel movements and the use of diphenoxylate hydrochloride with atropine sulfate (Lomotil) tablets were obtained by a research nurse (D.T.) using a standard questionnaire. Resting involuntary anal sphincter tone and the ability of the anal sphincters to contract voluntarily were assessed by two of the authors (T.A.R. and D.M.O.) at the time of follow-up. A subjective score was given to both the voluntary and involuntary anal tone: 1 (normal), 2 (fair = slight loss), and 3 (poor).

RESULTS

Twenty-four patients have been treated with a PSE of their rectal neoplasms, including 19 patients with T2 or T3 adenocarcinomas who have received postoperative XRT. Demographic and tumor characteristics of this cohort are summarized in Table 1. The median age of this group was 61 years, and there were 13 women and 11 men. Five patients had villous adenomas, one patient had a T1 adenocarcinoma, ten patients had T2 lesions, while eight had cancers that extended through the muscularis propria (T3). Two patients were noted to have perirectal lymph node metastasis at the time of operation. The tumors averaged 3.1 ± 1.6 cm (mean ± SD) in diameter and were situated an average 5.4 ± 2.5 cm from the anal verge. Five cancers were greater than 4 cm, and one cancer was poorly differentiated. All tumors were excised intact with microscopic-free margins.

The characteristics of those patients who underwent an APR during the same time period as those patients who had a PSE at our institution are also summarized in Table 1. This group is presented for comparison and was not randomized or matched to the prospectively evaluated group. While the median age of the patients who underwent an APR and the distance that their lesions were from the anal verge are similar to the group of patients who had PSE and XRT, the other parameters are indicative of more advanced lesions. The patients who were treated with APRs had significantly larger tumors (4.3 ± 1.8 cm) than those patients who were treated with PSEs ($P<.05$, t test), and there were more T3 tumors (18/26, 69%) than in those patients who underwent local excision (8/24, 33%).

No patient died after APR, but 50% (13/26) of the patients who underwent APRs experienced at least one complication (Table 2). There were four (three abdominal and one perineal) wound infections (15%), and four patients (15%) needed a second operation to revise their stomas (three hernia and one prolapse). Most complications were related to the genitourinary system. Four patients (15%) developed neurogenic bladders postoperatively that were treated with self-catheterization, and of 18 men, five (28%) developed impotence.

There were no operative deaths after PSE, but seven patients (29%) had a complication (Table 2). Three patients (12%) with adenocarcinomas developed wound infections, and radiation was delayed one to two weeks until the skin healed. There were four postoperative fistulas (17%); three required temporary diverting colostomies that were taken

Table 1.—Characteristics of Patients and Tumors Treated With PSE and Selective Radiotherapy (XRT) or APR*

	PSE With or Without XRT	APR
No. of patients (sex)	24 (13 F, 11 M)	26 (8 F, 18 M)
Median age (range), y	61 (43-81)	58 (23-81)
Lesion, No. (%)		
Villous adenoma	5 (21)	1 (4)
T1 adenocarcinoma	1 (4)	2 (8)
T2 adenocarcinoma	10 (42)	5 (19)
T3 adenocarcinoma	8 (33)	18 (69)
Mean ± SD distance from anal verge, cm	5.4 ± 2.5	5.4 ± 2.9
Mean ± SD size (maximum diameter), cm	3.1 ± 1.6	4.3 ± 1.8†
No. with poorly differentiated cancers	1	4

*PSE indicates parasacral excision; XRT, external-beam radiotherapy; and APR, abdominoperineal resection.
†APR vs PSE, $P<.05$, t test.

Table 2.—Postoperative Complications After PSE or APR*

	PSE	APR
Complication, No. (%)		
Impotence	0	5/18 M (28)
Neurogenic bladder	0	4/26 (15)
Wound infection	3/24 (12)	4/26 (15)
Stomal hernia/prolapse	0	4/26 (15)
Fistulas	4/24 (17)	0
No. (%) of patients with complications	7/24 (29)	13/26 (50)

*PSE indicates parasacral excision; APR, abdominoperineal resection; and M, males.

Table 3.—Subjective Assessment of Resting Anal Tone and Voluntary Anal Contraction Pressure Six Months After Completion of Treatment

	No. of Patients	
	Resting Anal Tone	**Voluntary Contraction**
Good	15	19
Fair	3	0
Poor	2	1
Total Available for Evaluation	**20**	**20**

Table 4.—Literature Review of Complications After PSE for Rectal Lesions*

Source, y	**No. of Cases**	**No. With Fistula**	**No. With Infection or Delayed Healing**
Wilson and Gordon,[15] 1969	20	4	2
Jorgensen and Ottsen,[16] 1975	10	2	1
Richard et al,[17] 1980	40	9	0
Thompson and Tucker,[18] 1987	26	7	2
Adloff et al,[19] 1983	41	5	5
Mason,[14] 1970	24	1	9
Allgower et al,[20] 1982	33	1	8
Total No. (%)	**194 (100)**	**29** (15)	**27** (14)

*PSE indicates parasacral excision.

down on completion of the radiotherapy, while one patient who had a villous adenoma removed was treated conservatively. All fistulas healed, and these patients have normal anal continence. There were no episodes of urinary retention, sexual dysfunction, or other complications. All patients had transient proctitis during radiotherapy that was manifested by a median of three (range, two to seven) bowel movements per day and was treated symptomatically.

Six months after completion of treatment (surgery and/or radiotherapy), bowel habits, resting anal tone, and the force of voluntary anal sphincter contraction were evaluated in 20 patients by history and physical examination. Nine patients (45%) experienced one bowel movement per day. The median for this group was two (range, one to nine) bowel movements per day. The resting anal sphincter tone was scored as normal in 15 patients, while three patients had a slight loss of tone, and two patients had poor tone. When asked to contract the anal sphincters, all but one patient had a "normal" squeeze pressure (Table 3).

There were two patients who required pads to prevent soiling. Both patients had poor resting anal tone and had postoperative radiotherapy. One of these patients had normal voluntary control of the sphincter but had eight to nine bowel movements per day. The second patient is the only one of the group who has not thoroughly regained control of the external sphincter.

The median follow-up for this cohort was 13 months, and there were no local recurrences. One patient developed metastatic disease to periportal lymph nodes, and another patient died of intractable congestive heart failure 11 months after resection without evidence of disease.

COMMENT

The results of this prospective study demonstrate that the postoperative morbidity after PSE of rectal neoplasms is comparable with the complication rates of a concurrent, nonrandomized group of patients undergoing APR. The addition of postoperative XRT did not preclude an acceptable rate of anal function, and when combined with complete excision of the primary rectal cancer, it may allow more patients to be safely treated without radical excision of the rectum and anus if these early results are maintained.

The complications following PSE reported in this study are similar to other series (Table 4). Rectocutaneous fistulas often present by the eighth postoperative day[14] and, if they are small and of low output, can be managed expectantly. Three patients with invasive cancers developed fistulas and were treated with a temporary colostomy so that radiotherapy could be started without significant delay. One patient with an excision of a villous adenoma was treated without fecal diversion. All fistulas have remained healed, and all patients have had good anal function.

Morbidity after APR in this retrospective analysis is also comparable with findings from previous reports.[21] The diagnosis of impotence and neurogenic bladder was made after urologic consultation, and only stomal complications that necessitated a second operation were included. Direct comparison between the patients who were treated with APR and those patients who received PSEs is limited because patients who were selected for APR generally had more advanced cancers. However, there is no evidence to suggest that PSE and radiotherapy were associated with excessive morbidity.

The majority of patients who have undergone a PSE and postoperative radiotherapy have had excellent anal function. Only two patients required protective pads. It is difficult to compare the anal function in our patients with those patients described in the literature because the number of bowel movements per day and the number of patients using pads is not always documented, but Westbrook et al[22] have reported incontinence in one of 19 patients. Even though diarrhea was experienced by all of the patients during radiotherapy, there was no evidence of anal function impairment after radiotherapy was completed. The subjective method of measuring resting anal sphincter tone and the force of voluntary contraction is admittedly crude and subject to bias, but it allowed us to document improvements during convalescence and suggested that most patients undergoing a PSE and radiotherapy will have full return of anal sphincter function.

Late morbidity in the rectum secondary to the radiation used in this study is expected to be minimal since doses below 60 Gy were used.[11] Small-bowel complications should also be very low since the small bowel is mobile (no laparotomy) and is generally excluded completely from the radiation fields.[13]

The excellent exposure provided by the posterior parasacral approach to the rectum facilitates a complete excision of the lesion for histologic study with microscopic-free margins. It also allows access to the mesorectum so that perirectal lymph nodes can be sampled, which is not feasible using the transanal approach. The choice between the transsphincteric or transsacral method depends on the distance of the lesion from the anal verge; the sphincters are not divided for higher lesions.

Although local excision has traditionally been restricted to small, well-differentiated, superficial, exophytic rectal cancers, this protocol has extended the indications to include neoplasms that have penetrated into the muscularis propria or through this layer. Postoperative radiotherapy was given to control any lymph node metastases and microscopic residual disease, but this combined modality regimen has little value if local recurrence and survival is not comparable with treatment with APR. The absence of any local failures in this cohort is encouraging, but the median follow-up has been only 13 months, and it is too soon to assess accurately recurrence and survival rates. However, these early results, combined with the relatively low complication rate, suggest that PSE and postoperative radiotherapy constitute a safe treatment regimen and may allow more patients to undergo anorectum-sparing surgery for distal rectal adenocarcinomas.

The authors acknowledge A. Pearse for help with data retrieval and Mae Reinauer for manuscript preparation.

References

1. Miles WE: A method of performing abdomino-perineal excision for carcinoma of the rectum and of the terminal portion of the pelvic colon. *Lancet* 1908;1:1812-1813 (reprinted, *Dis Colon Rectum* 1980;23:202-205).
2. Morson BC, Bussey HJR, Samoorian S: Policy of local excision for early cancer of the colorectum. *Gut* 1977;18:1045-1050.
3. Grigg M, McDermott FT, Pihl EA, et al: Curative local excision in the treatment of carcinoma of the rectum. *Dis Colon Rectum* 1984;27:81-83.
4. Mason AY: The place of local resection in the treatment of rectal carcinoma. *Proc R Soc Med* 1970;63:1250-1262.
5. Parks AG: Transanal technique in low rectal anastomosis. *Proc R Soc Med* 1972;65:975-976.
6. Kraske P: Extirpation of high carcinomas of the large bowel. *Verh Dtsch Ges Chir* 1885;14:464-473 (reprinted in English, *Dis Colon Rectum* 1984;27:499-503).
7. Stearns MW Jr, Sternberg SS, DeCosse JJ: Treatment alternatives: Localized rectal cancer. *Cancer* 1984;54:2691-2694.
8. Morson BC: Factors influencing the prognosis of early cancer of the rectum. *Proc R Soc Med* 1966;59:607-608.
9. Cohen AM, Wood WC, Gunderson LL, et al: Pathological studies in rectal cancer. *Cancer* 1980;45:2965-2968.
10. Nicholls RJ, Mason AY, Morson BC, et al: The clinical staging of rectal cancer. *Br J Surg* 1982;69:404-409.
11. Rich TA, Weiss DR, Mies C, et al: Sphincter preservation in patients with low rectal cancer treated with radiation therapy with or without local excision or fulguration. *Radiology* 1985;156:527-531.
12. Hoskins RB, Gunderson LL, Dosoretz DE, et al: Adjuvant postoperative radiotherapy in carcinoma of the rectum and rectosigmoid. *Cancer* 1985;55:61-71.
13. Mendenhall WM, Million RR, Bland KI, et al: Preoperative radiation therapy for clinically resectable adenocarcinoma of the rectum. *Ann Surg* 1985;202:215-222.
14. Mason AY: Surgical access to the rectum: A transsphincteric exposure. *Proc R Soc Med* 1970;(suppl)63:91-94.
15. Wilson SE, Gordon HE: Excision of rectal lesions by the Kraske approach. *Am J Surg* 1969;118:213-217.
16. Jorgensen SJ, Ottsen M: Posterior rectotomy for villous tumours of the rectum. *Acta Chir Scand* 1975;141:680-682.
17. Richard CA, Clot PH, Cohen Solal JC: L'abord postérieur du rectum: A propos de 40 cas. *Ann Chir* 1980;34:281-283.
18. Thompson BW, Tucker WE: Transsphincteric approach to lesions of the rectum. *South Med J* 1987;80:41-43.
19. Adloff M, Ollier JC, Arnaud JP, et al: L'abord postérieur du rectum: Technique, indications, complications: A propos de 41 observations. *J Chir* 1983;120:205-210.
20. Allgower M, Durig M, Hochstetter AV, et al: The parasacral sphincter-splitting approach to the rectum. *World J Surg* 1982;6:539-548.
21. Colcock BP, Jarpa S: Complications of abdominoperineal resection. *Dis Colon Rectum* 1958;1:90-96.
22. Westbrook KC, Lang NP, Broadwater JR, et al: Posterior surgical approaches to the rectum. *Ann Surg* 1982;195:677-685.

Discussion

Q Do you think that this is a more important question, ie, colostomy vs no colostomy in the T2 and maybe even early T3 lesions, than some of the chemotherapy adjuvant questions that are presently being asked? If you do, do you think that this is ever going to be amenable to a randomized trial of colostomy and no colostomy?

In light of the fact that the Gastro-Intestinal Study Group and the North-Central Cancer Treatment Group have shown that fluorouracil actually is synergistic with effect of radiation therapy, do you think that the best treatment in these T2 and early T3 lesions, which have anywhere from a 30% to 50% chance of microscopic perirectal nodal disease, might be the combination of radiation and fluorouracil rather than radiation alone?

A The first question really relates to the importance of this study, vis-à-vis the stated agenda of the large groups, in terms of asking the questions of chemoradiotherapy added to standard surgery. If one's goal is increasing survival, the goal of the National Cancer Institute, it would seem that a quality of life issue, as to whether or not you want to save the rectum, is not going to be as important politically as a chemoradiotherapy trial that may have survival advantage. I do believe that you will be able to show that local regional control will be as good with a lesser surgical procedure and radiotherapy as standard APR even with postoperative adjuvant radiotherapy.

The second question relates to the role of chemotherapy added to radiotherapy for these lesions. At the M. D. Anderson Cancer Center, we have a second prospective study now under way in which we are looking at those lesions that are greater than 4 cm and that are poorly differentiated. Within that context, the trial includes continuous infusion of fluorouracil with radiotherapy. I am not sure that for the small, well-defined rectal cancers, one necessarily has to add chemotherapy to radiation.

Dr Tyvin Rich's earlier study with radiotherapy alone for incompletely excised rectal cancers demonstrated excellent local control. We, at the M. D. Anderson Cancer Center, have a retrospective series of 16 patients treated with radiotherapy alone for T2 and T3 lesions who have 96% local control after a median follow-up of 18 months. I think that when we do this, we are doing basically a biopsy and then irradiating undisturbed tissue. That may be quite a bit different from doing postoperative therapy in patients who are recovering from the major dissection APR or a low anterior resection.

Q I am very interested to find out if any of your infectious or fistula complications were associated with presacral abscess or extension into retroperitoneal abscesses?

A No. They were not.

Q Do you have any experience with preoperative radiation therapy for these patients?

A Not in this setting. We have actually treated a couple of patients, and the morbidity has been markedly increased because with preoperative radiotherapy, you are performing surgery in an irradiated tissue that has difficulty healing.

Staging Renal Carcinoma

What Is Sufficient?

Mark A. Benson, MD; John R. Haaga, MD; Martin I. Resnick, MD

• We retrospectively reviewed the roentgenographic and pathologic staging of 64 patients with renal cell carcinoma to assess the role of the various staging modalities (ie, angiography, venacavography, bone scanning, ultrasound, computed tomography [CT], and magnetic resonance imaging). Specific attention was directed at detecting vena cava thrombus and metastatic bone disease, factors with a significant impact on the therapeutic approach. The findings support the role of CT as the principle tool for overall staging and the observation that venacavography is not indicated if CT has excluded caval thrombus. Similarly, routine bone scans are not warranted in the absence of an elevated alkaline phosphatase level or bone pain. The key to the more efficient utilization of imaging resources is understanding the capabilities of the technology available.

(*Arch Surg* 1989;124:71-73)

The development of several noninvasive imaging modalities (ie, ultrasound [US], computed tomography [CT], and magnetic resonance imaging [MRI]) has resulted in a debate over which or how many studies are indicated in the staging of patients with renal cell carcinoma.[1-5] Pressures to use resources more efficiently and contain medical costs argue against tests that provide redundant information, increase patient morbidity and expense needlessly, and do not have a significant impact on clinical management. Valid questions include (1) what is the role of former staging studies (ie, angiography or bone scanning), (2) when is venacavography indicated, and (3) will MRI replace CT as the current imaging standard? These issues require consideration to achieve a rational pattern of data collection before urologic intervention. No one study can possibly provide complete staging information in every instance. Prevention of wasted time and effort demands understanding the capabilities of the technology available to maximize study yield and facilitate appropriate evaluation and treatment.

In this study, we addressed these issues through a retrospective analysis of the radiographic staging of patients with renal cell carcinoma, comparing the preoperative clinical staging with the intraoperative and postoperative pathologic findings. The questions specifically asked were as follows: (1) Is venacavography indicated when CT has excluded caval thrombus? (2) Are routine bone scans warranted in the absence of chemical or clinical signs of metastatic disease? With respect to the diagnosis and delineation of caval thrombus, we also reviewed our experience with MRI, comparing the accuracy and correlation of its findings with the CT interpretation of the particular patient. The findings are discussed in light of previous studies and criteria suggested for imaging selection.

Accepted for publication July 8, 1988.

From the Division of Urology (Drs Benson and Resnick) and Department of Radiology (Dr Haaga), Case Western Reserve University School of Medicine, Cleveland.

Read before the Annual Meeting of the Society of Surgical Oncology, New Orleans, May 22, 1988.

Reprint requests to Division of Urology, University Hospitals of Cleveland, 2065 Adelbert Rd, Cleveland, OH 44106 (Dr Resnick).

METHODS

The medical charts of 64 patients with a discharge diagnosis of renal cell carcinoma were obtained from the records of University Hospitals of Cleveland, Cleveland Metropolitan General Hospital, and the Veterans Administration Hospital, Cleveland, from 1981 through 1987. The following information was retrieved and recorded: (1) patient age and sex; (2) type and interpretation of diagnostic studies; (3) admission laboratory values (including hematocrit, creatinine, serum urea nitrogen, aspartate aminotransferase, lactate dehydrogenase, alkaline phosphatase, and calcium); (4) presenting symptoms (including gross hematuria, pain, weight loss, and abdominal mass); (5) intraoperative findings; and (6) pathologic diagnosis (gross and microscopic). Only patients with complete pathologic, surgical, and radiologic reports were included to ensure uniformity of data collection and reporting. The information was tabulated and grouped according to pathologic stage (Robson classification)[6] to assess for trends with increasing volume of disease.

RESULTS

In Table 1, the characteristics of the patient population are depicted as outlined above. The findings correlate well with several documented features of renal cell carcinoma (ie, male sex preponderance, peak incidence in the sixth decade of life, broad distribution of presenting symptoms, and lack of a specific chemical indicator of disease).[7] No specific correlation between the number of diagnostic studies obtained and the pathologic stage was noted. Although fewer studies might be expected in patients with metastatic disease, the data reflect the inclusion of several patients who underwent planned chemotherapy following radical nephrectomy before its ineffectiveness was demonstrated. Significant positive correlations were noted between pathologic stage and symptoms of pain and alkaline phosphatase levels, and a negative correlation with hematocrit values.

The overall staging accuracy of CT in the study is depicted in Table 2, which gives the percentage of correctly identified staging measurements (ie, local extension, nodal disease, and renal vein and vena cava involvement), false-positive results, and false-negative results. In the 57 patients undergoing CT, vena cava and renal vein thrombus was excluded in 47 instances, nodal disease in 51, and local extension in 52. All eight vena cava and renal vein thrombi were identified, with only two false-positive results. For local extension and nodal spread determinations, there were three and five false-positive results and two and one false-negative results, respectively. The false-negative findings involved cases of focal microscopic extension and micrometastases only, not gross disease.

In the six patients undergoing MRI, the interpretation of the studies was equivalent to the CT diagnosis. No false-negative results were noted with respect to renal vein or vena cava thrombus. The same thrombus false-positive findings were encountered using both CT and MRI. Comparisons could not be made for false-positive or false-negative findings of local extension and nodal disease due to the limited number of studies.

Table 1.—Demographics of Patient Population: Presenting Symptoms, Admission Laboratory Values, and Diagnostic Studies

	Pathologic Stage			
	I	II	III	IV
Patient Population				
No. of patients	25	5	12	23
Mean age, y (range)	58 (32-88)	64 (54-79)	65 (54-76)	64 (30-79)
Sex, M/F	18/7	3/2	11/1	13/10
Presenting Symptoms				
Gross hematuria	11	2	5	7
Pain	10	2	4	16
Weight loss	2	2	1	4
Mass	3	. . .	2	2
Admission Laboratory Values, Mean (Range)				
Hematocrit	0.45 (0.28-0.50)	0.36 (0.28-0.46)	0.37 (0.32-0.47)	0.36 (0.21-0.48)
Creatinine, μmol/L	106 (62-150)	133 (88-168)	133 (106-256)	97 (80-168)
Serum urea nitrogen, mmol/L	6.1 (2.5-8.6)	5.7 (3.2-8.6)	6.8 (4.6-9.6)	5.7 (3.2-9.6)
Aspartate aminotransferase, U/L	20 (11-44)	22 (15-29)	16 (10-25)	28 (10-75)
Lactate dehydrogenase, U/L	211 (134-310)	213 (103-296)	212 (160-265)	250 (104-614)
Alkaline phosphatase, U/L	88 (41-177)	123 (63-145)	112 (97-174)	197 (40-760)
Calcium, mmol/L	2.37 (2.07-2.62)	2.39 (2.25-2.59)	2.30 (2.22-2.37)	2.47 (2.12-3.20)
Studies				
Angiography	12	5	9	9
Venacavography	7	3	5	5
Ultrasound	8	2	6	9
Computed tomography	25	5	12	16
Magnetic resonance imaging	2	. . .	3	1
Bone scan	17	3	10	20

Table 2.—Accuracy of CT Staging*

Pathologic Stage	Tumor Location (R/L)	No. of CT Scans	% Correct: Renal Vein	IVC	Nodes	Extended	False-Positive/False-Negative Results
I	13/12	25	100	100	100	91	2/0
II	3/2	5	100	90	60	60	3/2
III	7/4	11	100	91	82	100	2/1
IV	13/10	16	100	94	94	94	3/0

*CT indicates computed tomographic; IVC, inferior vena cava.

Table 3.—Bone Scan Findings Correlated With Alkaline Phosphatase Levels and Bone Pain

Pathologic Stage	No. of Scans	Elevated Alkaline Phosphatase Levels (n=115)	Bone Pain	Abnormal Bone Scan
I	17	3	10	0
II	3	3	3	0
III	10	5	3	. . .
IV	20	13	16	15

In the 35 patients undergoing invasive contrast studies (ie, angiography, venacavography, or both), thrombi were excluded in 25 instances and identified in six of eight patients. There were two false-positive and two false-negative results (involving renal vein thrombi). Local extension and nodal disease were not evaluated or mentioned in the majority of cases.

The bone scan findings correlated with the alkaline phosphatase levels and bone pain symptoms are illustrated in Table 3. Of the 50 patients undergoing study, no abnormal scans were found in patients with stage I and II disease. In the 15 instances of abnormal scans, all patients had either bone pain, an elevated alkaline phosphatase level, or both. The only equivocal case involved a patient with a small scapular hot spot suspicious for metastasis but not amenable to biopsy. This patient was followed up after radical nephrectomy, and the lesion remained unchanged for at least one year.

COMMENT

The staging techniques for patients with renal cell carcinoma have changed dramatically over the last decade with the evolution of the current imaging modalities. During the 1960s and 1970s, renal tumors were often identified by intravenous urography during the evaluation of patients with hematuria and abdominal masses. Nephrotomography, renal arteriography, and bone scans were typically performed to rule out local extension, nodal disease, and bone metastases in preparation for radical nephrectomy. Several studies, however, documented the deficiencies of arteriography with respect to identifying parameters other than vascularity. Bracken and Jonsson[8] and Futter et al[9] reported overall angiographic staging accuracies of only 36% to 44% and thought the use of the venous phase to determine the presence of thrombus was inadequate. Equivocal renal vein or vena cava involvement relied on venacavography for definitive confirmation. (Although occurring in only 3% to 7% of patients undergoing surgery for renal carcinoma, vena cava thrombus represents an important variable in determining the appropriate surgical approach, thereby helping decrease intraoperative morbidity.[4])

When US and CT ushered in the noninvasive imaging era in the mid-1970s, the roles of angiography and venacavography began to change. Although for many angiography arguably provided a preoperative road map, the overall staging accuracy of US and CT was clearly superior, generally in the range of 70% to 90%.[1,10] In addition to improved staging, morbidity secondary to bleeding, embolism, subintimal injection of contrast, vessel perforation and thrombosis, and catheter or wire breakage (total average incidence, 0.5%) could be avoided. Ultrasound represented a safe, inexpensive, rapid, radiation-independent imaging alternative with potential as a screening tool. Unfortunately, operator or machine dependency and imaging distortion secondary to bowel gas and fat have limited its generalized applicability.[5] Computed tomography became the staging standard by virtue of (1) clearer definition of local extension, nodal disease, and caval thrombus under most circumstances; (2) reproducibility of studies; and (3) ease of interpretation.[1,3,11] Despite these advantages, during the late 1970s and early 1980s several centers continued to advocate CT, arteriography, and venacavography for all patients with renal cell carcinoma.[4]

Through the 1980s, continued improvements in CT technology have further supported its role in staging. Most studies, including the current one, report an overall staging accuracy of 90% to 95%.[3] Such data question the need for routine angiography and venacavography in cases where the lesion is clearly confined by Gerota's fascia and enhances with contrast medium. Equivocal cases, involving avascular masses, questions of extension into the liver, and suggestion of vena cava thrombus, warrant further workup to guide management (ie, either using invasive studies with contrast medium or MRI).

With the advent of MRI in the mid-1980s, the role of CT has been challenged. Proponents have emphasized the superiority of MRI in the delineation of tissue planes, the detection of caval thrombus, and even tissue diagnosis, with a reported accuracy of 96%.[2,12] Their results for CT were only 70%, contrary to the prevailing data. Importantly, their series failed to control for study technique or contrast administration. By incorporating variable quality scans from several institutions for CT but not MRI, their figures may not be representative and their conclusions therefore are suspect. None of the known limitations of MRI were observed, including a 1% to 5% incidence of claustrophobia and artifact secondary to motion. Controlling for operational, technique, and machine variables, one would anticipate comparable accuracy for each modality. In our study, cases where CT and MRI were performed jointly had equivalent interpretations, including a false-positive reading for caval thrombus. Others have had similar experience. Further research is indicated before replacing CT with MRI as the initial staging modality.[13]

On the basis of availability of resources, overall staging accuracy, expense, noninvasiveness, low morbidity, and experience, CT remains the first choice in the initial evaluation of patients with known or suspected renal cell carcinoma. For masses detected on intravenous urography and suspected of being simple cysts, US confirmation with adherence to the specific criteria is sufficient (ie, through transmission, absence of internal echoes, and smooth wall with posterior enhancement).[7] Angiography by current consensus should be limited to (1) malignant neoplasms in a solitary kidney, where knowledge of the vascular anatomy before partial nephrectomy is essential; (2) equivocal cases where US, CT, or MRI is nondiagnostic, acknowledging that 10% of avascular masses represent tumor; and (3) extremely large tumors, where angioinfarction is contemplated before radical nephrectomy to aid in controlling the renal pedicle by allowing initial ligation of the renal vein. Is venacavography indicated when CT has excluded thrombus? The data suggest that CT is more than adequate in determining the presence of renal vein or caval thrombus, as no false-negative results were encountered. Venacavography, MRI, or both should be reserved for equivocal cases, studies with abnormal results, or in instances of suspected extension beyond the hepatic veins, where thorough delineation of the thrombus is critical in determining the appropriate surgical approach.

Bone scans have traditionally been part of the metastatic workup due to the importance of detecting spread before surgery, as the prognosis is not improved by radical nephrectomy in this setting. With increased sensitivity over plain film and the potential for earlier detection of disease, nuclear bone scans would seem to be an appropriate screening tool. Previous studies, however, have suggested that in the absence of bone pain or an elevated alkaline phosphatase level, bone scans provide a low yield.[14,15] Although useful for confirming clinically or roentgenographically suspected metastases, staging or treatment plans were not significantly altered. Our findings indicated no abnormal scans in lower stage disease and, using the criteria above for obtaining scans, no instances of metastatic disease would have been missed. We agree with the assertion that routine bone scans are not warranted and should be reserved for patients in whom spread is suggested on chemical or clinical grounds.

References

1. Cronan J, Feman R, Rosenfield A: Comparison of computerized tomography, ultrasound, and angiography in staging renal cell carcinoma. *J Urol* 1982;127:712-714.
2. Hricak H, Demas B, Williams R, et al: Magnetic resonance imaging in the diagnosis and staging of renal and perirenal neoplasms. *Radiology* 1985;154:709-715.
3. Richie J, Garnick M, Seltzer S, et al: Computerized tomography scan for diagnosis and staging of renal cell carcinoma. *J Urol* 1983;129:1114-1116.
4. Schefft P, Novick A, Straffon R, et al: Surgery for renal cell carcinoma extending into the inferior vena cava. *J Urol* 1978;120:28-31.
5. Webb J, Murray A, Bary P, et al: The accuracy and limitations of ultrasound in the assessment of venous extension in renal carcinoma. *Br J Urol* 1987;60:14-17.
6. Robson C, Churchill B, Anderson W: The results of nephrectomy for renal cell carcinoma. *J Urol* 1969;101:297.
7. Maldazys J, deKernion J: Current thoughts on the management of renal carcinoma. *Am Urol Assoc Update Series* 1985;28:2-7.
8. Bracken B, Jonsson K: How accurate is angiographic staging of renal cell carcinoma? *Urology* 1979;14:96-99.
9. Futter N, Collins J, Walsh W: Inaccuracies in angiographic staging of renal cell carcinoma. *Urology* 1979;14:629-630.
10. Jaschke W, vanKaik G, Peter S, et al: Accuracy of computed tomography in staging of kidney tumors. *Acta Radiol* 1982;25:593.
11. Sandler C, Raval B, David C: Computed tomography of the kidney. *Urol Clin North Am* 1985;12:657-676.
12. Choyke P, Kressel H, Pollack H, et al: Focal renal masses: Magnetic resonance imaging. *Radiology* 1984;152:471-477.
13. Lipuma J, Bryan P, Butler H, et al: Magnetic resonance imaging of the genitourinary tract. *Urol Clin North Am* 1986;12:531-550.
14. Blacher E, Johnson D, Haynie T: Value of routine radionuclide bone scans in renal cell carcinoma. *Urology* 1985;26:432-434.
15. Lindner A, Goldman D, deKernion J: Cost effective analysis of prenephrectomy radioisotope scans in renal cell carcinoma. *Urology* 1983;22:127-129.

Discussion

Q What are the indications for venography and angiography in evaluating patients?

A Generally it is well recognized that renal vein and, particularly, caval involvement are much more common with right-sided tumors. There have been reports in the literature that have placed criteria on when venocavography should be performed, particularly on right-sided tumors based on size and location in the kidney, ie, centrally located lesions; however, we did not find that and did not find it necessary to define our patients as having right- or left-sided tumors. We have obtained arteriograms in patients in whom we've had trouble diagnosing retroperitoneal tumors, but we generally have not found it to be useful. Many of these tumors have low vascularity. With renal tumors, I've mentioned angioinfarction, but I think many urologists today believe that angioinfarction is probably not that helpful in performing a radical nephrectomy, particularly for the larger tumors.

Photodynamic Therapy for Esophageal Tumors

James S. McCaughan, Jr, MD; Thomas A. Nims, MD; Jerry T. Guy, MD;
William J. Hicks, MD; Thomas E. Williams, Jr, MD; Leslie R. Laufman, MD

• Between 1982 and 1987, 40 patients with esophageal tumors (19 adenocarcinomas, 19 squamous carcinomas, and two melanomas) in whom conventional treatments were unsuccessful were treated with photodynamic therapy (PDT) after injection with either hematoporphyrin derivative or dihematoporphyrin ether. Patients underwent endoscopy again two to three days and one month after PDT and as needed when symptoms recurred. At one month, the average minimal diameter opening of 28 assessable tumors increased from 6 to 9 mm. Of the 35 patients who could be evaluated one month after PDT, the average improvement in food intake was from a liquid to a soft diet. Average survival time (from time of first treatment) was 7.7 months (n = 17) for adenocarcinoma, 5.8 months (n = 12) for squamous cell carcinoma, and 25 months (n = 2) for melanoma. Two patients with stage I adenocarcinoma were alive with no evidence of disease at 11 and 23 months. One patient with stage I squamous cell cancer died 18 months after PDT, with recurrence of tumor above the treated area noted eight months after treatment. One patient with stage I melanoma died of a synchronous colon cancer 31 months after PDT, with no evidence of residual melanoma.

(*Arch Surg* 1989;124:74-80)

Despite the various methods of treatment that have been attempted in patients with esophageal tumors, the prognosis remains poor. Regardless of the therapy, less than 4% of patients achieve five-year survival, and in 50% of these patients, the disease is unresectable when patients are first seen.[1] Chemotherapy, ionizing irradiation, or both may achieve some temporary relief, but the tumor frequently recurs with obstruction within six months.[2-5] Overall, surgical procedures carry an operative mortality approaching or exceeding 15% to 20%, with a mean survival frequently of less than six months.[6-9] Prosthetic intubation results in a mortality of 10% to 15%, with survival ranging only from two to four months. Solid foods usually cannot be eaten, and a complication rate of 25% can be expected.[10-14] Thus, most of our efforts are aimed at improving the ability of these patients to swallow and at improving their dietary intake for their few remaining months.

In 1978 Dougherty et al[15] reported success in treating cutaneous and subcutaneous malignant neoplasms with photodynamic therapy (PDT). The rationale for this treatment was that malignant neoplasms presensitized with hematoporphyrin derivative (HpD) can be selectively destroyed by exposing them to 630-nm light. Later, in 1984, Dougherty et al[16] reported that they had created a new dye by the fractionation of HpD and separation of a submixture. This product is designated dihematoporphyrin ether (DHE) (Photofrin II) and contains the active component of the HpD mixture. The efficacy of PDT has been demonstrated by several investigators treating many different kinds of malignant neoplasms, including melanomas of the choroid,[17-19] breast, skin, and subcutaneous metastases,[20,21] head and neck cancers,[19,22] bladder tumors,[23,24] gastric cancer,[25] tumors of the female genital tract,[19,21,26,27] primary skin cancers,[19,28] lung cancers,[19,29-31] and various other cancers.[21] In 1986, Dougherty's[32] review of the world literature stated that over 3000 patients had been treated with PDT.

We previously reported on our experience with HpD in the treatment of esophageal tumors.[33,34] This report is an update and expansion of those earlier studies, which employed both HpD and DHE as sensitizers.

Accepted for publication Sept 2, 1988.

From the Departments of Surgery (Drs McCaughan, Nims, and Williams) and Medical Oncology (Drs Guy, Hicks, and Laufman), Grant Medical Center, Columbus, Ohio.

Read before the Annual Meeting of the Society of Surgical Oncology, New Orleans, May 23, 1988.

Reprint requests to Laser Medical Research Foundation, 323 E Town St, Columbus, OH 43215 (Dr McCaughan).

PATIENTS AND METHODS

Forty patients (33 men and seven women) with esophageal malignant neoplasms (19 adenocarcinomas, 19 squamous cell carcinomas, and two melanomas) were treated with PDT between November 1982 and August 1987. The average patient age was 68 years (range, 54 to 88 years). All patients had received, were ineligible for, or had refused conventional surgery, ionizing radiation, or chemotherapy. The goal of the therapy was to facilitate swallowing; therefore, no patient was refused treatment because of their clinical status (Table 1).

All patients were hospitalized from at least the time of their injections until at least three days after their PDT sessions. Patient histories were obtained and patients underwent complete physical examinations. Barium esophagograms, computed tomographic scans of the chest and abdomen, liver and spleen scans, posteroanterior and lateral chest roentgenograms, complete blood cell count, blood chemistry studies, and urinalysis were performed. Clinical staging was done according to the *Manual for Staging of Cancer*,[35] which is related to tumor stage and presence of distal metastases, since regional nodes cannot be examined clinically. Staging was as follows: T1M0, stage I; T2M0, stage II; T3M0, stage III; and M1, stage IV.

A total of 85 PDT sessions were completed, 36 after a total of 28 injections of 3 mg/kg of HpD and 49 after a total of 45 injections of 2 mg/kg of DHE. After injection of the sensitizer, vital signs were taken every six hours, and daily complete blood cell counts, blood chemistry studies, and urinalyses were performed until the patient was discharged from the hospital. Daily chest roentgenograms were taken after PDT until the patient was discharged from the hospital.

Endoscopy

The PDT was performed usually on the third day after injection of the sensitizer (range, one to six days). Patients underwent endoscopy again two to three days and one month after PDT and as needed when symptoms recurred. All endoscopies were performed with topical anesthesia and intravenous sedation. Tumor length and the minimal diameter opening were estimated by direct flexible endoscopy. The tumor site and length were recorded as centimeters from the teeth. The diameter of the minimal opening was estimated with the use of open biopsy forceps of known diameter. Biopsies and brushings for cytologic examination were routinely performed. Still photographs were taken and videotapes made to document the effect of treatment. All PDT sessions and follow-up endoscopies were performed by one of us (J.S.M.).

Light Source and Dose

A tunable dye argon laser system (Spectra Physics) delivered 630 ± 2–nm light through a 400-μm quartz fiber inserted down the biopsy channel of the flexible endoscope. Initially rhodamine B dye was used for the dye laser, but for the past three years we have used kiton red dye.

Originally, we used a straight-tip fiber. The power output from these fibers was measured with a radiometer (Coherent 210). For surface treatment with straight-tip fibers, the light dose was

Table 1.—Patient Data*

Patient/ Age, y/Sex	Stage	Site, cm From Teeth	Previous Treatment	Survival, mo	Cause of Death or Status
			Adenocarcinoma		
1/76/M	I	25-30	Surgery (SGR), x-ray, chemotherapy	11	Alive, NED
2/71/M	I	41-43	YAG	23	Alive, NED
3/68/M	II	18-40	None	10	DOD; metastases
4/69/M	II	35-42	Dilation, YAG	6.5	DOD; ascites
5/68/M	II	28-40	Dilation	6.5	DOD; superior vena cava syndrome
6/71/M	II	40-44	YAG	11.5	Stroke; residual
7/68/M	II	34-45	None	11	DOD
8/55/M	II	35-40	X-ray, surgery (exploratory laparotomy), YAG	7	DOD
9/84/M	II	35-40	YAG	10	Alive; residual
10/58/M	II	35-45	None	1.5	DOD
11/65/F	II	35-42	Dilation	1	Aspiration pneumonia
12/84/M	II	31-35	X-ray, chemotherapy, YAG	5	Alive; residual
13/58/M	II	33-40	YAG	5	DOD; tracheoesophageal fistula
14/64/M	II	37-42	None	11	Myocardial infarction
15/88/M	III	18-26	YAG, dilation	4.5	DOD
16/64/M	IV	22-40	YAG	1	DOD
17/75/M	IV	30-36	Chemotherapy	2.5	DOD; pneumonia, pleural metastases
18/58/M	IV	40-45	Surgery (exploratory laparotomy), x-ray	2.2	DOD
19/58/M	IV	30-40	Surgery (SGR), x-ray, chemotherapy	2.7	DOD; gastrointestinal bleeding
			Melanoma		
20/69/M	I	38-40	None	31	Colon cancer; NED
21/88/M	II	31-38	None	19	DOD
			Squamous Carcinoma		
22/75/M	I	32-34	None	18	DOD
23/71/F	II	28-36	None	11	DOD
24/61/M	II	35-42	None	6	DOD
25/72/F	II	27-30	None	5	DOD
26/55/M	II	17-21	YAG	9.5	DOD; pneumonia, cirrhosis
27/59/F	III	27-32	YAG	0.5	Lung cancer
28/70/M	III	20-33	X-ray, chemotherapy	1.5	DOD
29/58/M	III	12-16	Surgery (laryngectomy), x-ray, chemotherapy	4	DOD
30/54/M	III	25-32	None	7	DOD; tracheoesophageal fistula
31/70/M	III	25-32	YAG	5.5	Aortic fistula, YAG
32/75/F	III	29-34	Chemotherapy, YAG	3	DOD
33/60/F	III	20-25	X-ray	4	DOD; tracheoesophageal fistula
34/57/M†	III	17-25	X-ray, chemotherapy	2.3	DOD; tracheoesophageal fistula
35/72/M	IV	18-23	X-ray, YAG	1.5	DOD
36/59/M	IV	17-23	None	2.5	DOD; pneumonia
37/70/M	IV	18-25	X-ray, dilation, jejunostomy	0.7	Peritonitis; J-tube leak
38/67/M	IV	28-36	None	0.13	Pulmonary saddle embolus; metastases
39/67/F	IV	30-42	Surgery (exploratory laparotomy)	1.3	DOD; pneumonia
40/76/M	IV	15-20	X-ray; YAG	0.5	Suicide

*SGR indicates subtotal gastric resection; NED, no evidence of disease; YAG, neodymium:YAG laser resection; and DOD, dead of disease.
†Dead of disease; tracheoesophageal fistula present before treatment.

estimated as joules per square centimeter of tissue from the time of exposure, the power delivered from the tip, and the area of the tumor exposed. Straight-tip fiber interstitial (inserted into the tumor) light dose could only be estimated as the total number of joules delivered from the power output and the time of insertion. Later, cylinder diffusing fibers were used to deliver the light perpendicular to the longitudinal axis over 1 to 2 cm. The power per centimeter was measured by dividing the total power measured with an integrating sphere radiometer by the length of the diffusing tip. Cylinder fiber light dose (surface and interstitial) was estimated as joules per centimeter of fiber from the power delivered per centimeter of diffusing fiber and the time of exposure. Tumors longer than the diffusing cylinder were treated by sequentially moving the fiber the length of the diffusing fiber.

Follow-up

Follow-up was achieved on 100% of patients. Each patient's ability to swallow was evaluated, and the cause of death was determined either by direct evaluation or by personal communication with the patient, family, and/or referring physician. Quality of life was evaluated by a comparison of baseline and one-month posttherapy measurements of Karnofsky performance status (KPS), weight, and diet. An esophageal grading system[36] was also used to evaluate the patient's quality of life. This system assigned a numerical grade based on the patient's swallowing ability (45%), pain type and severity (40%), ability to sleep (6%), leisure activity (5%), and work status (4%). The esophageal grades for swallowing ability were as follows: no ability to swallow, 0; clear fluids only, 15; blenderized foods, 25; most soft foods, 35; and regular food, 45.

RESULTS

Effect of Injection of Sensitizer

No clinical side effects were noted after injection of either HpD or DHE, including changes in vital signs or development of allergic responses.

Tumor Response

One month after treatment, 28 tumors (15 adenocarcinomas, 11 squamous cell carcinomas, and two melanomas) were assessable (Table 2). The remaining tumors could not be assessed either because of patient death or because the patient was doing well, lived several hundred miles away, and declined to return to our center for examination. At one month, the average length of the 15 adenocarcinomas had decreased from 9 to 7 cm, and the average minimum diameter opening had increased from 6 to 9 mm. The average length of the two melanomas had decreased from 5 to 3.5 cm, and the average minimum diameter opening had increased from 11 to 13 mm. The average length of the 11 squamous tumors had decreased from 6 to 5.3 cm, and the average minimum diameter opening had increased from 6 to 9 mm. Overall, the average length had decreased from 7.0 to 6.1 cm (not significant), but the average minimal diameter opening had increased from 6 to 9 mm ($P<.001$ by Student's t test).

Table 2.—Tumor Changes One Month After Photodynamic Therapy

	Tumor Length, cm		Minimal Diameter Open, mm		
Patient	Pretreatment	At 1 mo	Pretreatment	At 1 mo	Light Dose, J*
			Adenocarcinoma		
1	5	5	10	10	400/CF
2	2	0.5	9	12	500/CF
3	22	15	4	7	3150
4	7	5	8	4†	500/CF
5	12	7	6	10	400/CF; 500/CF; 400/CF
6	4	5	6	9	400/CF
7	11	6	8	8	420/CF
9	5	2	6	6	300/CF
10	10	10	2	10	1020
13	7	10	6	14	500/CF
14	5	5	0	5	420/CF
16	18	18	2	10	2340
17	6	4	4	8	630/CF
18	5	5	11	13	540/cm^2
19	10	8	10	13	450; 900/CF
			Melanoma		
20	2	2	14	14	420/CF
21	7	5	8	11	420/CF
			Squamous Carcinoma		
22	2	0	12	6	540/CF
23	8	5	8	12	660/CF
24	7	4	4	14	630/CF; 27/cm^2
25	3	3	8	9	500; 500; 400/CF
26	4	4	7	9	450/CF
29	4	8	0	8	600/CF
30	7	7	4	6	420/CF
31	7	5	7	7	500/CF
34	8	8	2	8	400; 700; 600/CF
35	5	5	5	10	500/CF
36	6	9	6	9	600/CF

*CF indicates centimeter of cylinder diffuser length; cm^2, square centimeter of tumor surface.

†Stricture.

Patient Survival

Thirty-one of 40 patients were assessable after the first PDT (17 adenocarcinomas, 12 squamous cell carcinomas, and two melanomas). Nine patients were excluded for the following reasons: three had preexisting tracheoesophageal fistulas (patients 28, 34, and 36); one committed suicide two weeks after PDT (patient 40); one with disseminated metastases had a saddle pulmonary embolus four days after PDT (patient 38); one had a mechanical perforation by the esophagoscope (patient 10); one patient who had previously had a complete obstruction died of aspiration pneumonia from gastrostomy tube feeding after PDT (patient 11); one patient died of synchronous obstructive lung cancer (patient 27); and one patient died of a preexisting leakage in the jejunostomy tube (patient 37) (Table 1). The average survival from the first PDT was 7.7 months for the 17 patients with adenocarcinoma, 5.8 months for the 12 patients with squamous carcinoma, and 25 months for the two patients with melanoma.

Figure 1 depicts the average survival time as a function of the clinical stage determined at the time of the first PDT session. The average survival for patients with stage I adenocarcinomas (two tumors) was 17 months. Two of these patients had complete response of the treated area and remained alive with no evidence of disease at 11 and 23 months. Survival for one patient with stage I squamous carcinoma was 18 months. This patient developed recurrence above the treated area eight months after the first PDT session but had no recurrence of the tumor in the treated area. Survival for one patient with stage I melanoma was 31 months. The patient died of synchronous carcinoma of the colon with no evidence of melanoma.

The average survival for patients with stage II adenocarcinoma (ten tumors) was 8.4 months. Two of these patients remained alive with residual disease five and 11 months after their first PDT sessions. Patient survival for

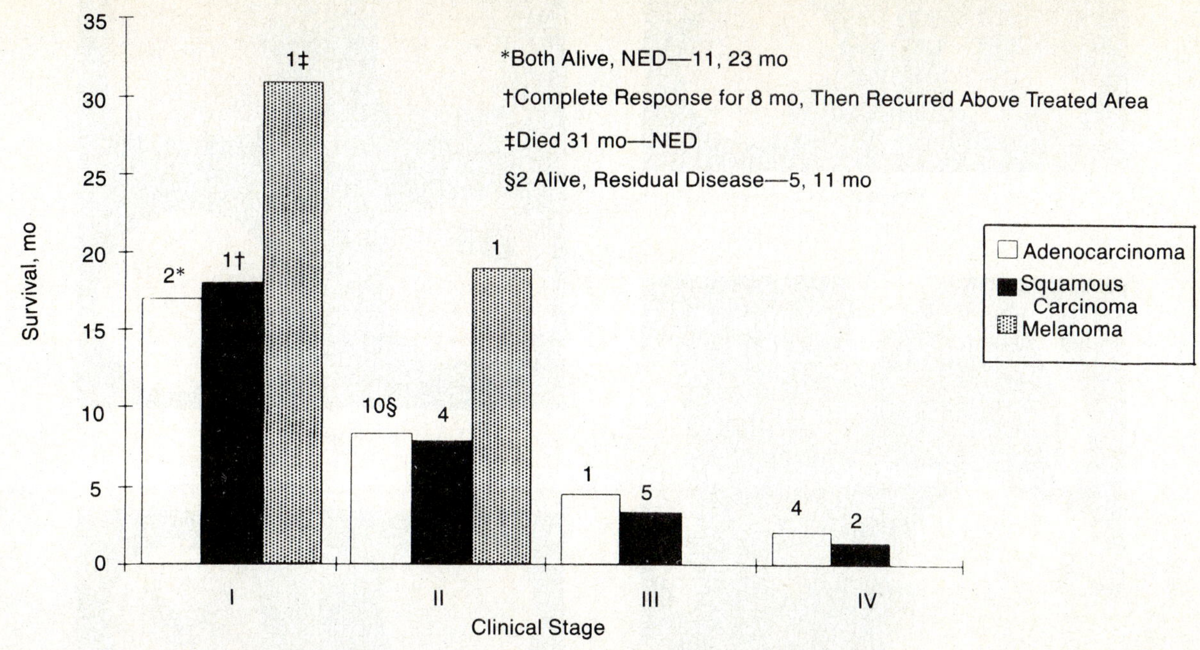

Fig 1.—Average survival time as related to clinical stage determined at time of first photodynamic therapy. NED indicates no evidence of disease.

stage II squamous carcinoma (four tumors) was 7.9 months; for stage II melanoma (one tumor) patient survival was 19 months.

Average survival for stage III tumors was 4.5 months for adenocarcinoma (one tumor) and 3.4 months for squamous carcinoma (five tumors). Stage IV survival was 2.1 months for adenocarcinoma (four tumors) and 1.4 months for squamous carcinoma (two tumors) (Figs 2 through 8).

Quality of Life

Thirty-five patients were assessable one month after their first PDT sessions. Quality of life was assessed according to changes in weight, KPS, esophageal grade, and diet. The KPS and weight remained essentially unchanged, the former increasing from an average of 62 to 66 and the latter decreasing from an average of 65.7 to 64.4 kg, but the esophageal grade and particularly the diet grade improved. The esophageal grade increased from an average of 59 to an average of 75. The average diet grade increased in one month from 16 to 32, which represents improvement from a liquid to a soft diet ($P<.001$ by Student's t test).

Nine patients had complete obstruction when first treated. They survived an average of three months (range, one to 11 months). One month after treatment, two patients had died, one was eating a regular diet, two were tolerating a soft diet, and four patients were tolerating a liquid diet, for an average diet grade of 23 (equal to a blended diet). At the time of their deaths, one patient was eating a regular diet, three patients were maintained on soft diets, four patients could tolerate liquid diets, and one patient could swallow only saliva.

Complications

There were no allergic responses to any of the injections. The highest average temperature at the time of PDT after injections in 58 afebrile patients was 36.9°C; the highest average temperature after PDT was 37.4°C, occurring an average of two days after therapy. The average white blood cell count of these patients before injection was 8×10^9/L and was 11×10^9/L one day after PDT. The average highest white blood cell count of 14×10^9/L occurred an average of three days after PDT.

The maximum amount of bleeding at any PDT endoscopy was characterized as oozing. One patient suffered a mechanical perforation of the esophagus by the esophagoscope at the junction of the proximal end of the tumor and the normal esophagus, but this was unrelated to the PDT.

Edema with decreased lumen was frequently noted at repeated endoscopy two to three days after PDT. This often was seen developing in areas at the end of the treatment. Occasionally, the edema exacerbated difficulty in swallowing, but the tumor was soft and easily dilated.

Nine of the 85 treatments caused pleural effusions in six patients. All cleared except in one patient (patient 20), who required bilateral chest tubes and a subsequent thoracotomy to ligate the thoracic duct for chylothorax.

Six strictures occurred in five patients. All were manageable by dilation. Three were associated with development of pleural effusion and three were not.

Three patients developed tracheoesophageal fistulas. In one case, this was probably unrelated to the PDT because the patient (patient 30) already had invasion of the trachea, and the fistula did not occur for several weeks. A second patient (patient 33) who developed a fistula had undergone a previous esophageal reconstruction skin graft and tracheostomy 12 years earlier for cancer of the larynx. The third patient to develop a fistula (patient 13) had an adenocarcinoma that had spread along the esophagus rapidly after the patient underwent radiation therapy.

In most patients, solar photosensitivity is a possible complication for at least one month after injection. Four

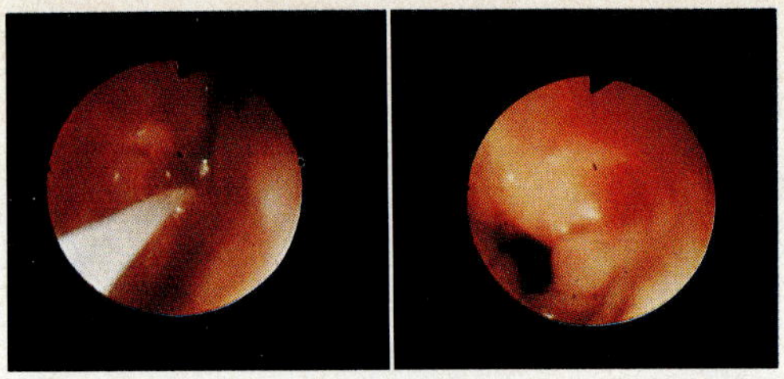

Figure 2.

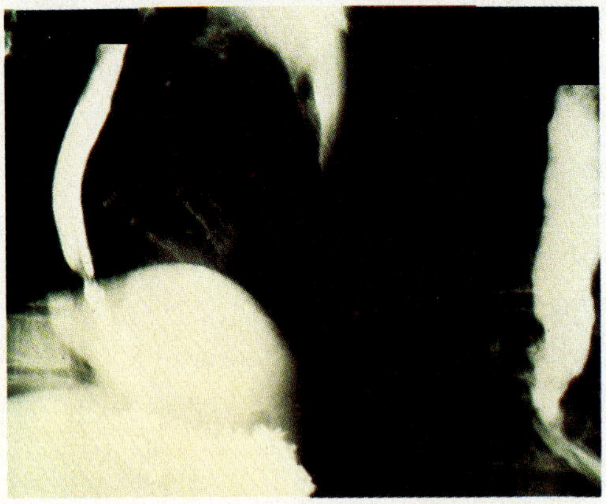

Figure 3.

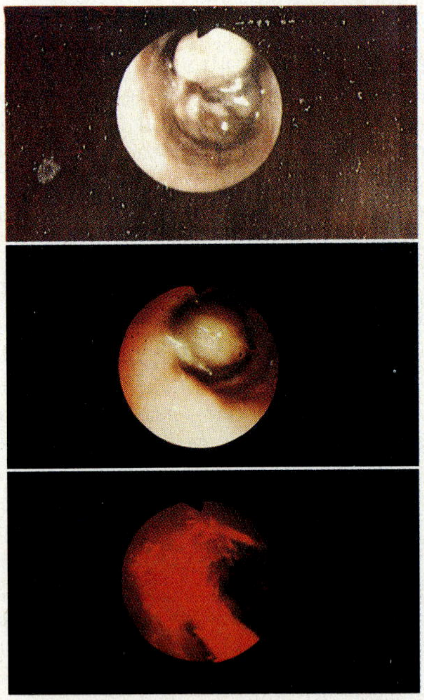

Figure 4.

Figure 5.

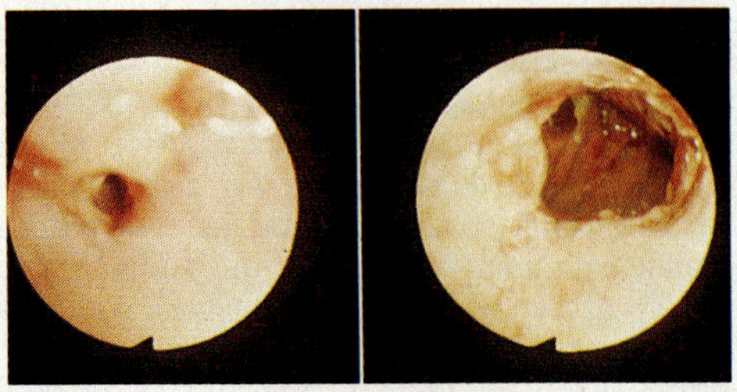

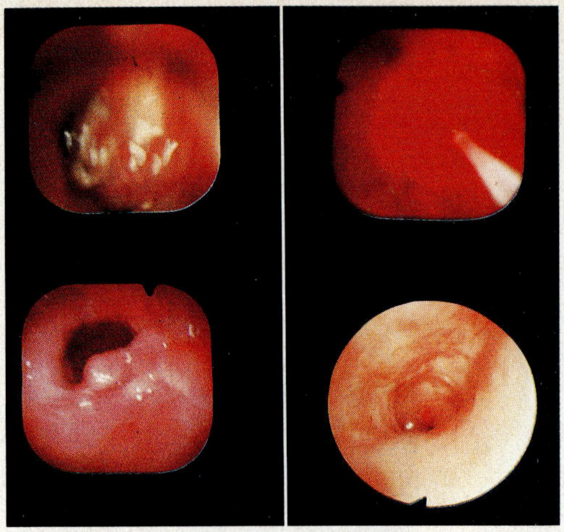

Figure 6.

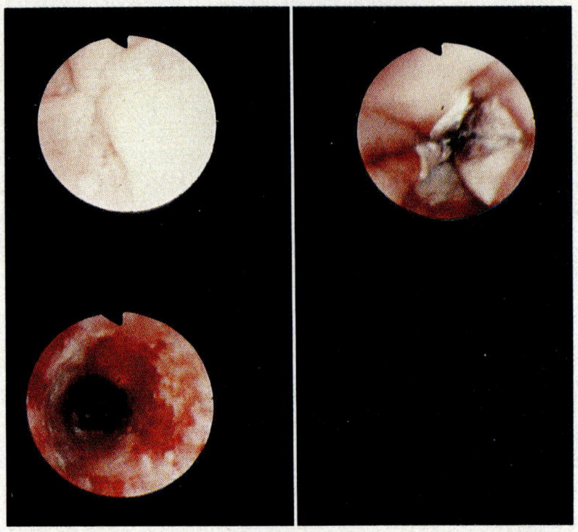

Figure 7.

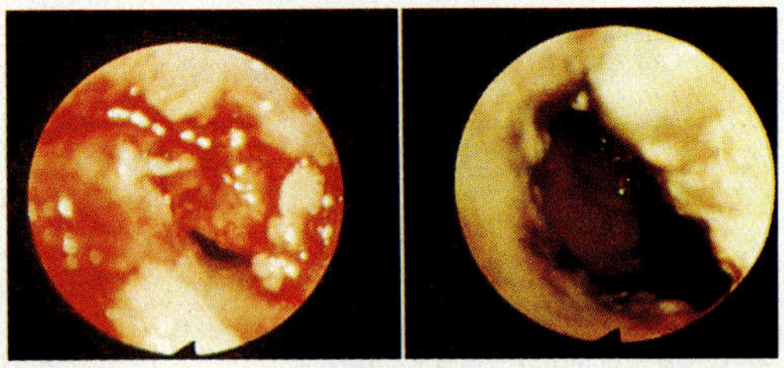

Figure 8.

patients developed gradual reddish brown discoloration of the exposed skin that lasted for several months. One patient sustained third-degree necrosis of a 2-cm-diameter area of his hand when he fell asleep with sun coming through the window eight weeks after his first injection of DHE. Nevertheless, these minor complications do not seem to offer too great a handicap for patients who are more than willing to trade the sunlight for the ability to swallow.

COMMENT

The survival rate of patients with cancer of the esophagus continues to be poor, regardless of the type of treatment. Morstyn et al[37] reported an average survival of three to four months in 71 patients with esophageal tumors who did not undergo surgery. In comparison, the average survival from the time of diagnosis of eight patients in our study with squamous carcinoma and adenocarcinoma who did not have any previous treatment was 11.4 months. Of 19 patients who had undergone previous forms of therapy (including six patients who had undergone x-ray therapy), average survival was 10.9 months. One patient with stage I melanoma died 31 months after his first treatment, with no evidence of disease. A patient with stage I squamous cell cancer had a complete response for eight months and then developed tumors similar to those previously treated above the treated area. A patient with stage I adenocarcinoma was alive with no evidence of disease 23 months after therapy. It should be noted that there was no correlation between length of survival and the length of the tumor or the minimal diameter opening before treatment. Survival was independent of histologic type for adenocarcinoma and squamous cell carcinoma when tumors in the same clinical stage were compared (Fig 1). Direct endoscopy should always be used to evaluate the opening because contrast roentgenograms are frequently misleading. Adenocarcinomas were noted to progress longitudinally over time.

The most important factor in palliation for these patients is the ability to swallow. In this regard, neither KPS nor the esophageal grade alone is a reliable measure of the patient's condition or prognosticator of survival. Patients who are able to swallow may have a high esophageal grade but a low KPS due to metastases. On the other hand, patients with a low esophageal grade due to obstruction may have a high KPS because the tumor is still localized. It should be emphasized, however, that no patient with a combined total score of less than 120 on both the KPS and esophageal grade scales lived longer than six months after PDT. Having observed desperate patients with complete obstruction, we believe that the ability to swallow even one's own saliva is sufficient to justify therapy. The PDT was particularly effective in achieving this goal. One month after PDT, of nine patients who had had complete obstruction, one was eating a regular diet, two were able to tolerate soft diets, and four patients were on liquid diets. Two patients had died, but both had improved their dietary intake at the time of their deaths, one to a soft diet and one to a liquid diet. It should be mentioned, however, that despite improvements achieved by the therapy, some patients will not have an increased dietary intake because of anorexia. Thus, we now recommend the use of feeding gastrostomies because we can frequently control the problems caused by obstructed saliva by treatment with PDT or the neodymium:YAG laser.

Although several patients developed complications related to PDT, many other patients treated with similar light doses did not develop problems. We believe that the development of these complications depends on whether the treated area was encased with concentric tumor, in which case complications did not develop.

Technically, it is difficult to treat segments of the esophagus sequentially without overlapping treated areas, and it is this overlap that may create the stricture. One patient developed two separate, discrete strictures after a treatment session, although the tumor area became smooth and tumor free (patient 22).

It is interesting that five patients in this study had a history of previous unrelated cancers. One patient had been diagnosed with cancer of the colon, one had developed cancer of the lung, and three patients had a history of cancer of the larynx. In addition, three patients developed synchronous, unrelated cancers, one patient developing cancer of the colon and two patients developing cancer of the vocal cord.

It is imperative that patients undergo bronchoscopy before treatment. In this series, six patients had malignant invasion of the respiratory tract at the time of PDT. Two patients (one with adenocarcinoma and one with squamous carcinoma) had invasion of the left main bronchus. Four patients with squamous carcinoma had invasion of the trachea. In addition, we urge that symptomatic patients undergo esophagoscopy, even if barium swallow examinations are normal. In this study, four patients with stage I disease and one patient with stage II disease were found to have esophageal cancer despite their "normal" findings on barium swallow examination. One patient with stage II disease was reported to have a "benign stricture." On the other hand, three patients who in reality developed benign strictures after PDT were diagnosed as having cancer. Obviously, a definitive diagnosis can be made only if patients undergo both bronchoscopy and esophagoscopy.

Fig 2.—Stage II squamous carcinoma in patient 24 before treatment (left) and two months after photodynamic therapy (right). Diet improved from clear liquids to regular food.

Fig 3.—Barium swallow study in patient 24 with squamous carcinoma before (left) and two months after (right) photodynamic therapy. Patient had gained 7.7 kg and was eating a regular diet.

Fig 4.—Esophageal melanoma in patient 21 before (left upper corner), during (right upper corner) (with the fiber in place), and three weeks after (left lower corner) photodynamic therapy. Patient improved from liquid to regular diet. He was treated seven times and survived 19 months after first treatment, during which time he ate a regular diet.

Fig 5.—Adenocarcinoma in patient 9 before (left) and three days after (right) treatment. Patient improved from clear liquid diet to soft diet. He received two treatments and was alive and on regular diet ten months after first treatment.

Fig 6.—Stage I adenocarcinoma in patient 2 before (left upper corner) and during (right upper corner) treatment with interstitial fiber and one month after first treatment (left lower corner). Patient was reinjected and retreated with surface technique and was alive 19 months after first treatment, with no evidence of disease (right lower corner).

Fig 7.—Adenocarcinoma in patient 14 causing complete obstruction before (left upper corner) and two days after (right upper corner) surface photodynamic therapy, showing opening of obstruction and reaction. Two months after (left lower corner) therapy, patient was eating a regular diet. He died 11 months later of myocardial infarction. He had received six treatments and was eating a regular diet at time of death.

Fig 8.—Adenocarcinoma in patient 12 before (left) and two days after (right) photodynamic therapy. Patient was alive five months after first treatment and continued to eat a soft diet.

References

1. McCaughan JS Jr, Williams TE Jr, Bethel BH: Palliation of esophageal malignancy with photodynamic therapy. *Ann Thorac Surg* 1985;40:113-120.
2. Belsey R, Hiebert CA: An exclusive right thoracic approach for cancer of the middle third of the esophagus. *Ann Thorac Surg* 1974;18:1-15.
3. Steiger Z, Franklin R, Wilson RF, et al: Complete eradication of squamous cell carcinoma of the esophagus with combined chemotherapy and radiotherapy. *Am Surg* 1981;47:95-98.
4. Newaishy GA, Read GA, Duncan W, et al: Results of radical radiotherapy of squamous cell carcinoma of the oesophagus. *Clin Radiol* 1982;33:347-352.
5. Earlam R, Cunha-Melo JR: Oesophageal squamous cell carcinoma: I. A critical review of surgery. *Br J Surg* 1980;67:381-390.
6. Cukingnan RA, Carey JS: Carcinoma of the esophagus (collective review). *Ann Thorac Surg* 1978;26:274-286.
7. Postlethwait RW: Complications and deaths after operations for esophageal carcinoma. *J Thorac Cardiovasc Surg* 1983;85:827-831.
8. Orringer MB, Orringer JS: Esophagectomy without thoracotomy: A dangerous operation? *J Thorac Cardiovasc Surg* 1983;85:72-80.
9. Rose JD, Smith PM: Fibre endoscopic insertion of palliative oesophageal tubes with the Nottingham introducer. *J R Soc Med* 1983;76:266-268.
10. Mannell A: Carcinoma of the esophagus. *Curr Probl Surg* 1982;19:553-647.
11. Payne WS: Palliation of esophageal carcinoma. *Ann Thorac Surg* 1979;28:208.
12. Graham DY, Dobbs SM, Zubler M: What is the role of prosthesis insertion in esophageal carcinoma? *Gastrointest Endosc* 1983;29:1-5.
13. Pfleiderer AG, Goodall P, Holmes GKT: The consequences and effectiveness of intubation in the palliation of dysphagia due to benign and malignant strictures affecting the oesophagus. *Br J Surg* 1982;69:356-358.
14. Angorn IB: Intubation in the treatment of carcinoma of the esophagus. *World J Surg* 1981;5:535-541.
15. Dougherty TJ, Kaufman JE, Goldfarb A, et al: Photoradiation therapy for the treatment of malignant tumors. *Cancer Res* 1978;38:2628-2635.
16. Dougherty TJ, Potter WR, Weishaupt KR: The structure of the active component of hematoporphyrin derivative, in Dorion DR, Gomer CJ (eds): *Porphyrin Localization and Treatment of Tumors*. New York, Alan R Liss Inc, 1984, pp 301-304.
17. Tse DT, Dutton JJ, Weingeist TA, et al: Hematoporphyrin photoradiation therapy for intraocular and orbital malignant melanoma. *Arch Ophthalmol* 1984;102:833-838.
18. Bruce RA: Evaluation of hematoporphyrin photoradiation therapy to treat choroidal melanoma. *Lasers Surg Med* 1984;4:59-64.
19. McCaughan JS Jr: Overview of experiences with photodynamic therapy for malignancy in 192 patients. *Photochem Photobiol* 1987;46:903-909.
20. Dahlman A, Wile AG, Burns RG, et al: Laser photoradiation therapy of cancer. *Cancer Res* 1983;43:430-434.
21. McCaughan JS Jr, Guy JT, Hawley P, et al: Hematoporphyrin derivative and photoradiation therapy of malignant tumors. *Lasers Surg Med* 1983;3:199-209.
22. Wile AG, Coffey J, Nahabedian MY, et al: Laser photoradiation therapy of cancer: An update of the experience at the University of California, Irvine. *Lasers Surg Med* 1984;4:5-12.
23. Benson RC, Kinsey JH, Cortese DA, et al: Treatment of transitional cell carcinoma of the bladder with hematoporphyrin derivative phototherapy. *J Urol* 1983;130:1090-1095.
24. Hisazumi H, Misaki T, Miyoshi N: Photoradiation therapy of bladder tumors. *J Urol* 1983;130:685-687.
25. Aida M, Kawaguchi M: Gastric cancer, in Hayata Y, Dougherty TJ (eds): *Lasers and Hematoporphyrin Derivative in Cancer*. Tokyo, Igaku-Shoin, 1983, pp 65-69.
26. Ward BG, Forbes IJ, Cowled PA, et al: The treatment of vaginal recurrences of gynecologic malignancy with phototherapy following hematoporphyrin derivative pretreatment. *Am J Obstet Gynecol* 1982;142:356-357.
27. Soma H, Nutahara S: Cancer of the female genitalia, in Hayata Y, Dougherty TJ (eds): *Lasers and Hematoporphyrin Derivative in Cancer*. Tokyo, Igaku-Shoin, 1983, pp 97-109.
28. Tokuda Y: Primary skin cancer, in Hayata Y, Dougherty TJ (eds): *Lasers and Hematoporphyrin Derivative in Cancer*. Tokyo, Igaku-Shoin, 1983, pp 88-96.
29. Hayata Y, Kato H, Konaka C, et al: Photoradiation therapy with hematoporphyrin derivative in early and stage 1 lung cancer. *Chest* 1984;86:169-177.
30. Balchum OJ, Doiron DDR, Huth GC: Photoradiation therapy of endobronchial lung cancer employing the photodynamic action of hematoporphyrin derivative. *Lasers Surg Med* 1984;4:13-30.
31. Vincent RG, Dougherty TJ, Rao U, et al: Photoradiation therapy in advanced carcinoma of the trachea and bronchus. *Chest* 1984;85:29-33.
32. Dougherty TJ: Photosensitization of malignant tumors. *Semin Surg Oncol* 1986;2:24-37.
33. McCaughan JS Jr, Williams TE, Bethel BH: Palliation of esophageal malignancy with photodynamic therapy. *Ann Thorac Surg* 1985;40:113-120.
34. McCaughan JS Jr, Hicks W, Laufman L, et al: Palliation of esophageal malignancy with photoradiation therapy. *Cancer* 1984;54:2905-2910.
35. Beahrs OH, Myers MH (eds): *Manual for Staging of Cancer: American Joint Committee on Cancer*, ed 2. Philadelphia, JB Lippincott Co, 1983.
36. Stoller JL, Samer KJ, Toppin DI, et al: Carcinoma of the esophagus: A new proposal for the evaluation of treatment. *Can J Surg* 1977;20:454-459.
37. Morstyn G, Thomas RJ, Mullerworth M, et al: Improved survival in esophageal cancer in the period 1978 to 1983. *J Clin Oncol* 1986;4:1062-1067.

Discussion

Q How long do you keep them out of the sun?

A We tell them to stay out of the sun for a month; we have a whole procedure we go through. We give them lectures and slide shows. Some of them don't believe us, and they go out and get a bad sunburn. We've had three patients of about 250 who have had to be admitted because of severe sunburn and are given corticosteroids, but most of the time it will subside, and we tell them to go out in the evening. They use factor 33, which will take care of the ultraviolet, but it won't protect them completely. Usually after a month, they can start going out slowly. The man who got sunburned in six months got it through his shirt, but he had recurrent disease in his bronchial stump that we treated and he is now almost three years, with no recurrence. He got sunburned playing golf six months after he had been treated, on a bright sunny day; maybe you figure, well, that's not much of a price to pay.

Q In operable esophageal cancer, does this have any role as initial therapy prior to surgery?

A The question is, would this be good preoperatively for somebody with cancer of the esophagus to try to open them? I think probably if you wanted to do that, you'd go ahead with a laser, but I don't know that there would be much point in doing it, myself.

Q Let's speak to the issue of using this treatment as primary therapy. You did have a patient or two in the esophageal group who went for a long period of time, and you also had some individuals, who died of other causes disease free. What about the use of the treatment as primary therapy?

A Well, this is investigational therapy, and we don't do this on anybody, unless they have had everything else. They're not candidates for it until it's approved by the Food and Drug Administration, for both legal and ethical reasons. Our patients, for example, a 77-year-old man who previously had a triple bypass, are not candidates for surgery. We have used PDT for patients with lung cancer who have had bilateral disease and small tumors. We treated one and got a complete response; then he had the other lobe out. That's been a year and there's no evidence of recurrence.

Q How do you decide on the dose of light?

A If you give enough light to any of the tissue, you will get a burn. You can think of this like x-ray therapy. You get too much, you get burned. Its just a different wavelength. And that is what we've been trying to figure out; what's the right light dosage?

Q On the basal cell carcinomas that you've previously treated on the face, do you treat them again, and how long do you have to wait?

A We have treated one patient with recurrence in his sacrum. We gave him a total of ten injections and 16 treatments over 2½ years, and we've had no problems with accumulation. Now, he has sort of a yellowish cast to his skin. I had another patient who had a Klatskin tumor. We put a U-tube in, and I treated her with endoscope. I went back for the third time. I passed my endoscope right into the tumor. She is now three years after treatment. The point is that you can inject this stuff over and over again and treat them over and over again.

Q Can you do this with oral cancer?

A Yes, it will work for small tumors. The one patient we treated had a previous laryngectomy. Then he had a tumor on his soft palate and we treated him, shining the light there for eight minutes. In two years there was no evidence of recurrence of that tumor. Again, these people had had every other treatment or we won't touch them. He died from his other metastases.

Effect of Timing of Lymphokine Presentation on Generation of Cytotoxic T Lymphocytes

Monica M. Stringfellow, MD; Richard E. Wilson, MD; Steven J. Burakoff, MD; Steven H. Herrmann, MD

• **Encouraging results of clinical trials with interleukin 2 therapy for advanced malignant neoplasms have led to efforts to reduce the toxicity and improve the efficacy of tumor immunotherapy. To begin to achieve this goal, we studied the lymphokine requirements for in vitro generation of polyclonal cytotoxic T lymphocytes (CTL) from C57BL/6 murine thymocytes. We found that both interleukin 2 and interleukin 6 are required for optimal generation of CTL from murine thymocytes. Timing studies show that neither lymphokine alone in culture will produce maximum CTL levels during the first 84 hours of culture. In addition, we found that thymocytes cultured with concanavalin A are unresponsive unless either interleukin 2 or interleukin 6 is present from the onset of culture.**

(*Arch Surg* 1989;124:81-84)

The encouraging results of clinical trials with interleukin 2 therapy for advanced malignant neoplasms raise the hope that exogenous lymphokines may be useful in augmenting host responses to tumor. Promising work in adoptive immunotherapy involves the in vitro generation of specifically sensitized T lymphocytes to mediate tumor regression in vivo.[1-4] It is important, therefore, to know the lymphokine requirements for generation of cytotoxic T lymphocytes (CTL) both in vitro and in vivo to reduce the toxicity and improve the efficacy of tumor immunotherapy.

The required sequence of molecular events leading to tumor-specific CTL development is unknown. The induction of CTL from precursor T cells requires transmembrane signals generated through both the antigen-specific T-cell receptor and lymphokine receptors.[5,6] Previous studies indicate that multiple lymphokines are required for T-lymphocyte activation. Depending on the assay system, interleukin 2 (IL-2), interleukin 6 (IL-6), interleukin 4 (IL-4), and interferon gamma have all been implicated in T-cell differentiation and activation.[7-12] Interleukin 2 is generally associated with T-cell proliferation, while IL-4 and IL-6 have been associated with the differentiation of B lymphocytes and with the differentiation of T cells, as indicated by the generation of a cytotoxic response and the expression of serine esterase activity.[8,12-14] The exact role of these lymphokines in CTL maturation and activation has not been established. The multiple lymphokine requirement for differentiation of thymocytes into CTL suggests that a cascade type of regulation may be involved. Signaling by one lymphokine may influence the effect of a second by inducing required lymphokine receptors or causing the production of final lymphokine mediators.[8,11,13]

In our assay system, a murine whole thymus preparation was cultured with concanavalin A (ConA) in the presence of various lymphokines; after a two- to four-day culture the polyclonal CTL response was measured by the lysis of P815 tumor cells in the presence of phytohemagglutinin. A first step in assigning lymphokine function is to define the lymphokine requirements under different culture conditions and to ask if there is a specific temporal order for addition of the necessary lymphokines. We have found evidence that, over a four-day incubation period, the cytotoxic response generated by thymocytes cultured in IL-2 plus IL-6 was greater than the response generated by culture in either alone; that thymocytes cultured in the absence of exogenous lymphokines rapidly lost the ability to generate a cytotoxic response; and that this exogenous lymphokine requirement could be fulfilled by either IL-2 or IL-6.

MATERIALS AND METHODS

Animals and Cell Lines

C57BL/6 and (BALB/c × DBA/2)F_1 female mice 6 to 8 weeks of age were purchased from The Jackson Laboratory, Bar Harbor, Me. P815 (H-2^d mastocytoma) was maintained by weekly passage as ascites in (BALB/c × DBA/2)F_1 mice.

Lymphokines

Human recombinant IL-2 was purchased from Amgen Biologicals, Thousand Oaks, Calif. Human recombinant IL-6 was produced in COS cells and purified to homogeneity.[15]

Accepted for publication Sept 21, 1988.
From the Department of Surgery, Brigham and Women's Hospital and Harvard Medical School (Drs Stringfellow and Wilson), and the Departments of Pediatrics and Pathology, Division of Pediatric Oncology, Dana Farber Cancer Institute and Harvard Medical School (Drs Burakoff and Herrmann), Boston.
Read before the Annual Meeting of the Society of Surgical Oncology, New Orleans, May 23, 1988.
Reprint requests to Department of Surgery, Brigham and Women's Hospital, 75 Francis St, Boston, MA 02115 (Dr Stringfellow).

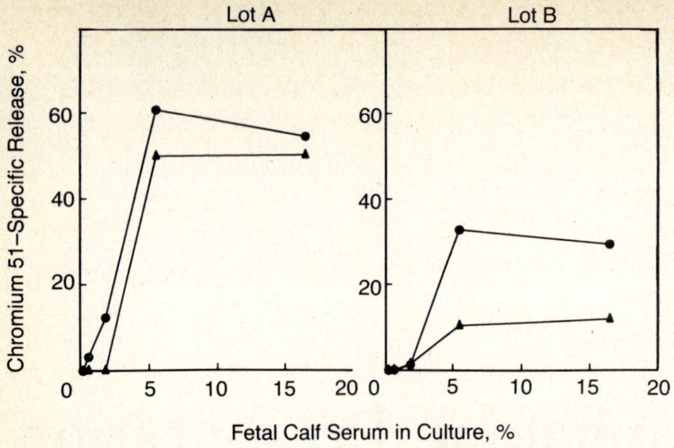

Fig 1.—Dependence of thymocytes on interleukin 6 for cytotoxic T-lymphocyte generation is function of fetal calf serum used in culture. Circles indicate cells cultured in interleukin 2 plus interleukin 6; triangles, cells cultured in interleukin 2 alone.

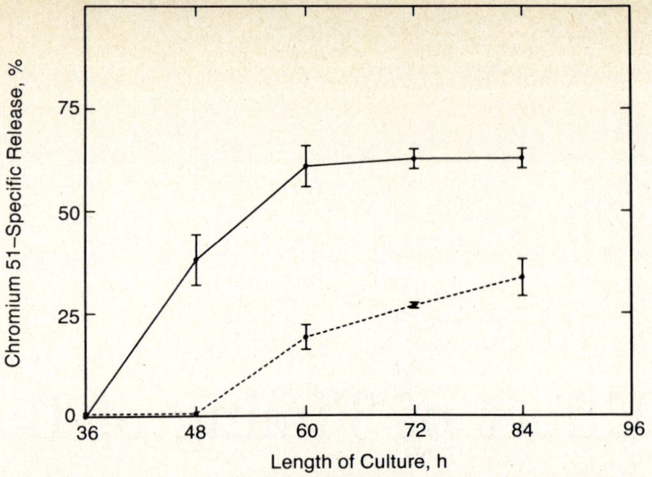

Fig 2.—Level of cytotoxic T lymphocytes generated by addition of interleukin 2 alone (broken line) compared with that generated by addition of interleukin 2 plus interleukin 6 (solid line). Effector cells were 8×10^5 per well C57BL/6 thymocytes plus 3 mg/L of concanavalin A. Bars indicate arithmetic mean ± SD ($P<.01$ for all points by Student's t test).

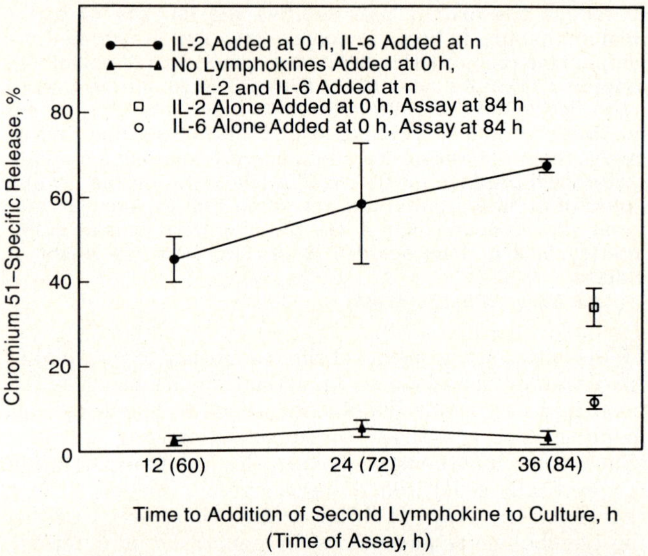

Fig 3.—Effect of delayed addition of lymphokine to C57BL/6 thymocytes plus concanavalin A. Total culture time in presence of interleukin 2 (IL-2) plus interleukin 6 (IL-6) was 48 hours. Total length of culture varied, as indicated in parentheses, from 60 to 84 hours. Bars indicate arithmetic mean ± SD ($P<.01$ for all points by Student's t test).

In Vitro Culture for CTL Generation

Whole thymocytes from 6- to 8-week-old C57BL/6 mice were prepared as described previously.[7] Eight hundred thousand thymocytes were cultured in 96-well, round-bottomed microtiter plates in the presence of 3 mg/L of ConA (Sigma Chemical Co, St Louis). Where indicated, IL-2 (20 U/mL) or IL-6 (100 ng/mL) were added either together or singly at defined intervals of time. Total culture time varied from 48 to 84 hours, as indicated. The culture medium consisted of RPMI 1640 supplemented with 100 U/mL of penicillin, 100 mg/L of streptomycin, 2 mmol/L of glutamine, and a selected lot of 5% heat-inactivated fetal calf serum (FCS).

It became apparent that the lymphokine requirements were dependent on the lot of FCS used in thymocyte culture. Figure 1 compares two different lots of FCS. In FCS lot A, at a concentration of 5%, the level of CTL generated by IL-2 alone was 50%, as compared with 61% for IL-2 plus IL-6. In 5% FCS lot B, 10% lysis resulted from culture in IL-2 alone, compared with 33% lysis from the addition of both IL-2 and IL-6. This FCS, from Hyclone Labs, Logan, Utah, lot 1111649, was used for all work presented. It is likely that FCS from lot A contains bovine lymphokines functional on murine thymocytes or products able to induce lymphokine production by thymocytes.

CTL Assay

After completion of the culture interval, microtiter plates were centrifuged at 1000 rpm for five minutes, the culture medium was decanted, and 10^4 chromium 51–labeled P815 target cells and 10 mg/L of phytohemagglutinin-P (Difco Laboratories Inc, Detroit) were added to each well in a final volume of 200 uL. After a four-hour incubation at 37°C, cells were pelleted and an aliquot of supernatant was removed and counted in a gamma counter. The percentage of specific lysis was calculated as follows: [100 × (chromium 51 released with effector cells) − (spontaneous chromium 51 release)]/[(maximal chromium 51 released with 5% Triton X-100) − (spontaneous chromium 51 release)].

RESULTS

The IL-6 requirement for generation of a CTL response was demonstrated in previous work using lectin-triggered thymocytes and a 48-hour in vitro culture.[7,8] To determine if thymocytes cultured for longer periods also require non–IL-2 lymphokines, the level of cytotoxicity was determined after 48, 60, 72, and 84 hours of culture. Thymocytes cultured with the IL-2 plus IL-6 combination reached the highest level of target cell lysis, 55%, at 60 hours and remained at this level (Fig 2). Target cell lysis was negligible by thymocytes cultured for 48 hours with added IL-2; however, with increasing lengths of culture the level of lysis increased until at 84 hours 34% of target cells were lysed (Fig 2). With longer periods of incubation, as predicted from Fig 2, the level of lysis by thymocytes cultured in the presence of IL-2 only was similar to that found for IL-2 plus IL-6 (data not shown). A maximal cytotoxic response, therefore, was generated if both lymphokines were present for at least 48 hours of thymocyte culture.

Next we asked if IL-6 and IL-2 must be present from the initiation of culture to generate a cytotoxic response. When the addition of IL-2 or IL-6 to culture was delayed

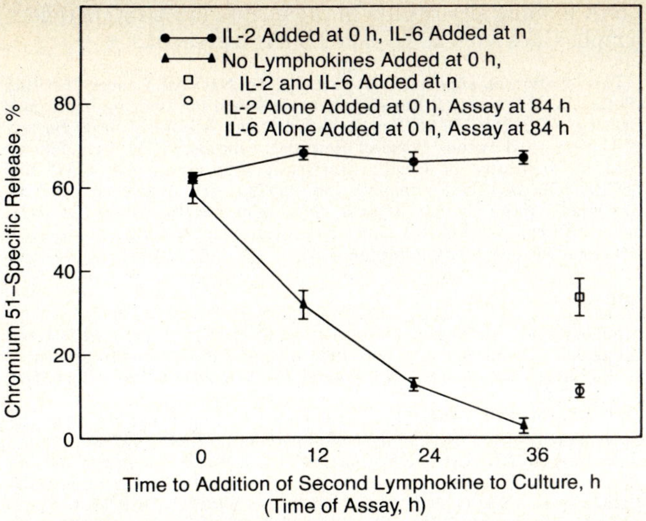

Fig 4.—Effect of delayed addition of lymphokine to C57BL/6 thymocytes plus concanavalin A. Assays measured lysis of chromium 51–labeled P815 tumor cells after 84 hours of total culture time. Bars indicate arithmetic mean ± SD; IL-2, interleukin 2; and IL-6, interleukin 6 ($P<.01$ for all points by Student's *t* test).

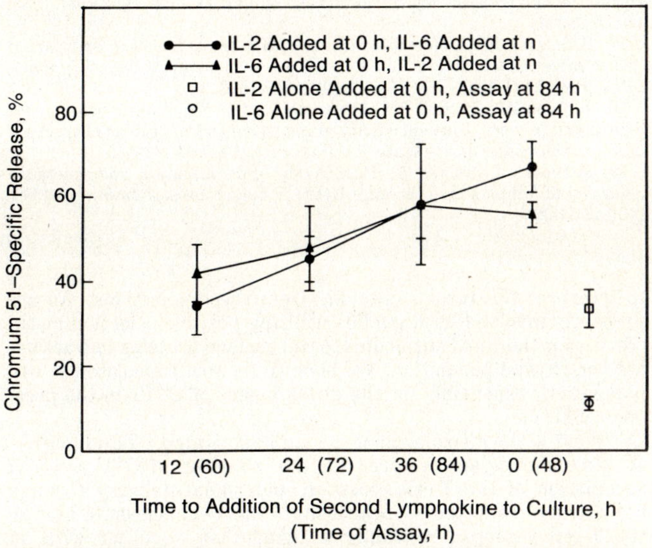

Fig 5.—Effect of sequence of lymphokine addition on cytotoxic T-lymphocyte generation. Total culture time in presence of interleukin 2 (IL-2) plus interleukin 6 (IL-6) was 48 hours. Total length of culture varied, as indicated in parentheses, from 48 to 84 hours. Bars indicate arithmetic mean ± SD ($P<.01$ for all points by Student's *t* test).

12 or more hours, and the level of response was determined 48 hours after lymphokine addition, a CTL response of less than 5% lysis was observed (Fig 3). Figure 4 shows that addition of IL-2 and IL-6 together at 0, 12, 24, or 36 hours after the onset of culture with assay of cytotoxic activity at 84 hours resulted in 59%, 32%, 13%, and 3% lysis, respectively. Thus, delay of lymphokine addition for 12 hours resulted in significantly diminished CTL response. We then asked if both lymphokines must be present during thymocyte culture to prevent loss of lytic ability. The addition of IL-2 at the initiation of culture with IL-6 added 12, 24, or 36 hours later resulted in a response ranging from 45% to 67% (Fig 3). Cultures incubated with IL-2 or IL-6 alone for 84 hours resulted in 34% and 11% lysis, respectively (Fig 3). The levels of cytotoxicity for thymocytes cultured with IL-2 from the onset of culture with IL-6 added 0, 12, 24, and 36 hours later were all approximately 66% when assayed at 84 hours (Fig 4). Thus, thymocytes cultured in the absence of lymphokine quickly became nonresponsive, while thymocytes cultured with IL-2 became maximally responsive provided that IL-6 was added 48 hours before assay for cytotoxicity (Fig 4).

Experiments completed to this point indicated that thymocytes cultured in the absence of IL-2 for more than 12 hours were unresponsive to the cytotoxicity-generating effects of subsequent culture in IL-2 plus IL-6. We asked if maintenance of the thymocyte's ability to respond was dependent on culturing in IL-2, or if IL-6 would also satisfy the requirement for added lymphokine. Thymocytes were cultured in IL-2 or IL-6 and the complementary lymphokine added at 0, 12, 24, or 36 hours, with cytotoxicity determined 48 hours after addition of the second lymphokine. The addition of the complementary lymphokine at the different time points resulted in a CTL response ranging from 40% to 60% (Fig 5). Thymocytes cultured for 84 hours with either IL-2 or IL-6 alone gave 34% and 11% lysis, respectively. Thus, either IL-2 or IL-6 maintained lectin-triggered thymocytes in an active state and these thymocytes were able to generate a CTL response, provided the complementary lymphokine was added (Fig 5).

COMMENT

Recent studies indicate that a differentiation factor is required for thymic precursors to respond to IL-2 and give rise to functional CTL.[6-10] The evidence that IL-6 can support the differentiation of T cells into active CTL was obtained using a 48-hour culture of thymocytes triggered with ConA.[7,8] A long-term goal of these studies is to define the lymphokine requirements controlling the T-cell response to antigen. In this investigation, our first question was to determine if IL-6 was required when thymocytes were cultured for more than 48 hours in the presence of IL-2. Our results show that the response generated by IL-2 (20 U/mL) plus IL-6 (100 ng/mL) added at the beginning of culture was greater than the response generated with IL-2 alone for all time points tested between 48 and 84 hours (Fig 2). With increasing lengths of culture time (≥96 hours), the response to IL-2 alone approached that found for the combination of IL-2 and IL-6 (data not shown). Thus, for short culture periods, a very limited CTL response was found unless IL-6 was added. The generation of CTL on longer culture in the presence of IL-2 alone may indicate that, given sufficient culture time, non–IL-2 lymphokines are generated when thymocytes are cultured with IL-2, or a small population of cells respond to IL-2 alone and these cells proliferate during longer cultures to match the cytotoxicity generated by adding the combination of lymphokines. In other studies we found that for 48-hour cultures, a half-maximal CTL response was obtained with approximately 250 pmol/L of IL-6. Since many different cell types are able to produce IL-6,[16] it is possible that during extended periods of incubation sufficient IL-6 is produced to support the generation of CTL. Defining the exact lymphokine requirements for CTL generation under all culture conditions will require the ability to block the effects of specific lymphokines through the use of blocking antibodies or the development of specific antagonists.

Culturing of cloned cytotoxic T cells in the presence of

ConA alone has been shown to result in blocking of both antigen-specific and lectin-dependent cytotoxicity.[17] Our results indicate that culture of thymocytes in the presence of ConA but in the absence of added lymphokines results in thymocytes that are unable to become cytotoxic. In contrast, culturing in either IL-2 or IL-6 alone, while unable to generate a high-level CTL response, prevents the unresponsiveness to later addition of the complementary lymphokine. It appears that triggering thymocytes through the antigen-specific T-cell receptor or some other ConA binding site results in thymocyte inactivation unless lymphokines such as IL-2 or IL-6 are present.[17-19]

This study was supported in part by the National Cancer Institute (Bethesda, Md) National Research Service Award for Training in Surgical Oncology, T32 CA09535-04 (Drs Stringfellow and Wilson); Ethicon–Society of University Surgeons Surgical Research Fellowship (Dr Stringfellow); National Institutes of Health (Bethesda, Md) grants CA 47831 and SO7RR05526-24 (Dr Herrmann) and AI17258 (Dr Burakoff); and the American Cancer Society (Atlanta, Ga) Junior Faculty Award (Dr Herrmann). Human recombinant IL-6 was provided by Steven C. Clark, PhD, Genetics Institute Inc, Cambridge, Mass.

References

1. Klarnet JP, Matis LA, Kern DE, et al: Antigen-driven T cell clones can proliferate in vivo, eradicate disseminated leukemia, and provide specific immunologic memory. *J Immunol* 1987;138:4012-4017.
2. Shu S, Chou T, Rosenberg SA: Generation from tumor-bearing mice of lymphocytes with in vivo therapeutic efficacy. *J Immunol* 1987;139:295-304.
3. Mulé JJ, Yang JC, Afreniere RL, et al: Identification of cellular mechanisms operational in vivo during the regression of established pulmonary metastases by the systemic administration of high-dose recombinant interleukin 2. *J Immunol* 1987;139:285-294.
4. Shu S, Chou T, Rosenberg SA: In vitro differentiation of T-cells capable of mediating the regression of established syngeneic tumors in mice. *Cancer Res* 1987;47:1354-1360.
5. Wagner H, Rollinghoff M: T-T cell interactions during in vitro cytotoxic allograft responses: I. Soluble products from activated Ly1⁺ cells trigger autonomously antigen primed Ly23⁺ T cells to cell proliferation and cytotoxic activity. *J Exp Med* 1978;148:1523-1538.
6. Kern DE, Gillis S, Okada M, et al: The role of interleukin-2 (IL-2) in the differentiation of cytotoxic T cells: The effect of monoclonal anti-IL-2 antibody and adsorption with IL-2 dependent cell lines. *J Immunol* 1981; 127:1323-1328.
7. Takai Y, Herrmann SH, Greenstein JL, et al: Requirements for three distinct lymphokines for the induction of cytotoxic T lymphocytes from thymocytes. *J Immunol* 1986;137:3494-3500.
8. Takai Y, Wong GG, Clark SC, et al: B cell stimulatory factor-2 is involved in the differentiation of cytotoxic T lymphocytes. *J Immunol* 1988; 140:508-512.
9. Raulet DH, Bevan MJ: A differentiation factor required for the expression of cytotoxic T-cell function. *Nature* 1982;296:754-757.
10. Takatsu K, Kikuchi Y, Kanatani T, et al: Generation of cytotoxic T lymphocytes from thymocyte precursors to trinitrophenyl-modified self antigens: I. Requirement of both killer-helper factor(s) and interleukin-2 for CTL generation from a subpopulation of thymocytes. *J Immunol* 1986; 136:1161-1170.
11. Widmer MB, Grabstein KH: Regulation of cytotoxic T-lymphocyte generation by B-cell stimulatory factor. *Nature* 1987;326:795-798.
12. Garman RD, Jacobs KA, Clark SC, et al: B-cell-stimulatory factor 2 (β_2 interferon) functions as a second signal for interleukin 2 production by mature murine T cells. *Proc Natl Acad Sci USA* 1987;84:7629-7633.
13. Uyttenhove C, Coulie PG, Van Snick J: T cell growth and differentiation induced by interleukin-HP1/IL-6, the murine hybridoma/plasmacytoma growth factor. *J Exp Med* 1988;167:1417-1427.
14. Wagner H, Hardt C, Rouse BT, et al: Dissection of the proliferative and differentiative signals controlling murine cytotoxic T lymphocyte responses. *J Exp Med* 1982;155:1876-1881.
15. Lotz M, Jirik F, Kabouridis P, et al: B cell stimulating factor 2/ interleukin 6 is a costimulant for human thymocytes and T lymphocytes. *J Exp Med* 1988;167:1253-1258.
16. Wong GG, Witek-Giannotti JS, Temple PA, et al: Stimulation of murine hemopoietic colony formation by human IL-6. *J Immunol* 1988; 140:3040-3044.
17. Sitkovsky MV, Pasternak MS, Lugo JP, et al: Isolation and partial characterization of concanavalin A receptors on cloned cytotoxic T lymphocytes. *Proc Natl Acad Sci USA* 1984;81:1519-1523.
18. Jenkins MK, Pardoll DM, Mizuguchi J, et al: T-cell unresponsiveness in vivo and in vitro: Fine specificity of induction and molecular characterization of the unresponsive state. *Immunol Rev* 1987;95:113-135.
19. Mizuochi T, Singer A: Intrathymic differentiation and tolerance induction of lymphokine-secreting Lyt2⁺ T helper cells. *J Immunol* 1988; 140:1421-1424.

Discussion

Q Is the IL-2 generating CTL in a maturation pathway separate from that of IL-6?

A It has been suggested that in low doses such as those used in this study, IL-2 is responsible for maintaining the viability and stimulating the proliferation of T cells in vitro. Interleukin 6 was initially found to be an inducer of B-cell differentiation, and it is possible this lymphokine is also responsible for the differentiation of CTL precursors. If CTL generation is best accomplished by proliferation of a precursor population as an initial step, and then secondary differentiation of these cells to functional CTLs, then we would expect cells cultured in IL-2, followed by IL-6 at a later time, to generate greater CTL response than the cells that were presented lymphokine in the reverse order. Our results suggest that a synergy exists between IL-2 and IL-6 in the production of CTLs from thymocytes.

Q Are there any ways of determining by phenotypic markers that individual subsets of cells are being driven to become functional CTLs?

A One of the most difficult problems in CTL research is the identification and purification of T-cell subsets on the basis of phenotypic markers. Methods of selection available at this time use antibodies to cell surface proteins such as CD4 and CD8, but as these molecules also play a role in T-cell activation it is difficult to interpret the results obtained from these selections. We are presently involved with studies utilizing positive selection methods with monoclonal antibodies to cell surface proteins to fractionate the thymic population. We hope to be able to isolate the cell population responsible for the development of CTLs in the presence of IL-6.

Q What is the mechanism of the lectin-activated CTL killing?

A Two signals are required for the induction of CTL activity: stimulation of the T-cell receptor, and signal delivery through lymphokine receptors. Concanavalin A has been shown to bind to the T-cell receptor, providing a signal that, together with an appropriate lymphokine, results in antigen nonspecific target cell lysis. Concanavalin A also binds many other cell surface molecules, and the importance of this for CTL generation is not known. We have shown in other studies that CTLs generated in this lectin-dependent manner release serine esterase during target cell lysis, therefore correlating with antigen-specific target cell lysis with esterase release. We have also found that when irradiated allogeneic murine thymocytes are used instead of ConA to stimulate the T-cell receptor, the pattern of CTL activity in response to IL-2 and IL-6 is similar to that seen with ConA stimulation. This indicates that the ability of IL-6 to support the generation of CTL is not limited to triggering the T-cell receptor through lectin.

Natural Killer Sensitivity of Colorectal Carcinoma Targets

Correlation With Degree of Differentiation

Darius J. Bägli, MD, CM; Glenn D. Steele, Jr, MD, PhD; Teresa Barlozzari, PhD

• Lymphocytes with natural killer (NK) ability recognize a wide range of target cells; however, the mediators of specific target recognition are still largely unknown. Despite the diversity of the NK target repertoire, it is typified by cells of relatively immature phenotype. The purpose of this study was to determine if colorectal carcinoma (CRC) targets were sensitive to spontaneous lysis by fresh human NK effector cells and to observe the role of CRC differentiation in this process. Results demonstrated that poorly differentiated CRC targets were susceptible to NK-mediated lysis whereas CRC targets with more differentiated structure were NK resistant. In addition, chemical induction of a more mature CRC phenotype confers NK resistance on a previously NK-susceptible target. This maturation-related modulation of NK sensitivity can provide a model with which to further study interaction between NK cells and CRC targets.

(*Arch Surg* 1989;124:89-93)

Lymphocytes possessing natural killer (NK) activity are unique in their ability to spontaneously lyse a wide range of normal, infected, or malignant and metastatic cell targets.[1] However, the structures mediating specific target recognition are still largely unknown, both for the NK cells and the targets themselves. Immunochemical techniques have demonstrated the importance of some molecules involved in NK activity. These include the glycoprotein LFA-1, a surface component of many different leukocytes involved in cell-cell adhesion. Monoclonal antibodies directed against LFA-1 on the surface of NK and cytotoxic T lymphocytes have been shown to abrogate the cytotoxic potential of these effector cells.[2] In humans and animals, molecules functionally related to the extracellular matrix glycoprotein laminin have been linked to processes of NK target recognition.[3-5] The implication of both these structures can be reconciled with their principal role as adhesion molecules, since the formation of a stable conjugate between the NK cell and its target is the first requirement for natural killing.[6] In addition, monoclonal antibodies against the T-200 glycoproteins[7] and GM_1 glycolipids have similarly implicated these molecules in NK function.

Despite the variety of NK-susceptible target cells and the heterogeneity of the molecules possibly involved in their recognition by NK cells, they do possess certain features in common. These include rapid growth and relatively immature phenotypes.[1,8] Indeed, these features are typical of tumor cells. However, they also describe some otherwise normal cells that constitute NK targets, such as immature thymocytes and bone marrow cells.[9] It is the NK susceptibility of these latter immature cells that has suggested a role for NK cells in regulating some hematopoietic processes in vivo.[10] On maturation, the NK susceptibility associated with human myeloid and lymphoid precursors is lost.[9] Similarly, in a study of murine teratoma, clones representing later stages of development with relative lack of embryonal surface antigens were virtually resistant to NK cytolysis.[11]

Developing this concept further, attempts to induce maturation of NK targets by chemical agents have met with successes. The well-studied NK target K-562 (a human erythroleukemia), when treated with the potent differentiating agent sodium butyrate, resulted in the induction of a number of differentiation markers. In addition, a striking resistance to NK lysis[12] was observed. Similar findings have been reported for other NK targets such as the human histiocytic lymphoma line U-937 treated with tetradecanoyl phorbol acetate, and the murine erythroid stem line GM-86 treated with hexametabisacetamide.[13] In both cases, significant native NK susceptibility was abrogated after treatment with unrelated agents that induced changes associated with a more mature phenotype.

In the case of solid tumors as well, chemical agents have been successfully employed to induce maturation. Agents such as sodium butyrate, tretinoin (retinoic acid), and polar solvents (dimethyl sulfoxide and dimethylformamide) have been used to differentiate murine melanoma,[14] mammary and rhabdomyosarcoma,[15] and human colorectal carcinoma (CRC) cell lines.[16-19] As a group, however, solid tumors have generally proved to be poor targets for natural unstimulated cytotoxicity.[20] The NK potential inherent in normal peripheral blood lymphocytes (PBLs) becomes significant against solid tumors only in the presence of interleukin 2.[21] Furthermore, little information about the relationship between the preexisting or induced maturational state of solid tumors and NK susceptibility is available.

The goals of the present study were to establish whether human CRC could act as targets for the spontaneous NK effectors, and whether the stage of CRC differentiation could influence their susceptibility to NK-mediated lysis. Results showed that the three CRC targets representing poor or early states of differentiation were sensitive to NK lysis, whereas the three CRC targets representing better or more mature stages of differentiation were insensitive to lysis by NK cells. Furthermore, the significant NK susceptibility of the poorly differentiated CRC targets

Accepted for publication Sept 15, 1988.

From the Laboratory of Cancer Biology, Department of Surgery, New England Deaconess Hospital and Harvard Medical School, Boston.

Read before the Annual Meeting of the Society of Surgical Oncology, New Orleans, May 23, 1988.

Reprint requests to Department of Surgery, Harvard Medical School, New England Deaconess Hospital, 50 Binney St, Boston, MA 02115 (Dr Bägli).

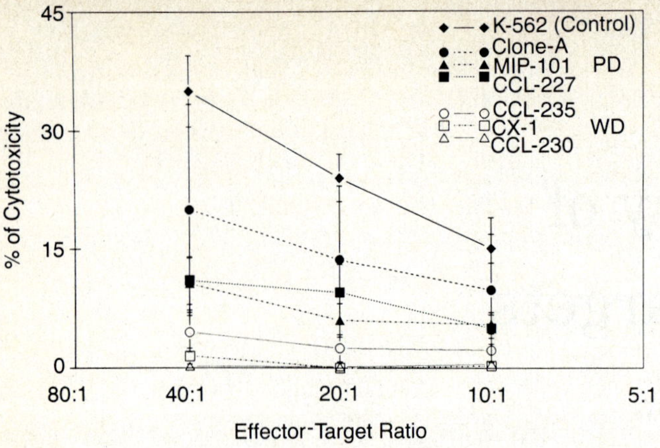

Fig 1.—Lysis of colorectal carcinoma (CRC) targets by peripheral blood lymphocytes. Results represent mean ± SD of four experiments performed in quadruplicate. WD indicates well-differentiated CRC; PD, poorly differentiated CRC (for K-562, $P<.01$).

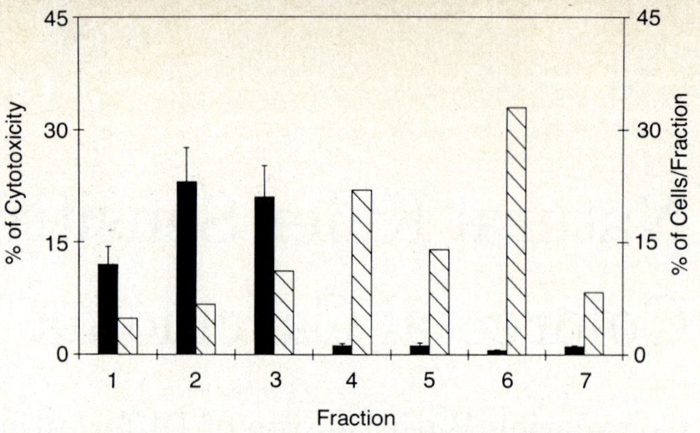

Fig 2.—Discontinuous inert silica compound (Percoll) gradient enrichment of large granular lymphocytes from peripheral blood lymphocytes. Lymphocytes harvested from each layer of Percoll gradients were employed in cytotoxicity assays with K-562. Striped bars indicate percent of total lymphocytes in fraction; solid bars, percent of specific cytotoxicity obtained from lymphocytes in each fraction at effector-target ratio of 40:1.

could be virtually eliminated after treatment of the targets with a chemical differentiating agent.

METHODS

Cell Lines

Colorectal carcinoma cell lines clone-A, MIP-101, CCL-227, CCL-235, CX-1, CCL-230, and the human erythroleukemia line K-562 were maintained in RPMI-1640 medium (GIBCO, Grand Island, NY) supplemented with 10% heat-inactivated fetal calf serum (Hazelton, Dutchland, Penn), 100 U/mL of penicillin (GIBCO), and 2 mmol/L of L-glutamine (GIBCO) referred to as "culture medium." Cells were passaged three times per week. All lines were tested free of mycoplasma by the Hoechst stain (Sigma Chemical Co, St Louis) for mycoplasmal RNA.

Preparation of PBLs and Large Granular Lymphocytes (LGLs)

Fresh human PBLs were obtained from the peripheral blood of healthy donors by Ficoll-Hypaque sedimentation. Cells were washed with Hanks' balanced salt solution (GIBCO) and monocyte/macrophage populations were removed by adherence on glass flasks. After passage through nylon wool columns, the nonadherent cells were fractionated by centrifugation on discontinuous gradients of an inert silica compound (Percoll, Pharmacia, Uppsala, Sweden) as described elsewhere.[22] Briefly, seven different fractions of Percoll (40.8%, 43%, 45.8%, 48.3%, 50.8%, 53.3%, and 66.6% in culture medium) were prepared. Lymphocytes harvested from the second and third low-density layers were pooled and used as LGLs throughout. The LGL structure was confirmed by Giemsa staining (Fischer).

Chemical Treatment With Differentiating Agent

The MIP-101 and clone-A cells were grown in culture medium in the presence or absence of 2 mmol/L of sodium butyrate (Sigma) for 14 days prior to placing in cytotoxicity assays. Cell viability for both the treated and untreated cells was assessed to be greater than 90% by trypan blue exclusion.

Cytotoxicity Assays

Target cells, 5×10^6, harvested by rubber policeman, were labeled with 300 μCi of sodium labeled with chromium 51 tetraoxide ($Na^{51}CrO_4$) (New England Nuclear, Boston) for 45 minutes at 37°C in medium with 5% fetal calf serum. Cells were washed twice, allowed to sit for 30 minutes at room temperature to reduce final spontaneous release, and washed again. Then 100 μL to labeled target cells per well at a concentration of 1×10^5/mL was plated in quadruplicate in 96-well, round-bottom, tissue culture plates (Costar); 100 μL of effectors was plated at effector-target (E/T) ratios of 40:1, 20:1, and 10:1. Plates were incubated for four hours at 37°C in 5% carbon dioxide/95% oxygen. Then 100 μL per well was harvested and counted. Spontaneous release and total release were determined by adding 100 μL of medium or 6 mol/L of hydrochloridic acid, respectively, in lieu of effectors, to target cell wells. Spontaneous release did not exceed 15%. Mean specific percent cytotoxicity was determined by the following formula:

Cytotoxicity = {[(Experimental cpm − Spontaneous Release cpm)]/[(Total Release cpm − Spontaneous Release)]} × 100.

Any target showing significant improvement in lysis (>15% cytotoxicity) with LGL as effectors was interpreted as being an NK-susceptible target.

Statistical Analysis

Data were analyzed using the Student *t* test.

RESULTS

PBL Cytotoxicity

Peripheral blood lymphocytes were tested for cytotoxicity against six different CRC cell lines (Fig 1). The human erythroleukemia cell line K-562, the classic target for NK cytotoxicity, was used as the control. The six CRC targets consisted of three poorly differentiated lines (clone-A, MIP-101, CCL-227) and three well-differentiated lines (CCL-235, CX-1, CCL-230). With fresh human PBLs, only the control line, K-562, was significantly killed (35% at an E/T ratio of 40:1 [Fig 1]). Even with an E/T ratio of 40:1, only low-level (<15%) cytotoxicity was seen for the CRC targets. However, all six targets showed significant cytotoxicity when PBL effectors were first stimulated with Hr–interleukin 2 (data not shown).

Effect of Enrichment for NK Activity on CRC Target Lysis (PBLs vs LGLs)

To test whether CRC could truly act as natural targets, as was suggested above by the small degree of lysis achieved with fresh unstimulated PBLs, LGLs were employed as effectors in cytotoxicity assays along with PBLs. The NK activity within the PBL population is known to exist predominantly in the subpopulation of LGLs. The effect of PBL enrichment for LGLs was demonstrated first in cytotoxicity assays against K-562, the classic NK target (Fig 2). Most of the NK activity was harvested as LGLs from the Percoll fractions of 43% and 45.8%, representing the second and third layers of the discontinuous Percoll gradients employed (Fig 2). This represents a significant improvement in cytotoxicity (PBLs alone, 16%; LGL fractions 2 and 3, 45% [Fig 3]). When PBLs and LGLs from the same donor were compared for their cytotoxic ability against the six CRC targets, an interesting stratification

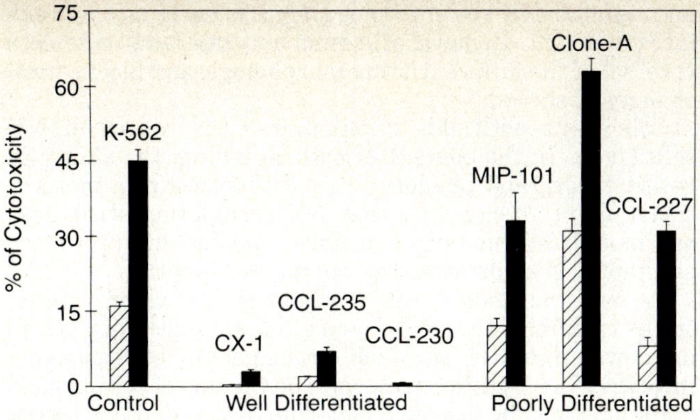

Fig 3.—Lysis of colorectal carcinoma by large granular lymphocytes (LGLs) and peripheral blood lymphocytes (PBLs). Effector-target ratio is 40:1. Peripheral blood lymphocytes and large granular lymphocytes (natural killer–enriched cells) were obtained from same donor for any single target cell line. Similar results were obtained for effector-target ratios of 20:1 and 10:1. Results (±SD) are representative of four assays in quadruplicate. Striped bars indicate percent of cytotoxicity by PBLs; solid bars, percent of cytotoxicity by LGLs (for poorly differentiated targets: PBLs vs LGLs, $P<.005$).

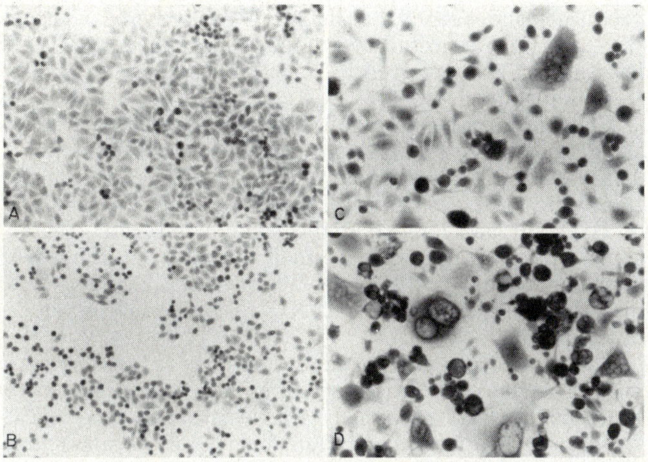

Fig 4.—Normal and sodium butyrate–treated MIP-101 and clone-A colorectal carcinoma. Top left, MIP-101; bottom left, clone-A; top right, MIP-101 after 14 day's culture in 2 mmol/L of sodium butyrate; bottom right, clone-A after 14 days' culture in 2 mmol/L of sodium butyrate (periodic acid–Schiff, ×250).

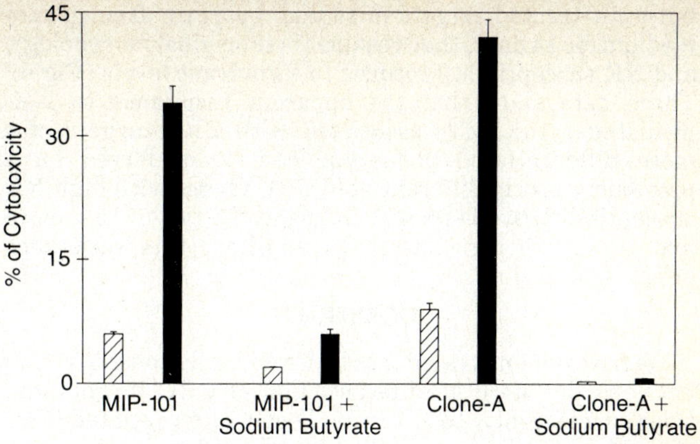

Fig 5.—Effect of sodium butyrate treatment on poorly differentiated colorectal carcinoma susceptibility to natural cytotoxicity; colorectal carcinoma cultures were supplemented with 2 mmol/L of sodium butyrate for 14 days, washed, and used in cytotoxicity assays. Effector-target ratio is 40:1. Similar results were obtained for effector-target ratios of 20:1 and 10:1. Results (±SD) are representative of four experiments in quadruplicate. Striped bars indicate percent of cytotoxicity by peripheral blood lymphocytes; solid bars, percent of cytotoxicity by large granular lymphocytes (for large granular lymphocytes, control vs sodium butyrate treatment, $P<.005$).

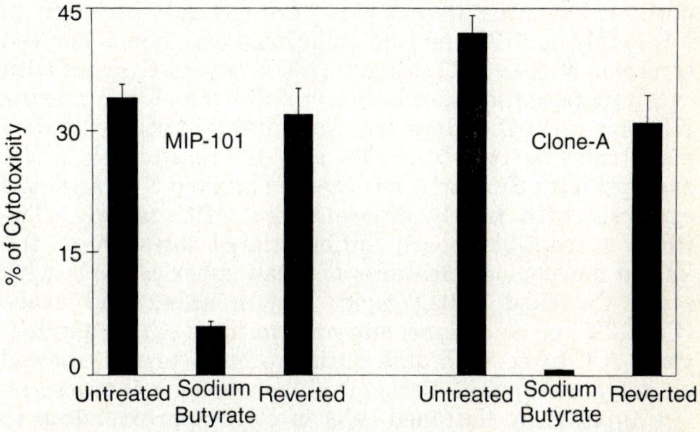

Fig 6.—Reversibility of sodium butyrate–induced natural killer resistance of poorly differentiated colorectal carcinoma treated with 2 mmol/L of sodium butyrate were grown in sodium butyrate–free medium for 14 days prior to use as targets in cytotoxicity assays. Effector-target ratio is 40:1. Similar results were obtained for effector-target ratios of 20:1 and 10:1. Solid bars indicate percent of cytotoxicity by large granular lymphocytes (large granular lymphocytes, control or reverted vs sodium butyrate treatment, $P<.005$).

was observed (Fig 3). Against all three poorly differentiated targets, the enrichment for NK activity produced LGL cytotoxicities that were significant. In contrast, none of the better differentiated targets showed any significant improvement in cytotoxicity with the use of LGLs as effectors, thus revealing them to be NK-resistant targets. These data suggest that an inverse relationship exists between the state of differentiation of CRC targets and their susceptibility to NK-mediated lysis by effector lymphocytes.

Effect of Chemically Induced Differentiation on NK Cytotoxicity

The following experiments determined whether the relationship between NK susceptibility and differentiation state of the targets observed could be preserved and demonstrated with targets in two different states of differentiation. The poorly differentiated targets MIP-101 and clone-A were treated with sodium butyrate, which is recognized as a potent inducer of differentiation in many cellular systems. After 14 days of treatment with 2 mmol/L of sodium butyrate, MIP-101 and clone-A cells underwent a number of characteristic maturational changes in growth rate, morphology, and metabolism (Fig 4 and "Comment" section). Also, sodium butyrate did not affect cell viability as confirmed by trypan blue exclusion. Both untreated and sodium butyrate–treated MIP-101 and clone-A cells were subjected to cytotoxicity assays with PBLs and LGLs (Fig 5). Neither the untreated nor the treated targets showed any significant cytotoxicity with PBLs as effectors. With LGLs as effectors, both untreated targets showed significant lysis as described earlier. After sodium butyrate treatment of the targets cells, however, no significant NK cytotoxicity remained for either target with LGLs as effectors (Fig 5). The pattern of killing of MIP-101 and clone-A cells after chemical differentiation by sodium butyrate now paralleled that of the well-differentiated lines described above. After culture of the sodium butyrate–treated targets in sodium butyrate–free culture medium for 14 days, they resume their original morphology, and NK susceptibility returns to significant levels (Fig 6). These data show that the apparent resistance to NK-mediated cytotoxicity associated with CRC targets of a more differentiated phenotype can be conferred on a previously poorly differentiated CRC target with high NK susceptibility by chemically inducing the target to a more mature morphologic state. In addition, this resistance effect is reversible.

COMMENT

We have demonstrated that an inverse relationship exists between the state of differentiation of CRC targets and their susceptibility to NK lysis. Poorly differentiated CRC showed marked susceptibility to NK cell-mediated lysis, whereas the well-differentiated CRC targets were NK resistant. Furthermore, the chemical induction of a more mature phenotype in two of these CRC also induces a resistance to NK cytolysis, implying that NK susceptibility is truly dependent on the phenotype of the target.

These observations are consistent with previous findings that have demonstrated that NK susceptibility is significantly influenced by the relative phenotype of the target. Murine thymocytes from very young animals (5 days old) showed maximal NK sensitivity in standard cytolytic assays. This sensitivity fell directly with increasing age until, at 7 months, thymocytes were virtually resistant to NK cytolysis.[13] The murine embryonal carcinoma–derived teratoma Nulli-SCC.1 is a highly NK-sensitive target with cytolytic potential approaching that of the classic murine NK target, YAC.[11] However, more differentiated endodermal strains derived from the same 129 teratoma lose NK susceptibility. Similarly, we observed marked NK-mediated cytolysis with poorly differentiated CRC targets. The three susceptible poorly differentiated lines share the known morphologic features of small spherical cells with some flattened cells, rapid growth rate, and trace (CCL-227) or no carcinoembryonic antigen (CEA) production. All three well-differentiated lines tested showed slower growth rates, recognized morphologic characteristics typified by flattened cells in close approximation to one another in monolayer cultures, and marked CEA production. These well-differentiated targets proved resistant to NK lysis.

This differentiation-related NK susceptibility was further analyzed by controlled differentiation of poorly differentiated NK-susceptible targets. When treated with sodium butyrate, the human NK target K-562 undergoes several maturational changes. K-562 is a leukemic stem line expressing few embryonic and fetal markers.[12] Culture in sodium butyrate increases endogenous peroxidaselike activity, slows growth rate, and significantly (50%) decreases NK-mediated lysis. The NK resistance was dose dependent and reversible. In addition, several K-562 subclones were also protected from NK lysis after sodium butyrate treatment, thus demonstrating that the differentiation-related changes in NK sensitivity were not an aberrant response of any single subclone.[12] Sodium butyrate treatment of the poorly differentiated CRC targets MIP-101 and clone-A produced similar results. Maturational changes included a decrease in growth rate, increase in cell size accompanied by increasingly fibroblastoid morphology and formation of mucin-containing vacuoles evidenced by periodic acid–Schiff staining. While neither target is a constitutive producer of CEA, this marker became detectable in culture medium after one to two weeks of sodium butyrate treatment (data not shown). When tested after two weeks of sodium butyrate treatment, NK sensitivity for both MIP-101 and clone-A was virtually lost. Similar NK resistance occurred as early as one week into treatment. Removal of sodium butyrate led to complete reversal of the differentiating morphologic and biochemical changes observed.

Coincident with this reversal was the return of NK sensitivity. In the context of natural killing, the ability to revert to original phenotype on withdrawal of a maturational agent[17,23] suggests that NK recognition structures are modulated on target surfaces during differentiation and that this modulation can be induced in vitro.

To our knowledge, the mechanism by which altered states of differentiation influence NK susceptibility is still unknown. However, any such mechanism must reasonably involve NK recognition molecules on the target cell surface. Sialic acid may be one such molecule involved in NK target recognition. Neuraminidase-accessible cell surface sialic acid shows an inverse correlation with NK sensitivity in sodium butyrate–differentiated K-562 cells.[24] Similar NK resistance correlating with increased sialic acid has been reported after interferon treatment of several murine cell targets.[25,26]

Chemical differentiation by sodium butyrate is known to affect cellular, membrane-associated,[16] and secreted[23] CEA levels. Surface CEA levels have been positively correlated with NK susceptibility in human carcinoma.[27] However, all three well-differentiated CRC in this study are CEA producers and were NK resistant. Furthermore, whether the trace CEA secreted by the butyrate-induced CRC cell line targets was involved in their NK resistance remains to be determined.

The involvement of major histocompatibility complex antigens in NK activity has recently been suggested.[28-30] These antigens are markers of cellular differentiation. In this study, the native clone-A target showed no expression of HLA-DR antigen while the sodium butyrate–treated clone-A targets showed a small increase in HLA-DR expression (data not shown). Whether this increase was directly associated with the NK resistance observed is unknown.

Finally, transfection techniques employing transforming oncogenes have demonstrated that NK cells are able to recognize and kill previously NK-resistant murine or rat fibroblasts that have been transformed to the malignant phenotype by c-Ha-*ras*[31] or v-Ki-*ras*,[32] respectively. Whether oncogene-associated NK sensitivity plays any role in the differentiation-related NK susceptibilities seen in this study remains to be determined. Investigation of a role for an activated or mutated *ras*-p21 protein product in this context would be of great interest.

In summary, we have shown that the NK susceptibility of CRC targets is dependent on the CRC state of differentiation. These observations are reconciled by similar descriptions in other tumor systems. Furthermore, the chemical differentiation of CRC targets to a more mature phenotype confers on them the NK resistance shared by well-differentiated CRC. As understanding of the NK target repertoire increases, the ability to induce reversible maturation-related alterations in NK sensitivity in this disease can provide a controlled model with which to study the processes that mediate interaction between NK cells and CRC.

This investigation was supported in part by grants P01 CA 44704-01 and CA-09280 from the National Institutes of Health, Bethesda, Md (Dr Bägli).

The authors wish to thank Barbara Wolf, MD, for assistance with the pathology review of the cell preparations.

References

1. Trichieri G, Perussia B: Biology of disease: Human natural killer cells: Biologic and pathologic aspects. *Lab Invest* 1984;50:489-513.

2. Schmidt R, Bartley G, Levine H, et al: Functional characterization of

LFA-1 antigens in the interaction of human NK clones and target cells. *J Immunol* 1985;135:1020-1025.
3. Hiserodt J: NK receptors and target antigens involved in cytotoxicity. *Nat Immun Cell Growth Regul* 1988;7:57-58.
4. Hiserodt J, Laybourn K, Varani J: Expression of a laminin-like substance on the surface of murine natural killer (NK) lymphocytes and its role in the NK recognition of tumor target cells. *J Immunol* 1985;135:1484-1487.
5. Hiserodt J, Reynolds C: Selective expression of laminin on rat large granular lymphocytes and its role in NK recognition of tumor cells, in Bonavide B, Collier RJ (eds): *Membrane Mediated Cytotoxicity.* New York, Alan R Liss Inc, 1987, pp 515-523.
6. Hiserodt J, Britvan L, Targan S: Characterization of the cytolytic reaction mechanism of the human natural killer (NK) lymphocyte: Resolution into binding, programming and killer-cell independent steps. *J Immunol* 1982;129:782-787.
7. Newman W, Fast L, Rose L: Blockade of NK cell lysis is a property of monoclonal antibodies that bind to distinct regions of T-200. *J Immunol* 1983;131:1742-1747.
8. Golden M, Dempsey RA, Mier JW, et al: The effect of differentiation inducers on the sensitivity of two myeloid cell lines to natural killer (NK) cell-mediated lysis. *Int J Immunopharmacol* 1983;5:411-419.
9. Hannson M, Kiessling R, Andersson B: Human fetal thymus and bone marrow contains target cells for natural killer cells. *Eur J Immunol* 1981;11:8.
10. Barlozzari T, Herberman RB, Reynolds C: Inhibition of pluripotent hematopoietic stem cells of bone marrow by large granular lymphocytes. *Proc Natl Acad Sci USA* 1987;84:7691-7695.
11. Stern P, Gidlund M, Orn A, et al: Natural killer cells mediate lysis of embryonal carcinoma cells lacking MHC. *Nature* 1980;285:341-342.
12. Dokhelar M-C, Testa U, Vainehenker W, et al: NK sensitivity of the leukemic K-562 cells: Effect of sodium butyrate and hemin induction. *J Immunol* 1982;129:211-216.
13. Gidlund M, Orn A, Pattergale PK, et al: Natural killer cells kill tumor cells at a given stage of differentiation. *Nature* 1981;292:848-850.
14. Deutsch V, Lotan R: Stimulation of sialyltransferase activity of melanoma cells by retinoic acid. *Exp Cell Res* 1983;149:237-245.
15. Calabresi P, Dexter D, Heppner G: Clinical and pharmacological implications of cancer cell differentiation and heterogeneity. *Biochem Pharmacol* 1979;28:1933-1941.
16. Tsao D, Shi Z, Wong A, et al: Effect of sodium butyrate on CEA antigen production by human colonic adenocarcinoma cells in culture. *Cancer Res* 1983;43:1217-1222.
17. Tsao D, Morita A, Bella A, et al: Differential effects of sodium butyrate, dimethyl sulfoxide and retinoic acid on membrane-associated antigen, enzymes and glycoproteins of human rectal adenocarcinoma cells. *Cancer Res* 1982;42:1052-1058.
18. Christensen TG, Burke B, Dextor D, et al: Ultrastructural evidence of dimethylformamide-induced differentiation of cultured human colon cancer cells. *Cancer* 1985;56:1559-1565.
19. Dexter D, Hager JC: Maturation-induction of tumor cells using a human colon carcinoma model. *Cancer* 1980;45:1178-1184.
20. Colotta F, Rambaldi A, Colombo N, et al: Effect of a streptococcal preparation (OK 432) on natural killer activity of tumor associated lymphoid cells in human ovarian carcinoma and on lysis of fresh ovarian tumor cells. *Br J Cancer* 1983;48:515-525.
21. Itoh K, Tilden A, Balch C: Lysis of human solid tumor cells by lymphokine-activated natural killer cells. *J Immunol* 1986;136:3910-3915.
22. Timonen T, Reynolds CW, Ortaldo JR, et al: *J Immunol Meth* 1982;51:269-277.
23. Niles RM, Wilhelm SA, Thomas P, et al: The effects of NB and retinoid acid on growth and CEA production in a series of human colorectal tumor cell lines representing different states of differentiation. *Cancer Invest* 1988;6:39-45.
24. Werkmeister JA, Pross HF, Roder JC: Modulation of K562 cells with sodium butyrate: Association of impaired NK sensitivity with sialic acid and analysis of other parameters. *Int J Cancer* 1983;32:71-78.
25. Yogeeswaran G, Gronberg A, Welsh R, et al: Interferon-induced increase in neuraminidase-releasable sialic acid and glycosphingolipid metabolism in mouse lymphoma and L1210 leukemia cell lines: Correlation with susceptibility to natural killer cell mediated lysis. *Int J Cancer* 1983;31:501-507.
26. Yogeeswaran G, Fujinami R, Kiessling R, et al: Interferon-induced alterations in sialic acid and glycoconjugates of L-929 cells. *Virology* 1982;121:363-371.
27. Clark D, McCulloch P, Lia S-K, et al: Sensitivity of human carcinoma cell lines to lysis by blood natural killer cells correlating with surface expression of CEA. *JNCI* 1984;72:505-512.
28. Storkus W, Howell D, Salter R, et al: NK susceptibility varies inversely with target cell class I HLA antigen. *J Immunol* 1987;138:1657-1659.
29. Kornbluth J, Spear B, Raab S, et al: Evidence for the role of class I and class II HLA antigens in the lytic function of a cloned line of human natural killer cells. *J Immunol* 1985;134:728-735.
30. Piontek G, Taniguchi K, Ljunggren H-G, et al: Yac-1 MHC class I variants reveal an association between decreased NK sensitivity and increased H-2 expression after interferon treatment or in vivo passage. *J Immunol* 1985;135:4281-4288.
31. Trimble W, Johnson P, Hozumi N, et al: Inducible cellular transformation by a metallothionein-ras hybrid oncogene leads to natural killer susceptibility. *Nature* 1986;321:782-784.
32. Johnson P, Baubock C, Roder J: Transfection of a rat cell line with the v-ki-*ras* oncogene is associated with enhanced susceptibility to natural killer cell lysis. *J Exp Med* 1985;162:1732-1737.

Discussion

Q Did you look at cell cycle distributions of your killer cells and of your well-differentiated and poorly differentiated tumor cells? In other words, could it be that your T cells in S phase are competing for a substrate and they die because they cannot?

A Yes, I see what you mean. We did not specifically look at the effect of cell cycle on the efficacy of killing by these cells, but in other tumor systems where sodium butyrate has been used to differentiate targets, particularly the classic NK target K-562, it was shown that the rate of growth, log phase vs plateau, did not affect the resistance that was conferred.

Q As everyone knows, in the NK lymphokine-activated killer area there are probably gradation effects, both quantitatively and qualitatively, of first the binding and then the killing event. Probably many of the functions we ascribe to lymphokine-activated killer cells are activated NK cells that are able to cross histocompatibility barriers to kill targets between different individuals or cells with different histologic types.

My question is: In comparing the cells that are poorly differentiated with those that are well differentiated, could part of the difference be related to the fragility of the poorly differentiated cells? I wonder if you saw some differences in the background lyses between these two groups of cells that may hint at least that those that are poorly differentiated may be more susceptible to lysis with less of a cytotoxic effect or less binding avidity of the cytotoxic cell. Have you tried these experiments with different doses of interleukin 2? Because, if this is simply a quantitative difference of receptor expression on the target that allows NK cells to bond to the more fragile cells, then you may be able to override that by preincubating the NK cells with interleukin 2 and see some degree of killing with the well-differentiated cells as well.

A In answer to the first question, we did not carry out specific studies measuring osmotic fragility of the targets. However, in terms of viabilities throughout the course of the experimental procedure, the ability to be labeled, the background spontaneous release of chromium, all of which indirectly speak to fragility, no differences were seen between the well-differentiated and poorly differentiated targets. Similarly, when the poorly differentiated targets were induced to differentiate chemically with sodium butyrate, they handled well and their viability was very good. With respect to interleukin 2, early on we did interleukin 2 activation in the experimental setup, both with the nonenriched PBL preparation as well as the LGLs, and in that case we did see significant lyses appearing for the well-differentiated targets. The poorly differentiated target lyses were even higher than the ones we saw herein. So certainly activation of these NK cells can render them more sensitive to a lower concentration of receptor on the surface of the target, as you mentioned.

Q It would appear paradoxic that if NK cells do have an in vivo role, then the cells that we would consider more of a problem, the poorly differentiated cells, would appear more susceptible to NK killing. Since we know that culture cells undergo a tremendous number of changes with time, have you looked at fresh tumor targets to see whether, in fact, these results are obtained in the natural situation?

A We have not looked at fresh tumor targets. That is an area that we would like to get into with this system. With respect to the apparent discrepancy between what is seen in terms of clinical prognosis with well-differentiated and poorly differentiated cells, it may be taking a great leap of faith to expect what is seen here to exactly mimic the clinical situation. However, you can see a parallel between these results and the incidence of the state of differentiation in pathologic specimens. The great minority of tumors are poorly differentiated, and this might be expected if you allow NK cells a role in early immune surveillance. The data that we showed today may parallel such a situation.

Cachectin Activity in the Serum of Cachectic, Tumor-Bearing Rats

Mark C. Stovroff, MD; Douglas L. Fraker, MD; Jeffrey A. Norton, MD

• Cachectin/tumor necrosis factor has been postulated to be a possible mediator of cancer cachexia. Using a sensitive bioassay, we attempted to detect circulating cachectin activity in the serum of sarcoma-bearing rats and to correlate levels with measurements of cachexia and the extent of disease. In addition, we resected the tumor to determine the time course of reversal of cachexia and the disappearance of cachectin activity in the serum. Circulating cachectin activity was not detectable in the serum of non–tumor-bearing rats or in tumor-bearing rats until 28 days after implantation. With evidence of food intake and body weight decline, cachectin activity became detectable in the serum and levels increased as cachexia and tumor burden increased. Serum cachectin activity levels correlated directly with tumor burden and inversely with food intake and body weight change. After resection of the tumor, food intake and body weight increased and serum cachectin activity became undetectable. Serum triglyceride levels were higher in cachectic tumor-bearing rats than in pair-fed non–tumor-bearing controls, and levels decreased after tumor resection as cachectin activity decreased. The results suggest that cachectin is a humoral mediator of cachexia in this rat-tumor model.

(*Arch Surg* 1989;124:94-99)

Cancer cachexia is a complex syndrome that includes anorexia and host tissue wasting. It is one of the most common manifestations of neoplasia and one that impacts negatively on the duration and quality of life of the cancer-bearing host.[1] Its cause is unknown, but is postulated to be a currently unidentified humoral factor.[2] Previous studies have demonstrated that the anorexia and cachexia of rats bearing a sarcoma was transferable via the circulation across a parabiotic anastomosis.[3]

Cachectin/tumor necrosis factor (TNF) may be a mediator of the cachexia associated with malignant neoplasms.[4] Initially isolated in the serum of trypanosomiasis-affected rabbits suffering paradoxically from both a profound hyperlipidemia and a wasting diathesis, cachectin was found to suppress the activity of lipoprotein lipase, a key enzyme in lipid biosynthesis.[5] Further studies have indicated that cachectin is a mediator of the metabolic derangements of chronic and acute infection.[4,6] The appearance of animals with chronic infectious diseases and cancer is similar, suggesting that cachectin may have a role in the pathophysiology of cancer cachexia as well. The results of studies to detect its presence in the serum of patients with cancer have been contradictory. Despite sensitive biologic and immunologic assays, studies by Scuderi et al[7] and Waage et al[8] failed to detect circulating cachectin/TNF levels in the serum of patients with cancer. More recently, Balkwill et al[9] were able to measure circulating levels of cachectin/TNF in the serum of some patients with cancer, but found no correlation between serum levels and clinical measures of cachexia.

In the present investigation, we attempted to detect circulating cachectin activity in the serum of sarcoma-bearing rats and to correlate levels with measurements of cachexia and extent of disease. In addition, we resected the tumor to determine the time course of reversal of cachexia and the disappearance of cachectin activity from the serum. The results suggest that cachectin is a humoral mediator of cachexia in this experimental rat-tumor model.

MATERIALS AND METHODS

General

The experiments were performed on male Fischer 344 rats initially weighing between 200 and 250 g. Animals were individually housed in wire-bottomed cages within a temperature- and humidity-controlled room. A 12-hour light/dark cycle was maintained. Rats were fed a casein-based semisynthetic diet (C-21, ICN, Cleveland) that allows accurate measurement of daily intake.[10]

The tumor was a transplantable methylcholanthrene-induced sarcoma. The tumor was transplanted in the subcutaneous space by either a sterile, viable, single-cell suspension (10^6 cells) or placement of 2-mm viable tumor fragments with the animal under intraperitoneal pentobarbital sodium (35 mg/kg) anesthesia. The sarcoma grows uniformly and the natural history has been previously reported.[11] It is locally invasive, does not metastasize, and causes anorexia and weight loss by 24 days after implantation. Death occurs from 30 to 40 days after transplantation.

The tumor was measured, using calipers, in three orthogonal linear dimensions three times weekly from the time it was first

Accepted for publication July 11, 1988.

From the Surgical Metabolism Section, Surgery Branch, National Cancer Institute, Bethesda, Md.

Read before the Annual Meeting of the Society of Surgical Oncology, New Orleans, May 23, 1988.

Reprint requests to Surgical Metabolism Section, Surgery Branch, National Cancer Institute, Bethesda, MD 20892 (Dr Norton).

palpable. At death, total body weight was recorded and the tumor was dissected free and weighed.

Blood Drawing

Fasting animals were anesthetized with intraperitoneal pentobarbital sodium (35 mg/kg); blood was collected in experiment 2 by aortic cannulation and in other experiments by retro-orbital puncture. Blood was allowed to clot at 4°C for two hours and serum was separated by centrifugation. Serum in experiment 2 underwent further separation via membrane filtration to isolate molecules of a molecular weight between 10 and 30 kilodaltons. Serum was then assayed immediately or frozen at −70°C until analyzed.

Tumor Resection

Tumor-bearing rats were anesthetized with intraperitoneal pentobarbital sodium (30 mg/kg) and the tumor was separated from the flank using blunt and sharp dissection. After all bleeding was controlled, the skin was reapproximated with clips. All non-tumor-bearing rats underwent similar anesthesia and a sham operation in which the skin was incised, a deep subfascial pocket was made, and skin was reapproximated.

L929 Bioassay

A standard cytotoxicity assay for cachectin/TNF activity using a TNF-sensitive L929 cell line was performed.[12] One hundred microliters of a suspension containing 2.5×10^5 cells/mL of L929 cells in RPMI 1640 medium supplemented with 10% fetal calf serum was plated on 96-well culture plates (Costar, Cambridge, Mass) and incubated overnight to establish a confluent monolayer. On parallel plates, serial dilutions of serum samples were made in complete medium with 2 mg/L of dactinomycin (Merck, Sharpe and Dohme, West Point, Pa) and 100-μL aliquots were transferred to the wells containing the L929 cells, giving a final concentration of 1 mg/L of dactinomycin. In addition, L929 cells incubated with dactinomycin-containing medium served as a control for cell viability. After an 18-hour incubation at 37°C the surviving cells were fixed and stained wtih 5% crystal violet (Sigma Chemical Co, St Louis). The dye uptake of each well was then determined by a titertak (Flow Laboratories, Helsinki) at 590 nm. One unit of activity was defined as the reciprocal of the dilution required to produce a 50% decrease in absorbance relative to control cells exposed to dactinomycin alone. Each sample was assayed in triplicate. In parallel assays employing a neutralizing antibody, samples were mixed with a 1:1 solution of a 1:25 dilution of a polyvalent TNF antibody (Endogen, Boston) for one hour at 4°C before the addition of the L929 cells. Each assay included an internal standard for reference using human recombinant TNF (Cetus, Emeryville, Calif).

Statistics

Data are presented as the mean ± SEM. Parametric results are analyzed by Student's independent t test and nonparametric results are analyzed by Wilcoxon's rank sum test. Percents are compared by Fisher's exact test.

Experiment 1

To verify the L929 cytotoxicity assay and the method of the collection and handling of serum specimens, cachectin activity was measured in the serum of nine F344 male rats before and after an intravenous, 200-μg/kg injection of recombinant human TNF. Serum was collected at 0, 30, 60, and 120 minutes, and was analyzed by the L929 bioassay.

Experiment 2

Experiment 2 was designed to determine the detectability of circulating cachectin activity in the serum of tumor-bearing rats. Fifty F344 male rats were acclimated to the C-21 diet and to individual cages. They were then randomized by a random-number method to receive either 5×10^6 viable sarcoma cells subcutaneously (n = 40) or saline solution (n = 10). Two rats did not develop tumor and were excluded from analysis. Food intake, body weight, and tumor size were measured daily. At weekly intervals after tumor implantation (beginning on day 14 when tumor became palpable) animals in a random group of tumor-bearing and non-tumor-bearing rats were killed and serum was collected. Cachectin activity was determined using the L929 bioassay. At death, tumor weight, body weight, and tumor burden (tumor weight/total body weight) were recorded for each rat.

Experiment 3

Seventy F344 male rats were acclimated to the C-21 diet and to individual cages. Forty tumor-bearing rats (28 days after implantation) underwent tumor resection when food intake in each animal was noted to have declined to less than 15% of normal rat food intake (<2 g/d). Thirty non–tumor-bearing rats were randomized to receive either normal food intake (ad libitum) or were paired to the tumor-bearing rats' food intake and each rat subsequently underwent a similar sham operation. Before and after resection, fasting-stage serum was collected and assayed for cachectin activity and triglyceride levels. Triglycerides were analyzed on an automated instrument (ABA 100, Abbott Laboratories, South Pasadena, Calif) by a spectrophotometric method. After resection, the survival, daily weight, and food intake were recorded.

RESULTS

Experiment 1

Recombinant human TNF given intravenously results in peak levels of detectable serum cachectin activity at 30 minutes, but high levels are still detectable at 120 minutes (Fig 1). Clearance of serum cachectin activity is rapid, with a half-life of less than 30 minutes. These results demonstrate that the L929 method that we used can reliably detect cachectin levels within the circulation.

Experiment 2

Food intake of non–tumor-bearing rats remained constant throughout the experimental period (15 g/d) (Table 1). The food intake of tumor-bearing rats remained constant until day 21, when it first declined significantly (Table 1 and Fig 2). From day 21 onward, the food intake of tumor-bearing rats progressively declined as the tumor burden progressively increased.

Circulating cachectin activity was not detectable in the serum of non–tumor-bearing rats or tumor-bearing rats at 21 days after implantation (Table 1). At 28 days after tumor implantation, cachectin activity was detectable in the serum of tumor-bearing rats (Fig 2 and Table 1) who were eating only 3 g/d and were losing weight (Table 1). With a greater tumor burden and further decline in food intake and body weight, cachectin activity levels became detectable in the serum of a greater proportion of tumor-bearing rats (Fig 2) and levels continued to increase significantly (Fig 2 and Table 1).

Serum cachectin activity levels correlated directly with tumor burden ($r = .72$; $P < .001$; Fig 3). Serum cachectin activity levels correlated inversely with food intake ($r = -.66$; $P < .001$; Fig 4) and body weight change ($r = -.75$; $P < .001$; Fig 5). These results correlated tumor-bearing serum cachectin activity levels with three important measures of cachexia: tumor burden, food intake, and body weight.

Experiment 3

Before tumor resection, tumor-bearing rats ate significantly less than non–tumor-bearing rats ($P < .005$). After tumor resection, tumor-bearing rats gradually increased their food intake and, by postoperative day 7, they were eating an amount similar to that of non–tumor-bearing rats (Fig 6). Non–tumor-bearing rats had a significant decline in food intake only on their operative and first postoperative days ($P < .01$), and their intake then returned quickly to baseline levels (Fig 6).

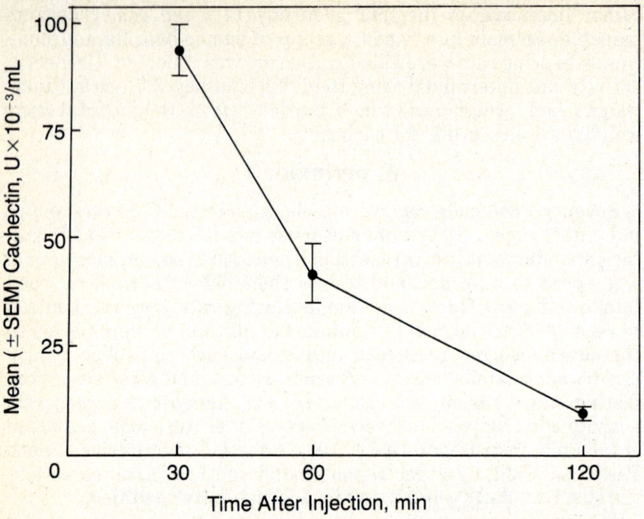

Fig 1.—Serum cachectin activity levels after intravenous injection of 200 μg/kg of recombinant human tumor necrosis factor. Activity levels were undetectable at time 0 before injection, were highest at 30 minutes, and decreased as time increased, indicating that sample collection methods and L929 assay could reliably detect serum cachectin activity levels.

Opposite to the increase in food intake of tumor-bearing rats after tumor resection were the level and presence of cachectin activity in the serum (Fig 7 and Table 2). Before tumor resection, 50% of the 28-day tumor-bearing rats assayed had detectable cachectin activity in the serum, with mean levels of 92±25 U/mL, vs consistently undetectable levels in non–tumor-bearing rats ($P<.01$). The level of cachectin activity in the serum of tumor-bearing rats before and soon after resection was not significantly different (Fig 7 and Table 2). However, by day 7 after tumor resection, when food intake returned to levels similar to those in non–tumor-bearing rats, cachectin activity was no longer detectable in the serum. In addition, low food intake itself did not cause cachectin activity in the serum because no pair-fed, non–tumor-bearing rat had detectable cachectin activity (Table 2).

Before tumor resection, tumor-bearing rats had significantly higher serum triglyceride levels than either non–tumor-bearing rats with normal food intake or non–tumor-bearing rats pair-fed to tumor-bearing rat food intake ($P<.005$) (Table 3). Following tumor resection, tumor-bearing rats' serum triglyceride levels decreased, and by postoperative day 7 these levels were significantly less than in either control group ($P<.005$). Pair-fed non–tumor-bearing rats exhibited a reverse pattern. Before sham operation and when consuming reduced levels of food, serum triglyceride levels of pair-fed non–tumor-bearing rats were significantly lower than levels in either the ad libitum-fed non–tumor-bearing rats or the tumor-bearing rats ($P<.005$). Postoperatively, as food intake returned to adequate levels, serum triglyceride levels also returned to normal levels. Non–tumor-bearing rats fed ad libitum maintained serum triglyceride levels within the normal range throughout the experiment.

Paralleling the changes in serum triglyceride levels after tumor resection were the changes in serum cachectin activity levels of tumor-bearing rats. Before tumor resection, tumor-bearing rats had high levels of both triglycerides and cachectin activity in the serum (Fig 7). After resection, levels of each substance declined in a similar manner (Fig 7). Serum cachectin activity was not detectable in either control group of non–tumor-bearing rats before or after sham operation.

Table 1.—Mean (±SEM) Food Intake, Body Weight Change, and Cachectin Activity Levels in Non–Tumor- and Tumor-Bearing Rats

Group	Days After Tumor Implant	n	Food Intake, g/d	Body Weight Change, g/wk	Cachectin Activity, U/mL
Non–tumor-bearing	0	10	15±1	31±2	0
Tumor-bearing	14	7	15±1	33±4	0
	21	5	12±2*	23±3	0
	28	8	3±1*†	−21±3*†	25±5*
	35	8	0±0.4*†	−41±3*†	43±9*‡
	42	4	0±0.3*†	−49±6*†	100±20*‡

*$P<.005$ vs non–tumor-bearing rats.
†$P<.005$ vs tumor-bearing rats on day 21.
‡$P<.05$ vs tumor-bearing rats on day 28.

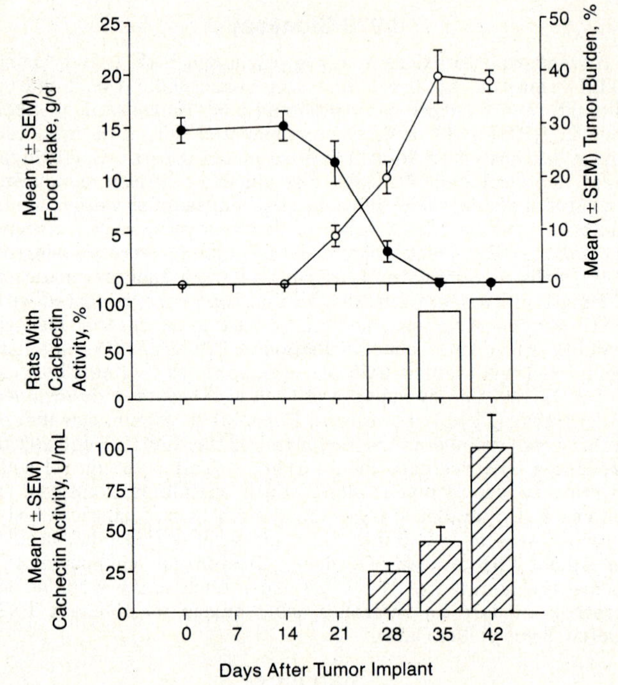

Fig 2.—Food intake, tumor burden, percent with serum cachectin activity detectable, and measured serum cachectin activity level of tumor-bearing rats as time from tumor implant increases. Food intake (closed circles) first significantly declined 21 days after implantation and tumor burden (open circles) of approximately 20%, and progressively declined as tumor burden progressively increased. Cachectin was detectable 28 days after tumor implantation, and levels significantly increased ($P<.05$) and percent of rats with detectable levels increased ($P<.01$) as time from tumor implantation progressed.

COMMENT

Cachectin, or TNF, is a macrophage-secreted peptide that circulates in the bloodstream and acts at distant sites via specific receptors present on a variety of metabolically important tissues such as muscle, adipose tissue, and

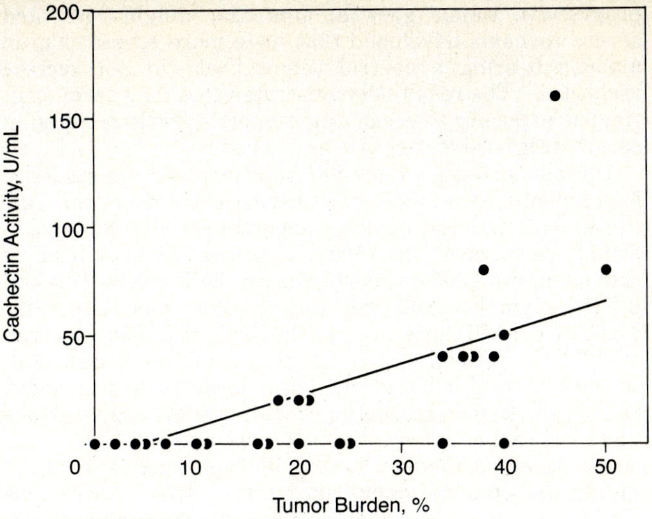

Fig 3.—Correlation of serum cachectin activity with tumor burden (tumor weight/total body weight). Serum cachectin activity increased directly with tumor burden ($r = .72$; $P < .001$).

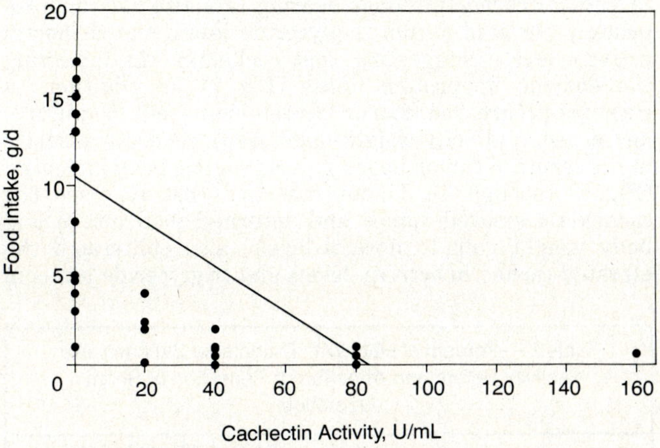

Fig 4.—Correlation of serum cachectin activity with tumor-bearing rat food intake. Serum cachectin activity correlated inversely with tumor-bearing rat food intake ($r = -.66$; $P < .001$).

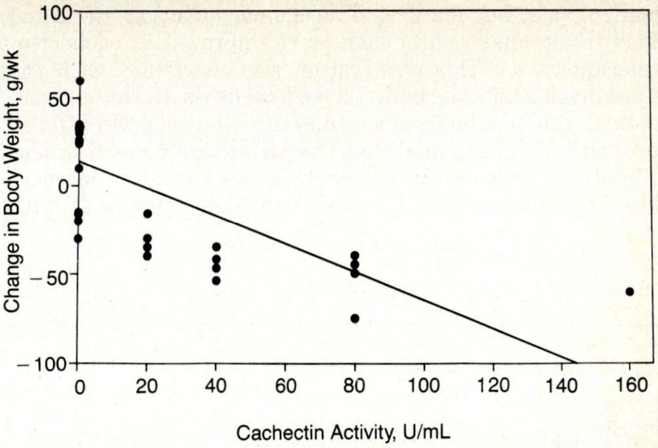

Fig 5.—Correlation of serum cachectin activity with tumor-bearing rat change in body weight. Serum cachectin activity levels correlate inversely with tumor-bearing rat change in body weight ($r = -.75$; $P < .001$).

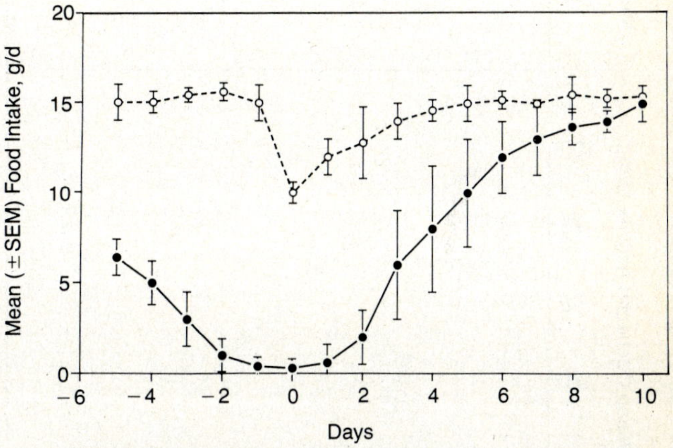

Fig 6.—Food intake of tumor-bearing (closed circles) and non–tumor-bearing (open circles) rats before and after tumor resection or sham operation. Food intake of cachectic tumor-bearing rats progressively declined as non–tumor-bearing rats consumed 15 g/d ($P < .05$). Tumor was resected or sham operation was performed on day 0.

liver.[13] It was recently isolated and purified as a result of two separate lines of research, one to isolate factors that cause the cachexia observed in wasting diseases and the other to isolate factors that cause tumor regression. It is now clear that cachectin is one of the mediators of the tissue and shocklike changes associated with endotoxin, bacteria, and other acute and chronic infectious diseases.[4,6,14] Although cachectin inhibits the synthesis and action of the enzyme lipoprotein lipase,[13,15] reduces body lipid stores,[4] and causes the necrosis of some tumors in animals,[16] investigations aimed at detecting its presence as a possible mediator of the host changes associated with cancer cachexia have been inconsistent. Aderka et al[17] demonstrated cytotoxic activity consistent with TNF activity spontaneously produced in vitro by peripheral blood mononuclear cells from patients with cancer, indicating that endogenous cachectin production may occur as part of the host response to cancer,[17] yet other studies have failed to detect circulating cachectin levels in the serum of tumor-bearing patients.[7,8] Moreover, a recent study using a sensitive enzyme-linked immunosorbent assay detected circulating cachectin levels in serum of some patients with advanced cancer, but levels did not correlate with the extent of disease or other measures of cachexia.[9]

Experimental work in animal models supports the notion that circulating factors cause cancer cachexia and that cachectin may be one of these factors. Previous studies with the sarcoma-bearing Fischer rat have supported the hypothesis that a circulating factor or factors caused the cachexia produced by the tumor. A parabiotic union that had a measured blood flow of 1.5% of the cardiac output per minute was able to transmit cachexia (anorexia and host weight loss) from a tumor-bearing rat to a non–tumor-bearing rat. Since the two rats were coupled only by the bloodstream and no tumor was present in the non–tumor-bearing animal at necropsy, it appeared likely that a stable circulating factor crossed the anastomosis and produced cachexia.[3] Recent work has indicated that non–tumor-bearing rats become tolerant to the anorectic and cachectic effects of recombinant human cachectin after repeated administration.[14,18] When tolerant non–tumor-bearing rats were given an inoculation of sarcoma, they lived substantially longer than animals previously unexposed to cachectin. Tumor growth was identical in cachectin-tolerant and control rats, but features of cachexia, including declining food intake and weight loss, were improved in cachectin-tolerant rats.[18] This observation was consistent with the hypothesis that cachectin caused cachexia in this experimental tumor model, since tolerance to cachectin offered protection to the animal from the cachectic effects of tumor. Finally, a transgenic tumor that persistently secretes human cachectin was injected into nude mice and, with progressive tumor growth, anorexia, weight loss, and severe cachexia developed that were more severe than in animals bearing a control tumor that did not secrete cachectin.[19] The results demonstrated that long-term, continuous exposure to escalating cachectin levels resulted in severe progressive cachexia and death.[19]

The present study provides additional strong evidence for cachectin as a mediator of cancer cachexia in this rat-tumor experimental model. Cachectin activity was reproducibly detected in the serum of cachectic tumor-bearing rats using the L929 bioassay. Only α-TNF (cachectin) and β-TNF (lymphotoxin) kill these L929 cells. No other cytokine can kill these cells, so the likelihood that cachectin or TNF is present is very high. In addition, cachectin activity was eliminated by high doses of a polyvalent antibody to human cachectin, providing additional evidence that true cachectin activity was measured, and the assay was further verified by measuring appropriate levels in the serum of non–tumor-bearing rats after intravenous administration of recombinant human TNF (Fig 1).

Cachectin activity was not present in the serum of non–tumor-bearing rats, nor in that of tumor-bearing rats, until 28 days after tumor implantation and the growth of the tumor burden to approximately 20% of body weight (Fig 2). Similar cachectic tumor-bearing rats also had inappropriately elevated serum triglyceride levels and cachectin activity levels, suggesting that cachectin was inhibiting the enzyme lipoprotein lipase (Fig 7). In addition, as cachexia progressed (tumor burden increased, food intake decreased, and body weight decreased), cachectin activity in the serum of tumor-bearing rats progressively increased (Figs 3 through 5). Tumor resection that reversed the cachexia (removed tumor and returned food intake and body weight gain to normal levels) also obliterated the elevated cachectin activity levels and triglyceride levels in

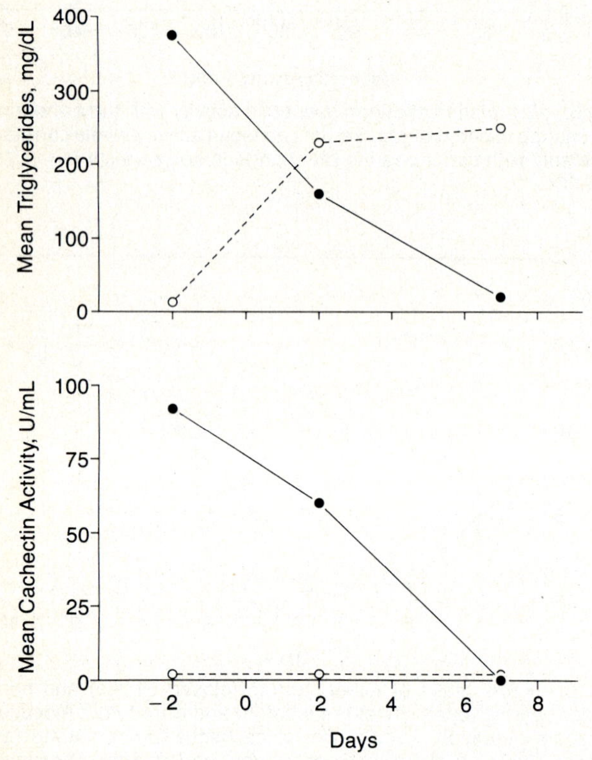

Fig 7.—Serum cachectin activity and triglyceride levels of tumor-bearing (closed circles) and pair-fed non–tumor-bearing (open circles) rats before and after tumor resection or sham operation, performed on day 0. Pair-fed non–tumor-bearing rats were given tumor-bearing rats' food intake. Tumor-bearing rats had significantly greater serum triglyceride and cachectin activity levels than pair-fed non–tumor-bearing rats ($P<.005$). Serum triglyceride levels of pair-fed non–tumor-bearing rats were significantly different from those of tumor-bearing rats on postoperative day 7 ($P<.005$).

Table 2.—Percent of Rats With Detectable Cachectinlike Activity Before and After Tumor Resection or Sham Operation

	Percent With Activity by Days From Resection or Sham Operation		
Group*	−2	+2	+7
Control non–tumor bearing	0	0	0
Pair-fed non–tumor bearing	0	0	0
Tumor-bearing	50†	57†	0

*Pair-fed non–tumor-bearing rats were fed the same amount of food daily that tumor-bearing rats consumed.
†$P<.05$ vs non–tumor-bearing rats by Fisher's exact test.

Table 3.—Daily Body Weight Change and Serum Triglyceride Levels Before and After Tumor Resection or Sham Operation

	Days From Tumor Resection or Sham Operation					
	Mean (±SEM) Daily Body Weight Change, g			Mean (±SEM) Triglycerides (mg/dL)		
Group*	−2	+2	+7	−2	+2	+7
Control non–tumor-bearing	3±0.2	2±0.2	2.5±0.3	110±20	96±20	210±30
Pair-fed non–tumor-bearing	−3±0.1†	−4±0.3†	2.5±0.2‡	13±5†	230±40‡	250±40‡
Tumor-bearing	−2.8±0.3†	−3.2±0.3†	2.6±0.2‡	375±60§	150±20‡	20±4‡§

*Pair-fed non–tumor-bearing rats were fed the same amount of food daily that tumor-bearing rats consumed.
†$P<.005$ vs control non–tumor-bearing rats.
‡$P<.005$ vs day −2.
§$P<.005$ vs control non–tumor-bearing and pair-fed non–tumor-bearing rats.

the serum of the tumor-bearing rat. Pair-fed non–tumor-bearing controls and standard non–tumor-bearing controls indicated that these findings were not due to reduced food intake or operative trauma.

This study demonstrates that experimental cancer cachexia in this rat model is mediated at least partially by a serum factor that has activity like that of recombinant human TNF. The serum factor's activity is blocked by an antibody to human recombinant cachectin and levels increase as cachexia progresses and decrease as cachexia regresses. The idea that an endogenous factor produced in response to an invasive stimulus such as a growing tumor can result in toxic effects on the host provides new insight into the potential pathophysiologic mechanisms of disease and may provide new approaches to disease treatment.

Catherine Gorschboth measured serum triglyceride levels, and Cetus Corp, Emeryville, Calif, provided recombinant human TNF.

References

1. Norton JA, Peacock JL, Morrison SD: Cancer cachexia. *CRC Crit Rev Oncol Hematol* 1987;7:289-327.

2. Theologides A: Pathogenesis of cachexia in cancer: A review and a hypothesis. *Cancer* 1972;20:484-488.

3. Norton JA, Moley JF, Green MV, et al: Parabiotic transfer of cancer anorexia/cachexia in male rats. *Cancer Res* 1985;45:5547-5552.

4. Beutler B, Cerami A: Cachectin and tumor necrosis factor as two sides of the same biological coin. *Nature* 1986;320:584-588.

5. Rouser CA, Cerami A: Hypertriglyceridemia associated with *Trypanosoma brucei* infection in rabbits: Role of defective triglyceride removal. *Mol Biochem Parasitol* 1980;2:31-38.

6. Tracey KJ, Beutler B, Lowry SF, et al: Shock and tissue injury induced by recombinant human cachectin. *Science* 1986;234:470-474.

7. Scuderi P, Sterling KE, Lam KS, et al: Raised serum levels of tumor necrosis factor in parasitic infections. *Lancet* 1986;2:1364-1365.

8. Waage A, Espivik T, Lamvik J: Detection of tumor necrosis factor like cytotoxicity in serum from patients with septicemia but not from untreated cancer patients. *Scand J Immunol* 1986;24:739-743.

9. Balkwill F, Burke F, Talbot D, et al: Evidence for tumor necrosis factor/cachectin production in cancer. *Lancet* 1987;2:1229-1232.

10. Peacock JL, Gorschboth CM, Norton JA: Impact of insulin on doxorubicin-induced rat host toxicity and tumor regression. *Cancer Res* 1987;47:4318-4322.

11. Popp MB, Morrison SD, Brennan MF: Total parenteral nutrition in a methylcholanthrene induced rat sarcoma model. *Cancer Treat Rep* 1981;65:137-143.

12. Flick DA, Gifford GE: Comparison of in vitro cell cytotoxic assays for tumor necrosis factor. *J Immunol Methods* 1984;68:167-175.

13. Beutler BJ, Mahoney N, LeTrang P, et al: Purification of cachectin, a lipoprotein lipase-suppressing hormone secreted by endotoxin-induced RAW 264.7 cells. *J Exp Med* 1985;161:984-995.

14. Cerami A, Beutler B: The role of cachectin/TNF in endotoxic shock and cachexia. *Immunol Today* 1988;9:28-31.

15. Kawakami M, Pekela PH, Lane MD, et al: Lipoprotein lipase suppression in 3T3-LI cells by an endotoxin-induced mediator from exudate cells. *Proc Natl Acad Sci USA* 1982;79:912-916.

16. Carswell EA, Old LS, Casse RL, et al: An endotoxin-induced serum factor that causes necrosis of tumors. *Proc Natl Acad Sci USA* 1975;72:3666-3670.

17. Aderka D, Fisher S, Levo Y, et al: Cachectin/tumor necrosis factor production by cancer patients. *Lancet* 1985;2:1190.

18. Stovroff MD, Norton JA: Cachectin: A mediator of cancer cachexia. *Surg Forum* 1987;38:413-415.

19. Oliff A, Defeo-Jones D, Boyer M, et al: Tumors secreting human TNF/cachectin induce cachexia in mice. *Cell* 1987;50:555-563.

Discussion

Q These rats normally have an elevated white blood cell count when their tumors enlarge, and at the same time they become anorexic. Tumor necrosis factor is also associated with an inflammatory response. Is there any way to decide whether this is part of the same inflammatory response or whether this is really something that is produced by tumor?

A These findings may be the result of an inflammatory response. Histopathologic analysis of the tumors showed substantial necrosis and a large number of infiltrating macrophages. This finding is consistent with those of other researchers who have suggested that the in vivo activation of macrophages that respond to tumor with TNF production is due to the tissue necrosis within the tumors.

Q What was body weight change in the non–tumor-bearing animals compared with that in the tumor-bearing animals? In most models, non–tumor-bearing animals that were pair-fed did not lose as much weight.

A We found that non–tumor-bearing pair-fed animals, not only in the present experiment but also in other studies, lost significantly more weight, although the body weight of a tumor-bearing animal includes a large growing tumor in addition to the host weight.

In both non–tumor-bearing rats given exogenous sublethal doses of cachectin/TNF and in anorectic sarcoma-bearing animals, compositional analysis disclosed a loss of total body protein and fat. Yet in the pair-fed control, host protein was saved as a normal physiologic response and only body fat deposits were reduced.

Q Is there any evidence of TNF production by the tumor itself?

A Cell culture of the tumor yielded no detectable cachectin activity, yet Balkwill et al[9] reported finding the message for TNF in two of six colorectal tumors by Northern blot analysis. Currently we have a C-DNA probe for TNF and we are looking for the message within the tumor, its infiltrating macrophages, and its circulating monocytes.

As many as five days after operation these rats still were relatively anorectic, suggesting that the animals still had activated monocytes with continued low levels of cachectin/TNF production. One study reported that only three months after a curative resection did isolated monocytes stop showing increased TNF production in response to a lipopolysaccharide in vitro.

Q What is the clinical importance of the negative TNF trials in patients who are losing weight? There is some evidence to suggest that the interferons may potentiate the effects of TNF.

A Cachectin/TNF is not the only factor responsible for the observed cachexia. We know that TNF induces the production of interleukin 1 and that it, along with other cytokines, can produce the changes we observed. In regard to clinical importance, almost 50% of patients with cancer die of cachexia or have some element of cachexia that plays a role in morbidity. We are studying the value of murine TNF antibodies and have developed a murine TNF antibody to try to reverse the cachexia in tumor-bearing animals. If we can reverse or at least ameliorate the cachexia present in patients with cancer they may have a better response to chemotherapy or operative intervention.

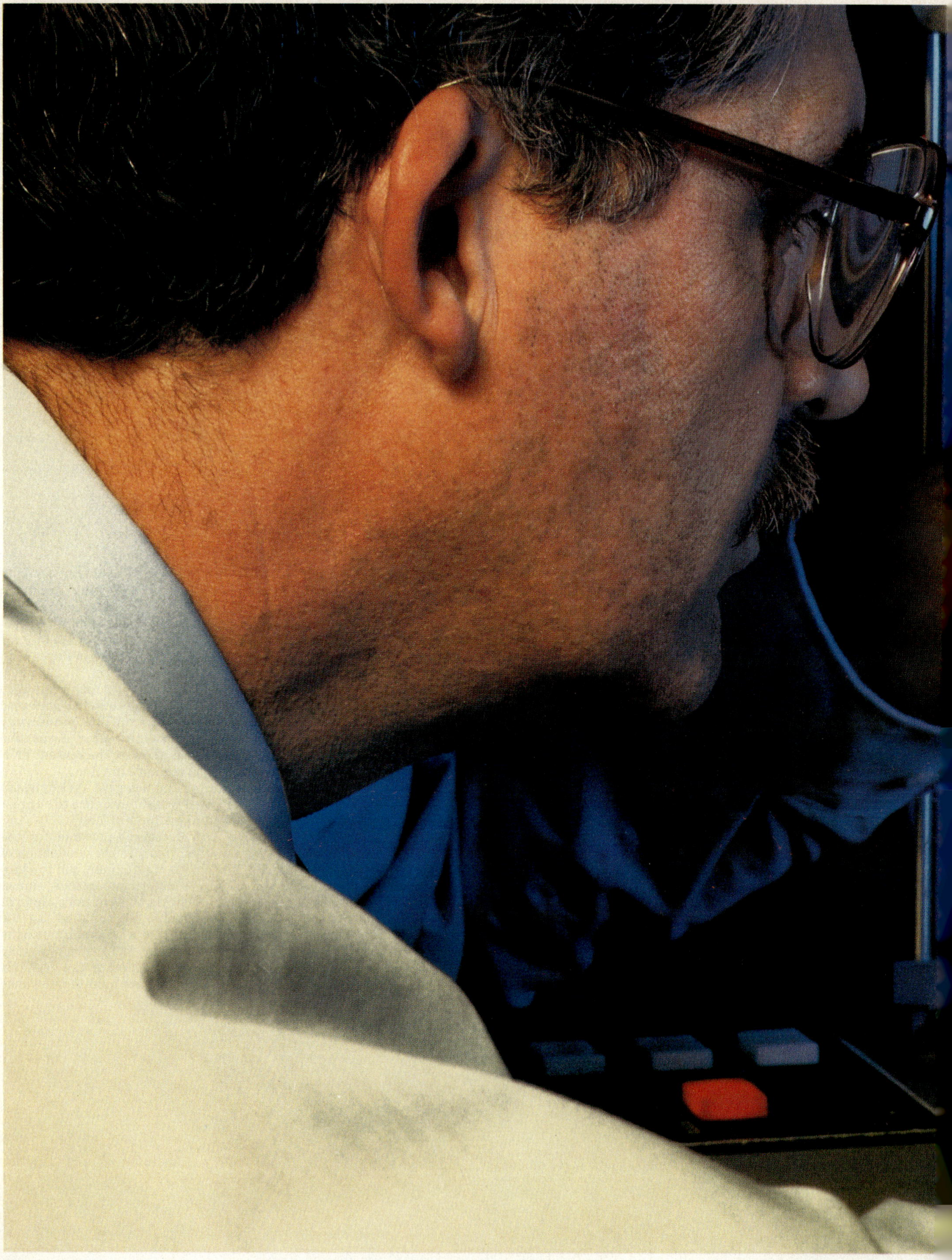

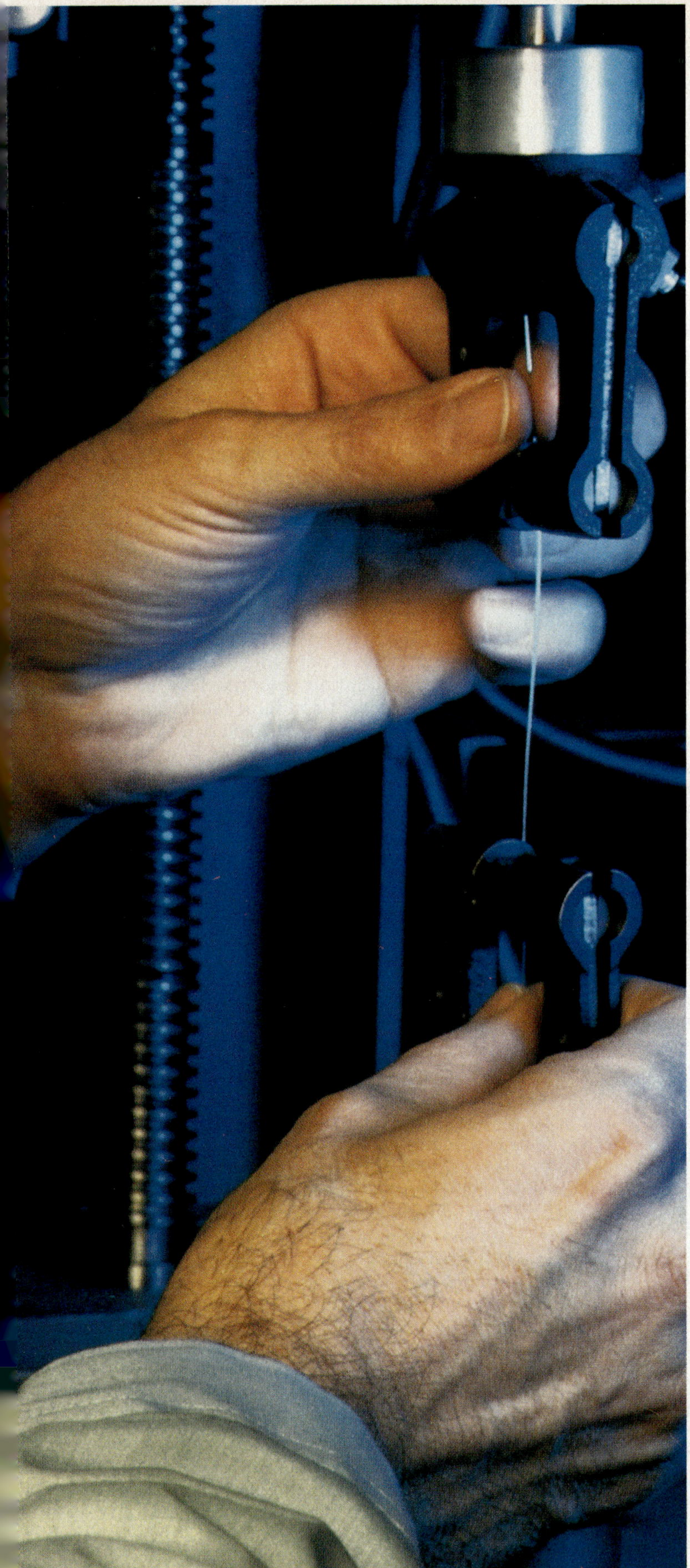

The Flip Side of Tumor Immunity

Richmond T. Prehn, MD, Liisa M. Prehn, MD

• A large amount of data suggest that tumors are, to some degree, dependent for their growth on a positive level of immune reaction, a level that is unique for each tumor. Each tumor gradually adjusts its immunogenicity to the level that will, in the immunologic context of its own particular host, maximize its growth. Thus, it follows that immunosuppression may be as likely as immunoaugmentation to have a therapeutic effect.

(*Arch Surg* 1989;124:102-106)

Some years ago, during the study of the immunogenic properties of hydrocarbon-induced tumors, a puzzling phenomenon was encountered. A number of sarcomas had been produced in mice by the subcutaneous implantation of paraffin pellets containing 3-methylcholanthrene. These tumors were found to vary widely in the strengths of their immunogenicities, some having virtually none while others would refuse to grow in specifically immunized syngeneic hosts.[1] When a variety of similar tumors had reached the size of 1 cm or more, a fragment of tissue was taken from each of two opposite poles of each tumor and transplanted to a different syngeneic recipient.[2] The resulting members of each pair of secondary tumors were compared, either at once or after five to seven transplant generations, for several characteristics, including growth rate, immunizing ability, and susceptibility to an established specific immunity. In a high percentage of cases, the sublines were found to differ, sometimes dramatically, in one or more of these attributes. What had been demonstrated was that each primary tumor, even when shown by antigenic specificity to be of clonal origin, contained within or soon developed, as judged by classic "immunization-challenge" tests, subclones of widely disparate immunogenic characteristics. Despite this heterogeneity, it has been repeatedly observed that tumors can remain highly immunogenic even after extensive in vivo passaging.[3] The change that sometimes does occur is more often a decline of immunizing capacity rather than a change of sensitivity to the immune response.[4] Although immunogenicity (which combines the immunizing ability and the sensitivity to immunity) can be altered by immunoselection,[5] the tumors are usually remarkably stable.[1,2]

Given the heterogeneity in the immunologic properties of the tumor cells, how can one explain, in the face of immune selection, the persistence of immunogenicity through many transplant generations? Why do highly immunogenic tumors tend to remain immunogenic and weakly or nonimmunogenic tumors persist as such? To us, the most satisfactory explanation is that the immunogenicity of a tumor is maintained by immunologic selection at a level close to that which is most conducive to the growth of that particular tumor. The implication is, of course, that the immune reaction is not always inhibitory to the tumor but that, for each tumor, there is a unique level of immune reaction that is optimal for its proliferation; levels of either a greater or a lesser degree would be relatively harmful to the tumor and less conducive to its growth. In other words, immunity has a tumor-facilitating flip side. Please note that what we are discussing is not suppression of tumor immunity, but a positive supportive effect of a certain level of immune reaction on tumor growth.

This theory is supported by the further observation that, among the tumors that had been passaged, there was a significant tendency for a subclone, if its response to a given level of immunity were low relative to that of the other member of the pair, to exhibit a relatively high immunizing capacity.[2] This relationship was not seen when the pairs of sublines obtained directly from the primary tumors were compared. Thus, it appears that the immunizing capacity of a tumor and its sensitivity to the immunity are independent variables; however, presumably because of immunologic selection during passaging, a change in one tends to be compensated by an opposing change in the other, thus tending to stabilize the overall immunogenicity of the tumor.[2]

This idea, that there exists for the growth of each tumor an optimal level of immune reaction peculiar to that tumor, we have called the "immunofacilitation theory"; it has been tested in a wide variety of ways in a large number of different contexts and, in aggregate, these tests have been supportive of the theory.[6] A seeming exception will be discussed after we have outlined the supporting evidence that has accrued, but first we will discuss some general implications of the facilitation theory.

It has been mentioned that, owing to the heterogeneity within each tumor, the immune properties of the tumor will be constantly adjusting to the immunologic environment. Nonetheless, in a vast variety of experimental tumor systems, it has been possible to inhibit tumor growth or to produce cures of established tumors by markedly enhancing antitumor immune reactions. However, these symptoms usually involve a transplanted tumor before it has

Accepted for publication Aug 26, 1988.
From the Department of Pathology, University of Washington, Seattle.
Read before the Annual Meeting of the Society of Surgical Oncology, New Orleans, May 24, 1988.
Reprint requests to Department of Pathology, University of Washington, Seattle, WA 98195 (Dr R. Prehn).

been able to undergo much expansion and consequent variation in its new host. In general, because of the problem of heterogeneity, the immunologic approaches to therapy may prove limited; how limited only time and experience will tell. Tumors that have undergone less progression, that are less malignant, and that are treated when small may be more homogeneous and so may offer a better opportunity for immunotherapy. It is also possible that some tumor types may adapt to changes in the immune environment less rapidly than do others.

It follows from the theory that, since each tumor tends to adjust its immunologic variables toward the optimum for that tumor, a therapeutic effect might be produced equally well by either raising or lowering the level of the immune reaction. We have suggested, not entirely facetiously, that chemotherapy may be the best form of immunotherapy[7]! Furthermore, the immunodepression that is often associated with cancer should, perhaps, be considered a host defense-mechanism to which the tumor, unfortunately, soon adapts.

If the tumor tends to be immunologically as well adjusted as we have suggested may be the case, how is it that some tumors will not grow well on transplantation unless the new host is immunosuppressed? The answer probably lies in the fact that the primary host may itself be relatively immunosuppressed by the carcinogen and/or by the tumor. More importantly, because of the manner of antigen presentation in the primary host, the primary autochthonous host is relatively difficult to immunize.[8,9] Consequently, the well-adjusted tumor will usually have a compensatingly higher immunogenicity than will be optimal for it in a new secondary host.

There is ample evidence that changes in the immune capacities of the animals can profoundly influence oncogenesis in many experimental systems[10,11]; how is this to be explained if tumors are immunologically so adaptable? In the instructive example of two-stage skin tumorigenesis, it has been shown that many initiated cells lie dormant for long periods and may never give rise to a tumor.[12] It has also been shown that the immunogenicity of tumors tends to be directly related to the concentration of carcinogen even in the absence of immunologic selection.[13] Therefore, whether an initiated cell progresses to overt tumor will depend, at least in part, on the antigenicity of the clone in relation to the immunologic characteristics of the host. Adaptation, via selection, cannot occur until after cellular proliferation has produced heterogeneity among the tumor cells.

The incidence of some tumors in the human may also be markedly altered by altering the immunocompetences of the hosts. Thus, when humans are immunosuppressed for kidney grafting, the incidence of skin tumors is increased.[14] Presumably, this is a different spectrum of tumors, with a compensatingly different sensitivity to immune reactions, than that which occurs in the skins of immunologically normal people. The fact that the tumor incidence is increased suggests, however, that the skin of a normal person is overly reactive for optimal growth of the average clone of potential skin tumor cells; the tumors that are actually realized in normal skin are probably derived from an immunologically selected minor subpopulation of less immunogenic clones. The remainder remain dormant, presumably because of the lack, for them, of a sufficiently propitious immune environment.

In the human, the observation of an increased cancer incidence among patients with immunodeficiency has been confined to a relatively few tumor types, most notably ultraviolet-induced skin tumors, among patients immunosuppressed for allografting, and Kaposi's sarcoma among patients with acquired immunodeficiency syndrome.[14,15] (The increased incidence of tumors of the immune system per se, ie, lymphoid tumors, may have little to do with a changed immune reaction against the tumors and thus should probably not be considered in the present context.) Why is it that the incidences of a greater variety of human tumors are not overtly influenced by an immunodepressed state? A likely explanation is that those few tumor types whose incidences are increased by immunodepression are, indeed, the only human tumors of which most of the originally transformed precursors were so immunogenic that they were not immunologically stimulated to grow in the absence of immunodepression (classic immunosurveillance?). The remaining less immunogenic types would actually, according to the facilitation hypothesis, tend to appear less often in immunodepressed patients or more often if immunity were augmented rather than reduced. According to the theory, both the more and the less immunogenic types are dependent on the immune reaction, but the optimal level of the immunity differs. For example, although Kaposi's sarcoma is a common feature of the acquired immunodeficiency syndrome, it is apparently associated with the less severe cases.[16,17] This probably means that the tumor, although it grows best in the immunologically compromised patient, is, nonetheless, dependent on the presence of an immune reaction, albeit a level of reaction less than that which can be mounted by a normal person.

It has been observed in some human tumor systems that the degree of local immunologic reactivity at the tumor site is directly correlated with a good prognosis. This has been especially noted in breast cancer.[18] How is this to be explained in terms of the immunofacilitation hypothesis? Perhaps in some cases the immune reaction does become greater than is optimal for tumor growth. In others, however, we suggest that the tumor, which is actually dependent on the immune reaction, loses its dependency during its biologic progression, much as a hormonally dependent tumor tends with time to lose its dependence on the relevant hormone.[19] The lack of leukocytic reactions around melanoma metastases, for example, is in striking contrast to the usually heavy infiltrations around early lesions. The good prognosis that is associated with an immunologic reaction may, therefore, be an association and nothing more; the reaction may be merely a marker of a tumor that is still early in its biologic progression and still in its dependent phase. A tumor that is early in its progression would have a relatively good prognosis because of this fact, not because of the immune reaction that is also associated with the early stages of progression.

Recently a seemingly paradoxical set of observations was published concerning the biology of human malignant melanomas. It was found that the prognosis of superficial cutaneous lesions was relatively poor if these lesions underwent substantial spontaneous regression. Similar lesions, if they did not show regression, seldom metastasized and were not dangerous.[20] Apparently, the stronger the host's reaction to the primary lesion in the skin, the more likely the growth of metastases. While a number of hypotheses could probably be advanced to explain the paradox, we are intrigued by how well it may be explained by the immunofacilitation theory.

Recent work from other laboratories with different tumor systems suggest that the cells that metastasize may not always differ in any significant way from the cells that remain in the primary lesion.[21,22] Therefore, different behaviors, such as simultaneous growth of a metastasis and regression at the primary site in the skin, may be due to differences in the anatomic sites rather than to differences in the tumor cells. To explain the paradox of the behavior of cutaneous melanomas, one has simply to add the fact, which few immunologists would dispute, that the skin probably has a much more potent intrinsic immunologic mechanism than do most other organs. Therefore, the melanoma, which evolved to grow within the strong immunologic environment of the skin, would grow poorly, if at all, in the relatively deficient immunologic environment of one of the internal organs. However, if, by chance or immune manipulation,[23] the host became more reactive than was optimal for the melanoma's in situ growth, the host might be so reactive that the melanoma could grow in a more immunologically deficient site.

A second and not mutally exclusive explanation of the paradoxical growth of melanomas is that the vigorous immune response in the skin causes, either by selection and/or actual mutation,[24] the development of variant clones that are less dependent on the immune response and can, therefore, grow in more immunologically deficient internal organs.

In our laboratory, we have made four distinctly different types of experimental challenges to the immunofacilitation theory.[6] The first was to attempt titrations of the immune reaction, both in vivo and in vitro, and then to determine the effect on tumor growth and/or on oncogenesis. For example, it was found that mice that had undergone thymectomy as adults, exposed to 450 rad of whole-body radiation, and then immunologically restored to varying extents by giving various dosages of normal syngeneic spleen cells were most susceptible to sarcogenesis with 3-methylcholanthrene when the spleen-cell dosage was at an intermediate level.[25] In other words, the mice that had been restored to a modest extent were more susceptible than were those that had been restored either minimally or maximally. Numerous other experiments along similar lines were done with similar results, both in our own laboratory and by others.[19,26-33] Perhaps the nicest work was done by Shearer and Parker,[30] who showed that a similar result could be found by titrating specific antibody against the growth of tumor cells both in vivo and in vitro. The conclusion from these studies was that a modest, rather than a minimal, immune reaction was usually most conducive to tumor growth; a larger reaction could, of course, be inhibitory.

The second and quite different method of challenging the hypothesis was based on the observation, in the mouse, that there exists a relationship between the original latency of a chemically induced tumor in the primary autochthonous host and its immunogenicity as shown by subsequent transplantation tests in syngeneic animals. A detailed reexamination of this relationship showed that the tumors of shortest latencies had intermediate levels of immunogenicity.[34] Tumors that had had longer latencies in the original hosts tended to have either higher or lower immunogenicities. Ancillary work suggested that the differing latencies among the tumors were a direct consequence of the differing levels of immune reactivity.[34] Thus, it again could be concluded that the optimal level of immune reaction for rapid oncogenesis was not minimal but intermediate.

The third method was based on the previously established fact that, even among mice genetically able to metabolize the carcinogen to its active form, there exist, among different strains, large differences in susceptibilities to tumor induction. Most remarkably, it was found that the mouse strain most susceptible to tumor formation by a large concentration of 3-methylcholanthrene, in subcutaneously placed paraffin wafers, was the strain least susceptible to a low concentration, and vice versa.[35] The rank order of susceptibilities, across as many as ten different genotypes, was found to reverse when the concentration of carcinogen was changed from high to low. Subsequent work suggested that the rank-order–reversal phenomenon was dependent on an intact immune system,[36] and it was already known that, when the chemical was administered in paraffin wafers, the immunogenicities of the tumors tended to be directly related to the concentration of carcinogen.[37] The most reasonable interpretion of these findings seems to be that optimal oncogenesis was produced by combining high tumor immunogenicities, as produced by high concentrations of carcinogen, with a strain of mouse with relatively low immune capacity, and vice versa. Thus, oncogenesis was favored by an intermediate level of antitumor immune reaction.

The fourth and last method of challenging the hypothesis that a modest immune reaction is a positive aid to tumor formation is the observation that thymectomy of the 3-day old mouse, which, in contrast to thymectomy at birth or at 7 days of age, causes hyperplastic autoimmune lesions,[38] increases susceptibility to subsequent chemical carcinogenesis.[39] It was observed that this increase in susceptibility occurred only with low concentrations of chemical; with higher concentrations, thymectomy at 3 days of age inhibited tumor formation.[39] Once again it seems that an elevated immune capacity, as evidenced by the tendency to the development of autoimmune lesions, aided oncogenesis only when the tumors were of the relatively low immunogenicity type that are characteristic of low concentrations of carcinogen. The parallels with the "reversal phenomenon" are striking.

The apparent correlation between experimental autoimmunity and susceptibility to low-dose oncogenesis[39] and the association of many autoimmune diseases in the human with an increased risk of cancer[6] suggest the hypothesis that increased autoimmune reactivity may often be a causative factor in oncogenesis. It appears that partial immunologic crippling, whether produced by aging,[40] radiation,[41,42] or a variety of other factors,[43,44] may sometimes result in a decline of the suppressor cells that is greater than the decline of the effectors; this differential decline may be especially true of the suppressors of various antiself reactions. The resulting autoimmunity is apparently conducive to oncogenesis with low dosages of carcinogen.[39] In other words, cancer may be, at least in part, an autoimmune disease.[6]

The hypothesis that immunity can be a positive aid to tumor growth is not new, but it is only within the last decade that the evidence supporting it has become persuasive. The consistency of the results obtained with such disparate approaches as we have described seems, to us, to make a virtually conclusive case in favor of the hypothesis, but the mechanisms are not clear. Recent evidence has implicated the macrophage, which is now known to be capable of secreting growth-promoting factors.[45-47] Recently, work by Tsuda et al[48] has shown that the slower growth of tumors in aged mice is caused, at least in part, by a deficiency of certain tumor-facilitating lymphocytes. However, the work of Shearer and Parker[30] with antibody suggests to us that perhaps any immune effector can facilitate tumor growth if the quantitative relationships are correct.

Although the evidence for the immunofacilitation theory seems, for the most part, strong and consistent, there is one set of observations that was at first troubling. It has been observed repeatedly, and in a number of different tumor systems, that many transplanted tumors do not grow well in nude mice.[49] This is not because of a lack of an immune system, as the facilitation theory would, at first consideration, probably suggest; immunogenic, and only immunogenic, tumors grow better if the nude mice are first irradiated or otherwise presumptively further immunodepressed.[50] This is so despite the fact that nude mice are, without irradiation, already incapable of rejecting a nonmalignant allograft or zenograft.[49] Tumors that exhibit this behavior include methylcholanthrene-induced sarcomas of the type that were used to demonstrate that there is, for each tumor, some positive level of immune reaction that is conducive to tumor growth.

One possible explanation for the behavior of transplanted tumors in nude mice, which is consistent with the immunofacilitation theory, assumes that immunity to normal-tissue xenografts and allografts is, per se, qualitatively different from some facet of antitumor immunity and that the nude mouse has an excess of the latter.[49] Although the antitumor facet of the immune reaction in nude mice is excessive for many transplanted tumors, it is suboptimal for skin carcinogenesis with 3-methylcholanthrene,[51] a fact that again probably illustrates the profound importance of the manner of antigen presentation. The antitumor reaction of the nude mice could be dependent in part on natural killer cells, which nude mice have been shown to possess,[52] but since the radiosensitive resistance in the nude mice correlates with the presence in the tumors of specific immunogenicity (in normal mice), a role for tumor-specific antigens is implied.[50] This explanation suggests that irradiation of the nude mouse reduces a putative antitumor immunity nearer to an optimum, but possibly still positive, level for tumor growth. Even were the antitumor immunity completely abolished by irradiation, the transplanted tumor might still be expected to grow better than it would in the face of the excessive amount of antitumor activity that is postulated to exist in the unirradiated adult nude mouse.

The apparent fact that immunity can be either stimulatory or inhibitory to tumor growth, depending on quantitative factors—that immunity has a flip side—is, in our minds, a serious complication to immunologic approaches to therapy and may help to explain why immunologic approaches have not as yet lived up to their seeming potential. Hopefully, the knowledge of the existence of this complication will make the creation of more successful immunologic strategies feasible. Progress would seem to depend on developing a way of assessing the individual tumor's sensitivity to immunity and whether the host's response is higher or lower, in vivo, than is optimal for the growth of that tumor. We think it encouraging that tumors of little immunogenicity that are induced by very low dosages of carcinogen, and therefore perhaps most human tumors, can be influenced, albeit not as yet to the host's advantage, by immunomodulation[39]; we are encouraged to believe that when tumor immunity can be abrogated specifically, a therapeutic effect may be achieved with many tumors, especially early in their progression. Until that time, cautious trials of less ideal immunosuppressants, such as cyclosporine, might be useful. Presently available data suggest that cyclosporine may not be more harmful to the cancer patient than to the transplant patient[53]; it has been shown, under some conditions, to be a successful adjunct to chemotherapy[54] and to interfere with experimental metastases, perhaps by a direct cytotoxic effect on tumor cells.[55,56] The fact that cyclosporine increases the incidence of some types of tumor[14] and can, under some conditions, produce autoimmunity[43] does not necessarily mean that it cannot be used for therapy. In its favor is the fact that it can be of benefit in the hyperplasia of psoriasis, although its efficacy in that disease may be attributable to a direct cytotoxic effect on keratinocytes rather than to immunologic effects.[57] In any case, immunosuppressive therapy seems fully as rational as immunoaugmentive; we would anticipate some striking successes, but many tumors will probably adapt and thus escape from either immunosuppression or immunoaugmentation.

References

1. Prehn RT, Main JM: Immunity to methylcholanthrene-induced sarcomas. *JNCI* 1957;18:769-778.
2. Prehn RT: Analysis of antigenic heterogeneity within individual 3-methylcholanthrene-induced mouse sarcomas. *JNCI* 1970;45:1039-1045.
3. Srivastava PK, DeLeo AB, Old LJ: Tumor rejection antigens of chemically induced sarcomas of inbred mice. *Proc Natl Acad Sci USA* 1986;83:3407-3411.
4. Globerson A, Feldman M: Antigenic specificity of benzo(a)pyrine-induced sarcomas. *JNCI* 1964;32:1229-1243.
5. Bubenik J, Adamcova B, Kolkovsky P: Changes in the antigenicity of tumours passaged against immunoselective pressure, in Klein J, Vojtbiiskovba M, Zelenby B (eds): *Genetic Variations in Somatic Cells, Proceedings of the Symposium on the Mutational Process.* Prague, Czechoslovakia, Academia Publishing House, Czechoslovak Academy of Sciences, 1967, pp 403-408.
6. Prehn RT, Prehn LM: The autoimmune nature of cancer. *Cancer Res* 1987;47:927-932.
7. Prehn RT: Immunotherapy by chemotherapy. *Inserm* 1980;97:297-303.
8. Klein G, Sjogren HO, Klein E, et al: Demonstration of resistance against methylcholanthrene-induced sarcomas in the primary autochthonous host. *Cancer Res* 1960;20:1561-1572.
9. Basombrio MA, Prehn RT: Immune status of autochthonous and adoptively protected mice toward spontaneous and chemically induced tumors. *Cancer Res* 1972;32:2545-2550.
10. Prehn RT: Function of depressed immunologic reactivity during carcinogenesis. *JNCI* 1963;31:791-805.
11. Dorsch SE, Cook EP: Neoplasia in adoptively immunosuppressed rats: A possible model for tumorigenesis in transplant recipients. *Transplantation* 1983;36:68-72.
12. Reddy AL, Caldwell M, Fialkow PJ: Sequential studies of skin tumorigenesis in phosphoglycerate kinase mosaic mice: Effect of resumption of promotion on regressed papillomas. *Cancer Res* 1987;47:1947-1951.
13. Lawler EM, Prehn RT: Influence of immune status of host on immunogenicity of tumors induced with two doses of methylcholanthrene. *Cancer Immunol Immunother* 1982;13:194-197.
14. Penn I: Cancers following cyclosporine therapy. *Transplantation* 1987;43:32-35.
15. Fisher BK, Warner LC: Cutaneous manifestations of the acquired immunodeficiency syndrome. *Int J Dermatol* 1987;26:615-630.
16. Rivin BE, Monroe JM, Hubschman BP, et al: AIDS outcome: A first follow-up. *N Engl J Med* 1984;311:857.
17. Moss AR, McCallum G, Volberding PA, et al: Mortality associated with mode of presentation in the acquired immune deficiency syndrome. *JNCI* 1984;73:1281-1284.
18. Black MM, Zachrau RE, Hankey BF, et al: Skin window elasticity to autologous breast cancer. *Cancer* 1988;62:72-83.
19. Prehn RT: Immunostimulation of the lymphodependent phase of neoplastic growth. *JNCI* 1977;59:1043-1049.
20. Ronan SG, Eng AM: Thin malignant melanomas with regression and metastases. *Arch Dermatol* 1987;123:1326-1330.
21. Vaage J: The metastasizing potentials of mouse mammary tumors and their metastases. *Int J Cancer* 1988;41:855-858.
22. Fødstad O, Aamdal S, McMenamin M, et al: A new experimental metastasis model in athymic nude mice, the human malignant melanoma LOX. *Int J Cancer* 1988;41:442-449.
23. West WH, Tauer KW, Oldham RK, et al: Immunotherapy of advanced cancer. *N Engl J Med* 1987;316:275.
24. Fulton AM, Loveless SE, Heppner GH: Mutagenic activity of tumor-associated macrophages. *Cancer Res* 1984;44:4308-4311.
25. Prehn RT: Immunostimulation of chemical oncogenesis in the mouse. *Int J Cancer* 1977;20:918-922.
26. Prehn LM: Immunostimulation of highly immunogenic target tumor cells by lymphoid cells in vitro. *JNCI* 1976;56:833-838.
27. Prehn RT: The immune reaction as a stimulator of tumor growth.

Science 1972;176:170-171.
28. Fidler IJ: In vitro studies of cellular-mediated immunostimulation of tumor growth. *JNCI* 1973;50:1307-1312.
29. Medina D, Heppner G: Cell-mediated immunostimulation induced by mammary tumor virus-free BALB/c mammary tumors. *Nature* 1973;242:329-330.
30. Shearer WT, Parker CW: Antibody and complement modulation of tumor cell growth in vitro and in vivo. *Fed Proc* 1978;37:2385-2389.
31. Prehn RT: Do tumors grow because of the immune response of the host? *Transplant Rev* 1976;28:34-42.
32. Murasko DM, Prehn RT: Stimulatory effect of immunization on tumor induction by Moloney murine sarcoma virus. *JNCI* 1978;61:1323-1327.
33. Outzen HC: Development of carcinogen-induced skin tumors in mice with varied states of immune capacity. *Int J Cancer* 1980;26:87-92.
34. Prehn RT, Bartlett GL: Surveillance, latency, and the two levels of MCA-induced tumor immunogenicity. *Int J Cancer* 1987;39:106-110.
35. Prehn LM, Lawler EM: Rank order of sarcoma susceptibility among mouse strains reverses with low concentrations of carcinogen. *Science* 1979;204:309-310.
36. Prehn LM, Lawler EM: The immune basis of dosage-induced reversal of the rank-order of strain susceptibility to MCA. *Int J Cancer* 1987;39:240-243.
37. Prehn RT: Relationship of tumor immunogenicity to concentration of the oncogen. *JNCI* 1975;55:189-190.
38. Kojima A, Prehn RT: Genetic susceptibility to post-thymectomy autoimmune disease in mice. *Immunogenetics* 1981;14:15-27.
39. Prehn LM, Kojima A: Paradoxical effect of three-day thymectomy on sarcogenesis in the mouse with different dosages of methylcholanthrene. *Cancer Res* 1986;46:4921-4926.
40. Thoman ML, Weigle WO: Deficiency in suppressor T cell activity in aged animals: Reconstitution of this activity by interleukin-2. *J Exp Med* 1983;157:2184-2189.
41. North RJ: Radiation-induced, immunologically mediated regression of an established tumor as an example of successful immunomanipulation: Preferential elimination of suppressor T cells allows sustained production of effector T cells. *J Exp Med* 1986;164:1652-1660.
42. Hellstrom I, Hellstrom KE: Antitumor effect of whole-body x-irradiation: Possible role of an x-ray sensitive T suppressor cell population. *Transplant Proc* 1979;11:1073-1076.
43. Sakaguchi S, Sakaguchi N: Thymus and autoimmunity. *J Exp Med* 1988;167:1479-1485.
44. Berd D, Maguire HC Jr, Mastrangelo MJ: Potentiation of human cell-mediated and humoral immunity by low-dose cyclophosphamide. *Cancer Res* 1984;44:5439-5443.
45. DeLustro F, Mackel AM, DeLustro B, et al: Human monocyte regulation of connective tissue growth. *Am Zool* 1983;23:213-220.
46. Evans R: Macrophage requirement for growth of a murine fibrosarcoma. *Br J Cancer* 1978;37:1086-1089.
47. De Groot JW, Compier-Spies PI, Wilbrink B, et al: Tumor growth stimulatory macrophages induced by a subclinical bacterial infection in vivo. *J Leukocyte Biol* 1986;40:433-443.
48. Tsuda T, Kim YT, Siskind GWW, et al: Role of thymus and T-cells in slow growth of B16 melanoma in old mice. *Cancer Res* 1987;47:3097-3100.
49. Welsch CW, O'Connor DH, Aylsworth CF, et al: Normal but not carcinomatous primary rat mammary epithelium: Readily transplanted to and maintained in the athymic nude mouse. *JNCI* 1987;78:557-565.
50. Prehn LM, Outzen HC: Primary tumor immunity in nude mice. *Int J Cancer* 1977;19:688-691.
51. Outzen HC: A preliminary analysis of skin tumor induction in immunomodulated mice, in Houchens D, Overjera A (eds): *Proceedings of the Symposium on the Use of Athymic (Nude) Mice in Cancer Research.* New York, Gustav Fisher Verlag, 1978, pp 93-99.
52. Hanna N: Role of natural killer cells in control of cancer metastasis. *Cancer Metastasis Rev* 1982;1:45-64.
53. Pichlmayr R: Is there a place for liver grafting for malignancy? *Transplant Proc* 1988;20(suppl 1):478-482.
54. Meador J, Sweet P, Stupecky M, et al: Enhancement by cyclosporin A of daunorubicin efficacy in Ehrlich ascites carcinoma and murine hepatoma 129. *Cancer Res* 1987;47:6216-6219.
55. Twentyman PR: Modification of cytotoxic drug resistance by non-immunosuppressive cyclosporins. *Br J Cancer* 1988;57:254-258.
56. Barbera-Guillem E, Canavata ML, Lopez de Tejada I, et al: Influence of host defenses on the hepatic colonization of B6F10 melanoma cells. *Exp Metastasis* 1988;6:153-169.
57. Nickoloff BJ, Fisher GJ, Mitra RS, et al: Additive and synergistic antiproliferative effects of cyclosporin A and gamma interferon on cultured human keratinocytes. *Am J Pathol* 1988;31:12-18.

In Other AMA Journals

ARCHIVES OF INTERNAL MEDICINE

Tetracycline for Sclerosis of Thyroid Cysts: A Randomized Study

Laszlo Hegedüs, MD; Jens Mølhom Hansen, MD; Steen Karstrup, MD; Søren Torp-Pedersen, MD; Niels Juul, MD

In a prospective study, 53 consecutive patients with solitary thyroid cysts were randomized to ultrasonically guided cyst aspiration and subsequent flushing with isotonic saline (n=30) or tetracycline hydrochloride (n=23). The patients were followed up clinically and ultrasonically 1, 3, 6, and 12 months after treatment. If the cyst recurred, a repeated treatment was offered. Cure was defined as the absence of any residual nodule and an ultrasonic cyst volume of less than 1 mL 12 months after the last treatment. During follow-up, two patients without recurrence after saline treatment and six patients without recurrence after tetracycline treatment developed solid cold nodules. Fourteen (47%) of 30 patients in the saline group and ten (43%) of 23 patients in the tetracycline group were cured (not statistically significant). Tetracycline does not seem to offer any advantage over isotonic saline in the treatment of thyroid cysts, and some of these patients still need thyroid surgery (*Arch Intern Med* 1988;148:1116-1118).

Reprint requests to Department of Internal Medicine and Endocrinology F, Herlev Hospital, DK-2730 Herlev, Denmark (Dr. Hegedüs).

Recombinant Human Tumor Necrosis Factor Alone and With Chemotherapeutic Agents

Effect on Nude Mouse–Supported Human Bladder Cancer Heterografts

Anurag K. Das, MD; Philip J. Walther, MD, PhD; Niall J. Buckley, MD; Susan H. M. Poulton

• Although studies done in tissue culture (in vitro) have shown synergism between recombinant human tumor necrosis factor (rhTNF) and chemotherapeutic agents, whether such synergism exists in a complex in vivo environment with acceptable toxic side effects has not been determined, to our knowledge. The effect of rhTNF alone and in combination with cisplatin, etoposide, doxorubicin, or dactinomycin on the growth of heterotransplants of human bladder transitional cell carcinoma was studied using a modified subrenal capsule assay in athymic nude mice. Only etoposide potentiated rhTNF cytotoxicity; no increase in host toxicity was noted. Variably enhanced toxic side effects were seen with other combinations. It is concluded that rhTNF combined with etoposide may have potential clinically exploitable therapeutic "synergism" in the treatment of advanced bladder cancer.

(*Arch Surg* 1989;124:107-110)

Tumor necrosis factor (TNF) is a polypeptide found in the serum of animals sensitized to an immunopotentiator such as BCG and then challenged with endotoxin.[1] Tumor necrosis factor is produced by macrophages both in vivo and in vitro and has been shown to cause hemorrhagic necrosis of some tumors when passively transferred to tumor-bearing animals.[1,2] With the availability of relatively pure recombinant human TNF (rhTNF), in vivo and in vitro chemosensitivity studies have been carried out testing the effectiveness of rhTNF alone and in combination with chemotherapeutic and immunotherapeutic agents.[3-6] While in vivo assays against some syngeneic mouse tumors have resulted in complete tumor regression after TNF therapy, treatment of animals with human tumor xenografts has not been as effective. Although intralesional injections of TNF directly into the tumor have provided significant tumor regression and an occasional complete cure,[7] this is not a particularly valuable method for measuring antineoplastic agent effectiveness. Intravenous or intraperitoneal TNF alone has some cytotoxic effect on human tumor xenografts but seldom results in significant tumor regression.[3,5,7,8] Since rhTNF alone is believed to have few toxic side effects,[3,9] it would seem to be an ideal agent to use in combination with chemotherapeutic agents if it enhanced the tumor cytotoxicity–host toxicity ratio.

In vitro studies have shown TNF effectiveness against a variety of human transformed and nontransformed cell lines.[4,9,10] Dactinomycin has long been known to modify the cytotoxicity of TNF and this combination has become the standard to define TNF activity. Why dactinomycin significantly enhances TNF cytotoxicity is not known, although inhibition of RNA synthesis is postulated to be the major mechanism.[11] Recently, synergistic enhancement by TNF of the in vitro cytotoxicity of chemotherapeutic agents targeted at DNA topoisomerase II has been reported[6]; the most commonly used agents targeted at DNA topoisomerase II include dactinomycin, doxorubicin, and etoposide (VP-16). To our knowledge, the mechanism of this enhanced cytotoxicity remains unknown. However, whether any potentiation of either tumoricidal efficacy or host toxicity (two components of the "therapeutic index") occurs when these drugs are combined with TNF in the complex in vivo pharmacologic milieu is not known; such issues require the use of an animal model.

We studied the effects of purified rhTNF alone and in combination with three drugs targeted at DNA topoisomerase II—dactinomycin, doxorubicin, and etoposide—and one drug that is not—cisplatin, but that has known efficacy in the therapy of bladder carcinoma. Both the cytotoxicity and the toxicity of each agent alone and in combination were examined using tumor xenografts of human bladder transitional cell carcinoma—a tumor believed to be biologic response modifier sensitive. To perform the testing we used our modified nude mouse subrenal capsule assay (MSRCA)—a precise, rapid, in vivo chemosensitivity assay.

MATERIALS AND METHODS

Cytotoxic Agents

Patient grade sterile preparations of cisplatin (Platinol), doxorubicin hydrochloride (Adriamycin), etoposide (VePesid), and dactinomycin D (Cosmegen) were utilized for this study and prepared fresh using the manufacturer's recommendations. The rhTNF used had a purity of 95% by sodium dodecyl sulfate/polyacrylamide gel electrophoresis. Endotoxin contamination was minimal, 0.058 ng/0.29 mg of protein by *Limulus* amebocyte lysate assay, and the bioactivity was 22 413 U/μg of protein. It was prepared using bovine serum albumin (BSA) as a carrier protein according to the manufacturer's recommendation and stored at −20°C before reconstitution and −70°C after reconstitution.

Human Tumor Xenografts

Human tumor heterotransplants of a bladder transitional cell carcinoma tumor line (DU-4284) have been maintained by serial subcutaneous passages in nu/nu athymic nude mice. Nude mice were all from our inbred breeding colony designated BALB/c AnBom Urd and were maintained in the Animal and Laboratory Isolation Facility (a true barrier facility) of Duke University Medical Center, Durham, NC. The tumor line was established from a lymph node metastasis in a patient with high-grade transitional cell carcinoma and was used in its 18th passage. It has a subcutaneous doubling time of four days. Tumor was removed from mice and kept bathed in RPMI-1640 until it was implanted in mice, usually within two to three hours.

MSRCA

Eight-week-old nude mice from our breeding colony were used for all experiments. Since the subrenal capsule in mice is transparent, implanted tumors can be measured in situ. The implantation technique has been previously described.[12] A system that employs a stereoscopic zoom microscope (Olympus model SZH, Olympus Corporation, Lake Success, NY) with an ocular micrometer was used at ×11.4 magnification such that 1 mm was equivalent to 11.4 ocular units. The length and width of each implant were recorded in ocular units. Briefly, the following protocol was observed.

Day 1.—Initial body weight was taken after mice were anesthetized with pentobarbital sodium. Using sterile technique, a 1.5-cm incision was made over the left flank and the kidney was exteriorized. A small incision was then made in the transparent

Accepted for publication July 8, 1988.

From the Departments of Surgery (Urology) (Drs Das, Walther, and Buckley and Ms Poulton) and Pathology (Dr Walther), Medical Research Service, Durham Veterans Administration Medical Center and Duke University School of Medicine (Dr Walther), Durham, NC.

Read before the Annual Meeting of the Society of Surgical Oncology, New Orleans, May 23, 1988.

Reprint requests to Box 3314, Duke University Medical Center, Durham, NC 27710 (Dr Walther).

Table 1.—Morbidity and Mortality With rhTNF* Alone and in Combination With Chemotherapeutic Agents

Drug	Dose	Weight Change, %	Mortality, %
Control (none)	...	+3.0	0
Control (2% BSA†)	...	+1.0	0
rhTNF	50 μg/kg × 2	+4.0	0
rhTNF	50 μg/kg × 3	+7.0	12.5
rhTNF	100 μg/kg × 3	+3.0	0
Etoposide alone	45 mg/kg × 2	−10.3	0
Etoposide + rhTNF	45 mg/kg × 2 50 μg/kg × 2	−11.3	0
Cisplatin alone	6 mg/kg × 2	−1.4	0
Cisplatin + rhTNF	6 mg/kg × 2 50 μg/kg × 2	−3.5	0
Doxorubicin alone	12 mg/kg	−1.9	0
Doxorubicin + rhTNF	12 mg/kg 50 μg/kg × 2	−15.0	12.5
Dactinomycin alone	0.5 mg/kg	−7.6	0
Dactinomycin + rhTNF	0.5 mg/kg 50 μg/kg × 2	...	100

*rhTNF indicates recombinant human tissue necrosis factor.
†BSA indicates bovine serum albumin.

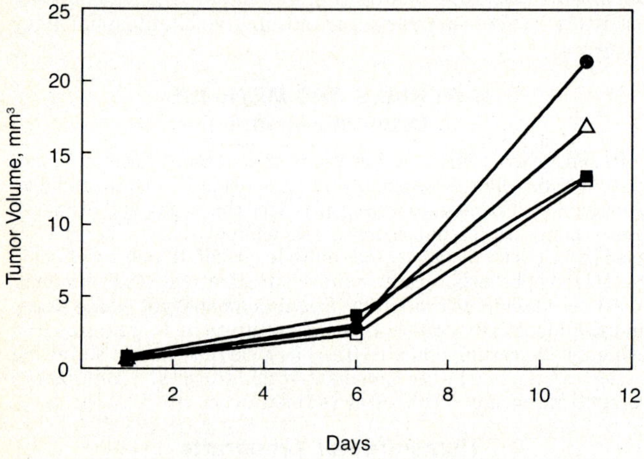

Fig 1.—Effect of multiple-dose intravenous (IV) recombinant human tumor necrosis factor (rhTNF) on DU-4284 in nu/nu athymic nude mice. In all figures each point represents mean tumor volume of seven to ten mice. Solid circles indicate control (2% bovine serum albumin) IV on days 7 and 8; open squares, rhTNF 50 μg/kg IV on days 7 and 8; open triangles, rhTNF 50 μg/kg IV on days 7, 8, and 9; and solid squares, rhTNF 100 μg/kg IV on days 7, 8, and 9.

Table 2.—Relative Tumor Survival Values for rhTNF* Alone and in Combination With Chemotherapeutic Agents

Drug	Relative Tumor Survival, %‡
Control (BSA†)	100 ± 73
rhTNF, 50 μg/kg × 2	58 ± 35
rhTNF, 50 μg/kg × 3	59 ± 33
rhTNF, 100 μg/kg × 3	44 ± 29
Etoposide alone	59 ± 19
Etoposide + rhTNF	28 ± 9
Cisplatin alone	47 ± 15
Cisplatin + rhTNF	41 ± 19
Doxorubicin alone	59 ± 23
Doxorubicin + rhTNF	49 ± 55
Dactinomycin alone	73 ± 70

*rhTNF indicates recombinant human tumor necrosis factor.
†BSA indicates bovine serum albumin.
‡Values are mean ± SD.

capsule; fine forceps were used to place a 0.75-mm³ piece of tumor, and exact measurements were determined using the ocular micrometer. The kidney was then replaced and the incision closed with clips.

Day 6.—Mice were anesthetized, clips were removed, kidneys were exteriorized, and, using the ocular micrometer, precise measurements of tumor length and width were noted before reclosure. Volume determinations of the tumor at day 1 and day 6 were made using the formula for a spheroid. Any mice whose tumors had regressed from day 1 to day 6 were rejected at this point. The remaining mice were then randomized into groups of eight.

Days 7 Through 9.—Therapy was administered according to the doses shown in Table 1. Controls received 0.1 mL of intravenous 2% BSA. When a combination of TNF and chemotherapeutic agents was used, the chemotherapeutic agent was always given approximately one hour before the TNF. The TNF was always given intravenously (volume, 0.1 mL), while chemotherapeutic agents were always given intraperitoneally in a volume of 0.2 to 0.3 mL.

Day 11.—Mice were killed, weighed, and tumor-bearing kidneys were excised. Final length and width measurements were determined before samples of tumor-bearing kidneys were sectioned and stained for microscopic examination.

Analysis of Data

Analysis of Tumor/Cohort Consistency.—After tumor volume determinations at days 1, 6, and 11 had been made, day 6/day 1 and day 11/day 6 growth ratios were calculated. These were analyzed using the nonparametric Kruskall-Wallis one-way analysis of variance.[13] This analysis confirmed that all cohorts were not statistically significantly different (text statistic [T] = 10.40, $P = .49$) prior to therapy (day 6/day 1), while after therapy (day 11/day 6), there were statistically significant differences among the cohorts (T = 23.51, $P = .01$).

Relative Tumor Survival (RTS).—This was calculated using the formula $(R_T/R_C) \times 100$ where R_T is the day 11/day 6 ratio of a treated cohort and R_C is the day 11/day 6 ratio of the control (BSA) cohort. By definition, then, the controls (BSA) have 100% tumor survival. To determine if there were any statistically significant differences between certain cohorts, the nonparametric Mann-Whitney U test[13] was used since the data include percentages and are not normally distributed.

Analysis of Potential Synergism.—To determine possible synergism, the actual RTS values for chemotherapeutic drug plus rhTNF were compared with predicted relative survival values. Predicted relative survival values were determined by multiplying the RTS values of rhTNF alone and the chemotherapeutic drug alone. For example, the RTS for etoposide alone is 59%, for rhTNF alone is also 59%, and the predicted RTS for etoposide plus rhTNF is then 34%.

All data were analyzed using a statistical graphics system (STATGRAPHICS, Statistical Graphics Corporation, Rockville, Md).

RESULTS

Host Toxic Side Effects

Table 1 shows the mortality and weight loss for mice treated with combinations of chemotherapeutic agents and rhTNF. There was no significant mortality or weight loss from rhTNF therapy alone. There was also no significant change in mortality of cohorts treated with etoposide alone and etoposide plus rhTNF and cisplatin alone and cisplatin plus rhTNF. However, the weight loss in doxorubicin alone cohorts was only 1.9% compared with 15% in doxorubicin plus rhTNF cohorts, signifying increased morbidity. While dactinomycin *alone* had a mortality of 0% and a weight loss of 7.6%, dactinomycin plus rhTNF had 100% mortality. This suggests that the lethal toxicity is by a mechanism not related to cachexia.

Dose/Schedule Analysis of rhTNF Cytotoxicity

Figure 1 shows the actual growth curves of different rhTNF treatment regimens assessed using the MSRCA. Relative tumor survival defined above is tabulated in Table

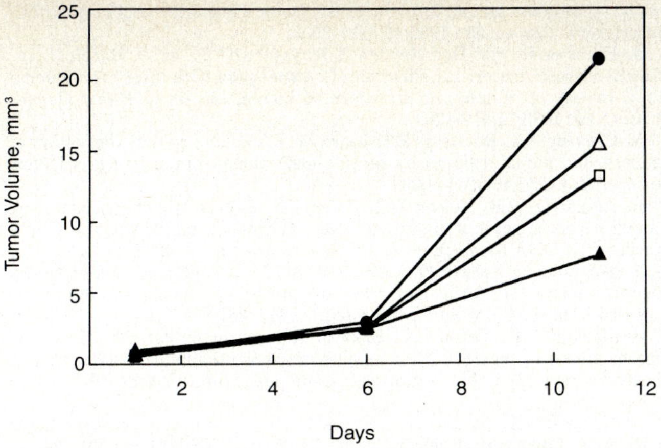

Fig 2.—Effect of etoposide and recombinant human tumor necrosis factor (rhTNF) alone and in combination with DU-4284 in nu/nu athymic nude mice. Solid circles indicate control (2% bovine serum albumin); open triangles, etoposide 45 mg/kg intraperitoneally (IP) on days 7 and 8; open squares, rhTNF 50 μg/kg on days 7 and 8; and solid triangles, etoposide 45 mg/kg IP on days 7 and 8 and rhTNF 50 μg/kg intravenously on days 7 and 8.

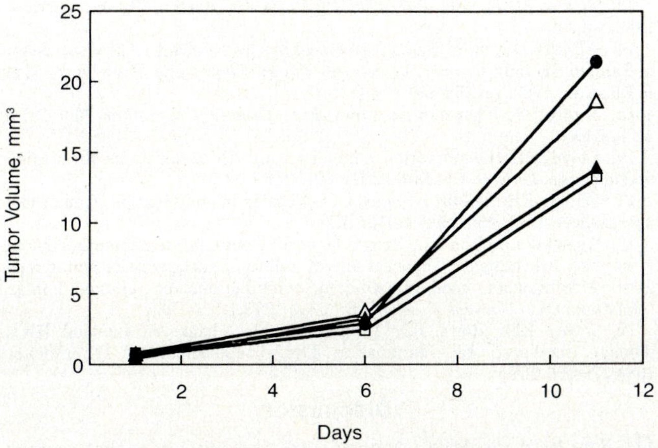

Fig 3.—Effect of doxorubicin and recombinant human tumor necrosis factor (rhTNF) alone and in combination on DU-4284 in nu/nu athymic nude mice. Solid circles indicate control (2% bovine serum albumin); open triangles, doxorubicin 12 mg/kg intraperitoneally (IP) on day 7; open squares, rhTNF 50 μg/kg intravenously (IV) on days 7 and 8; and solid triangles, doxorubicin 12 mg/kg IP on day 7 and rhTNF 50 μg/kg IV on days 7 and 8.

2. Multiple-dose rhTNF was moderately effective alone in doses that caused no significant toxic side effects.

Analysis of Single Antineoplastic Agent Cytotoxicity Alone and in Combination With rhTNF

Figures 1 through 4 depict the actual growth curves for etoposide, cisplatin, and doxorubicin alone and in combination with rhTNF. The RTS values are shown in Table 2. Cisplatin was the most effective drug (RTS, 41%), while dactinomycin was the least effective (RTS, 73%). The Mann-Whitney *U* test revealed a statistically significant difference between the etoposide only and etoposide plus rhTNF cohorts ($P=.0019$). No statistically significant differences were noted in the cisplatin alone and cisplatin plus rhTNF cohorts ($P=.52$) or in the doxorubicin alone and doxorubicin plus rhTNF cohorts ($P=.12$).

Analysis of Synergism

To determine possible synergism, the predicted RTS of rhTNF in combination with a particular chemotherapeutic agent was compared with the actual RTS. The actual and

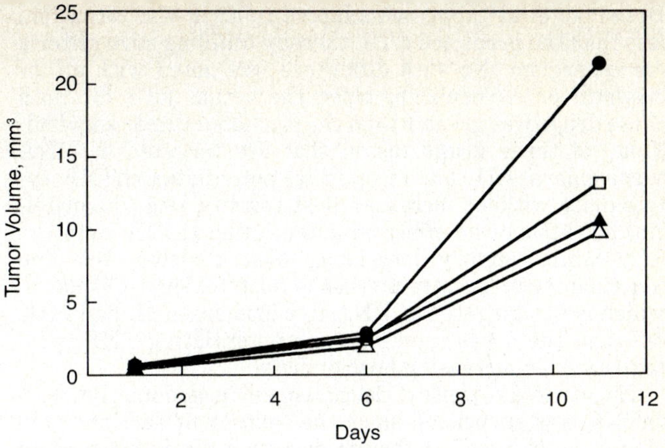

Fig 4.—Effect of cisplatin and recombinant human tumor necrosis factor (rhTNF) alone and in combination on DU-4284 in nu/nu athymic nude mice. Solid circles indicate control (2% bovine serum albumin); open triangles, cisplatin 6 mg/kg intraperitoneally (IP) on days 7 and 8; open squares, rhTNF 50 μg/kg intravenously (IV) on days 7 and 8; and solid triangles, cisplatin 6 mg/kg IP on days 7 and 8 and rhTNF 50 μg/kg IV on days 7 and 8.

Table 3.—Predicted and Actual Relative Tumor Survivals

	Relative Tumor Survival, %	
	Predicted	Actual
Etoposide + rhTNF*	34	28
Cisplatin + rhTNF	27	41
Doxorubicin + rhTNF	34	49

*rhTNF indicates recombinant human tumor necrosis factor.

predicted RTS values for the three agents are shown in Table 3. Only etoposide demonstrated an actual RTS (28%) that was less than the predicted RTS (34%), thus fulfilling the definition of therapeutic "synergism."

COMMENT

While chemotherapeutic agents exert direct cytotoxic metabolic effects on dividing cells, biologic response modifiers as a class usually exert a tumor cytotoxic effect via a receptor either directly and/or by activation of host cells.[4] While normal cells seem to be immune to the cytotoxic effects of rhTNF, the exact mechanism of tumor cytotoxicity remains unclear.

Although potentiation of rhTNF tumor cytotoxicity has been reported in in vitro experiments, particularly when used in conjunction with chemotherapeutic agents targeted at DNA topoisomerase II, in vitro assays do not provide any measure of the possible increased toxic side effects when combinations of agents are used ("therapeutic index"). Alexander et al[6] demonstrated enhanced cytotoxic activity of rhTNF in combination with dactinomycin over a wide variety of concentrations. However, doxorubin enhanced rhTNF cytotoxicity only at concentrations above 10 mg/L. The peak achievable plasma concentration of doxorubicin is believed to be 0.6 to 1 mg/L,[14] suggesting that doxorubicin potentiation of rhTNF may not be clinically applicable; our results would confirm this.

Our nude mouse in vivo assay demonstrated a statistically significant difference between the etoposide plus rhTNF and the etoposide alone cohorts. The extent of this difference would suggest potentiation, ie, synergism of tumor cell kill. While the definition of drug synergism in an in vivo system is a difficult question,[15-17] our actual RTS for the etoposide plus rhTNF cohort was, using the

Drewinko et al[18] approach adapted to an in vivo situation, less than the predicted RTS, thereby fulfilling such criteria for synergism. No such difference was noted with either cisplatin or doxorubicin, since the actual RTS for both these drugs was greater than the predicted tumor survival. Thus, of three drugs tested that are targeted at DNA topoisomerase II, one (etoposide) potentiates rhTNF cytotoxicity without increased host toxicity, one (doxorubicin) has little or no effect on potentiating rhTNF cytotoxicity while slightly increasing host toxicity, and one (dactinomycin) greatly increases host toxicity. Cisplatin, which is not targeted at DNA topoisomerase II, had little effect at the doses used either in potentiating TNF cytotoxicity or in increasing host toxicity.

The marked toxicity of dactinomycin in combination with rhTNF was surprising since the toxicity of dactinomycin alone was minimal. Although dactinomycin is believed to inhibit RNA synthesis as well as act on DNA topoisomerase II,[11,19] its primary mechanism of increased toxicity in combination with rhTNF remains poorly understood. This suggests the possibility that "toxic synergism" may also exist where the therapeutic index could conceivably be worsened. Thus, whether dactinomycin is of any value in combination with TNF (as assessed in this assay system) is still unknown to our knowledge, although further efforts in addressing the toxicity of dactinomycin plus rhTNF are presently ongoing.

Doxorubicin did not potentiate rhTNF activity at the dose used while it did cause some increase in host toxicity. However, we had carefully chosen our clinically relevant doses based on previous toxicity studies such that drug-alone doses would have minimal toxic side effects while achieving some tumor kill, and thus either increased toxic side effects or increased tumor kill would be easily identifiable when drugs were used in combination with rhTNF. Therefore, although doxorubicin may enhance the effectiveness of rhTNF at higher doses, it will probably do so only at unacceptable toxicity levels.

Of the four, etoposide, a nonintercalating epipodophyllotoxin, shows promise as an agent to be used in combination with rhTNF, since its increased tumor cell kill without any increase in host toxicity in the doses studied. Since in vitro studies had shown that the drug must precede treatment with rhTNF,[6] the drugs were always administered one hour prior to therapy with rhTNF. Further dose- and time-related studies with the etoposide and rhTNF combination seeking to arrive at optimal dose and time schedules will be necessary and are ongoing.

In conclusion, we have developed an in vivo animal system that would appear to be an excellent model for the study of potential synergism of cytotoxic agents with rhTNF for the treatment of human bladder carcinoma. It also may be applicable for the study of other human malignant neoplasms that have been adapted into an athymic nude mouse host. Using this approach, the combination of etoposide and rhTNF appears promising for potential clinical utilization. In vivo studies to determine ideal time and dose schedules in this animal model may assist in the design of clinical trials.

This investigation was supported in part by a grant from Merit Review, Veterans Administration Research Service, Durham, NC, and the CURED Foundation, Duke University, Durham.

Human RhTNF was provided by Cetus Corp, Emeryville, Calif.

References

1. Ruff MR, Gifford GE: Tumor necrosis factor, in Pick E (ed): *Lymphokines.* Orlando, Fla, Academic Press Inc, 1981, vol 2, pp 235-275.

2. Carswell EA, Old LJ, Kassel RL, et al: An endotoxin-induced serum factor that causes necrosis of tumors. *Proc Natl Acad Sci USA* 1975;72:3666-3770.

3. Balkwill FR, Lee A, Aldam G, et al: Human tumor xenografts treated with recombinant human tumor necrosis factor alone or in combination with interferons. *Cancer Res* 1986;46:3990-3993.

4. Fransen L, Van Der Heyden J, Ruysschaert R, et al: Recombinant tumor necrosis factor: Its effect and its synergism with interferon-gamma on a variety of normal and transformed human cell lines. *Eur J Cancer Clin Oncol* 1986;22:419-426.

5. Creasey AA, Reynolds MT, Laird W: Cures and partial regression of murine and human tumors by recombinant human tumor necrosis factor. *Cancer Res* 1986;46:5687-5690.

6. Alexander RB, Nelson WG, Coffey DS: Synergistic enhancement by tumor necrosis factor of in vitro cytotoxicity from chemotherapeutic agents targeted at DNA topoisomerase II. *Cancer Res* 1987;47:2403-2406.

7. Sohmura Y, Nakata K, Yoshida H, et al: Recombinant human tumor necrosis factor: II. Antitumor effect on murine and human tumors transplanted in mice. *Immunopharmacology* 1986;8:357-368.

8. Haranaka K, Satomi N, Sakurai A: Antitumor activity of murine tumor necrosis factor (TNF) against transplanted murine tumors and heterotransplanted human tumors in nude mice. *Int J Cancer* 1984;34:263-267.

9. Haranaka K, Satomi N: Cytotoxic activity of tumor necrosis factor (TNF) on human cancer cells in vitro. *Jpn J Exp Med* 1981;151:191-194.

10. Helson L, Greene S, Carswell E, et al: Effect of tumor necrosis factor on cultured human melanoma cells. *Nature* 1975;258:731-732.

11. Ostrove JM, Gifford GE: Stimulation of RNA synthesis in L929 cells by rabbit tumor necrosis factor. *Proc Soc Exp Biol Med* 1979;160:354-358.

12. Bogden AE, Kelton DE, Cobb WR, et al: A rapid screening method for testing chemotherapeutic agents against human xenografts, in Houchens DP, Ovejira AA (eds): *Proceedings of the Symposium on the Use of Athymic (Nude) Mice in Cancer Research.* New York, Gustar Fischer, 1978, pp 231-250.

13. Rosner B: *Fundamentals of Biostatistics.* Boston, Duxbury Press, 1986, pp 288-472.

14. Alberts DS, chen HSG: Pharmacokinetics relevant to in vitro assay, in Salmon SE (ed): *Cloning of Human Tumor Stem Cells.* New York, Alan R Liss Inc, 1980, pp 352-356.

15. Mantel N: Therapeutic synergism. *Cancer Chemother Rep* 1974; 4:147-149.

16. Lloyd HH: Combination chemotherapy: Considerations for design and analysis. *Cancer Chemother Rep* 1974;4:157-165.

17. Wittes RE, Goldin A: Unresolved issues in combination chemotherapy. *Cancer Treat Rep* 1986;70:105-125.

18. Drewinko B, Loo TL, Brown B, et al: Combination chemotherapy in vitro with Adriamycin: Observations of additive, antagonistic, and synergistic effects when used in two-drug combinations on cultured human lymphoma cells. *Cancer Biochem Biophys* 1976;1:187-195.

19. Tewey KM, Rowe TC, Yang L, et al: Adriamycin-induced DNA damage mediated by mammalian DNA topoisomerase II. *Science* 1984;226:466-468.

Discussion

Q Your data show that etoposide was the only agent that seemed to be effective and the others were not. How might you explain your observation?

A Well, the initial in vitro data published by Alexander et al[6] showed that dactinomycin, doxorubicin (Adriamycin), and etoposide (VP = 16) were all effective. However, if you look at their data closely they show that only dactinomycin is really effective at low doses and doxorubicin is effective at doses that are not clinically achievable. It may well be that doxorubicin is effective at higher doses, but these doses would probably cause so many toxic side effects that one would not see the effectiveness.

Q I was interested in your very distinct toxic reactions with dactinomycin. In the older literature, in some of the in vitro assays dactinomycin was used to supplement the TNF effect. These studies would try to set the stage by sensitizing cells with dactinomycin and then check for TNF activity. It is very intriguing that you are showing such a dramatic synergism between the two, even though it is a lethal synergism, and one would wonder if whether it's just the dosage that you use. Maybe with a lesser dose you might get antitumor activity.

A Dr Buckley, one of our coauthors, is going to be presenting a paper at the American Association for Cancer Research that looks at full-dose response curves of dactinomycin and TNF, starting at much lower dose levels and progressing upward. His data essentially show that there is a dose-response curve and if you drop the dactinomycin dose down to levels of 0.1 and 0.25 mg/kg, there is much less toxic reaction, but the toxic side effects are more dependent on the dactinomycin than the TNF. With this particular dose of dactinomycin, even with much lower doses of TNF, you still get significant toxic reactions. Since we did not see much response to dactinomycin at this dose alone, we doubt that with much lower doses of dactinomycin plus TNF one would see any kind of a tumor response.

Squamous Cell Carcinoma Arising in Previously Burned or Irradiated Skin

Michael J. Edwards, MD; Rose M. Hirsch, MD; J. Ralph Broadwater, MD; David T. Netscher, MD; Frederick C. Ames, MD

• Squamous cell carcinoma (SCC) arising in previously burned or irradiated skin was reviewed in 66 patients treated between 1944 and 1986. Healing of the initial injury was complicated in 70% of patients. Mean interval from initial injury to diagnosis of SCC was 37 years. The overwhelming majority of patients presented with a chronic intractable ulcer in previously injured skin. The regional relapse rate after surgical excision was very high, 58% of all patients. Predominant patterns of recurrence were in local skin and regional lymph nodes (93% of recurrences). Survival rates at 5, 10, and 20 years were 52%, 34%, and 23%, respectively. Five-year survival rates in previously burned and irradiated patients were not significantly different (53% and 50%, respectively). This review, one of the largest reported series, better defines SCC arising in previously burned or irradiated skin as a locally aggressive disease that is distinct from SCC arising in sunlight-damaged skin. An increased awareness of the significance of chronic ulceration in scar tissue may allow earlier diagnosis. Regional disease control and survival depend on surgical resection of all known disease and may require radical lymph node dissection or amputation.

(*Arch Surg* 1989;124:115-117)

Squamous cell carcinoma (SCC) arising in previously injured skin (Marjolin's ulcer) is a rare entity. We reviewed two subsets of patients with Marjolin's ulcers, those having previously burned skin and those having previously irradiated skin as the site of malignant transformation. The natural history, patterns of recurrence, and survival were analyzed for both groups. We hypothesized that injured skin, complicated by chronic ulceration, undergoes malignant transformation, and that the natural histories of the resulting carcinomas are similar and independent of the initial injury. We also compared these patients with a published analysis of all patients with SCC of the skin treated in our institution to determine whether patients with scar carcinomas had a poorer prognosis than patients with SCC arising in sunlight-damaged skin.

PATIENTS AND METHODS

The medical records of all patients treated at the M. D. Anderson Cancer Center, Houston, for SCC arising in previously burned or irradiated skin were reviewed. Records of 66 patients treated between 1944 and 1986 were analyzed for demographic data, clinical presentation, treatment, patterns of treatment failure, and survival.

Demographic data analyzed included age, gender, and factors related to the initial cutaneous injury. Factors believed to be important included age at the time of injury, cause and anatomic site of injury, wound treatment, time required for wound healing, and epithelial ulceration after initial healing.

Data analyzed relating to the clinical presentation of SCC included presenting signs and symptoms, stage of disease, and interval from the time of initial injury to the development of SCC. The extent of surgical procedures required for local disease control and the use of other treatment modalities were included in the analysis. Subsequent recurrence was analyzed by site (local skin, regional nodes, and distant metastasis) and time from surgical excision to recurrence. Differences between groups were analyzed using the two-sample t test and the χ^2 test where appropriate. Survival analysis was by the Kaplan-Meier method. Differences in survival rates were analyzed by the Wilcoxon test.

RESULTS

Twenty patients developed radiation-induced SCC and 46 patients developed squamous carcinoma after a thermal injury. At the time of diagnosis, the average age of all patients was 58 years; the majority (38 [58%]) were men. Mean age at the time of initial injury was 37 years in patients with radiation-induced injury and only 13 years in patients with thermal injury ($P<.01$).

The wounds in both groups were often (36 [55%]) allowed to heal by secondary intention. However, for 24 patients (36%), we found no clear record of initial wound management. The majority of patients (47 [71%]) experienced recurrent ulceration or prolonged wound healing. Only eight patients (12%) had primary wound healing without complications. The presence or absence of complications during healing could not be determined for 11 patients (17%).

The mean interval from initial injury to diagnosis of SCC was 37 years (range, 1.5 to 82 years). Squamous cell carcinoma developed earlier in irradiated skin than in burned skin (24.8 ± 15.7 compared with 43.7 ± 20.4 years, $P<.01$). During the last two decades, the incidence of both burn- and radiation-induced carcinomas decreased. At the time of diagnosis of carcinoma, most patients complained of a chronic fissure or ulcer for several months or years (Table 1). Presenting signs and symptoms were similar for irradiated and burned patients except that a greater number of burned patients presented with suspicious regional adenopathy (37% vs 5% [17 vs one]).

The head and neck and upper extremity were the most commonly involved anatomic sites. The hand was the most frequently involved site in patients who had radiation-induced cancers. Most carcinomas developed in sites considered to be predisposed to repeated trauma: the flexor (16 [34%]) and extensor (eight [17%]) surfaces over joints and areas overlying bony prominences (nine [19%]).

Initial surgical treatment was determined by extent of disease at presentation. Forty-two patients were initially treated with wide local excision alone. However, many patients required extensive resection to achieve adequate surgical margins. Eight had wide local excision and regional lymphadenopathy. Regional lymph nodes were dissected for patients presenting with suspicious adenopathy and for lesions directly overlying regional nodal basins. Prophylactic node dissection was not generally done. A major extremity amputation was required as initial treatment in seven patients. Locally advanced unresectable disease was treated by arterial chemotherapy (four patients) and radiation therapy (one patient). Systemic chemotherapy was used as initial therapy in one patient with metastatic disease. No treatment was given to one patient with extensive local and metastatic disease. The initial treatment of three patients at other institutions could not be determined.

Accepted for publication Sept 2, 1988.

From the Division of Surgery, Department of General Surgery, University of Texas M. D. Anderson Cancer Center, Houston.

Read before the Annual Meeting of the Society of Surgical Oncology, New Orleans, May 24, 1988.

Reprint requests to University of Texas M. D. Anderson Cancer Center, 1515 Holcombe Blvd, Box 106, Houston, TX 77030 (Dr Edwards).

Table 1.—Presenting Signs and Symptoms of 66 Patients

Complaint	No. (%) of Irradiated Patients	No. (%) of Patients With Burns	Total No. (%)
Chronic ulceration/fissure	20 (100)	45 (96)	**65 (98)**
Pain	13 (65)	22 (48)	**35 (54)**
Chronic infection	5 (25)	19 (40)	**24 (36)**
Adenopathy	1 (5)	17 (37)	**18 (27)**
Distant metastasis	0 (0)	3 (6)	**3 (5)**

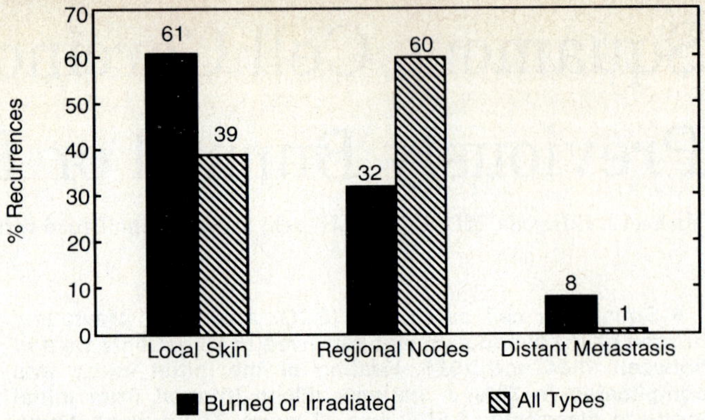

Fig 2.—Recurrence rates and locations are compared between those of 1224 patients with squamous cell carcinoma of all types (106 recurrences, 8.7%) and 66 patients with previously irradiated or burned skin (38 recurrences, 58%).

Table 2.—Sites of Initial Recurrence of Squamous Cell Carcinoma

Site	No. (%) of Irradiated Patients	No. (%) of Patients With Burns	Total No. (%)
Local skin	6 (30)	17 (37)	**23 (35)**
Regional nodes	7 (35)	5 (11)	**12 (18)**
Distant metastasis	1 (5)	2 (4)	**3 (5)**
Total	**14 (70)**	**24 (52)**	**38 (58)**

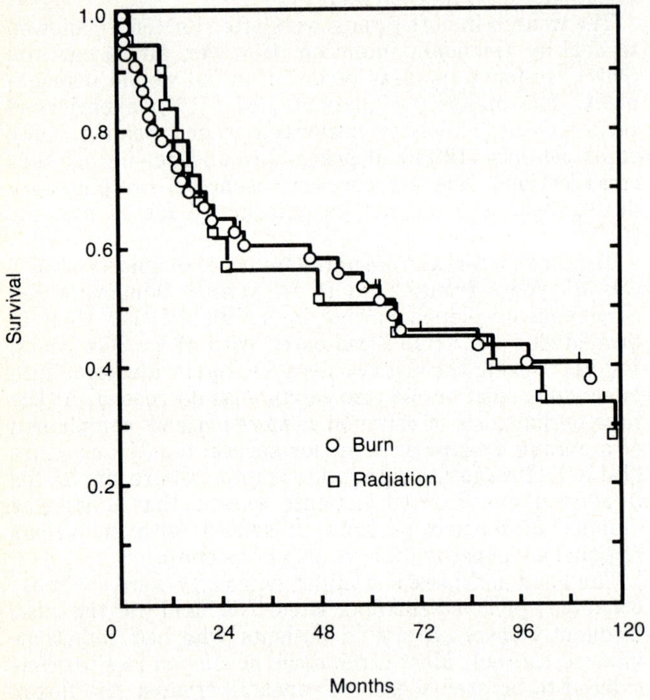

Fig 1.—Survival rates of previously burned and irradiated patients ($P = .99$, Wilcoxon test).

Recurrent disease developed in 58% (38) of all patients. Of 42 patients who presented with apparent local disease, five (12%) subsequently developed regional nodal metastasis as their initial site of recurrence. The incidence of recurrent disease was higher for SCCs arising in irradiated skin (14 [70%]) compared with those arising in previously burned skin (24 [52%]). The time from the surgical treatment of cancer to recurrence ranged from two months to 28 years (median, 13 months for each subset). Most recurrences were in local skin and regional lymph nodes (Table 2). Median survival after local or regional recurrence was 21 and 12 months, respectively. Distant metastases eventually occurred in only 17% of patients (11) and were most often found in bone, followed by lung and distant skin.

Survival rates for all patients at 5, 10, and 20 years after their initial diagnosis of carcinoma were 52%, 34%, 23%, respectively. Five-year survival rates were similar for both groups of patients: 53% at five years when carcinoma originated in previously burned skin and 50% where previously irradiated skin was the source ($P = .99$, Fig 1). Patients presenting with regional adenopathy had a particularly poor prognosis. Their median survival was 16 months; patients who had no adenopathy had a median survival of 66 months.

COMMENT

This review shows that patients with SCC arising in previously burned or irradiated skin have similar natural histories and survival. The age at initial injury was significantly lower for patients who were burned. The frequency of burns occurring in children and the older age at which patients or medical personnel usually received radiation therapy or exposure are the most likely reasons for this age difference.

The incidence of SCC arising from both irradiated and burned skin has declined over the past two decades. All patients in our series who had radiation-induced carcinoma were treated before 1959. Many of the radiation-induced upper-extremity and hand burns (nine patients [45%]) were the result of cutaneous injuries incurred by physicians and other medical personnel using now-outmoded radiation oncology or diagnostic radiologic equipment. Improvements in radiation technology and an improved understanding of radiation risks have made treatment safer and practically eliminated the risk of radiation-induced carcinoma.[1] The declining incidence of carcinomas arising in burned skin may be due to early, complete, and durable coverage of wounds. Improved methods of wound closure promote primary wound healing and reduce chronic wound problems that may predispose to malignant change.

These SCCs most frequently originate in areas of exposed skin most susceptible to burn or radiation injury: the head, neck, and extremities.[2] Repeated ulceration and prolonged healing of severe burn wounds have been noted as potential risk factors for the development of invasive carcinoma.[3] Wound sites where repeated trauma occurs are prone to chronic ulceration and potentially increase the risk of malignant transformation. In this series, 70% (33 patients) of cancers originated in scars over joints or bony prominences, which are sites susceptible to repeated trauma. The potential for chronic ulceration and delayed wound healing as risk factors for malignant transformation, especially in these areas prone to trauma, should be considered during initial wound management; complete wound healing should be achieved in these areas.

Ulcers and fissures that arise in areas of scarring that

fail to respond promptly to therapeutic measures should have biopsy specimens taken. A malignant lesion may appear as a benign chronic ulcer or fissure and be neglected for a long time. The patient often does not consult a physician until late in the course of the disease. Even then, many physicians may not recognize the significance of ulceration, which is why diagnosis late in the natural history of the disease is common.

Surgical excision is the most effective treatment for scar carcinomas. Where technically feasible, the entire area of previously injured skin should be excised with the carcinoma since residual burned or irradiated skin may be the site of future recurrent disease. Whether prophylactic node dissection would be useful is speculative. Among the 42 patients in our series with local disease initially treated by wide local excision alone, only five (12%) developed subsequent nodal metastasis. Our policy is to follow up regional nodes closely in these patients with localized primary carcinomas. We do not recommend routine prophylactic regional node dissection for localized scar carcinomas.

For patients who present with locally advanced disease and metastases to regional lymph nodes, extensive surgical procedures including regional lymph node dissection, extremity amputation, or resection of other vital tissues may be required.[4] Postoperative radiation therapy may be useful in previously burned patients with narrow surgical margins or nodal metastasis with extranodal extension into connective tissue.

Our high rate of overall recurrence (58% of all patients) is consistent with other reports but also may reflect a selection bias caused by the referral of patients with more advanced disease to the M. D. Anderson Cancer Center. A comparison with a previously reported series of all patients with cutaneous SCCs treated at our institution[5] shows that the rate of recurrence in the subset of patients with scar carcinomas was notably higher (58% vs 9%). Patterns of recurrence, however, were similar, with very few of the patients developing distant metastasis as the initial site of recurrence (Fig 2). A comparative review of the timing of the failures revealed that though approximately two thirds (24 of 38) of recurrences developed within the first 36 months after diagnosis (median, 13 months), approximately one fourth (eight of 38) developed after five years. This is in contrast to the timing of recurrences seen in patients with squamous carcinoma arising in sunlight-damaged skin, where recurrences after five years were rare.[5]

This study confirms that scar carcinomas are aggressive. Five-year survival was only 52%. In comparison, patients with sunlight-induced SCCs have a five-year survival of 90%.[6] The exact reason for the poor prognosis in patients with Marjolin's ulcers is unknown. Theoretical explanations of this poor prognosis have included an inherent biologic aggressiveness of scar carcinomas and the possibility that areas of scarring provide an immunologically privileged site for tumor growth.[7] Advanced disease at the time of diagnosis may be the primary factor. Patients with scar carcinomas have a high incidence of nodal involvement at initial presentation (27%). In contrast, patients with SCC due to actinic injury infrequently have nodal involvement (0.5% to 3.3%).[8,9]

In this study, the biologic behavior of carcinomas arising in irradiated and burned skin was similar. The prolonged course and neglect of lesions arising in scarred skin may be the primary factor responsible for their advanced stage at initial presentation and ultimately poor prognosis.[10] Early recognition and biopsy may be the most important management principle.

The appropriate control of radiation exposure and the current treatment of thermal injuries will prevent the majority of these aggressive cancers. An awareness of the etiologic factors and aggressiveness of these infrequent cancers is necessary to diagnose them promptly and provide optimal treatment.

References

1. Hood IC, Young JEM: Late sequela of superficial irradiation. *Head Neck Surg* 1984;7:65-72.
2. Treves N, Pack GT: The development of cancer in burn scars. *Surg Gynecol Obstet* 1930;6:749-782.
3. Bowers RF, Young MO: Carcinoma arising in scars, osteomyelitis, and fistulae. *Arch Surg* 1960;80:564-570.
4. Maillard GE, Landolt A: Penetrating Marjolin's ulcer of scalp involving bone and dura mater treated by wide excision and direct application of a split-skin graft on the brain: A ten year follow-up. *Br J Plast Surg* 1984; 37:463-467.
5. Ames FC, Hickey RC: Metastasis from squamous cell skin cancer of the extremities. *South Med J* 1982;75:920-924.
6. Stoll HL Jr: Squamous cell carcinoma, in Fitzpatrick TB, Eisen AZ, Wolff K, et al (eds): *Dermatology in General Medicine*, ed 2. New York, McGraw-Hill International Book Co, 1979, pp 362-377.
7. Bostwick J, Pendergrast WJ, Vasconery LO: Marjolin's ulcer: An immunologically privileged tumor? *Plast Reconstr Surg* 1976;57:66-69.
8. Lund HZ: How often does squamous cell carcinoma of the skin metastasize? *Arch Dermatol* 1965;92:635-637.
9. Moller R, Reymann F, Klaus HJ: Metastases in dermatological patients with squamous cell carcinoma. *Arch Dermatol* 1979;115:703-705.
10. Nancarrow JD: Cicatrial cancer in the south-west of England: A regional plastic surgery unit's experience over a 20-year period. *Br J Surg* 1983;70:205-208.

Discussion

Q I was unaware in the past of the higher incidence of lymph node metastases in irradiated scar recurrences or malignant neoplasms as opposed to the burned ones. Perhaps burned patients have had split-thickness skin grafts and do not have much dermis, whereas in irradiated patients the skin was full thickness, with dermis, which allowed for lymphatic spread to regional nodes. Have the authors given this some thought?

A We had a higher percentage of burned patients with lymph nodes at the initial presentation. Thirty-seven percent of the people who were burned had positive nodes when they presented, whereas people who were irradiated had a much lower incidence of positive nodes. I do not know if this relates to the primary biology of the disease. However, the nodes were more likely to be dissected in the patients who were previously burned, and therefore, when disease recurred, it tended to recur not at the site of the regional nodes but in the local skin. People who were irradiated, on the other hand, did not as often have palpable nodes at initial presentation, and subsequently developed recurrences in the local nodes that had not been dissected. The radiation-induced carcinomas also tended to recur a bit earlier than the burn scar carcinomas.

Q As a radiotherapist, I can assure you that radiation fibroses lymphatics and markedly impairs the lymphatic drainage in that part, and this might explain why patients with radiation burns did not have such a high incidence of lymph nodal metastases.

Q I thought you said that about 17% of your entire series had distant disease. What did these patients die of?

A The vast majority died of an extensive tumor burden and complications related to locally advanced disease. Only 17% of the patients developed distant metastases at any time during the course of the disease. These metastases tended to occur in bone and lung and a few in distant skin.

Q Many of the tumors were much larger than the squamous carcinomas that occur in sun-damaged skin. Did you look at size as possibly related to prognosis? Did you compare them with the subset of patients with sun-related SCCs larger than 2 cm, which I believe is also a relatively poor prognostic group?

A We compared for size of lesions arising in the burned scalp compared with carcinomas that occurred in the scalp due to other causes, and we found a similar survival.

Q Ryan and Krementz did some interesting work with injection of fluorouracil into such tumors as you described, with the idea that this might immunologically protect the patient, and they had some interesting results. We have tried that ourselves, in a small number of cases. What is your feeling about that?

A That has been tried in a small number of patients, and there have been some interesting anecdotal experiences. However, no convincing scientific data currently exist that would make us want to change from our present standard therapy of surgical excision.

Is Limb-Sparing Surgery Applicable to Neurogenic Sarcomas of the Extremities?

John S. Bolton, MD; Jean-Nicolas Vauthey, MD; Gist H. Farr, Jr, MD; Edward I. Sauter, MD; John C. Bowen III, MD; David G. Kline, MD

• The presentation, treatment, and outcome of 12 patients with high-grade neurogenic sarcoma (NS) of the extremity were compared with those of 21 patients with high-grade extremity soft-tissue sarcoma of nonneural origin in a retrospective study from January 1976 to January 1988. Pain and neurologic deficit were more common in the NS group. Limb-sparing surgery was carried out with equal frequency in both groups. Local recurrence was six times more frequent in the NS group at three-year follow-up (59% vs 10%). Width of resection margin was the dominant prognostic variable bearing on local control after limb-sparing surgery. Anatomic and functional constraints tended to limit resection margin in patients with NS arising from mixed motor-sensory or predominantly motor nerves.

(*Arch Surg* 1989;124:118-121)

Within the past decade, limb-sparing surgery has become the treatment of choice for most extremity soft-tissue sarcomas (STSs). A multidisciplinary approach to these lesions has evolved, combining a function-sparing resection with adjuvant irradiation and/or chemotherapy. Reports from multiple institutions using a variety of multidisciplinary approaches have documented limb salvage rates in excess of 90% in selected patients, with no significant adverse effects of limb-sparing surgery on local control, distant disease-free, and overall survival rates.[1-4]

These reported series have included a variety of histotypes of STS. Tumor grade, size, and location have been viewed as the important tumor-related prognostic variables predictive of local control with limb-sparing surgery, and histotype has been viewed as relatively unimportant. However, to our knowledge, no series has analyzed the various histotypes of STS in sufficient detail to determine whether histotype has a bearing on the outcome of limb-sparing surgery.

Neurogenic sarcoma (NS) of the extremity may present unique anatomic and functional problems to the surgeon attempting to carry out limb-sparing surgery, especially when the tumor arises from a mixed motor-sensory nerve and is of high grade. Because of the relative rarity of these lesions, previous reported series of NS have often included cases accumulated over a long period during which treatment approaches have varied considerably.[5] Other series have combined truncal and extremity lesions in their analysis and have not reported treatment results separately by grade, relationship of the tumor to nerve, width of the resection margin, or type of primary surgical treatment.[6,7]

Because of referral patterns to our institution, we see a relatively large number of NSs involving nerves of the extremity. For this reason, we reviewed our recent experience and analyzed our results with limb-sparing surgery in this group of patients as compared with our overall experience with limb-sparing surgery in patients with high-grade STS of the extremity.

Accepted for publication Aug 26, 1988.

From the Departments of Surgery (Drs Bolton, Vauthey, Sauter, and Bowen) and Pathology (Dr Farr), Ochsner Clinic and Alton Ochsner Medical Foundation, and the Department of Neurosurgery, Louisiana State University School of Medicine (Dr Kline), New Orleans.

Read before the Annual Meeting of the Society of Surgical Oncology, New Orleans, May 24, 1988.

Reprint requests to Ochsner Clinic, 1514 Jefferson Hwy, New Orleans, LA 70121 (Dr Bolton).

PATIENTS AND METHODS

Records of patients treated at our institution between January 1976 and January 1988 for STSs of the upper and lower extremity were reviewed. For this study, "extremity" STS included any lesion for which amputation was a therapeutic alternative, so that lesions of the shoulder and pelvic girdle were included. Patients judged to have metastatic disease at presentation such that treatment was not of curative intent were excluded from further review. The remaining cases were subjected to histologic review by one of us (G.H.F.) without knowledge of the clinical outcome. Lesions classified as low-grade (grade 1) on histologic review were excluded from further study. Twelve cases of high-grade NS of the extremity were identified. Eleven of these cases exhibited characteristic histologic features of peripheral nerve sheath tumors and, in addition, had prominent areas of high-grade sarcoma. Tumors were so designated if mitoses were abundant (more than ten per ten high-power fields), cells showed marked pleomorphism of nuclei and marked variation of nuclear/cytoplasmic ratios, and there were areas of necrosis. Areas were also seen in which the mitotic activity was high and tumor cells were small and uniform with little cytoplasm. These areas of primitive or undifferentiated sarcoma were used as additional evidence of highly aggressive tumors but were not used to make the diagnosis of NS per se. Heterotopic elements or epithelioid differentiation were occasionally seen. Seven patients had a well-established diagnosis of von Recklinghausen's disease. In all but one case of NS, the microscopic features were reinforced by a clear-cut origin of the tumor from a major nerve. The one exception was believed unequivocably to be an NS by virtue of histologic criteria alone. In addition, one

Table 1.—Patient and Tumor Characteristics at Presentation			
	Neurogenic Sarcoma (N=12)	Soft-Tissue Sarcoma (N=21)	P*
Pain, No. (%)	12 (100)	2 (10)	<.01
Neurologic deficit, No. (%)	7 (58)	1 (5)	<.01
Associated von Recklinghausen's disease, No. (%)	7 (58)	0 (0)	<.01
Recurrent tumor at presentation, No. (%)	0 (0)	5 (24)	NS
Tumor size (mean), cm	9.3	9.2	NS
Tumor grade 3, No. (%)	10 (83)	17 (81)	NS
Proximal extremity location, No. (%)	10 (83)	16 (76)	NS
Below fascia, No. (%)	11 (92)	18 (86)	NS

*NS indicates not significant.

case of neuroepithelioma arising in the posterior tibial nerve was identified and included in the review. Cases identified as STS other than NS were classified and graded according to standard histopathologic criteria.

Thus, initial clinical and histologic review identified 12 patients with high-grade extremity NS and 21 patients with high-grade extremity STS (other than NS) treated with curative intent. These cases underwent intensive clinical review, and the following information was collected: size, grade (2 or 3), and location of the lesion within the extremity; presenting symptoms and signs, including the presence or absence of pain and neurologic deficit; functional status before and after treatment; type of resection employed, with particular attention to the gross and microscopic margins; type of adjuvant treatment; and the local disease-free, distant disease-free, and overall survival.

Follow-up was obtained by patient examination in most instances. When this proved impossible, follow-up was obtained by telephone contact with the local physician or directly with the patient. Median follow-up for survivors was 26 months. Local and distant disease-free survival curves and overall survival curves were generated by life-table analysis. Comparisons between survival curves were done by the Breslow test (generalized Wilcoxon statistic),[8] and a multivariate analysis of factors that significantly affected local recurrence was performed by means of the Cox proportional hazards regression model.[9] Additional comparisons between groups was done by χ^2 analysis.

RESULTS

Of the 12 patients identified with high-grade NS of the extremity, in ten the NS arose from a mixed motor-sensory nerve. The nerves of origin were as follows.

Nerve	No.
Brachial plexus element	5
Sciatic	1
Posterior tibial	1
Ulnar	1
Median	1
Obturator	1

The 21 patients in the STS group had a variety of histotypes, as follows.

Histotype	No.
Neurogenic sarcoma	12
Malignant fibrous histiocytoma	8
Leiomyosarcoma	2
Synovial sarcoma	2
Liposarcoma	2
Epithelioid sarcoma	2
Malignant mesenchymoma	2
Malignant giant-cell tumor	2
Rhabdomyosarcoma	1

Table 1 details the clinical features of each group. Significant differences were apparent in the presence of pain, neurologic deficit, and association with von Recklinghausen's disease, all of which were more common in the NS group. However, the two patient groups were similar in regard to tumor size, percentage of grade 3 lesions, frequency of proximal and deep (below fascia) location, and presence of recurrent disease on presentation for treatment at our institution. Median patient age was 37 years for the NS group and 66 years for the STS group.

Table 2.—Treatment Characteristics			
	No. (%)		
	Neurogenic Sarcoma (N=12)	Soft-Tissue Sarcoma (N=21)	P*
Primary amputation	3 (25)	2 (9.5)	NS
Limb-sparing resection	9 (75)	19 (90.5)	NS
<1-cm margin	7 (78)	8 (42)	NS
>1-cm margin	2 (22)	11 (58)	NS
Adjuvant radiation therapy	5 (56)	11 (58)	NS
Adjuvant chemotherapy	3 (33)	8 (42)	NS

*NS indicates not significant.

All patients in this series underwent an attempt at definitive resection with curative intent. Table 2 details the surgical and adjuvant treatment given in each group. The primary amputation rate was slightly higher in the NS group, but this difference was not significant. Amputation achieved an adequate margin (minimum of 1 cm) in all cases in which it was employed. Among the patients treated with limb-sparing surgery, a higher proportion of patients with NS had less than a 1-cm margin; however, this difference was not significant. Adjuvant radiation therapy and chemotherapy were used with equal frequency in each group.

Local disease-free survival at 36 months was 41% for the NS group and 90% for the STS group (Fig 1). This difference was significant ($P<.03$). Distant disease-free survival and overall survival rates were not significantly different between the two groups; however, the trend clearly favored the STS group, and the difference approached significance for overall survival (Fig 2). For the 33 patients as a whole, margin width was examined as a prognostic factor predictive of local disease-free survival. A highly statistical significant advantage in favor of the group having margin width greater than 1 cm was demonstrated ($P=.009$; Fig 3). Cox regression analysis was used to compare the relative contribution of the histotype (NS vs all other) and the margin width in determining the local disease-free survival. Both variables contributed significantly ($P=.024$

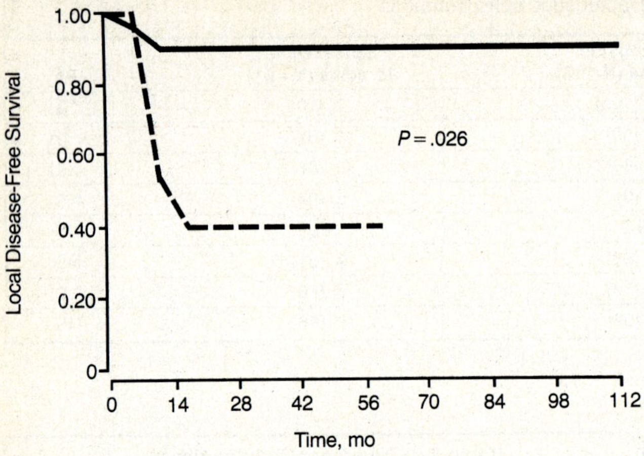

Fig 1.—Local disease-free survival in neurogenic sarcoma (dashed line) and soft-tissue sarcoma (solid line) groups.

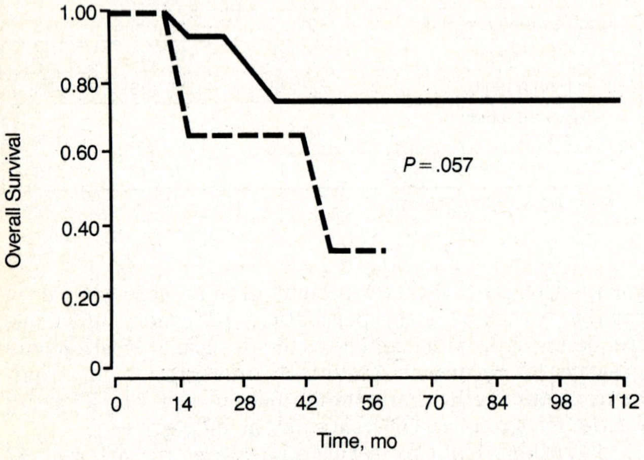

Fig 2.—Overall survival in neurogenic sarcoma (dashed line) and soft-tissue sarcoma (solid line) groups.

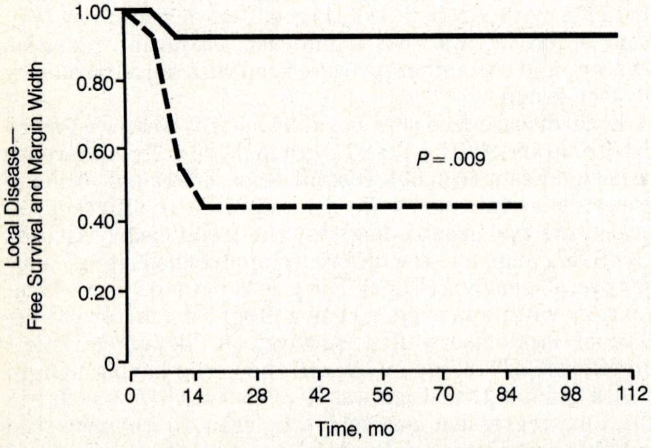

Fig 3.—Local disease-free survival as function of resection margin width greater than 1 cm (solid line) or less than 1 cm (dashed line).

and $P = .005$, respectively); however, margin width appeared to be the dominant variable in predicting local disease-free survival. The significance of the combination was $P = .0016$.

Although the primary amputation rate was only slightly higher for the NS group, the ultimate amputation rate was significantly higher in that five patients in the NS group required amputation for recurrent disease, while only one patient in the STS group did so. Only two of 12 patients in the NS group retained an anatomically and functionally intact extremity until death or termination of the study as compared with 16 of 21 patients in the STS group ($\chi^2 = 4.96$, $P < .05$).

COMMENT

This study demonstrated that patients with high-grade NS of the extremity had a significantly higher risk of local recurrence after limb-sparing surgery than did patients with high-grade STS of other histologic type. While significant differences in distant disease-free survival and overall survival were not manifest between these two groups, the strong trend toward decreased overall survival in the NS group suggests that this difference will become significant with longer follow-up or with larger sample size.

In our NS group, the tumor arose from a mixed motor-sensory nerve of the extremity in ten of 12 patients. The two patients whose tumor did not arise from such a nerve had favorable outcomes in regard to local and distant disease-free status and functional result, suggesting that the adverse outcome noted in this study is largely confined to the group with involvement of mixed motor-sensory nerve. Thus, the results of this study cannot be extrapolated to NSs of the extremity that are of low grade or that do not involve mixed motor-sensory nerves. In our overall institutional experience (data not shown), management of these latter groups has not posed difficulties greater than those seen with STS in general.

With covariate analysis, the width of resection margin emerged as the dominant variable predictive of local disease-free survival. Anatomic and functional constraints tended to limit margin width in the NS group, as less than total nerve ablation was done in the majority of cases in the hope of preserving nerve function. Thus, although all gross tumor was thought to have been removed by the operating surgeon, microscopic, and in some cases even a small amount of macroscopic, disease may have persisted. Others have noted the importance of adequate margin in limb-sparing surgery for extremity STS,[10,11] and recurrence after inadequate resection is not unique to patients with NS. When the NS involves mixed motor-sensory nerves, however, the extent of functional loss encountered in adequate resection is extensive. Thus, the problems posed by NS of the extremity relate more to functional and anatomic considerations that bear on margin size with limb-sparing surgery than to any different biologic behavior per se of these lesions.

The 36% incidence of NS among our overall group of patients with high-grade extremity STS was higher than that reported in most series, but this is explained by referral patterns to one surgeon at our institution (D.G.K.), not by the histologic criteria used to diagnose NS in this study.

In a recent review of localized STS of the lower extremity, Collin et al[12] noted neurofibrosarcomas to have a significantly higher risk of local recurrence than did other histotypes of STS. This analysis included grade 1 lesions; moreover, the histologic criteria for diagnosis of neurofibrosarcoma and the relationships of the tumors to motor nerve were not detailed in this study. Therefore, no direct comparison can be drawn between our study and that of Collin et al; however, it is likely that an even higher local recurrence rate would have been noted in the earlier study had attention been focused on high-grade tumors involving major nerves.

Despite the findings of this study, it is possible that a significant proportion of patients with NS of the extremity can undergo limb-sparing surgery. However, the provision of adequate proximal, distal, and radial margins remains the paramount consideration bearing on local control of tumor with limb-sparing surgery, since, in this study as in others, adjuvant therapy could not ensure local control if the initial surgical margin was inadequate.[13,14] Thus, for high-grade NS involving motor nerve, segmental nerve resection will be required in virtually every case along with wide radial resection. When this can be accomplished with anticipation of acceptable extremity function postoperatively, limb-sparing surgery should be carried out in preference to amputation. Nambisan et al,[7] for example, reported sciatic nerve sacrifice as an adjunct to limb-sparing surgery for an NS involving the sciatic nerve, resulting in moderate functional impairment but with an overall acceptable functional result.

By contrast, high-grade NSs arising from the brachial plexus are especially difficult to control with limb-sparing surgery, because adequate longitudinal and radial resection entails sacrifice of a large portion of the innervation of the upper extremity and possibly the axillary artery and vein. The current study included five patients with high-grade NS of the brachial plexus. In each of these cases, the tumor was located at or distal to the cord level, such that interscapulothoracic amputation could have achieved an adequate proximal margin. Three patients who were initially treated with limb-sparing resection and adjuvant chemoradiotherapy rapidly had recurrences. In each case, only a limited initial resection was done in an attempt to preserve neurologic function. The two remaining cases were initially managed with interscapulothoracic amputation and remain free of disease, with good functional status, at 21 and 24 months.

Neurogenic sarcomas involving the brachial plexus at the root or truncal level are not included in this review. For lesions at this level, neither wide local resection nor interscapulothoracic amputation proximal to the tumor is possible. Only subtotal resection followed by irradiation and/or chemotherapy is possible in these cases.[15]

References

1. Eilber FR, Guiliano AE, Huth J, et al: Limb salvage for high-grade soft-tissue sarcomas of the extremity: Experience at the University of California Los Angeles. *Cancer Treat Symp* 1985;3:49-57.
2. Suit HD, Mankin HJ, Schiller AL, et al: Results of treatment of sarcoma of soft tissue by radiation and surgery at Massachusetts General Hospital. *Cancer Treat Symp* 1985;3:43-47.
3. Rosenberg SA, Tepper J, Glatstein E: The treatment of soft-tissue sarcoma of the extremities: Prospective randomized evaluation of (1) limb-sparing surgery plus radiation therapy compared with amputation and (2) the role of adjuvant therapy. *Ann Surg* 1982;196:305-315.
4. Enneking WF, McAuliffe JA: Adjunctive preoperative radiation therapy in treatment of soft-tissue sarcomas: A preliminary report. *Cancer Treat Symp* 1985;3:37-42.
5. Ducatman BS, Scheithauer BW, Piepgras DG: Malignant peripheral nerve sheath tumors: A clinical pathologic study of 120 cases. *Cancer* 1986;57:2006-2021.
6. Storm FK, Eilber FR, Mirra J: Neurofibrosarcoma. *Cancer* 1980;45:126-129.
7. Nambisan RN, Rao U, Moore R: Malignant soft tissue tumors of nerve sheath origin. *J Surg Oncol* 1984;25:268-272.
8. Breslow N: A generalized Kruskal-Wallis test for comparing K samples subject to unequal patterns of censorship. *Biometrika* 1970;57:579-594.
9. Cox DR: Regression models and life tables. *J R Statist Soc* 1972;34:187-220.
10. Collin C, Godbold J, Hajdu S, et al: Localized extremity soft tissue sarcoma: An analysis of factors affecting survival. *J Clin Oncol* 1987;5:601-612.
11. Markhede G, Angervall L, Stener B: A multivariate analysis of the prognosis after surgical treatment of malignant soft-tissue tumors. *Cancer* 1982;49:1721-1733.
12. Collin C, Hajdu S, Godbold J, et al: Localized, operable soft tissue sarcoma of the lower extremity. *Arch Surg* 1986;121:1425-1433.
13. Bojsen-Moller M, Myhre-Jensen O: A consecutive series of 30 malignant schwannomas: Survival in relation to clinical pathologic parameters and treatment. *Acta Pathol Microbiol Immunol Scand* 1984A;92:147-155.
14. Thomas J, Piepgras D, Scheithauer B, et al: Neurogenic tumors of the sciatic nerve: A clinicopathologic study of 35 cases. *Mayo Clin Proc* 1983;58:640-647.
15. Lusk M, Kline D, Garcia C: Tumors of the brachial plexus. *Neurosurgery* 1987;21:439-453.

Discussion

Q Did you break down your analysis by tumors arising from the plexus vs peripheral nerves, and was there any difference in recurrence rates?

A We had five patients with brachial plexus tumors; two of them were treated with primary amputation and they had no recurrence; three patients had an attempt at limb-sparing surgery with inadequate primary resection; they had recurrences and eventually died.

Q I think your conclusions are essentially correct. However, I think that because of the numbers of the patients, it is hard to draw detailed conclusions. In general, if only one nerve of the extremity can be resected, this is preferable to an amputation. This includes the sciatic nerve. In other words, if one has to resect the sciatic nerve because of tumor involvement, the result is far superior to an amputation. If you're dealing with the brachial plexus, then it is altogether a different situation. The other point is, as true of other STSs, postoperative radiation is helpful to provide local control if you have removed all the gross tumor, but the surgical margin may be inadequate.

Q What I am interested in is whether you think that the radiation therapy that was used was adequate or if you might have had better results with the limb-sparing surgery. In the original abstract, for instance, some of the patients didn't receive radiation therapy as an adjuvant at all.

A I think the message is to obtain adequate margins in all cases. You can see that we obtained good results in nonneurogenic STSs with 90% local disease-free survival, and this compares well with other series. During the same period we made the same progress in high-grade NSs arising from major motor nerves. Radiation therapy was used mainly as an adjuvant, and with a small number of patients. I don't think that we can draw a conclusion. I don't think radiation therapy can make up for positive margins.

Patterns of Recurrence After Resection of Osteosarcoma of the Extremity

Strategies for Treatment of Metastases

James F. Huth, MD, Frederick R. Eilber, MD

• We studied recurrence patterns in 255 patients with high-grade osteosarcoma of the extremity and the efficacy of the treatment of these recurrences. One hundred seven patients developed metastatic disease: 77 had isolated pulmonary metastases, 17 had simultaneous metastases to lung and elsewhere, and 13 had metastases to other sites. Of the 77 patients with metastases confined to the lung, 51 (66%) underwent thoracotomy for resection of the metastases, and 13 (17%) are long-term disease-free survivors. Patients with simultaneous metastases to lung and other sites, and patients with metastases to sites other than lung, have a poor prognosis with only one long-term disease-free survivor in these groups. Thoracotomy has a limited role in the treatment of metastatic disease. Improvements in aggressive, systemic chemotherapy are essential for improving the prognosis in these patients.

(*Arch Surg* 1989;124:122-126)

Osteosarcoma is a relatively uncommon malignant neoplasm that commonly affects individuals in the second decade of life. The majority of these tumors involve the long bones of the extremity that are the most actively growing areas of bone at this stage of life. These tumors have a propensity for local recurrence, as well as hematogenous spread. Metastases to the regional lymph nodes are uncommon. Pulmonary metastases are the most common initial manifestation of disseminated disease.

At the time of diagnosis, most patients with osteosarcoma of the extremity do not have detectable distant metastatic disease. Until recently, therapy was directed toward removal of the primary lesion, usually by means of an amputation.[1] Most patients went on to develop metastatic disease and eventually died of uncontrolled disseminated disease.[2] Recent advances in multimodality treatment of osteosarcoma have resulted in (1) better local control with a significant decrease in the rate of local recurrence and (2) improvement in overall survival.[3-5]

We have treated 162 patients with high-grade osteosarcoma of the extremity from 1974 through 1986. Our study examines the patterns of recurrence in these patients and the efficacy of the various treatment modalities used to treat metastatic disease to various sites.

PATIENTS AND METHODS

Eligibility Criteria

One hundred sixty-two patients with a diagnosis of high-grade osteosarcoma of the extremity seen in the division of surgical oncology from 1974 through 1986 were included in this study. The criteria for inclusion were as follows:

1. The tumor was localized to the primary site (femur, tibia, fibula, humerus, radius, or ulna) with no evidence of metastatic disease. Preoperative workup included a complete physical examination, blood chemistry determinations, chest roentgenogram, computed tomographic (CT) scan of the lung or whole-lung tomography, CT scan of the primary site to assess the extent of the tumor, and bone scan.

2. Preoperative confirmation that the tumor was high grade (Enneking stage II)[6] was made by the Pathology Department at UCLA.

3. After giving informed consent, all patients underwent resection of the tumor at our institution. An attempt was made to perform an en bloc excision of the tumor and involved bone with at least an 8-cm proximal margin (from the most proximal area of bone marrow involvement) and reconstruction of the excised segment with allograft or endoprosthesis. An amputation was performed when ability to achieve a satisfactory margin was not possible or when the patient did not desire a limb-salvage procedure.

Preoperative Therapy

Chemotherapy.—Preoperative chemotherapy was offered to all patients before surgery. Patients choosing the limb-salvage program were offered intra-arterial doxorubicin hydrochloride (Adriamycin) infusion. Intra-arterial catheters were placed percutaneously by the Seldinger technique under fluoroscopic guidance

Accepted for publication Sept 21, 1988.

From the Department of Surgery, Division of Oncology, UCLA School of Medicine. Dr Huth is now with the University of North Carolina at Chapel Hill.

Read before the Annual Meeting of the Society of Surgical Oncology, New Orleans, May 25, 1988.

Reprint requests to Department of Surgery, The University of North Carolina at Chapel Hill, Burnett-Womack Clinical Sciences Building 229H, Chapel Hill, NC 27514 (Dr Huth).

in the department of radiology. Doxorubicin was given by continuous infusion at the rate of 30 mg/d for three days (total dose, 90 mg). Patients who refused intra-arterial therapy received preoperative intravenous chemotherapy (T-10 Rosen protocol).[7]

Radiotherapy.—Radiation therapy was given at 3.5 Gy fractions for five or ten days using a 10-meV linear accelerator to patients who received intra-arterial doxorubicin. The dosages were changed over time to maximize the therapeutic advantage while minimizing local complications of this therapy.

Surgery

We attempted an en bloc excision of the primary tumor with an 8-cm proximal margin and confirmation that other margins were also free of tumor at the time of excision in each case. Reconstruction was achieved with either a cadaveric allograft or a custom-designed metallic endoprosthesis. Amputation was performed when a functional reconstruction was not feasible or when the patient refused a limb-salvage procedure.

Postoperative Therapy

Beginning in 1978, patients were offered adjuvant chemotherapy as part of a prospective, randomized study comparing the T-10 Rosen protocol (doxorubicin, methotrexate sodium, vincristine sulfate, bleomycin sulfate, cyclophosphamide, dactinomycin) vs no therapy. Patients treated before this time received doxorubicin and high-dose methotrexate with leucovorin calcium rescue.

Patient Follow-up

Patients were examined one week and one month after discharge from the hospital, and then at three-month intervals. Follow-up examination included a physical examination, blood chemistry determinations, and chest roentgenogram. Lung tomography or chest CT scan was performed at six months. If recurrence was suspected, appropriate additional examinations were performed, and therapeutic options including chemotherapy, radiation therapy, or additional surgery were considered.

RESULTS

Patient Enrollment

One hundred sixty-two (105 male, 57 female) patients were included in this study. The patients ranged in age from 3 to 75 years (median, 20 years). The age and sex distribution is shown in Fig 1.

Location and Histologic Findings

All tumors in this study arose in the long bones of the extremity. All tumors were high-grade osteosarcoma (Enneking stage II). The Table gives a complete listing of the location of the primary tumor and the operation performed to remove the tumor.

Preoperative Therapy

Ninety-one patients received preoperative intra-arterial doxorubicin followed by preoperative radiation therapy. Forty-five patients received 17.5 Gy, and 46 received 35 Gy of preoperative radiation. Forty-three patients received multimodality preoperative chemotherapy without radiation therapy. The remaining 28 patients, all of whom underwent extremity amputation, elected not to receive preoperative radiation therapy.

Surgical Procedures

Of the 134 patients receiving preoperative therapy, 117 were able to undergo limb-sparing surgery. As listed in the Table, these procedures included (1) replacement of the excised segment with a cadaveric allograft, 20 patients; (2) replacement of the excised segment with a custom-fit metallic endoprosthesis, 90 patients; and (3) other procedure (excision without reconstruction, excision and fusion), seven patients. The remaining 45 patients underwent amputation because they did not want a limb-salvage procedure (28 patients) or because of inability to perform an adequate excision and spare a functional extremity (18 patients).

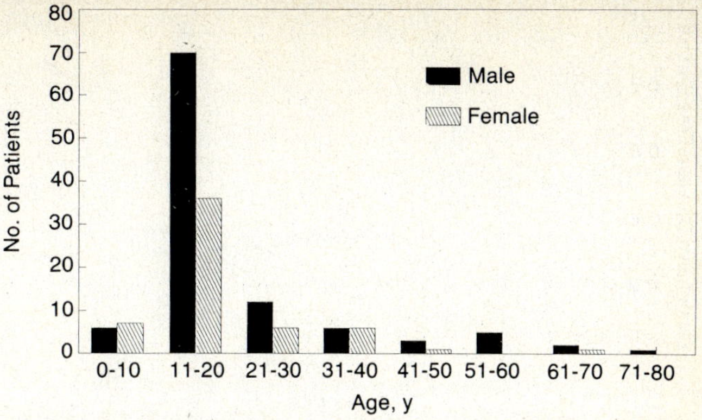

Fig 1.—Age and sex distribution of patients. There were 105 male patients and 57 female patients, ranging in age from 3 to 75 years. Median age was 20 years. Over 65% of patients were between ages of 11 and 20 years.

Site of Primary Tumor and Operation Performed

Primary Tumor Location	No. of Patients: Amputation	Excision and Cadaver Graft	Excision and Endoprosthesis	Other
Femur Distal	21	11	70	2
Proximal	1	1	9	0
Tibia	17	0	2	2
Fibula	2	0	0	1
Humerus	2	8	9	1
Radius	2	0	0	1
Total	**45**	**20**	**90**	**7**

Complications of Therapy

Fifty-eight postoperative complications occurred in 45 patients. Patients undergoing amputation had only three complications (6.6%), and all three were wound sloughs that required reoperation. Twenty-seven patients (30%) who underwent excision and reconstruction with an endoprosthesis had 33 postoperative complications, and 18 required further surgery, including three amputations. These complications included five wound sloughs, six infections, four loosenings, five fractures, four stiffnesses of the extremity, two nerve palsies, three positive operative margins, one extrusion of the prosthesis, one instability of the prosthesis, one phlebitis, and one flexion contracture. Fourteen patients (70%) who had an excision and cadaver allograft had 23 complications, all requiring reoperation. These included six loosenings, four extrusions, four fractures, two infections, one instability, one arterial thrombosis, and one positive surgical margin. Four of these patients required subsequent amputation. One hundred seventeen patients (72%) had no postoperative complications.

Postoperative Therapy

Fifty-one patients received a combination of doxorubicin and high-dose methotrexate postoperatively, 63 received the T-10 protocol as described by Rosen, ten received other

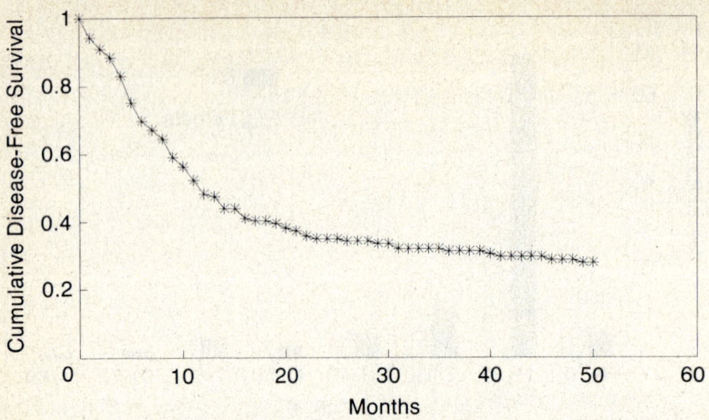

Fig 2.—Disease-free survival of all patients. One hundred seven patients (66%) developed recurrent disease. Actuarial disease-free survival was 48%, 35%, 31%, and 28% at 1, 2, 3, and 4 years, respectively, after original surgery.

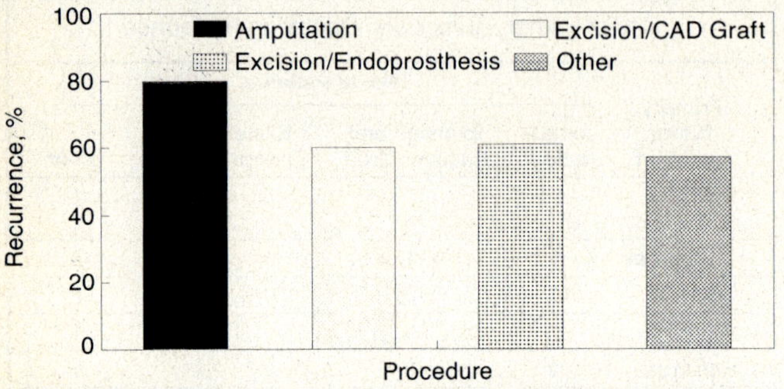

Fig 3.—Procedure vs recurrence. Procedure performed on primary tumor had no significant effect on incidence of metastatic disease. CAD indicates cadaver.

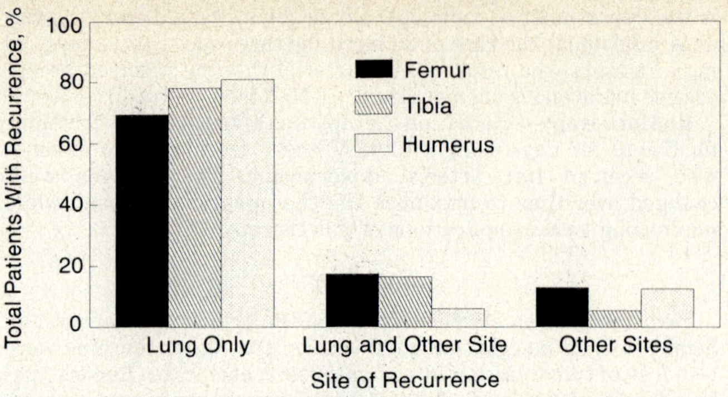

Fig 4.—Site of primary tumor vs recurrence. Site of primary tumor (femur, tibia, or humerus) had no significant effect on incidence of metastatic disease.

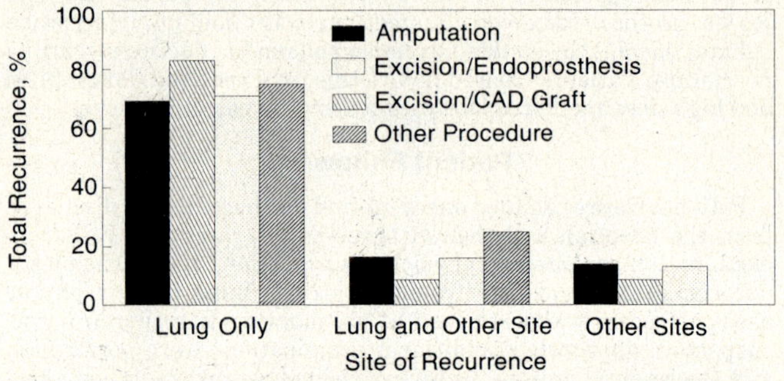

Fig 5.—Procedure vs pattern of recurrence. Procedure performed on primary tumor had no significant effect on distribution of metastatic disease. CAD indicates cadaver.

doxorubicin-containing regimens, and 38 received no postoperative adjuvant chemotherapy.

Recurrence

One hundred seven (66%) of 162 patients developed recurrent disease during the follow-up period. Actuarial analysis of disease-free survival (DFS) is shown in Fig 2. Disease-free survival was 48%, 35%, 31%, and 28% at 1, 2, 3, and 4 years, respectively. Median time to recurrence was 12 months. Patients who received adjuvant chemotherapy had an improved DFS (median DFS, 14 months) compared with those who did not receive postoperative chemotherapy (median DFS, six months). There was no significant difference in survival between those who received doxorubicin–high-dose methotrexate vs those who received the T-10 protocol.

Patterns of Recurrence

The lung was the sole site of metastases in 77 (72%) of the 107 patients who developed recurrent disease. An additional 17 patients (16%) developed recurrent disease simultaneously in the lung and one additional site: six local, five bone, and six central nervous system. The remaining 13 patients (12%) had recurrence at isolated sites distant from the primary site: ten bone, two soft tissue, and one central nervous system.

Patients who underwent an amputation had a slightly higher incidence of recurrence (80%) compared with those undergoing limb-salvage surgery (60%), as shown in Fig 3. However, these differences were not statistically significant. Neither the location of the primary tumor (Fig 4) nor the procedure performed on the primary tumor (Fig 5) had any effect on the distribution of metastatic disease. The pattern of metastatic disease was similar for patients who received adjuvant chemotherapy compared with those who received no postoperative therapy.

Management of First Recurrence

Metastases Confined to the Lung.—Seventy-seven patients had lung metastases as the only manifestation of recurrence, and 51 (66.2%) of 77 were candidates for pulmonary resection based on the size and number of metastases as well as the interval of time from resection of the primary tumor to recurrence. Additional criteria for resectability included (1) no evidence of recurrent disease at the primary site, (2) no evidence of hilar disease on chest roentgenogram or lung CT scan, and (3) no pleural effusion. The median time to recurrence in those patients who underwent thoracotomy was nine months (range, one to 46 months) compared with a median of five months (range, one to 11 months) for those who did not undergo throacotomy.

Of the 77 patients with metastases isolated to the lung, 51 (66%) underwent thoracotomy. Forty-six (90%) of these 51 patients were able to have all their disease resected. This included 21 patients with bilateral disease and 25 patients with unilateral disease. Twelve patients remained free of disease after their first thoracotomy, nine of whom had unilateral disease, and three of whom had bilateral disease. (Patients with bilateral disease underwent median

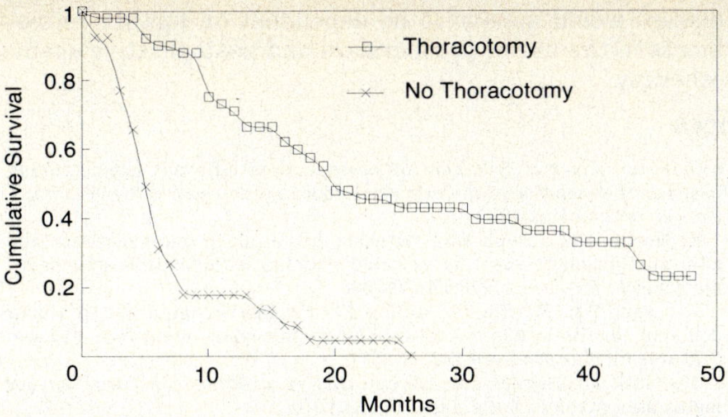

Fig 6.—Survival of patients with metastases confined to lung. Seventy-seven patients had metastases confined to lung. Fifty-one underwent thoracotomy for resection of metastases, and 26 had no further surgery. Actuarial survival for patients who underwent thoracotomy was 71%, 45%, 36%, and 23% at 1, 2, 3, and 4 years, respectively, following *diagnosis* of recurrence.

sternotomy or staged thoracotomy, which for purposes of discussion is considered one operation for metastatic disease.) Survival for patients after thoracotomy was 71% at one year, 45% at two years, 36% at three years, and 23% at four years after diagnosis of recurrence (median survival, 20 months).

Of the 26 patients who were not considered candidates for resection of their pulmonary metastases, 24 died with a median survival of five months after diagnosis of their first recurrence (Fig 6).

Metastases to the Lung and Another Site.—Seventeen patients developed metastases to the lung and another site. Six developed a local recurrence in addition to pulmonary metastases, five developed simultaneous metastases to lung and bone, and six developed simultaneous metastases to lung and the brain. Despite attempts to control disease in this group (with 11 thoracotomies, one amputation, and two excisions), 16 died; the remaining patient is alive and free of disease 47 months after undergoing a thoracotomy and excision of a local recurrence. The median survival for this group is ten months.

Metastases to Sites Other Than the Lung.—Thirteen patients developed recurrent disease at a site other than the lung. Ten patients developed bony metastases, two developed a recurrence in soft tissue of the pelvis, and one developed a brain metastasis. Twelve died, and one remains alive 17 months after diagnosis of bone metastases receiving chemotherapy. Further surgery failed to permanently control disease in the four patients in whom it was attempted. The median survival for this group was nine months.

Management of Second Recurrence

Thirty-four patients had recurrence after thoracotomy for resection of isolated lung metastases. The site of recurrence was limited to the lung in 30, involved the lung and other sites in two, and involved bone and soft tissue in the remaining two. In all patients with extrapulmonary recurrences, disease was unresectable. The 30 patients with recurrent metastases confined to the lung represent 16 patients whose initial lung involvement was bilateral and 14 patients whose initial involvement was unilateral. Of the 14 patients whose previous pulmonary disease was unilateral, six had recurrence in the ipsilateral lung, four had recurrence in the contralateral lung, and four had recurrence in both the lung that was operated on and the lung that was not operated on. Twelve of the 30 patients underwent another thoracotomy.

Management of Third Recurrence

All 12 patients who underwent a second thoracotomy for metastatic disease had recurrence. All but one of these recurrences were confined to the lung. Seven patients underwent a third thoracotomy, and one patient remains free of disease 14 months after his most recent operation.

COMMENT

Our study was undertaken to examine the metastatic patterns in patients with osteosarcoma of the extremity and the role that surgery plays in the further management of patients in whom primary treatment fails. There have been several studies examining the role of thoracotomy in the treatment of metastatic disease.[8-10] These studies examined a highly select population of patients, many referred because they met certain criteria of resectability. Our study avoids this selection criteria, because we have included all patients with extremity osteosarcomas who have had all their initial treatment at our institution.

Metastatic disease in the lung accounted for the overwhelming majority of recurrences. The overall incidence of metastases to the lung was 94 (58%) of 162, which included 77 patients with metastases only to the lung and 17 patients with metastases to the lung and another site. This represents 88% (94/107) of all the metastatic disease encountered. Surgery only had an impact in patients with metastases confined solely to the lung: 13 (25%) of 51 patients undergoing thoracotomy are long-term, disease-free survivors. However, this represents only 17% (13/77) of all patients with metastases confined to the lung and only 12% (13/107) of all patients who developed metastatic disease. Thus, the impact of resection of pulmonary metastases on improving survival of patients with osteosarcoma is minimal.

The overall prognosis in the treatment of osteosarcoma appears to be improving because of the development of more rigorous and effective adjuvant chemotherapy programs. These programs have evolved to include preoperative neoadjuvant chemotherapy. The purpose of this therapy is twofold: (1) to begin systemic treatment earlier in the course of the disease without the two- to four-week delay required for surgery and subsequent postoperative recovery and (2) to examine the effect of the preoperative therapy on the primary tumor to better plan postoperative treatment. Rosen et al[7] have demonstrated that switching the therapy regimen postoperatively in patients who failed to show a good response to the preoperative regimen results in a better disease-free survival.

Although we believe that surgery still has a role in the treatment of metastatic disease, our study suggests that the impact of surgical resection is small, approximating a 10% improvement in overall survival. Because the lung is the primary site of initial recurrence, it is tempting to try to focus additional therapy at this site. At this point, however, the therapeutic options are limited. Zaharia et al[11] have described a series of patients treated with adjuvant radiation therapy to the lung parenchyma in conjunction with systemic chemotherapy after resection of the primary tumor. These patients received 20 Gy whole-lung irradiation postoperatively in an attempt to control micrometastases to the lung. All seven patients treated only with irradiation to the lung had recurrence in the lung, and 19 (65.5%) of 29 patients who received radiation and chemotherapy had recurrence. Thus, it would appear that radiation at this dosage is insufficient to control pulmonary metastatic disease. Pulmonary tolerance to radiation therapy prohibits the use of higher doses of radiation. Future progress in the control of metastatic disease would appear to be dependent on further refinements in the use of preoperative and postoperative chemotherapy.

References

1. Dahlin DL, Coventry MB: Osteogenic sarcoma: A study of 600 cases. *J Bone Joint Surg Am* 1967;49:101-110.
2. Friedman MA, Carter SK: The therapy of osteogenic sarcoma: Current status and thoughts for the future. *J Surg Oncol* 1972;4:481-510.
3. Sim FH: Musculoskeletal oncology: State of the art. *Orthopedics* 1987;10:1673-1684.
4. Eilber FR, Mirra JJ, Grant TT, et al: Is amputation necessary for sarcomas? A seven year experience with limb salvage. *Ann Surg* 1980;192:431-438.
5. Malawar M: Surgical technique and results of limb sparing surgery for high grade sarcomas of the knee and shoulder. *Orthopedics* 1985;8:597-607.
6. Enneking WF: A system of staging musculoskeletal neoplasms. *Clin Orthoped* 1986;204:9-24.
7. Rosen G, Caparros B, Huvos AG, et al: Preoperative therapy for osteogenic sarcoma: Selection of postoperative adjuvant chemotherapy based on the response of the primary tumor to preoperative chemotherapy. *Cancer* 1982;49:1221-1230.
8. Morton DL, Joseph WL, Ketcham AS, et al: Surgical resection and adjuvant immunotherapy for selected patients with multiple pulmonary metastases. *Ann Surg* 1973;178:360-366.
9. Joseph WL, Morton DL, Adkins PC: Prognostic significance of tumor doubling time in evaluating operability in pulmonary metastatic disease. *J Thorac Cardiovasc Surg* 1971;61:23.
10. Huth JF, Holmes EC, Vernon SE, et al: Pulmonary resection for metastatic sarcoma. *Am J Surg* 1980;140:9-16.
11. Zaharia M, Caceres E, Valdivial S, et al: Postoperative whole lung irradiation with or without Adriamycin in osteogenic sarcoma. *Int J Radiat Oncol Biol Phys* 1986;12:907-910.

Discussion

Q The topic that has been of interest to many individuals and institutions through the years is the role of thoracotomy and resection of metastases, either osteosarcoma or other diseases. I am curious about whether or not you believe that you have identified any subgroup of patients that you would not take to surgery. What were the criteria of inoperability in the patients who never made it to surgery and on the patients who did undergo resection? Are there any that you would not do again? Do you still advise second and third operations for resection of metastases? Is there a number of metastases beyond which all patients had a recurrence?

A I think our indications for a thoracotomy have become more restrictive over the years and in this series we were certainly generous in our indications for a thoracotomy, as it dates back to 1974. We do have certain criteria. We like to see a disease-free interval of a year or a tumor doubling time of greater than 40 days, and certainly solitary vs multiple metastases have been shown in several series to do better, although it is not to the extent where you would exclude multiple metastases only on that basis. If patients present with a short disease-free interval or a rapid tumor doubling time, we tried to manipulate their chemotherapy to slow down the growth of the tumors before we subjected them to thoracotomy. We have ruled out for thoracotomy patients who present with a pleural effusion with malignant cells or patients who present with significant disease in the hilum. You can argue that the number of metastases makes a difference, but one patient stands out in my memory. He was a 20-year-old man who on CT scan appeared to have four metastases; at the time of exploration he had over 50. He had only one resection of these and has not had a recurrence after five years. The data also show that recurrent disease in the lung carries a very poor prognosis. Operating two or three times has diminishing returns, although the one patient who survived after three thoracotomies would probably disagree with me.

Q What have we accomplished when we fail? That is, in all of these patients who are heavily pretreated with "big-gun" chemotherapy or experimental agents, how much have you extended their life span for those who eventually die of their disease?

A That is a very difficult question to answer. Obviously, we select patients for thoracotomy now because they have a slow-growing tumor and a long disease-free interval. If you just set them aside and do not operate on them, they are going to have a better survival than those that you exclude from thoracotomy.

The bottom line, I guess, has to be how many patients undergo resection who never have a recurrence. I do not think this is at odds with previous data that we presented because those were selected patients and there were a lot of patients we treated who were sent in for a thoracotomy because they were at good risk. The percentages get better then; up to 40% of those patients are disease free, as opposed to 25%.

In this series, we have looked only at patients who came to us with their primary tumor intact, who were then operated on with no evidence of metastatic disease at that time and then were followed up through the course of their disease until they had a recurrence or not. So it is an unselected group and the statistics look worse.

Q In these young patients, it seems that basically each resection has provided about one year of palliation for very little morbidity and no operative mortality.

A Yes, I think we may be helping the young patient who will bounce back from the surgery very quickly. Even though he or she goes on to experience recurrence, I suspect we have prolonged his or her life. It is difficult to evaluate prolongation of life because we really have no basis for comparison since these patients are already highly selected.

In Other AMA Journals

ARCHIVES OF OTOLARYNGOLOGY–HEAD & NECK SURGERY

The Pitfalls of Technetium Tc 99m/Thallium 201 Parathyroid Scanning

G. Scott Voorman, MD; George H. Petti, Jr, MD; Eloy Schulz, MD; George D. Chonkich MD; Gerald A. Kirk, MD

Technetium Tc 99m/thallium 201 parathyroid scanning has been proved to be effective by multiple researchers. A review of 54 patients who underwent scanning and operations at an institution showed the scans to be accurate in 83%. There were 15% false-negative and 2% false-positive scans. The pitfalls of parathyroid scanning can be related to false-positives and false-negatives (*Arch Otolaryngol Head Neck Surg* 1988;114:993-995).

Reprint requests to Department of Head and Neck Surgery, Loma Linda University Medical Center, 11234 Anderson St, Suite 2576, Loma Linda, CA 92354 (Dr Petti).

Clinical Experience With Regional Pancreatectomy for Adenocarcinoma of the Pancreas

William F. Sindelar, MD, PhD

• Twenty patients with adenocarcinoma of the pancreas underwent a regional pancreatectomy, including resection of the pancreas, regional lymphadenectomy, duodenectomy, antrectomy, and sleeve resection of the portal vein. Three patients required mesenteric arterial reconstruction. Adjunctive radiotherapy was administered to 17 patients, with 11 patients receiving intraoperative radiation and six patients receiving postoperative external-beam–radiation. Complications developed in 11 patients (55%), including infectious and septic events (five patients), biliary or enteric fistulas (two patients), mesenteric vascular thrombosis (two patients), and other complications (two patients). Four patients (20%) suffered treatment-related deaths. The overall median survival was 12.0 months. Survival at one year was 50% and, at three years, 10%. Two patients died of causes unrelated to cancer at 18 and 39 months, and one patient remains alive and free of disease 50 months following therapy. Morbidity and survival did not differ among patients who received intraoperative, conventional postoperative, or no radiation therapy. Although occasional patients may benefit with survivals of longer than three years, regional pancreatectomy carries major morbidity and produces little survival benefit for most patients with pancreatic cancer.

(*Arch Surg* 1989;124:127-132)

Surgical resections for adenocarcinoma of the pancreas carry considerable mortality and morbidity and only rarely result in long-term survival.[1] Although resection is the only potentially curative treatment modality for pancreatic cancer, typically fewer than 10% of all patients with pancreatic adenocarcinoma have disease sufficiently localized to permit surgical extirpation.[1] Traditionally, pancreatduodenectomy (Whipple's operation) has been utilized to resect localized disease in patients, although some surgeons have advocated total pancreatectomy. However, with either pancreatduodenectomy or total pancreatectomy, less than 10% of patients have been long-term survivors, and at least 50% of patients have local recurrences within the resection bed.[1,2]

In attempts to extend the limits of resectability, to improve local control rates, and to improve survival, Fortner[3] developed the regional pancreatectomy, an extirpative procedure that removes en bloc the pancreas, regional lymph nodes, duodenum, gastric antrum, and intrapancreatic portal vein. The technically complex procedure was proposed as a method of surgically removing tissues in the region of pancreatic neoplasms to afford wide margins in all directions. The morbidity and mortality of the regional pancreatectomy in experienced hands were reported to be comparable with Whipple's resections or total pancreatectomies, and the procedure was suggested to improve survival.[4] A 62% one-year survival rate was achieved at Memorial Sloan-Kettering Cancer Center, New York, in 1977.[4] Fortner[5] reported a series of 61 patients in 1984, who had undergone regional pancreatic resections, with median survivals of 13 months for patients having pancreatic adenocarcinomas and 40 months for patients with periampullary or islet cell tumors of the pancreas.

Regional pancreatectomy has generated controversy among surgeons.[6] The procedure has been suggested by some to extend resectablity and to promote disease control, while others have criticized the operation as being highly morbid and technically difficult without a meaningful impact on overall survival. Relatively few institutions have performed the regional resection, and its use, at present, must be considered investigational.[1]

The present article describes the experience with regional pancreatic resections performed at the National Cancer Institute, Bethesda, Md, in a population of patients with adenocarcinomas of the pancreas. Patients who were entered on to studies of intraoperative or conventional radiation therapy used as adjuncts to surgical resection.[7,8] The morbidity, mortality, and efficacy of disease control are analyzed.

Accepted for publication July 11, 1988.

From the Surgery Branch, National Cancer Institute, National Institutes of Health, Bethesda, Md.

Read before the Annual Meeting of the Society of Surgical Oncology, New Orleans, May 25, 1988.

Reprint requests to Surgery Branch, National Cancer Institute, National Institutes of Health, Bethesda, MD 20892 (Dr Sindelar).

Table 1.—Clinical Results in 20 Patients Who Underwent Regional Pancreatectomy*

Patient/ Age, y/Sex	Type of Resection	Type of Adjunctive Radiation	Stage†	Complications: Early	Complications: Late	Time to Recurrence, mo	Time to Local Recurrence, mo	Survival, mo
1/42/F	RT	IORT	III	None	None	5	5	12
2/71/M	RT	IORT	III	Chylous ascites	Malnutrition; stroke	18‡	18‡	18
3/74/F	RT	None	II	Chylous ascites	Breast cancer; myocardial infarction	24	26	26
4/58/M	RT	EBRT	III	Bacterial peritonitis	None	9	9	12
5/54/M	RTA	None	IV	Biliary fistula, intestinal fistulas, abscesses, sepsis, hepatic failure; death	...	2	2	2
6/49/M	RT	EBRT	III	None	None	7	7	7
7/66/M	RT	IORT	III	Abscess	None	7	7	7
8/54/F	RT	EBRT	III	Abscess	None	12	12	12
9/58/F	RT	IORT	III	None	None	9	9	9
10/44/M	RT	IORT	II	None	Bezoar	31	31	31
11/56/F	RT	IORT	II	Mesenteric infarction, sepsis, respiratory failure, hepatic failure; death	...	2‡	2‡	2
12/67/M	RT	IORT	III	None	Renal calculi; stroke	39‡	39‡	39
13/60/M	RTA	EBRT	III	None	None	8	8	9
14/60/F	RT	EBRT	III	Abscess, wound infection	None	10	10	19
15/59/F	RTA	IORT	III	Portal thrombosis, biliary fistula, intestinal fistulas, sepsis, hepatic failure; death	...	2‡	2‡	2
16/59/F	RT	IORT	III	None	None	6	12	12
17/66/M	RT	IORT	IV	None	Colonic hemorrhage	50‡	50‡	50§
18/52/M	RT	None	III	Myocardial infarction	...	1‡	1‡	1
19/53/F	RT	EBRT	III	None	None	8	8	10
20/57/F	RS	IORT	III	Ileus	Malnutrition	7	7	8

*RT indicates regional total pancreatectomy; IORT, intraoperative radiation therapy; EBRT, external-beam radiation therapy; RTA, regional total pancreatectomy with arterial resection; and RS, regional subtotal pancreatectomy.
†Staging: I indicates confined to pancreas; II, peripancreatic or vascular invasion; III, nodal involvement; and IV, visceral or peritoneal spread.
‡No disease recurrence at time of death or last follow-up.
§Alive at time of last follow-up.

PATIENTS AND METHODS

Patients

Twenty patients had a regional pancreatectomy performed at the National Cancer Institute. The patients were among groups that were accrued into prospective pilot studies that investigated the role of intraoperative radiotherapy in treating various malignant neoplasms and into prospectively randomized studies that compared adjunctive intraoperative therapy with conventional postoperative radiotherapy in treating patients with resectable pancreatic cancers.[7] Patients with biopsy-proved adenocarcinomas of the pancreas who, on exploration, were found to have localized disease without visceral or peritoneal metastases underwent a pancreatic resection. Most patients received either intraoperative radiation of the resection bed or postoperative external-beam fractionated radiation. Patients with tumor involvement of the portal vein or of the peripancreatic major visceral arterial tree underwent a regional resection. The patients with pancreatic cancer who had a regional pancreatectomy form the basis of this report (Table 1).

The 20 patients who underwent a regional pancreatectomy included 11 men and nine women. The median age was 58 years, with a range of 42 to 74 years. No patient had stage I disease (confined to the pancreas), three patients had stage II disease (local extension into the duodenum or peripancreatic vasculature), and 15 patients had stage III disease (regional lymph node involvement). Two patients had stage IV disease (metastatic spread); both patients with stage IV disease were considered intraoperatively to have localized disease, but on pathologic review of the resected specimen, they were found to have microscopic discontinuous peritoneal implants.

Surgery

Patients who underwent a regional pancreatectomy had operative procedures performed according to the methods described by Fortner.[3,5] Patients had resections that included a total pancreatectomy (19 patients) or a subtotal pancreatectomy that removed the pancreatic head and neck (one patient), extirpation of the extrahepatic bile duct below the bifurcation with incontinuity cholecystectomy, subtotal distal gastrectomy, total duodenectomy, splenectomy (19 patients), complete regional lymph node dissection (peripancreatic, hepatic, celiac, superior mesenteric, upper para-aortic, and upper paracaval), and removal of the intrapancreatic portion of the portal vein. The portal vein was reconstructed by an end-to-end anastomosis in all patients; this was performed without portal venous shunting or systemic heparinization. Visceral arterial resections and reconstructions were performed in three patients: one patient had an aberrant common hepatic artery arising from the superior mesenteric artery that was resected from its origin to the hepatic bifurcation and that was replaced with an arterial bypass constructed from the splenic artery; and two patients required resection of the origin of the superior mesenteric artery that was reconstructed with an anastomosis of the residual artery to the aorta. Biliary reconstruction was performed by an end-to-side choledochojejunostomy. An end-to-side gastrojejunostomy was performed in all patients. An end-to-side, double-layer pancreaticojejunostomy was constructed in the single patient who had a subtotal pancreatectomy.

Radiotherapy

Radiotherapy was administered to 17 patients. Patients received, after informed consent, either intraoperative radiation at the time of surgery to the resection bed or conventional fractionated external-beam radiation postoperatively to the upper region of the abdomen. Patients with negative regional lymph nodes did not receive radiation therapy. Three patients were part of a pilot study in which all patients received intraoperative radiation, while 17 patients were entered into a protocol that randomly assigned participants to receive either intraoperative radiation or conventional therapy (defined as no radiation for tumors confined to the pancreas and as fractionated postoperative external-beam radiation for tumors with extrapancreatic or nodal spread).

Intraoperative radiation was delivered following resection and vascular reconstruction but before gastrointestinal anastomosis. Patients received 20 Gy of radiation in a single dose using 9 to 11 meV delivered by a linear accelerator.[8] Patients typically received intraoperative radiotherapy to the pancreatic bed, celiac and superior mesenteric axes, porta hepatis, upper abdominal aorta and vena cava, and base of the left diaphragm. Conventional external-beam radiotherapy was delivered using 6- to 10-mV photons in anterior-posterior opposed fields to the upper region of the abdomen. Patients received a total of 45 to 50 Gy in 1.2 to 1.8 Gy/d fractions delivered five days per week during five to seven weeks.

Eleven patients received intraoperative radiotherapy, and six patients received external-beam radiotherapy. Three patients were not irradiated, one patient because of pathologically negative lymph nodes and two patients because of early postoperative deaths.

Analysis

All patients who underwent a regional pancreatectomy were scored for the type and severity of postoperative complications. All deaths that occurred within the initial hospitalization for surgery were considered to be related to treatment. All patients were followed up clinically at monthly intervals until recurrence or death. Pathologic documentation of local or distant recurrent disease was obtained in all patients by autopsy or by surgical exploration performed at the time of suspected recurrence. The time to disease recurrence, the time to local recurrence (defined as a recurrence anywhere within the peritoneum or retroperitoneum exclusive of isolated metastases to the liver), and the overall survival times were determined by life-table analysis.

RESULTS

Overall Results

Twenty patients underwent a regional pancreatectomy, with the patient characteristics, type of resection, type of adjunctive radiotherapy, treatment complications, and outcome detailed in Table 1. The overall results are summarized in Table 2.

Table 2.—Complications and Disease Control in 20 Patients Who Underwent Regional Pancreatectomy

Category	No. (%)
Complications	11 (55)
Infections and abscesses	5 (25)
Multiple-system failure	3 (15)
Enteric or biliary fistulas	2 (10)
Mesenteric or portal thrombosis	2 (10)
Other	3 (15)
Mortality	4 (20)
Survival	
1-y	10 (50)
2-y	4 (20)
3-y	2 (10)
Median, mo	12.0 (. . .)
Disease-free interval (median), mo	9.0 (. . .)
Local tumor control	4 (20)

Surgery

One patient received a subtotal resection of the pancreatic head, while 19 patients had a total pancreatectomy. The median operative time was ten hours (range, five to 20 hours). The median operative blood requirement was 10.5 U (range, 3 to 40 U).

Portal vein resection with an end-to-end reanastomosis was performed in all patients. The median length of portal vein that was resected was 4.0 cm (range, 2 to 6 cm), and the median duration of portal vein clamp time was 18 minutes (range, eight to 25 minutes).

Pancreatic visceral arterial resections were performed in three patients. One patient had a resection of an aberrant hepatic artery that was reconstructed by an anastomosis of the celiac stump of the splenic artery to the hepatic arterial remnant. Two patients had sleeve resections of the base of the superior mesenteric artery that were reconstructed by an anastomosis of the superior mesenteric arterial remnant to the aorta. No prosthetic arterial grafts were used in any patient.

Disease Control

Survival of the 20 patients who underwent a regional pancreatectomy was 50% at 12 months, 20% at 24 months, and 10% at 36 months. The median survival was 12.0 months. One patient remains alive at 50 months. Three patients died of postoperative complications, free of cancer. Two patients died of cerebrovascular accidents, free of malignant neoplasms, during follow-up (at 18 and 39 months). Figure 1 illustrates the actuarial survival curve for all patients.

The median time to disease recurrence was 9.0 months. Two patients died without recurrence at 18 and 39 months, and one patient is alive, free of disease at 50 months. Three patients died in the postoperative period without pathologic evidence of residual or recurrent disease, while one patient who died of complications at two months had recurrent disease at the time of death. The actuarial plot of disease recurrence is given in Fig 2.

Local disease failure occurred in 14 patients (70%), defined as failure within the retroperitoneum or on the peritoneal surfaces. Of the 16 patients who survived surgery, three patients (19%) had local disease control at the time of death or at last follow-up. The median time to local disease recurrence was 9.0 months.

Treatment Mortality

Four patients (20%) died of complications of treatment. One patient who manifested no immediate clinical postop-

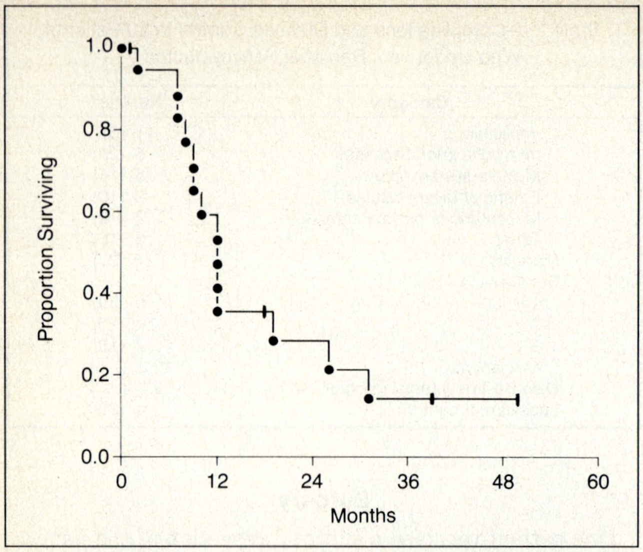

Fig 1.—Life-table plot of survival of 20 patients who underwent regional pancreatectomy at National Cancer Institute, Bethesda, Md. Patients alive or patients who died free of cancer are censored and are represented as tic marks at time of death or last follow-up.

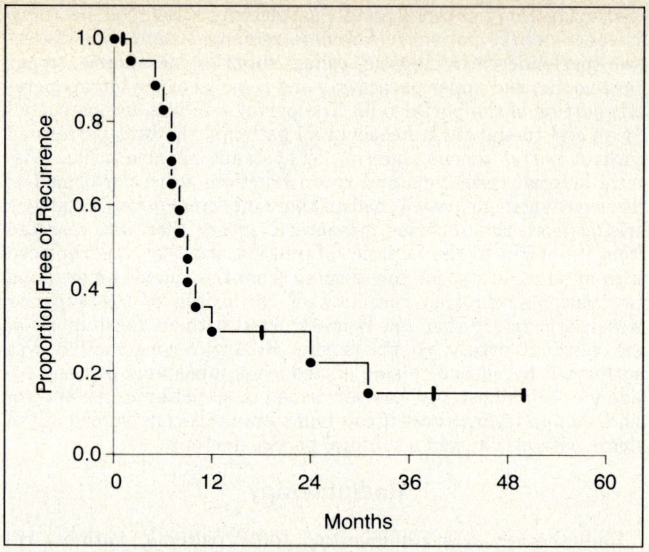

Fig 2.—Life-table plot of disease-free survival of 20 patients who underwent regional pancreatectomy at National Cancer Institute, Bethesda, Md. Patients free of recurrence are censored and are represented as tic marks at time of death or last follow-up.

erative complications died suddenly of a myocardial infarction one month after treatment. One patient who underwent an extensive extirpation that required resection of a substantial segment of the superior mesenteric artery developed a biliary fistula with intra-abdominal abscesses one week postoperatively. The patient developed episodes of sepsis, small intestinal fistulas, and multiple-organ failure. The patient died two months following surgery. One patient developed mesenteric arterial thrombosis two weeks postoperatively that resulted in infarction of most of the small intestine. The patient developed multiple gastrointestinal fistulas, sepsis, and multiple-organ failure. The patient died two months postoperatively. One patient developed portal venous thrombosis one week postoperatively and went on to develop multiple gastrointestinal fistulas; this patient died of hepatic failure two months postoperatively.

Treatment Complications

Postoperative complications developed in 11 patients (55%), and these are summarized in Tables 1 and 2. Infectious complications were frequent, with five patients (25%) developing bacterial peritonitis, intra-abdominal abscesses, or wound infections. Sepsis with multiple-organ failure occurred in three patients (15%). Enteric or biliary fistulas developed in two patients (10%) and were associated with intra-abdominal sepsis. Mesenteric vascular thrombosis and infarction occurred in two patients (10%), with one patient having thrombosis of the superior mesenteric artery and with the other patient having portal venous occlusion. Persistent chylous ascites developed in two patients (10%); this condition spontaneously resolved by three months postoperatively in one patient and required peritoneovenous shunting in the other patient. One patient had a prolonged postoperative ileus (14 days). One patient suffered a cardiac arrest and could not be resuscitated; autopsy revealed a myocardial infarction with no intra-abdominal pathologic condition.

Late Events

Sixteen patients survived a regional pancreatectomy and were discharged from the hospital. No patients suffered from intractable diabetes or malabsorption that required hospitalization for control. All patients required insulin (4 to 60 U/d, typically in two divided doses). All patients required pancreatic enzyme replacement (4 to 10 capsules with each meal), including the single patient in the series with a subtotal pancreatic resection. All patients suffered some weight loss (5% to 15% of the discharge weight) initially on leaving the hospital; this weight loss typically stabilized or was reversed within three months of hospital discharge.

Late complications developed in some patients (Table 1). Two patients were considered to have alimentation and nutritional problems that were severe enough to require special dietary supplements. One patient developed a gastric bezoar that was composed of vegetable material two years postoperatively and required endoscopic removal. One patient suffered repeated bouts of lower gastrointestinal tract bleeding, beginning two years postoperatively and eluding diagnostic attempts at localization. Arteriography ultimately suggested scattered areas of arteriovenous ectasia in the colon, and the bleeding episodes resolved following a subtotal colectomy. No malignant disease was present at the time of laparotomy.

In some patients, late events developed that were considered to be unrelated to the treatment undertaken for pancreatic cancer. One patient developed a localized primary adenocarcinoma of the breast 18 months after a pancreatectomy and underwent a mastectomy. The patient ultimately died of a myocardial infarction and was found to have metastatic pancreatic cancer in the liver at the time of death. One patient with a history of renal stones developed renal calculi that required lithotripsy and endoscopic removal one year after a pancreatectomy. Two patients died of strokes, free of recurrent pancreatic cancer, at 18 and 39 months following a pancreatectomy.

Adjuvant Radiotherapy

Intraoperative radiotherapy was delivered to 11 patients, and conventional postoperative external-beam radiation was given to six patients. Three patients received no radiation therapy. There were no significant differences in

Table 3.—Comparison of Results of Patients Who Underwent Regional Pancreatectomy for Adenocarcinoma of Pancreas

		No. (%)					
				Survival, mo			
Series Study, y	No. of Patients	Mortality	Morbidity	12	24	36	Median Survival, mo
Fortner,[5] 1984	35	9 (26)	41 (67)	14 (40)	3 (9)	1 (3)	12.5
Present study, 1988	20	4 (20)	11 (55)	10 (50)	4 (20)	2 (10)	12.0

overall survival between the patient group that received intraoperative irradiation (12-month median survival) and the patient group that received either no radiation or conventional radiotherapy (ten-month median survival). Although not reaching statistical significance, there was a trend toward earlier disease recurrence among patients who received no radiation or conventional irradiation (75% recurrence at any site and 75% local recurrence at 12 months), compared with the patients who received intraoperative irradiation (56% recurrence at any site and 44% local recurrence at 12 months).

COMMENT

Adenocarcinoma of the pancreas is an aggressive visceral malignant neoplasm, claiming nearly 25 000 lives yearly in the United States.[1] Pancreatic carcinoma is a highly lethal disease, with only approximately 1% of patients successfully cured by surgical intervention.[1] Surgical removal of the neoplasm is the only treatment modality that potentially can result in cure, but only about 15% of all patients with pancreatic cancers are found at operation to have lesions sufficiently localized to permit resection. The expected five-year survival rates of patients with resected adenocarcinoma of the pancreatic parenchyma is under 10%, and about 50% of patients who undergo resection have local recurrences within the tumor bed.[1,2] A pancreatduodenectomy (Whipple's operation) has been the surgical procedure traditionally utilized for pancreatic resections, although a total pancreatectomy has been advocated by some surgeons.

The regional pancreatectomy was initially described in 1973, by Fortner[3] as a resective procedure potentially applicable to locally advanced pancreatic cancers. The procedure was considered to enhance disease control possibly by extirpating all tissues in the region of the pancreas that could harbor residual neoplastic cells that were spread from the primary tumor. The regional pancreatectomy consists of en bloc resection of the pancreatic head or entire gland, the duodenum, the regional lymph nodes (peripancreatic, celiac, hepatic, superior mesenteric, upper para-aortic, and upper para-caval), much of the extrahepatic bile duct, and the intrapancreatic portion of the portal vein. The procedure involves reconstuction of the sleeve-resected portal vein by an end-to-end anastomosis. The regional pancreatectomy also involves visceral arterial resection in patients with neoplastic involvement of the celiac, hepatic, or superior mesenteric arteries.

The initial report of the regional pancreatectomy described four patients. There was a 25% operative mortality and a six-month survival of 25%.[3] In 1977, Fortner and colleagues[4] reported on a series of 18 patients who had undergone a regional pancreatectomy at Memorial Sloan-Kettering Cancer Center, with a mortality of 17% and a 62% one-year actuarial survival rate. It was suggested that the regional pancreatectomy improved the resectability rate of patients with pancreatic neoplasms, allowed the resection of large lesions that were considered untreatable by the conventional Whipple's operation or by a total pancreatectomy, and resulted in improved survival, compared with patients who undergo conventional pancreatic resections.

By 1984, Fortner[5] accumulated a series of 61 patients with regional pancreatic resections, including 35 patients with adenocarcinoma of the pancreas, 21 patients with periampullary tumors, islet cell tumors, or other malignant pancreatic lesions, and five patients with benign conditions. The overall treatment-related mortality was 23%. The mortality decreased to 8% during the three years that immediately preceded the report. For patients with adenocarcinoma of the pancreas who underwent a regional resection, the median survival was 13 months. The longest surviving patient died with cancer at 53 months following surgery. Patients who underwent a regional pancreatectomy for periampullary malignant neoplasms or islet cell tumors had a median survival of 40 months.

The utility of the regional pancreatectomy has been debated by pancreatic surgeons.[6] Proponents of regional resections have claimed that the procedure allows resection of lesions that were too extensive for conventional Whipple's or total pancreatic resections and that the regional procedure produces long-term survival in some patients. Critics of the regional pancreatectomy point out that, while the operation requires considerable technical skill and hospital resources, it does not substantially enhance survival in most patients with pancreatic cancer. Most centers that perform large numbers of surgical procedures for pancreatic adenocarcinoma consider the regional pancreatectomy to be an experimental procedure. Few institutions have amassed any experience with the regional pancreatectomy. The present series reports the experience with regional resection at the National Cancer Institute and attempts to interpret the utility of the procedure in patients with locally advanced pancreatic adenocarcinoma.

Twenty patients underwent a regional pancreatectomy at the National Cancer Institute. The overall morbidity was 55%, and the treatment mortality was 20%; these rates are consistent with those reported by Fortner[5] for patients who undergo regional resections for adenocarcinoma of the pancreatic parenchyma (Table 3). Although some isolated series have shown highly favorable mortality and complication rates for pancreatic resections, the morbidity and mortality of regional resections correspond closely to the average complication rates of multiple series of conventional pancreatic resections for cancer. Whipple's operations show an average 20% mortality and 52% morbidity in collected series, and total pancreatectomies demonstrate 22% mortality and 53% morbidity.[1] Consequently, it may be suggested that the regional resection can be performed with an overall risk that does not substantially exceed that of Whipple's or total pancreatic resections. The morbidity of the regional pancreatectomy may be reduced as surgical experience increases. In the present series, complications developed in seven (47%) of 15 patients whose operations were performed by experienced attending surgeons (defined as surgeons who had performed at least five pancreatic resections of any type for malignant disease), but complications occurred in four (80%) of five patients who had resections performed by less-experienced attending surgeons (defined as surgeons who had performed fewer than five pancreatic resections).

The survival rates in the present series were 50% at 12 months and 10% at 36 months, closely approximating the results of Fortner's[5] series (Table 3). In combined series of pancreatic resections for pancreatic adenocarcinomas, the average three-year survival has been reported as 13% for Whipple's operations and as 18% for total pancreatectomies.[1] There is no substantial difference, therefore, in the expected survivals of patients who undergo a regional pancreatectomy as compared with pancreatic resections that do not involve the portal vein or regional nodes. Direct comparisons of survival rates may be misleading, however, since patients who undergo a regional pancreatectomy typically have disease that is considered too advanced to allow a conventional Whipple's resection or a total pancreatectomy. The population of patients with regional resections represents a group with advanced disease and a poor prognosis. In the present series, there were no patients with stage I disease confined within the pancreas who would be considered as candidates for resection by a conventional Whipple's operation or a total pancreatectomy. Consequently, some patients may be salvaged by a regional pancreatectomy who could not be resected by a conventional pancreatectomy.

In the present series, no significant differences developed in morbidity, mortality, or disease control between the patient groups that received intraoperative radiotherapy and those that received conventional external-beam therapy or no radiotherapy. There was, however, a trend toward delayed disease recurrence in the patients who received intraoperative irradiation. Since the overall morbidity and mortality rates in the present series were similar to those reported by Fortner[5] in patients who received a regional resection without radiation, it can be reasonably suggested that adjunctive radiotherapy does not substantially increase the risk of treatment-related morbidity following a regional pancreatectomy.

General conclusions may be drawn from the present experience and from the literature reporting on regional pancreatectomy. Regional resections may be performed on selected patients with locally advanced adenocarcinomas of the pancreas with an expected morbidity of at least 50% and an expected mortality of at least 20%. Complications may be diminished in the hands of surgeons who are experienced in pancreatic resections. The expected median survival of 12 months suggests that a regional pancreatectomy offers no substantial benefit for most patients with pancreatic cancer. However, since approximately 10% of patients may enjoy long-term survival, a regional pancreatectomy should be considered as a treatment option in selected patients at centers with considerable experience in pancreatic surgery. Further investigation appears to be warranted into the possible utility of radiation therapy in conjunction with resection for pancreatic cancer.

References

1. Sindelar WF, Kinsella TJ, Mayer RJ: Cancer of the pancreas, in DeVita VT, Hellman S, Rosenberg SA (eds): *Cancer: Principles and Practice of Oncology*, ed 2. Philadelphia, JB Lippincott Co, 1985, pp 691-739.
2. Tepper J, Nardi G, Suit H: Carcinomas of the pancreas: Review of MGH experience from 1963 to 1973: Analysis of surgical failure and implications for radiation therapy. *Cancer* 1976;37:1519-1524.
3. Fortner JG: Regional resection of the pancreas: A new surgical approach. *Surgery* 1973;73:307-320.
4. Fortner JG, Kim DK, Cubilla A, et al: Regional pancreatectomy: En bloc pancreatic, portal vein and lymph node resection. *Ann Surg* 1977;186:42-50.
5. Fortner JG: Regional pancreatectomy for cancer of the pancreas, ampulla, and other related sites: Tumor staging and results. *Ann Surg* 1984;199:418-425.
6. Brooks JR: Cancer of the pancreas, in Brooks JR (ed): *Surgery of the Pancreas*. Philadelphia, WB Saunders Co, 1983, pp 263-298.
7. Sindelar WF: Intraoperative radiotherapy in carcinoma of the stomach and pancreas, in Schlag P, Hohenberger P, Metzger U (eds): *Combined Modality Therapy of Gastrointestinal Tract Cancer.* New York, Springer-Verlag NY Inc, 1988, pp 226-243.
8. Sindelar WF, Hoekstra HJ, Kinsella TJ: Surgical approaches and techniques in intraoperative radiotherapy for intra-abdominal, retroperitoneal, and pelvic neoplasms. *Surgery* 1988;103:247-256.

In Other AMA Journals

ARCHIVES OF OTOLARYNGOLOGY–HEAD & NECK SURGERY

Bacteriologic Analysis of Wound Infection Following Major Head and Neck Surgery

Jennifer Rubin, MD; Jonas T. Johnson, MD; Robin L. Wagner; Victor L. Yu, MD

Wound infection was studied prospectively in 23 (6.5%) of 354 patients who participated in a series of antibiotic trials during major contaminated head and neck surgical procedures. Polymicrobial infection was identified in 22 (96%) of 23 cases. The most commonly encountered organisms were aerobic bacteria (91%), anaerobes (74%), and fungi (48%). All fungal infections resolved without systemic antifungal therapy. It was, therefore, concluded that the presence of fungus represented colonization. The primary treatment of an infected wound is surgical drainage accompanied by broad spectrum antibiotic therapy to prevent sepsis. The value of postoperative wound cultures is unclear. The majority of patients who developed wound infection had a variety of organisms that appeared to be unrelated to the prophylactic antibiotic used, as well as to the particular surgery performed (*Arch Otolaryngol Head Neck Surg* 1988;114:969-972).

Reprint requests to Department of Otolaryngology, Eye and Ear Hospital, Suite 500, 203 Lothrop St, Pittsburgh, PA 15213 (Dr Johnson).

Débridement of Wounds With Dakin's Solution

To the Editor.—The article in the April 1988 issue of the ARCHIVES by Kozol and colleagues[1] recommended that we abandon the use of Dakin's solution in open, dirty, necrotic wounds. Unfortunately, this article, like many other reports based on laboratory studies in rats and rabbits, ignores the observations and lessons learned in clinical surgery over many years. A wound that is covered with dead, infected tissue must be débrided one way or another. Any technique, whether it is surgical débridement or frequent dressing changes, will damage normal underlying tissue. The purpose of using frequent dressing changes with half-strength Dakin's solution is to débride rapidly the dead, necrotic, infected tissue. Once this is done, healing can take place regardless of where the neutrophils migrate. Once the wound is clean, application of the dressings with Dakin's solution is stopped and the wound either is allowed to epithelialize or is surgically closed. Furthermore, even though Kozol et al recommend the abandonment of Dakin's and saline solutions and the use of normal saline solution, where are the controls to show that normal saline solution is the solution of choice? Where are the controls to show that surgical débridement does not hurt normal tissue? Finally, why do surgical journals continue to publish these silly little studies that have no bearing on clinical surgery?

JOHN G. RAFFENSPERGER, MD
Department of Surgery
Childrens Memorial Hospital
2300 Children's Plaza
Chicago, IL 60614

1. Kozol RA, Gillies C, Elgebaly SA: Effects of sodium hypochlorite (Dakin's solution) on cells of the wound module. *Arch Surg* 1988;123:420-427.

To the Editor.—Kozol et al conclude that the adverse effects of hypochlorites on various cell lines in their wound module argue against the use of Dakin's solution in open wounds. Unfortunately, extrapolations from cell culture or other "wound facsimiles" to the surgical wound are tenuous at best. Both hypochlorite itself, as well as compounds that generate hypochlorous acid (the active species of all hypochlorite microbicidal formulations), have enjoyed long-term clinical popularity principally because of their efficacy and safety.[1-3]

The apparently contradictory results obtained by Kozol et al may, in part, be explained by the wound module, which bears little similarity to a real wound milieu. The cell culture environment lacks the organic substances (principally proteinaceous components of serum, fibrin, and collagen) of the clinical wound. It is well known that hypochlorites are consumed by organic matter.[4,5] The absence of these organic substances in the wound module precludes consumption, as normally occurs in the clinical wound. Consumption and buffering of hypochlorites by organic matter in the clinical wound accounts for the requirement of higher concentrations of hypochlorites to achieve effective antimicrobial activity in clinical wounds. It also explains wound tolerance of these higher levels of hypochlorite concentration.

Kozol et al do not detail the composition of the Dakin's solution used in their study. Specifically, they do not state whether the hypochlorite was buffered and, if so, what the pH was. Dakin himself modified the formulation, first buffering it with boric acid and then with carbonate.[5] Buffering serves two important functions. First, it reduces the alkalinity of hypochlorite. Even very dilute solutions of unbuffered hypochlorite (laundry bleach) in saline solution have a pH in excess of 10. Second, by reducing the pH, the solution's equilibrium is shifted toward generation of hypochlorous acid: $NaOCl + H^+ \rightleftharpoons HOCl + Na^+$. As noted above, hypochlorous acid is the actual microbicidal species in all hypochlorite formulation. Hence, lower pH translates to greater efficacy and this allows lower concentrations to be used.[5-7]

Hypochlorites have an excellent antimicrobial spectrum and act rapidly against gram-positive and gram-negative bacteria, viruses (including human immunodeficiency virus), fungi, and spores. Resistant organisms do not develop. No adverse local effect has been determined in the clinical wound and no systemic toxicity has been found no matter what the duration of use in recommended concentrations. Actual clinical use has proven to us that hypochlorites are effective tools in wound management.

SALVATORE BARESE, MS, PA
CHARLES B. CUONO, MD, PHD
Yale University School of Medicine
Department of Surgery
PO Box 3333, 4 YPB
New Haven, CT 06510

1. Swanker WA: The use of chlorpactin WCS 90 as an antiseptic in surgery. *Am J Surg* 1955; 90:44-46.
2. Rudolph R, Noe J: *Chronic Problem Wounds.* Boston, Little Brown & Co Inc, 1983.
3. Gilman AG, Goodman LS, et al: *The Pharmacological Basis of Therapeutics,* ed 7. New York, Macmillan Publishing Co Inc, 1985, pp 963-964.
4. Block SS: *Disinfection, Sterilization, and Preservation,* ed 3. Philadelphia, Lea & Febiger, 1983, pp 157-179.
5. Barese S, Fichandler B, Cuono C: Important considerations in the use of hypochlorites as antimicrobials. *Proc Am Burn Assoc* 1985;17:59.
6. Cotter J, Fader R, Herndon D: Development of a 0.1% sodium hypochlorite solution for possible use in burn therapy. *Proc Am Burn Assoc* 1985;17:60.
7. Cotter J, Fader R, Lilley C, et al: Chemical parameters, antimicrobial activities, and tissue toxicity of 0.1 and 0.5% sodium hypochlorite solutions. *Antimicrob Agents Chemother* 1985; 28:118-122.

In Reply.—I would like to thank Drs Raffensperger and Cuono and Mr Barese for their interest in our work. They bring up the dilemma of the applicability of animal and in vitro models to clinical surgery. To this issue, Claude Bernard, the father of experimental medicine, said the following:

I not only conclude that experiments made on animals from the physiological, pathological and therapeutic points of view have results that are applicable to theoretical medicine, but I think that without such comparative study of animals, practical medicine can never acquire scientific character.[1]

The fact that a practice or ritual has been used in surgery for decades does not diminish the value of further scientific evaluation of that practice.

Mr Barese and Dr Cuono point out that organic matter in wounds consumes the hypochlorites. Nobel Prize winner Alexander Fleming addressed this very issue about Dakin's solution and commented that "It loses its antiseptic action so quickly. In ten minutes, it can't do much damage and, after that, nature has two hours' rest in which to recuperate without being interrupted."[2]

Peacock noted that "The history of wound surgery is, in large measure, the history of military surgery."[3] Dakin's solution was popularized during World War I as an alternative to surgical débridement because of logistical problems of wound care in the battlefield. Grossly infected, necrotic wounds should be surgically débrided. Clean, open wounds are most safely cared for with normal saline solution, which in general is not toxic to native cells.

ROBERT A. KOZOL, MD
Department of Surgery
University of Connecticut
School of Medicine
Farmington, CN 06032

1. Baker HJ, Hunt CE, Lindsey JR: Animal experimentation in wound healing research, in Menaker L (ed): *Biologic Basis of Wound Healing.* Hagerstown, Md, Harper & Row Publishers Inc, 1975, p 312.

2. Maurois A: *The Life of Alexander Fleming.* New York, EP Dutton, 1968.

3. Peacock E: Wound healing and wound care, in Schwartz SI (ed): *Principles of Surgery,* ed 3. New York, McGraw-Hill International Book Co, 1978, p 316.

Cancer Surveillance After Augmentation Mammoplasty

To the Editor.—The major point of the article by Silverstein et al[1] in the June 1988 issue of the ARCHIVES entitled "Breast Cancer in Women After Augmentation Mammoplasty" seems to be that augmentation mammoplasty with silicone-gel–filled implants make film-screen mammography, our best diagnostic tool, less sensitive. I must politely disagree.

In conjunction with our mammographer, G. William Ecklund, MD, we have shown that state-of-the-art mammographic cancer surveillance is possible in augmented breasts if specialized techniques are utilized.

Selected patients who have undergone augmentation mammoplasty during the past several years have demonstrated to us the advantages of modified patient positioning and compression techniques to optimize breast tissue visualization (Figure). Five views are routinely utilized for each breast: the standard mediolateral oblique and vertical craniocaudal repeated standard views with anterior compression and a 90° mediolateral compression view. Magnified views, focal compressed magnified views, and the use of lead markers have also helped us in identifying suspicious masses and/or calcifications. A videotape is available to demonstrate these techniques.

By modifying the mammographic examination and supplying appropriate counseling and reassurance about the procedure to both patients and physicians, patient cooperation and improved image quality have been obtained. It is incumbent on the referring physician to convey to the mammographer as much information about the patient as possible, including the type and location of the clinical concerns prompting this study.

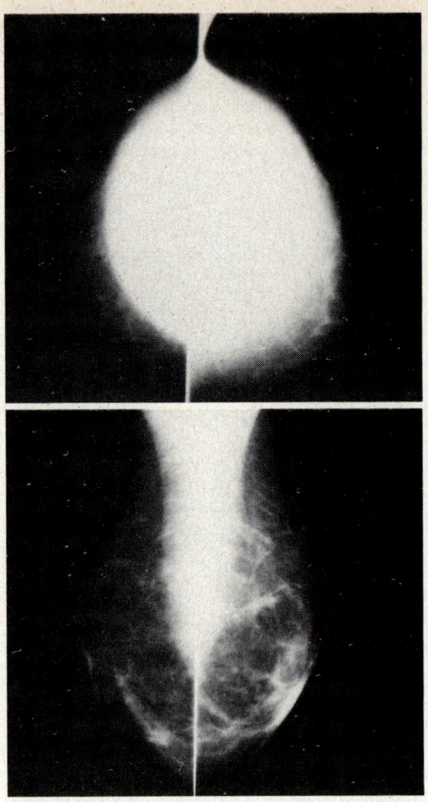

Standard (top) and modified (bottom) compressions of mediolateral oblique view of same patient, who had significant capsular contracture in addition to augmentation.

STEPHEN H. MILLER, MD
La Jolla, Calif

1. Silverstein MJ, Handel N, Gamagami P, et al: Breast cancer in women after augmentation mammoplasty. *Arch Surg* 1988;123:681-685.

Books

Surgery of the Liver and Biliary Tract, edited by L. H. Blumgart, 1552 pp, $350, New York, Churchill Livingstone Inc, 1988.

Surgery of the Liver and Biliary Tract is destined to become the classic reference for surgeons and students of surgical disease of the right upper quadrant. Professor Blumgart has assembled a host of Western authorities on a wide range of subjects germane to the surgical treatment of diseases of the liver, gallbladder, and bile ducts. The range of this work far surpasses other contemporary works on this subject as witnessed by the sheer mass of this two-volume endeavor.

Divided into 18 major sections, this book encompasses the entire gamut of surgical liver disease beginning with anatomy and pathophysiology and including diagnostic techniques, both radiology and endoscopy, as well as a section on preoperative and postoperative anesthetic and metabolic considerations for the patient with a diseased liver. More mundane problems are also addressed, with more than 150 pages devoted to stone disease of the gallbladder and biliary ducts. Extensive sections on bile duct tumors, bile duct and liver cysts, and liver tumors are complemented by rigorous treatment of hepatic resection techniques as well as radiological and endoscopic palliative procedures. Cirrhosis and portal hypertension, both in the adult and child, and hepatic transplantation round out the final volume.

Unlike many multiauthored texts,

this work exhibits a surprising homogeneity between chapters that reflects both careful editorial supervision and the quality of the individual contributors. Multiple black-and-white photographs and clearly constructed line drawings by a single artist contribute to easy readability.

Priced at $350, this work is not a casual purchase. Nevertheless, it represents very good value considering its scope and breadth. *Surgery of the Liver and Biliary Tract* will certainly take its place as one of the premiere reference works for surgeons who deal with both straightforward and complex disorders of the liver and biliary system. This work is a must for all reference libraries and will be a handsome and often-used addition to the collection of both the experienced hepatobiliary surgeon as well as those entering the field.

Greg Van Stiegmann, MD
Denver

Cancer of the Breast, ed 3, edited by William L. Donegan and John S. Spratt, 752 pp, with illus, $99, Philadelphia, WB Saunders Co, 1988.

A spate of new textbooks on breast disease have been published during the past few years. The field may now be overpopulated. A good update of an earlier book, however, is always welcome.

In the third edition of *Cancer of the Breast,* editors William Donegan and John Spratt have assembled 29 other authors, half of them from Louisville, who write of relevant, timely changes in the approach to breast cancer. New material is frequent. The full spectrum of clinical care and much of the related basic science are covered. Controversy has not been covered up. One of the editors, for instance, challenges the widely held belief that screening mammography will reduce the risk of dying of breast cancer.

One of the best chapters in the book is not about new developments. It is a history of breast cancer written by Dr Donegan. The alternating views of breast cancer as primarily systemic vs local are traced over centuries. The classic radical mastectomy, one learns, was described more than 100 years before Halsted. The rise and fall of theories and procedures over the course of 5000 years makes good reading.

The strength of this text is its emphasis on aspects of breast cancer that concern the surgeon. This is not surprising, because both editors are surgical oncologists. The chapter on diagnosis reviews extensively the classic signs of breast cancer and devotes considerable space to biopsy techniques. The section on needle localization biopsy is complete in terms of technique, although one can disagree with the author that an immediate specimen roentgenogram is useful for occult masses as well as for microcalcifications.

The chapters on staging and primary treatment and on surgical management, each among the longest in the book, actually constitute a single description of primary therapy for breast cancer. Illustrations of particular operations are clear, and the accompanying legends are detailed. The book may be worth its $99 price as a surgical atlas of breast procedures alone. Although surgeons may quibble over fine points, the techniques shown are current and acceptable. Best of all, operative techniques are kept in proper perspective with the greater demands of the disease.

The last chapter, on statistical methods in cancer research, is an unexpected bonus. In a day when treatment is dictated primarily by results of randomized studies, it is useful to know the means by which studies should be judged. One section of the chapter is entitled "Principles to Remember." It lists 13 guidelines to be used in designing protocols or interpreting data. For the occasional statistician, the criteria are eye-opening. Another surprise is a review of common statistical methods for determining significance. The commonly used Student's *t* test never seemed so understandable.

Cancer of the Breast does not have as many distinguished contributors as some other recently published texts, but it is unusually clear and to the point. In the final analysis, it may prove to be more useful.

Lawrence Norton, MD
Denver

Calendar of Events

1989

January

Southeastern Surgical Congress, Jan 24-27, Innisbrook Conference Center, Tampa, Fla.

February

Society of University Surgeons, Feb 9-11, The Johns Hopkins University, Baltimore, Local Coordinator: Dr Greg B. Bulkey, The Johns Hopkins Hospital, 600 N Wolfe St, Blalock 685, Baltimore, MD 21205.

March

Central Surgical Association, March 8-11, Calgary, Alberta, Canada.

April

American College of Surgeons (Spring), April 2-6, Boston.

Association for Surgical Education, April 5-8, Tampa, Fla.
Local Coordinator: Dr Charles Cox, University of South Florida.

Society for Clinical Vascular Surgery, April 5-9, Innisbrook, Tarpon Springs, Fla.

American Surgical Association, April 10-12, Broadmoor, Colorado Springs, Colo.

Surgical Infection Society, April 13-14, The Broadmoor, Denver.

May

American Association for Thoracic Surgery, May 8-10, Sheraton/Hynes, Boston.

The Society of Surgical Oncology Inc, May 21-24, Westin St Francis, San Francisco.

June

Society for Vascular Surgery/International Cardiovascular Society, June 18-21, Hilton, New York.

Western Thoracic Surgical Association, June 21-25, Hyatt Regency, Monterey, Calif.

September

Society of Thoracic Surgeons, Sept 10-13, Convention Center, Baltimore.

October

American Association for the Surgery of Trauma, Oct 5-7, Chicago.

American Society of Anesthesiologists, Oct 14-18, New Orleans.

American College of Surgeons (Congress), Oct 15-20, World Congress Center, Atlanta.

American College of Chest Physicians, Oct 30-Nov 3, Boston.

November

Western Surgical Association, Nov 11-14, St Louis.

American Heart Association, Nov 13-16, New Orleans.

THE SURGERY BOARDS REVIEW COURSE

January 23-29, 1989 – Houston
March 6-12, 1989 – Portland, Oregon
April 24-30, 1989 – Chicago

Now, a special update for your written or recertification or oral exam

OBJECTIVES:
- To increase knowledge of surgical principles and practice
- To prepare candidates to take written and oral board exams
- To provide a comprehensive review for recertification

METHODS:
- HOME STUDY MATERIALS consisting of a syllabus of questions and answers with assignments
- SEMINAR with projection slides and syllabus

*"The faculty was outstanding. The most pleasant thing was learning a tremendous amount, not only from world-famous authorities but from people who are relatively unknown as well."**

BASIC SURGERY

Anatomy
Embryology

Physiology
Body Fluids
Electrolytes
Acid-Base
Blood Gasses
Metabolic Response
Wound Healing

Anesthesiology

Shock
Resuscitation
Bleeding
Transfusion

Neoplasia

Transplantation

Trauma
Burns
Head Injuries

Surgical Care
Pre- and post-op
Nutrition
Patient Monitoring
Complications
Medical Problems
Infections

GENERAL SURGERY

Alimentary Tract
Esophagus
Stomach
Appendix
Colon
Rectum and Anus

Endocrine
Thyroid
Parathyroid
Pituitary
Adrenal

Abdomen
Liver and Gallbladder
Pancreas and Spleen
Peritonitis
Abdominal Abscess
Abdominal Wall
Retroperitoneum
Abdominal Hernias

Breast

Skin

Head and Neck
Anatomy
Tumors
Trauma

SPECIAL SURGERY

Thoracic Surgery
Chest Wall/Pleura
Lung/Mediastinum

Cardiac Surgery
Congenital Heart
Acquired Heart

Vascular Surgery
The Great Veins
Peripheral Arteries
Veins and Lymphatics

Orthopedic Surgery
Bone Disease
Fractures
Joint Disorders
Amputations

Hand Surgery
Hand Anatomy
Hand Injuries
Hand Infections

Pediatric Surgery

Urologic Surgery

Gynecologic Surgery

Neurosurgery

Plastic Surgery

Limited Enrollment: SURGERY BOARDS REVIEW REGISTRATION

Name ______________________
Address ______________________
City/State/Zip ______________________
Phone ______________________

For:
☐ January 23-29, 1989 – Houston
☐ March 6-12, 1989 – Portland
☐ April 24-30, 1989 – Chicago
☐ October 4-10, 1989 – Chicago
☐ Check is enclosed for $ ______
☐ Please send more information.

Mail today to:
1094 Dawn Lane, Dept. S12
P.O. Box 2218
Terre Haute, IN 47802

*"Accommodations were comfortable..."**

GOALS AND LOCATION: The course is to help you pass your written and oral, or recertification exams. Home study questions are sent upon registration. Your best buy is to repeat the course just before written and oral board exams. The Houston course will be held at the Doubletree at Houston Intercontinental Airport, 15747 John F. Kennedy Blvd., Houston, Texas 77032. The Doubletree has an outdoor pool, whirlpool spa, fine dining and free parking and airport transportation. Rates are $69 single and $88 double. Please wait for instructions before buying travel tickets.

*"...and those little extras...."**

LOWEST AIR FARES: Reliable Travel offers you the lowest air fare – often below super-saver rates. Please call toll-free 1-800-645-6504 ext. 10 and identify yourself with this Osler course for special group fares.

*"...remarkably complete and pleasant."**

PLACEMENT SERVICE: For a practice opportunity write or call (800) 356-7537.

*"...the most education for the money."**

FEES AND C.M.E. CREDITS:
- **C.M.E. Credits Hours: 65 hrs.**
- Practicing Surgeon: $690
- Resident or Fellow: one third off
- Repeating course within 3 years: half price
- **Add 10% for Houston after Jan. 15, 1989.**
- Attendees not in course hotel add $8/day.
- Fees include no lodging or meals.
- $50.00 will reserve your position.
- Most home study materials will be mailed after half of registration fee is received.

*"...home study material was extremely helpful."**

CANCELLATIONS: Refunds subject to $50 fee, will be made until the seminar begins.
- Cancellation after mailing home study material requires retention of half of the fee.

*"I feel [the course] helped me pass the boards."**

INFORMATION:
Joseph H. Selliken Jr., M.D.
THE SURGERY REVIEW COURSE
1094 Dawn Lane, Terre Haute, IN 47802
(800) 356-7537 or (812) 299-5658

**Comments by participants of our courses*

Papers Read Before the Annual Meeting of the Society of Surgical Oncology, New Orleans, La, May 22 to May 25, 1988—Part II

Conservative Surgery and Radiation Therapy for Early Breast Cancer

Long-term Cosmetic Results

Mary Ann Rose, MD; Ivo Olivotto, MD; Blake Cady, MD; Clinton Koufman, MD; Robert Osteen, MD; Barbara Silver; Abram Recht, MD; Jay R. Harris, MD

• To evaluate the cosmetic outcome of conservative surgery (CS) and radiation therapy (RT) for early-stage breast cancer and its stability over time, we reviewed the records of 593 patients treated from 1968 to 1981. The breast appearance was scored as "excellent," "good," "fair," or "poor." Median follow-up was 76 months (range, 37 to 186 months). Cosmetic results were generally excellent or good. The percents of excellent, good, fair, and poor results at three years were 65%, 25%, 7%, and 3%, respectively. Patients not receiving adjuvant chemotherapy were more likely than those receiving chemotherapy to have excellent scores at five years (71% vs 40%). Tumor size also influenced cosmetic outcome: 73% of patients with T1 tumors vs 55% with T2 tumors had excellent scores at five years. Our results were stable over time: of 36 patients assessable at seven years whose cosmetic scores were good or excellent at three years, 34 (94%) continued to have good or excellent scores, and only two (5%) deteriorated to fair. We conclude that the cosmetic results achieved with CS and RT are good to excellent in approximately 90% of patients and that these results remain stable for at least seven years.

(*Arch Surg* 1989;124:153-157)

In recent years, the combination of conservative surgery (CS) and radiation therapy (RT) has gained increasing acceptance as an alternative to modified radical mastectomy for the treatment of early-stage breast carcinoma. The results of retrospective studies have shown excellent local tumor control with breast-conserving treatment,[1-6] and prospective randomized trials have demonstrated equivalent survival rates for patients treated with mastectomy or CS and RT.[7,8] In the setting of comparable local control and survival, the issue of long-term cosmetic outcome following the conservative approach has become increasingly important to the patient and to the treating physician.

Most reports of cosmetic results have shown that the majority of patients treated conservatively have a satisfactory breast appearance.[9-14] In an earlier report from our institution, 86% of patients had a good to excellent overall cosmetic score at five years.[9] Breast retraction, telangiectasia, and breast edema were the major factors determining the physician's long-term assessment of cosmetic outcome. These results are typical of those described by other researchers.[10-14]

The purpose of the present study was to enlarge and update our earlier observations to assess the long-term cosmetic outcome in patients treated with CS and RT. Our results indicate that good to excellent results are maintained over many years.

PATIENTS AND METHODS

Seven hundred thirty-three women with clinical stage I or II invasive breast carcinoma were treated with CS and RT at the Joint Center for Radiation Therapy, Boston, between July 1968 and December 1981. Fourteen women had bilateral tumors treated during that period for a total of 747 treated breasts. One hundred fifty-four patients were excluded from the analysis because cosmetic follow-up was not undertaken at this institution. A total of 593 patients were therefore assessable for the analysis of cosmetic outcome.

Follow-up was generally performed at six-month intervals after completion of treatment. Patients were censored from cosmetic follow-up at the time of local, distant, or opposite breast recurrence. The range of follow-up was 37 to 186 months, with a median of 76 months. The presence and severity of breast edema, retraction, fibrosis, telangiectasia, and arm edema were noted and a score of none, minimal, moderate, or severe was assigned by the physician for each factor on a standard follow-up form.[15] A score of "none" reflected no radiation sequelae; a score of "slight" reflected a change in the breast observable only by the trained eye; a score of "moderate" denoted an obvious change or defect in the breast; and a score of "severe" indicated a serious deformity or functional impairment, such as the need for a prosthesis to compensate for size difference between the breasts or the use of a sleeve to control arm edema. The overall cosmetic result was classified by the physician as excellent, good, fair, or poor. An "excellent" score was assigned when the treated breast looked essentially the same as the opposite breast. A "good" cosmetic score was used to describe minimal but identifiable effects of radiation on the treated breast. A "fair" cosmetic score was given when significant effects of radiation on the breast were noted. A "poor" cosmetic score was used to describe severe normal tissue sequelae. Both the scoring system for the individual radiation sequelae and that for the overall cosmetic outcome were subject to some physician bias and were not quantified by measurements of breast size, density, or nipple displacement. However, these

Accepted for publication Nov 7, 1988.

From the Joint Center for Radiation Therapy and Department of Radiation Therapy, Harvard Medical School (Drs Rose, Recht, and Harris and Ms Silver), the Departments of Surgery, New England Deaconess Hospital (Dr Cady), Beth Israel Hospital (Dr Koufman), and Brigham and Women's Hospital (Dr Osteen), Boston; and the Cancer Control Agency of British Columbia (Dr Olivotto), Vancouver, Canada. Dr Rose is now with St Anne's Hospital, Fall River, Mass.

Read before the Annual Meeting of the Society of Surgical Oncology, New Orleans, May 25, 1988.

Reprint requests to St Anne's Hospital, 795 Middle St, Fall River, MA 02721 (Dr Rose).

scores did reflect both the degree to which these sequelae were obvious to the examiner and the degree of functional adjustment required by the patient. Several different physicians examined these patients over the time course of the study, a factor that also may have introduced some bias. In general, a physician's evaluation of a fair or poor result was harsher than the patient's perception of her result.

Results were plotted graphically by grouping observations into six-month time intervals. Not all patients were evaluated during every six-month interval. If more than one observation was made per patient per time interval, the worst score was used. The midpoint of each time interval was used in all curves; thus, individual observations ranged up to three months on either side of each time point. Analysis of results and comparisons between subgroups at specific time points of 3, 5, and 7 years were also undertaken.

The entire group of 593 patients was analyzed according to the following factors: (1) overall cosmetic score and time course, and the extent of (2) breast retraction, (3) breast edema, and (4) telangiectasia. The group was then subdivided and analyzed according to (1) whether or not an axillary dissection was performed, (2) use of adjuvant chemotherapy, (3) tumor size, (4) tumor location in the breast, and (5) age of the patient.

A description of our "standard" three-field technique to treat the breast and regional nodes has been previously reported.[16] The dose to the breast, and draining nodes when treated, was generally 4600 to 5000 cGy in 4½ to five weeks. Of 593 assessable patients, 550 (93%) received an additional boost (497 by iridium implant) to bring the total dose to 6000 cGy or more to the primary tumor area. Radiotherapy technical factors that had an impact on cosmetic outcome are addressed in a subsequent article.[17]

Axillary dissection was performed in 419 patients. In general the dissections were limited to level I and II lymph nodes to determine the need for adjuvant chemotherapy. "Complete" axillary dissections, including stripping of the axillary vein, were rarely performed in these patients.

One hundred thirty-four patients received some form of adjuvant chemotherapy, a factor previously reported to influence cosmetic outcome.[18,19] In 77 patients RT was completed before initiation of chemotherapy; in 49 patients RT and chemotherapy were delivered concurrently; seven patients received "sandwich" treatment that consisted of chemotherapy-radiotherapy-chemotherapy; and one patient completed her chemotherapy before beginning radiotherapy. The effect of sequencing of RT and adjuvant chemotherapy has been the subject of a separate report from our institution.[19]

Of the 593 patients, 340 had tumors measuring 2 cm or less (T1) and 253 had tumors between 2 and 5 cm (T2). It was not possible in this retrospective study to relate tumor size to breast size. Two hundred three patients had tumors located in "medial" portions of the breast, defined as the upper inner quadrant, the lower inner quadrant, and the 12-o'clock position. Three hundred twenty-seven patients had tumors located in "lateral" portions of the breast, defined as the upper and lower outer quadrants and at the 6-o'clock position. Fifty-five patients had tumors located centrally, defined as within 1 cm of the areola. In eight patients the primary location was unrecorded.

To determine the effect of age on cosmetic outcome, patients were divided into four age groups: age less than 35 years, 46 patients; age 35 to 50 years, 252 patients; age 51 to 65 years, 199 patients; and older than 66 years, 96 patients.

Statistical comparisons between groups and proportions were calculated at fixed time points using Fisher's exact test. *P* values of .05 or less were considered statistically significant.

RESULTS

The overall cosmetic scores for treated patients over time are shown in Fig 1. At three years, 62% of patients were scored as excellent, 26% as good, 9% as fair, and 3% as poor. At five years, 65% of patients had excellent scores, 25% good, 7% fair, and 3% poor. The results at seven years were similar to those at five years, with 54% scored as excellent, 24% as good, 15% as fair, and 7% having a poor score. To document further the stability of cosmetic results over time, we examined the outcome at seven years for two subsets of patients: those who had excellent scores at three years and those who had good scores at three years. Of 188 patients with excellent scores at three years, 25 were evaluated at seven years. Of those 25, 20 (80%) continued to have excellent results, four (16%) deteriorated to good, and one (4%) deteriorated to fair. Of 78 patients with good scores at three years, 11 were evaluated at seven years. Of those 11, six (55%) continued to have good scores, four (36%) improved to excellent, and one (9%) deteriorated to fair by seven years. No patient with either an excellent or good score at three years who was reevaluated at seven years had results that deteriorated to poor.

Overall cosmetic scores most closely paralleled the degree of breast retraction (Fig 2). Twenty-eight (78%) of 36 patients with fair or poor results three years after treatment showed evidence of moderate or severe retraction, while only 15 (6%) of 266 patients scored as good or excellent had moderate or severe retraction ($P<.0001$). The development of breast retraction generally occurred in the first three years and remained stable thereafter. At three years, 50% of 303 patients evaluated had no retraction, 35% had slight, 13% had moderate, and 2% had severe evidence of retraction. At seven years, 23 (43%) of 53 patients evaluated had no retraction, 21 (40%) had slight, seven (13%) had moderate, and two (4%) had severe retraction.

The development of telangiectasia occurred more slowly than breast retraction with the onset in most patients at 12 to 18 months (Fig 3). Moderate or severe telangiectasia was unusual, occurring in only 8% of patients at three and five years. At seven years eight (15%) of 53 assessable patients had moderate or severe telangiectasia (seven moderate, one severe).

Breast edema was most pronounced in the first year after treatment with 33% of patients exhibiting mild edema and 6% exhibiting moderate or severe edema at that time (Fig 4). Twenty percent of patients had some edema beyond three years that tended to resolve slowly between the fourth and eighth years. The incidence of breast edema was closely related to the use of axillary nodal dissection. Moderate and severe edema were significantly more common at one year in patients who underwent axillary dissection (8%) than in those who did not (<1%, $P=.002$). Beyond one year, the likelihood of persistent moderate and severe edema was close to zero; however, the likelihood of having any degree of breast edema was significantly greater after axillary dissection. Three years after treatment, 24% of patients who had an axillary dissection had some degree of breast edema compared with 11% of those who had no dissection ($P=.007$). At seven years the percentages were identical to those at three years but the difference was no longer statistically significant due to smaller numbers of evaluated patients.

The influence of the factors analyzed on cosmetic outcome is summarized in the Table. The use of an axillary dissection was associated with a decrease in the percentage of overall excellent outcomes in the first two years. There were significantly fewer excellent results six months after treatment among women who had an axillary dissection than among those who did not: 71% vs 86% ($P=.0005$). This difference persisted up to 18 months, at which time 75% of patients who did not have an axillary dissection had an excellent result compared with 61% of those treated with dissection ($P=.005$). Beyond two years, however, there was no difference in the overall cosmetic result. At five years, both groups had a 65% incidence of excellent results.

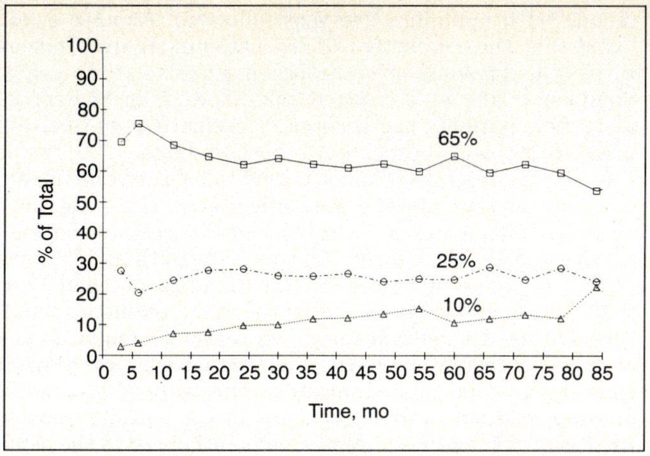

Fig 1.—Overall cosmetic results, 1968 to 1981. Numbers of patients assessable at 3, 5, and 7 years were 302, 179, and 54, respectively. Squares indicate percent excellent; circles, percent good; and triangles, percent fair/poor.

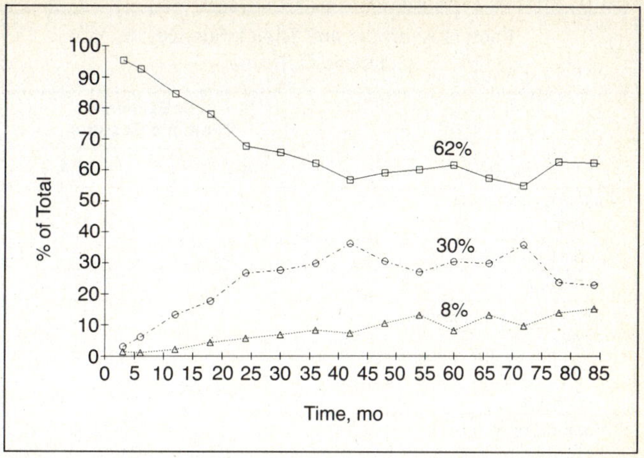

Fig 3.—Time course and extent of telangiectasia. Squares indicate percent none; circles, percent minimal; and triangles, percent moderate/severe.

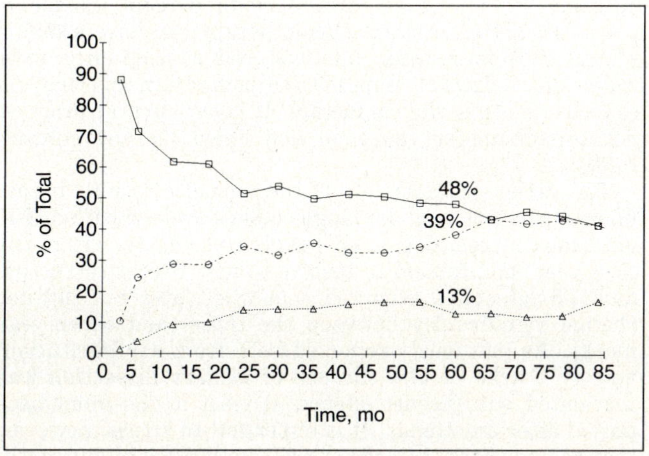

Fig 2.—Time course and extent of breast retraction. Squares indicate percent none; circles, percent minimal; and triangles, percent moderate/severe.

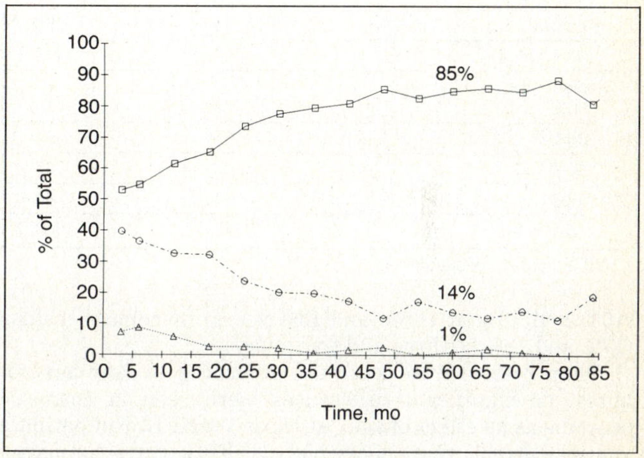

Fig 4.—Time course and extent of breast edema. Squares indicate percent none; circles, percent minimal; and triangles, percent moderate/severe.

Patients who received adjuvant chemotherapy were significantly less likely to have excellent cosmetic scores and significantly more likely to have fair or poor scores at three and five years. Sixty-eight percent of patients who did not receive chemotherapy had excellent scores at three years compared with 37% of patients who did receive chemotherapy ($P<.0001$). At five years, the corresponding figures were 71% and 40%, respectively ($P=.001$). Conversely, 9% of patients who did not receive chemotherapy had fair or poor scores at three years compared with 24% of those who did receive chemotherapy ($P=.004$). At five years, these figures were 8% and 20%, respectively ($P=.09$). These differences persisted to seven years but the number of patients evaluated at that time was small.

Patients with tumors measuring 2 cm or smaller (T1) had a greater proportion of excellent cosmetic results compared with patients whose tumors were larger than 2 cm (T2). At three years, 70% of patients with T1 tumors were scored as having excellent results compared with 52% of patients with T2 tumors ($P=.002$). At five years, 73% of patients with T1 tumors had excellent results compared with 55% of those with T2 tumors ($P=.02$). When the comparison was restricted to patients who did not receive adjuvant chemotherapy, a similar trend was observed. At five years, 76% of patients with T1 tumors treated without chemotherapy had excellent results compared with 64% of patients with T2 tumors treated without chemotherapy ($P=$not significant [NS]). There were significantly more fair and poor results among patients with T2 tumors at both three and five years. Eighteen percent of patients with T2 tumors had fair or poor scores at three years compared with 8% of those with T1 tumors ($P=.01$). At five years, 16% of patients with T2 tumors had fair or poor scores compared with 6% of those with T1 tumors ($P=.05$). When the analysis was restricted to patients who received adjuvant chemotherapy, 14% of patients with T2 tumors had fair or poor scores at five years compared with 5% of patients with T1 tumors ($P=$NS).

Overall, the location of the primary tumor did not significantly influence the cosmetic outcome. At three years, 56% of patients with medial primary tumors had excellent outcomes compared with 66% of those with lateral tumors and 61% of those with central primary tumors ($P=$NS). At five years, the results were similar with 64%, 67%, and 56% having excellent results, respectively (all, $P=$NS). Patients with lateral primary tumors were somewhat less likely to have fair or poor results (10% and 8% at three and five years) than patients with medial lesions

Factors Analyzed and Their Influence on Cosmetic Outcome

Factor	% of Excellent Cosmetic Results* 3 y	5 y
Axillary dissection		
Yes	60	65
No	67	65
P value	NS	NS
Adjuvant chemotherapy		
Yes	37	40
No	68	71
P value	<.001	.001
Tumor size		
T1	70	73
T2	52	55
P value	.002	.02
Tumor location		
Medial	56	64
Central	66	67
Lateral	61	56
All *P* value	NS	NS
Patient age, y		
<35	73	75
35-50	61	64
51-65	63	67
≥66	61	58
All *P* value	NS	NS

*NS indicates not significant.

(15% and 13% at three and five years) or central lesions (17% and 19% at three and five years).

When results were analyzed according to four age cohorts, no significant differences were seen in cosmetic outcome as an effect of age. At three years, 73% of patients younger than 35 years of age had excellent scores compared with 61% of women 35 to 50 years old, 63% of women 51 to 65 years old, and 61% of women 66 years old or older. At five years, the percents of excellent scores for these age groups were 75%, 64%, 67%, and 58%, respectively.

COMMENT

The results of this study with more patients and longer follow-up corroborate the earlier reports from our institution that 90% of patients treated with CS and RT have a good or excellent cosmetic outcome. Moreover, we have not observed detectable deterioration of the cosmetic outcome over time. Excellent scores at three years were likely to remain excellent and good results were more likely to become excellent than to deteriorate by seven years. Few patients were found to have an unsatisfactory cosmetic appearance even as late as seven years after treatment.

In the literature there has been controversy over the stability of the cosmetic results of CS and RT over time. Danoff et al[12] reported that two- to three-year follow-up was adequate to assess cosmetic outcome in patients treated with radiation alone but that longer follow-up was necessary in patients receiving chemotherapy. Ray and Fish[10] reported significant deterioration in the cosmetic results over the first three years after treatment, but they have published no subsequent report. Several centers in France have assessed their cosmetic results at five to ten years. Pierquin[2] reported that 90% (65/72) of patients with T1 lesions treated conservatively had very good cosmetic results with minimum five-year follow-up. Amalric et al[13] found that three quarters of 288 patients treated conservatively had modest or no radiation sequelae at ten years. Similarly, Calle et al[14] found that more than 95% of 99 assessable patients had acceptable cosmetic results at ten years. Our results corroborate these findings.

In this analysis, we did not intend to focus on the impact of chemotherapy on the cosmetic result since we have described this in detail elsewhere.[18,19] Our results continue to show that the use of adjuvant chemotherapy has a significant adverse effect on the cosmetic outcome, but that this is primarily true when the two treatment modalities are used simultaneously. We recently compared the cosmetic outcome of 41 patients treated with concurrent radiotherapy and chemotherapy (cyclophosphamide, methotrexate sodium, and fluorouracil in conventional doses) with that of 41 patients treated sequentially with the same regimen.[19] Among patients treated concurrently, 12% had an excellent, 58% had a good, 19% had a fair, and 11% had a poor cosmetic outcome two years after treatment. Among patients treated sequentially, 52% had an excellent, 38% had a good, 10% had a fair, and none had a poor cosmetic outcome at two years (difference in percent excellent, $P=.004$). Since adjuvant chemotherapy can have a major effect, especially when administered concurrently with radiation, we have attempted to adjust for it in this analysis to focus on other clinical factors. It is our current practice not to administer radiation and chemotherapy concurrently.

The various components of the cosmetic result—breast edema, retraction, and telangiectasia—evolved with different time courses. Breast edema occurred early (within the first year) and tended to resolve slowly. Breast retraction and telangiectasia occurred somewhat later but did not change significantly between the three- and seven-year marks. As previously reported both from our institution[9] and by Clarke et al,[20] the use of axillary dissection was associated with breast edema, at least in the immediate period after treatment. It is important to stress, however, that at five years the cosmetic result was not significantly influenced by the use of axillary node dissection, and in our view the benefits from such surgery far outweigh this transient cosmetic concern. Axillary dissection is useful in establishing more accurately the patient's prognosis, assuring local tumor control in the axilla, and simplifying the radiotherapy approach to treatment of the breast itself. It is our practice at this time to recommend a level I and II axillary dissection in all but elderly or debilitated patients.

We found that tumor size was an important factor in determining the cosmetic outcome. This is likely related to the necessity of more extensive breast surgery for larger tumors but may also reflect an unfavorable tumor to breast size ratio. In a separate report we have analyzed the technical factors of both the radiotherapy and the surgery to determine their impact on the cosmetic outcome.[17] This report clearly identifies the extent of breast surgery as a major factor influencing the cosmetic outcome. The results presented herein show the location of the tumor in the breast and the age of the patient to have no significant impact on the cosmetic outcome.

Our results provide support for the use of breast-conserving treatment by demonstrating satisfactory cosmetic results that appear to remain stable over time. While we are encouraged by the stability of the cosmetic results observed over the study time period, we realize that it is still possible to observe cosmetic deterioration over longer periods and we plan to continue to monitor our treated patients to assess this.

References

1. Calle R, Vilcoq JR, Zafrani B, et al: Local control and survival of breast cancer treated by limited surgery followed by irradiation. *Cancer* 1986;12:873-878.

2. Pierquin B: Conservative treatment for carcinoma of the breast: Experience of Creteil—ten-year results, in Harris JR, Hellman S, Silen W (eds): *Conservative Management of Breast Cancer.* Philadelphia, JB Lippincott, 1983, pp 11-14.

3. Clarke DH, Le MG, Sarrazin D, et al: Analysis of local-regional relapses in patients with early breast cancer treated by excision and radiotherapy: Experience of the Institut Gustave Roussy. *Int J Radiat Oncol Biol Phys* 1985;11:137-145.

4. Clark RM: Alternatives to mastectomy—the Princess Margaret Hospital experience, in Harris JR, Hellman S, Silen W (eds): *Conservative Management of Breast Cancer.* Philadelphia, JB Lippincott, 1983, pp 35-46.

5. Montague ED, Ames FC, Schell SR, et al: Conservative surgery and irradiation as an alternative to mastectomy in the treatment of clinically favorable breast cancer. *Cancer* 1984;54:2668-2672.

6. Recht A, Silver B, Schnitt S, et al: Breast relapse following primary radiation therapy for early breast cancer: I. Classification, frequence and salvage. *Int J Radiat Oncol Biol Phys* 1985;11:1271-1276.

7. Veronesi U, Zucali R, Luini A: Local control and survival in early breast cancer: The Milan trial. *Int J Radiat Oncol Biol Phys* 1986;12:717-720.

8. Fisher B, Bauer M, Margolese R, et al: Five-year results of a randomized clinical trial comparing total mastectomy and segmental mastectomy with or without radiation in the treatment of breast cancer. *N Engl J Med* 1985;312:665-673.

9. Beadle GF, Silver B, Botnick L, et al: Cosmetic results following primary radiation therapy for early breast cancer. *Cancer* 1984;54:2911-2918.

10. Ray Gr, Fish VJ: Biopsy and definitive radiation therapy in stage I and II adenocarcinoma of the female breast: Analysis of cosmesis and the role of electron beam supplementation. *Int J Radiat Oncol Biol Phys* 1983;9:813-818.

11. Clarke D, Martinez A, Cox RS: Analysis of cosmetic results and complications in patients with stage I and II breast cancer treated by biopsy and irradiation. *Int J Radiat Oncol Biol Phys* 1983;9:1807-1813.

12. Danoff BF, Goodman RL, Glick JH, et al: The effect of adjuvant chemotherapy on cosmesis and complications in patients with breast cancer treated by definitive irradiation. *Int J Radiat Oncol Biol Phys* 1983;9:1625-1630.

13. Amalric R, Santamaria F, Robert F, et al: Conservation therapy of operable breast cancer—results at five, ten and 15 years in 2216 consecutive cases, in Harris JR, Hellman S, Silen W (eds): *Conservative Management of Breast Cancer.* Philadelphia, JB Lippincott, 1983, pp 15-21.

14. Calle R, Vilcoq JR, Pilleron JP, et al: Conservative treatment of operable breast carcinoma by irradiation with or without limited surgery—ten year results, in Harris JR, Hellman S, Silen W (eds): *Conservative Management of Breast Cancer.* Philadelphia, JB Lippincott, 1983, pp 3-9.

15. Harris JR, Levene MB, Svensson G, Hellman S: Analysis of cosmetic results following primary radiation therapy for stages I and II carcinoma of the breast. *Int J Radiat Oncol Biol Phys* 1979;5:257-261.

16. Siddon RL, Buck BA, Harris JR, et al: Three-field technique for breast irradiation using tangential field corner blocks. *Int J Radiat Oncol Biol Phys* 1983;9:583-588.

17. Olivotto IA, Rose MA, Silver B, et al: Long-term cosmetic outcome after conservative surgery and radiotherapy for early breast cancer: Causes of cosmetic failure, abstracted. *Int J Radiat Oncol Biol Phys* 1988;15:154-155.

18. Beadle GF, Harris JR, Come S, et al: The effect of adjuvant chemotherapy on the cosmetic results after primary radiation treatment for early stage breast cancer: A preliminary analysis. *Int J Radiat Oncol Biol Phys* 1984;10:2131-2137.

19. Gore SM, Come SE, Griem K, et al: Influence of the sequencing of chemotherapy and radiation therapy in node-positive breast cancer patients treated by conservative surgery and radiation therapy, in Salmon SE (ed): *Adjuvant Therapy of Cancer.* New York, Grune & Stratton, 1987, vol 5, pp 365-373.

20. Clarke D, Martinez A, Coe RS, et al: Breast edema following staging axillary dissection in patients with breast carcinoma treated by radical radiotherapy. *Cancer* 1982;49:2295-2299.

Discussion

Q Dr Rose, did you compare your group of patients who were treated with the iridium implantation with those who received no boost or electron boost?

A Yes we did. It will be the subject of an article that is coming out by Dr Olivotto concerning the technical aspects of treatment. When we compared patients who received iridium boosts with those who received no boost or electron boosts, 80% were excellent without a boost or with electron boosts vs only 60% who were excellent with iridium. At the present time, we are not using iridium implants routinely, and that is one of the reasons.

Q Did the size of breasts influence results?

A As you know, when you read a patient's chart and try to get this information, all you have is some subjective comment about large breasts or pendulous breasts and it is really difficult to quantitate that. In our experience, patients with very large breasts may have more retraction, but only if they are treated on a low-energy machine such as the 4-mV linear accelerator or with cobalt. If the appropriate energy machine is used, you should get a good cosmetic result. Those patients probably do less well in terms of symmetry and cosmetics with mastectomy and reconstruction, so it is all relative.

Q Could you comment on the correlation between posttreatment mammography and the clinical appearance of the breast?

A On mammography you may see diffuse increased density throughout the breast. You may also see skin edema. Usually the appearance stabilizes at about one year. We do not get mammograms until six months after treatment, but we believe that the mammographic appearance of the breast is beginning to stabilize at about one year and certainly by three years. It is not a normal-appearing mammogram, but I think that it is important in terms of follow-up of the patients. A mammographer has to be used to read mammograms of a radiated breast. You can see microcalcifications as a result of the implant. You can also see puffy popcorn-looking calcification as a result of fat necrosis.

Q What is the incidence of arm edema after the treatment?

A The incidence of arm edema after a level I and II dissection was only about 5% in patients who did not have the axilla and supraclavicular areas treated. We noticed that there is more arm edema and breast edema when the axilla and supraclavicular areas are treated. In recent years we have tended to get away from treating the third field. We let the surgeons dissect the axilla, and that is it for control in the axilla.

Q I see the major limitation of this treatment being that you cannot make the breast look any better than it started out looking. The most excellent results leave the breast looking identical, and in Atlanta, where I am working, that does not seem to be good enough for most women. We have seen requests for this treatment drop from 67% in 1982 to 20% in 1987. Do you see a trend like this?

A Absolutely not. A reconstructed breast, which is what you are talking about, is not a normal breast. Even if the breast does not look perfect, in my experience, women still generally prefer a breast that feels like a breast than a breast that looks perhaps a little bit better than our poor results.

Q I also want to ask about breast size. I know you said that you did not have that information, but some people have a subjective impression that the small breast does not do as well with radiation because, since the dose is fairly uniform regardless of the size of the breast, the skin changes are more intense. I wanted to ask you if you had any subjective impression about that? Others, for instance the Mayo Clinic, have reported much less satisfactory cosmetic results with radiation; the factor that they looked at was patient satisfaction. Did you have any information on patient satisfaction? Did you let the patient evaluate the cosmetic result rather than the physician?

A Yes. A point that I would like to make is that the cosmetic outcome really depends on the technique used. We are treating 400 new breast cases per year. The technique has gone through incredible refinements over the last 20 years. I do not see any difference at this time related to breast size, because the machine on which we treat the patient is chosen for that particular patient's breast size, so that we do not have these problems of more dose to the skin of smaller breasts and more dose to the subcutaneous tissue of larger breasts. We make every effort to avoid that problem by treating the patient on the right machine. Second, we tried to score patient satisfaction, but with a chart review it is very difficult to get a sense of that. Also, I think that there is a range of levels of patient satisfaction. However, in general it is fair to say that the physicians have been more critical of the results than have the patients themselves.

Local Recurrent Mammary Carcinoma Failing Multimodality Therapy

A Solution

Patricia M. McCormack, MD; Manjit S. Bains, MD; Michael E. Burt, MD, PhD; Nael Martini, MD; Ted Chaglassian, MD; David A. Hidalgo, MD

• Chest wall recurrence following radiation and hormonal therapy is an uncommon but serious and disabling condition. A chest wall ulcer secondary to treatment for recurrence also presents the same dilemma. Over the past 35 years, the Thoracic Service at our institution has treated 35 patients for these problems by surgical resection and reconstruction. Eight patients were seen after the first recurrence, six after the second, ten after the third, and ten after the fourth. One patient had chest wall resection with mastectomy when recurrence followed radiation therapy. Following resection of the tumor, 21 patients had reconstruction using mesh or a mesh "sandwich." There were no operative deaths and no respirator need. Twenty patients are alive from five to 120 months, with a median of 50 months. One of 35 patients had chest wall rerecurrence. Surgical resection of recurrent mammary carcinoma resistant to all other therapy is a viable alternative for both palliation and cure.

(*Arch Surg* 1989;124:158-161)

Local recurrence following initial treatment of primary operable mammary carcinoma varies from 1% to 2% for stage I to 10% to 12% for stage II. Major factors relating to relapse include type and extent of operation and the status of the lymph nodes.[1,2] Factors of lesser importance are the size and histologic grade of the primary tumor, the presence of invasion of the skin, and the length of free interval since primary treatment.[3-5] Hormone receptor status as a factor remains equivocal.[6] With the recent change to less radical surgery, an increase in local recurrence rates is being observed.

Postoperative radiation therapy decreases the incidence of local recurrence in high-risk patients but does not increase the overall cure rate.[7,8] Adjuvant chemotherapy *alone* does not decrease the incidence of local recurrence.[9]

Accepted for publication Sept 21, 1988.

From the Departments of Thoracic Surgery (Drs McCormack, Bains, Burt, and Martini) and Plastic Surgery (Drs Chaglassian and Hidalgo), Memorial Sloan-Kettering Cancer Center, and the Cornell University Medical College (Dr McCormack), New York.

Read before the Annual Meeting of the Society of Surgical Oncology, New Orleans, May 23, 1988.

Reprint requests to 1275 York Ave, New York, NY 10021 (Dr McCormack).

Local recurrence of tumor on the chest wall is usually treated with simple excision, where possible, followed by radiation therapy and chemotherapy in the presence of metastatic disease. In most instances, although specific percentages are not available, this suffices to control the tumor. There is a small group of patients, however, in whom the recurrence is not eradicated. This is usually related to tumor invasion of the underlying bony structures. These are the patients who need excision of the involved areas of the chest wall for control of the recurrent disease.

A second subgroup includes the patients who develop an ischemic ulceration following surgery and radiation therapy. These ulcerations can also be excised in a similar manner with equally good results.

SUBJECTS, MATERIALS, AND METHODS

From 1954 to 1987 the Thoracic Service at Memorial Sloan-Kettering Cancer Center, New York, performed 250 chest wall resections for tumor. Thirty-five of these were for mammary carcinoma, locally recurrent. The pathology material and patient charts were reviewed. The data were analyzed and results are presented herein.

Locally recurrent breast cancer for the purpose of this study is defined as the reappearance of cancer in the ipsilateral breast, the skin of the chest wall, or the parasternal area in the internal mammary lymph node chain.

The goal of the surgery is to resect all tumor with clear margins and to reconstruct the chest wall to provide physiologic integrity and a normal outward appearance, as most patients have already had radiation therapy to the area of recurrence. The blood supply to the skin of this area is compromised. This must be considered in the planning of skin and soft-tissue replacement. The plastic surgeon is consulted preoperatively to plan the most appropriate method for replacement of soft tissue and skin to restore as closely as possible a normal external appearance.

An intact thoracic cage is a prerequisite for adequate respiration. Any defect 5 cm or smaller will usually not interfere with pulmonary function. However, a larger defect should be repaired with a rigid prosthesis to prevent a "flail chest" with resultant pulmonary compromise. A defect directly over the heart and great vessels also requires a rigid replacement to protect these vital structures from inadvertent contusion. Since 1974, we have used a polyethylene template (Marlex) mesh–methyl methacrylate composite for this replacement.[10,11] The advantages it offers are (1)

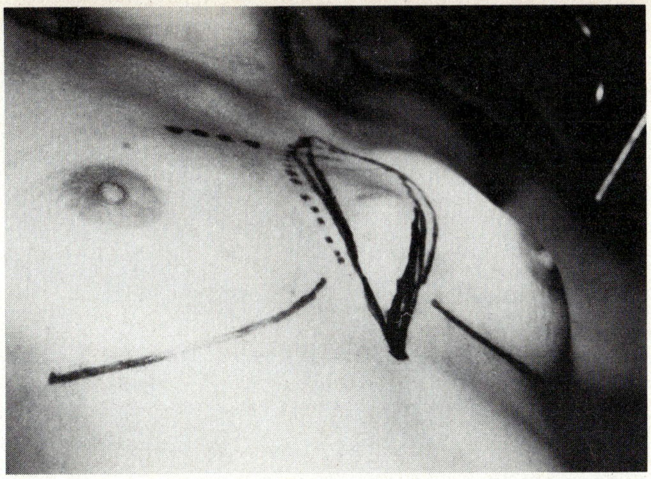

Fig 1.—Incision placed wide of recurrent tumor.

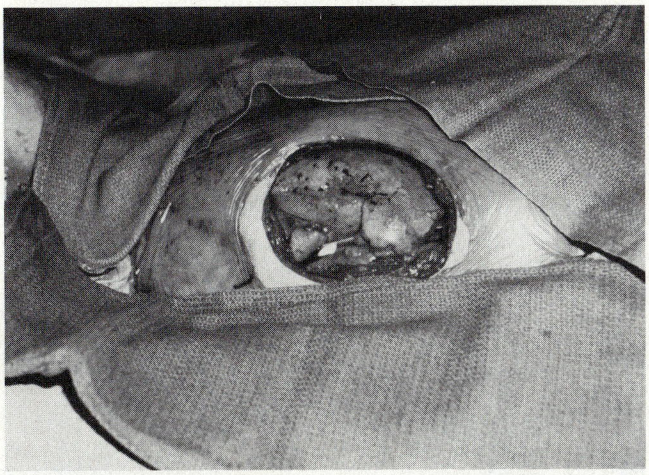

Fig 2.—Defect resulting from four-rib resection. Lung forms base of defect.

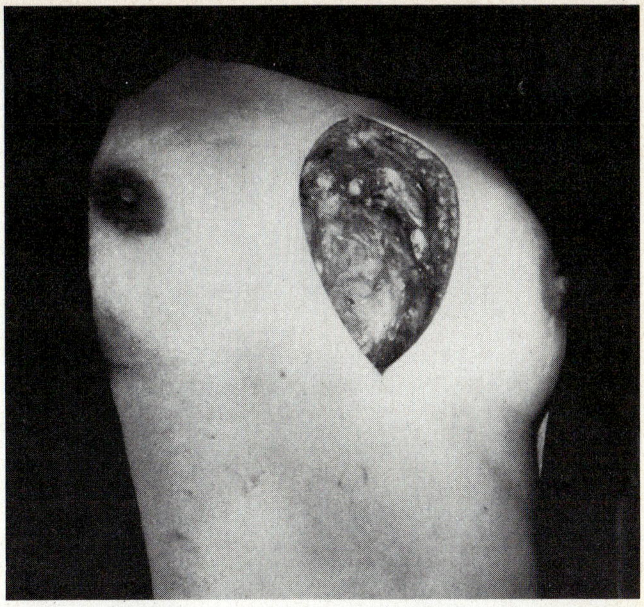

Fig 3.—Body of sternum and costal cartilages have been resected.

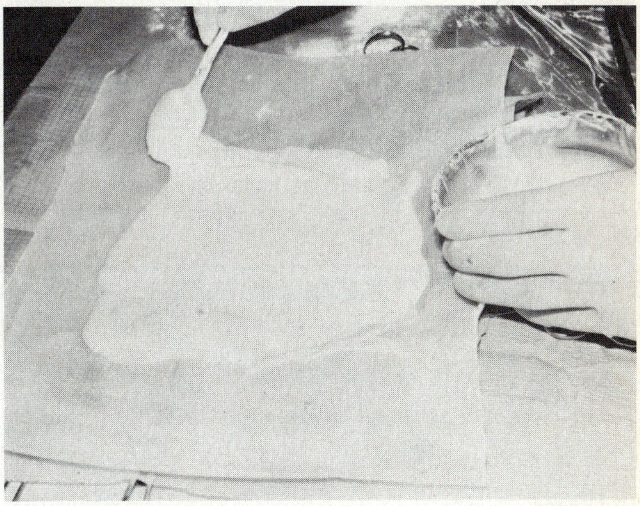

Fig 4.—Methyl methacrylate composite is spread over polyethylene template (Marlex) mesh.

ready availability in the operating room, (2) the ability to construct a prosthesis to fit any size defect with any contour, and (3) resistance to wound infections because of tissue ingrowth into the mesh interstices. No patient has needed respirator support with this prosthesis in place.

Chest wall resection included sternum alone in five patients, ribs alone in 11, sternum plus ribs in ten, and a wedge resection of the adherent lung in eight. One patient required a forequarter amputation for neurovascular invasion that resulted in a painful paralytic arm.

Repair of the resultant defect in the thoracic cage consisted of a mesh-methyl methacrylate composite in the majority of the patients (26 [74%] of 35). Polyethylene template mesh alone was used in four patients and no replacement was necessary in five patients.

Soft-tissue coverage was not necessary in five patients where adjacent skin involvement was minimal. Twenty patients had a myocutaneous flap raised and transferred to cover the rigid repair with a soft-tissue replacement. This has been the most frequent type of tissue transfer used in the past decade and the most successful. A free myocutaneous flap can also be used and gives an excellent result. The microvascular technique required for a free flap lengthens operating time but provides an alternative when lesser options are not possible. The site of origin of the flap was based on the size and location of the defect as well as prior surgical scars and radiation treatment portals. Twenty patients had a myocutaneous flap, six had skin alone, in four the opposite breast was used, and in five no soft tissue was needed.

There was one rerecurrence among the 35 resections. There were two major infections that required drainage and irrigation of the wound and extended the hospital stay two weeks. Twenty-eight percent (10/35) of the patients are alive with disease at a median survival time of 36 months, while an equal number of patients are free of disease at a median time of 52 months.

TECHNIQUE

Initially, the skin incision should be made 2 cm wider than any visible tumor. It is then deepened to the rib level (Fig 1). An interspace is entered below the known tumor recurrence and the pleural cavity is explored with a finger. Adherence of the lung and the depth and size of the tumor can be readily assessed. If tumor invasion into lung is found, the adherent lung is wedged, using a stapler, and removed en bloc with the specimen.

One normal rib above and below the involved rib(s) and a 5-cm clearance laterally are the bone resection margins (Fig 2). When the sternum is involved, it is recommended to remove a "sleeve" of sternum rather than a lateral portion only (Fig 3). The internal

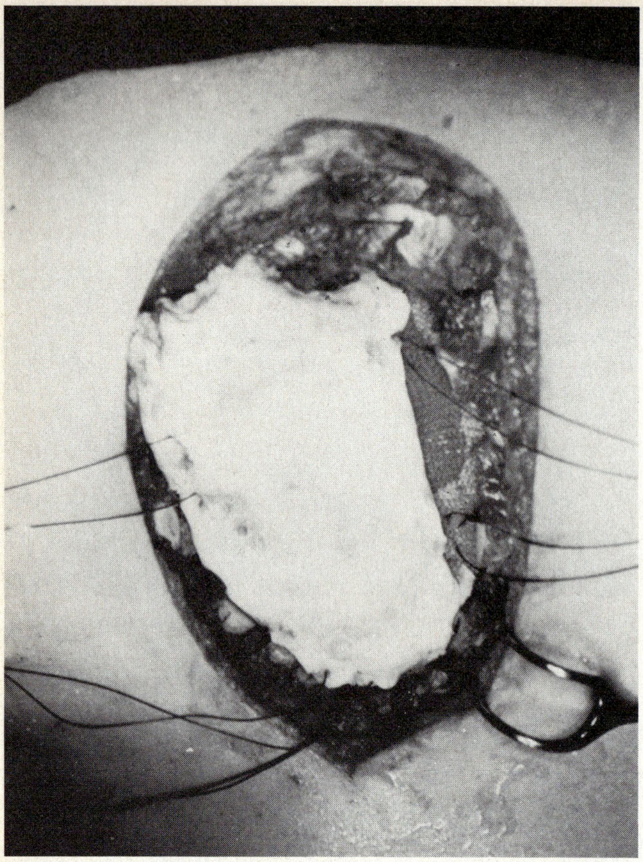

Fig 5.—Mesh–methyl methacrylate composite sutured in place.

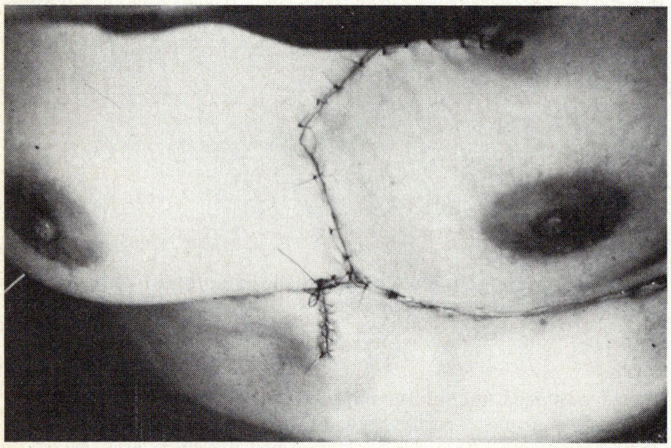

Fig 6.—Sliding flaps of both breasts bridged the soft-tissue defect.

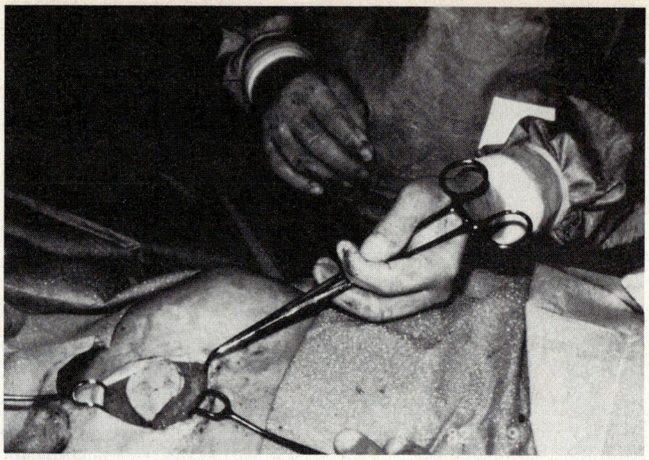

Fig 7.—Latissimus dorsi myocutaneous flap, after being tunneled under axilla, is placed on top of methyl methacrylate composite.

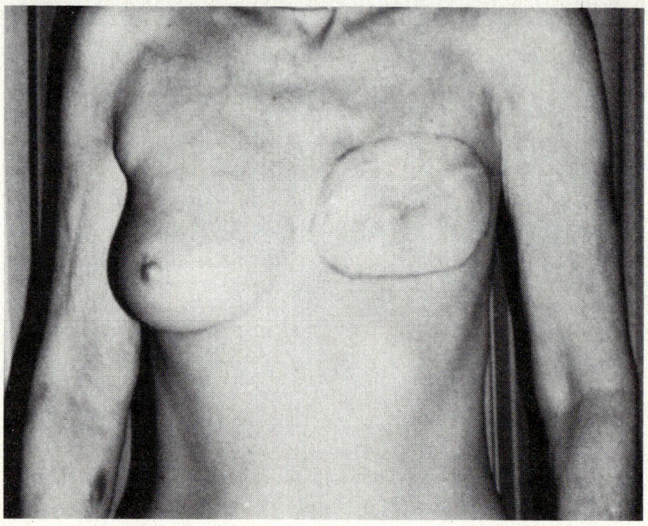

Fig 8.—Myocutaneous flap on sixth postoperative day.

mammary artery and intercostal neurovascular bundles are identified and secured under direct vision.

After the resection is complete, when hemostasis is secured and the chest tubes have been placed, a clean lap pad is placed over the defect, creating a red-on-white pattern illustrating the size and contour to be followed in making the new insert. A piece of mesh is placed over this, and the methyl methacrylate is spread on the mesh according to the pattern (Fig 4). A second layer of mesh is then placed on top of the methyl methacrylate. It takes five minutes to harden. During this time, the composite is shaped to assume the contour of the resected chest wall. Excess mesh is trimmed to allow an approximately 2-cm sewing ring. Any heavy nonabsorbable suture material can be used to secure the composite to the skeletal rim of the defect (Fig 5).

The plastic surgeon then restores the soft-tissue deficit (Fig 6). Skin flaps or the remaining breast can be used when the cosmetic result is not paramount. The myocutaneous or free flaps give superior results and were used in the majority of our patients (Figs 7 and 8). The patient is ready to be discharged from the hospital between the seventh and tenth postoperative days.

RESULTS

The ages of the patients ranged from 28 to 72 years, with a median age of 55 years. One patient had chest wall resection included with the radical mastectomy when the tumor was found to involve the ribs. Eight patients had one recurrence, six had two recurrences, ten had three recurrences, and ten had four recurrences before chest wall resection was done. The disease-free interval from treatment of the primary tumor to the first local recurrence varied from one to 30 years. The median was six years.

Most recurrences are located in or near the operative scar. Eighty percent are apparent within five years after surgery, and the remainder occur within the first ten years. In our series, there was one recurrence 30 years later. This is rare.

Half of the patients with local recurrence have this as

the only evidence of their cancer. Twenty-five percent have had metastases elsewhere preceding the development of chest wall tumor and the other 25% will develop metastases within a few months of the chest wall resections.

COMMENT

Locally recurrent breast cancer should first be treated by one or any combination of the usual therapeutic modalities, namely, local surgery, radiation therapy, chemotherapy or hormonal therapy, or any appropriate combination of these.[8,9,12] If recurrence persists despite their use, chest wall resection presents an alternative treatment possibility.

The survival results of this procedure reflect the stage of the disease rather than the chest wall surgery. In patients with local recurrence as the only residual carcinoma, a median survival approaching five years was seen in this series. There were no operative deaths. The wound infections were managed with local care. A single patient had a tumor recurrence that was re-excised; however, the patient died six months later of overwhelming metastatic cancer.

Respirator support was not needed for any patient following recovery from anesthesia when a methyl methacrylate composite was used.

Chest wall resection had a role to play in intractable locally recurrent breast cancer. It offers significant palliation even in the presence of recurrent tumor elsewhere.

References

1. Haagensen CD: *Disease of the Breast*, ed 2. Philadelphia, WB Saunders Co, 1971.
2. Valagussa P, Bonadonna G, Veronesi U: Patterns of relapse and survival following radical mastectomy: Analysis of 716 consecutive patients. *Cancer* 1978;41:1170-1178.
3. Donegan WL, Perez-Mesa CM, Watson FR: A biostatistical study of locally recurrent breast carcinoma. *Surg Gynecol Obstet* 1966;122:529-540.
4. Zimmerman KW, Montague ED, Fletcher GH: Frequency, anatomical distribution and management of local recurrences after definitive therapy for breast cancer. *Cancer* 1966;19:67-74.
5. Carter RL: Significance of local recurrence, in Stoll BA (ed): *Secondary Spread in Breast Cancer.* London, Heinemann Medical Books Ltd, 1977, pp 31-44.
6. Rosenman J, Bernard S, Kober C, et al: Local recurrences in patients with breast cancer at the North Carolina Memorial Hospital (1970-1982). *Cancer* 1986;57:1421-1425.
7. Aberizk WJ, Silver B, Hellman S, et al: The results of radiation therapy for locally recurrent breast carcinoma after mastectomy. *Int J Radiat Oncol Biol Phys* 1984;10(suppl):78-79.
8. Aberizk WJ, Silver B, Henderson IC, et al: The results of radiotherapy in patients with isolated local-regional recurrence of breast carcinoma after mastectomy. *Cancer* 1986;53:1214-1218.
9. Bonadonna G, Valagussa P, Rossi A, et al: Ten-year experience with CMF-based adjuvant chemotherapy in resectable breast cancer. *Breast Cancer Res Treat* 1985;5:95-115.
10. McCormack PM, Bains MS, Beattie ED Jr, et al: New trends in skeletal reconstruction after resection of chest wall tumors. *Ann Thorac Surg* 1981;31:45-52.
11. Boyd AB, Shaw WW, McCarthy JG: Immediate reconstruction of full-thickness wall defects. *Ann Thorac Surg* 1981;32:337-346.
12. Beck TM, Hart NE, Woodard DA, et al: Local or regionally recurrent carcinoma of the breast: Results of therapy in 121 patients. *J Clin Oncol* 1983;1:400-405.

Discussion

Q I wonder if you could comment on the treatment of these patients after chest wall resection. I think most of us believe that this is a lethal sign and the probability of these patients dying of their disease shortly is quite high. How do you manage them postoperatively?

A It depends on whether they have evidence of any disease elsewhere.

Q Let's say they are free of disease elsewhere.

A Then they just get followed up expectantly.

Q Do you still use this technique for patients who have infected chest walls and in cases of ulcerated wounds on the chest wall?

A Yes we do, with the provision that preoperatively they get appropriate antibiotics and local wound care. Even if you get an infection that is superficial above the mesh sandwich, you can irrigate it without having to remove the sandwich. We have done this in the two instances related herein and in two since this report was written.

Q While at M. D. Anderson Hospital and Tumor Institute (Houston) we used that in patients who did not have infections, but I just used myocutaneous flaps in patients who did have infections, and I did not find any significant flail chests. We measured the preoperative and postoperative vital capacity and the forced expiratory volume at 1 s in a number of patients. Just using myocutaneous flaps for massive chest wall resections up to 450 cm^2, we were able to show there was no significant difference in the preoperative and postoperative pulmonary functions without any Richard's support for the chest wall.

A That is very interesting, thank you.

Q Can I ask you why you left using the mesh alone and went to the methyl methacrylate, because when we went to the stiffeners, we found that there was really no advantage, even with a very large chest wall deficit, over using polyethylene template and pulling it taut. I want to know why you abandoned the use of mesh alone and went to the stiffeners.

A One of the main reasons was cosmetic. With mesh alone, you are left with a flat chest. With polyethylene template mesh–methyl methacrylate composite you can shape it to the contour that you like. Frequently these patients are women who are very conscious of what they look like, particularly after mastectomy. We find that it is easy to use. If the patient is improved cosmetically, I think it is worth doing.

In Other AMA Journals

ARCHIVES OF INTERNAL MEDICINE

The Alveolar-Arterial Oxygen Gradient in Patients With Documented Pulmonary Embolism

David T. Overton, MD, Joseph J. Bocka, MD

It has been reported that the finding of a normal Pao_2 level on arterial blood gas analysis does not exclude the diagnosis of acute pulmonary embolism. We wished to determine whether a more thorough evaluation of the blood gases would prove more helpful; specifically, whether it is possible for a patient with acute pulmonary embolism to have a normal alveolar-arterial (A-a) oxygen gradient. We studied this question in a patient population in which the diagnosis was definitively made via pulmonary arteriography. Sixty-four patients met all study criteria. In these patients, the A-a gradient ranged from 11.6 to 83.9 mm Hg (mean, 41.8 mm Hg). In three patients, the A-a gradient was normal for age. We conclude that a normal A-a oxygen gradient does not exclude the diagnosis of acute pulmonary embolism, and should not preclude further diagnostic procedures if there is a high index of suspicion (*Arch Intern Med* 1988;148:1617-1619).

Reprint requests to Department of Emergency Medicine, William Beaumont Hospital, 3601 W 13 Mile Rd, Royal Oak, MI 48072 (Dr Overton).

Extent of Lymph Node Dissection in Melanoma of the Trunk or Lower Extremity

Daniel G. Coit, MD, Murray F. Brennan, MD

• The extent of lymph node dissection necessary to optimize survival and minimize local recurrence in patients with melanoma of the trunk or lower extremity is not well defined. We reviewed the records of 420 patients undergoing superficial or combined superficial and deep groin dissection for melanoma. Prognosis depended on the extent of lymph node involvement rather than the extent of surgery performed. Node-positive patients undergoing elective lymph node dissection had an improved survival over those undergoing therapeutic lymph node dissection. In no subgroup of patients was more extensive lymphadenectomy associated with significant improvement in survival or alteration in pattern of recurrence. Dissection of the deep pelvic nodes in patients with melanoma appears to be of more prognostic than therapeutic value.

(*Arch Surg* 1989;124:162-166)

There are a number of issues that remain controversial in the management of the regional lymph nodes in patients with malignant melanoma. The role of elective lymphadenectomy (ELND) remains a matter of debate, polarized on the one hand by a number of retrospective reviews,[1-5] which suggest a survival advantage in high-risk patients, and on the other hand by two prospective randomized studies reported by Sim et al[6] and Veronesi et al,[7] which report no survival advantage in any subgroup of patients undergoing ELND over those offered therapeutic lymphadenectomy (TLND) when pathologic lymph nodes become clinically evident.

Furthermore, in patients with melanoma metastatic to or potentially metastatic to groin nodes, the extent of groin dissection necessary to achieve optimal locoregional control and survival is not well defined. Many investigators have suggested that the superficial inguinofemoral lymphadenectomy (SILND) is sufficient for patients with clinically and histologically negative groin nodes, reserving combined superficial and deep inguinofemoral and ileo-obturator lymphadenectomy (CILND) for patients with either clinically or histologically positive superficial groin nodes.[8-11] Others have suggested that deep pelvic node involvement is indicative of disseminated disease and that deep groin dissection does not have an impact on survival.[12]

Accepted for publication Aug 26, 1988.

From the Department of Surgery, Memorial Sloan-Kettering Cancer Center, New York.

Read before the Annual Meeting of the Society of Surgical Oncology, New Orleans, May 25, 1988.

Reprints not available.

We undertook our study to clarify the management of groin nodes in patients with melanoma of the trunk or lower extremities. We addressed such issues as the role of ELND and the extent of surgery necessary in these patients, with regard to both survival and patterns of recurrence.

PATIENTS AND METHODS

We reviewed the records of 420 patients with malignant melanoma of the trunk and lower extremities undergoing either SILND or CILND at Memorial Sloan-Kettering Cancer Center, New York, between 1974 and 1984. Elective lymphadenectomy during that period was generally recommended for patients with lesions that were Clark level III or deeper or had a Breslow thickness of 1.5 mm or more, and clinically negative nodes. Therapeutic lymphadenectomy was undertaken for palpable, clinically involved nodes in the absence of distant metastatic disease. Node dissection was defined as palliative if the patient had evidence of distant metastatic disease and the procedure was performed for locoregional control of disease only.

Because the period of study embraced an evolution in the assessment of the primary lesions, with Breslow thickness available only in the latter years, all patients' tumors were staged according to the current American Joint Committee on Cancer staging system (Table 1). Records were analyzed for patient age and sex, clinical and pathologic disease stage, extent of surgery, extent of nodal involvement, pattern of recurrence, and status at last follow-up. Intervals to recurrence and survival were calculated from the time of lymph node dissection to the time of recurrence or last follow-up, respectively. Survival curves were calculated, using the method of Kaplan and Meier.[13] Survival distributions were compared using the log rank test.[14] Patterns of recurrence were compared, using the χ^2 test.

There were 175 male patients and 245 female patients. The median age of the patients was 51 years (range, 15 to 94 years). The distribution of clinical and pathologic disease stages is shown in the following tabulation and in Table 2.

	Clinical Stage	Pathologic Stage
IA	8	10
IB	68	69
IIA	112	91
IIB	50	31
III	148	161
IV	34	58

As can be seen, the intent of operation was elective in 238 patients (57%), therapeutic in 148 patients (35%), and palliative in the remaining 34 patients (8%). An SILND was performed in 269 patients—191 elective, 62 therapeutic, and 16 palliative. A CILND was performed in 151 patients—47 elective, 86 therapeutic, and 18 palliative.

Pathologically positive nodes were recovered in 203 patients (48%), in 53 (22%) after ELND, in 119 (80%) after TLND, and in

Table 1.—American Joint Committee on Cancer Melanoma Staging System

TX	Unknown, cannot assess
T0	Atypical melanocytic hyperplasia, in situ, Clark I
T1	Clark II, ≤0.75 mm
T2	Clark III, 0.76-1.50 mm
T3	Clark IV, 1.51-4.0 mm
T4	Clark V, >4.0 mm or satellites within 2 cm of primary tumor
NX	Unknown, cannot assess
N0	Negative
N1	One regional node station, nodes mobile, <5 cm diameter, or negative nodes and <5 intransit metastases
N2	More than one node station positive, nodes >5 cm or fixed, >5 intransit metastases, or any intransit metastases with positive nodes
MX	Unknown, cannot assess
M0	None
M1	Skin or subcutaneous tissue beyond primary nodal area
M2	Visceral

Stage Grouping

Stage IA	T1, N0, M0
Stage IB	T2, N0, M0
Stage IIA	T3, N0, M0
Stage IIB	T4, N0, M0
Stage III	Any T, N1, M0
Stage IV	Any T, N2, M0
	Any T, any N, M1-2

31 (91%) after palliative lymphadenectomy.

Complete follow-up data were available for 415 patients (99%). The median follow-up of patients alive at the time of this review was 86 months. The median time to death in patients dying of disease was 20 months.

RESULTS

The estimated five-year survival was related to extent of lymph node involvement (Fig 1). For patients with histologically uninvolved nodes, the five-year survival was 80%. For patients with only positive superficial inguinofemoral nodes, the five-year survival was 37% (median, 36 months; $P<.001$ vs none). For patients with both superficial and deep nodes (iliac, obturator, or both) involved, the median survival was 12 months with only one patient in this series surviving five years ($P<.001$ vs superficial node involvement only).

In patients with negative nodes, there was no difference in survival between those undergoing SILND and those undergoing CILND (Fig 2). The trend favoring SILND in node-negative patients was not significant and correlated with prognostic variables of the primary lesions being slightly more favorable in the SILND group.

Elective Lymphadenectomy

Fifty-three (22%) of 238 patients undergoing ELND were found to have histologically positive nodes. A significant survival advantage was observed in these patients when compared with 119 patients undergoing TLND with histologically positive nodes (Fig 3), with a five-year survival of 53% (median, 64 months) in the former group vs a five-year survival of 31% (median, 32 months) in the latter group ($P<.005$).

Superficial nodes only were involved in 48 (91%) of these 53 patients. In these 48 patients, there was a trend toward a survival advantage after CILND (67%) compared with SILND (44%) (Fig 4), but this difference was not statistically significant ($P>.05$). Three patients undergoing elective CILND were found to have microscopic deep node involvement. Two of these patients died of disease at 32 and 59 months after lymphadenectomy, respectively, and

Table 2.—Clinical and Pathologic Stages in 420 Patients Undergoing Groin Dissection for Melanoma Between 1974 and 1984: Clinical Understaging

Clinical Stage	No. (%) of Patients With Occult Positive Nodes
Stage IA	0/8 (0)
Stage IB	4/68 (6)
Stage IIA	28/112 (25)
Stage IIB	21/50 (42)
Total	**53/238** (22)

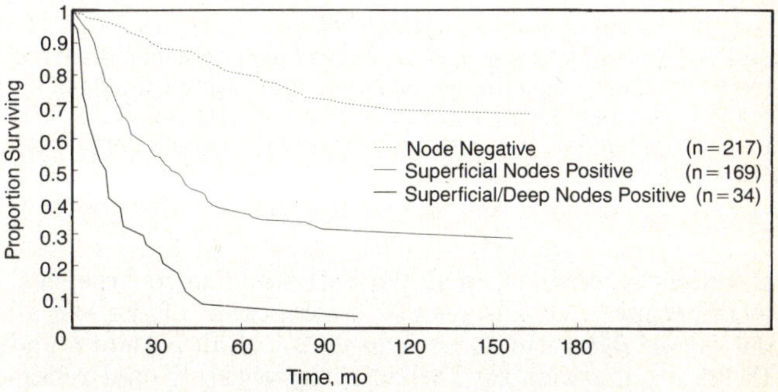

Fig 1.—Survival by extent of lymph node involvement in 420 patients after groin dissection for melanoma.

one remains alive with intransit disease at 44 months after lymphadenectomy.

Therapeutic Lymphadenectomy

Of the 148 patients undergoing TLND, positive nodes were recovered in 119 (80%). In this group, the overall five-year survival was 31%, 37% for patients with only superficial nodal involvement (median, 39 months), and 5.6% for patients with superficial and deep nodal involvement (median, 12 months). One hundred nine patients undergoing TLND had only superficial nodes involved. The CILND conferred no survival advantage over SILND in this group of patients (38% vs 34%; median, 40 months for both groups; P, not significant) (Fig 5).

Palliative Lymph Node Dissection

Thirty-four patients underwent palliative lymphadenectomy for clinical stage IV disease. All patients in this group were dead of disease by 50 months after lymphadenectomy (median, 12 months). The extent of surgery had no impact on the length of survival in this group.

Patterns of Recurrence

The patterns of nodal recurrence are shown in Table 3. Recurrence was documented in 198 (47%) of 420 patients, in 97 (36%) of 269 patients after SILND, and in 101 (67%) of 151 patients after CILND ($P<.001$). Node-negative patients had recurrences more frequently after CILND than after SILND—12 (39%) of 32 vs 34 (18%) of 185, respectively ($P<.02$). This reflects the slightly worse prognostic characteristics of the primary lesions in the node-negative patients undergoing CILND. Node-positive patients had recurrences with equal frequency after either procedure—63 (75%) of 84 after SILND and 89 (75%) of 119 after CILND.

Nodal recurrence, defined as recurrence in the groin that was operated on, either superficial or deep, was observed as the first site of failure in 12 patients, 2.9% of

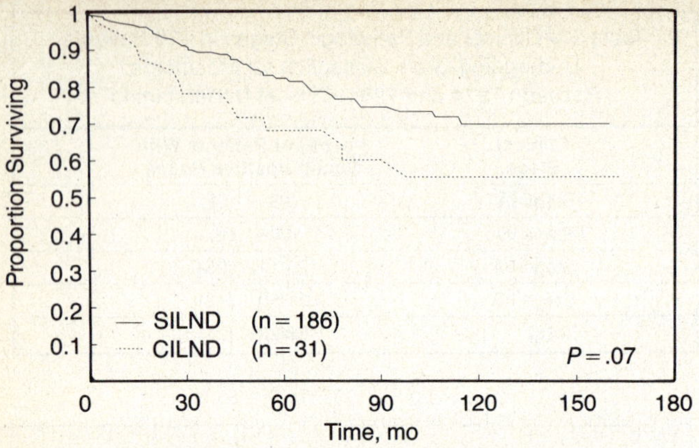

Fig 2.—Survival by extent of surgery in 217 patients with melanoma and histologically negative lymph nodes after superficial inguinal-femoral lymphadenectomy (SILND) vs combined superficial and deep inguinalfemoral and ileo-obturator lymphadenectomy (CILND).

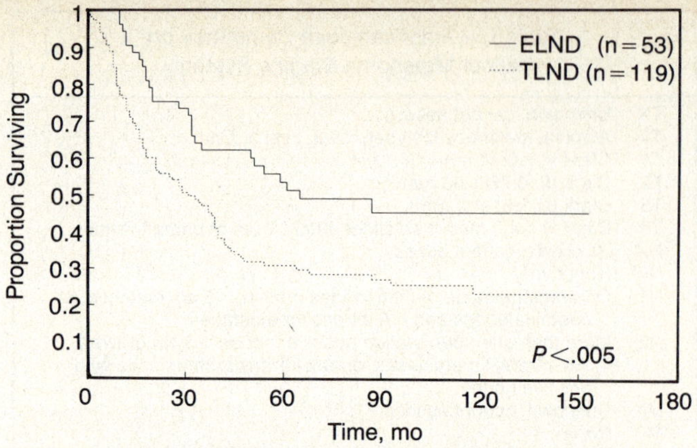

Fig 3.—Survival by intent of surgery in 172 patients with melanoma and histologically positive lymph nodes after elective lymphadenectomy (ELND) vs therapeutic lymphadenectomy (TLND).

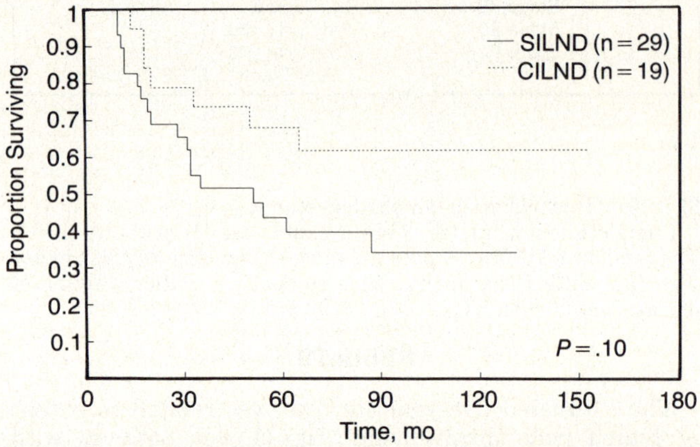

Fig 4.—Survival by extent of surgery in patients with melanoma and histologically positive superficial lymph nodes only after elective superficial inguinalfemoral lymphadenectomy (SILND) vs combined superficial and inguinalfemoral and ileo-obturator lymphadenectomy (CILND).

all patients, and 6.1% of all patients who had recurrences. Nodal recurrence was seen as a component of the overall pattern of failure in 26 patients, 6.2% of all patients, and 13.1% of all patients who had recurrences. Nodal recurrence was no more common after SILND than after CILND, either as the first site of failure or as a component of the overall pattern of failure. This was true whether the nodes at the original lymphadenectomy were positive or negative.

Prediction of Deep Node Positivity

Clinical and pathologic factors of the 150 patients who underwent CILND were further analyzed to see what might predict deep node positivity. Factors that were important included positive Cloquet's node, the number of positive superficial nodes, the clinical stage of the patient's disease, and, of borderline significance, whether the superficial nodes were microscopically or macroscopically positive (Table 4). Factors that were not significant included site of the primary tumor and the sex and age of the patient.

Morbidity and Mortality

One patient in this series died after SILND, for an overall operative mortality of 0.24%. The median length of stay in the hospital was 13.5 days after SILND and 17 days after CILND. No attempt was made to define short-term or long-term morbidity, as estimates of these from retrospective reviews are notoriously conservative. Nonetheless, it is generally acknowledged that the complications after CILND are as great or, in most series, greater than those associated with SILND.[7,8,10,11]

COMMENT

It is quite clear that histologic involvement of groin nodes by malignant melanoma is associated with a guarded prognosis, with only 20% to 30% of patients surviving five years free of disease after aggressive surgery.[7,9-11,15] It is also apparent that survival correlates with extent of lymph node involvement: those patients with microscopic superficial node involvement fare better than those with grossly positive superficial nodes,[9,11,16] and survival with positive deep nodes is uniformly poor (Table 5). Less clear is the impact that more-extensive surgery has on improving the outcome in patients with melanoma metastatic or potentially metastatic to the groin nodes. In our study, there was no significant survival advantage in any subgroup of patients undergoing CILND when compared with those undergoing SILND.

Node-Negative Patients

In node-negative patients, the survival distributions were no different (Fig 2). This would imply that in the setting of histologically negative superficial nodes, the likelihood is small of microscopic spread confined to the deep nodes that could be encompassed by more extensive surgery. In fact, only one of the 150 patients undergoing CILND was found to have positive deep groin nodes with negative superficial groin nodes, and this patient died of systemic disease 44 months after lymphadenectomy. This low incidence of "skip metastases" reflects that reported by other investigators.[8-10] Furthermore, nodal recurrence in node-negative patients was no more common either as the first site of recurrence or as a component of the overall pattern of failure in patients undergoing SILND over those subjected to CILND.

Node-Positive Patients

In node-positive patients, no survival advantage of CILND over SILND could be demonstrated. When analyzed by intent of operation, survival distributions for

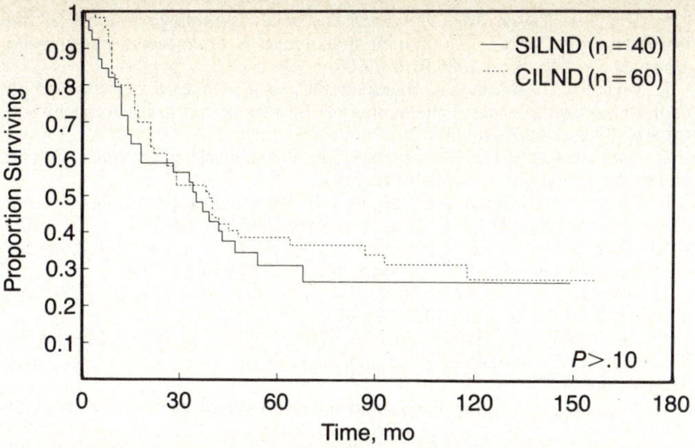

Fig 5.—Survival by extent of surgery in patients with melanoma and histologically positive superficial lymph nodes only after therapeutic superficial inguinalfemoral lymphadenectomy (SILND) vs combined superficial and deep inguinalfemoral and ileo-obturator lymphadenectomy (CILND).

Table 3.—Patterns of Recurrence After Groin Dissection for Melanoma*

Nodal Status	No. (%) of Patients With Recurrence	No. (%) of Patients With Nodes as First Site of Recurrence	No. (%) of Patients With Nodes as a Component of Recurrence
Node-positive patients			
SILND	63/84 (75)	4 (6)	9 (14)
CILND	89/119 (75)	3 (3)	10 (11)
Node-negative patients			
SILND	34/185 (18)	4 (11)	6 (18)
CILND	12/32 (38)	1 (8)	1 (8)
All patients			
SILND	97/269 (36)	8 (8)	15 (15)
CILND	101/151 (67)	4 (4)	11 (11)

*SILND indicates superficial inguinofemoral lymphadenectomy; CILND, combined superficial and deep inguinofemoral and ileo-obturator lymphadenectomy.

patients undergoing TLND were nearly identical for the two procedures. The same was true if only the superficial node–positive patients undergoing CILND, ie, a favorable subset of patients most likely to benefit from removal of microscopic deep nodal metastases, were compared with node-positive patients undergoing the more conservative operation.

Positive nodes were recovered in 53 (22%) of 238 patients undergoing ELND—6% of patients with clinical stage IB disease, 25% of patients with clinical stage IIA disease, and 42% of patients with clinical stage IIB disease (Table 2). The survival at five years in this group was 24% better than in the group of patients undergoing TLND with positive nodes. These data once again confirm the retrospective observations of other investigators[1-3,8-10] who advocate ELND in patients at risk for occult nodal metastases before they become clinically apparent.

This survival increment must be viewed in perspective, however. If we accept that the survival impact of ELND in node-negative patients is less important, then applying that 22% survival advantage to the 22% of patients undergoing ELND who are node-positive yields a net impact on survival of all patients undergoing ELND of about 5%. If this is so, it may be impossible, even in the current

Table 4.—Factors Predictive of Deep Groin Node Positivity in 150 Patients Undergoing Combined Superficial and Deep Groin Dissection for Melanoma Between 1974 and 1984

Factor	No. of Patients With Factor	No. (%) of Patients With Positive Deep Nodes	P
Cloquet's node			
Negative	60	2 (3)	...
Positive	24	19 (79)	<.001 vs negative
No. of Positive superficial nodes			
0	33	1 (3)	...
1-3	65	8 (12)	.11 vs 0
>3	25	11 (44)	.001 vs 1-3 <.001 vs 0
Clinical stage			
I-II	47	3 (6)	...
III	85	19 (22)	.01 vs I-II
IV	18	10 (56)	.005 vs III <.001 vs I-II
Superficial nodes			
Microscopically positive	17	2 (12)	...
Macroscopically positive	100	29 (29)	.08 vs microscopically positive

Table 5.—Five-Year Survival in Patients With Melanoma and Histologically Positive Deep Groin Nodes

Source, y	No. of Patients With Positive Deep Nodes	No. of Patients Alive >5 y	5-y Survival, %
Fortner et al,[10] 1964	46	4	9
McCarthy et al,[12] 1974	4	0	0
Haagensen,[16] 1976	20	0	0
Finck et al,[9] 1982	24	3	12
Dasmahapatra and Karakousis,[8] 1983	10	4	40
Karakousis et al,[11] 1986	18	1	6
Present study, 1988	34	1	3
Total	**156**	**13**	**8.4**

Intergroup Melanoma randomized trial, to prove that ELND has a role in the management of primary melanoma in patients at high risk for occult nodal metastases.

Nineteen patients underwent elective CILND for clinically negative groin nodes and were found to have only superficial nodes involved. There was a trend toward improved survival in this group when compared with patients undergoing elective SILND who were found to have superficial positive nodes (Fig 4), but this was not significant. This trend can be explained in part by the fact that, based on the predictive factors of number of positive superficial nodes and macroscopic appearance of the superficial nodes, some of the patients in the elective SILND group may have had positive deep nodes, thus adversely affecting survival in this group.

Significance of Deep Node Positivity

The reason that deep pelvic node dissection cannot be shown to improve survival lies in the very poor prognosis of those patients in whom the deep nodes are positive. While there are a number of long-term survivors with positive deep nodes after CILND reported in the literature, the collective five-year survival is no more than 10% (Table 5). In this review, of 34 patients with histologically positive deep nodes, only two are alive, one with intransit disease 40 months after lymphadenectomy and one free of disease 102 months after lymphadenectomy. Of 23 patients with macroscopically positive deep nodal disease, 22 died of disease two to 46 months after lymphadenectomy. Of 11 patients with microscopic deep nodal disease, ten died of disease four to 59 months after lymphadenectomy. Of 19 patients who underwent therapeutic CILND for clinically positive nodes, 18 with positive deep nodes died of disease four to 44 months after lymphadenectomy. Three patients undergoing elective CILND were found to have microscopic positive deep nodes; two of these patients died of disease 32 and 59 months, respectively, after lymphadenectomy, and one patient is alive with intransit disease 44 months after lymphadenectomy. In summary, involvement of deep groin nodes in this series was associated with systemic spread of disease in at least 32 (94%) of 34 patients in whom it was found.

Nodal Recurrence

One of the arguments in support of CILND is that it will result in improved locoregional control, especially in patients with clinically positive nodes, avoiding the difficult problem of deep pelvic nodal recurrence. Data from our study do not support this position. It is of interest, however, that of the 13 patients in whom nodal recurrence was the first site of relapse, two (15%) are currently alive and free of disease at 42 and 146 months, respectively, after recurrence—one after surgery and one after chemotherapy and surgery.

CONCLUSION

A proportion of patients with melanoma metastatic to groin nodes have disease that is locoregional only and will be rendered long-term disease free by aggressive surgery. However, the ultimate prognosis appears to depend more on the extent of the disease than on the extent of surgery performed. Patients harboring occult metastases who undergo ELND have an improved chance of survival compared with those patients undergoing TLND for clinically positive nodes. Patients with only superficial nodes involved have a substantially better survival than those with positive superficial and deep nodes. In no subgroup of patients was more extensive lymphadenectomy associated with a significant improvement in survival or alteration in the pattern of recurrence in those patients who had recurrences. We conclude that dissection of the deep pelvic nodes in patients with melanoma may be more of prognostic than therapeutic value in the majority of patients.

References

1. Koh HK, Sober AJ, Day CL, et al: Prognosis of clinical stage I melanoma patients with positive elective regional node dissection. *J Clin Oncol* 1986;4:1238-1244.
2. Balch CM: The role of elective lymph node dissection in melanoma: Rationale, results, and controversies. *J Clin Oncol* 1988;6:163-172.
3. McCarthy WH, Shaw HM, Milton GW: Efficacy of elective lymph node dissection in 2347 patients with clinical stage I malignant melanoma. *Surg Gynecol Obstet* 1980;161:575-580.
4. Illig L, Aigner KR, Biess B, et al: Diagnostic excision of the Rosenmuller's node—screening for occult metastases before elective regional node dissection in patients with lower limb melanoma. *Cancer* 1988;61:1200-1206.
5. Fortner JG, Woodruff J, Schottenfeld D, et al: Biostatistical basis of elective lymph node dissection for malignant melanoma. *Ann Surg* 1977;186:101-103.
6. Sim FH, Taylor WF, Pritchard DJ, et al: Lymphadenectomy in the management of stage I malignant melanoma: A prospective randomized study. *Mayo Clin Proc* 1986;61:697-705.
7. Veronesi U, Adamus J, Bandeira DC, et al: Delayed regional lymph node dissection in stage I melanoma of the skin of the lower extremities. *Cancer* 1982;49:2420-2430.
8. Dasmahapatra KS, Karakousis CP: Therapeutic groin dissection in melanoma. *Surg Gynecol Obstet* 1983;156:21-24.
9. Finck SJ, Giuliano AE, Mann BD, et al: Results of ileoinguinal dissection for stage II melanoma. *Ann Surg* 1982;196:180-186.
10. Fortner JG, Booher RJ, Pack GT: Results of groin dissection for malignant melanoma in 220 patients. *Surgery* 1964;55:485-494.
11. Karakousis CP, Emrich LJ, Rao U: Groin dissection in malignant melanoma. *Am J Surg* 1986;152:491-495.
12. McCarthy JG, Haagensen CD, Herter FP, et al: The role of groin dissection in the management of melanoma of the lower extremities. *Ann Surg* 1974;179:156-159.
13. Kaplan EL, Meier P: Nonparametric estimation from incomplete observation. *J Am Stat Assoc* 1958;53:457-481.
14. Peto R, Pike MC, Armitage P: Design and analysis of randomized clinical trials requiring prolonged observations of each patient: II. Analysis and examples. *Br J Cancer* 1977;35:1-39.
15. Roses DF, Provet JA, Harris MN, et al: Prognosis of patients with pathologic stage II cutaneous malignant melanoma. *Ann Surg* 1985;201:103-107.
16. Haagensen CD: Surgical management of melanomas of the trunk and extremities, in Najarian JS, Delaney JP (eds): *Advances in Cancer Surgery.* New York, Stratton Intercontinental Medical Book Co, 1976.

Discussion

Q I do not think it can be as categorical as you stated that the deep node dissection does not offer suvival advantage, at least in our experience. We had 117 patients who had groin dissection, 56 of whom had positive nodes, and 43 patients had palpable nodes as well. Of these 43 patients who had palpable nodes, 18 (44%) also had deep inguinal nodes involved. In all the patients who had TLND, we performed a radical or ileo-inguinal node dissection, and the estimated five-year survival two years ago was 48% for patients who had only inguinal nodes involved and 30% for patients who had inguinal and deep nodes involved.

I have updated the survival for the 56 patients with positive nodes. All patients now have had at least a five-year follow-up, and the five-year survival for the patients who had only inguinal nodes involved was 42%. The five-year survival for the patients who had positive inguinal as well as deep nodes was 33%. Therefore, I think that we have to look at this issue more extensively because our experience differs from yours. I am not sure whether we see a different kind of population. The mean number of nodes involved in our patients with positive lymph nodes was 5.3, with a median of two positive nodes.

I feel, however, that it is important that a complete node dissection be performed in patients who have palpable nodes in the groin to realize the full potential of this operation. I think that there is a survival advantage with an ileo-inguinal node dissection, and not simply a diagnostic staging.

A One of the concerns that we had about your earlier report was the short median follow-up and the fact that only two of those patients with deep positive nodes were actually known to survive beyond five years. The fact that you are able to tell us today that 33% of those patients are alive and free of disease is an important addition.

Q You say the ELNDs seem to have a survival advantage of some 20 months over the TLNDs. Could it also be that you are comparing apples and oranges? Perhaps you are picking up the disease at two different times in its course so there is a greater time between treatment and death but death still happens in August 1988. If you left the patients alone they might have a 20-month period before they develop clinically positive nodes.

A I think that is a very good question, and the answer is very clearly no. It is not lead time bias for two reasons. First of all, we know that the median time from diagnosis to the development of clinically positive nodes is 16 months in this group of patients. We have looked at about 1000 patients to find these disease intervals. If this were a matter of lead time bias, what we would see is these two curves coming together, plateauing at the same survival, but we do not see that. We see a sustained survival advantage beyond ten years of follow-up. This is clearly not a phenomenon of lead time bias. We were very concerned about that, but I think this is clearly a sustained survival difference.

Hepatectomy Prolongs Survival of Mice With Induced Liver Metastases

Manuel H. Castillo, MD; Ralph J. Doerr, MD; Norman Paolini, Jr, MS;
Stephen Cohen, PhD; Martin Goldrosen, PhD

• Resection of hepatic metastases from colorectal cancer has been shown to prolong survival in some patients. Whether this results from a reduction of tumor burden or is an indirect effect mediated by hepatectomy is questionable. Male C57BL/6Ros 8-week-old mice underwent ileocolic vein injection of a suspension of 0.3 mL of 2×10^5 viable liver-derived murine (MCA-38) colonic adenocarcinoma cells. This model produces hepatic metastases in all lobes of the liver. At 7, 14, or 21 days after tumor injection, mice were randomized to receive either 42% resection of the liver or laparotomy alone. Survival in the animals with hepatectomy was significantly prolonged when the hepatectomy was performed 14 or 21 days after tumor injection.

(*Arch Surg* 1989;124:167-169)

Liver metastases represent the most important cause of death for patients with colorectal cancer.[1] Laboratory data suggest that partial hepatectomy (HEP) might benefit this patient population by inducing an immune response capable of producing regression of micrometastases or by retarding progression of established macrometastases.[2]

Data regarding the effect of partial HEP on tumor systems are controversial. Both tumor progression and regression or disappearance of metastases have been reported following partial HEP.[2-4] A proved metastatic model using the ileocolic vein (ICV) was selected to study these observations.[5] Animals were injected with syngeneic liver-derived MCA-38 colonic adenocarcinoma cells. Liver metastases were successfully induced and partial HEP (42%) was performed on these tumor-bearing mice at 7, 14, and 21 days following ICV injection. In this study, we report our results on the effect of partial HEP on survival and the reliability of the ICV injection as an excellent metastatic model.

Accepted for publication Oct 13, 1988.
From the Department of Surgery, State University of New York at Buffalo (Drs Castillo and Doerr), and Roswell Park Memorial Institute, Buffalo (Mr Paolini, and Drs Cohen and Goldrosen).
Read before the Annual Meeting of the Society of Surgical Oncology, New Orleans, May 23, 1988.
Reprint requests to Department of Surgery, Veterans Administration Medical Center, 3495 Bailey Ave, Buffalo, NY 14215 (Dr Castillo).

MATERIAL AND METHODS

Animals

Male C57BL/6Ros mice (West Seneca Laboratories, West Seneca, NY), 6 to 8 weeks old, were maintained on a standard mouse diet of pellets and water ad libitum.

Tumor Cells

The C57BL/6Ros tumor-bearing mice were killed and pinned to a dissecting board. Abdominal and chest walls were resected and HEP was performed. The liver was placed into a sterile Petri dish containing 10 mL of 0.25% trypsin–edetic acid (EDTA) maintained at 4°C. Tumor nodules were dissected from normal liver tissue using scalpel and fine-tissue forceps. The tumor was divided into 2-mm fragments. Disaggregation was done by 15 minutes of trypsinization (10 mL of fresh 0.25% trypsin–edetic acid). The enzyme tumor suspension was diluted up to 50 mL with RPMI 1640 and 10% heat-inactivated fetal calf serum plus antibiotics (complete tissue culture media), filtered through a four-layer No. 200 nylon mesh, and spun at 200 g. The pellet was washed once in complete tissue culture medium and resuspended to a final concentration of 2×10^5 cells per milliliter. Viability of injected cells was determined by trypan blue exclusion technique ranging between 90% and 95%.

ICV Injection

Male C57BL/6Ros mice, 6 to 8 weeks old, were fasted overnight. They were anesthetized by intraperitoneal (IP) injection of pentobarbital sodium, 55 mg/kg. The cecum was exteriorized through a low midline limited laparotomy (LAP). The ICV was identified in the mesentery. With a 30-gauge needle and 1-mL tuberculin syringe, 0.3 mL of the cell suspension was injected into the vein. Gentle pressure with a cotton-tipped applicator over the injection site for one minute achieved hemostasis. The cecum was returned to the peritoneal cavity, care being taken to prevent torsion. The wound was closed in layers.

HEP

Animals were fasted overnight and reanesthetized by IP pentobarbital, 50 mg/kg. An upper abdomen midline incision was used. The liver was freed of all fibrous attachments and exteriorized. The lateral portions of the median and right lobes were dissected. A 4-0 silk tie was used for mass ligation. The lobes were resected and hemostasis was obtained. The liver was returned to the peritoneal cavity and the wound was closed in layers. The operative mortality for the hepatectomy was 4%.

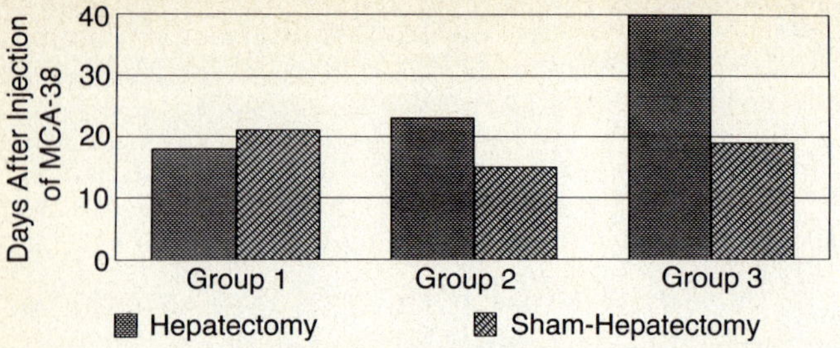

Survival after ileocolic vein injection (ICV) of MCA-38. Group 1 mice received their hepatectomy or sham laparotomy seven days after ICV injection. Group 2 mice received it 14 days after injection. Group 3 received it 21 days after injection. Survival is shown as total days of survival after injection of ICV with MCA-38. There is significant difference in survival in hepatectomized mice when compared with sham-operated-on controls (χ^2, $P=.05$). In both groups 2 and 3, hepatectomized mice survived significantly longer than their sham-operated-on controls (*t* test, $P=.05$).

LAP

Animals were fasted overnight and anesthetized by IP pentobarbital sodium, 50 mg/kg. Through an upper midline incision, liver was dissected free from all fibrous attachments and eviscerated. After gentle manipulation, it was returned to the peritoneal cavity and the wound was closed in layers.

Survival

All experimental animals had their ears marked, and were inspected twice a day until their death. Date of death was recorded in all animals.

RESULTS

The 8- to 10-week-old C57BL/6Ros mice had a 0.3-mL suspension containing 2×10^5 viable liver-derived MCA-38 cells from a syngeneic donor injected into the portal circulation, using the ICV. In 99% of those injected, foci of liver metastases were obtained in all lobes with an operative mortality of 2%. Survivors (49 animals) were randomly assigned to a HEP group or LAP control group on days 7, 14, or 21 following injection. All animals were observed twice a day and followed up until their death.

Survival in the HEP group was significantly prolonged ($P=.05$) over LAP controls when HEP was performed 14 or 21 days after injection (Figure). When HEP was performed seven days after ICV injection, no difference ($P=.05$) in survival was noted (Figure).

Survival of HEP mice vs LAP mice alone was analyzed by the χ^2 method. Separate survivals on days 7, 14, and 21 following injection were analyzed by *t* test.

COMMENT

Dissemination of the tumor via the portal vein has been shown to be the route of spread to the liver[6-8] for colonic carcinoma. Multiple modalities of therapy have been tried to control the disease and improve survival. Resection of the primary tumor without treatment of the metastases yields a median survival of 4.1 to 12 months.[1] In a 1984 report, Wagner et al[9] identified the fate of hepatic metastases from colorectal carcinoma that were left unresected: 50% of the patients with solitary metastases were alive at two years, but only 20% were alive at three years. As expected, those patients with multiple metastases did considerably worse.[9]

The limited tolerance of the liver to radiation therapy curtails external beam or internal radiotherapy for curative purposes. Multiple chemotherapeutic agents and routes of administration have been investigated: partial responses, short duration of response, lack of complete responses, and high toxic reactions are the most important mitigating factors of this treatment modality.[10] The search continues for new drugs and biologic response modifiers capable of inducing complete response with acceptable toxicity.

Woodington and Waugh[11] reported that 20% of 25 patients who sustained partial HEP as therapy for liver metastases survived five or more years with an operative mortality of 4%. As more experience with this approach was gained, an improvement in five-year survival was noted.[9,12-14] Presently, five-year survival rates up to 45% have been obtained.[15]

In vivo and in vitro experimental data on the effect of partial HEP have been controversial. Craddock et al[16] reported that partial HEP triggers DNA synthesis in the liver and lymphoid organs. Ono et al[17] found activation of effector lymphocytes following partial HEP. Natural killer cells and autoreactive cytotoxic T cells were present. Ono et al[2] also demonstrated regression and disappearance of inoculated mouse ascitic hepatoma (MH-B4) after HEP.

Others have reported progression of disease following HEP.[3,4,18] A limiting factor in this area of research has been the lack of a reproducible model of liver metastases in animals with intact immune systems. The model utilizing intraportal vein injection, described by Koike et al,[19] resulted in an unacceptable mortality rate. Intrasplenic injection followed by splenectomy was also reported.[20,21] The changes in the immune system subsequent to splenectomy alone add an important variable in this model that cannot be disregarded.

Goldrosen et al[5] described an experimental model to induce liver metastases in a single-stage procedure, simulating the natural history of the disease. Using the ICV, a 98% success rate was obtained with an acceptable 6.1% mortality. They described the metastatic process in this model to be in three stages. The covert stage is from one day after injection to ten days. Micrometastases can be identified beginning on day 11. By 21 days after injection palpable and visible macrometastases are found. An average survival of 53.3 days was reported.

Utilizing this tumor-bearing model, we found partial HEP significantly prolonged survival. We investigated this beneficial effect and believe that modulation of the immune response[22] by partial HEP may account for this improved survival. This phenomenon is believed to be separate from simple tumor burden reduction.

It remains to be proved that this mechanism is present in humans after HEP for colorectal metastasis to the liver. Further studies will also address the amount of resection needed to trigger this immune response and whether formal lobectomy is necessary or the effect can be seen after metastasectomy alone.

References

1. Hughes KS, Sugarbaker PH: Resection of the liver for metastatic solid tumor, in Rosenberg SA (ed): *Surgical Treatment of Metastatic Cancer.* Philadelphia, JB Lippincott, 1987, pp 125-128.
2. Ono M, Tanako N, Kunzo O: Complete regression of mouse hepatoma transplanted after partial hepatectomy: The immunological mechanism of such regression. *Cancer Res* 1986;46:5049-5053.
3. Paschkis KE, Canatarow A, Stasney J: Tumor growth in partially hepatectomized rats. *Cancer Res* 1955;15:579-582.
4. Stolar CJ, Anderson KD: Growth of mouse hepatoma following liver resection. *J Pediatr Surg* 1980;15:513-516.
5. Goldrosen MH, Paolini N, Holyoke ED: Description of a murine model of experimental hepatic metastases. *JNCI* 1986;77:823-828.
6. American Cancer Society: *1985 Cancer Facts and Figures.* New York, American Cancer Society, 1985, p 9.
7. Taylor FW: Cancer of the colon and rectum: A study of routes of metastases and death. *Surgery* 1962;52:305-308.
8. Rosenberg SA, Spiess P, Lafreniere R: A new approach to the adoptive

immunotherapy of cancer with tumor-infiltrating lymphocytes. *Science* 1986;233:1318-1321.

9. Wagner JS, Adson MA, van Herrden JA, et al: Natural history of hepatic metastases from colorectal cancer: Comparison with resective treatment. *Ann Surg* 1984;199:502-508.

10. Kemeny MM, Goldberg DA, Browning S, et al: Experience with regional chemotherapy and hepatic resection as treatment of hepatic metastases from colorectal primaries: A prospective randomized study. *Cancer* 1985;55:1265-1270.

11. Woodington GF, Waugh JM: Results of resection of metastatic tumors of the liver. *Am J Surg* 1963;105:24-29.

12. Kortz WJ, Meyers WC, Hanks JB, et al: Hepatic resection for metastatic cancer. *Ann Surg* 1984;199:182-186.

13. Fortner JG, Silua JS, Golbey RB, et al: Multivariate analysis of a personal series of 247 consecutive patients with liver metastases from colorectal cancer. *Ann Surg* 1984;199:306-324.

14. Cady B, McDermott WV: Major hepatic resection for metachronous metastases from colon cancer. *Ann Surg* 1985;201:205-209.

15. Iwatsuki S, Esquivel CO, Gorden R, et al: Liver resection for metastatic colorectal cancer. *Surgery* 1986;100:804-810.

16. Craddock CG, Nakai GS, Fukuta H, et al: Proliferative activity of the lymphocytic tissues of rats as studied with tritium-labeled thymidine. *J Exp Med* 1964;120:389-412.

17. Ono M, Tanaka N, Orita K: Activation of NK activity and autoreactive cytotoxicity after hepatectomy. *Acta Med Okayama* 1984;38:207-213.

18. Fisher B, Fisher ER: Experimental studies of factors influencing hepatic metastasis: II. Effect of partial hepatectomy. *Cancer* 1959;12:929-931.

19. Koike A, Sahyun S, Long ML: The fate of Ehrlich cells injected into the portal system. *Cancer Res* 1963;16:716-720.

20. Lafreniere R, Rosenberg SA: Successful immunotherapy of murine experimental hepatic metastases with LAK cells and IL-2. *Cancer Res* 1985;45:3735-3741.

21. Kopper L, Van Hanh T, Lapis K, et al: Experimental model for liver metastases formation using Lewis lung tumor. *J Cancer Res Clin Oncol* 1982;103:31-38.

22. Doerr RJ, Castillo MH, Paolini N, et al: Induction of cytokines in murine non-parenchymal liver cells by partial hepatectomy. Abstract of the Society of Surgical Oncology, New Orleans, May 22-25, 1988.

Discussion

Q It is clearly a surgical feat to be able to do HEPs on mice and have them survive. (1) Do you get tumor implants at your injection site? (2) If in fact you do not believe that the reason for prolonged survival is decreased tumor burden, what is it due to?

A The answer to this second question is going to be our next report. Dr Abdul will explain why this phenomenon is happening, so if you stay for the next 15 minutes you are going to receive the answer. We have been looking at the injection site and there is no seeding in the mesentery. Why, we do not know, but we do not get seeding in the site of the injection.

Q Did any of the animals in the surgical group die as a result of the operation, or are you only looking at those that survived the operation?

A Yes, about 4% of our animals die during the HEP or during the first 24 hours after the HEP. When we started trying to define the 42% HEP in the model, we had a pretty high mortality, so then we went through the operating microscope and we found out that if we avoid the hepatic biliary vein, we decreased the mortality to 4%; we do not use the operating microscope now.

Q Although you say that there was no change or no reduction or no effect of the change in the tumor burden, have you actually tried to measure the tumor burden in the residual left lobe at the time of partial HEP and again at subsequent times?

A Yes indeed, we have been doing this. We do not have the data, but we considered that whatever is happening is related to changes in the immune system.

Q Was there any weight loss following the HEP in the animals?

A Not that we observed.

Q Two questions: When you operated on these animals, you did not totally remove all the tumors. Is that correct?

A That is correct; they had tumors in all lobes.

Q So you essentially removed what is considered to be 47%.

A Forty-two percent.

Q Forty-two percent of the tumor. There was remaining tumor so you are invoking that these animals had prolonged survival, not only from the cytoreductive surgery, but also because there is something else in play. So now the magic question is what else? This is an interesting model. What are you going to do to study what comes into play or what do you think comes into play from this point?

A We have been interested in what is going on in the nonhepatic liver cells in response to the HEP. At the University of Yokahama (Japan), they showed that when you do HEPs, you have increased natural killer cell activity.

Q I think this is very important because over the last five years we have become much more aggressive with hepatic metastases and the point is, are we doing more than just cytoreductive surgery or ridding the liver of metastases, or is something else in play? It is possible that there is something else in play and I think that this model may help to delineate that something. I like this approach.

In Other AMA Journals

ARCHIVES OF INTERNAL MEDICINE

Clinical Symptoms and Length of Survival in Patients With Terminal Cancer

David B. Reuben, MD; Vincent Mor, PhD; Jeff Hiris

Planning terminal care for patients with malignant neoplasms is difficult, in part, because accurate measures of prognosis have not been defined. Using data from the National Hospice Study, we examined the correlation of 14 easily assessable clinical symptoms with survival in patients with terminal cancer. Performance status was the most important clinical factor in estimating survival time, but five other symptoms had independent predictive value as well (shortness of breath, problems eating or anorexia, trouble swallowing, dry mouth, and weight loss). We generated four parametric accelerated time survival models to estimate survival in patients with combinations of these symptoms and validated the log-normal model on the entire data set. This model was unaffected by patient age, sex, primary tumor type, or site. Our findings illustrate the value of biologically "soft" clinical data in predicting survival in patients with terminal cancer. The prevalence of similar symptoms among patients with cancer of various primary and metastatic sites also supports the concept of a common final clinical pathway in patients with advanced malignant neoplasms (*Arch Intern Med* 1988;148:1586-1591).

Reprint requests to Division of General Internal Medicine, Rhode Island Hospital, 593 Eddy St, Providence, RI 02903 (Dr Reuben).

Partial Hepatectomy Augments the Liver's Antitumor Response

Ralph Doerr, MD; Manuel Castillo, MD; Paul Evans, MS;
Norman Paolini, MS; Martin Goldrosen, PhD; Stephan A. Cohen, PhD

• Despite adequate locoregional control, colorectal metastasis to the liver remains a significant cause of death. Resection of hepatic metastasis improves five-year survival 18% to 34%. A study of the impact of 40% partial hepatectomy on cytokine production in the liver was undertaken. Nonparenchymal liver cells (NPCs) were prepared by collagenase perfusion and metrizamide gradient from partially hepatectomized and laparotomized control C57BL/6Ros mice. Nonparenchymal cell from partially hepatectomized mice compared with laparotomized mice showed a twofold to threefold increase in interferon (IFN) activity. Both interferon alpha/beta and supernatants from cultured NPCs of partially hepatectomized mice suppressed the proliferation of liver-derived MCA-38 colon adenocarcinoma cells in vitro. This tumor has been shown to metastasize to the liver of C57BL/6Ros mice. The production of various cytokines by NPCs induced by partial hepatectomy may provide a possible antimetastatic mechanism.

(*Arch Surg* 1989;124:170-174)

Sinusoidal or nonparenchymal liver cells (NPCs) play an important protective role in clearing potentially pathogenic substances such as viruses, bacteria, and endotoxin.[1] Recent reports[2-6] have demonstrated that these same cells may have the potential to eliminate metastatic tumors that arise from the colon. Both cell-cell contact and the production of cytotoxic or cytostatic factors are suggestive mechanisms. Colon-derived tumors in humans have been shown to metastasize to the liver at a high rate.[7] Recently, this laboratory developed a model system in mice that simulates the hepatic metastasis of human colon carcinoma.[8] The resection of metastatic colorectal cancer of the liver has been shown to prolong survival in some patients.[9-13] Our study is designed to determine whether this therapeutic effect is due to reduction of the tumor burden or the result of the surgery on the liver's antitumor system.

Evidence is presented herein that partial hepatectomy can augment the liver's host defense system by enhancing cytostatic or cytotoxic antitumor activity of NPCs.

Accepted for publication Oct 12, 1988.

From the Departments of Surgery (Drs Doerr and Castillo) and Medicine, Division of Gastroenterology and Hepatology (Dr Cohen and Mr Evans), State University of New York at Buffalo, Buffalo General Hospital, and the Department of Cell and Tumor Biology, Roswell Park Memorial Institute (Dr Goldrosen and Mr Paolini), Buffalo.

Read before the Annual Meeting of the Society of Surgical Oncology, New Orleans, May 23, 1988.

Reprint requests to Department of Surgery, Buffalo General Hospital, 100 High St, Buffalo, NY 14203 (Dr Doerr).

MATERIALS AND METHODS

Animals

Adult 8- to 10-week-old male C57BL/6Ros mice received a standard mouse diet of pellets and water ad libitum.

Medium

Tissue culture medium consisted of RPMI 1640 medium supplemented with 25 mmol/L of HEPES, gentamicin (50 μg/mL), and 10% fetal bovine serum.

Reagents

Collagenase type IV, bovine serum albumin, and murine interferon (IFN) alpha/beta were used in the study.

Preparation of NPCs

Nonparenchymal liver cells were isolated by modifying a previously described method.[3,14] Briefly, mice were killed by cervical dislocation, the skin over the abdomen and chest was reflected, and the inferior vena cava was ligated above the diaphragm. The inferior vena cava below the liver was cannulated with a heparinized 20-gauge needle. The liver was preperfused at 37°C with 40 mL of Hank's balanced salt solution (HBSS) without Ca^{++} and Mg^{++} (pH 7.2) delivered over two minutes with the outflow through an incision in the portal vein. The liver was then perfused with 100 mL of sterile HBSS (pH 7.6) and supplemented with 0.05% type IV collagenase delivered over five minutes. The distended and blanched liver was removed, rinsed with HBSS, teased apart with a rubber policeman, and passed through a 100-μm nylon mesh screen.

Five milliliters of a single liver cell suspension was mixed with 7 mL of 30% wt/vol metrizamide dissolved in HBSS (without sodium chloride), then gently overlaid with 1 mL of HBSS (with sodium chloride) and centrifuged at 550 g for 15 minutes at 23°C. The NPCs were collected from the interface, washed twice in HBSS, and resuspended in tissue culture medium. The NPCs obtained were greater than 95% viable by this method.

Assay of Cytotoxic Activity

The target cells were adapted to continuous growth in tissue culture medium and labeled with sodium chromate ($^{51}Na_2CrO_4$) for one hour at 37°C (100 mCi/10^6 cells). The chromium phosphate Cr 51–release assay was performed in 96-well, flat-bottomed tissue culture plates. The NPCs were mixed with 2×10^4 tumor target cells in triplicate in a total volume of 100 μL and incubated for 18 hours in a humidified atmosphere of 5% carbon dioxide in air. Supernatants were harvested and counted in a gamma counter. The results were expressed as the percentage of specific release calculated by using the following equation: % specific release $= 100 \times (A/B/CB)$, where A indicates counts per minute from experimental cells; B, counts per minute from spontaneous release; and C, counts per minute from target cells. YAC-1 target cells were used in this study and were free of mycoplasma.

Assay of Murine IFN Activity

Interferon samples were prepared by incubation of cells in 96-well, flat-bottomed tissue culture plates. Interferon in cell-free supernatants was measured by inhibition of the cytopathic effect of vesicular stomatitis virus against a mouse fibroblast L cell line (L929) using the method of Finter.[15] Briefly, L cells were seeded into 24-well tissue culture plates (6×10^4 cells per well) and allowed to form confluent monolayers. The cells were then overlayed with serial dilutions of the test supernatant or reference IFN and incubated overnight at 37°C. After removal of the IFN, the cells were challenged with vesicular stomatitis virus (≈40 plaque-forming units per well). After 24 hours, the cells were stained with a 1% solution of crystal violet, and the percentage of lysis was determined. One unit of IFN was defined as the highest dilution causing a 50% reduction in cytopathic effect and is reported in National Institutes of Health reference units per milliliter. The lower limit of detection in this assay was 20 U/mL.

Rabbit antimouse IFN alpha/beta was used in the study. A 1:140 dilution of anti-IFN neutralized 100 U of IFN alpha/beta.[16]

Preparation of Liver-Derived (LD) MCA-38 Tumor Cells

Mice bearing liver tumors between the sixth and eighth week after ileocolic vein injection were killed and pinned to a dissecting board. The liver was exteriorized by a midline incision. A lobe-by-lobe hepatectomy was performed into a glass Petri dish containing 10 mL of 0.25% trypsin–edetic acid maintained at 4°C.

Tumor nodules were carefully dissected from normal liver tissue, and nonnecrotic tissue and nonnecrotic portions were cut into 2- to 3-mm fragments using a scalpel blade and fine forceps. These fragments were collected into a 50-mL plastic tube containing 10 mL of fresh 0.25 trypsin–edetic acid and rotated for 15 minutes. The resulting tumor enzyme suspension was diluted up to 50 mL using RPMI 1640 medium with 10% fetal bovine serum plus gentamicin, filtered through a four-layer No. 200 nylon mesh, and spun at 200 g. This pellet was washed once in medium and resuspended to a final concentration of 2×10^4 cells/mL. Viability of cells was determined by trypan blue dye exclusion and usually was greater than 90%.

Laparotomy

Experimental mice were fasted overnight and anesthetized by intraperitoneal injection of pentobarbital sodium (60 mg/kg). A 3-cm midline incision was made from the tip of the sternum to the pubis. All lobes of the liver were carefully examined anteriorly and posteriorly using a small stainless steel retractor and saline-moistened cotton-tipped applicator. The abdomen was closed using a 5-0 nylon monofilament suture and stainless steel clips.

Hepatectomy

Experimental mice were fasted overnight and anesthetized with intraperitoneal pentobarbital sodium (60 mg/kg). An upper abdominal incision was made. The liver was freed of all fibrous attachments and eviscerated. The right lobe and lateral portion of the median lobe were dissected, avoiding injury to the gallbladder, extrahepatic biliary tree, or major vessels. A 4-0 silk tie was used for mass ligation; the lobes were resected, constituting a 42% hepatectomy by weight. Hemostasis was obtained. The liver was returned to the peritoneal cavity, and the wound was closed in layers.

Survival

All experimental animals were palpated beginning at the fourth week until death to assess hepatic tumor growth. The day of death was recorded.

RESULTS

Augmentation of Anti–YAC-1 and IFN Activity of NPCs After Hepatectomy

The NPCs from laparotomized mice were assayed for their ability to display natural cytotoxicity against the standard natural killer target, YAC-1 tumor cells. The NPCs either directly or after culture displayed little cytotoxicity (Table 1). In contrast, NPCs from mice hepatectomized seven days previously had significant natural cytotoxicity. As also shown in Table 1, IFN was detected in the culture supernatant of NPCs from hepatectomized mice.

Augmentation of Cytostatic Antitumor Activity of NPCs After Hepatectomy

Inhibition of tumor growth or cytostasis is another method to measure effector cell function. The results in Table 2 demonstrate that NPCs from hepatectomized mice were cytostatic against YAC-1 tumor cells (natural killer sensitive).[17]

Cytostatic Antitumor Activity of Culture Supernatants From NPCs After Hepatectomy

To determine if NPCs from hepatectomized mice can produce antitumor cytostatic factor(s), cells were cultured overnight and supernatants were tested for their antiproliferative activity. As in Table 3, NPCs from hepatectomized mice produced a cytostatic factor against YAC-1 tumor cells. Anti-IFN alpha/beta did not affect the cytostatic activity of these supernatants. Furthermore, IFN alpha/beta did not directly inhibit the proliferation of YAC-1 tumor cells (Figure). The NPCs contain a mixed population that includes Kupffer's cells and large granular lymphocytes or natural killer cells.[4,5,18,19] In other experiments (data not shown), the cytotoxic and cytostatic activity was confined to the lymphocyte population.

Syngeneic murine colon adenocarcinoma cells (LD-MCA-38) have been previously shown to form metastatic foci in the liver if injected into the ileocolic vein.[8] Furthermore, hepatectomy seems to increase the liver span of hepatectomized mice previously injected with LD-MCA-38 through the ileocolic vein. Therefore, experiments were carried out to determine if hepatectomy of mice could induce cytostatic antitumor factors by NPCs against this freshly excised tumor. Table 4 shows that culture supernatants from

Table 1.—Effect of Hepatectomy of C57BL/6 Mice on Anti–YAC-1 Cells and Interferon Activity of Nonparenchymal Liver Cells

Treatment In Vivo*	% Specific Release, No Preincubation†	YAC-1 Cells ± SD, Preincubation	Interferon, U/mL‡
Laparotomy	3±1	1±3	<20
Hepatectomy	16±1	16±2	20

*C57BL/6 mice were either laparotomized or hepatectomized seven days before being killed, and nonparenchymal liver cells were obtained as described in the "Materials and Methods" section.

†Cytotoxicity of nonparenchymal liver cells was determined either with no preincubation or after 18 hours of preincubation in 10% fetal bovine serum at an effector-to-target ratio of 20:1 against chromium phosphate Cr 51–YAC-1 for 18 hours.

‡Nonparenchymal liver cells were incubated for 18 hours in 10% fetal bovine serum and assayed for interferon activity.

Table 2.—Effect of Hepatectomy of C57BL/6 Mice on Cytostatic Antitumor Activity of NPCs*

Cells	Tritiated Thymidine Incorporation, cpm ± SD†	% Inhibition‡
YAC-1	40 437 ± 9000	0
Lap-NPCs§	308 ± 56‖	. . .
Hep-NPCs§	762 ± 189‖	. . .
Lap-NPCs + YAC-1	40 619 ± 6939	0
Hep-NPCs + YAC-1	3791 ± 1836‖	92

*NPCs indicates nonparenchymal liver cells.
†Cytostasis was determined by incubation of 2×10^4 tumor cells, 4×10^5 NPCs, or both in 10% fetal bovine serum for 60 hours, pulsed with 0.5 μCi of tritiated thymidine for 18 hours, and harvested.
‡Percentage of inhibition = 1 − cpm [NPCs + tumor cells]/cpm [tumor cells].
§C57BL/6 mice were either laparotomized (Lap) or hepatectomized (Hep) seven days before being killed, and NPCs were obtained as described in the "Materials and Methods" section.
‖The 95% confidence intervals do not overlap. The true means are significantly different, with a type 1 error rate of alpha = .05.

Table 4.—Effect of Hepatectomy of C57BL/6 Mice on the Generation of a Cytostatic Antitumor Factor by NPCs*

Experimental Cells	Tritiated Thymidine Incorporation, cpm ± SD†	% Inhibition
LD-MCA-38	9616 ± 1298	. . .
Lap-NPCs‡ + LD-MCA-38	8545 ± 516	12
Lap-NPCs/anti-IFN§ + LD-MCA-38	7589 ± 453	21
Hep-NPCs‡ + LD-MCA-38	4679 ± 1045‖	52
Hep-NPCs/anti-IFN§ + LD-MCA-38	7030 ± 1871	27

*NPCs indicates nonparenchymal liver cells; LD, liver derived; and IFN, interferon.
†Cytostasis was determined by incubation of 2×10^4 MCA-38 cells and various dilutions of culture supernatants in 10% fetal bovine serum for 60 hours, pulsed with 0.5 μCi of tritiated thymidine for 18 hours, and harvested. Percentage of inhibition = 1 − cpm [NPC supernatant + tumor cell]/cpm [tumor cells].
‡C57BL/6 mice were either laparotomized (Lap) or hepatectomized (Hep) seven days before being killed. The NPCs were isolated, 4×10^5 cells were cultured in 10% fetal bovine serum for 18 hours, and culture supernatant was obtained.
§The NPCs were treated with 100 neutralizing units of anti–IFN alpha/beta before being cultured.
‖The 95% confidence intervals do not overlap. The true means are significantly different, with a type 1 error rate of alpha = .05.

laparotomized mice have antiproliferative effects against freshly excised LD-MCA-38 tumor cells. Moreover, supernatants of NPCs from hepatectomized mice exert an even greater antiproliferative effect. Anti–IFN alpha/beta partially neutralized some of this cytostatic activity. As shown in the Figure, IFN alpha/beta can also directly inhibit the proliferation of MCA-38 tumor cells.

In this study, we observed that NPCs from hepatectomized mice can induce cytolytic and cytostatic activity against the natural killer–sensitive tumor YAC-1 cells.

Statistical Analysis

Ninety-five percent confidence intervals were calculated by parameter interval estimation and compared for experimental and control groups.

COMMENT

Despite adequate local and regional control of colorectal carcinoma, metastasis to the liver remains directly or indirectly the most frequent cause of death.[9] Numerous

Table 3.—Effect of Hepatectomy of C57BL/6 Mice on the Generation of a Cytostatic Antitumor Factor by NPCs*

Experimental Cells	Tritiated Thymidine Incorporation, cpm ± SD†	% Inhibition
YAC-1	37 424 ± 1189	. . .
Lap-NPCs‡ + YAC-1	35 900 ± 2694	6
Lap-NPCs/anti-IFN§ + YAC-1	37 400 ± 980	0
Hep-NPCs‡ + YAC-1	3046 ± 184‖	92
Hep-NPCs/anti-IFN† + YAC-1	4527 ± 631‖	88

*NPCs indicates nonparenchymal liver cells; IFN, interferon.
†Cytostasis was determined by incubation of 2×10^4 YAC-1 cells and various dilutions of culture supernatants in 10% fetal bovine serum for 60 hours, pulsed with 0.5 μCi of tritiated thymidine for 18 hours, and harvested. Percentage of inhibition = 1 − cpm [NPC supernatant + tumor cell]/cpm [tumor cells].
‡C57BL/6 mice were either laparotomized (Lap) or hepatectomized (Hep) seven days before being killed. The NPCs were isolated, 4×10^5 cells were cultured in 10% fetal bovine serum for 18 hours, and culture supernatant was obtained.
§The NPCs were treated with 100 neutralizing units of anti–IFN alpha/beta before being cultured.
‖The 95% confidence intervals do not overlap. The true means are significantly different, with a type 1 error rate of alpha = .05.

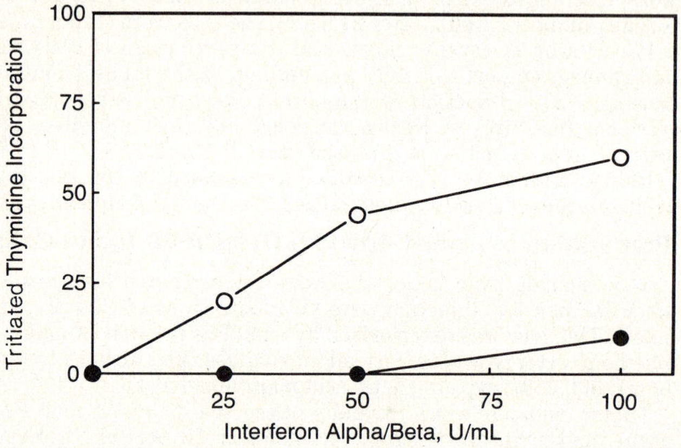

Cytostatic effect of interferon alpha/beta on liver-derived MCA-38 and YAC-1 cell lines.

studies have established that resection of liver metastases from colorectal carcinoma substantially improves five-year survival from 18% to 34%.[13,20] It seems unlikely that the resected metastases are the only sites of disease in the liver.

Prior studies on the effect of hepatectomy on tumor growth in experimental animals have yielded conflicting results. Paschis et al[21] transplanted Morris hepatomas and found that the feedback mechanism for growth inhibition was disrupted by the same process that permits liver regeneration following partial hepatectomy. Increased hepatic metastases were noted in the Walker 256 carcinosarcoma system if hepatectomy was performed at the time of tumor transplantation.[22,23] This effect was lost if hepatectomy preceded tumor implantation by 48 hours. In contrast, Ono et al[24] recently observed complete regression of a transplanted mouse hepatoma (MH-134) growing under the dorsal skin in syngeneic hosts after hepatectomy.

Part of the difficulty in studying the effect of hepatectomy on metastasis has been the lack of a reproducible colon-derived hepatic metastasis model. Recently, our laboratory developed a technique for induction of murine hepatic metastases through vascular seeding. Goldrosen et al[8] injected LD-MCA-38 tumor cells into the ileocolic vein of C57BL/6 mice and obtained metastatic liver foci.

The advantage of this system is a staged progression of metastasis. Utilizing this model, we determined that partial hepatectomy imparts significant improvement in survival in the tumor-bearing host.[25] Fourteen days after injection of the tumor, the time corresponding to the establishment of micrometastases in the liver, partial hepatectomy resulted in 34% improvement in survival. Partial hepatectomy 21 days after tumor inoculation, a phase that corresponds to visible macroscopic foci, improved survival by 52.5%. The mechanism by which this therapeutic effect of partial hepatectomy remains is unclear.

The liver's antitumor immune activity has been under intense scrutiny.[24-27] It has been noted that the liver regeneration that follows partial hepatectomy is characterized by an oncofetal antigen expression capable of immunizing the host. The Kupffer cells have been postulated as the stimulators of this response.[26] These liver-derived macrophages, which constitute 30% of the total cell population of the liver and up to 50% of the total fixed macrophages in the body, undergo intense DNA synthesis during the liver regeneration phase following partial hepatectomy. Furthermore, nonspecific lymphocyte proliferation with high rates of differentiation and mitosis has also been identified following hepatectomy.[27]

Partial hepatectomy triggers DNA synthesis in other lymphoid organs besides the liver. Ono et al[24] demonstrated that following hepatectomy of syngeneic mice, natural killer activity is substantially increased in the spleen if measured five to seven days after hepatectomy. More recently, this same group[28] described augmentation of lymphokine-activated killer precursors in the spleen five to seven days after hepatectomy. Hellstrom et al[29] found lymph nodes from hepatectomized mice cytotoxic for tumor cells in culture. However, few studies on the antitumor studies have been carried out with isolated NPCs after hepatectomy.

We observed that NPCs from mice hepatectomized seven days previously can induce cytolytic activity against the natural killer–sensitive tumor YAC-1. Furthermore, these same cells can produce cytostatic factor(s) against YAC-1 as well as freshly excised colon-derived MCA-38 tumor cells. The cytostatic activity of NPCs against YAC-1 seems to be independent of IFN alpha/beta, since this cytokine has no direct cytostatic effect on this tumor (Figure). However, the antiproliferative effect against LD-MCA-38 may be partly due to the direct effect of IFN on these cells, since some IFN was detected in the culture supernatants of NPCs from hepatectomized mice (data not shown). In addition, IFN alpha/beta can directly inhibit the proliferation of MCA-38 cells at concentrations produced by the NPCs (Figure).

Since Kupffer's cells (AdNPC) from hepatectomized mice did not exert any antitumor activity, it seems that the cell population from C57BL/6 mice responsible for cytolysis and cytostasis against YAC-1 is the natural killer. We have previously shown that natural killer/large granular lymphocytes in the liver from normal C3HeB/FeJ mice and Wistar rats can exert cytotoxicity against YAC-1 cells. However, NPCs from C57BL/6 mice have little cytotoxicity and little detectable IFN.[2,30] It seems that hepatectomy may induce the production of IFN that augments in situ natural killer activity.

Partial hepatectomy performed at the time of resection for colorectal metastases exerts a profound immune effect both on remaining liver tissue and possible occult metastasis. Further studies should be carried out to understand better the biology of hepatectomy to take advantage of this procedure in the treatment of colorectal liver metastasis.

This work was supported by grant R01-28835 from the National Institutes of Health, Bethesda, Md (Dr Cohen), by a Veterans Administration Merit Review (Dr Cohen), and by the Margaret Duffy and Robert Cameron Troup Fund, Buffalo General Hospital (Drs Doerr and Cohen).

References

1. Nolan JP: The role of endotoxin in liver disease. *Gastroenterology* 1975;69:1346-1352.

2. Cohen SA, Goldrosen MH: Interferon α/β produced by nonparenchymal liver cells from C57B1/6.NU/NU mice modulates MCA-38 colon adenocarcinoma. *Proc Am Assoc Cancer Res* 1988;29:414.

3. Cohen SA, Salazar D, von Muenchhausen W, et al: Natural anti tumor defense system of the murine liver. *J Leukocyte Biol* 1985;37:559-564.

4. Kaneda K, Dan C, Wake K: Pit cells as natural killer cells. *Biomed Res* 1983;4:567.

5. Leung K, Salazar D, Ip M, et al: Characterization of natural cytotoxic effector cells isolated from rat liver. *Nat Immun Cell Growth Regul* 1987; 5:150-152.

6. Roos E, Tulp A, Middlekoop O, et al: Interaction between liver metastasizing lymphoid tumor cells and hepatic sinusoidal endothelial cell, in Knook C, Wisse E (eds): *Sinusoidal Liver Cells.* Amsterdam, Elsevier Science Publishers, 1982, p 461.

7. Havelarr IJ, Sugarbaker PH, Vermess M, et al: Rate of growth from intra-abdominal metastases from colorectal cancer. *Cancer* 1984;54:163-171.

8. Goldrosen MH, Paolini N Jr, Holyoke ED: Description of a murine model of experimental hepatic metastases. *JNCI* 1986;77:823-828.

9. Wagner JS, Adson MA, van Herrden JA, et al: Natural history of hepatic metastases from colorectal cancer: Comparison with resective treatment. *Ann Surg* 1984;199:502-508.

10. Kortz WJ, Meyers WC, Hanks JB, et al: Hepatic resection for metastatic cancer. *Ann Surg* 1984;199:182-186.

11. Fortner JG, Silva JS, Golbey RB, et al: Multivariate analysis of a personal series of 247 consecutive patients with liver metastases from colorectal cancer. *Ann Surg* 1984;199:306-324.

12. Cady B, McDermott WV: Major hepatic resection for metachronous metastases from colon cancer. *Ann Surg* 1985;201:204-209.

13. Iwatsvki S, Sunzaburo E, Carlos O, et al: Liver resection for metastatic colorectal cancer. *Surgery* 1986;100:804-810.

14. Richman LK, Klingenstein RJ, Richman JA, et al: The murine Kupffer cell: I. Characterization of the cell serving accessory function in antigen-specific T cell proliferation. *J Immunol* 1979;123:2602.

15. Finter NB: Standardization of assay of interferons. *Methods Enzymol* 1978;78:14.

16. Senik A, Gresser I, Maury C, et al: Enhancement of mouse NK cells by interferon. *Transplant Proc* 1979;11:993.

17. Roder JC, Lohman-Matthes M, Domzig W, et al: A functional comparison of tumor killing by activated macrophages and natural killer cells. *Eur J Immunol* 1979;9:283.

18. Bouwens L, Remel K, Baekland M, et al: Large granular lymphocytes or 'pit cells' from rat liver: Isolation, ultrastructural characterization and natural killer activity. *Eur J Immunol* 1987;17:37.

19. Praaning-van-Dalen DP, Brouwer A, Knook DL: Clearance capacity of rat liver Kupffer, endothelial, and parenchymal cells. *Gastroenterology* 1981;81:1036-1044.

20. Hughes KS, Members of the Registry of Hepatic Metastases: Resection of the liver for colorectal carcinoma metastases: A multi-institutional study of patterns of recurrence. *Surgery* 1986;100:278-284.

21. Paschis KE, Canatarow A, Stasney J, et al: Tumor growth in partially hepatectomized rats. *Cancer Res* 1955;15:579-582.

22. Stolar CJ, Anderson KD: Growth of mouse hepatoma following liver resection. *J Pediatr Surg* 1980;15:513-516.

23. Fisher B, Fisher ER: Experimental studies of factors influencing hepatic metastasis: II. Effect of partial hepatectomy. *Cancer* 1959;12:929-931.

24. Ono M, Tanaka N, Kunzo O: Complete regression of mouse hepatoma transplanted after partial hepatectomy: The immunological mechanism of such regression. *Cancer Res* 1986;46:5049-5053.

25. Castillo MH, Doerr RJ, Paolini N, et al: Partial hepatectomy prolongs survival of mice with experimentally induced liver metastases. Read in part before the 41st annual meeting of the Society of Surgical Oncology, New Orleans, May 23, 1988.

26. Miyahara S, Yokomuro K, Takahaski H, et al: Regeneration and the immune system: I. In vivo and in vitro activation of lymphocytes in liver regeneration and the role of Kupffer cells in stimulation. *Eur J Immunol* 1983;13:878-883.

27. Yokomuro K, Miyahara S, Takahaski H, et al: Regeneration of the

immune system: II. Suppressor activities of lymphocytes activated in vivo by liver regeneration and their genetic control. *Eur J Immunol* 1983;13:883-889.

28. Ono M, Tomaka N, Orita K: Activation of NK activity and auto reactive cytotoxicity after hepatectomy. *Acta Med Okayama* 1984;38:207-213.

29. Hellstrom I, Hellstrom KE, Nishioka M: Reactivity to tumor associated antigens detected in mice undergoing liver regeneration. *Nature* 1975;243:744-746.

30. Werner-Wasik M, Muenchhauser W, Nolan J, et al: Endogeneous interferon α/β produced by murine Kupffer cells augments liver associated natural killing activity, in Mihick E (ed): *Cancer Immunology Immunotherapy.* New York, Springer-Verlag New York Inc, in press.

Discussion

Q This is a stimulating paper for me. You could not have picked a better mouse system. The C57 black mouse has a super immune system. If you would have used the DBA or the C3H mouse, you might have found a different result. But this particular immune system is super, and when you begin to look at some of the immune stimulatory mechanisms that you saw, this reflects on some information that was discovered a number of years ago when we started to look at antithymocyte serum and antilymphocyte serum in this particular strain of mouse and then induced polyoma tumors. We found that C57 black mice had tremendous resistance against those tumors when compared with the C3H or the DBA mice, so strain selection may have worked in your favor.

A I think that's one thing of interest, but I do not think that it makes a tremendous difference what the size of the resection is. Whether it's large or small, you are going to get that immune response.

Q I am quite surprised by these results. When I was at the National Cancer Institute, Bethesda, Md, we looked at an intraperitoneal tumor model where we performed a laparotomy three days, 14 days, or five weeks after tumor inoculation, and we would see tremendous promotion of tumor growth intraperitoneally, especially at the laparotomy site, that could not be overcome with interleukin 2 lymphokine-activated killer treatment. So, in the discussion of these results, we hinted that growth factors such as B-cell growth factor and cell growth factor (TGF) beta might be one of the reasons why we saw this tremendous growth promotion of tumor. The TGF beta, being an interleukin 2 inhibitor or neutralizer, would offer an explanation for the tumor promotion we saw, which would wear off by 14 days.

I noted that in the seven-day model herein, you did not see a favorable outcome by day 14, and by day 21 you did. Are you monitoring growth factors that should be present after hemihepatectomy and that are responsible for liver regeneration?

A We are looking at TGF beta at this point. We have the probes for that. Interestingly enough, we have antiproliferative activity in the supernatants from the MCA-38s so that so far it's had an inhibitory effect, which I know is paradoxical. I really do not have an explanation at this point. We're not doing anything with the prostaglandins.

Q I looked at a rat model back in the late 1960s. When you do a partial hepatectomy, it's the best-known model for synchronization of protein synthesis, DNA synthesis, and everything, so it makes it much easier to study different pathways. I think you are just activating multiple different pathways by doing a partial hepatectomy. The other thing that I think is probably important is the activation of the complement cascade.

A Unfortunately, the rat is a much better model for the ileocolic vein injection, but we have not been able to get the tumors to grow in the liver.

Q I am disturbed by one major thing: there does not seem to be a dose response to this. In other words, you said it does not matter how much liver you remove. Did you really study that carefully? Did you find out if removing half the liver produces more of a cytokine response than taking out a little?

A No, we have not done that. All we have done is removed 42% of the liver.

Q If this is really a biologic phenomenon, there should be some sort of dose response.

Q You comment that on these patients you are asking for interleukin 1, and I presume you are doing a routine laboratory cytokine proliferation assay. Have you thought to look for hepatocyte stimulatory factors, recently described as interleukin 6, that cross-react in that assay and probably is the active agent in promonocytes? I wonder if you have had a chance to check for that. That might be contaminating your assessment of the interleukin 1 levels after hepatectomy.

A I think the interleukin 6 is something that we have been calling leukoregalin. Yes, we are looking at it, but to date, we do not have the data.

In Other AMA Journals

ARCHIVES OF INTERNAL MEDICINE

National Study of Internal Medicine Manpower: XII. The Future of Graduate Medical Education in Internal Medicine: What Do Program Directors Predict?

Lu Ann Aday, PhD; Ronald M. Andersen, PhD; Gerald S. Levey, MD; Christopher S. Lyttle, MA; Llewellyn J. Cornelius, MA; Catherine F. Glen

The 1985-1986 National Study of Internal Medicine Manpower asked directors of residency and fellowship programs about their plans to change the size of their programs in the near future. The vast majority (71% to 76%) of the directors expected their programs to remain about the same size for the next couple of years. For fellowship directors, this reflects a decline in the number planning to increase their program size since 1976-1977 from 32% to 18%. Directors of programs that are principal affiliates of medical schools are more likely to plan a decrease, while Veterans Administration directors are more likely to plan an increase in program size. The reason residency directors cited most frequently as important to their plans to increase program size was a perceived shortage of internists. Fellowship directors most frequently cited the need for fellows in clinical research. Stipend availability was the most important factor that influenced plans to decrease program size. Overall, residency and fellowship directors planned to increase the size of their programs around 1%. Program directors and others in the internal medicine community should consider how they can change the stipend availability, admissions criteria, and other incentives to channel trainees into the areas of greatest potential need and demand for the profession (*Arch Intern Med* 1988;148:1509-1514).

Reprint requests to Center for Health Administration Studies, The University of Chicago, 1101 E 58th St, Suite 111, Chicago, IL 60637 (Dr Andersen).

Prolongation of Survival of Nude Mice Bearing Human Colon Cancer

Treatment With Yttrium 90–Labeled Anti–Carcinoembryonic Antigen Antibody

David M. Hyams, MD; Jose M. Esteban, MD; Barbara G. Beatty, PhD; Philip M. Wanek, RPh; J. David Beatty, MD

• Nude mice bearing diffuse intraperitoneal carcinomatosis of the human colon cancer cell line LS174T were treated with an anti–carcinoembryonic antigen monoclonal antibody (MAB) that was labeled with yttrium 90 (^{90}Y-ZCE025). Control animals were either untreated or treated with nonspecific ^{90}Y-MAB (^{90}Y-96.5c). The median survival (MS) for untreated animals was 26 days. The MS for specific and nonspecific therapy that consisted of 120 μCi of ^{90}Y-MAB was 69 and 34 days, respectively. No significant improvement in the MS was observed with a second 120-μCi administration of ^{90}Y-MAB given two weeks later. A decreased MS was observed with 80 μCi of ^{90}Y-MAB given every four days for three cycles. In each category, specific therapy had a significant advantage over nonspecific therapy in increased effectiveness and decreased toxicity. The ^{90}Y-ZCE025 therapy gave an increased life span of almost 200%. The therapeutic effects with different dosing regimens have important implications for treatment planning.

(*Arch Surg* 1989;124:175-179)

The curative treatment of colorectal adenocarcinoma consists of surgical resection and radiation therapy. However, both of these modalities are limited by the anatomic location of the disease, as well as its degree of dissemination. At the present time, systemic chemotherapy offers no curative hope for afflicted patients.

Monoclonal antibodies (MABs) have the potential to improve on nonsurgical therapies by enabling tumor-directed delivery of high-dose pharmacologic or radiation therapy. Such tumor "targeting" could increase the therapeutic index by providing more toxic therapy to malignant cells, while minimally affecting normal tissues.[1,2]

In a previous publication, we described a nude mouse model for human colon carcinomatosis, successfully treated with yttrium 90–labeled anti–carcinoembryonic antigen (CEA) antibody.[3] Doses of the potent beta emitter ^{90}Y ranged from 40 to 160 μCi. Treated animals that were killed 12 days after therapy had consistently lower tumor burdens than untreated animals, or than animals that were undergoing treatment with a ^{90}Y-labeled nonspecific MAB.

The present study was designed to elaborate on these findings by determining whether such therapy might offer a significant survival advantage. In addition, the search for an optimal dosing scheme for the administration of ^{90}Y-labeled anti–CEA antibody in a CEA-producing tumor-bearing animal has been commenced.

MATERIALS AND METHODS

Tumor Cell Line

The LS174T cells, derived from a CEA-producing human colon cancer, were maintained in a monolayer culture in low-glucose Dulbecco's modified Eagle's medium and HAM's F-12 (1:1) containing 7.5% fetal calf serum, 1% glutamine, 1.5% HEPES buffer, and 100 000 U of penicillin-streptomycin (Irvine Scientific, Santa Ana, Calif). To prevent culture-induced phenotypic drift, cell cultures were restarted from frozen stock every three months. Using this technique, CEA production by the LS174T cell line, as measured by enzyme immunoassay (Roche Diagnostics, Nutley, NJ), was stable. Before inoculation, cells were washed with phosphate-buffered saline solution (PBSS)–0.1 mmol/L of edetic acid (EDTA), trypsinized with 0.25% trypsin, washed once in complete media, and resuspended to the appropriate concentration in PBSS.

Animal Model

Six-week-old female nu/nu BALB/c mice, weighing 20 to 25 g (University of California, San Diego), were maintained in a closed colony, as previously described.[4] Animals received an intraperitoneal (IP) injection of 0.2 mL of rabbit anti–mouse lymphocyte

Accepted for publication Nov 29, 1988.

From the Departments of General Oncologic Surgery (Drs Hyams, B. G. Beatty, and J. D. Beatty) and Anatomic Pathology (Dr Esteban), City of Hope National Medical Center, Duarte, Calif, and Hybritech Inc, San Diego (Mr Wanek).

Read before the Annual Meeting of the Society of Surgical Oncology, New Orleans, May 23, 1988.

Reprint requests to Department of General Oncologic Surgery, City of Hope National Medical Center, 1500 E Duarte Rd, Duarte, CA 91010 (Dr J. D. Beatty).

Dose Schedule	Treatment	No. of Animals Studied	No. (%) of Animals: Treatment Death	Disease Death	Survival, d: 25th Percentile	50th Percentile	75th Percentile	Mean ± SEM
No treatment	Control	39	0	39 (100)	27	26	24	25.9 ± 0.10
120 μCi, 1 cycle	Nonspecific	8	3 (37.5)	5 (62.5)	49	34	22	35.13 ± 7.90
	Specific	8	0	8 (100)	90	69	67	74.75 ± 6.69
120 μCi, 2 cycles every 2 wk	Nonspecific	12	4 (33.3)	8 (66.7)	54	36	25	37.08 ± 6.39
	Specific	12	1 (8.3)	11 (91.7)	80	76	67	72.67 ± 7.01
80 μCi, 3 cycles every 4 d	Nonspecific	8	8 (100)	0	23	22	22	22.25 ± 0.72
	Specific	8	3 (37.5)	5 (62.5)	48	43	31	40.00 ± 4.60

Toxicity and Survival Benefit of Yttrium 90–Labeled Antibody in Mice With Peritoneal Carcinomatosis of LS174T Xenografts*

*Control animals received no treatment; nonspecific treatment was with ^{90}Y-labeled 96.5c monoclonal antibody; and specific treatment was with ^{90}Y-labeled ZCE025 monoclonal antibody.

serum (cytotoxic titer, 1:6400; M. A. Bioproducts, Walkersville, Md). Simultaneously, 8×10^5 cells of LS174T were injected IP in 1 mL of PBSS. As described previously, random autopsy seven days after inoculation consistently demonstrated multiple macroscopic tumor nodules of 0.2 to 2 mm that lined that peritoneal surface.

Antibodies

The term ZCE025 refers to a murine IgG1 MAB directed to an epitope of CEA. The MAB, 96.5c, is a murine IgG2a with specificity for the p97 antigen of melanoma (Hybritech Inc, San Diego). Purification of ZCE025 and 96.5c, and labeling with ^{90}Y was accomplished through a modified proprietary diethylenetriamine pentaacetic acid technique.[3]

Each antibody dose was calibrated by making a 1:100 dilution of stock, radiolabeled MAB and counting 10 μL in 5 mL of aqueous counting scintillant. The ^{32}P channel of a liquid scintillation counter (Beckman LS150, Beckman Instruments, Fullerton, Calif) was used for each measurement. This channel was calibrated to a standard traceable to the National Bureau of Standards. Appropriate dilutions of the stock solution was made in PBSS. All of the antibody was used within 72 hours of preparation and diluted immediately before injection.

Therapeutic Regimen

Seven days after tumor inoculation, animals for each experiment were randomized into three groups that received either no therapy, therapy with nonspecific ^{90}Y-labeled MAB (96.5c), or therapy with ^{90}Y-labeled specific anti–CEA MAB (ZCE025). A 1-mL injection of radiolabeled MAB in PBSS was given IP to the animals in the treatment groups. Three different ^{90}Y-MAB treatment regimens were studied: one cycle of 120 μCi given on day 7, two cycles of 120 μCi given on days 7 and 21, and three cycles of 80 μCi given on days 7, 11, and 15. Radiolabeled MAB was administered with a specific activity of 30 μCi/μg. In the dose range used, unlabeled MAB had previously been shown to be nontherapeutic.

Animals were maintained four to a cage with ad libitum food and water. Deaths were recorded as they occurred, noting whether the death was due to treatment toxicity (treatment death) or malignant disease progression (disease death). Survival (treatment and disease deaths combined) was plotted using the Kaplan-Meier technique, while statistical analysis was accomplished using the generalized Wilcoxon method.

RESULTS

The animal model utilized was chosen for its reliability and reproducibility. Seven days after inoculation, animals undergoing random autopsy had multiple tumor nodules of 0.2 to 2.0 mm over the peritoneal surface. Each of these nodules consistently demonstrated the characteristic histologic pattern of a human adenocarcinoma, with exuberant CEA production as shown by immunohistochemical studies. Vascular ingrowth consistent with established tumor was readily seen. Furthermore, the pattern of spread mimicked the transperitoneal carcinomatosis of human colorectal tumor growth. As in humans, tumor growth resulted in the death of the animals.

A total of 39 animals served as concurrent no treatment controls. Mean survival ± SEM for these animals was 25.9 ± 1.0 days. Untreated tumor growth consistently resulted in ascites by days 16 to 18, bulky tumor by day 22, and death with hemorrhagic ascites by days 24 to 27. Tumor burdens appeared to be consistent with those seen in earlier studies (4 to 5 g). An examination of the tight clustering of the 25th, 50th, and 75th percentile "days of survival" demonstrates the consistency of the model (Table).

Our previous report demonstrated the greatest inhibition of tumor growth with doses of 120 and 160 μCi. However, 160 μCi of ^{90}Y-ZCE025 (specific treatment) also produced extensive depletion of bone marrow and treatment-associated death. Therefore, in the first series of these survival experiments, we examined the effect of 120 μCi of ^{90}Y-labeled MAB given as a single dose. There was a significant ($P<.001$) prolongation of the mean survival to 35.1 ± 7.9 days with nonspecific therapy. With the specific anti–CEA radioconjugate, a much longer mean survival of 74.8 ± 6.7 days was documented ($P<.001$). Kaplan-Meier plots demonstrating this effect on Fig 1 show an increased life span of 165%. Postmortem examination of animals allowed identification of the cause of death, whether due to disease or treatment. Animals with empty bone marrows, depleted spleens, and minimal tumor were classified as treatment deaths. Animals with extensive tumor growth were considered to be disease deaths, irrespective of the hematologic status. Treatment death was significant (3/8, 37.5%) in the animals that received 120 μCi of ^{90}Y-labeled nonspecific MAB (96.5c). No toxic deaths were noted in the animals treated with the specific MAB (ZCE025) that was labeled with 120 μCi of ^{90}Y.

Pilot investigations of a single 120-μCi dose of MAB demonstrated that the bone marrow depletion was greatest during the first week after injection of the radionuclide. Recovery was 80% of control appearance by 14 to 21 days. Therefore, we felt that a second dose of equal activity, aimed at eliminating any residual tumor, might be tolerated satisfactorily 14 days after the initial therapeutic dose. With the 120-μCi two-cycle regimen (total dose, 240 μCi), the survival advantage of nonspecific (mean ± SEM = 37.1 ± 6.4 days) over no treatment, and specific (mean ± SEM = 72.7 ± 7.0 days) over nonspecific treatment were again significant ($P<.001$) (Fig 2). Although the specific treatment group had an increased life span of 192%, the survival advantage for the two-cycle regimen compared with the single-dose regimen was not significant.

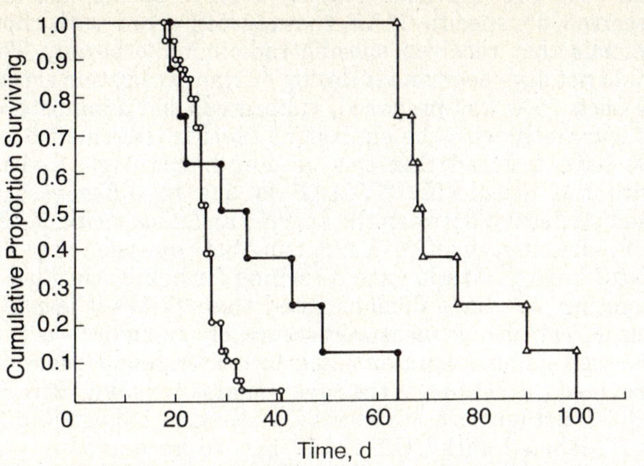

Fig 1.—Comparison of specific treatment (open triangles, 120 μCi for one dose) with identical dose regimen of nonspecific treatment (closed circles) and untreated control animals (open circles).

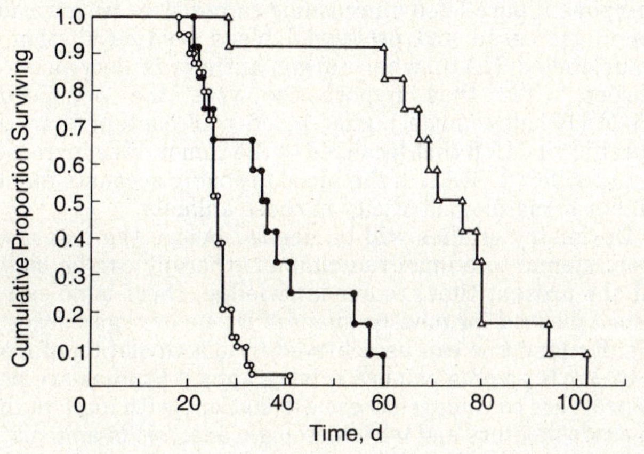

Fig 2.—Comparison of specific treatment (open triangles, 120 μCi every two weeks for two doses) with identical dose regimen of nonspecific treatment (closed circles) and untreated control animals (open circles).

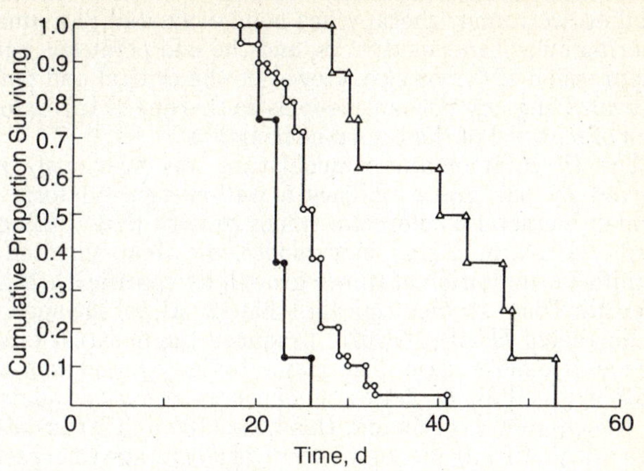

Fig 3.—Comparison of specific treatment (open triangles, 80 μCi every four days for three doses) with identical dose regimen of nonspecific treatment (closed circles) and untreated control animals (open circles).

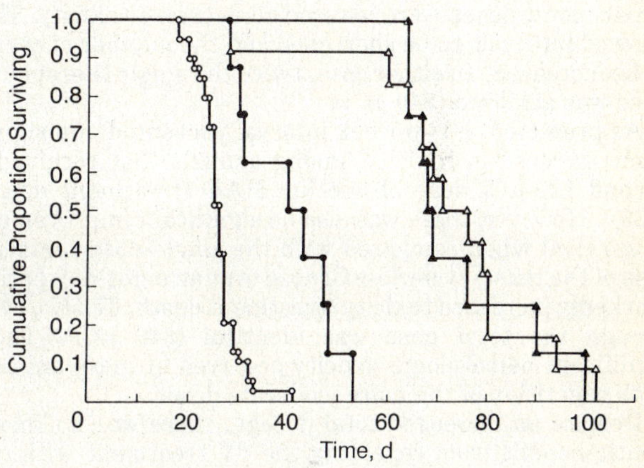

Fig 4.—Comparison of all specific treatment regimens (closed triangles, 120 μCi for one dose; open triangles, 120 μCi every two weeks for two doses; closed circles, 80 μCi every four days for three doses) with untreated control animals (open circles).

Toxicity (treatment death) was marginally increased to 33.3% (4/12) for animals that received nonspecific MAB therapy (96.5c) and 8.3% (1/12) for animals that received specific MAB therapy (ZCE025) by the 120-μCi two-cycle regimen (Table).

The final experiments examined more frequent administration of lower doses of ^{90}Y-MAB. This regimen was designed to accomplish a higher dose of ^{90}Y-MAB over a shorter period of time without increase of toxicity. The schedule consisted of 80 μCi of ^{90}Y-labeled MAB administered every four days for three cycles (days 7, 11, and 15), to a total activity of 240 μCi. This three-cycle regimen resulted in a marked increase in toxicity without the survival benefit of the previous regimens. Toxicity accounted for 100% (8/8) of the deaths among animals that received nonspecific ^{90}Y-MAB (96.5c) treatment (Table). Indeed, survival among untreated controls (mean ± SEM = 25.9 ± 1.0 days) was significantly better ($P<.001$) than survival of animals that received nonspecific MAB (mean ± SEM = 22.3 ± 0.7 days) (Fig 3). Toxicity accounted for 37.5% (3/8) of the deaths among animals that received specific ^{90}Y-MAB (ZCE025) treatment. While survival of all animals that received specific radioimmunotherapy (mean ± SEM = 40 ± 4.5 days) was significantly better ($P<.001$) than that of untreated tumor-bearing animals (increased life span, 65%), it was significantly poorer ($P<.001$) than that of animals that received specific therapy in either of the two preceding regimens (Fig 4).

It should be noted that all animals in this study that did not die as a result of treatment toxicity did eventually die of disease progression. No animal was "cured" of disease.

COMMENT

Since the time of their development, MABS have been proposed as antitumor agents by a number of authors.[5-7] They have since been tested in animals and humans, with a variety of conjugates designed to identify or treat malignant tumors.[8-10] While the clinical utility of MABs for radiolocalization already shows promise,[11] their greatest potential is for clinical cancer treatment.[12] A variety of studies have demonstrated a specific antineoplastic effect of tumor-directed radiolabeled MABs.[13,14] In most of these studies, antitumor therapy has been evaluated in animals bearing subcutaneous tumors, and the end point has been suppression of tumor size. However, the critical end point in evaluating any new antineoplastic therapy is the extension of survival of the tumor-bearing host.

The IP carcinomatosis model that was previously reported by our group[3] mimics a well-recognized form of human metastatic colorectal tumor growth that routinely leads to death. Using this model, we demonstrated a significant inhibition of tumor growth by specific ^{90}Y-MAB therapy. Those studies indicated that 120 μCi of the specific radiolabeled MAB (ZCE025) produced the greatest effectiveness-toxicity ratio. The major toxicity noted was hematologic cellular depletion of bone marrow and the spleen. In the current experiment, this dose (120 μCi) translated into a dramatically increased survival advantage (increased life span, 165%). In most human colon cancer xenograft experiments, an increased life span of 30% for systemic chemotherapy is considered to be very good.

Multiple-dosing schemes were investigated to determine whether residual tumor could be eradicated and survival could be further enhanced. In the 120-μCi two-cycle experiment, intervals were chosen that would allow significant bone marrow recovery. In the 80-μCi three-cycle experiment, doses were lowered to decrease toxicity. This allowed intervals to be shortened and the number of cycles to be increased. In either case, twice the single therapeutic dose was achieved (240 μCi).

As predicted, a two-week interval prevented any significant increase in toxicity among animals that received a second 120-μCi dose of specific MAB (treatment death, 8.3%). However, there was also no significant improvement in survival when compared with the single-dose regimen. Use of the three-cycle 80-μCi dose over an eight-day period markedly increased toxicity (treatment death, 37.5%), even though the total dose was identical (240 μCi). Thus, significant hematologic toxicity occurred in these animals with repetition of the more moderate doses.

Despite an increased total dosage, there was no therapeutic benefit from repeating the ^{90}Y treatment with the specific MAB once, or even twice. Histopathologic studies in our laboratory, stimulated by the failure of the multiple-dose regimens to increase survival, have shown that the tumor, which regrows after ^{90}Y-MAB treatment, does not express CEA.[15] This loss of CEA expression may be due to clonal selection or antigenic modulation. Further studies are in progress to understand the cause of this change of antigen expression. However, the immediate therapeutic implication of the loss of CEA in ^{90}Y-MAB–treated LS174T tumor is that higher first-treatment doses of ^{90}Y-MAB will need to be administered. Examination of higher ^{90}Y-MAB doses will necessitate hematologic support (eg, bone marrow transplantation) to counteract the hematologic toxicity.

One interesting finding, consistent in all of our studies, has been the increased toxicity seen in all animals that received nonspecific MAB therapy compared with those animals that received specific radioimmunotherapy. This could not have been due to dosing or standardization errors, as each dose was prepared, calibrated, and administered concurrently with the equivalent specific treatment dose. We have deduced that this greater hematologic toxicity with the nonspecific ^{90}Y-MAB is due to differences in biodistribution between the specific and nonspecific MAB.

Biodistribution of ^{90}Y-MAB using beta emission requires tissue homogenization and bleaching for liquid scintillation counting. We have demonstrated that ^{90}Y-MAB levels in tissues can also be measured accurately and more easily in the well gamma counter using bremsstrahlung emission, provided the volume in the tube remains constant (B.G.B., 1986). Furthermore, we have shown that the biodistribution of ^{90}Y-labeled anti–CEA MAB that we have used is very similar to the biodistribution of indium 111–labeled anti–CEA MAB (B.G.B., 1986). Published biodistribution studies from our laboratory have demonstrated an inverse correlation between the tumor uptake, expressed as percent injected dose per gram, and the tumor size when specific ^{111}In-labeled anti–CEA antibody was administered.[16] A concomitant increase in the ^{111}In-MAB blood pool component paralleled diminishing tumor size. We have also found increased and prolonged blood pool circulation of radiolabeled MAB, when target antigen is decreased or absent.[17] We thus hypothesize that the nonspecific ^{90}Y-MAB had a much higher blood pool content than the specific ^{90}Y-MAB that localized to the tumor. This increased nonspecific ^{90}Y-MAB in the blood probably accounts for the higher hematologic toxicity in these animals.

Dosimetry studies will be needed before the transition from animal to human radioimmunotherapy can be made. At the present time, to our knowledge, there is no established method for measurement of tissue or organ doses of ^{90}Y. Estimations can be achieved by extrapolation of from ^{111}In-MAB gamma camera scintigraphy.[18] Studies are now in progress to compare these estimations with implantable microdosimeters and with histologic analysis in animals.

In these animal studies, we have demonstrated that anti–CEA antibodies, labeled with ^{90}Y, can kill human colon cancer cells and that they can dramatically extend survival. With continued careful studies of labeled antibody dosing, biodistribution, and tissue interaction, this modality has the potential to be an effective contributor in the management of patients with colon cancer.

This study was supported in part by a grant from the Margaret Early Foundation, Los Angeles; by Health Training Grant CA 09477, Cancer Center Core Grant CA 33572, and Program Project Grant CA 43904 from the National Institutes of Health, Bethesda, Md; and by a grant from Hybritech Inc, San Diego.

The authors wish to thank Robert Hill, PhD, Department of Biostatistics, City of Hope National Medical Center, Duarte, Calif, for his kind assistance and statistical review.

References

1. Cobb LM, Humm JL: Radioimmunotherapy of malignancy using antibody targeted radionuclides. *Br J Cancer* 1986;54:863-870.

2. Schlom J, Weeks MO: Potential clinical utility of monoclonal antibodies in the management of human carcinomas, in DeVita VT, Hellman S, Rosenberg SA (eds): *Important Advances in Oncology 1985*. Philadelphia, JB Lippincott Co, 1985, chap 9.

3. Hyams DM, Esteban JM, Lollo CP, et al: Therapy of peritoneal carcinomatosis of human colon cancer xenografts with yttrium 90–labeled anti-carcinoembryonic antigen antibody ZCE025. *Arch Surg* 1987;122:1333-1337.

4. Giovanella BC, Stehlin JS: Heterotransplantation of human malignant tumors in 'nude' athymic mice: I. Breeding and maintenance of 'nude' mice. *JNCI* 1973;51:615-619.

5. Schlom J: Basic principles and applications of monoclonal antibodies in the management of carcinomas: The Richard and Hinda Rosenthal Foundation award lecture. *Cancer Res* 1986;46:3225-3238.

6. Baldwin RW, Byers VS: Monoclonal antibodies in cancer treatment. *Lancet* 1986;1:603-605.

7. Larson SM, Carrasquillo JA, Reynolds JC: Radioimmunodetection and radioimmunotherapy. *Cancer Invest* 1984;2:363-381.

8. Begent RH: Recent advances in tumor imaging: Use of radiolabelled antitumor antibodies. *Biochim Biophys Acta* 1985;780:151-166.

9. Freeman AI, Mayhew E: Targeted drug delivery. *Cancer* 1986;58(suppl 2):573-583.

10. Thorpe PE, Brown AN Bremner JA Jr, et al: An immunotoxin composed of monoclonal anti-Thy 1.1 antibody and a ribosome-inactivating

protein from *Saponaria officinalis:* Potent antitumor effects in vitro and in vivo. *JNCI* 1985;75:151-159.
11. Beatty JD, Hyams DM, Morton BA, et al: Impact of radiolabeled antibody imaging on management of colon cancer. *Am J Surg,* in press.
12. Rosen ST, Zimmer AM, Goldman-Leikin R, et al: Radioimmunodetection and radioimmunotherapy of cutaneous T cell lymphomas using an ^{131}I-labeled monoclonal antibody: An Illinois Cancer Council Study. *J Clin Oncol* 1987;5:562-573.
13. Esteban JM, Schlom J, Mornex F, et al: Radioimmunotherapy of athymic mice bearing human colon carcinomas with monoclonal antibody B72.3: Histological and autoradiographic study of effects on tumors and normal organs. *Eur J Cancer Clin Oncol* 1987;23:643-655.
14. Anderson-Berg WT, Squire RA, Strand M: Specific radioimmunotherapy using ^{90}Y-labeled monoclonal antibody in erythroleukemic mice. *Cancer Res* 1987;47:1905-1912.
15. Esteban JM, Hyams DM, Beatty BG, et al: Effect of ^{90}Y-labeled anti-CEA monoclonal antibody on the morphology and phenotype of human tumors grown as peritoneal carcinomatosis in athymic mice. *Cancer Res,* in press.
16. Philben VJ, Jakowatz JG, Beatty BG, et al: The effect of tumor CEA content and tumor size on tissue uptake of indium 111–labeled anti-CEA monoclonal antibody. *Cancer* 1986;57:571-576.
17. Jakowatz JG, Beatty BG, Vlahos WG, et al: High-specific-activity ^{111}In-labeled anticarcinoembryonic antigen monoclonal antibody: Biodistribution and imaging in nude mice bearing human colon cancer xenografts. *Cancer Res* 1985;45:5700-5706.
18. Williams LE, Beatty BG, Beatty JD, et al: Estimation of administered Y-90 activity needed to achieve certain tumor radiation doses in colorectal cancer patients. *Cancer Res,* in press.

Discussion

Q The first question that I was going to ask is about the yttrium itself. What is the distance of effective radiation? Is it a very short distance?

A Yttrium is a high-energy beta emitter that emits approximately 80% of its radiation over a 3-mm distance. However, for 100% of the beta radiation, you have to go out to almost 1 cm, which is a difficult problem in a small mouse model. As you increase the dose of yttrium that you want to use for tumor control, you increase the toxicity to other areas of the animal.

Q That would be one thing that you could modify, because you could use another radioisotope, depending on what kind of model you are going to treat. For example, I do not know how iodine 125 stacks up with ^{90}Y. I imagine it must be shorter, but I am not sure about that.

A Well, iodine 131 is probably a better alternative. One of the advantages of ^{90}Y is that its path length is excellent for human use, which is, of course, the ultimate aim of the studies. All of the animal studies of radioconjugates directed against human tumor markers are somewhat crippled by the need to use a human tumor. Right now, there are no models using large animals in which you can use human tumor xenografts.

Q The second question that I had refers to antigenic modulation; at least, this is implied by the altered immunohistology after ^{90}Y therapy. Did you get the same thing in vitro with this line? Have you tried incubating with unlabeled monoclonal antibody because it is a little surprising that you had such a distinct loss of CEA after ^{90}Y therapy?

A Actually many authors have described changes in antigen expression after therapy. We have not done the in vitro studies that you suggest, but we are interested in studies that will help to distinguish between antigenic modulation and clonal selection.

Q In exactly the same tumor model with the nude mice, using the same cell line, our experience with treating them with adoptive immunotherapy with human monocytes and gamma interferon, was that a lot of the nude mice would waste away, whereas other nude mice would develop bulky IP tumor masses. So, we would see two different patterns of mortality. I am very surprised by the nice curves that you have. They start dying in the most effective treatment group, around day 80, and they are all dead by day 100. It is very surprising that you did not see any cures. Apparently, your animal facilities must be very good, because to keep them out for 80 days under these conditions is already good. However, did you see the two different patterns of dying? I ask this because the animals that wasted away practically had no tumor at all, but they still died. So, what is the cause of dying? Did you perform autopsies on all your animals?

A Autopsies were performed whenever feasible. In this study, we did not see many animals waste away. The early deaths of animals with minimal tumor we attributed to radiation toxicity. In other studies in animals without tumor, we see the same effect with toxic doses of radiation; the animals waste away. They get thin and scrawny, and they die.

Regarding the absence of cures, we share your concern. We have tried to decrease the number of cells to get a longer living model, so that we would have more time for bone marrow recovery and could give subsequent doses, but we have found that we get less consistent tumor growth. With 800 000 cells, we have a highly consistent tumor on repetitive trials, but the rate of tumor growth is very rapid. Perhaps this explains the absence of cures.

In Other AMA Journals

ARCHIVES OF INTERNAL MEDICINE

The 'Do Not Resuscitate' Order: A Profile of Its Changing Use

Palmi V. Jonsson, MD; Michael McNamee, MD; Edward W. Campion, MD

The "do not resuscitate" (DNR) order has wide-ranging ethical, legal, and economic implications. We reviewed the course of 244 patients who died during two three-month periods, in 1982 and 1986. We found that 68% of patients who died had a DNR order written, including 94% with malignancy and half of patients with cardiovascular disease. Most orders (61%) were written within three days of death, with 64% written on medical-surgical floors and 34% in critical care units. Even among patients under the age of 60 years, 57% had a DNR order written by the time of death. Ninety-one percent of DNR orders were written by attending physicians, with accompanying explanatory note in 84%. Documentation showed only 14% of patients but 77% of families being consulted. In 1983 a new two-level DNR order system defined two levels of intensity: "all but cardiopulmonary resuscitation" and "comfort measures only." Equal numbers of patients received each order in the 1986 sample. No patient was transferred to the critical care units after a DNR order had been written. The prevalence of DNR orders written for patients dying of cardiovascular disease increased from 27% to 64% over the four years. We conclude, from study of deaths in this representative community hospital, that an explicit DNR order is now the rule rather than the exception, but decisions are made late and involve family far more than the patient (*Arch Intern Med* 1988;148:2373-2375).

Reprint requests to Hebrew Rehabilitation Center for the Aged, 1200 Center St, Roslindale, MA 02131 (Dr Jonsson).

Survival of Patients With Stage B2 Colon Carcinoma

The Gastrointestinal Tumor Study Group Experience

Russell Nauta, MD; Donald M. Stablein, PhD; E. Douglas Holyoke, MD

• The Gastrointestinal Tumor Study Group, a multispecialty collaborative clinical research program, executed two studies of surgically resected colon carcinoma, including patients with serosal penetration but no positive regional lymph nodes (stage B2). In the first study, 232 patients with stage B2 disease were operated on and survival was unaffected by therapy. In the stage B2 group, survival was 78% at five years, and is estimated to be 64% ten years after surgery. A second study, begun in 1979, compared survival and recurrence data on patients who underwent surgical resection and were treated postoperatively with fluorouracil and hepatic irradiation vs those who were observed. Hematologic toxicity of the regimen and accumulation of data from the first study caused the termination of randomization of patients with stage B2 disease with continued registration to observation only. One hundred twenty-four untreated patients with stage B2 carcinoma had a five-year survival rate of 77%, confirming the relatively high survival of this group of patients who are treated with surgery alone. Our patients' five-year survival of 78% corresponds favorably to the 87% survival rate anticipated in an age-, sex-, and race-matched cohort of Americans not specifically diagnosed as having cancer. Adjuvant trials, in seeking improved survival, should recognize that our review of 356 patients implies a considerably higher-than-anticipated five-year survival for the patient with stage B2 disease who undergoes surgical resection. Toxicity of the marginally effective agents currently available and the large numbers of patients necessary to demonstrate an advantage in a treatment arm suggests that patients with stage B2 disease should be excluded from many adjuvant trials of colon cancer treatments.

(*Arch Surg* 1989;124:180-182)

All staging systems for colorectal carcinoma attempt to group patients with similar prognoses based on symptomatology, metastatic behavior, or mural growth patterns.[1] Such systems quantifying the depth of wall penetration of the primary tumor and the presence or absence of nodal metastases do so to determine whether these morphologic characteristics alter prognosis.

The treatment of established metastatic disease with chemotherapy in patients with colon cancer has not been demonstrated to prolong survival and such therapies usually have substantial toxicity. To offer experimental, marginally effective modalities as adjuvant treatment one is obliged to test a population at high risk to justify the toxicity of the therapy.

PATIENTS AND METHODS

Patients

The Gastrointestinal Tumor Study Group, a collaborative research organization sponsored by the Clinical Therapy Evaluation Program of the Division of Cancer Treatment, National Cancer Institute, Bethesda, Md, in 1975 began a study to compare the effects of no postoperative therapy, chemotherapy, immunotherapy, and a combination of chemotherapy and immunotherapy in patients with surgically resected colonic cancer with either serosal penetration (stage B2) or involved regional lymph nodes (stage C). The results of this protocol, GI 6175, failed to substantiate significant treatment differences, but disclosed a 78% survival after five years in patients with stage B2 disease.[2] In 1979, protocol GI 6179 began the accrual of patients who were prospectively randomized in a phase III clinical trial designed to compare combined therapy of hepatic irradiation and fluorouracil chemotherapy with a surgery-only control arm. As in the previous study, all patients had undergone potentially curative surgery with en bloc resection and negative resection margins for stage B2 or stage C colon cancers. Patients entering the study were required to have histologic proof of a colon cancer extending either through the serosa or pericolonic fat or to have positive nodes. Patients were randomly assigned to a control arm or to a combined radiotherapy/chemotherapy arm.

Because of toxicity, several reductions in protocol therapy were required.[3] On Dec 31, 1981, a treatment-related death in this study was reported, and combined with the good survival results of the patients with stage B2 disease in the prior study, we decided to exclude any more patients with stage B2 disease from therapy.

In an effort to substantiate the survival experience of patients with stage B2 disease who were observed in the first study, an additional series of 100 patients with stage B2 disease were registered and assigned to the surgery-only arm of the study.

Methods

Survival experience from all eligible patients with stage B2 disease (surgically resected colon cancer with penetration of the serosa and negative regional lymph nodes) in protocol GI 6175 and untreated patients in protocol GI 6179 with stage B2 disease was collected and analyzed. Product-limit estimates of survival distributions were calculated and log-rank tests of equality of survival curves were performed. Expected survival was calculated annually

Patient Characteristics by Protocol*

	Protocol		
	GI 6175 (n=232)	GI 6179 (n=124)	Total (N=356)
Sex, % male	61	56	59
Age, %			
≤50	12	15	13
51-60	25	29	26
61-70	44	29	39
>70	19	27	22
No. of nodes examined ≥10, %	48	56	51
Stage, contiguous organ involvement (stage B3), %	20	22	21
Median follow-up of survivors, y	9.5	4.1	8.5

*See text for explanation of protocols.

Accepted for publication Nov 1, 1988.

From the Department of Surgery, Georgetown University, Washington, DC (Dr Nauta); and the Surgical Oncology Department, Roswell Park Memorial Institute, Buffalo, NY (Dr Holyoke). Dr Stablein is with the EMMES Corp, Potomac, Md.

Read before the Annual Meeting of the Society of Surgical Oncology, New Orleans, May 23, 1988.

Reprint requests to GITSG Statistical Center, The EMMES Corp, 11325 Seven Locks Rd, Suite 214, Potomac, MD 20854 (Dr Stabelin).

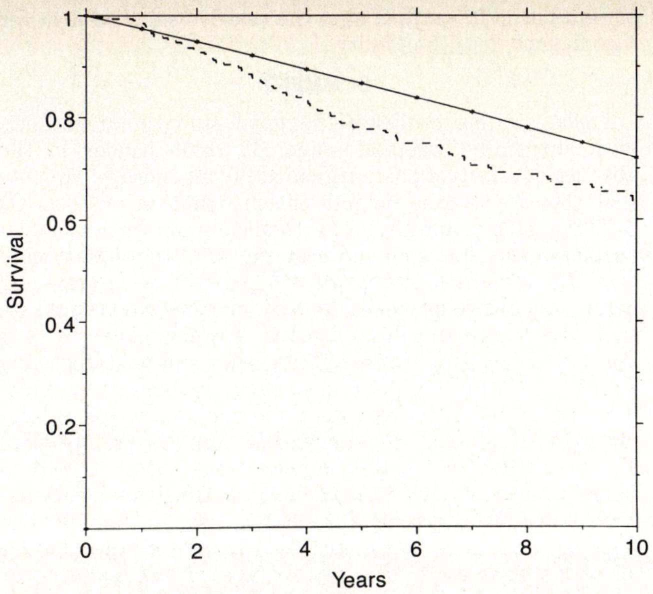

Fig 1.—Broken line represents survival of patients with stage B2 colon cancer in protocol groups GI 6175 and GI 6179 combined. Solid line represents survival of age, sex, and race-matched controls.

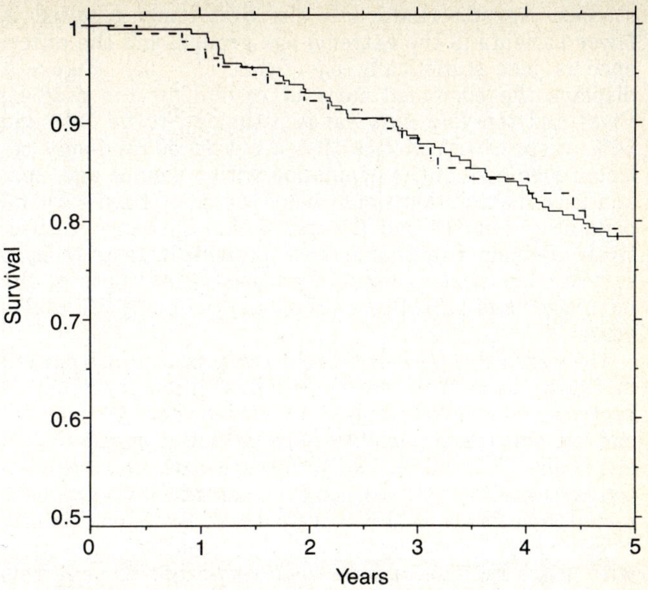

Fig 2.—Survival experience of patients with stage B2 colon cancer patients. Solid line represents protocol group GI 6175; broken line, group GI 6179.

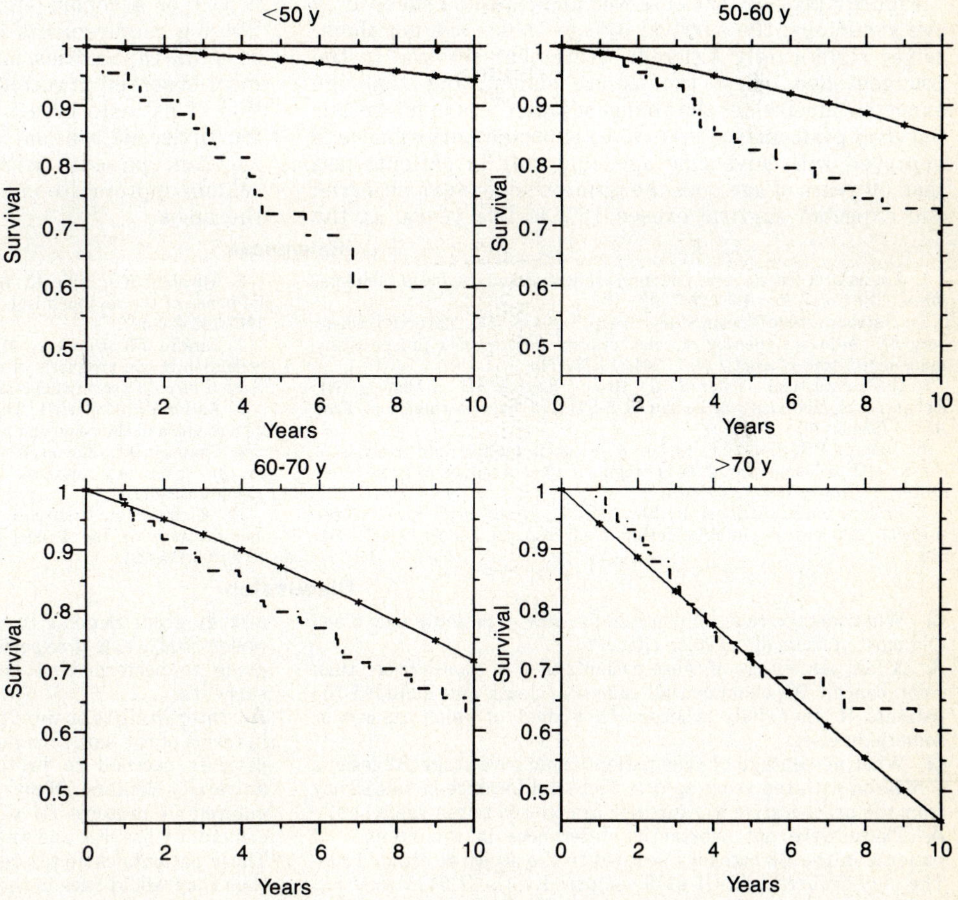

Fig 3.—Observed (broken line) and expected (solid line) survival by age groupings in protocol groups GI 6175 and GI 6179.

for cohorts with identical age, sex, and race distribution using the Cancer Survival System software developed by the End Results Section of the National Cancer Institute. Relative survival is the ratio of observed actuarial survival to the expected survival of a cohort of randomly selected subjects with identical age, sex, and race composition.

RESULTS

The Table displays the characteristics of the 356 patients analyzed in this report. Sex, the number of pathologically negative nodes reported, and the percentage of patients with contiguous organ involvement were similar in the two studies. Age distribution in the first study resulted in fewer patients in the extreme age groups, and the difference is just statistically significant ($P=.05$). Figure 1 displays the combined survival results for the studies. Five- and ten-year survival is estimated to be 78% and 64%, respectively. Notice that a cohort of randomly selected members of the population with a similar age, sex, and race distribution would be expected to have survival percentages of 87% and 72% at five and ten years, respectively. Beyond five years, these patients appear to have survival identical to randomly selected members of the population and have an excess mortality of only 9% at five years.

The survival experiences of the two protocols are plotted in Fig 2. Note that, since the follow-up on the GI 6179 protocol is not as long, only the first five years are plotted, and the survival probabilities are plotted from 0.5 to 1 to emphasize differences. No differences are observed between these two studies, as five-year survivals are estimated to be 78% and 77% in protocols GI 6175 and GI 6179, respectively. Thus, the first study's results for patients with stage B2 disease have been replicated through this time period. We have further examined sex, number of nodes examined, and contiguous organ involvement. None was statistically significant, although a large number of negative nodes and the lack of other organs involved were both protective.

Figure 3 provides the observed and expected survival by age groupings; the survival by age values are not themselves significantly different. Note that survival in the youngest and oldest groups are similar, but that the expected survival for the youngest patients is much better. Survival performance relative to expected performance is improved with advancing age, and only in patients less than 50 years of age does the difference between observed and expected survival exceed 12% at five years. In the patients over 70 years of age, the relative survival is never significantly less than unity.

COMMENT

These studies replicate the good survival of patients with surgically resected stage B2 colon cancer in the absence of effective postsurgical adjuvant therapy. We note that this is the case despite the inclusion in protocol GI 6179 of a larger number of participating institutions and a surgical base that included academic and community centers. Long-term follow-up of 356 patients with stage B2 carcinoma in two prospective randomized studies suggests that the survival achieved with surgery alone is only approximately 10% worse at five years and is statistically similar to that of the general population thereafter. While it is recognized that treatment and control groups did not differ with respect to survival in the Gastrointestinal Tumor Study Group, it is demonstrated after a median follow-up of 8.5 years that the overall survival of patients with stage B2 cancer is 78% at five years. This survival does not appear to be extensively affected by the number of nodes examined, the sex or age of the patient, or contiguous organ invasion. In historical series, rather than among trial participants, other authors[4-9] have reported five-year survivals ranging from 52% to 85%, while the National Surgical Adjuvant Breast and Bowel Project reported a 70% five-year survival rate in a preliminary report of a cohort of patients with stage B2 disease.[10] Staging requirements for trial entry, along with modern scanning capabilities, may account for much of the improvement observed in recent studies. With the possible exception of patients presenting with stage B2 disease in the fourth decade, we conclude that, because of their excellent survival, patients with stage B2 colon carcinoma are seldom appropriate candidates for adjuvant trials of toxic therapies.

References

1. Zinkin D: A critical review of the classification and staging of colorectal cancer. *Dis Colon Rect* 1983;26:37-43.
2. Gastrointestinal Tumor Study Group, Lessner HE, Mayer RJ, Ellenberg SS: Adjuvant therapy of colon cancer: Results of a prospectively randomized trial. *N Engl J Med* 1984;310:737-743.
3. Gastrointestinal Tumor Study Group, Kaplan RS, Steinberg SM: Enhanced myelotoxicity of combined 5-FU and hepatic radiation. *Proc ASCO* 1984;3:557.
4. Chapuis PH, Dent OF, Fisher R, et al: A multivariate analysis of clinical and pathologic variables in prognosis after resection of large bowel cancer. *Br J Surg* 1985;72:698-702.
5. Phillips RKS, Hittinger R, Blesovsky L, et al: Large bowel cancer surgical pathology and its relationship to survival. *Br J Surg* 1984;71:604-610.
6. Turnbull RB, Kyle K, Watson FR, et al: Cancer of the colon: The influence of the no touch isolation technique on survival rates. *Ann Surg* 1967;166:420-427.
7. Kirklin JW, Dockerty MB, Waugh JM: The role of the peritoneal reflection in the prognosis of carcinoma of the rectum and sigmoid colon. *Surg Gynecol Obstet* 1949;88:326-331.
8. Astler VB, Coller FA: The prognostic significance of direct extension of carcinoma of the colon and rectum. *Ann Surg* 1954;139:846-851.
9. Simpson WC, Mayo CW: The mural penetration of the carcinoma cell in the colon: An anatomic and clinical study. *Surg Gynecol Obstet* 1939;61:872-877.
10. Wolmark N, Fisher B, Wieand HS: The prognostic value of the modifications of the Dukes' C class of colorectal cancer. *Ann Surg* 1986;203:115-121.

Discussion

Q What was the cause of death in the 25% of patients who died? Did most of them die of colon cancer?

A A fair percentage of these patients died of causes other than colon cancer. We examined all causes of death and included the patients in the study whether they died of colon cancer or something else.

Q What percentage of your patients now have stage B2 lesions compared with ten years ago? Is there a difference in selectivity from the preoperative workup now, as opposed to ten years ago?

A There were not substantial differences in the number of patients in the B2 category accrued to the study at either time. The only difference in GI 6179 compared with GI 6175 was that we recognized that the patients with stage B2 disease appeared to be doing well and had some treatment-related toxicity; we ultimately elected in the latter study to register all of the patients with stage B2 disease rather than randomize them to therapy or no therapy.

Q Why did your patients do so well? The control group always does better than what has been generally reported. Does the quality of the initial surgical procedure have something to do with it? Obviously, any surgeon who is interested enough to be part of a study group is going to have a special interest in the neoplasm under study, and if experience means anything, that surgeon is going to perform that particular operation better than most surgeons.

A Interesting to us were the differences between the two studies in terms of the surgeons performing the procedures. Many of the patients accrued to protocol GI 6175 were accrued through university centers. Many of the patients who were ultimately entered in protocol GI 6179 were entered after surgery in a community hospital and were referred by their medical oncologist. These patients came to protocol GI 6179 by a more diverse route than they would have in the first study. Despite that, the survival curves for patients with stage B2 disease in the two studies are virtually impossible. We looked for variables to explain why our patients did better than others have reported, but found nothing.

Q Was there increased long-term morbidity in the group that received hepatic irradiation?

A The amount of radiation delivered, which was approximately 21 Gy, did not result in extraordinary toxicity. Therapy-related deaths were not related to radiation hepatitis, but to leukopenia.

Interactions of Human Colorectal Carcinoma Cells With Basement Membranes

Analysis and Correlation With Differentiation

George W. Daneker, Jr, MD; Andrew J. Piazza; Glenn D. Steele, Jr, MD, PhD; Arthur M. Mercurio, PhD

• The abilities of colorectal carcinoma cell lines to adhere and invade through a basement membrane were examined. The four poorly differentiated cell lines studied were three to four times more adherent and spread to a greater extent following adherence to a basement membrane matrix than the three moderately well-differentiated (MWD) lines. One exception was the MWD cell line DLD-2, whose histologic features resembled a signet ring carcinoma. The ability of these cells to invade through a basement membrane model was measured. This assay showed that the poorly differentiated cell lines as well as DLD-2 were three times more invasive than the remaining MWD cell lines. These data indicate that tumor cell adherence can be correlated with invasion through basement membranes. In addition, the ability of colorectal carcinoma cells to interact with the basement membrane seems, in general, to be inversely related to the degree of cytodifferentiation.

(*Arch Surg* 1989;124:183-187)

A correlation between the histologic grade and the clinical behavior of colorectal carcinomas has long been appreciated.[1] Poorly differentiated tumors are observed to have a more advanced stage at diagnosis, an earlier progression to metastasis, and a poorer prognosis per stage than moderately well-differentiated tumors.[2,3] This correlation has recently been confirmed in a multi-institutional study by the Gastrointestinal Tumor Study Group.[4] While the relationship between tumor grade and clinical behavior has been well documented, the cellular properties related to differentiation that determine biological behavior are not well understood.

One biological property that merits close examination is the interaction of carcinoma cells with the extracellular matrix or, more specifically, the basement membrane.[5-7] The adherence of these cells to basement membrane components has been proposed to be an initiating step in the processes of tumor invasion and subsequent metastases.[8,9] Adherence may also induce or modulate cellular functions, such as synthesis and secretion of degradative enzymes, and it may promote cell motility.[10,11]

Carcinoma cells adhere to basement membranes by receptor-mediated mechanisms that involve receptor binding to the glycoprotein laminin.[5-7] In a previous study, we analyzed the ability of human colorectal carcinoma cell lines to interact with this basement membrane component.[12] The results of this study demonstrated that the interaction of colorectal carcinoma cells with laminin varied according to the degree of cytodifferentiation. Poorly differentiated cell lines were able to adhere and spread on laminin to a substantially greater extent than moderately well-differentiated lines. Both adherence and spreading were shown to be mediated by a peptide sequence in the laminin molecule that is recognized by a specific cell surface receptor.[13]

In our study, we expanded the scope of our observations from cellular interactions with purified basement membrane components to interactions with an intact basement membrane. A murine sarcoma basement membrane preparation, matrigel, was used in these experiments as a basement membrane model.[14] Matrigel contains all the components of intact basement membranes, and it is able to form a solid basement membrane matrix in vitro. Initially, the ability of established colorectal carcinoma cell lines to adhere and spread on matrigel was determined. We then measured the ability of these cells to adhere, penetrate, and then migrate through a matrigel barrier in response to a soluble attractant. Finally, these data were compared with data from an assay measuring cell migration in response to soluble attractants in the absence of matrigel.

MATERIALS AND METHODS

Cell Lines

Human colorectal carcinoma cell lines that were initiated from tumor tissue and are now established in serial subculture were used. CCL 222, CCL 228, CCL 235, CCL 238,[15] Clone A, and DLD-2 were used.[16,17] CX-1 was isolated from the cell line HT-29 at the National Institutes of Health, Bethesda, Md. MIP 101 was also used.[18] Cells were routinely maintained in 45% RPMI 1640 and 45% Dulbecco's modification of Eagle's essential medium (DMEM) supplemented with 10% fetal bovine serum (FBS), 1% L-glutamine, streptomycin sulfate (50 μg/mL), and penicillin G potassium (50 U/mL). Confluent cultures were subcultured by detachment with 0.1% trypsin–0.5 mmol/L of edetic acid in phosphate-buffered saline (PBS) for five minutes at 37°C. This suspension was replated at a density that yielded single cells in a logarithmic growth phase for their use in the assays described below. The cell lines were subcultured at least 24 to 48 hours before these assays were performed. Cells were routinely screened for mycoplasmal DNA by staining with Hoescht stain 33258 and were determined to be free of mycoplasmal contamination on this basis.

Accepted for publication Oct 14, 1988.

From the Laboratory of Cancer Biology, New England Deaconess Hospital, and Harvard Medical School, Boston. Dr Daneker is now with the University of Cincinnati Medical Center.

Read before the Annual Meeting of the Society of Surgical Oncology, New Orleans, May 24, 1988.

Reprint requests to Department of Surgery, University of Cincinnati Medical Center, ML 558, 231 Bethesda Ave, Cincinnati, OH 45267 (Dr Daneker).

Preparation of Matrigel

The basement membrane extract matrigel was prepared from Englebreth-Holm-Swarm sarcoma.[14] The sarcoma was grown as allografts in C57/BL16 mice. After harvesting, the tumor tissue was washed in 3.4 mol/L of sodium chloride and 0.05 mol/L of Tris hydrochloride (HCl), pH 7.4, containing protease inhibitors. The tissue was extracted with 2.0 mol/L of urea and 0.05 mol/L of Tris HCl, pH 7.4 (1 mL per gram of tissue), at 4°C overnight. This mixture was then centrifuged at 10 000 g for 30 minutes at 4°C. The extract was collected, and the pellet was washed once with an equal volume of the urea buffer. The extract and the wash were then combined and dialyzed against 0.05 mol/L of Tris HCl, pH 7.4, containing 0.15 mol/L of sodium chloride at 4°C overnight. The dialyzed extract was centrifuged at 15 000 rpm for 20 minutes at 4°C, and the supernatant (matrigel) was stored at −20°C.

Adherence Assays

Multiwell (11.3-mm) tissue culture plates were coated with either matrigel or bovine serum albumin (BSA) by incubation with a 20-μg/mL solution of these proteins in PBS at 4°C overnight. The wells were then washed twice with Hank's balanced salt solution (HBSS) and incubated with serum-free DMEM at 37°C for 30 minutes before their use in the assays.

For the assays, a cell suspension (see above) was added to DMEM containing 10% FBS to inactivate the trypsin and centrifuged at 1000 rpm for five minutes. The cell pellet was resuspended in DMEM containing 1.0% BSA. Cells were counted visually using a hemocytometer. Viability was assessed by trypan blue dye exclusion and only suspensions with more than 95% viability were used. An aliquot (200 μL) of the cell suspension containing 5×10^5 cells per milliliter was added to the protein-coated wells. The plates were incubated at 37°C in a humidified atmosphere of 95% air and 5% carbon dioxide (CO_2) for 75 minutes. The nonadherent cells were then removed by two gentle washes with warm HBSS. Adherent cells were fixed with methanol and stained with a 10% (vol/vol) solution of Giemsa stain in PBS. These cells were viewed using brightfield optics with a microscope (Nikon Diaphot) equipped with a 16-square reticle. With a 20× objective, the surface area of this grid was 0.25 mm². For each adhesion assay, the number of cells in the reticle was determined in triplicate. Results for these experiments are expressed as the mean number of adherent cells per reticle. The extent of cell spreading was also evaluated in these assays. Spreading was defined as an extension of cytoplasmic processes resulting in a deviation from the rounded morphologic features seen immediately after the addition of the cells to the tissue culture plates.

Adherence assays performed in the presence of the protein synthesis inhibitor cycloheximide were carried out in a similar manner. Cyclocheximide was added immediately after resuspension of cells in DMEM containing 1.0% BSA. The final concentration of cycloheximide in the cell suspension was 75 μg/mL.

Cells destined for use in delayed plating assays were incubated for one hour at 37°C in a humidified atmosphere of 95% air and 5% CO_2 after resuspension in DMEM containing 1.0% BSA. After this incubation period, the cell suspension was added to wells containing matrigel or BSA.

Assays of Migration in Response to a Soluble Attractant (Chemotaxis)

Assays for chemotaxis and chemoinvasion were performed in a modified microchamber apparatus (Boyden) (Fig 1).[19] Polyvinylpyrrolidone-free polycarbonate filters with 12-μm pores were placed between the upper and lower chambers. Conditioned medium, obtained by incubating the murine fibroblast cell line 3T3 isolated at the National Institutes of Health in serum-free DMEM containing 50 μg/mL of ascorbate overnight, was added to the lower chamber.[20] A cell suspension was prepared as described above, and an aliquot of this suspension containing 2.5×10^5 cells was added to the upper chamber. The apparatus was then incubated at 37°C in a humidified atmosphere of 95% air and 5% CO_2 for five hours. At the end of this period, the cells on the upper surface were mechanically removed with a cotton swab. The filters were then fixed in methanol and stained with a 10% solution of Giemsa stain. Cells that had migrated through the pores in the filters and were present on the lower surface were counted using the method described for adherence assays.

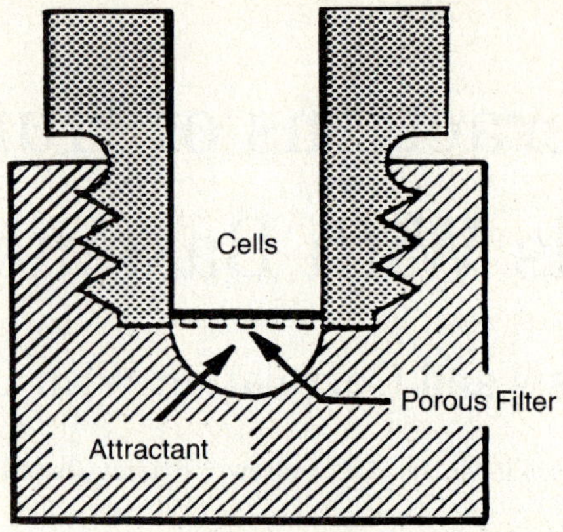

Fig 1.—Microchamber apparatus (Boyden). Cell suspension is added to upper chamber and chemoattractant is added to lower chamber. For invasion assays, perforated filter coated with matrigel is placed between chambers; uncoated filter is used in chemotaxis assays.

Assay for Adherence, Penetration, and Migration Through a Matrigel Barrier in Response to a Soluble Attractant (Chemoinvasion)

For chemoinvasion assays, the polyvinylpyrrolidone-free filters were coated with matrigel diluted to a final concentration of 500 μg/mL in cold distilled water.[20] The matrigel solution (100 μL) was applied to the filters, air-dried, and then reconstituted with serum-free DMEM for 30 minutes at 37°C. The filters were then placed in the microchamber apparatus with the matrigel layer facing the upper chamber. Assays were otherwise carried out as described above for chemotaxis. Cells that were present on the lower surface of the filter at the end of the assay were considered to have invaded.

Data were analyzed using the Student *t* test.

RESULTS

Characteristics of Colorectal Carcinoma Cell Lines

Eight established human colorectal carcinoma cell lines were employed in this study. These cell lines have been classified on the basis of criteria that relate to their degree of differentiation (Table). These criteria include carcinoembryonic antigen (CEA) expression, ability to form tumors in nude mice, histologic features of xenografts, and in vitro morphology (see Table for references). Poorly differentiated cell lines express little CEA, form tumors readily in nude mice, and exhibit the amorphous morphologic features characteristic of poorly differentiated tumors when grown as xenografts. In contrast, the moderately well-differentiated cell lines express abundant CEA, form tumors less readily in nude mice, and display an organized glandular morphologic condition when grown as xenografts. After evaluating the data presented in the Table, we classified the cell lines Clone A, MIP 101, CCL 222, and CCL 228 as poorly differentiated and the cell lines

Characteristics of Colorectal Carcinoma Cell Lines

	Clone A	MIP 101	CCL 222	CCL 228	CX-1[d]	DLD-2	CCL 235	CCL 238
Tissue source	Colon[16]	Colon[18]	Colon[23]	Colon[23]	Colon[23]	Colon[17]	Rectum[24]	Colon[23]
Tumor site	1°[16]	Liver[18]	Ascites[23]	1°[23]	1°[23]	1°[17]	1°[24]	1°[23]
Xenograft grade	Poor[23]	Poor[18]	Poor[23]	Poor[23]	Moderate/well[25]	Moderate/well[25]	Moderate/well[25]	Not determined
In vitro morphology*	Fusiform	Fusiform	Spherical/ fusiform	Fusiform/ cuboidal	Cuboidal	Cuboidal	Cuboidal	Cuboidal
Tumor incidence, cells subcutaneously injected	100%,[23] 10^6	100%,[18] 10^7	90%,[23] 10^6	90%,[23] 10^6	100%,[25] 10^7	100%,[25] 10^7	100%,[25] 10^7	0%,[23] 10^6
Agar plating efficiency	16%[23]†	8%[18]‡	32%[23]†	32%[23]†	Not determined	7%[17]‡	Not determined	4%[23]†
Carcinoembryonic antigen, ng/10^6 cells§	0	0	2.5	0.7	70	120	523	362
Doubling time, h	22[23]	22[18]	27[23]	22[23]	Not determined	48[17]	169[24]	30[23]

*Assessed by phase-contrast microscopy.
†Colonies >20 μm.
‡Colonies >50 cells.
§Determined on conditioned cell media using radioimmunoassay.

CX-1, DLD-2, CCL 235, and CCL 238 as moderately well differentiated. The cell line DLD-2 is distinct from the other moderately well-differentiated cell lines because its xenograft histologic features resemble a signet ring carcinoma and it synthesizes large amounts of mucin in vivo and in vitro (G.W.D. and A.M.M., unpublished data, 1987).

Interactions of Colorectal Carcinoma Cell Lines With Matrigel

We examined the ability of the colorectal carcinoma cell lines described in the Table to interact with the reconstituted basement membrane matrix matrigel. The data obtained for the adherence of tumor cell lines on matrigel-coated surfaces are presented in Fig 2. The difference in adherence between the two differentiation classifications was striking. Adherence of the poorly differentiated cell lines Clone A, MIP 101, CCL 222, and CCL 228, as well as the moderately well-differentiated line DLD-2, was three to four times greater than adherence to the moderately well-differentiated cell lines CX-1, CCL 235, and CCL 238. The actual adherence values for the poorly differentiated cell lines were 186 ± 4.5 (mean $\pm$ SEM) and for the moderately well-differentiated lines, 65 ± 1.9. This difference was significant to a P value of .0001. The signet ring cell line DLD-2 adhered avidly to matrigel (228 ± 6.3). These numerical values for adherence were obtained from a larger number of experiments than the values reported in Fig 2.

To exclude the possibility that trypsin removed cell surface proteins that are involved in matrix interactions, we performed several additional experiments. Specifically, we observed that incubation of the cells for one to two hours at 37°C after trypsinization and before use in these assays did not produce a change in adherence as compared with their use immediately after trypsinization. Furthermore, similar adherence data were obtained when a divalent cation chelator, edetic acid, rather than trypsin, was used to detach the cells (data not shown). These observations confirm that trypsin treatment did not selectively remove surface-binding proteins for basement membrane components.

Pretreatment of tumor cells with cycloheximide before their use in the assays had no effect on adherence (data not shown). The difference in adherence between the cell lines presented in Fig 2, therefore, cannot be attributed to differences in their rates of de novo protein synthesis, especially the synthesis of basement membrane component–binding proteins. Nonspecific adherence to proteins by the tumor cells was determined in an assay using wells coated with BSA. For all cell lines, fewer than 1% of the number of cells that adhered to matrigel adhered to BSA.

The ability of colorectal tumor cells to adhere to matrigel correlated with their ability to spread on this substratum. The poorly differentiated cell lines Clone A and MIP 101 showed extensive cytoplasmic spreading following adherence. Fusiform elongation after adherence was seen for the poorly differentiated lines CCL 222 and CCL 228. Less-extensive spreading was noted following adherence of the moderately well-differentiated cell lines CX-1, CCL 235, and CCL 238. The moderately well-differentiated cell line DLD-2 did, however, spread extensively following adherence.

Motility of Colorectal Carcinoma Cells in Response to Chemical Attractants

We examined the ability of the colorectal carcinoma cell lines to migrate through a porous barrier in response to conditioned fibroblast medium as a chemoattractant (Fig 3). This chemoattractant was chosen because of its reproducible activity on a broad range of cell lines.[20] The cell lines Clone A and MIP 101 showed the greatest motility in this assay, although the remaining poorly differentiated and all the moderately well-differentiated cell lines were motile to some degree. The difference in motility between the moderately well-differentiated cell lines compared with Clone A and MIP 101 was significant (mean $\pm$ SEM, 9 ± 0.9 moderately well differentiated, 25 ± 1 Clone A, MIP 101, $P = .001$); however, the difference in motility between the moderately well-differentiated cell lines and the remaining poorly differentiated cell lines CCL 222 and CCL 228 was not significant (mean $\pm$ SEM, 7 ± 0.9 moderately well differentiated, 10 ± 1 CCL 222 and 228).

Invasion of Colorectal Carcinoma Cells Through a Matrigel Barrier in Response to a Soluble Attractant

These assays were performed to measure the ability of tumor cell lines to invade through matrigel in response to a chemoattractant. Invasion in this model is defined as the

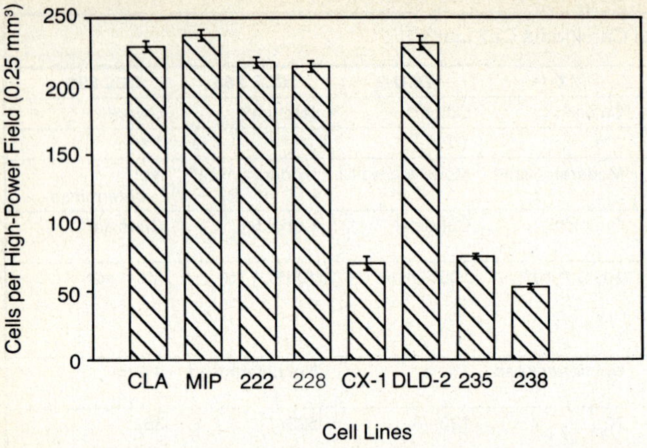

Fig 2.—Adherence of cell lines to matrigel-coated surfaces. Matrigel was coated on tissue culture wells overnight and then reconstituted with media before use. Data were obtained from at least five separate experiments. Error bars represent standard error of mean.

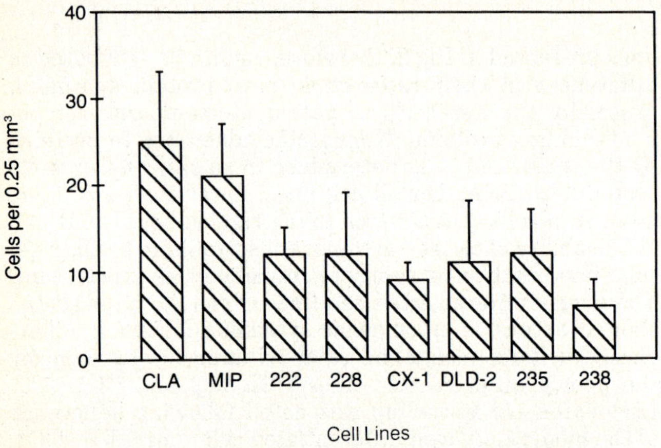

Fig 3.—Migration of cell lines toward chemoattractant (chemotaxis). Chemotaxis assays were performed in microchamber apparatus (Boyden) using perforated filter between chambers. Conditioned 3T3 medium from National Institutes of Health, Bethesda, Md, was used as chemoattractant. Data were obtained from at least five separate experiments. Error bars represent standard error of mean.

ability of cells to adhere, penetrate, and migrate through a barrier layer of matrigel in response to a chemoattractant. Important parameters such as the thickness of the matrigel layer and time of the assay were determined empirically to yield the optimal resolution of invasion potential among the cell lines.[20] From the data presented in Fig 4, it is evident that all cell lines were invasive to some extent. The poorly differentiated cell lines Clone A, MIP 101, CCL 222, and CCL 228, however, were two to three times more invasive than the moderately well-differentiated cell lines CX-1, CCL 235, and CCL 238 (mean ± SEM, 30 ± 0.9 poorly differentiated vs 9 ± 0.7 moderately well differentiated, $P = .001$). DLD-2, which resembled the poorly differentiated cell lines in its ability to interact with matrigel, was also able to invade through a matrigel barrier in numbers similar to the poorly differentiated cells (mean ± SEM, 37 ± 3.0).

COMMENT

Recent studies have postulated that the ability of malignant cells to interact with basement membrane components

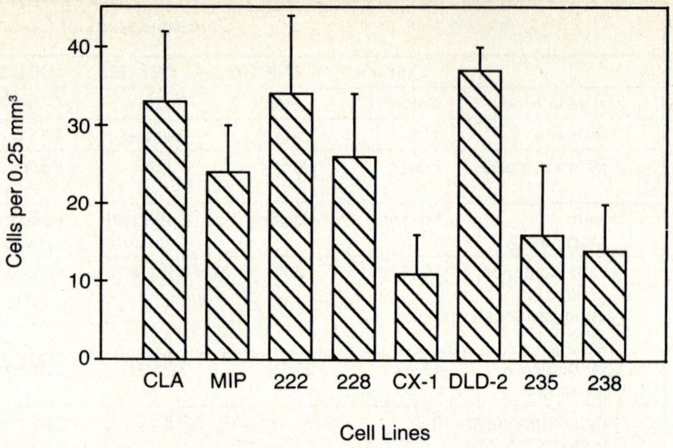

Fig 4.—Adherence, penetration, and migration through matrigel layer toward chemoattractant (invasion). Invasion assays were performed in microchamber apparatus (Boyden) using matrigel-coated filter between chambers. Conditioned 3T3 medium from National Institutes of Health, Bethesda, Md, was used as chemoattractant. Data were obtained from at least five separate experiments. Error bars represent standard error of mean.

is an important determinant of their invasive and metastatic behavior.[5-9] On the basis of these postulates, we were interested in determining whether the degree of differentiation is a factor that influences the ability of colorectal carcinoma cells to interact with the basement membrane. In our study, we have shown that the ability of colorectal carcinoma cell lines to adhere to and spread on matrigel, a basement membrane matrix, is related to their degree of cytodifferentiation.[14] The poorly differentiated colorectal carcinoma cell lines were two to three times more adherent and spread to a greater extent on matrigel than the moderately well-differentiated cell lines. An exception to this correlation was the moderately well-differentiated cell line DLD-2. This line, whose xenograft morphologic features resemble the notoriously aggressive signet ring carcinoma, adhered and spread on matrigel to the same extent as the poorly differentiated cell lines. This exception indicates that factors other than cytodifferentiation may contribute to the interaction of cells with the basement membrane. From these data, we can conclude that adherence to matrigel may effect a morphologic change, although this change does not seem to be mandatory for adherence to this material. Any potential significance of the extent and rate of spreading in vivo, however, may not be appreciated under the conditions chosen for thse assays.

The chemoinvasion assay developed by Albini et al[20] was used to measure the ability of the colorectal carcinoma cell lines to adhere, penetrate, and migrate through a matrigel layer in response to a chemoattractant. In this assay, the poorly differentiated cell lines, as well as the moderately differentiated line DLD-2, were two to three times more invasive than the other moderately well-differentiated lines. From these data, combined with the adherence data, we conclude that the ability of a tumor cell to adhere to the basement membrane correlates with its ability to invade through a basement membrane matrix. In contrast, the ability to invade through a basement membrane did not correlate with the ability of these cells to migrate toward a chemoattractant (chemotaxis) in the absence of the basement membrane. Chemotaxis by these cells, therefore, may be a reflection of their intrinsic motility but it does not seem to be a relevant measure of their motility following adherence to the basement membrane.

The data presented in this study complement one currently accepted model for tumor invasion.[8,9] In this model, the initial requisite step for invasion is tumor cell adherence, via cell surface receptors, to a basement membrane component such as laminin. This attachment may prompt the synthesis and secretion of proteolytic enzymes that are necessary for degradation of the basement membrane. Migration through the degraded basement membrane may also be stimulated by adherence to basement membrane components as well as by soluble motility factors.[21,22] On the basis of this model, we believe that the increased invasive potential of the poorly differentiated colorectal carcinoma cell lines, as well as the moderately well-differentiated line DLD-2, is, in part, related to their increased ability to adhere and spread on basement membranes. In addition, their ability to migrate through the basement membrane is enhanced by adherence to basement membrane components regardless of their degree of differentiation.

We believe it is premature to establish the correlation between adherence and invasion too strongly. Invasion is a complex, multivariable process. Other basic tenets of the invasion model need to be evaluated for these cell lines. For example, it is important to determine whether adherence-related enzyme secretion or stimulated motility vary with cytodifferentiation. Nevertheless, the ability of the colorectal carcinoma cells to interact with basement membranes may, in part, explain the more aggressive clinical behavior of poorly differentiated colorectal carcinomas as compared with well-differentiated tumors. Furthermore, reagents that identify differences in cell surface receptors for basement membrane components may be useful for distinguishing more clinically aggressive tumors among those with a similar histopathologic appearance.

This work was supported by grant CA 44707 from the National Institutes of Health. Henry Sears, MD, provided editorial assistance and Laura Edwards provided the statistical analysis involved in preparation of this manuscript. Dr Mercurio is the recipient of an American Cancer Society Junior Faculty Award.

Daniel Dexter, PhD, from E. I. DuPont DeNemours & Co, Wilmington, Del, provided the Clone A and DLD-2. The MIP 101 was provided by Richard Niles, PhD, Mallory Gastrointestinal Research Laboratory, Boston. The Englebreth-Holm-Swarm sarcoma was a gift from Herbert Kupchuck, PhD, Boston University.

References

1. Dukes CE: The surgical pathology of rectal cancer. *Proc R Soc Med* 1943;37:131-140.
2. Klimpfinger M, Benham A, Denk H: Pathological findings in colorectal cancers and discussion of their significance for tumor therapy according to stage. *Wien Klin Wochenschr* 1987;99:488-493.
3. Mentges B: Colon carcinoma: Preoperative CEA, tumor differentiation, and prognosis. *Dtsch Med Wochenschr* 1987;112:1245-1249.
4. Steinberg SM, Barwich KW, Stablein DM: Importance of tumor pathology and morphology in patients with surgically resected colon cancer: Findings from the Gastrointestinal Tumor Study Group. *Cancer* 1986;58:1340-1345.
5. Martin GR, Timpl R: Laminin and other basement membrane components. *Ann Rev Cell Biol* 1987;3:57-85.
6. Timpl R, Dziadek M: Structure, development, and molecular pathology of basement membranes. *Int Rev Exp Pathol* 1986;29:1-112.
7. Von der Mark K, Kuhl U: Laminin and its receptor. *Biochim Biophys Acta* 1985;823:147-160.
8. Liotta LA, Rao CN, Weiner VM: Biochemical interactions of tumor cells with the basement membrane. *Ann Rev Biochem* 1986;55:1037-1055.
9. Terranova VP, Hujanen ES, Martin GR: Basement membrane and invasive activity of metastatic tumor cells. *JNCI* 1986;77:311-316.
10. Turpeenniemi-Hujanen T, Thorgeivsson VP, Liotta LA: Laminin increases the release of type IV collagenase from malignant cells. *J Biol Chem* 1986;261:1883-1889.
11. Goodman SL, Newgreen D: Do cells show an inverse locomotory response to fibronectin and laminin substrates? *EMBO J* 1985;4:2769-2771.
12. Daneker GW, Steele GD, Mercurio AM: The ability of human colorectal carcinoma cells to interact with the extracellular matrix in vitro is related to their degree of differentiation. *Cancer Res*, in press.
13. Graf J, Iwamoto Y, Sasaki M, et al: Identification of an amino acid sequence in laminin mediating cell attachment, chemotaxis and receptor binding. *Cell* 1987;48:989-996.
14. Kleinman HK, McGarvey ML, Hassell JR, et al: Basement complexes with biological activity. *Biochemistry* 1986;25:312-318.
15. Hay R, Macy M, Corman-Weinblatt A, et al (eds): *American Type Culture Collection Catalogue of Cell Lines and Hybridomas.* Rockville, Md, American Type Culture Collection, 1985.
16. Dexter DL, Barbosa JA, Calabresi P: *N,N*-dimethylformamide-induced alteration of cell culture characteristics and loss of tumorigenicity in cultured human colon carcinoma cells. *Cancer Res* 1979;39:1020-1025.
17. Crabtree GW, Dexter DL, Stoeckler JD, et al: Activities of purine-metabolizing enzymes in human colon carcinoma cell lines and xenograft tumors. *Biochem Pharmacol* 1981;30:793-798.
18. Niles RM, Wilhelm SA, Steele GD, et al: Isolation and characterization of an undifferentiated human colon carcinoma cell line (MIP-101). *Cancer Invest* 1987;5:545-552.
19. McCarthy JB, Furcht LT: Laminin and fibronectin promote haptotactic migration of B16 mouse melanoma cells in vitro. *J Cell Biol* 1984;98:1474-1480.
20. Albini A, Iwamoto Y, Kleinman HK, et al: A rapid in vitro assay for quantitating the invasive potential of tumor cells. *Cancer Res* 1987;47:3239-3245.
21. Liotta LA, Mandler R, Murano G, et al: Tumor autocrine motility factor. *Proc Natl Acad Sci USA* 1986;83:3302-3306.
22. Wewer UM, Taraboletti G, Sobel ME, et al: Role of laminin receptor in tumor cell migration. *Cancer Res* 1987;47:5691-5698.
23. Trainer DL, Kline T, McCabe FL, et al: Biological characterization and oncogene expression in human colorectal carcinoma cell lines. *Int J Cancer* 1988;41:287-296.
24. Leibovitz A, Stinson JC, McCombs WB, et al: Classification of human colorectal adenocarcinoma cell lines. *Cancer Res* 1976;36:4562-4569.
25. Daneker GW, Mercurio AM, Guerra L, et al: Laminin expression in colorectal carcinomas varying in degree of differentiation. *Arch Surg* 1987;122:1470-1474.

Discussion

Q I think your results that evaluate adherence and invasiveness in vitro correlate with generally accepted principles of histology and aggressiveness. I had several questions; the first relates to the agents that may identify these cell surface receptors. Do you have monoclonal antibodies or other agents that you can use to identify these receptors or correlate them with other products of these cells, such as CEA, for example?

A There are a few polyclonal antibodies made against the receptors that are available at the National Institutes of Health. In addition, Yumada's group there has cloned some of the sequence in the receptor. They've actually made a monoclonal antibody to fusion protein, so reagents are there and potentially useful.

Q The second question is can you correlate these in vitro results with in vivo results, for example, a cecal injection model or other models using these particular cell lines?

A That's a good question. We've wanted to use some of the antibodies we have on some of our xenograph sections to see whether we can. Leota has done some preliminary work at the National Institutes of Health and showed in pathologic specimens from human tumors that there is increased expression of receptors in some metastatic deposits in more invasive tumors.

Q Back in October at the forum, your group reported on human tumors and epidermal growth factor-receptor activity in primary and metastatic sites. Have you looked at any of the primary or metastatic tumors from patients as to their ability to adhere?

A We have not. Actually, we limited our work to using only commercially available cell lines, but that's a good point. Everyone knows the obvious limitations of in vitro cell lines.

Q Do you have any information on proteases, collagenases, plasmin, or plasminogen in the systems?

A No. Some other groups have looked at it, and there was a report in 1986 in which adherence stimulated the production of type 4 collagenase by tumor cells, so there is some work done. There are difficulties with experimental design in looking at proteases. I think that is why we haven't seen more about that.

Q One more thing—it's not just chemoattraction, is it? Is there any chemokinetic activity? Is it increased penetration in general or is it specific in response to a chemoattractant?

A It's hard to say. Some of it is a response to chemoattractant. Some of the laminin lysis fragments are very active as chemoattractants.

DEFINING A NEW STANDA

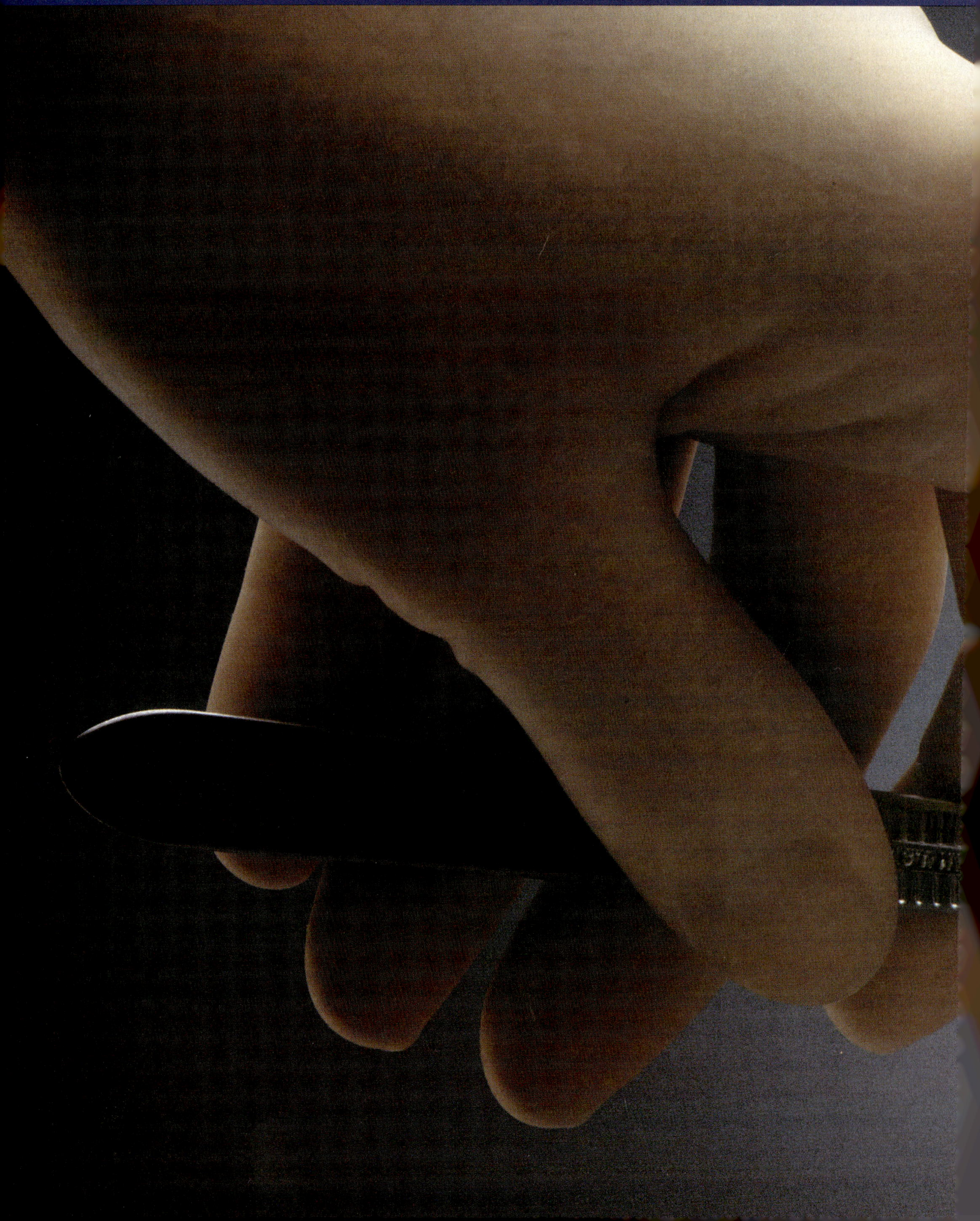

The Desmoid Tumor

Not a Benign Disease

Mitchell C. Posner, MD; Man H. Shiu, MD; James L. Newsome, MD;
Steven I. Hajdu, MD; Jeffrey J. Gaynor, PhD; Murray F. Brennan, MD

• The necessity of aggressive therapy for desmoid tumors has not been clearly established. To evaluate the therapeutic value of adequate resection and radiation therapy, we conducted a retrospective study of 138 patients treated from 1965 through 1984. Univariate analysis revealed five factors predictive of local failure: (1) age between 18 and 30 years, (2) presentation with recurrent disease, (3) partial or limited margin excision, (4) tumor at or close to the microscopic margin of resection, and (5) radiation therapy not administered for gross residual disease. Multivariate analysis identified two of these factors as having independent predictive value for recurrence: (1) presentation with recurrent disease and (2) less-than-adequate margins of resection. The five-year survival probability was 92%, but 11 of the 138 patients died as a consequence of locally uncontrolled tumor. These findings confirm that desmoid tumors are malignant soft-tissue neoplasms that warrant aggressive therapy.

(*Arch Surg* 1989;124:191-196)

Desmoid tumors are relatively rare malignant soft-tissue neoplasms derived from fascial or musculoaponeurotic structures.[1] Their classification as low-grade fibrosarcomas is based primarily on a marked propensity for local invasion.[2-6] In contrast to other soft-tissue sarcomas, the necessity for aggressive therapy of desmoid tumors has not been clearly established. Failure to recognize their malignant local behavior has led to conflicting recommendations regarding surgical management. The role of radiation therapy in the management of this neoplasm is poorly defined. In an attempt to evaluate the therapeutic value of adequate resection and the potential benefit of adjunctive radiation therapy and to define factors that influence local tumor control, a retrospective analysis was undertaken.

PATIENTS AND METHODS

Examination of the tumor registry at Memorial Sloan-Kettering Cancer Center, New York, between the years 1965 and 1984 identified 185 patients with a presumptive diagnosis of desmoid tumor or low-grade fibrosarcoma. Following histologic review of all slides, 144 were classified as desmoid tumors. One hundred thirty-eight charts were available for review. Seven patients were excluded due to a lack of follow-up information. The remaining 131 patients form the basis for this report.

Accepted for publication July 15, 1988.

From the Departments of Surgery (Drs Posner, Shiu, and Brennan), Pathology (Drs Newsome and Hajdu), and Biostatistical Epidemiology (Dr Gaynor), Memorial Sloan-Kettering Cancer Center, New York.

Read before the Annual Meeting of the Society of Surgical Oncology, New Orleans, May 23, 1988.

Reprint requests to Memorial Sloan-Kettering Cancer Center, 1275 York Ave, New York, NY 10021 (Dr Brennan).

Clinicopathologic Data

Patient demographics extracted from chart analysis included the following: age, sex, symptoms, possible causal factors, previous surgical or adjuvant treatment, and presentation (untreated or recurrent). Tumor characteristics examined were the site, size, depth, and invasion of bone or major neurovascular structures. Tumor size was determined by measurement of either a pathologic specimen or an intraoperative lesion. The classification of tumor penetration as either superficial or deep was dependent on the tumor's anatomic relationship to the superficial fascia. Bone or neurovascular invasion was considered present when identified on gross examination and confirmed microscopically.

The pathologic diagnosis of desmoid tumor in all patients was established following critical review of the available tissue slides by one of the authors (S.I.H.). Histologically, desmoid tumors are composed of uniform collagenous fibrocytes in broad bundles and fascicles. The neoplastic cells are arranged in a one-directional spreading pattern without interruption or necrosis (Fig 1). The intercellular matrix is abundant, is often scarlike, and stains uniformly positive with trichrome stain. The overall appearance of desmoid tumors is that of a well-differentiated "mature" fibrous neoplasm that shows no cellular pleomorphism or mitotic activity. Direct invasion of contiguous structures by fingerlike projections of tumor is frequently demonstrated (Fig 2).

Surgical Treatment

Treatment data obtained included the surgical procedure, scope of resection, margins of resection, and adjuvant therapy. The *scope of resection* was determined by careful review of the operative note and categorized as follows: (1) Partial excision refers to incomplete resection or intralesional debulking. (2) Limited margin resection describes removal of all gross tumor with only a scant margin (millimeters) of uninvolved surrounding tissue. Although the surgeon's intent was complete tumor excision, microscopic examination invariably demonstrated disease at or close to the margin following limited margin resection. (3) Wide margin and compartment resection entails monobloc soft-tissue resection encompassing the entire tumor and its ramifications, with a variable margin of normal surrounding tissue and no exposure of the tumor during extirpation.

The *margin of resection* was then classified as adequate, marginal, or inadequate based on pathologic examination. Adequate resection referred to a wide margin of uninvolved tissue on all sides and no evidence of tumor on microscopic examination of the margin. The resection was deemed marginal if the tumor approximated the surgical margin (ie, was within millimeters). Microscopic evidence of tumor at the resection margin confirmed an inadequate resection.

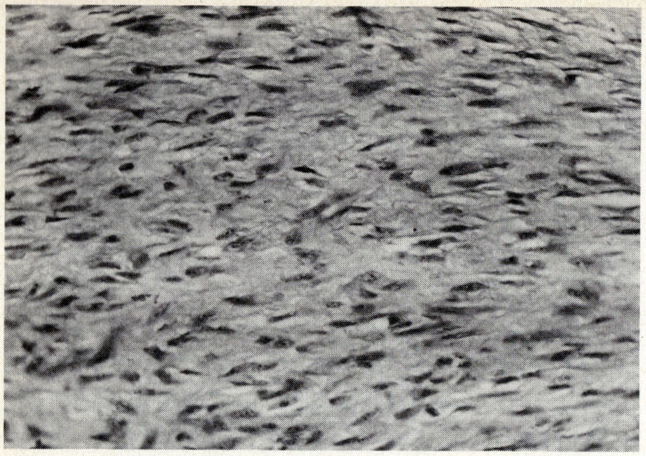

Fig 1.—Desmoid tumor (low-grade fibrosarcoma) composed of uniform collagenous fibrocytes (hematoxylin-eosin, original magnification ×450).

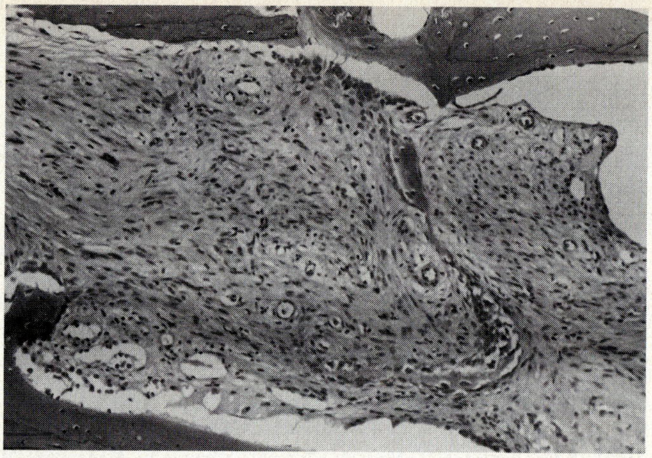

Fig 2.—Desmoid tumor (low-grade fibrosarcoma) invading medullary cavity of bone (hematoxylin-eosin, original magnification ×170).

Radiation Therapy

The intent of radiotherapy was categorized as either primary therapy or as an adjunct to surgery. The following techniques were used for delivery of radiation therapy during the study period: (1) external beam, (2) temporary implant of iridium 192 sources via afterloading catheters, and (3) permanent interstitial implant of iodine 125 seeds (brachytherapy). The brachytherapy technique has been previously described.[7-9] In selected patients, multiple techniques were employed.

Statistical Analysis

The study end points were local recurrence and death. Follow-up was obtained from recent chart documentation, when available, or by personal contact with the patient or responsible physician. The probability of local recurrence and overall survival curves were generated according to the method of Kaplan and Meier.[10] Univariate analysis comparing recurrence rates between patient subgroups was performed using the log-rank test of statistical significance.[11] Multivariate analysis using the Cox model of stepwise linear regression[12] was applied to identify independent factors that significantly influenced local recurrence.

Patients

There were 80 females (61%) and 51 males (39%), a female-to-male ratio of 1.6:1. The median age was 29 years (range, 6 to 73 years). Seventy-eight patients were referred for treatment of their initial tumor, 67 with their tumor intact or biopsied and 11 who had recently undergone resection, with residual disease on either microscopic or gross examination. Fifty-three patients presented with locally recurrent disease. Administration of radiotherapy some time prior to presentation at our center was documented in 11 patients.

Sixty-seven patients (51%) had tumors located at an extremity site, 19 (15%) at a retroperitoneal site, 16 (12%) in the abdominal wall, 13 (10%) in the chest wall, and ten (8%) in the head and neck. Gardner's syndrome was described in four patients, and two patients had visceral desmoid tumors.

One hundred twenty-eight patients had curative attempts at resection of their primary tumor, two had biopsy only, and one patient with Gardner's syndrome who had extensive tumor involvement of the abdominal wall and small-bowel mesentery underwent palliative resection. The *scope of resection* was categorized as wide margin or compartmental in 64 patients, limited margin in 40 patients, and partial excision in 24 patients. The *resection margin* was considered adequate in 47 patients (37%) and less than adequate in 81 patients (63%). Of those whose resection margin was deemed less than adequate, 41 showed tumor approximating the surgical margin, albeit microscopically negative, and 40 showed tumor at the resection margin. Radiotherapy was administered to 15 patients with positive margins. Five patients were given radiation therapy as an adjunct to complete tumor extirpation.

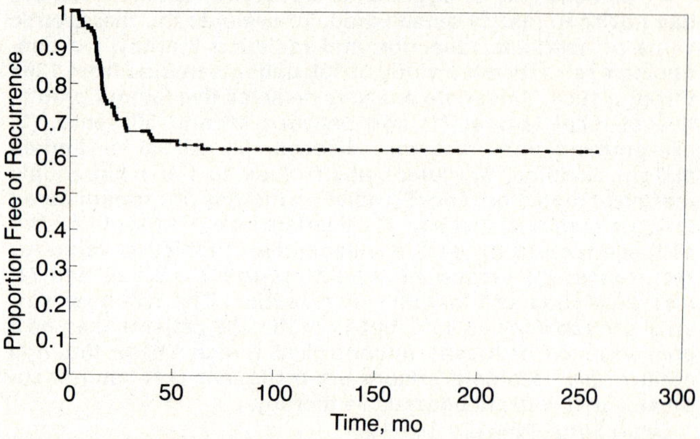

Fig 3.—Probability of local recurrence in patients treated with curative intent (n = 128). Kaplan-Meier plot. Local failure rate was 37% at five years.

RESULTS

Analysis of local recurrence and survival data is based only on patients who underwent resection for cure. The median follow-up for the 128 patients who underwent curative attempts at resection was 7.3 years.

Local Tumor Control

Eighty-two of the 128 tumors were successfully controlled following definitive surgical treatment with or without radiation therapy at our center. The probability of local failure is estimated to be 37% at five years (Fig 3). Local recurrence occurred in 46 patients, with a median time to recurrence of 15 months (range, three to 64 months). Approximately 80% of the recurrences were observed to occur within the first two years following resection (Fig 3). Distant failure in conjunction with locally recurrent disease was seen in one patient with a large retroperitoneal lesion that was unsuccessfully resected multiple times. Pathologically confirmed lung metastases developed eight years following the initial attempt at resection, and the patient died one year later as a result of disease progression.

Table 1.—Univariate and Multivariate Analysis of Influence of Prognostic Variables on Rate of Local Recurrence

Prognostic Variable	Favorable Characteristic	Unfavorable Characteristic	Analysis: Univariate P*	Multivariate: P†	Multivariate: Cox Model Coefficient‡
		Clinicopathologic Factors			
Age	<18 or >30 y	18 to 30 y	.006	...	...
Sex	F	M	NS	...	...
Symptoms	None	Painful mass or other	NS	...	...
Presentation	Untreated	Recurrent disease	.01	.02	0.70±0.30
Site	Extremity	Nonextremity	NS	...	...
Size (diameter)	<10 cm	>10 cm	NS	...	...
Depth	Superficial	Deep	NS	...	...
Vital structure invasion	Absent	Present	NS	...	...
		Treatment Factors			
Scope of resection	Wide margin/ compartmental	Partial excision or limited margin	.02	...	...
Margins of resection	Adequate	Marginal or inadequate	.0002	.0002	1.40±0.41
Radiation for gross residual disease	Yes	No	.02	...	...
Radiation for minimal residual disease	Yes	No	NS	...	...

*Based on log-rank test; NS indicates not significant.
†Based on score test.
‡The Cox model coefficient permits evaluation of the additive influence of one or more adverse prognostic factors for comparison with patients without these factors. In coding for the model, the covariate was scored as 1 if unfavorable and 0 if otherwise.

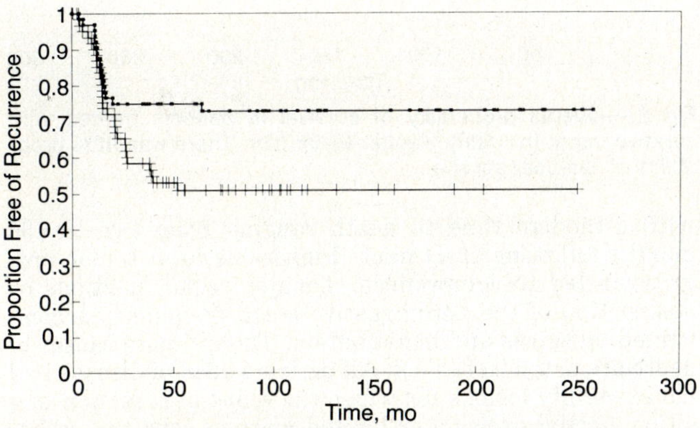

Fig 4.—Rate of local recurrence in patients with wide margins or compartment resection (squares, n=64) and limited margins or partial excision (hatch marks, n=64). $P=.02$. Kaplan-Meier plots.

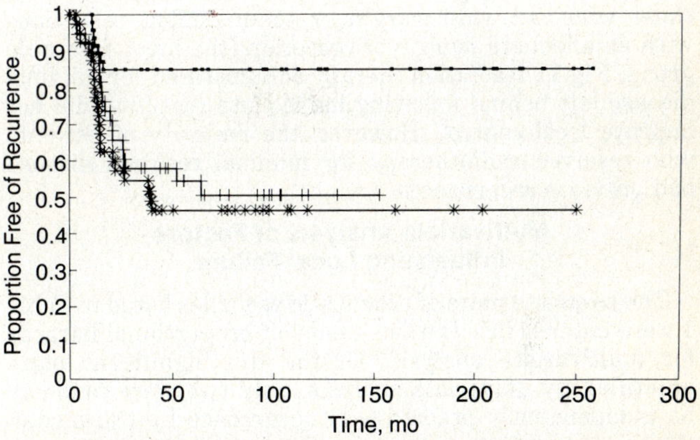

Fig 5.—Rate of local recurrence in patients with adequate margins (squares, n=47), marginal resection margins (hatch marks, n=41), and inadequate margins (asterisks, n=40) of resection. $P=.0002$ for patients with adequate margins compared with those with less-than-adequate margins. Kaplan-Meier plots.

Clinicopathologic and Treatment Factors Influencing Local Failure

Univariate analyses of the influence of clinicopathologic and treatment variables on the rate of local recurrence are depicted in Table 1.

Of the clinicopathologic factors, only age and presentation with or without locally recurrent disease significantly influenced the rate of local recurrence. Desmoid tumors predominate in young age groups (70% under 45 years), and those less than 30 years of age have an increased rate of local recurrence (43% vs 27%). When this variable is analyzed with respect to three chronologic groups (<18, 18 to 30, and >30 years), patients who are between 18 and 30 years of age are at significantly increased risk of local failure ($P=.006$). The presence of symptoms, sex, tumor size or location, depth of penetration, and bone or neurovascular invasion had no demonstrable impact on local recurrence.

Of the treatment factors, *scope of resection* significantly influenced subsequent local recurrence (Fig 4). Wide margin or compartment resection was associated with a prolonged disease-free interval compared with less extensive procedures ($P=.02$). As expected, conservative resection was more likely to result in less-than-adequate margins of resection than wide margin or compartment resection (100% vs 27%).

An adequate *resection margin,* as determined by path-

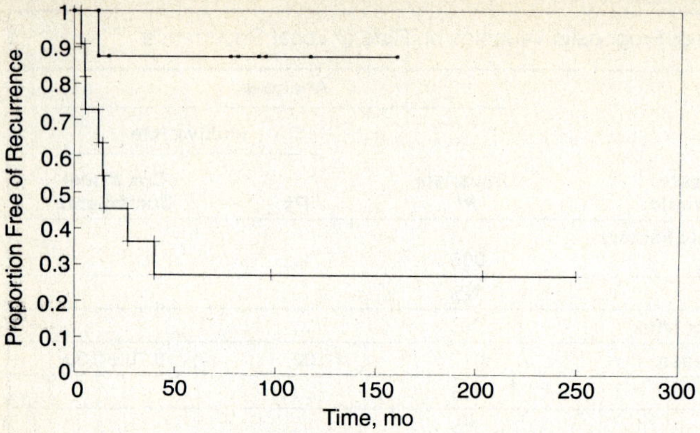

Fig 6.—Effect of radiation therapy on rate of local recurrence of gross residual disease in patients with (squares, n = 9) and without (hatch marks, n = 11) radiation therapy. *P* = .02. Kaplan-Meier plots.

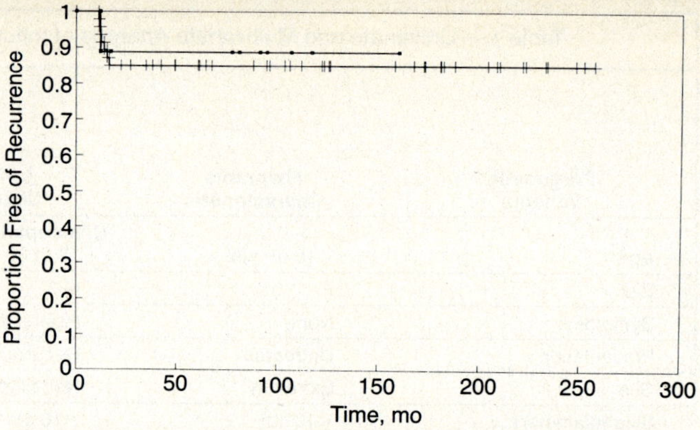

Fig 7.—Effect of radiation therapy on rate of local recurrence in patients who underwent partial tumor excision (squares, n = 9) compared with patients who underwent wide margin or compartment resection with adequate margins (hatch marks, n = 47). *P* = .8.

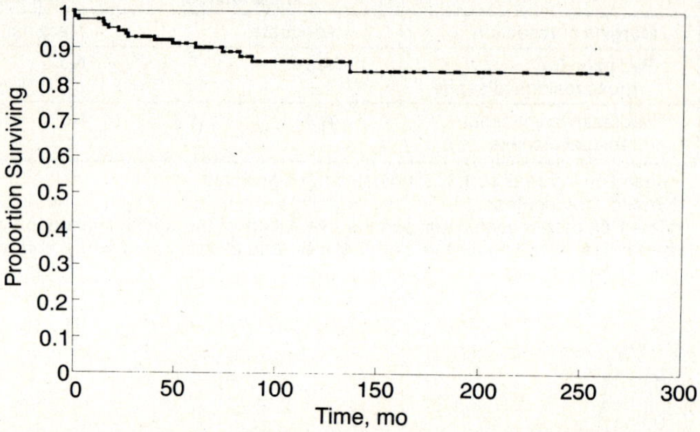

Fig 8.—Overall probability of survival in patients treated with curative intent (n = 128). Kaplan-Meier plot. There was 92% probability of five-year survival.

ologic examination, significantly reduced local recurrence compared with less-than-adequate resection margins (Fig 5), either marginal or inadequate. However, no difference in local recurrence rates was demonstrated between the marginal and inadequate margin subsets (*P* = .6).

Although the numbers are small, radiotherapy appeared to improve local control following incomplete tumor excision. Radiation therapy for gross residual tumor following inadequate resection significantly reduced the rate of local recurrence (Fig 6). In fact, there was no significant difference in local failure for patients who underwent radiation therapy following partial tumor excision compared with those who had wide margin or compartment resections with an adequate margin of resection (the most favorable group, Fig 7). Radiation therapy administered for minimal disease left behind following inadequate resection did not improve local control. However, the majority of patients who received radiotherapy for minimal residual disease had previous recurrences.

Multivariate Analysis of Factors Influencing Local Failure

The covariate pairs of prognostic variables listed in Table 1 were entered into the Cox model of proportional hazards for multivariate analysis. Of the five significant pairs identified by univariate analysis, only two were found to be independently predictive of recurrence by the model: (1) less-than-adequate margin of resection (*P* = .0002) and (2) presentation with recurrent disease (*P* = .02). The Cox model coefficients predict a fourfold increase in the rate of local failure with a less-than-adequate margin of resection and a twofold increase due to presentation with recurrent disease. If both unfavorable factors are present, the model predicts an eightfold increase in the rate of local recurrence.

Treatment of Local Failure

Thirty-three of the 46 patients with failed initial treatment at Memorial Hospital underwent further resection with curative intent. Nine patients received radiotherapy in addition in surgery. Twenty-eight patients (85%) reresected for cure are alive without evidence of disease, with a median follow-up of 70 months (range, two to 236 months).

Survival

The overall five-year survival probability of patients treated with curative intent was 92% according to the Kaplan-Meier curve (Fig 8). Four patients died of causes unrelated to their tumors. Eleven patients died of disease, with a median time to death ranging from two to 136 months following treatment. Inexorable local tumor progression led to compromise of major organ functions or obstruction of the aerodigestive tract, frequently accompanied by sepsis and malnutrition. The ultimate causes of death are listed in Table 2. All patients dead of disease had nonextremity lesions for which the scope of resection was either partial excision or limited margins, and the pathologic margins of resection were less than adequate in all. Only one patient who died received radiotherapy as a method for control of residual disease visible on gross or microscopic examination. The tumor site was retroperitoneal in four patients, the abdominal wall in two patients, the head and neck in two patients, and the chest wall in one patient. The two remaining patients had Gardner's syndrome with extensive involvement of the abdominal wall and small-bowel mesentery.

COMMENT

The desmoid tumor remains a poorly understood neoplasm as a result of disparate reports regarding pathologic classification, tumor biology, and treatment alternatives. Many early reports documented the relentless local invasion of these tumors.[2,5,6,13,14] The term *aggressive fibromatosis* has, however, been applied as a diagnostic label for these neoplasms. At times, such a diagnosis may give an erroneous sense of security to the treating physician. Desmoid tumors are considered at our institution to be malignant soft-tissue tumors that have a predilection for

Table 2.—Causes of Death Following Treatment

Patient No.	Site	Initial Treatment	Cause of Death
1	Tonsillar fossa, neck	Commando procedure	Local disease progression, tracheal compression
2	Neck, shoulder girdle	Local excision	Local disease progression, intrathoracic invasion, superior vena cava syndrome
3	Chest wall	Chest wall resection	Local disease progression, intrathoracic and intra-abdominal invasion, tracheal compression
4	Abdominal wall, pelvis	Abdominal wall resection, hemipelvectomy	Local disease progression, fecal fistula, sepsis
5	Abdominal wall	Abdominal wall resection	Local disease progression, intra-abdominal invasion, small-bowel and colonic fistulas, pulmonary fibrosis secondary to bleomycin therapy
6	Abdominal wall, retroperitoneum	Abdominal wall resection of retroperitoneal mass, right-sided hemicolectomy, partial gastrectomy, small-bowel resection	Local disease progression, intra-abdominal invasion, malnutrition
7	Retroperitoneum	Resection of retroperitoneal mass, external beam and interstitial radiation	Local and distant disease progression, intra-abdominal invasion, pulmonary metastases
8	Retroperitoneum	Resection of retroperitoneal mass, partial cystectomy, sigmoid colectomy	Fistula, sepsis
9	Retroperitoneum	Resection of entire small bowel, small-bowel transplant	Sepsis, malnutrition, homograft rejection
10	Gardner's syndrome, abdominal wall	Abdominal wall resection, small-bowel resection	Local disease progression, chest wall and intra-abdominal invasion, duodenal fistula, sepsis, hepatic and renal failure
11	Gardner's syndrome, abdominal wall	Subtotal colectomy, resection of abdominal wall	Local disease progression, small-bowel fistula, malnutrition

aggressive local behavior and that rarely metastasize.[1,15] This classification, although not universally accepted, is corroborated by this in-depth retrospective analysis. The Task Force for Soft Tissue Sarcomas of the American Joint Committee for Cancer Staging and End Results Reporting also regarded these tumors as malignant neoplasms, referring to them as nonmetastasizing low-grade fibrosarcomas.[16] In addition, the American Cancer Society lists the desmoid tumor as a low-grade soft-tissue sarcoma,[17] and an expert panel[18] agreed on its behavior as such. The pronounced tendency toward local failure and potential for subsequent mortality, especially when managed inappropriately, confirms that the desmoid tumor is not a benign disease.

The natural history of untreated desmoid tumors, in general, is slow, relentless growth with invasion of contiguous structures. However, a small number of patients with inadequate excision may have stabilization and/or regression of their tumors. In the present series, 29% of patients who underwent partial excision were without evidence of disease at last follow-up. As mentioned above, distant tumor dissemination is uncommon[1] but did occur in a single patient. Transformation to a different histologic type, a process described by others, was not observed.

Aggressive resection in an effort to obtain as wide a margin of uninvolved surrounding tissue as possible is clearly the single most important determinant of a successful outcome. This finding, based on a retrospective analysis of 131 patients, corroborates our previous conviction[1,2,3,6] and that of others.[19,20] A recommendation of wide margin resection is in direct contradistinction to that of other authors, who do not recognize the malignant behavior of desmoid tumors and espouse conservative simple excision.[21-24] However, it is clear that marginal resection in the present series offered no advantage over surgical excision that was inadequate on gross examination. The resection should therefore be considered inadequate when the margin of resection on microscopic examination either is involved by tumor or approximates tumor. Presumably, undetected residual microscopic disease is present at the tumor bed site following excision with "minimal" surgical margins. Similarly, when a desmoid tumor recurs, attempts at curative resection of locally recurrent disease are warranted; observations in this study indicate that these patients can still be salvaged by appropriate surgery.

The use of radiotherapy either as a primary definitive treatment for control of residual disease or as an adjunct to surgical excision is less clear. There are conflicting reports regarding the efficacy of this treatment modality. Control of residual tumor visible on both microscopic and gross examination by radiation delivered by either the brachytherapy technique or external beam has been demonstrated.[20,25] In addition, partial or complete tumor regression when radiation is used as an alternative to surgery has been reported.[20,26] Other reports showed no benefit or a deleterious effect with the use of radiotherapy.[22] Our data suggest the possibility of prolonged local control in patients who undergo radiation following incomplete tumor extirpation. However, the numbers are small and further evaluation is necessary.

Standard chemotherapeutic agents have been sporadically used, but reports are anecdotal and results inconclusive. The role of hormonal therapy and other unconventional chemotherapeutic agents (nonsteroidal anti-inflammatory drugs, theophylline, chlorothiazide, etc) are similarly ill defined.

Controversy regarding the appropriate management of desmoid tumors may have resulted from misconceptions regarding their pathologic classification and clinical behavior. Benign fibromatoses do not have the histologic characteristics of desmoid tumors described in this study. We believe desmoid tumors should be recognized as low-grade soft-tissue sarcomas with a marked tendency toward local invasion. Failure to acknowledge this malignant behavior leads to conservative and inadequate surgical therapy with resultant local failure and the potential for subsequent mortality. Aggressive attempts at resection are warranted not only for initial definitive treatment but also to salvage patients who have recurrences. When an adequate margin of resection cannot be obtained due to the need to preserve vital anatomic structures, the addition of radiation therapy may provide the necessary "margin" to prevent local failure. The desmoid tumor is not a benign disease, and clinicians as well as pathologists should make every effort to distinguish it from fibromatoses. Proper management of desmoid tumors requires aggressive resectional techniques and, in select instances, adjunctive therapy to ensure a favorable outcome.

References

1. Hajdu SI: *Pathology of Soft-tissue Tumors.* Philadelphia, Lea & Febiger, 1979.
2. Das Gupta TK, Brasfield RD, O'Hara J: Extra-abdominal desmoids: A clinicopathological study. *Ann Surg* 1969;170:109-121.
3. Shiu MH, Flancbaum L, Hajdu SI, et al: Malignant soft tissue tumors of the anterior abdominal wall. *Arch Surg* 1980;115:152-155.
4. Suit HD, Russell WO: Radiation therapy of soft tissue sarcomas. *Cancer* 1975;36:759-764.
5. Gonatas NK: Extra-abdominal desmoid tumor. *Arch Pathol Lab Med* 1961;71:214-221.
6. Brasfield RD, Das Gupta TK: Desmoid tumors of the anterior abdominal wall. *Surgery* 1969;65:241-246.
7. Ellis F: Connective tissue sarcoma, in Hilaris BS (ed): *Handbook of Interstitial Brachytherapy.* Acton, Mass, Publishing Services Group Inc, 1975, pp 263-273.
8. Shiu MH, Turnbull AD, Nori D: Control of locally advanced extremity soft tissue sarcomas by function-saving resection and brachytherapy. *Cancer* 1984;53:1385-1392.
9. Shiu MH, Collin C, Hilaris BS, Nori D, et al: Limb preservation and tumor control in the treatment of popliteal and antecubital soft tissue sarcomas. *Cancer* 1986;57:1632-1639.
10. Kaplan EL, Meier P: Non-parametric estimation from incomplete observations. *Am Stat Assoc J* 1958;53:457-481.
11. Mantel N: Evaluation of survival data and two new rank order statistics arising in its consideration. *Cancer Chemother Rep* 1966;40:163-170.
12. Cox DR: Regression models and life tables. *J R Stat Assoc* 1972;34: 187-220.
13. Hunt RT, Morgan HC, Ackerman LV: Principles in management of extra-abdominal desmoids. *Cancer* 1960;13:825-836.
14. Pack GT, Ehrlich HE: Neoplasms of the anterior abdominal wall with special consideration of desmoid tumors: Experience with 391 cases and a collective review of the literature. *Int Abst Surg* 1944;79:177-198.
15. Hajdu SI: *Differential Diagnosis of Soft Tissue and Bone Tumors.* Philadelphia, Lea & Febiger, 1985.
16. Russell WO, Cohen J, Enzinger F, et al: A clinical and pathologic staging system for soft tissue sarcomas. *Cancer* 1977;40:1562-1570.
17. Hajdu SI: Soft tissue sarcomas: Classification and natural history. *Cancer* 1981;31:271-280.
18. Fine G, Hajdu SI, Morton DL, et al: Soft tissue sarcomas: Classification and treatment. *Pathol Ann* 1982;17:155-195.
19. Khorsard J, Karakousis C: Desmoid tumors and their management. *Am J Surg* 1985;149:215-218.
20. Kiel KD, Suit HD: Radiation therapy in the treatment of aggressive fibromatoses (desmoid tumors). *Cancer* 1984;54:2051-2055.
21. Reitamo JJ, Sheinin TM, Hayry P: The desmoid syndrome: New aspects in the cause, pathogenesis and treatment of the desmoid tumor. *Am J Surg* 1986;151:230-237.
22. Reitamo JJ: The desmoid tumor: IV. Choice of treatment, results and complications. *Arch Surg* 1983;118:1318-1322.
23. Rock MG, Pritchard DJ, Neiman HM, et al: Extra-abdominal desmoid tumors. *J Bone Joint Surg* 1984;66A:1369-1374.
24. Cole NM, Guiss LW: Extra-abdominal desmoid tumors. *Arch Surg* 1969;98:530-533.
25. Assad WA, Nori D, Hilaris BS, et al: Role of brachytherapy in the management of desmoid tumors. *Int J Radiat Oncol Biol Phys* 1979;5:1951-1956.
26. Wara WM, Phillips TL, Hill DR, et al: Desmoid tumors: Treatment and progress. *Radiology* 1977;124:225-226.

Discussion

Q I would like to present a different viewpoint of this disease and its treatment. We have spent a lot of time reviewing its pathologic characteristics in our hospital. Low grade fibrosarcoma does have up to one mitosis per ten high-power fields. One virtually never sees mitoses in a desmoid tumor, but the difference is that desmoid tumors are much much more vascular than low-grade fibrosarcomas. Low-grade fibrosarcomas rarely respond to radiation, but desmoid tumors respond beautifully to radiation. There have been several reports of radiotherapists treating desmoid tumors without any surgery at all with excellent long-term results. We do as wide an excision as we can, but we never mutilate the patient, and we do not worry about free margins. We always use radiotherapy after primary resection, and we rarely if ever see any recurrences in our own patients.

The real problem is that people undergo limited resections and then get recurrence after recurrence after recurrence and only then get radiation in tissues that are difficult to treat, and then these patients are in trouble. Patients with this disease who get radiation after the first treatment do the best, especially those with Gardner's syndrome, who have the bowel problems that most of your complications and deaths were associated with. I agree that desmoid tumor is not a benign disease, but it should never be overtreated with surgical resection, because this is unnecessary.

A The desmoid tumor appears to be very ubiquitous. Our data show that in some patients radiotherapy does have some value. However, there was a subset of patients who had minimal disease left behind following resection who did not respond at all to radiotherapy. I agree that our intent should be to avoid mutilating patients, and in patients with extremity lesions, one can continue to do resections with limb salvage without any possibility of death. In patients with lesions at other sites, such as the head and neck and abdominal wall, desmoid tumors appear to need aggressive resection with or without radiotherapy.

Q Regardless of how skillful or aggressive you are, there will occasionally be a desmoid tumor that is nonresectable. I have had two such patients under my care, and both responded to the administration of tamoxifen citrate. You did not mention this possibility, and it may not be common knowledge. Both patients were women, and neither had undergone irradiation before the administration of tamoxifen was started.

A There are anecdotal reports in the literature of the use of various nontraditional chemotherapeutic agents, such as tamoxifen, theophylline, and hydrochlorothiazide, with differing results. In this analysis I could not find any pattern, and that is why I did not mention it.

Q What about spontaneous regression? This is the mysterious thing about desmoid tumors, and it has been reported before. One of my patients had an advanced desmoid tumor that involved the brachial plexus and the intervertebral foramina that disappeared completely, and it has been gone for over 12 years. This boy did not take anti-inflammatory drugs. Two other patients had a marked decrease in the size of their tumors associated with the use of nonsteroidal anti-inflammatory drugs. Have you had any experience with spontaneous regression?

A There is no question that desmoid tumors can act very strangely. Approximately 20% of our patients who had a resection that was inadequate on gross examination did not have recurrences after long-term follow up. Some patients do have spontaneous regression. I do not know what is behind that.

Scar or Recurrent Rectal Cancer

Positron Emission Tomography Is More Helpful for Diagnosis Than Immunoscintigraphy

Peter Schlag, MD; Burkhard Lehner, MD; Ludwig G. Strauss, MD; Peter Georgi, MD; Christian Herfarth, MD

• We used positron emission tomography and fludeoxyglucose F 18 to assess metabolic activity of a pelvic mass in 18 patients who had suspected recurrent rectal cancer. Computed tomography could not differentiate tumor from scar. All patients presenting increased uptake of fludeoxyglucose F 18 by the mass were proved by histologic studies to suffer from recurrent tumor. Six of seven patients with low fludeoxyglucose uptake had nonmalignant lesions. Using immunoscintigraphy in 14 patients with elevated carcinoembryonic antigen levels, only four of ten recurrences could be identified by increased antibody accumulation in the mass. On the other hand, two of four benign lesions were interpreted as being recurrent tumor because of high uptake. Therefore, only positron emission tomography seems to be a useful diagnostic tool in the differentiation of recurrent rectal cancer and scar by providing information about the metabolic activity of a mass.

(*Arch Surg* 1989;124:197-200)

After curative surgical resection of rectal cancer, local tumor recurrence has been observed in 30% of patients.[1] When patients present with clinical signs of recurrence during follow-up, computed tomography (CT) of the pelvis is performed. In the case of a suspicious pelvic soft-tissue mass, however, differentiation between recurrent tumor and scar often is a problem. Needle biopsy guided by CT is an invasive procedure that cannot be used as a standard procedure and is reliable only in the case of a positive finding. To solve the problem of differentiation between scar and cancer, we investigated the feasibility and utility of two new diagnostic tools: positron emission tomography (PET) (for measurement of metabolism in the suspicious mass) and immunoscintigraphy. It has been demonstrated that neoplastic tissue has an augmented metabolic rate with increased glycolysis and lactate production that result in a high glucose consumption rate.[2,3] After the intravenous injection of fludeoxyglucose F 18, increased accumulation of this positron emitter in neoplastic tissue can be measured by PET.[4,5] Since the time monoclonal antibodies were developed, there have been efforts to use them for diagnosis and therapy.[6-8] A high percentage of colorectal tumors produce carcinoembryonic antigen (CEA) and carboanhydrate antigen 19-9 (Ca 19-9) and serial CEA/Ca 19-9 measurements have been used in postoperative follow-up studies.[9-11] In the case of an unexplained increase in CEA/Ca 19-9 levels, immunoscintigraphy has been performed to localize the tumor.[12] Therefore, we performed immunoscintigraphy with radioactive-labeled CEA/Ca 19-9 antibodies in the patients who had a suspicious pelvic mass and elevated CEA/Ca 19-9 levels. We investigated the hypothesis that antibody accumulation in the pelvic mass might give additional information and help to differentiate scar and cancerous tissue.

Accepted for publication July 6, 1988.

From the Departments of Surgery (Drs Schlag, Lehner, and Herfarth) and Nuclear Medicine (Dr Georgi), University of Heidelberg, and the Department of Nuclear Medicine, German Cancer Research Center (Dr Strauss), Heidelberg, Federal Republic of Germany.

Read before the Annual Meeting of the Society of Surgical Oncology, New Orleans, May 25, 1988.

Department of Surgery, University of Heidelberg, Im Neuenheimerfeld 110, 6900 Heidelberg, Federal Republic of Germany (Dr Schlag).

PATIENTS AND METHODS

After curative resection of rectal cancer, 18 patients showed clinical signs of recurrent disease during follow-up. Eleven of the patients had undergone anterior resection and seven had undergone abdominoperineal extirpation of the rectal tumor. Histologic staging of the primary tumor disclosed a pT2 tumor in four cases, a pT3 tumor in ten cases, and a pT4 tumor in four cases. The median disease-free interval was 15 months. In all patients a pelvic mass could be demonstrated by CT (Fig 1, top). All patients underwent PET to evaluate the potential of metabolic measurements for differentiating benign from malignant lesions. All patients were required to have a lesion diameter exceeding 1.5 cm to be included in the study (Table). After identification and marking of the CT section showing the greatest tumor diameter, PET was performed using a whole-body PET scanner (Scanditronix Co, Uppsala, Sweden, PC 2048-7 WB). The fludeoxyglucose F 18 (FDG), with an activity ranging from 115 to 440 megabecquerels, was injected intravenously and sequential images were acquired at five-minute intervals for a total of one hour. The PET cross-sectional images were compared with the corresponding CT images to permit positive identification of the lesion. For quantification of FDG uptake, a region-of-interest technique was used and time-activity curves were calculated from each series. Quantitative uptake of the radionuclide was measured in the suspicious mass as well as in the region of the gluteal muscles, which were

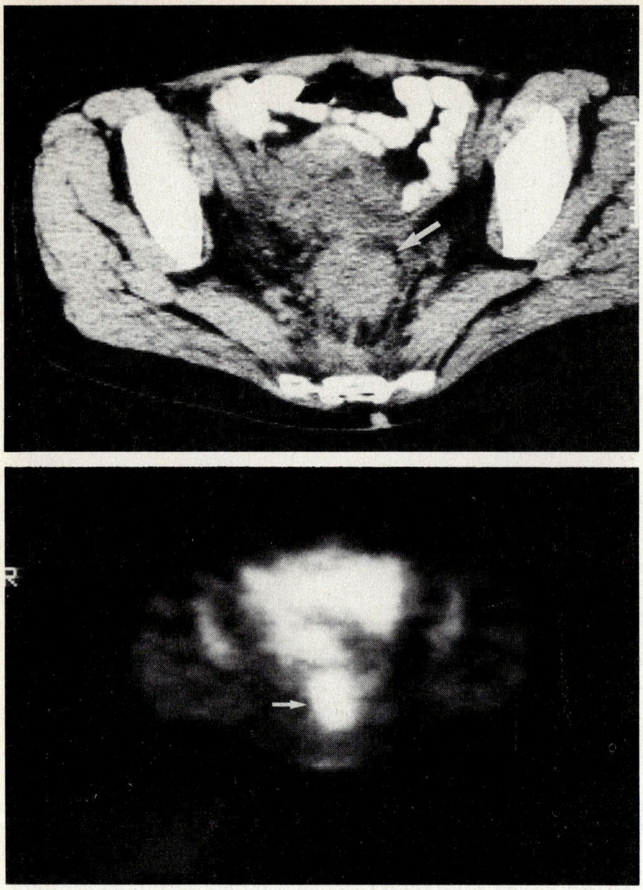

Fig 1.—Top, Pelvic mass (arrow) representing recurrent rectal cancer demonstrated in computed tomographic cross section. Bottom, Representative positron emission tomographic image (57.5 minutes after injection of fludeoxyglucose F 18) of same patient with high fludeoxyglucose F 18 accumulation in pelvic mass (arrow), indicating recurrent rectal cancer.

used as a normal soft-tissue reference. Tracer uptake was expressed as a differential absorption ratio (DAR), as follows: tissue concentration (nanocuries/gram)/[injected dose (nanocuries)/body weight (grams)]. Fourteen of the 18 patients had elevated CEA (>5 ng/mL) or Ca 19-9 (>35 U/L) levels. In these patients, immunoscintigraphy using a cocktail of J-131–labeled F(ab′)$_2$-fragments of monoclonal antibodies specific against CEA and Ca 19-9 (IMA CIS Firma CIS, Dreieich, Federal Republic of Germany) was performed. After intravenous administration of the labeled antibodies with a maximal dose of 72 megabecquerels, planar scintigraphic images in the anterior, posterior, and right lateral positions with as many as 100 kilocounts for each image were obtained on days 1, 3, 5, and 7 using a gamma scintillation camera (Ohio Nuclear, Sigma 410, Wiesbaden, Federal Republic of Germany; parallel hole collimator). Tracer accumulation in the pelvic area was assessed and tumor recurrence was assumed in the case of increased tracer uptake in the suspicious pelvic mass. For confirmation of the diagnosis made by PET and immunoscintigraphy, histologic studies of resected tumor specimens or serial biopsy specimens were used. In addition, the patient's clinical course and the change in the size of the mass that was judged to be benign were observed for at least four months using CT.

RESULTS

Increased uptake of FDG corresponding to an increased metabolic rate in the suspicious pelvic mass, as compared with reference soft tissue, could be seen by PET in 11 of the 18 patients (Fig 1, bottom). All of these patients were

Activity of Fludeoxyglucose F 18

Tissue	Mean (±SD) DAR, Time After Infusion*			
	7.5 min	17.5 min	37.5 min	57.5 min
Recurrent cancer (n=11)	2.35±0.4	2.05±0.5	1.90±0.6	2.05±0.7
Scar (n=6)	1.1±0.2	1.0±0.3	0.8±0.3	0.75±0.3
Soft tissue (n=18)	0.75±0.3	0.75±0.3	0.7±0.3	0.75±0.3

*DAR indicates differential absorption ratio.

shown by histologic studies to have recurrent rectal cancer. In these patients a rapid FDG uptake could be measured in the pelvic mass, followed by a slight decrease of the DAR up to 40 minutes after injection (Fig 2). At the end of the PET measurement (57.5 minutes after FDG injection), the tracer concentration was nearly three times as high as in normal soft tissue (Fig 3), with a FDG tumor-to–soft tissue ratio of 2.7. Therefore, the tumor region could clearly be discriminated from normal soft tissue. Six of the 14 patients with elevated CEA/Ca 19-9 levels manifested increased labeled antibody uptake in the pelvic mass. However, in only four of these six patients could a recurrence of rectal cancer be proved. Eight of the 14 patients with elevated tumor marker levels did not show any substantial antibody accumulation within the area of the pelvic mass that would falsely indicate a benign lesion. Histologic findings disclosed scar tissue only in two of these eight patients. Using PET, normal FDG uptake in the pelvic mass could be measured in seven of the 18 patients. In these patients a moderate increase in the FDG concentration up to 15 minutes after injection could be observed in the lesion by PET. This was followed by a continuous decrease in DAR values (Fig 3). Mean DAR values at the end of the measurement were identical for both nonmalignant scar tissue and normal reference soft tissue, with a scar tissue–to–soft tissue ratio of 1.0. Histologic examination could verify the presence of scar tissue in six of the seven patients with normal FDG uptake. One of these seven patients showed a recurrent malignant tumor. Therefore, there only was one false-negative result in 18 cases, indicating that a clear discrimination between cancer and soft tissue, as well as scar tissue, could be obtained by measurement of the metabolic rate using PET. Differentiation between scar tissue and cancer was best 57.5 minutes after injection of FDG. Sensitivity in differentiation was 92%, with a specificity of 100%, resulting in a positive predictive value of 100% and a negative predictive value of 86%. Immunoscintigraphy, however, only detected four of ten recurrences and two of four benign lesions. These four patients with elevated CEA/Ca 19-9 levels were later found to have liver metastases from the rectal cancer. In six cases false-negative results and in two cases false-positive results were seen. Sensitivity, therefore, was only 40% and specificity was 50%, resulting in a low negative predictive value of 25% and a positive predictive value of 67%.

COMMENT

Measurement by PET of FDG metabolism in malignant tumors has already been described earlier: an increased FDG uptake has been seen in gliomas. A correlation between FDG uptake and differentiation of the tumor has even been observed.[13] In pulmonary neoplasms there was a substantially increased FDG accumulation compared with normal pulmonary tissue.[14] In the present

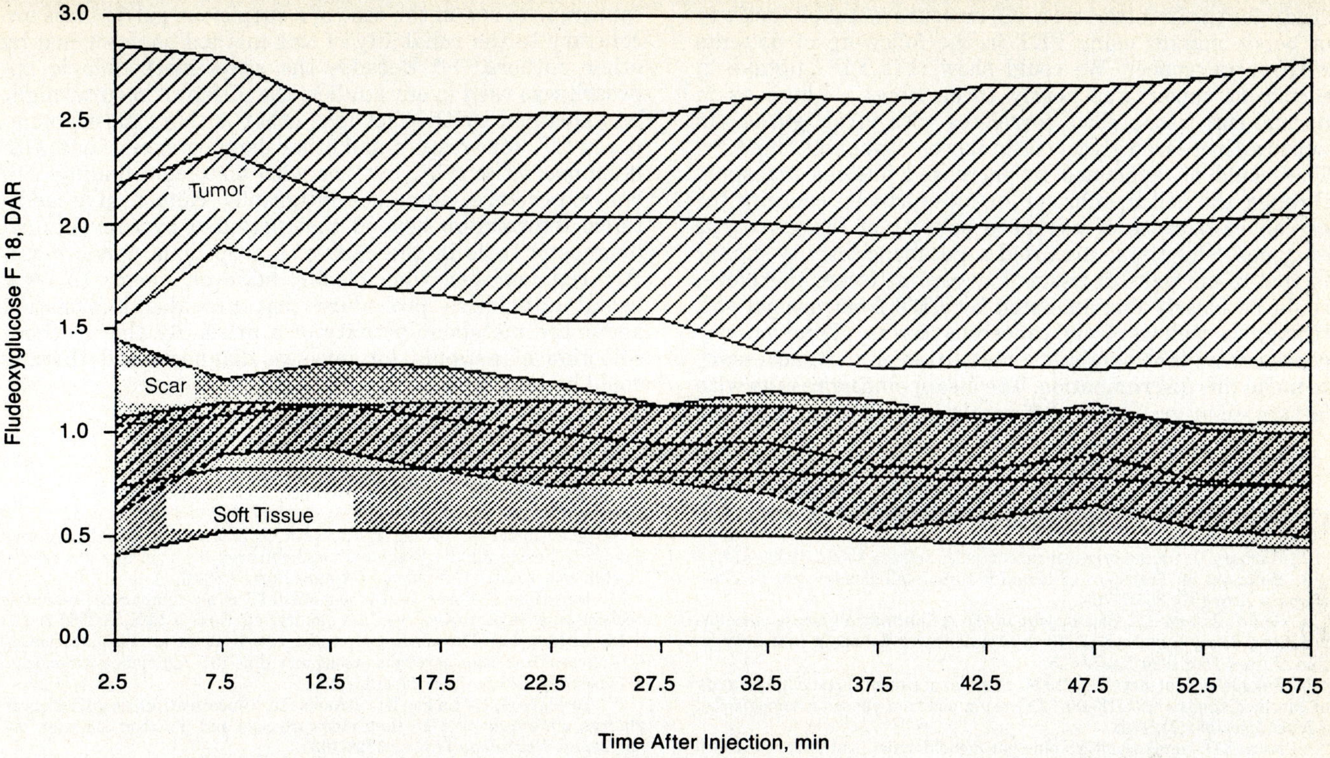

Fig 2.—Mean time-activity curve and SD for colorectal tumor, scar tissue, and reference soft tissue after intravenous injection of fludeoxyglucose F 18. DAR indicates differential absorption ratio.

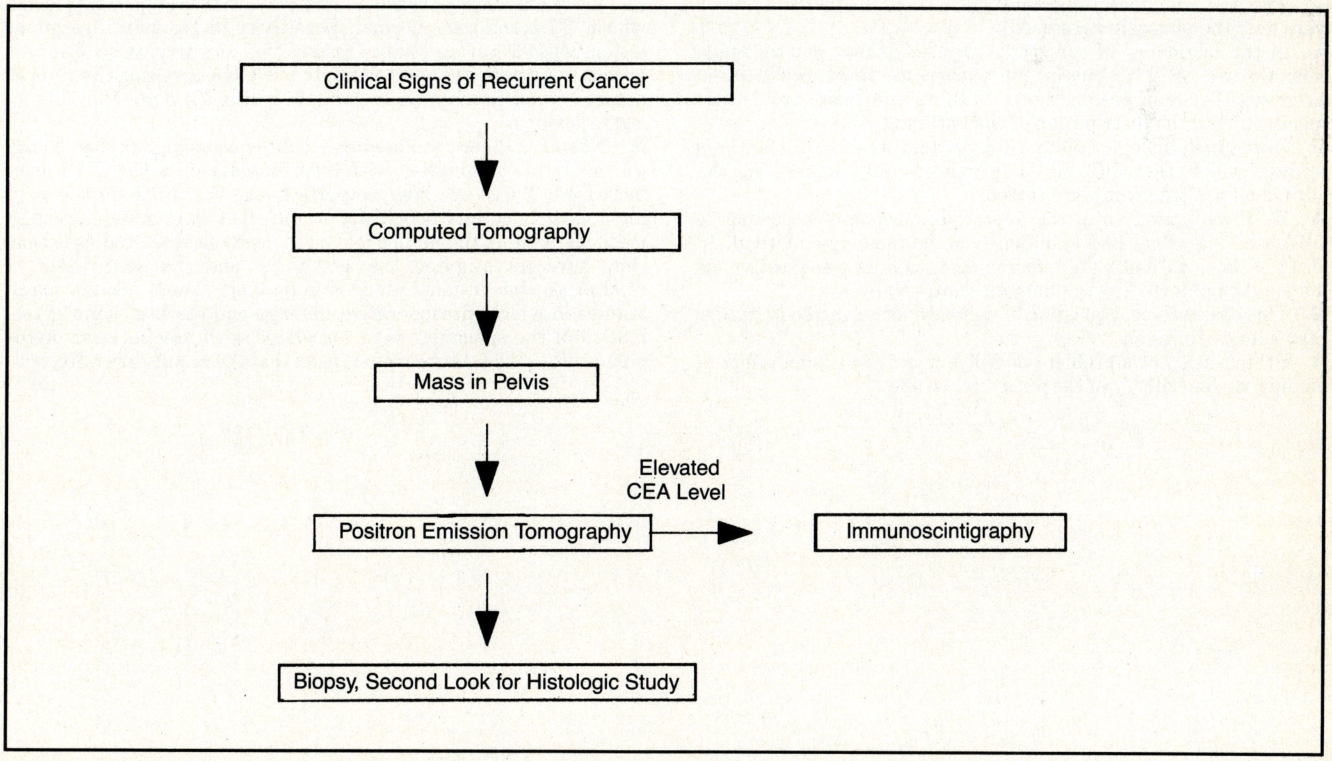

Fig 3.—Study design. CEA indicates carcinoembryonic antigen.

study, for the first time we could measure metabolic activity of pelvic masses using PET in the follow-up of patients with rectal cancer. We could show that FDG uptake in recurrent tumor was nearly three times as high as in normal soft tissue. This correlates with investigations in which an increased glycolysis in cancer tissue was found.[13,14] This could be explained by increased glucose transport through the cell membrane[3] or an enhanced capacity for glycolysis because of increased activity of the glycolytic enzymes. Scar tissue disclosed a metabolic activity similar to that of normal soft tissue. Cancerous tissue, therefore, could be clearly discriminated by PET from normal soft tissue, as well as from cancerous tissue. Time-activity curves show that only a few measurements are necessary to make this discrimination. The disappointing results with immunoscintigraphy in differentiating between scar and cancerous tissue in the case of a suspicious pelvic mass are contrary to the reliability of this method as described by other authors.[3,15,16] Because the same methodologic approach was used in our studies, the different results might be explained by the fact that other authors mostly compared CT, sonography, and other diagnostic methods with immunoscintigraphy, but not with histologic findings. In our experience, immunoscintigraphy cannot give additional information beyond that provided by conventional diagnostic tools in the case of a suspicious pelvic mass. Positron emission tomography, however, seems to be a useful adjunctive procedure that provides information about the metabolic activity of a mass. By this method, selection of patients for invasive diagnosis and therapy could be improved.

References

1. Herfarth C, Schlag P, Hohenberger P: Surgical strategies in locoregional recurrences of gastrointestinal carcinoma. *World J Surg* 1987;11:504-510.
2. Warburg O: On the origin of cancer cells. *Science* 1956;123:309-314.
3. Hatanaka M: Transport of sugars in tumor cell membranes. *Biochem Biophys Acta* 1974;355:77-104.
4. Som P, Atkins HL, Bandoypadhyay D: A fluorinated glucose analogue 2-fluoro-2-deoxy-D-glucose (F-18): Nontoxic tracer for rapid tumor detection. *J Nucl Med* 1980;21:670-675.
5. Fukuda H, Matsuzawa T, Ito M, et al: Experimental and clinical study of cancer diagnosis with (F-18) FDG using positron emission tomography. *J Nucl Med* 1984;25:50-51.
6. Munz LD: Immunszintigraphie mit monoklonalen Antikörpern. *Dtsch Med Wochenschr* 1987;112:649-654.
7. Biersack HJ, Bockisch A, Vogel J, et al: Szintigraphischer Malignomnachweis mit radioaktiv markierten Tumorantikörpern. *Dtsch Med Wochenschr* 1987;112:341-344.
8. Mach JP, Carrel S, Forni N, et al: Tumor localization of radiolabeled antibodies against carcinoembryonic antigen in patients with carcinoma. *N Engl J Med* 1980;303:5-10.
9. Abel U, Quentmeier A, Herfarth C: Monitoring plasma CEA in the follow-up of colorectal cancer: The validation of a class of diagnostic criteria for early detection of local recurrence and metastases. *Theor Surg* 1986;1:136-141.
10. Quentmeier A, Schlag P, Herfarth C: Bestätigung der Bedeutung des CEA: Testes für die Diagnostik und chirurgische Therapie des rezidivierten colorectalen Carcinoms. *Chirurg* 1986;57:83-87.
11. Denstman F, Rosen L, Khubchandani IT, et al: Comparing predictive decision rules in postoperative CEA monitoring. *Cancer* 1986;58:2089-2095.
12. Leyden MJ, Thompson CH, Lichtenstein M, et al: Visualization of metastases from colon carcinoma using an iodine 131–radiolabeled monoclonal antibody. *Cancer* 1986;57:1135-1139.
13. Di Chiro G, De La Paz RL, Brooks RA: Glucose utilization of cerebral gliomas measured by F-18 fluorodeoxyglucose and positron emission tomography. *Neurology* 1982;32:1323-1329.
14. Nolop KB, Rhodes CG, Brudin LH, et al: Glucose utilization in vivo by human pulmonary neoplasms. *Cancer* 1987;60:2682-2689.
15. Chatal JF, Herry JY, Laneche B, et al: Immunoscintigraphic localization of gastrointestinal carcinomas and their recurrences, in Schmidt HAE, Ell PJ, Britton KE (eds): *Nuclear Medicine in Research and Practice.* New York, Schattauer, 1986, pp 424-426.
16. Begnet RHJ, Keep PA, Searle F, et al: Radioimmunolocalization and selection for surgery in recurrent colorectal cancer. *Br J Surg* 1986;73:64-67.

Discussion

Q Was the immunoscintigraphy performed using SPECT or were only the planar images used?

A In the beginning of our study we used planar scintigraphy. Now we use SPECT, but in our experience there really is no difference between the methods. I think the main problem is specificity and the distribution of the antibody.

Q In the immunologic studies, did you test whether the antigen against which the antibody is prepared was present in the individual patients who were tested?

A We investigated all of the operative specimens according to CEA staining or Ca 19-9 staining by an immunologic method. In all 14 of these patients, the immunologic staining was positive, so it should be detected by the immunoscintigraphy.

Q This seems to be a question of delivery of the antibody, rather than a lack of antigen.

A I think it is not a problem of delivery only but is an effect of binding and specificity of the antibody we used.

Q We studied recurrence in patients with rising CEA levels whose CT scans were normal. Sensitivity in the identification of lesions was 85% in our study. Perhaps this sensitivity was different because our patients had relatively low CEA levels at the time of detection and perhaps your patients had much higher levels and larger lesions.

A No, all of these patients had CEA levels no higher than 50 ng/mL. Only in combination with liver metastases is the CEA level increased. There are many reports in the literature on the very high sensitivity and specificity of different immunoscintigraphy methods. I think the main problem in most of these studies is that they have investigated the sensitivity and specificity only in relation to conventional diagnostic findings. There are not many studies in which intraoperative findings and the histologic examination of the specimen were correlated with preoperative metabolic studies. This is the main reason that the results are different.

Meeting the surgical challenge: hernia repair.

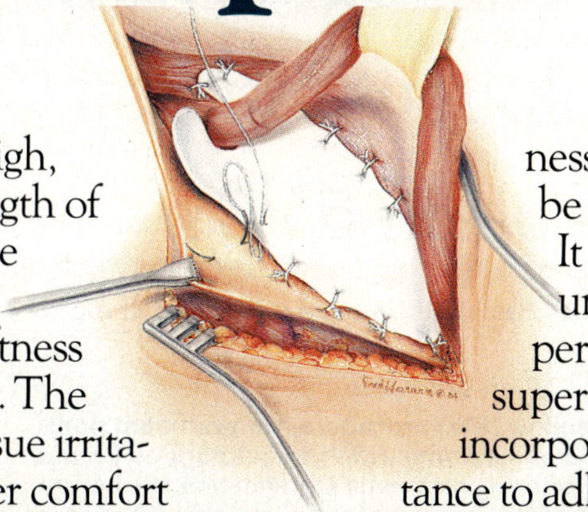

This remarkable surgical patch, capable of tissue incorporation and possessing both strength and superior handling, is used in even the most demanding soft tissue repairs.

Clinical experience shows that the GORE-TEX™ Soft Tissue Patch provides dependable reinforcement and suture retention, low levels of complications, and conforms easily to the contours of the natural tissue.

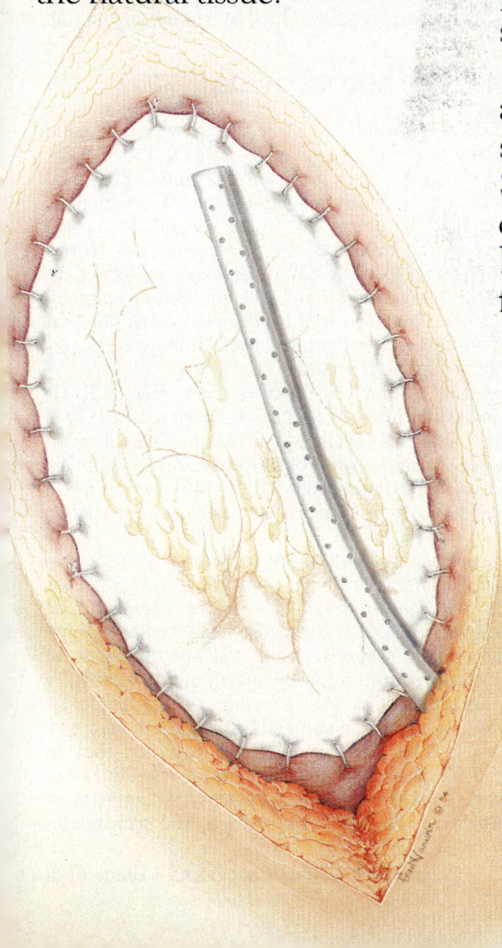

And yet, the high, balanced strength of the Soft Tissue Patch does not sacrifice the softness of the material. The result is less tissue irritation and greater comfort for the patient postoperatively.

Also, it is highly versatile. It is widely used in clinical applications ranging from hernia repairs, including large abdominal wall defects, to prolapse, banding and reconstruction of tissue deficiencies.

Tissue ingrowth is encouraged by the microporous structure of the GORE-TEX Soft Tissue Patch, unlike other prostheses that can become encapsulated by fibrous scar tissue. Recent clinical publications and experience support greater tissue acceptance and a significantly lower incidence of visceral adhesions in the experimental model.

Packaged sterile, the GORE-TEX Soft Tissue Patch comes in both 1.0mm and 2.0mm thicknesses and can be resterilized. It provides unmatched performance: superior handling, incorporation, resistance to adhesion formation and treatability in the presence of infection.

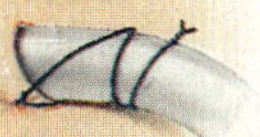

For more information, use the coupon or call, toll free, 800/638-4804.

GORE-TEX™ Soft Tissue Patch

AOS-289

☐ Please have your sales representative call for an appointment.

☐ Send detailed information concerning clinical results.

☐ I'm interested in a free sample of the GORE-TEX™ Soft Tissue Patch.

Name ______

Address ______

City ______

State ______ Zip ______

Surgical Specialty ______

Phone ______

Hospital Affiliation ______

W.L. Gore & Associates, Inc.
Post Office Box 1220, Route 213 North
Elkton, MD 21921

GORE

CREATIVE TECHNOLOGIES WORLDWIDE

Prognostic Significance of Cellular Immunity to Autologous Breast Carcinoma and Glycoprotein 55

Maurice M. Black, MD; Reinhard E. Zachrau, MD; Roy H. Ashikari, MD; Benjamin F. Hankey, ScD

• Using a skin window (SW) procedure, we evaluated postoperative cell-mediated immunity (CMI) to autologous breast cancer with reference to its prognostic significance, the nature of the immunogen, and the therapeutic implications. It appears that SW reactivity to autologous breast cancer is prognostically favorable per se and is independent of the prognostic significance of the nuclear grade of the cancer cells; SW reactivity to autologous breast cancer reflects CMI to a determinant(s) that is expressed by glycoprotein 55, the principal envelope glycoprotein of the RIII-murine mammary tumor virus; the glycoprotein 55–like CMI determinant(s) is more regularly expressed by preinvasive than by invasive breast cancers; tumor antigenicity and host reactivity may vary independently; and postoperative monitoring of CMI to autologous breast cancer is prognostically and therapeutically important.

(*Arch Surg* 1989;124:202-206)

Numerous studies have demonstrated that the biological behavior of breast cancer reflects interactions between the aggressive potential of the cancer and tumor-retarding influences of the host. The aggressive potential is inversely correlated with the microscopically demonstrable differentiation of the cancer cell nuclei (nuclear grade [NG]).[1,2] More recently, automated cytophotometry has been utilized to provide numerical representations of the microscopically demonstrable variations in the NG.[3] The salient point is that variations in the NG are associated with highly significant differences in survival. However, the survival characteristics are also influenced by immunological host responses to the tumor. Such prognostically significant responses are microscopically evident in the primary cancer and in the regional lymph nodes as lymphoreticuloendothelial cellular reactions that are consistent with cell-mediated immunity (CMI).[2,4,5] Manifestations of such CMI are also demonstrable by means of in vitro[6-8] and in vivo[9-11] measurements. Each of these indexes demonstrates that immunogenicity develops during the preinvasive phase of breast cancer and that immunologically mediated tumor retardation depends on both, the retention of the specific antigenicity of the cancer cells and the specific CMI of the host.[12,13]

We now report on expanded observations on the prognostic significance of specific immunity against NG-characterized autologous breast cancer, as evaluated in vivo by the skin window (SW) procedure. We shall demonstrate that the prognostically favorable SW reactivity in patients with breast cancer is directed against a CMI determinant(s) that is similar to a determinant(s) expressed by glycoprotein 55 (gp55), the principal envelope glycoprotein of the RIII-murine mammary tumor virus, and that is more regularly expressed by preinvasive than by invasive breast cancers.

PATIENTS AND METHODS

Our study population included those patients with operable breast cancer characterized in our previous report on SW reactivity to autologous breast cancer.[11] In addition to expanded clinical follow-up data, this report includes results on the SW responses of these patients to gp55. We also report on the responses to gp55 in a series of patients with breast cancer who were not tested against autologous breast cancer. All SW tests were performed on patients who had no evidence of metastases or second primary cancers. Informed consent, as approved by the New York Medical College (Valhalla) Committee for Protection of Human Subjects, was obtained from all study participants.

The gp55 was isolated from virus derived from milk of RIII-strain mice. The isolation procedure has been described in a previous publication.[14] For SW testing, 2 μg of gp55 was applied to the center of 25-mm-diameter round glass coverslips. After air drying, the coverslips were immersed for 15 minutes in a 1:1 mixture of ether and 95% ethanol, air dried again, and stored at −20°C until use.

The SW test procedure involved the application of a target-containing (gp55 or autologous tumor) coverslip to an abraded area of skin for approximately 30 hours. After removal, the coverslip was stained with Wright's stain and evaluated as to type and extent of the cellular response. The various patterns of responses and their classification have been defined previously.[9,11] In essence, the stained coverslips were examined microscopically for focal aggregations of mononuclear cells of the histiocytic or lymphoblastoid type, having nonvacuolated cytoplasm that is typically basophilic. The histiocytic-type aggregates may be monolayered or multilayered. In the lymphoblastoid-type aggregates, the cells may be spherical or hand-mirror–shaped, and multinucle-

Accepted for publication Nov 3, 1988.

From the Departments of Pathology (Drs Black and Zachrau) and Surgery (Dr Ashikari), New York Medical College, Valhalla, and Surveillance and Operations Research Branch, Division of Cancer Prevention and Control, National Cancer Institute, Bethesda, Md (Dr Hankey).

Read before the Annual Meeting of the Society of Surgical Oncology, New Orleans, May 25, 1988.

Reprint requests to Department of Pathology, New York Medical College, Valhalla, NY 10595 (Dr Black).

Table 1.—Skin Window (SW) Reactivity Against Autologous Carcinoma Among Unselected Patients With In Situ and Invasive Breast Cancer, One to 24 Months Postoperatively, and Among Patients With Invasive Breast Cancer Known to Have Subsequently Developed Systemic Metastases (MET)

	SW 1-24 Months Postoperatively, No. (%)		SW Tests 1->120 Months Postoperatively, No. (%)	
			Interval From SW to MET, mo	
SW Response Intensity*	In Situ Breast Cancer	Invasive Breast Cancer	<30	≥30
Tests				
≥3	51 (46)†	153 (19)†	6 (5)‡	40 (21)‡
2	14	85	5	16
1	47 (42)	566 (70)	105 (91)	131 (70)
Total	**112 (100)**	**804 (100)**	**116 (100)**	**187 (100)**
Patients§				
≥3	21 (60)‖	87 (31)‖	...	...
2	7	42	...	...
1	7 (20)	150 (54)	...	...
Total	**35 (100)**	**279 (100)**	...	...

*See "Patients and Methods" section for explanation.
†$P<.0001$ for the difference in relative frequency of an SW response intensity of 3 or more by stage.
‡$P<.0001$ for the difference in relative frequency of an SW response intensity of 3 or more by interval between SW test and development of metastasis.
§By the maximal SW response during the interval.
‖$P<.001$ for the difference in relative frequency of an SW response intensity of 3 or more by stage.

Table 2.—Skin Window (SW) Reactivity Against RIII-Glycoprotein 55 (gp55) Among Unselected Patients With In Situ and Invasive Breast Cancer, One to 24 Months Postoperatively, and Among Patients With Invasive Breast Cancer Known to Have Subsequently Developed Systemic Metastases (MET)

	SW 1-24 Months Postoperatively, No. (%)		SW Tests 1->120 Months Postoperatively, No. (%)	
			Interval From SW to MET, mo	
SW Response Intensity*	In Situ Breast Cancer	Invasive Breast Cancer	<30	≥30
Tests				
≥3	37 (43)†	98 (30)†	18 (26)‡	30 (34)‡
2	9	49	9	14
1	41 (47)	179 (55)	43 (61)	43 (49)
Total	**87 (100)**	**326 (100)**	**70 (100)**	**87 (100)**
Patients§				
≥3	16 (62)‖	38 (52)‖	...	...
2	2	13	...	...
1	8 (31)	22 (30)	...	...
Total	**26 (100)**	**73 (100)**	...	...

*See "Patients and Methods" section for explanation.
†$P<.05$.
‡Not significant.
§By the maximal SW response during the interval.
‖Not significant.

ated Langhans' giant cells may be present. Less commonly, the cellular response is in the form of aggregates of elongated and multipolar histiocytic cells (stellate type) or of lymphoblastoid cells with associated neutrophilic, eosinophilic, and basophilic polymorphonuclear leukocytes. Basophils and/or eosinophils may also be scattered among the other types of responses. None of these response patterns is found when either blank coverslips or coverslips with normotypic breast tissue are applied to patients with breast cancer or to control subjects.

Numerical values were assigned in relation to the size of aggregates of any of the above described types, namely, 1 for less than 25%, 2 for 25%, 3 for 50% to 75%, and 4 for more than 75% occupation of a low-power (×100) microscopic field. The collective designation "positive" is given to any of the described response patterns when the aggregates occupy 50% or more of a low-power field (SW response of 3 or higher). Skin window responses with aggregates occupying 25% to less than 50% of a low-power field are designated as "borderline positive." The designation "negative" is given to SW responses with aggregates occupying less than 25% of a low-power field (SW response of 1), those with larger aggregates showing prominent cytonecrosis, and those without distinct types of aggregates.

The data were evaluated by one of us (B.F.H.), utilizing the statistical methods cited in our prior report.[11]

RESULTS

Skin Window Reactivity Against Autologous In Situ and Invasive Breast Cancer

The results of the SW tests against autologous stage 0 in situ breast cancer and against invasive breast cancer during the one- to 24-month postoperative interval are listed in Table 1. As judged by the total number of tests, positive (≥3) responses were proportionately more frequent among patients with in situ (46%) than those with invasive (19%) breast cancer ($P<.0001$). A similar difference in SW reactivity between patients with in situ and those with invasive breast cancer was found in terms of the maximal response per patient during the one- to 24-month postoperative interval, namely, 60% vs 31% ($P<.001$). Table 1 also lists the distribution of SW responses of those patients with invasive breast cancer who developed systemic metastases less than 30 or 30 months or more after SW tests that had been performed at diverse postoperative intervals. Positive (≥3) SW responses against autologous invasive breast cancer were uncommon (5%) among patients who developed metastases less than 30 months after testing and significantly less frequent than among patients who developed metastases 30 months or more after testing (21%) ($P<.0001$).

Skin Window Reactivity Against gp55 Among Patients With In Situ and Invasive Breast Cancer

As shown in Table 2, the relative frequency of positive (≥3) SW responses against gp55, one to 24 months postoperatively, was greater among patients with in situ than patients with invasive breast cancer. This difference is statistically significant for the total number of positive tests. Evaluation by maximal response per patient during this interval shows the same trend, but that difference is not statistically significant.

Comparison of the observations (Tables 1 and 2) reveals that, among patients with invasive breast cancer, positive reactivity was more frequently found against gp55 than against the autologous carcinoma, namely, 30% vs 19% ($P<.0005$), by total number of tests, and 52% vs 31% ($P=.002$), by maximal response per patient during the one- to 24-month postoperative interval. The proportion of positive SW responses to gp55 was also significantly greater than that to autologous carcinoma among patients with invasive breast cancer who subsequently developed

Table 3.—Simultaneous Skin Window (SW) Reactivity Against RIII–Glycoprotein 55 (gp55) and Autologous Carcinoma Among Unselected Patients With In Situ and Invasive Breast Cancer Tested One to 120 or More Months Postoperatively

SW vs gp55: Response Intensity*	SW vs Autologous Breast Cancer: Response Intensity, No. (%)† ≥3	2	1	Total
In Situ				
≥3	32 (78)‡¶ [37]‖	6	3	**41** (100)
2	7 (41)	7	3	**17** (100)
1	1 (3)‡	1	27 [31]#	**29** (100)
Total	**40**	**14**	**33**	**87** [100]
Invasive				
≥3	68 (52)§¶ [14]‖	28	36	**132** (100)
2	5 (6)	42	30	**77** (100)
1	6 (2)§	13	266 [54]#	**285** (100)
Total	**79**	**83**	**332**	**494** [100]

*See "Patients and Methods" section for explanation.
†Numbers in brackets are percentages related to bracketed total.
‡$P<.0001$.
§$P<.0001$.
‖$P<.0001$.
¶$P<.005$.
#$P<.0005$.

Table 4.—Qualitative and Quantitative Characteristics of Skin Window (SW) Reactivity Against Autologous Carcinoma Among Patients With In Situ and Invasive Breast Cancer With Positive SW Reactivity Against RIII–Glycoprotein 55 (gp55) in Simultaneous Tests, One to 120 or More Months Postoperatively

SW vs gp55 Positive (≥3) Response Type*	SW vs Autologous Breast Cancer, No. (%): Positive (≥3) Type: Same	Different	All Types: 2	1	Total
In Situ					
Lymphoblastoid	14 (82)†	0	2	1	**17** (100)
Histiocytic	15 (63)‡	3	4	2	**24** (100)
Other types	0	0	0	0	0
Total	**29** (71)§	**3**	**6**	**3** (7)‖	**41** (100)
Invasive					
Lymphoblastoid	19 (39)†	4	11	15	**49** (100)
Histiocytic	35 (49)‡	5	16	16	**72** (100)
Other types	3	2	1	5	11
Total	**57** (43)§	**11**	**28**	**36** (27)‖	**132** (100)

*See "Patients and Methods" section for explanation.
†$P<.005$.
‡Not significant.
§$P<.005$.
‖$P<.02$.

systemic metastases. This was particularly evident among patients who developed metastases more than 30 months after SW testing (26% vs 5%, $P<.0005$), but to a lesser extent also among those who developed metastases 30 months or more after testing (34% vs 21%, $P<.05$). All of these differences in reactivity against autologous breast cancer and gp55 indicated the need to examine the reactivity against both targets by simultaneous testing in individual patients.

Simultaneous SW Reactivity Against Autologous Breast Cancer and gp55

Quantitative Features.—As shown in Table 3, among both patients with in situ and those with invasive breast cancer, failure to respond to gp55 was characteristically associated with failure to respond to the autologous carcinoma in simultaneous tests. This was observed in tests performed over a wide range of postoperative intervals, ie, from one month to more than ten years. However, the proportions of simultaneous tests that were negative to both gp55 and autologous carcinoma differed between the in situ and the invasive breast cancer series, ie, 31% vs 54% ($P<.0005$).

Patients with in situ and patients with invasive breast cancers differed also in regard to the relative frequency of simultaneous reactivity against gp55 and autologous carcinoma: in the in situ cancer patient series, positive reactivity against gp55 was associated with positive reactivity against autologous cancer in 78% of the tests, compared with 52% in the invasive cancer patient series ($P<.005$). It should also be noted that simultaneous positive reactivity against both gp55 and autologous cancer was found in 37% of the in situ cancer patient series in contrast to only 14% of the invasive cancer patient series ($P<.0001$).

These observations suggest that positive SW reactivity against autologous breast cancer reflects host reactivity against a CMI determinant(s) that is expressed by gp55, *and* the presence of such a gp55-like CMI determinant(s) in the breast cancer cells. It further appears that host reactivity and breast cancer antigenicity may vary independently.

Qualitative Features.—As mentioned above, the SW responses to autologous breast cancer may show qualitative as well as quantitative variations among different patients and in the same patient at different times. Analogous variations in SW responses have been observed in tests against gp55. It was, therefore, of interest to examine the qualitative characteristics of *simultaneous* SW responses to gp55 and autologous breast cancer in those instances in which the SW reactivity against gp55 was positive (≥3) at any postoperative interval.

As shown in Table 4, the qualitative SW characteristics were divided into the following three groups: lymphoblastoid, histiocytic, and other types. The simultaneous responses to the autologous carcinoma were grouped according to the quantitative features, ie, 3 or more (positive), 2 (borderline positive), and 1 (negative). In addition, positive (≥3) responses to the autologous cancer were subdivided into those with the same and those with a different type of response. The in situ breast cancer patient series revealed a particularly striking similarity between the simultaneous SW responses to gp55 and autologous cancer, ie, 71% were both qualitatively and quantitatively similar. This degree of similarity was significantly ($P<.005$) greater than that found in the invasive breast cancer patient series (43%).

Considered in toto, the data of Tables 3 and 4 support the view that immunogenic human breast cancers express a CMI determinant(s) that is similar to a CMI determinant(s) expressed by RIII-gp55. It further appears that such antigenicity regularly accompanies the preinvasive phase of mammary carcinogenesis but is less regularly expressed by invasive breast cancers.

Prognostic Significance of SW Reactivity Against Autologous Invasive Breast Cancer and gp55

The prognostic influence of SW reactivity against autologous breast cancer, per se and in relation to the NG of the

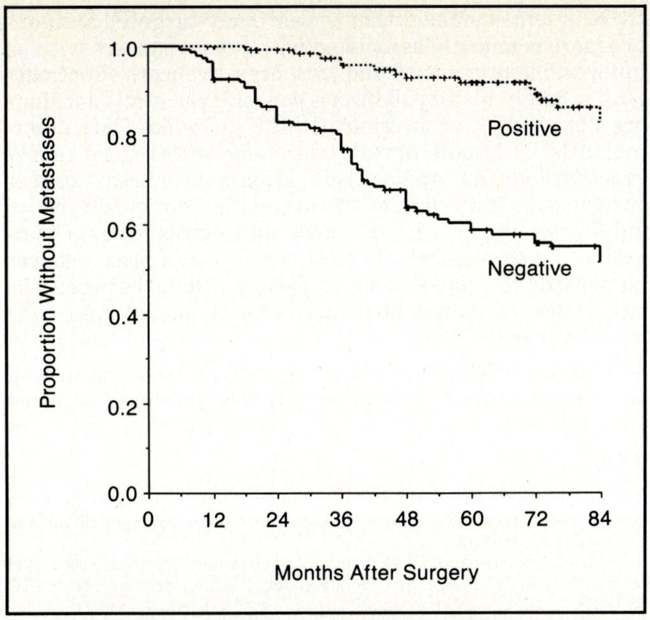

Fig 1.—Proportion of patients with invasive breast cancer free of metastases at increasing postoperative intervals, in relation to maximal skin window (SW) reactivity against autologous carcinoma, one to 24 months postoperatively. Positive (SW response, ≥2) includes 129 patients; negative, (SW response, <2) 150 patients.

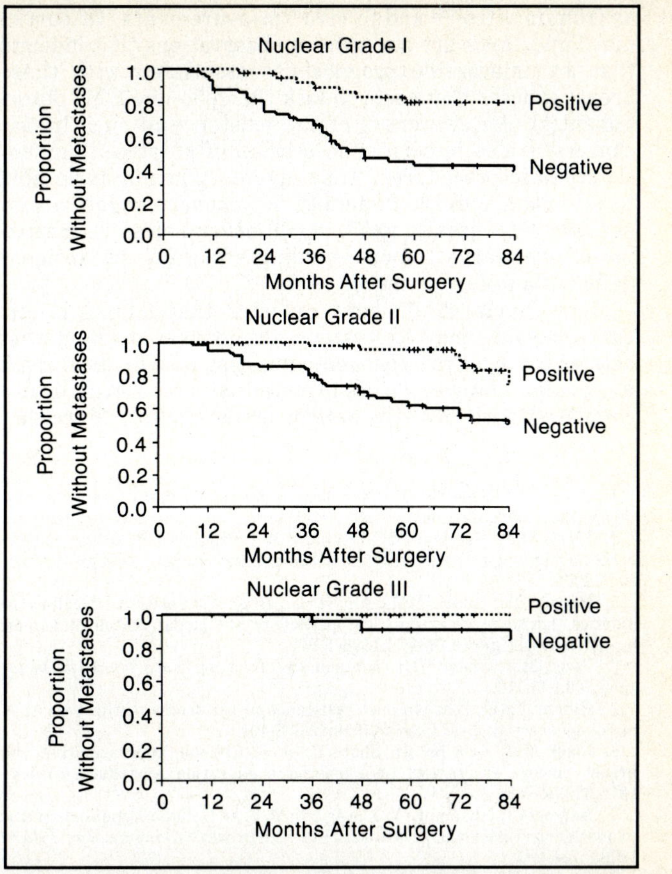

Fig 2.—Proportion of patients with invasive breast cancer free of metastases at increasing postoperative intervals, in relation to nuclear grade (NG) and maximal skin window (SW) reactivity against autologous carcinoma, one to 24 months postoperatively. Patient numbers by category were as follows: NG I: SW positive, 43, and SW negative, 63; NG II: SW positive, 54, and SW negative, 62; NG III: SW positive, 32, and SW negative, 25.

cancer, is depicted in Figs 1 and 2, respectively. The Kaplan-Meier survival curves are consistent with those reported previously[11] and demonstrate the prognostic significance of SW reactivity. Figure 2 also illustrates the independent prognostic significance of the NG. The prognostic significance of the differences between the SW-positive and SW-negative Kaplan-Meier survival curves was evaluated by adjusted and unadjusted Mantel-Haenszel χ^2 tests.[15] In addition, the Cox proportional hazards model was used to analyze the joint effects on prognosis of clinical and pathologic variables in conjunction with the SW test status.[16] These procedures demonstrate the prognostic significance of SW reactivity *after* adjustment for the variables patient age, lymph node status, and NG of the cancer.

With respect to the prognostic significance of SW reactivity against gp55, it is noteworthy that 15 of our patients with negative SW responses to autologous invasive breast cancer, one to 24 months postoperatively, showed positive (≥3) reactivity in simultaneous tests against gp55 on at least one occasion. Eleven of these patients, however, had shown positive SW reactivity against autologous breast cancer at least once before or after the discrepant responses. Only one of these 11 patients so far has developed systemic metastases that occurred 76 months postoperatively. Ten of these 11 patients are free of recurrent disease at 24, 28, and 61 to 80 months postoperatively. The remaining four patients were consistently nonreactive against their autologous cancer in four to eight tests, despite one or more positive SW responses to gp55 in simultaneous tests. In contrast to the aforementioned 11 patients, all four of the latter group developed systemic metastases less than 36 months postoperatively. These findings indicate that breast cancer antigenicity and specific host CMI may vary independently and that the prognostic significance of SW reactivity against gp55 depends on the expression of the gp55-like CMI determinant(s) by the cancer cells.

COMMENT

Our study provides further evidence of the prognostic significance of SW reactivity against autologous breast cancer, as a single variable and in association with the NG of the cancer cells. Since the prognostic significance of CMI to autologous breast cancer is maintained over a wide range of postoperative intervals, agents or procedures that are capable of inducing a negative-to-positive change in SW reactivity against autologous breast cancer should reduce the development and/or progression of metastatic disease over a broad range of postoperative intervals. It is important that studies of putative immunotherapeutic agents include measurements of specific reactivity against autologous cancer before and after treatment.[10] The failure to perform such measurements makes it difficult, if not impossible, to determine whether the treatment in question has immunostimulatory capabilities, let alone therapeutic benefits.

Among patients with in situ breast cancers, there is a striking similarity in the responses to gp55 and autologous cancer, both qualitatively and quantitatively. Thus, it appears that a gp55-like CMI determinant(s) is regularly expressed during the preinvasive phase of breast cancer. A significant minority may cease to express this determinant(s) during the invasive phase of the disease. This conclusion follows from our microscopic findings[12] as well as from in vitro[17,18] and in vivo[10] measurements. Of particular importance are our current observations that indicate that an unfavorable prognosis is associated with those breast cancers that seem to lack the gp55-like CMI determinant(s). An awareness of the existence of such breast cancers is also important in studies of putative immunotherapeutic procedures. Thus, agents that might be able to stimulate specific immunity, ie, convert negative into positive responses to gp55, would nevertheless be incapable of exerting a tumor-retarding effect on the antigen-deficient autologous cancer cells.

Mesa-Tejada et al[19] have reported that human breast cancer tissues may express an antigenic component that acts as a target for xenogenic anti-gp55 antibodies. Such antibodies, however, do not preferentially react with in situ compared with invasive human breast cancer. Moreover, there is some evidence that the antibody-targeted antigens are more commonly associated with breast cancers with an unfavorable prognosis[20] and with breast cancers of patients with a family history of breast cancer.[21] Such relationships are not evident with regard to the gp55-like CMI determinant(s) of human breast cancer nor with regard to SW reactivity against gp55. Also, patients with breast cancer rarely manifest circulating antibodies to gp55[22] or to autologous breast cancer. These differences in the observations on serological and CMI responses to breast cancer emphasize the importance of distinguishing between the two types of immunological reactivity in patients with breast cancer.

The authors thank Arnold S. Dion, PhD, Center for Molecular Medicine and Immunology, Newark, NJ, for the isolation of gp55 from RIII-murine mammary tumor virus.

References

1. Black MM, Speer FD: Nuclear structure in cancer tissue. *Surg Gynecol Obstet* 1957;105:97-102.

2. Black MM, Barclay THC, Hankey BF: Prognosis in breast cancer utilizing histologic characteristics of the primary tumor. *Cancer* 1975;36:2048-2055.

3. Moran RE, Black MM, Alpert L, et al: Correlation of cell-cycle kinetics, hormone receptors, histopathology and nodal status in human breast cancer. *Cancer* 1984;54:1586-1590.

4. Black MM, Speer FD: Immunology of cancer. *Surg Gynecol Obstet* 1959;109:105-116.

5. Hamlin IME: Possible host resistance in carcinoma of the breast: A histological study. *Br J Cancer* 1968;22:383-401.

6. Black MM, Leis HP Jr, Shore B, et al: Cellular hypersensitivity to breast cancer: Assessment by a leukocyte migration procedure. *Cancer* 1974;33:952-958.

7. Akiyoshi T, Nakamura Y, Kawaguchi M, et al: Cellular hypersensitivity to autologous tumor extracts in patients with breast carcinoma. *Jpn J Surg* 1978;8:236-241.

8. Cannon GB, Dean JH, Herberman RB, et al: Lymphoproliferative responses to autologous tumor extracts as prognostic indicators in patients with resected breast cancer. *Int J Cancer* 1981;27:131-138.

9. Black MM, Leis HP Jr: Human breast carcinoma: III. Cellular responses to autologous breast cancer: Skin window procedure. *NY State J Med* 1970;70:2583-2589.

10. Black MM, Zachrau RE: Immune mechanisms: Prognostic, therapeutic and preventive significance, in: Ariel IM, Cleary JB (eds): *Breast Cancer: Diagnosis & Treatment.* New York, McGraw-Hill International Book Co, 1986, pp 128-142.

11. Black MM, Zachrau RE, Hankey BF, et al: Skin window reactivity to autologous breast cancer: An index of prognostically significant cell mediated immunity. *Cancer* 1988;62:72-83.

12. Black MM, Kwon CS: Precancerous mastopathie: Structural and biological considerations. *Pathol Res Pract* 1980;116:491-514.

13. Black MM, Zachrau RE: Stepwise mammary carcinogenesis: Immunological considerations, in Zander J, Baltzer J (eds): *Advances in Early Detection and Treatment of Breast Cancer.* New York, Springer Publishing Co Inc, 1985, pp 64-72.

14. Dion AS, Williams CJ, Pomenti AA: The major structural proteins of murine mammary tumor virus: Technique for isolation. *Anal Biochem* 1977; 82:18-28.

15. Mantel N: Evaluation of survival data and two new rank order statistics arising in its consideration. *Cancer Chemother Rep* 1966;50:163-170.

16. Cox DR: Regression models and life tables (with discussion). *J R Stat Soc B* 1972;34:187-220.

17. Black MM, Zachrau RE, Shore B, et al: Cellular immunity to autologous breast cancer and RIII-murine mammary tumor virus preparations. *Cancer Res* 1978;38:2068-2076.

18. Zachrau RE, Black MM, Dion AS, et al: Specificity of the simultaneous cell-mediated immune reactivity to RIII-murine mammary tumor virus glycoprotein 55 and human breast cancer tissues. *Cancer Res* 1978; 38:3414-3420.

19. Mesa-Tejada R, Keydar I, Ramanarayanan M, et al: Detection in human breast carcinoma of an antigen immunologically related to a group-specific antigen of mouse mammary tumor virus. *Proc Natl Acad Sci USA* 1978;75:1529-1533.

20. Keydar I, Selzer G, Chaitchik S, et al: A viral antigen as a marker for the prognosis of human breast cancer. *Eur J Cancer Clin Oncol* 1982; 18:1321-1328.

21. Mesa-Tejada R, Branwood AM, Keydar I, et al: Increased incidence of immunohistochemically detectable mouse mammary tumor virus-related antigen in breast carcinoma tissues of patients with a family history of this disease. *Proc Annu Meet Am Assoc Cancer Res Am Soc Clin Oncol* 1979; 20:276.

22. Dion AS, Girardi AJ, Williams CJ, et al: Responses of serum from breast cancer patients to murine mammary tumor virus: Fact or artifact? *J Natl Cancer Inst* 1987;79:207-211.

Discussion

Q Have you taken patients with some of the precursor lesions, such as carcinoma in situ, and atypical hyperplasias to see if they react?

A Well, it depends on your definition. Yes, when I said in situ to preinvasive lesion, that includes lesions that I call precancerous mastopathy, a lesser degree of atypia than overt in situ carcinoma. They are immunogenic in a high proportion of cases.

Q Do you think that late-stage lesions go through the same early reactivity or do you think that these tumors are predestined and bypass this early reactivity? Also, do you have any kind of evidence to discuss that biology?

A In our invasive group there is a wide range of individuals whose disease is merely considered to be operable. But as I showed you, even if you consider those patients who are known to have developed metastases, you have this same relationship. The behavior will be a function not of cure but of survival free of clinically evident metastases. I differentiate metastases from local recurrence; local recurrence is a different bird entirely. You can always measure tumor immunity, host immunity, and tumor antigenicity, and the behavior will always be the same and predictable at any stage, at any interval postoperatively.

Q Do you feel that the early immune response stimulates a tumor when it progresses, and can it actually make a contribution to tumor progression?

A No, it is quite the reverse. If you have immunity to the tumor in terms of a definite response to the tumor, by leukocyte migration test, or by any other immunological procedure you wish, it is always associated with a favorable prognosis.

Q Have you had a chance to look at this with flow cytometry to see if you are possibly duplicating the same thing? Did Fig 1 show anything that you could relate to estrogen receptors?

A I introduced nuclear differentiation in 1950, so it has been here a little longer than flow cytometry. Flow cytometric measurements correlate well with NG determinations.[3] Regarding estrogen receptors, I really think that that is after the fact. Patients who have estrogen receptor positivity tend to have well-differentiated nuclei and that is the basis of its prognostic significance,[3] but you do not have to take that into account at all. In fact, it is immaterial after you have taken care of the NG. I think that the NG is a very powerful measurement, and I must emphasize that NG and histological grade are not the same thing. They may sometimes be, but they may be decidedly different. If you rely on histological grade only, you get the most bizarre types of interpretation.

Photodynamic Therapy for Cutaneous and Subcutaneous Malignant Neoplasms

James S. McCaughan, Jr, MD; Jerry T. Guy, MD; William Hicks, MD; Leslie Laufman, MD; Thomas A. Nims, MD; John Walker

• Twenty-seven patients with cutaneous and subcutaneous malignant neoplasms were treated with photodynamic therapy. Therapy was administered to 248 areas during a total of 72 separate treatment sessions after patients received a total of 45 injections of sensitizer. Seven patients had basal cell carcinoma, three had squamous cell carcinoma, three had malignant melanoma, one had liposarcoma, and 12 had breast cancers. One patient had Bowen's disease. Treatment was given either by surface radiation or interstitially. One month after treatment, 48 (67%) of the treatment sessions resulted in a complete response (no clinical evidence of tumor), and 19 (26%) resulted in a partial response (>50% reduction in the number or size of tumors). Fifteen patients were examinable 12 months after treatment, and in this group, 31 treatment sessions were evaluated as a complete response one month after therapy, 15 (48%) of which retained this status at one year after treatment. By comparing the ability of different light-delivery instrumentation, it was concluded that the Yellow Springs radiometer (Yellow Springs Instruments, model 65A, Yellow Springs, Ohio) provided the most reliable spot power density readings. Straight-tipped fibers are nonhomogeneous and can result in overtreatment of the central area with necrosis and pain and in undertreatment of the periphery.

(*Arch Surg* 1989;124:211-216)

It has been known since 1924[1] that the presence of endogenous porphyrins causes some tumors to give off a red-orange fluorescence when exposed to ultraviolet light. Subsequent studies in rats showed that systemic injections of hematoporphyrin gave the characteristic red-orange fluorescence in tumors but not in normal tissue.

In 1961, Lipson and Baldes[2] reported using a hematoporphyrin derivative that was prepared by treating hemoglobin with an acetic acid–sulfuric acid solution. The derivative from this process produced a higher degree of fluorescence to the tumors than the original hematoporphyrin.

Original work was aimed at using fluorescence of tumors as a diagnostic technique. In 1968, Gregorie and Horger[3] found a 75% to 85% correlation of fluorescence with positive biopsy specimens of squamous carcinomas and adenocarcinomas in 226 patients who were treated with intravenous hematoporphyrin derivative.

In 1972, Diamond and Granelli[4] reported destruction of experimental tumors by exposing them to white light after systemic injection of hematoporphyrin derivative. Subsequently, Dougherty and his group at Roswell Park Memorial Institute, Buffalo, NY, began their laboratory animal experimentation by using hematoporphyrin derivative and various light systems to administer photodynamic therapy (PDT).

In 1984, Dougherty et al[5] extracted an active mixture from hematoporphyrin derivative called dihematoporphyrin ether, which is given intravenously and disseminates throughout the entire body. Because it begins to clear rapidly from normal cells while remaining in tumor tissue, after several days, the concentration of hematoporphyrin derivative is greater in tumor tissue relative to adjacent normal tissue. As a dye, hematoporphyrin derivative absorbs light at certain wavelengths. Although the greatest absorption occurs in the 405-nm range (blue-green), another absorption peak occurs in the 630-nm (red) range of wavelengths and is preferred for this treatment because it penetrates tissue better. When the light is absorbed, the dye is activated, and singlet oxygen[6] is produced, causing death to tumor tissue. Normal tissue remains relatively unharmed because it no longer contains sufficient dye to cause a reaction at the light doses employed.

Since 1978, numerous investigators have used PDT to treat patients with a variety of tumors by using various light sources, methods of delivery, and dose measurements.[7-17] In 1982, we treated five patients with skin cancers by using projectors (Kodak) and red filters as the light source.[18]

This report details the results of PDT administered during a five-year period to patients with various skin and subcutaneous malignant neoplasms. A tunable dye argon laser system was used for the light source. The report also compares the ability of different light-delivery instrumentation to estimate the light doses delivered and the relationship of power density and temperature.

PATIENTS AND METHODS

All patients had received, refused, or were ineligible for conventional surgery, chemotherapy, or ionizing radiation therapy. All patients were informed of the investigational nature of the treatment. Patients and their relatives watched a slide presentation and received pamphlets from an oncologic nurse specialist who described the technique. The nurse also emphasized the need for patients to avoid direct sunlight exposure for one month after treatment. Patients were further counseled to limit their sunlight exposure during the second posttreatment month.

Twenty-seven patients received a total of 45 injections of sensitizer and underwent a total of 72 separate treatment sessions. Most patients underwent treatment of multiple lesions; in all, a total of 248 cutaneous or subcutaneous areas were treated. Seven patients had basal cell carcinoma, three had squamous cell carcinoma, three had malignant melanoma, one had liposarcoma, and 12 had breast cancers. One patient had Bowen's disease.

The photosensitizer was injected through a running intravenous line of 5% glucose in Ringer's lactate solution as a single bolus. Initially, patients were given 3.0 mg/kg of hematoporphyrin derivative (Photofrin I, Photofrin Medical Inc, Cheektowaga, NY). Later, 2.0 mg/kg of dihematoporphyrin ether (Photofrin II, Photofrin Medical Inc, Cheektowaga, NY, or Johnson & Johnson Products Inc, Raritan, NJ) was used.

Two to six days after injection of the sensitizing agent, the tumor areas were treated with 630 ± 2 nm of light, delivered through 400- or 600-μm quartz fibers. The 630-nm therapeutic light was generated by a 20-W argon laser (Spectra Physics, model

Accepted for publication Sept 2, 1988.
From the Laser Medical Research Foundation, Columbus, Ohio.
Read before the Annual Meeting of the Society of Surgical Oncology, New Orleans, May 23, 1988.
Reprint requests to 323 E Town St, Columbus, OH 43215 (Dr McCaughan).

Table 1.—Clinical Results in Patients Treated With PDT*

Diagnosis	No. Patients	No. Injections	No. Treatment Areas	No. Treatment Sessions	Tumor Response at Each Treatment Session at 1 mo: CR	PR	SR	NR	PROG	No Recurrence: 6 mo	12 mo
Basal cell carcinoma	7	13	36	27	16	10	–	–	–	11	4
Squamous cell carcinoma	3	5	5	5	3	1	1	–	–	2	2
Malignant melanoma	3	5	27	7	5	0	1	1	–	2	1
Liposarcoma	1	2	3	2	1/?	?	?	?	–	1	1
Breast cancer	12	18	174	29	21	8	–	–	–	7	6
Bowen's disease	1	2	3	2	2	–	–	–	–	2	1
Total	**27**	**45**	**248**	**72**							

*PDT indicates photodynamic therapy; CR, complete response; PR, partial response; SR, some response; NR, no response; PROG, progression; and minus sign, unassessable.

171, Mt View, Calif) that pumped a tunable dye laser (Spectra Physics, model 375), initially circulating rhodamine-B dye without the tuning wedge and later with Kiton Red using a single plate birefrigent filter. The wavelength was monitored before, during, and after each treatment with a spectrometer (SA Instruments, model H-20, Metuchen, NJ).

The treatment was given either by surface radiation or interstitially. Originally, fiber tips were straight cut and polished for both surface and insertion techniques. Later, fibers with a microlens on the tip were used for surface irradiation (Laser Guide, Santa Barbara, Calif, or Laser Medical Research Foundation, Columbus, Ohio), and cylinder-diffusing fibers were used for interstitial therapy when the tumor was large enough. Interstitial insertion was made through a suitable hypodermic needle or directly into the tumor. The quarts fibers were coupled to the dye laser either directly or through a beam splitter (Photofrin Medical Inc, Cheektowaga, NY) to allow us to use simultaneously up to four fibers for interstitial implantation.

All patients were observed daily in the hospital for at least four days after PDT. After discharge, they were seen at least weekly for one month, at least every two to three months for one year, and periodically thereafter. Interim contact and follow-up were made by the primary physician and by telephone calls to the patients.

Tumor response to treatment was evaluated as follows: complete response, no clinical evidence of tumor; partial response, more than a 50% reduction in the number or size of tumors; some response, tumor reduction of 20% to 50%; no response, tumor reduction of 0% to 20%; and progression.

The adjacent skin was evaluated for erythema, edema, blisters, necrosis, and pain. The time and location of residual tumor and the development of new tumors were recorded. Photographs were taken routinely for more accurate comparison.

This study also investigated the accuracy with which power densities are currently measured, thereby affecting the ability to estimate light doses delivered. Surface power densities were measured with three different techniques: (1) the Coherent radiometer (Coherent, model 210, Palo Alto, Calif) placed on the surface; (2) the Yellow Springs radiometer (Yellow Springs Instruments, model 65A, Yellow Springs, Ohio) placed on the surface; and (3) the total power measured at the tip of the fiber with the Coherent 210 radiometer divided by the area of the circle of light at the surface of the plane being irradiated. The power density at many treatment sites was measured with all three techniques for later comparison.

For interstitial therapy, the total power was measured from the fiber tip with a Coherent 210 radiometer for straight-tipped fibers. When a cylinder fiber was used, the length of the diffusing tip was measured, and the total power output was determined by using an integrating sphere radiometer (United Detector Technology, model 61, Hawthorne, Calif). The power was recorded on a "per centimeter of length of diffusing fiber" basis.

The number of joules per centimeter squared for surface irradiation was calculated from the power density and the time of exposure. The interstitial treatment dose was measured by the total number of joules from straight-tipped fibers or from the joules per centimeter of diffusing length when cylinder fibers were used.

The power density configuration of the output from the different fiber types was also measured. With the fiber held at a fixed distance from the radiometer, the power density was measured with the Yellow Springs radiometer at 1.0-cm distances along the x and y axes through the center of the light circle. Changes in the power densities at varying distances from the fiber tips were also measured.

RESULTS

Clinical Findings

Clinical results are presented in Table 1. One month after treatment, 48 (67%) of 72 treatment sessions resulted in complete responses, and 19 (26%) resulted in partial responses. Fifteen patients were examinable 12 months after treatment. In this subgroup, one month after therapy, 31 treatment sessions were evaluated as complete responses, 15 (48%) of which retained this status at one year after treatment. (Some patients developed obvious new lesions in the field of treatment many months after the treatment, although the original lesions remained as complete responses. These are not included in the list of areas reported, showing no recurrence at six or 12 months.)

Many patients had multiple lesions in the treated areas, and many had end-stage disease and died before the six- or 12-month evaluation could be made. Nevertheless, several of these patients' lesions were categorized as complete responses at the time of patient death. Three patients who

Fig 1.—Left, Squamous cell cancer of eyelid. Right, Two years after two 8-minute surface treatments of photodynamic therapy. Five years after treatment, there has been no evidence of disease. Patient continues to have no disease.

Fig 2.—Top left, Metastatic breast cancer metastases to skin. Entire areas outlined were treated with 630-nm light. Top right, Four days after photodynamic therapy, tumors were reddish brown and necrotic. Bottom, Six months after photodynamic therapy, there was no clinical evidence of disease in treated areas.

Fig 3.—Left, Basal cell metastases to neck. Right, Three months after surface and interstitial photodynamic therapy, tumor has been completely eradicated.

Fig 4.—Left, Skin and subcutaneous metastatic breast cancer. Right, Twenty-four hours after photodynamic therapy, tumors were black and necrotic, while adjacent skin areas were only hyperemic.

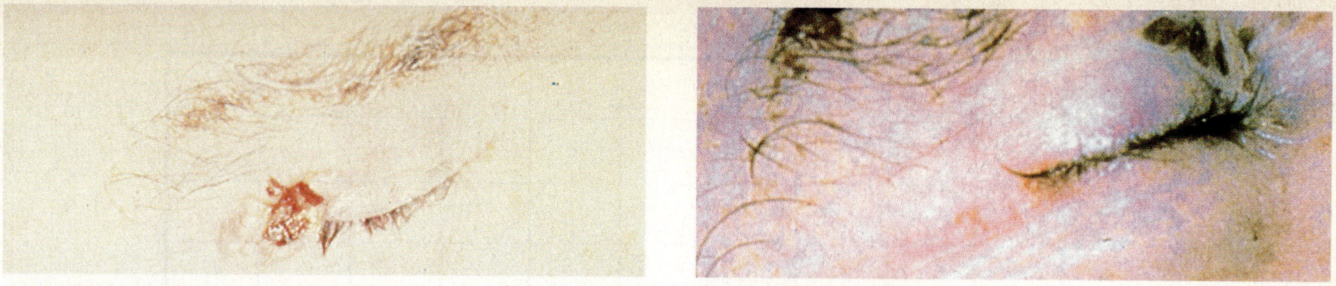

Figure 1.

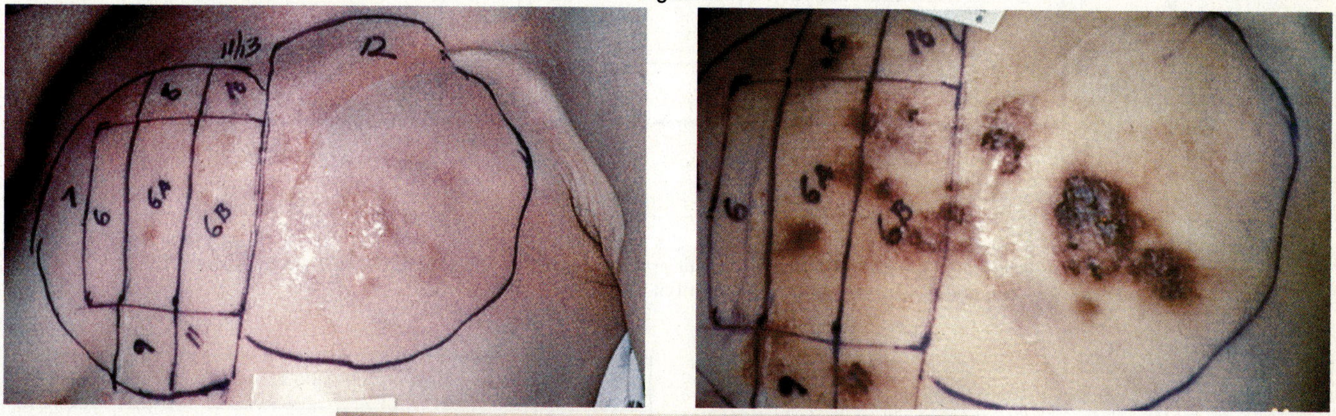

Figure 2.

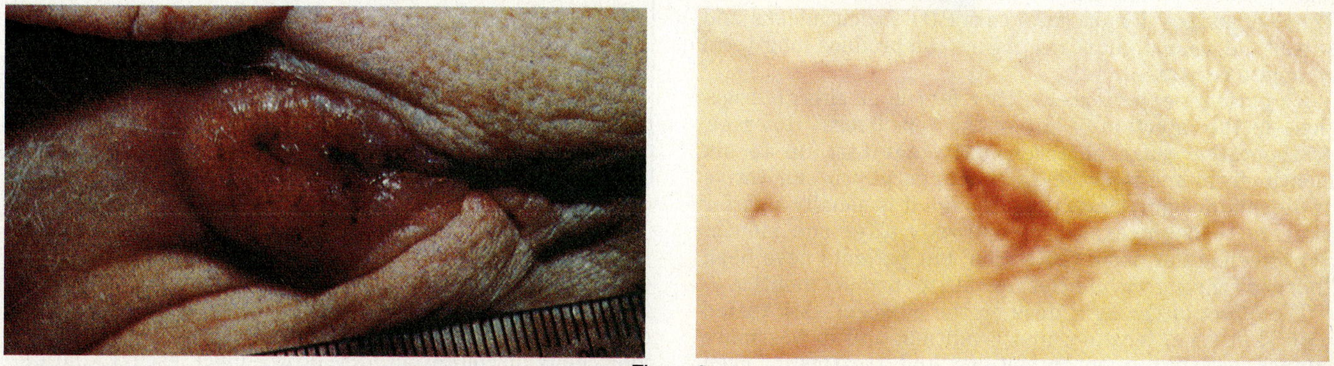

Figure 3.

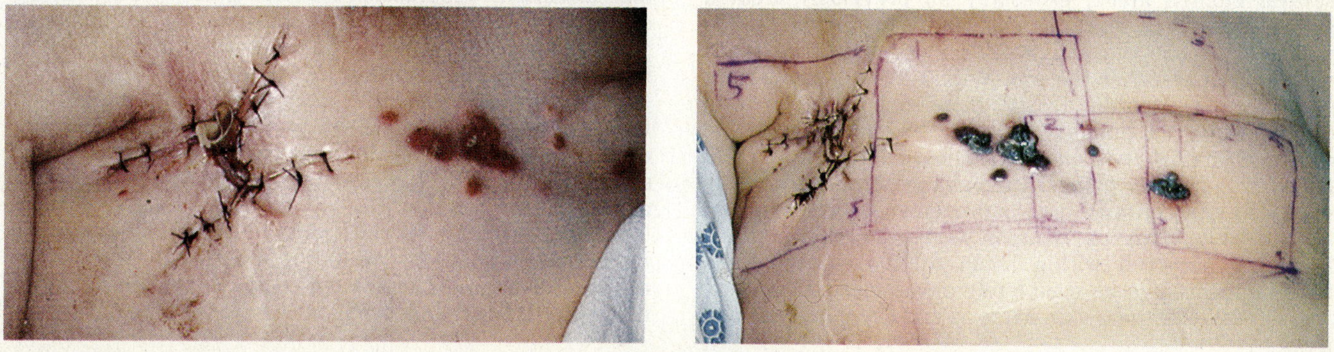

Figure 4.

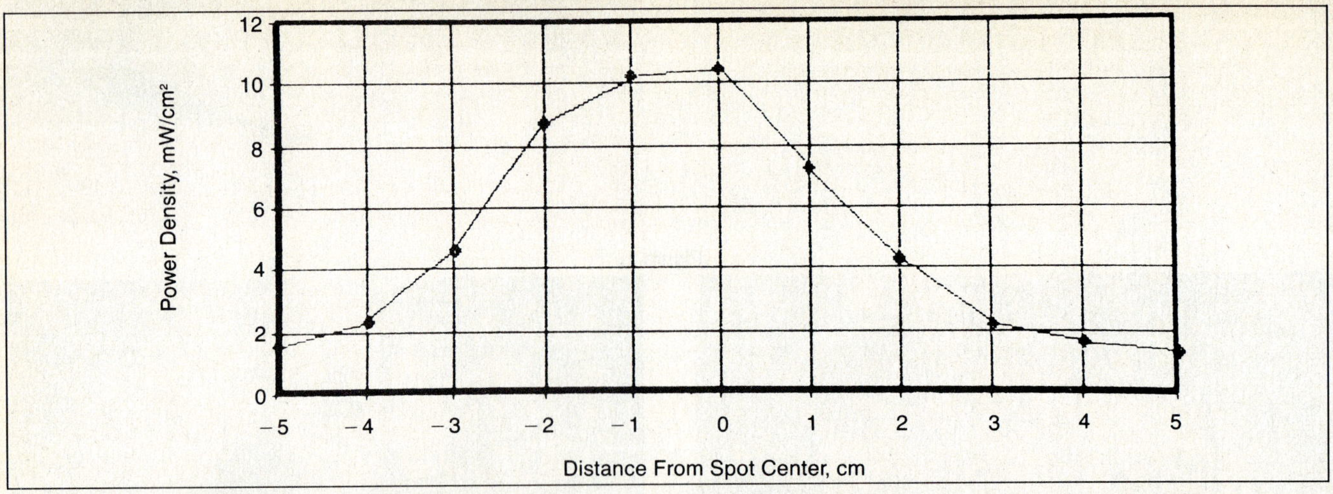

Fig 5.—Graph shows power densities delivered by straight-tipped fiber (polished) with 630-nm light, as measured with Yellow Springs radiometer. Output from this type of fiber tip is nonhomogeneous and results in overtreatment of central area with necrosis and pain and in undertreatment of periphery.

had severe chronic pain obtained relief within three weeks after treatment. Two patients with adjuvant PDT at the time of surgical excision of their tumor had histologically proved tumors at the margins of the resections. After PDT, these lesions achieved complete responses, lasting up to 24 and 12 months.

Figure 1 shows a squamous cell cancer before PDT (left) and two years after two 8-minute surface treatments (right). The patient is still alive five years after treatment with no evidence of disease. Figure 2 shows metastatic breast cancer to skin (top left); four days after PDT, the tumors were reddish brown and necrotic (top right); and six months after PDT, no tumors were visible or palpable (bottom). Figure 3 shows metastatic basal cell cancer before (left) and three months after two treatments (right). Figure 4 shows metastatic breast cancer before PDT (left) and 24 hours after treatment (right). The nodules are black and necrotic, while the adjacent skin is not damaged. These examples demonstrate that PDT for cutaneous and subcutaneous malignant neoplasms can produce long-term complete responses.

No patients experienced either febrile or allergic reactions to the injection of any of the sensitizers. However, postoperative solar photosensitivity can last up to six months from one injection of hematoporphyrin derivative or dihematoporphyrin ether, although it is usually safe for patients to begin exposure cautiously after one month. Sunscreens offer some protection, but patients have been "burned" through white clothing at two and six months.

The effect of the light dose on the adjacent skin varied with skin type, location, and condition, and it was more intense on subsequent injections and treatment, even several months apart, especially on previously treated areas. The ideal reaction was slight erythema to the adjacent skin, no pain, and blue-black necrosis of the tumor within 48 hours after therapy. With a homogeneous light source and the power density measured from the total output delivered divided by the area of the spot, we obtained complete responses with doses in the range of 20 to 30 J/cm.[2] Doses greater than this range almost invariably produced unacceptable pain and necrosis of the adjacent skin in white patients. If areas were overtreated, tissue blanching occurred within hours after treatment, and tissue appeared to be completely devascularized and developed full-thickness skin necrosis and dry gangrene and eschar formation. Essentially, whatever became white turned black soon after. Other sequences of reaction to overtreatment of the skin were erythema and/or edema, violaceous discoloration, dry brown-black eschar, and demarcation. This progression took two to 14 days, depending on the light dose and was accompanied by a "burning" pain. Three patients had to be readmitted to the hospital because of this complication.

Table 2.—Power Densities at Treatment Sites

Power Density Using Radiometer, mW/cm²		
Yellow Springs (Center)	**Coherent (Power/Area)**	**Coherent Surface (Center)**
Nonhomogeneous fiber		
30-44*	41	52
36	41	60
15	18	24
12	16	18
16	11	20
13	11	20
25	27	41
Homogeneous fiber		
23-25*	28	41
30	32	41
25	24	40
60	65	106
23	21	−†
24	23	−†
40	−†	69
75	−†	110

*Spot readings.
†Minus sign indicates unassessable.

The skin reaction to PDT given two days after injection was greater than when given on day 3. The reaction on days 3 through 6 clinically appeared to be the same for similar high doses. The color, density, and size of the tumor also affect the reaction.

Tumors over 2.0 cm thick are only partially destroyed by surface irradiation. We feel it is better to "debulk" or excise these larger tumors and treat the remaining tissue bed with PDT, either subsequently or at the time of surgery

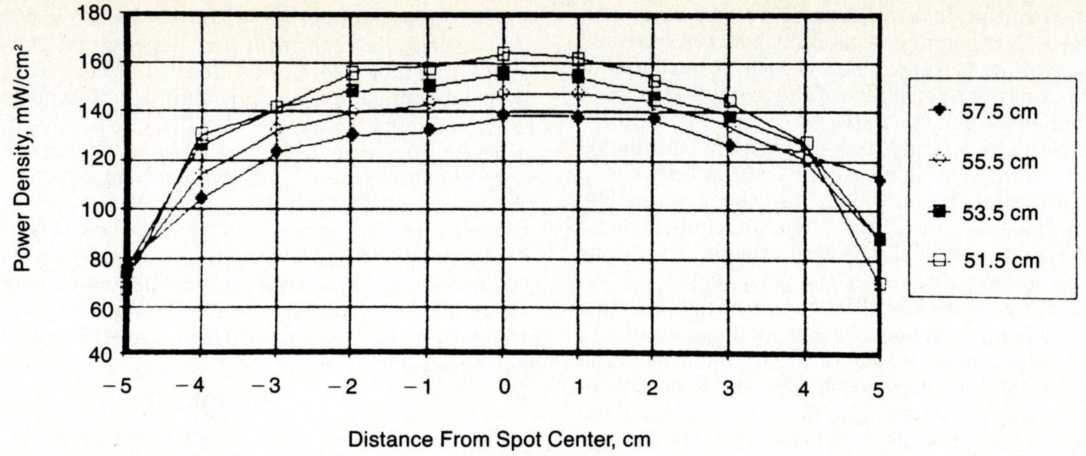

Fig 6.—Effect of varying distance from lens fiber (1.6 W of 630 nm) that has angle of divergence of 20° on power density. Power density decreases approximately 4% for each centimeter of distance.

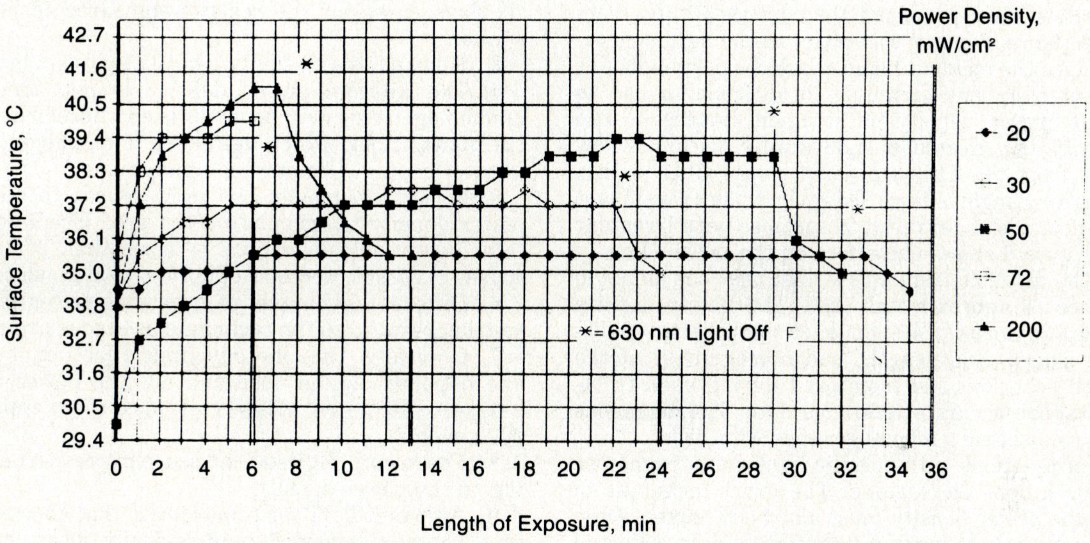

Fig 7.—Skin surface temperatures using different power densities during photodynamic therapy.

while the area is exposed. The use of PDT as an adjuvant in this setting may be an aid in decreasing the amount of surgery required to "get around" the lesion. Two patients who underwent tumor excision with concomitant PDT had no recurrence of tumor for over one year, although the margins of the resected specimen showed pathologic evidence of tumor.

Due to the inflammatory reaction, it is difficult to evaluate the response only one month after treatment. Two tumors evaluated as partial responses at one month were reevaluated to be complete responses at six months. One patient with a clinical complete response at one month had histologic viable tumor subcutaneously when the area was excised for pain relief. The only way to evaluate the reaction truly would be to excise the areas treated and examine them histologically; obviously, for these patients, that was generally not feasible or purposeful. Since the cancerous periphery of malignant ulcers necrosed, some actually became larger by the end of one month, although the edges became sharply demarcated as though excised with a scalpel. Large, noncancerous ulcers require several months to heal. Thus, prolonged follow-up is necessary to evaluate the treatment results truly. Early re-treatment should be done as soon as residual or recurrent cancer is identified. We were able to obtain long-term complete responses (over two years) in some patients after only one re-treatment.

Power Density Measurements

Currently, investigators are using different techniques to measure power densities. As demonstrated in this study, these techniques produce differences in power density measurements. Powers from straight-tipped fibers or from lens-tipped fibers, measured with the integrating sphere, were 10% to 20% greater than powers that were measured with the Coherent 210 radiometer. Even powers of two different Coherent radiometers gave different power readings, varying from 5% to 15%. It is extremely important, therefore, to calibrate these instruments periodically. Especially problematic is the nonhomogeneity of many delivery sources that gives a higher power density in the center of the target, resulting in an undertreated periphery and central necrosis. Nonhomogeneous light sources have led several investigators to report recurrence or incomplete tumor destruction in the periphery of the treated area.[10,11,19] This phenomenon is demonstrated in Fig 5. The power densities delivered by a straight-tipped fiber, as measured with a Yellow Springs radiometer, are plotted on the x axis. A similar graph can be made for the y axis. The output from a straight-tipped fiber is nonhomogeneous and results in overtreatment of the central area with necrosis and pain and in undertreatment of the periphery.

Table 2 compares power densities measured at the time of treatment by using a Yellow Springs or a Coherent 210 radiometer for direct measurements and by the area of the circle technique for a homogeneous lens and a nonhomogeneous fiber tip light source. The most convenient technique to measure the power density is from the total power output at the tip and the area of the circle of light at the treated surface, especially for intraoperatively sterile areas. This requires a homogeneous lens light source. The Yellow Springs radiometer provided the most convenient spot power density readings. By holding the Coherent 210 radiometer on the surface that was being irradiated, higher power densities were produced than by the other techniques since the radiometer was closer to the light source. Moreover, since the incident beam should be perpendicular to the radiometer, this technique is difficult to use to measure the power density on irregular surfaces. The power density can decrease significantly within a few centimeters from the fiber tip when a lens fiber with a rapidly diverging angle is used. This may cause a significant difference in the dose delivered to surfaces with irregular contours. Figure 6 shows the effect on the power density of varying the distance from a lens fiber that has an angle of divergence of approximately 20°. The power density decreases approximately 4% for each centimeter of distance. The output, wavelength, and homogeneity of the light must be checked and monitored during each treatment to establish accurate reference data. Homogeneous lens fibers can become nonhomogeneous with use.

Reports of reactions with specific light doses cannot be compared on a dose basis alone. The exact technique of measuring the power density must also be reported. Only then will we be able to compare accurately data collected from various centers that conduct PDT studies.

Temperature Changes

With power densities in the 10- to 200-mW/cm² range, the reaction is reciprocal and depends on the total dose given and not the power density. Above this, however, thermal changes may occur, and these temperature elevations are due to power density. Hyperthermia can be produced from the laser light itself if the power density is high enough. When PDT was performed three days after the injection of 2.0 mg/kg of dihematoporphyrin ether, the temperature 2.0 mm under the surface of a skin cancer rose from 28.8°C to 31.6°C when the surface was exposed to a power density of 29 mW/cm². The temperature returned to 29.4°C immediately when the light was turned off. Figure 7 shows the skin surface temperatures with different power densities during PDT.

COMMENT

Based on this study, we were able to draw the following conclusions regarding PDT.

1. Photodynamic therapy for cutaneous and subcutaneous cancers provides a complete response in some patients that lasts up to five years.
2. The reaction to PDT two days after injection of the sensitizer was greater than at three days. From three to six days, however, the reaction appeared to be clinically similar.
3. Solar photosensitivity can last up to six months.
4. The average power density is not adequate if a nonhomogeneous light source is used; therefore, a straight-cut quartz fiber, which delivers a nonhomogeneous light, is not acceptable for surface irradiation.
5. Using a homogeneous light source to measure the power density by calculating the area irradiated and the total power output, a dose of more than 20 to 30 J/cm² causes excessive necrosis of normal skin in white patients.
6. Different techniques of measuring power density yield varying results, so the technique used must be reported.
7. Clinically, the photodynamic reaction is reciprocal and depends on the dose and not the power density, as long as the power density is less than approximately 200 mm/cm².
8. The laser light itself can cause hyperthermia, depending on the power density.
9. Adjuvant PDT for tumor areas that showed a "tumor in a resected margin" pathologically gave complete responses that lasted up to 24 months.

References

1. Policard A: Etudes sur les aspects offerts par des tumeur experimentales examinee a la lumiere de woods. *CR Soc Biol* 1924;91:1423-1428.
2. Lipson RL, Baldes EJ: The use of hematoporphyrin in tumor detection. *Nat Cancer Inst* 1961;26:1-8.
3. Gregorie HB Jr, Horger EO: Hematoporphyrin-derivate fluorescence in malignant neoplasms. *Ann Surg* 1968;167:829.
4. Diamond I, Granelli S: Photodynamic therapy for malignant tumors. *Lancet* 1972;2:1175-1177.
5. Dougherty TJ, Potter WR, Weishaupt KR: The structure of the active component of hematoporphyrine derivative, in Dorion DR, Gomer CJ (eds): *Porphyrin Localization and Treatment of Tumors.* New York, Alan R Liss Inc, 1984, pp 301-314.
6. Weishaupt KR, Gomer CJ: Identification of singlet oxygen as the cytologic agent in photoradiation of a murine tumor. *Cancer Res* 1976;36:2326-2329.
7. Dougherty TJ, Kaufman JE: Photoradiation therapy for the treatment of malignant tumors. *Cancer Res* 1978;38:2628-2635.
8. Dougherty TJ, Lawrence G: Photoradiation in the treatment of recurrent breast carcinoma. *J Nat Cancer Inst* 1979;62:231-237.
9. Dougherty TJ: Photoradiation therapy for cutaneous and subcutaneous malignancies. *J Invest Dermatol* 1981;77:122-124.
10. Carruth JAS, MacKenzie AL: Preliminary report of a pilot study of photoradiation therapy for the treatment of superficial malignancies of the skin, head and neck. *Eur Soc Surg Oncol* 1985;11:000-000.
11. Forbes IJ, Ward AD: Multidisciplinary approach to phototherapy of human cancers, in Dorion DR, Gomer CJ (eds): *Porphyrin Localization and Treatment of Tumors.* New York, Alan R Liss Inc, 1984, pp 693-708.
12. Dahlman A, Wile AG: Laser photoradiation therapy of cancer. *Cancer Res* 1983;43:430-434.
13. Tokuda Y: Primary skin cancer, in Hayata Y, Dougherty TJ (eds): *Lasers and Hematoporphyrine Derivative in Cancer.* New York, Igaku-Shoin Medical Publishers Inc, 1983, pp 88-95.
14. Tse DT, Dutton JJ: Hematoporphyrin photoradiation therapy for intraocular and orbital malignant melanoma. *Arch Ophthalmol* 1984;102: 833-838.
15. Wile AG, Dahlman A: Laser photoradiation therapy of recurrent human breast cancer and cancer of the head and neck, in Kessel D, Dougherty TJ (eds): *Porphyrin Photosensitization.* New York, Plenum Press, 1983, pp 47-52.
16. Zhonghe G, Yingcai H: Evaluation of photoradiation therapy (PRT) in 20 cases of cancer, in Andreoni A, Cubeddu R (eds): *Porphyrins in Tumor Phototherapy.* New York, Plenum Press, 1984, pp 375-380.
17. Zorat PL, Tomio L: Hematoporphyrin phototherapy of malignant tumors, in Andreoni A, Cubeddu R (eds): *Porphyrins in Tumor Phototherapy.* New York, Plenum Press, 1984, pp 381-387.
18. McCaughan JS, Guy JT: Hematoporphyrin derivative and photoradiation therapy of malignant tumors. *Lasers Surg Med* 1983;3:199-209.
19. Bandieramonte G, Marchesini R: Hematoporphyrin-derivative and phototherapy in extensive basal cell carcinoma of the dorsal skin, in Adrenoni A, Cubeddu R (eds): *Porphyrins in Tumor Phototherapy.* New York, Plenum Press, 1984, pp 389-394.

Antioxidants vs Carotenoids

Inhibitors or Promoters of Experimental Colorectal Cancers

Thomas A. Colacchio, MD; Vincent A. Memoli, MD; Laurie Hildebrandt

• The organospecific, 1,2-dimethylhydrazine-induced murine tumor model was used to test the effects on tumor formation of the following dietary supplements: (1) ascorbic acid, 7% per weight; (2) alpha tocopherol, 1% per weight; (3) beta carotene, 1% per weight; and (4) canthazanthin, 1% per weight. Following a four-week dietary acclimation, a 16-week 1,2-dimethylhydrazine induction, and a four-week hiatus, the animals were killed, underwent autopsies, and tumor formation was recorded. The antioxidant supplements of ascorbic acid and alpha tocopherol resulted in a significant decrease in tumor formation when compared with control groups. In contrast, the beta carotene group showed no difference in tumor formation, and canthazanthin, a non-provitamin A carotenoid, resulted in an increase in tumor formation when compared with controls. In addition, the K-gel powder control diet (a carrier medium for alpha tocopherol acetate) had a significantly higher rate of tumor formation than the regular chow and placebo beadlet control diets. In sum, ascorbic acid and alpha tocopherol demonstrated a clear chemopreventive effect, whereas beta carotene had no effect, and canthazanthin appeared to function as a promoter in this organospecific tumor model.

(*Arch Surg* 1989;124:217-221)

Colorectal carcinoma is the most common visceral cancer in the United States, with a rising annual incidence and mortality that are predicted to be 147 000 new cases and more than 60 000 deaths for the year 1988.[1] Despite the increasing efforts of educational programs to improve early diagnosis, there has been little change in survival, and these incidence figures represent an increase of more than 25% over the past three decades. Although the etiology of this disease is multifactorial, environmental factors with specific reference to regional dietary habits play a major role.[2] In addition, high-risk populations in North America have been found to harbor fecal mutagenic substances,[3-5] and some studies have suggested that dietary factors may influence these by affecting either the actual amount of carcinogen intake or the formation of mutagenic substances in vivo.[6,7]

A broad range of compounds has been used in various tumor models to study the potential inhibition of chemical carcinogenesis. As a result of these studies and the available epidemiologic data, several prospective trials are currently under way to evaluate the effect of certain dietary supplements on the presence and level of fecal mutagens and the formation of metachronous colorectal neoplasms. The antioxidants, ascorbic acid and alpha tocopherol, and the provitamin A carotenoid, beta carotene, are among the supplements currently being evaluated. Unfortunately, the reported efficacy of these compounds as chemopreventive agents in various tumor models is inconclusive. This study reports a series of experiments designed to test the chemopreventive efficacy of ascorbic acid, alpha tocopherol, beta carotene, and canthazanthin in preventing tumor formation in an organospecific murine model utilizing symmetric 1,2-dimethylhydrazine.

MATERIALS AND METHODS

Tumor Model

Weanling male Holtzman rats (Holtzman Company, Madison, Wis) were housed in individual cages in the Dartmouth Medical School Animal Care Facility, Hanover, NH, using a standard 12-hour light/dark cycle. After a four-week dietary acclimation period, weekly subcutaneous injections of 1,2-dimethylhydrazine were begun. (Symmetric 1,2-dimethylhydrazine, Sigma Chemical Co, St Louis, was dissolved in phosphate-buffered saline solution and corrected to a pH of 7.0 with 10N sodium hydroxide.) The dose schedule was 30 mg/kg per week injected subcutaneously for 16 weeks, resulting in a total dose of 480 mg/kg.

Four weeks after the final injection, the animals were killed and autopsies were performed. At necropsy, the thoracic and abdominal cavities were examined for evidence of ascites and primary or metastatic tumor formation. In addition, the entire intestinal tract from the duodenum to the anus was removed, opened, and examined for tumor formation. Biopsy specimens of all suspected lesions were prepared and stained using standard histologic techniques with hematoxylin-eosin. The biopsy slides were then evaluated microscopically and diagnosed as adenoma, carcinoma, or other (nonneoplastic). In addition, biopsy specimens of suspected metastatic lesions were similarly analyzed histopathologically. The number of primary lesions, their location, and the presence of metastatic deposits were then recorded for each animal. Only tumors confirmed histopathologically were included.

Accepted for publication Oct 13, 1988.
From the Departments of Surgery (Dr Colacchio and Ms Hildebrandt) and Pathology (Dr Memoli), Dartmouth Medical School, Hanover, NH.
Read before the Annual Meeting of the Society of Surgical Oncology, New Orleans, May 25, 1988.
Reprint requests to Department of Surgery, Dartmouth Medical School, Hanover, NH 03755 (Dr Colacchio).

Table 1.—Results of 1,2-Dimethylhydrazine Induction in Ascorbic Acid Supplement and Nonsupplement Groups

	Dietary Supplement		
	Ascorbic Acid (N=30)	Regular Chow (N=26)	*P* Value* (NS>.01)
No. of rats with tumors	23	26	.0001†
No. of rats with cancers	20	24	.0001†
No. of tumors	1.43	3.35	.0001‡
No. of cancers	1.20	2.88	.0001‡
Colon			
No. of rats with tumors	19	25	.0001†
No. of rats with cancers	16	21	.0001†
No. of tumors	0.93	2.08	.0002‡
No. of cancers	0.70	1.61	.0008‡
Small bowel			
No. of rats with tumors	11	18	.0001†
No. of rats with cancers	11	18	.0001†
No. of tumors	0.50	1.27	.0164‡
No. of cancers	0.50	1.27	.0164‡

*NS indicates not significant.
†χ^2 (1 *df*).
‡Student's *t* test.

Table 2.—Results of 1,2-Dimethylhydrazine Induction in Alpha Tocopherol Supplement and Nonsupplement Groups

	Dietary Supplement		
	Alpha Tocopherol (N=23)	K-Gel Powder (N=14)	*P* Value* (NS>.01)
No. of rats with tumors	22	14	.0001†
No. of rats with cancers	21	14	.0001†
No. of tumors	2.30	5.00	.0001‡
No. of cancers	2.13	4.43	.0001‡
Colon			
No. of rats with tumors	19	13	.0006†
No. of rats with cancers	19	12	.0136†
No. of tumors	1.39	2.00	.0079‡
No. of cancers	1.35	1.79	NS‡
Small bowel			
No. of rats with tumors	15	13	.0001†
No. of rats with cancers	13	13	.0001†
No. of tumors	0.91	3.43	.0003‡
No. of cancers	0.87	2.93	.0008‡

*NS indicates not significant.
†χ^2 (1 *df*).
‡Student's *t* test.

Table 3.—Results of 1,2-Dimethylhydrazine Induction in Beta Carotene Supplement and Nonsupplement Groups

	Dietary Supplement		
	Beta Carotene (N=28)	Placebo Beadlets (N=28)	*P* Value* (NS>.01)
No. of rats with tumors	28	28	NS†
No. of rats with cancers	28	28	NS†
No. of tumors	4.54	4.04	NS‡
No. of cancers	3.79	3.71	NS‡
Colon			
No. of rats with tumors	28	27	NS†
No. of rats with cancers	28	27	NS†
No. of tumors	3.29	3.21	NS‡
No. of cancers	2.64	2.96	NS‡
Small bowel			
No. of rats with tumors	18	17	NS†
No. of rats with cancers	17	15	NS†
No. of tumors	1.29	0.82	NS‡
No. of cancers	1.14	0.75	NS‡

*NS indicates not significant.
†χ^2 (1 *df*).
‡Student's *t* test.

Table 4.—Results of 1,2-Dimethylhydrazine Induction in Canthazanthin Supplement and Nonsupplement Groups

	Dietary Supplements		
	Canthazanthin (N=27)	Placebo Beadlets (N=28)	*P* Value* (NS>.01)
No. of rats with tumors	27	28	NS†
No. of rats with cancers	27	28	NS†
No. of tumors	5.89	4.04	.0060‡
No. of cancers	5.67	3.71	.0039‡
Colon			
No. of rats with tumors	26	27	NS†
No. of rats with cancers	26	27	NS†
No. of tumors	4.67	3.21	.0178‡
No. of cancers	4.44	2.96	.0145‡
Small bowel			
No. of rats with tumors	20	17	NS†
No. of rats with cancers	20	15	.0352†
No. of tumors	1.22	0.82	NS‡
No. of cancers	1.22	0.75	NS‡

*NS indicates not significant.
†χ^2 (1 *df*).
‡Student's *t* test.

Supplemental Diets

The animals were divided into groups and placed on prescribed diets with water ad libitum during the initial four-week acclimation period and they were maintained on these for the entire course of the study. There were four supplemental diets studied: (1) regular powdered chow (Purina) with 7% per weight ascorbic acid (J. T. Baker Chemical Co., Phillipsburg, NJ); (2) regular pelleted chow (Dyets Inc, Bethlehem, Pa) with 1% per weight alpha tocopherol (1.49% per weight racemic DL-alpha tocopherol acetate in K-gel powder carrier medium, Hoffmann-LaRoche Inc, Nutley, NJ); (3) regular pelleted chow with 1% per weight beta carotene (in beadlet form, Hoffmann-LaRoche Inc); and (4) regular pelleted chow with 1% per weight canthazanthin (in beadlet form, Hoffmann-La Roche Inc). These were matched with control diets containing the appropriate carrier compounds: (1) regular chow (pelleted and powdered); (2) regular pelleted chow with 1.49% per weight K-gel powder; and (3) regular pelleted chow with 10% per weight placebo beadlets (beta carotene and canthazanthin are prepared as 10% per weight beadlets).

Statistical Analysis

The results were analyzed by group according to the presence or absence of tumor formation, the location of the tumor (small bowel vs colon), and the histologic characteristics of the tumor (adenoma vs carcinoma). Group means with SDs were then calculated. These means were compared using the χ^2 test and Student's *t* test, with statistical significance being a *P* value less than .01.[8]

Table 5.—Reports of Ascorbic Acid Dietary Supplements

Source, y	Carcinogen*	Animal/Site	Effects
Soloway et al,[12] 1974	FANFT	Dog/bladder	None
Mirvish et al,[18] 1972	NMOR	Rat/liver and forestomach	None in forestomach; decreased in liver
Jones et al,[20] 1981	1,2-dimethylhydrazine	Mouse/colon	None alone; decreased with butylated hydroxyanisole
Reddy et al,[13] 1982	1,2-dimethylhydrazine/methylnitrosourea	Rat/colon with multiple dose	Decreased with single dose; none
Dunham et al,[14] 1982	UV light	Mouse/skin	Decreased incidence
Abul-Hajj and Kelliher,[15] 1982	DMBA/transplant	Rat/mammary	Increased incidence
Fukushima et al,[16] 1983	BBN	Rat/bladder	Increased incidence
Khar'Kovaskaya et al,[17] 1982	PHPLA	Mouse/multiple	Decreased incidence
Fukushima et al,[19] 1983	BBN	Rat/bladder	None with 1%; increased with 5%
Tsuda et al,[21] 1984	Methylnitrosourea	Rat/multiple	Increased in bladder
Colacchio and Memoli,[9] 1986	1,2-dimethylhydrazine	Rat/colon	Decreased incidence

*FANFT indicates nitrofurylthiozolyforamide; UV, ultraviolet; DMBA, dimethylbenzanthracene; BBN, butylhydroxybutylnitrosamine; PHPLA, *p*-hydroxyphenyl lactic acid; and NMOR, nitrosomorpholine.

Table 6.—Reports of Alpha Tocopherol Dietary Supplements

Source, y	Carcinogen*	Animal/Site	Effect
Shamberger,[29] 1970	DMBA	Mouse/skin	Decreased incidence
Cook and McNamara,[22] 1980	1,2-dimethylhydrazine	Mouse/colon	Decreased incidence
Smalls and Patterson,[23] 1982	BP	Hamster/chromosome aberration	Decreased incidence
Shklar,[24] 1982	DMBA	Hamster/oral	Decreased incidence
Ip,[28] 1982	DMBA	Rat/mammary	None
Toth and Kashinath,[25] 1983	1,2-dimethylhydrazine	Mouse/colon	Increased incidence
Horvath and Ip,[26] 1983	DMBA	Rat/mammary	None alone; decreased incidence with selenium
Odukoya et al,[27] 1984	DMBA	Hamster/oral	Decreased incidence

*DMBA indicates dimethylbenzanthracene; BP, benzo(a)pyrene.

RESULTS

The mean weight gain over the 24-week period varied somewhat between the various supplement groups (279.8 to 339.9 g); generally, animals in 1,2-dimethylhydrazine–induced groups have a lower weight gain than those in noninduced groups.[9] The only significant difference noted between the supplement and nonsupplement 1,2-dimethylhydrazine–induced groups was between the canthazanthin–1,2-dimethylhydrazine (279.8 g) and placebo beadlet–1,2-dimethylhydrazine (325.6 g) groups ($P = .0013$).

The results of 1,2-dimethylhydrazine induction on tumor formation in the control groups (regular chow, placebo beadlet, and K-gel powder) are shown in Tables 1 through 3. Although there is no spontaneous intestinal tumor formation in these animals, this relatively high-dose induction schedule resulted in 100% tumor formation in the control groups at 20 weeks. Almost all these animals have cancers and the majority of these tumors are in the colon. There were significantly more tumors found in both the colon and small intestine of the K-gel powder group when compared with the regular chow and placebo beadlet groups. In addition, there were significantly more colon tumors found in the placebo beadlet group when compared with the regular chow group.

A comparison of the results of 1,2-dimethylhydrazine induction in the ascorbic acid supplement and regular chow groups is shown in Table 1. There was a highly significant difference in the number of animals with tumors and the number of tumors per animal between these two groups. This was noted in both the colon and, although less striking, in the small bowel. A similar trend was found when the alpha tocopherol group was compared with the K-gel powder group (Table 2). In this instance, however, the differences were more pronounced in the small bowel rather than in the colon.

Table 3 shows the comparison between the beta carotene supplement group and the placebo beadlet group. There was no difference in the numbers of animals with tumors or cancers or in the number of tumors or cancers per animal noted. Similarly, no differences were found either in the colon or small bowel. In contrast to this, Table 4 shows the difference between the canthazanthin supplement group and the placebo beadlet group; there is a striking increase in both the number of tumors and the number of cancers found in the canthazanthin group. The breakdown shows that there are more tumors and cancers in both the colon and small bowel, but these individual comparisons fall short of statistical significance.

COMMENT

Many compounds of varying toxicity have been used as chemopreventive agents in several animal tumor models, but the results of these studies have often been inconclusive or contradictory. Two basic mechanisms of action have

Table 7.—Reports of Beta Carotene and Canthazanthin Dietary Supplements			
Source, y	**Carcinogen***	**Animal/Site**	**Effect**
Beta carotene			
Epstein,[37] 1977	UV light	Mouse/skin	Decreased incidence
Seifter et al,[30] 1982	Maloney sarcoma virus	Mouse	Decreased incidence; increased regression
Mathews-Roth,[31] 1982	UV light/DMBA	Mouse/skin	Decreased and delayed incidence
Rettura et al,[32] 1982	C3HBA adenocarcinoma cells	Mouse/implant	Decreased incidence; increased survival
Seifter et al,[33] 1983	C3HBA adenocarcinoma cells	Mouse/implant	Increased effect of radiation therapy; increased survival
Alam and Alam,[34] 1983	DMBA	Rat/salivary gland	Slight decreased incidence
Colacchio and Memoli,[9] 1986	1,2-dimethylhydrazine	Rat/colon	None
Canthazanthin			
Mathews-Roth,[31] 1982	UV light	Mouse/skin	Decreased and delayed incidence
Santamaria et al,[35] 1983	Benzo(a)pyrene	Mouse/skin	Decreased incidence

*UV indicates ultraviolet; DMBA, dimethylbenzanthracene.

been proposed for these agents: (1) an alteration of the metabolism of the carcinogen by decreased activation and/or increased detoxification; and (2) the scavenging of active molecular species of the carcinogens to prevent them from reaching critical target sites in the cells.[10] The exertion of this scavenging effect thereby protecting the cells from attack has been the rationale for the chemopreventive use of antioxidant compounds such as ascorbic acid and alpha tocopherol. The ability to inhibit the formation of free radicals and to quench singlet-excited oxygen has led some to postulate the potential for a chemopreventive effect by the carotenoids beta carotene and canthazanthin.[11] In addition, the provitamin A activity of beta carotene might also inhibit tumor formation (1) by exerting hormonelike effects on the cells later in the genesis of cancer, thus returning them to a more differentiated state or (2) possibly by increasing the immunocompetence of the host.

Ascorbic acid has been an extensively studied compound for its potential as a chemopreventive agent (Table 5).[9,12-21] It has been evaluated by several authors in various tumor models with conflicting results. In two studies that used the organospecific carcinogen 1,2-dimethylhydrazine in a murine model, the authors showed no protective effects when it was used as a single agent in a multidose induction model.[13,20] These results clearly differ from the dramatic protective effects reported herein that are highlighted by the complete absence of tumor formation in almost seven (25%) of the animals in the supplement group. Possible explanations for this include the following: (1) differences in the dose and form of ascorbic acid used (0.25% and 1.0% per weight of sodium ascorbate as reported by Reddy et al[13] and 25 to 500 mg/kg per day as reported by Jones et al[20]); (2) inherent differences in the animal model used or in the schedule and total dose of 1,2-dimethylhydrazine given; (3) differences in the length of the preinduction acclimation period (ten days in the study of Jones et al and two weeks in the study of Reddy et al).

Fewer studies have been done using alpha tocopherol (Table 6),[22-29] but the results have also been conflicting, especially in the 1,2-dimethylhydrazine murine model. Cook and McNamara[22] found that a vitamin E–supplemented diet (0.06% per weight) resulted in a decrease in tumor formation when compared with an alpha tocopherol–deficient diet (0.0001% per weight); however, these groups were not compared with a control group receiving a regular diet. Using a mammary model, Ip[28] found that alpha tocopherol deficiency led to an increase in tumor formation, whereas alpha tocopherol supplements resulted in no difference from the control group (0.0003% per weight vs 0.000075% per weight and 0.1% per weight). In contrast, Toth and Kashinath[25] found that a high-dose alpha tocopherol–supplemented diet (4% per weight) actually resulted in an increase in tumor formation in a 1,2-dimethylhydrazine mouse model. Once again, inherent differences in the model used, the dose of alpha tocopherol supplementation, and/or the composition of the diet in the control group are the likely explanations for the differences between these other studies and the findings reported herein. Although the reason for the increase in tumor formation occurring in the group receiving the K-gel powder placebo diet is unclear, there was a marked decrease in tumor formation in the group maintained on the diet supplemented with K-gel powder containing 1% per weight alpha tocopherol.

The carotenoids beta carotene and canthazanthin have been less extensively tested as chemopreventive agents (Table 7),[9,30-37] and, to our knowledge, there has been only one report on the use of beta carotene in a 1,2-dimethylhydrazine murine model.[8] In this initial study, it was noted that the supplemental diet containing 1% per weight of beta carotene had no effect on the induction of tumor formation. This was despite the relatively high dose of beta carotene used and the uniformly preventive effects noted by other authors in several different tumor models. In this case, the cause for the lack of efficacy may be due to the inability of beta carotene to affect the genesis of malignant transformation of mucosal intestinal cells, in addition to the factors stated previously in regard to the reported discrepancies with the study of ascorbic acid and alpha tocopherol.

Similar to beta carotene, the non–provitamin A carotenoid, canthazanthin, has been shown to be effective in preventing the photocarcinogenic enhancement of benzo(a)pyrene on skin cancer development in animals[31,35,36] and also to be photoprotective for patients with erythropoietic protoporphyria.[38,39] The effects on the organospecific 1,2-dimethylhydrazine model of a diet supplemented with 1% per weight of canthazanthin are reported herein. These results clearly demonstrate an enhancement of both tumor and cancer formation in the supplement group when compared with the placebo group. The reasons for this apparent promotional effect of canthazanthin are unknown but may well be due to specific differences in the interaction between carotenoids and various tissues (ie, squamous epithelium vs columnar epithelium) or possibly a direct effect on the luminal surfaces of the intestine by the high concentrations of this agent, as the majority is cleared in the feces.

In summary, this report would support the continued and expanded study of the antioxidants ascorbic acid and alpha tocopherol as chemopreventive agents of colorectal neoplasms based on the effects seen in this organospecific tumor model. However, more studies need to be performed in these specific tumor model systems to justify the continued use of carotenoids in human chemopreventive studies of colorectal neoplasms.

This investigation was supported by Public Health Service grant CA35860, Washington, DC.

References

1. Silverberg E: Cancer statistics 1988. *CA* 1988;38:5-22.
2. Enstrom JE: Assessing human epidemiologic data on diet as an etiologic factor in cancer development. *Bull NY Acad Med* 1982;58:313-322.
3. Bruce WR, Varghesse AJ, Furrer R, et al: A mutagen in the feces of normal humans, in Hiatt HH, Watson JD, Winston JA (eds): *Origins of Human Cancer.* Cold Spring Harbor, NY, Cold Spring Harbor Laboratory, 1977, pp 1641-1646.
4. McCann J, Ames BN: Detection of carcinogens as mutagens in the salmonella/microsome test. *Proc Natl Acad Sci USA* 1976;73:950.
5. Hendricks DG, Cornforth DP, Bartholomew DT, et al: Influence of dietary fiber and method of meat cookery upon human fecal microflora and mutagenicity of stool extracts. Read before the First Conference of Radioprotectors and Anticarcinogens, Gaithersberg, Md, June 21-24, 1982.
6. Mower HL, Ichinotsubo D, Wang LW, et al: Fecal mutagens in two Japanese populations with different colon cancer risks. *Cancer Res* 1982;42:1164-1169.
7. Wilkins TD, Lederman M, VanTassell AL, et al: Characterization of a mutagenic bacterial product in human feces. *Am J Clin Nutr* 1980;33:2513-2520.
8. Colten T: *Statistics in Medicine.* Boston, Little Brown & Co Inc, 1975, pp 99-150.
9. Colacchio TA, Memoli VA: Chemoprevention of colorectal neoplasms. *Arch Surg* 1986;121:1421-1424.
10. Wattenberg LW, Lam LKT, Loub WD, et al: Inhibitors of chemical carcinogenesis, in Hiatt HH, Watson JD, Winston JA (eds): *Origins of Human Cancer.* Cold Spring Harbor, NY, Cold Spring Harbor Laboratory, 1977, pp 785-789.
11. Krinsky NI, Deneke SM: Interaction of oxygen and oxy-radicals with carotenoids. *JNCI* 1982;61:201-209.
12. Soloway MS, Cohen SM, de Kernion JB, et al: Failure of ascorbic acid to inhibit FANFT-induced bladder cancer. *J Urol* 1974;113:483-486.
13. Reddy BS, Hiroto N, Katayame S: Effect of dietary sodium ascorbate on 1,2-dimethylhydrazine or methylnitrosourea induced colon carcinogenesis in rats. *Carcinogenesis* 1982;3:1097-1099.
14. Dunham WB, Zuckerhandle E, Reynolds R, et al: Effects of intake of L-ascorbic acid on the incidence of dermal neoplasms induced in mice by ultraviolet light. *Proc Natl Acad Sci USA* 1982;79:7532-7536.
15. Abul-Hajj YJ, Kelliher M: Failure of ascorbic acid to inhibit growth of transplantable and dimethylbenzanthracene induced rat mammary tumors. *Cancer Lett* 1982;17:67-73.
16. Fukushima S, Imaida K, Sakata T, et al: Promoting effects of sodium L-ascorbate on two-stage urinary bladder carcinogenesis in rats. *Cancer Res* 1983;43:4454-4457.
17. Khar'Kovaskaya NA, Khrustalev SA, Zharova EI, et al: Effect of ascorbic acid on carcinogenicity of *p*-hydroxyphenylacetic acid. *Bull Eksp Biol Med* 1982;93:64-66.
18. Mirvish SS, Wallcave L, Eagen M, et al: Ascorbate-nitrate reaction: Possible means of blocking the formation of *N*-nitroso compounds. *Science* 1972;177:65-68.
19. Fukushima S, Hagiwara A, Ogiso T, et al: Promoting effects of various chemicals in rat urinary bladder carcinogenesis. *Food Chem Toxicol* 1983;21:59-68.
20. Jones FE, Komorowski FA, Condon RE: Chemoprevention of 1,2-dimethylhydrazine induced large bowel neoplasms. *Surg Forum* 1981;31:435-437.
21. Tsuda H, Sakata T, Shirai T, et al: Modification of MNU initiated carcinogenesis in the rat by subsequent treatment with antioxidants, phenobarbital, and ethinyl estradiol. *Cancer Lett* 1984;24:19-27.
22. Cook MG, McNamara P: Effects of vitamin E on dimethylhydrazine induced colonic tumors in mice. *Cancer Res* 1980;40:1329-1331.
23. Smalls E, Patterson RM: Reduction of benzo(a)pyrene induced chromosomal aberrations by DL-alpha-tocopherol. *Eur J Cell Biol* 1982;28:92-97.
24. Shklar G: Oral mucosal carcinogenesis in hamsters: Inhibition by vitamin E. *JNCI* 1982;5:791-793.
25. Toth P, Kashinath P: Enhancing effect of vitamin E on murine intestinal tumorigenesis by 1,2-dimethylhydrazine hydrochloride. *JNCI* 1983;6:1107-1111.
26. Horvath P, Ip C: Synergistic effect of vitamin E and selenium in the chemoprevention of mammary carcinogenesis in rats. *Cancer Res* 1983;43:5335-5341.
27. Odukoya O, Hawach F, Shklar G: Retardation of experimental oral cancer by topical vitamin E. *Nutr Cancer* 1984;6:98-104.
28. Ip C: Dietary vitamin E intake and mammary carcinogenesis in rats. *Carcinogenesis* 1982;3:1453-1456.
29. Shamberger RJ: Relationship of selenium to cancer. *JNCI* 1970;44:931-936.
30. Seifter E, Rettura G, Padawer J, et al: Maloney murine sarcoma virus tumors in cba/j mice: Chemoprevention and chemotherapeutic actions of supplemental beta-carotene. *JNCI* 1982;68:835-840.
31. Mathews-Roth MM: Antitumor activity of beta-carotene, canthaxanthine and phytoene. *Oncology* 1982;39:33-37.
32. Rettura G, Stratford F, Levenson SM, et al: Prophylactic and therapeutic actions of supplemental beta-carotene in mice inoculated with C3HBA adenocarcinoma cells: Lack of therapeutic action of supplemental ascorbic acid. *JNCI* 1982;59:73-77.
33. Seifter E, Rettura G, Padawer J, et al: Regression of C3HBA mouse tumor due to X-ray therapy combined with supplemental beta-carotene or vitamin A. *JNCI* 1983;71:409-417.
34. Alam SQ, Alam BS: Chemopreventive effects of beta-carotene and 13-*cis*-retinoic acid on salivary gland tumors. *Fed Proc* 1983;42:1313.
35. Santamaria L, Bianchi A, Arnaboldi A, et al: Dietary carotenoids block photocarcinogenic enhancement by benzo(a)pyrene and inhibit its carcinogenesis in the dark. *Experientia* 1983;39:1043-1045.
36. Santamaria L, Bianchi A, Arnaboldi A, et al: Prevention of the benzo(a)pyrene photocarcinogenic effect by beta-carotene and canthaxanthine: Preliminary study. *Boll Chim Farm* 1980;119:745-748.
37. Epstein JH: Effects of beta-carotene on ultraviolet induced cancer formation in the hairless mouse skin. *Photochem Photobiol* 1977;25:211-213.
38. Goerz G, Ippen H: Treatment of photodermatoses with carotenoids. *Dtsch Med Wochenschr* 1977;102:1051-1055.
39. Goerz G: Erythropoietic protoporphyria. *Fortschr Med* 1979;97:1625-1630.

Discussion

Q How applicable to the treatment of human tumors do you think this is? I am not familiar with the trials of colorectal cancer but I certainly am with melanoma and I have participated in some of those trials. People would come with what appeared to be very interesting prehuman data, yet so far it has not proved to be of any benefit in randomized trials of humans that I am aware of with regard to melanoma.

A The information we have to date is that in the studies done at Memorial-Sloan Kettering, New York, by J. DeCosse, on the patients with familial polyposis, some decrease in both the numbers of polyps and the size of the polyps following treatment with ascorbic acid was observed. In addition, the group from Toronto has looked at mutagens in the stool that have been found in higher numbers and frequency in "high-risk groups" relative to low-risk groups. In this group they did find that there was a decrease in mutagen content. Whether that will translate into actual decrease in the risk for developing colorectal cancer is unclear. Our own study of mutagens with ascorbic acid and alpha tocopherol is just finishing and we hope to have that information available soon.

Finally, the most important part of what I was trying to say was my concern about the rapid transition of agents from animal and epidemiologic data into human trials. I am worried about the possibility of beta carotene being used as a promoter as opposed to its use as an inhibitor. It seems to work in skin cancer, but I am not sure the preventive effect will be carried over in humans. The caution we need to take away from this is not to be too quick to rush agents into clinical trials.

Plasma Ultrafiltration as Cancer Therapy

Alan Wile, MD

• Studies of cancer-related immunosuppression reveal the presence of low-molecular-weight (<10 kilodaltons) serum factors capable of in vitro lymphocyte suppression. Removal of suppressor factors by ultrafiltration (UF) prolongs survival in tumor-bearing rabbits. This study determined the prevalence of low-molecular-weight suppressor factors in patients with cancer and normal volunteers and evaluated safety and feasibility of UF in patients with cancer. Intact serum and serum ultrafiltrate from 32 patients with cancer and 24 normal volunteers was examined with mitogen-induced lymphocyte blastogenesis. Eleven (34%) of serum samples from patients with cancer suppressed blastogenesis, while ultrafiltrate was suppressive in 25 (78%). None of the ultrafiltrate from normal volunteers was suppressive. Six patients with cancer underwent UF in a phase I trial, completing 82 sessions. There were no therapy-related complications, and high-performance liquid chromatography showed significant (>90%) posttreatment reduction in serum suppressor factors.

(*Arch Surg* 1989;124:222-224)

Defects in cellular immune function are well documented in patients with cancer. These patients are observed to develop lymphopenia,[1] which correlates with poor prognosis.[2] Inability to mount a delayed cutaneous hypersensitivity reaction to skin test antigens with adequate numbers of lymphocytes is a frequent and grave prognostic sign, representing loss of lymphocyte function.[3] The cause of impaired lymphocyte function associated with cancer has been speculated on and is the subject of numerous articles.[4]

Of interest are reports of impaired lymphocyte function when normal lymphocytes obtained from healthy donors are placed in serum obtained from patients with cancer.[5-7] Furthermore, lymphocytes from patients with cancer regain function when placed in media devoid of these patients' serum.[8] These observations suggest that a portion of the defect in cellular immune function associated with cancer is a reversible phenomenon mediated by humoral factors.

To increase understanding of cancer-related immunosuppression, I investigated soluble immunosuppressor factors (SIFs) elaborated by tumor-bearing animals. The presence of immunosuppressive factors was observed in rats inoculated with a transplantable tumor.[9] These SIFs were secreted by host tissues associated with immune function and were not tumor products. It was determined that there were multiple low-molecular-weight (<10 kilodaltons [kd]) and several high-molecular-weight (>10 kd) factors.[10] Three of the low-molecular-weight factors were heat labile (100°C) and are presumed to be polypeptides.

The temporal sequence of elaboration of SIFs was determined by obtaining serial blood samples from tumor-bearing animals.[11] A biphasic response was observed, with serum obtained shortly after tumor inoculation enhancing splenocyte response while serum obtained later was suppressive. The suppressor effect was confined to that portion of serum passing through a filter with a molecular weight cutoff of 10 kd. The enhancing effect resided in the portion of serum retained by the ultrafilter. This observation suggested that removal of low-molecular-weight SIFs by ultrafiltration (UF) might unmask sufficient endogenous lymphocyte-enhancing activity to alter favorably the host-tumor interaction.

This hypothesis was tested by conducting continuous plasma UF in rabbits inoculated with the VX-2 carcinoma.[12] Two plasma volumes were removed with the aid of an ultrafilter (Diafilter 20; Amicon Corp, Danvers, Mass; molecular weight cutoff, 10 kd). Prolongation of survival was observed in animals undergoing a single UF therapy, especially when UF was combined with an immunoadjuvant (Detox; RIBI Immunochem Research Inc, Hamilton, Mont).

With the knowledge obtained from the animal models, a search was made for low-molecular-weight SIFs associated with human cancer. That effort comprises the substance of this article and describes the prevalence of SIFs in normal volunteers and patients with cancer, techniques used to quantitate SIFs, and a phase I trial of continuous plasma UF to remove SIFs as cancer therapy.

SUBJECTS AND METHODS

Thirty-two patients undergoing therapy for metastatic cancer consented to be blood donors for the initial portion of this study. Eleven had lymphoma, eight had breast cancer, seven had colon cancer, and two had lung cancer. Prostatic cancer, leukemia, stomach cancer, and nasopharyngeal cancer each accounted for one patient. No patient received a cytotoxic drug, including prednisone, the week before blood drawing. Twenty-four normal volunteers also donated blood.

Blood samples remained at room temperature for two hours to facilitate clotting. Serum was removed after centrifugation at 1500 rpm for ten minutes. Serum was divided into aliquots and frozen at −70°C. Aliquots of serum underwent UF by means of membranes (Amicon PM-10; Amicon Corp) with a molecular weight cutoff of 10 kd under a positive pressure of 30 psi of nitrogen. Serum ultrafiltrate was frozen at −70°C. Serum and ultrafiltrate were numerically coded and assayed in blinded fashion with normal subjects and patients with cancer mixed in sequence.

The effect of serum and ultrafiltrate on lymphocyte function was ascertained by means of a mitogen-induced lymphocyte blastogenesis assay using normal human lymphocytes as targets. Sixty milliliters of blood from a volunteer was defribrinated by mechanical means with removal of clot within five minutes of blood drawing. Remaining serum was diluted with 60 mL of phosphate-buffered saline. Aliquots were placed in centrifuge tubes containing 15 mL of Ficoll-Hypaque (Histopaque 1077; Sigma Chemical, St Louis), with care taken not to mix the serum and Ficoll-Hypaque layers. The mixture was centrifuged for 40 minutes at 1500 rpm (20°C). After centrifugation, the lymphocyte-rich interface between serum and Ficoll-Hypaque was aspirated. The interface from multiple tubes was pooled and centrifuged at 2000 rpm for ten minutes, and the supernatant was removed. The lymphocyte pellet was resuspended in 10 mL of RPMI 1640 tissue culture medium with 10% fetal calf serum. The final cell suspension was adjusted so that 180 μL contained 1×10^6 viable lymphocytes with a mitogen concentration (phytohemagglutinin; Burroughs Wellcome, Beckenham, England) of 2.5 to 5.0 mg/L.

The blastogenesis assay was conducted in microtiter test plates. Twenty microliters of serum or ultrafiltrate were added to 180 μL of the lymphocyte suspension and incubated at 37°C for 72 hours in 95% oxygen–5% carbon dioxide. After 72 hours, 10 μL of tritiated thymidine (100 mCi/L; Amersham Corp, Arlington Heights, Ill) was added to each well and incubated for an additional 18 hours. After the second incubation, the contents of the wells were aspirated, deposited on filter paper, and placed in vials containing scintillation cocktail, and radioactivity was counted in a liquid scintillation counter (one minute per sample). Samples were assayed in sextuplicate. Mean and SD were calculated. Controls included lymphocytes in normal human serum with and without phytohemagglutinin. Percentage inhibition of lymphocyte blastogenesis was calculated by dividing the results obtained with

Accepted for publication Sept 30, 1988.

From the Division of Surgical Oncology, Department of Surgery, University of California Irvine Medical Center, Orange, Calif.

Read before the Annual Meeting of the Society of Surgical Oncology, New Orleans, May 25, 1988.

Reprint requests to Division of Surgical Oncology, Department of Surgery, University of California Irvine Medical Center, 101 City Dr S, Orange, CA 92668 (Dr Wile).

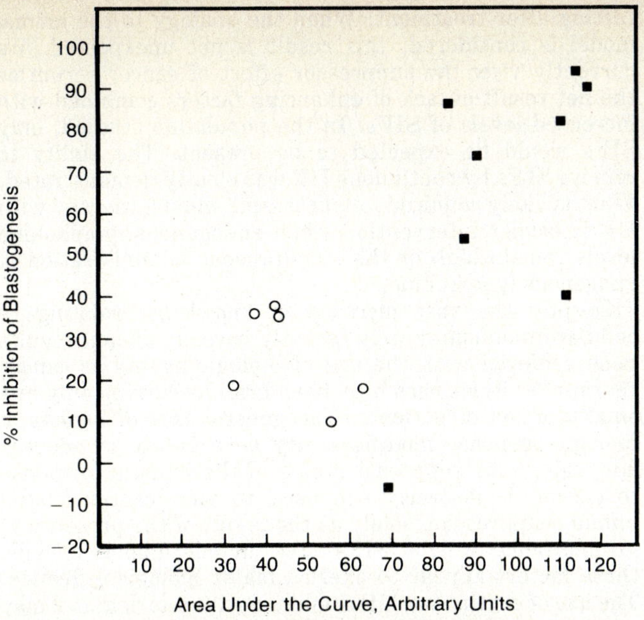

Fig 1.—Close correlation of low-molecular-weight soluble immunosuppressor factors when quantitated by blastogenesis assay and high-performance liquid chromatographic assay (area under curve). Patients with cancer (closed squares) could be distinguished from normal volunteers (open circles) on basis of area under curve.

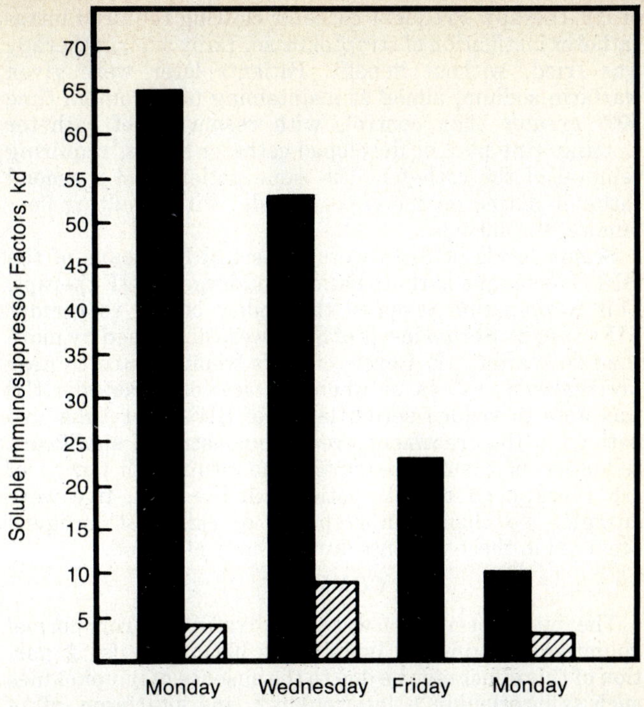

Fig 2.—Changes in serum levels of low-molecular-weight soluble immunosuppressor factors in single patient over time during course of ultrafiltration therapy. Although soluble immunosuppressor factors returned to high levels between treatment sessions, general trend was toward diminution in serum levels. Closed bars indicate pretreatment values; hatched bars, posttreatment values; kd, kilodaltons.

the experimental sample by the normal serum control, subtracting results from 1, and multiplying by 100.

Low-molecular-weight SIFs were quantitated by means of a high-performance liquid chromatography (HPLC) device coupled to a molecular seiving column (GPC 100 7u; Alltech Assoc Inc, Deerfield, Ill). The presence of SIFs was detected and plotted on graph paper. The area under the curve was measured with the use of a planimeter, with results expressed in arbitrary units. Comparisons were made with an external standard using known amounts of bovine insulin. Six normal individuals and eight patients with cancer underwent simultaneous quantitation of SIFs by means of the blastogenesis assay and the HPLC technique.

Six patients with cancer underwent plasma UF as a phase I trial; all failed conventional therapy and consented to participate in an experimental program approved by the University of California Irvine Human Subjects Committee (Orange, Calif). A double-lumen dialysis (Quinton) catheter was placed via the saphenous vein into the iliac vein. Delayed cutaneous hypersensitivity was ascertained before therapy and at monthly intervals.

Plasma UF was conducted in an outpatient setting. The dialysis catheter was connected to a custom UF controller (COBE Laboratories, Lakewood, Colo) mated to an ultrafilter (Amicon Diafilter 30). Ultrafiltration was achieved by withdrawing blood through the filter from heparinized patients. A negative transmembrane pressure was applied (0 to 350 mm Hg) to facilitate UF. The volume of ultrafiltrate was precisely matched with replacement saline returned to the patient with blood components retained by the filter. The goal of each treatment session was removal of three plasma volumes of ultrafiltrate. This was determined for each patient by means of a nomogram based on height, weight, hematocrit, and gender.

Blood samples were obtained from each patient before and after UF sessions for determination of SIF levels. Serum from these samples was ultrafiltered in the laboratory (Amicon PM-10 filter). The ultrafiltrate was frozen at −70°C for quantitation of SIFs by the HPLC technique.

RESULTS

The effect of intact serum from normal volunteers on mitogen-induced lymphocyte blastogenesis was averaged and used as a reference point. Ultrafiltrate from normal volunteers was suppressive (34.0%±31.41%; maximum, 75%). In comparison, intact serum from patients with cancer resulted in a mean suppression of 49.0%±38.3%, with mean suppression by ultrafiltrate of 86.8%±11.9%. Based on these observations, abnormal suppression was defined as 80% or greater inhibition of lymphocyte blastogenesis. Using this definition, the intact serum of 11 (34%) of the 32 patients with cancer was suppressive. Twenty-five (78%) of 32 patients with cancer possessed abnormal suppressor activity in serum ultrafiltrate, compared with none of 24 normal volunteers.

Dilution of suppressive ultrafiltrate to 1% with tissue culture medium resulted in loss of significant suppressor activity in six of 14 samples assayed in the blastogenesis assay. An additional four samples became less suppressive but did not fall below the 80% level.

Analysis of serum ultrafiltrate by HPLC methods revealed a single peak eluting at four minutes. Simultaneous examination of ultrafiltrate with the blastogenesis assay and the HPLC method demonstrated good correlation between the quantity of SIFs present as calculated by the area under the curve and the degree of inhibition of blastogenesis. It was observed that patients with cancer could be separated from normal volunteers on the basis of HPLC analysis of serum ultrafiltrate (Fig 1). In addition, values derived by the HPLC method were reproducible, while there was variability in the bioassay.

The six patients with cancer completed 82 sessions of UF, during which it was usually possible to remove three plasma volumes (5 to 10 L) in three to four hours. Flow through the system was limited by the size of the catheter lumen, but rates as high as 250 mL/min were reached. On occasion, patients experienced muscle cramps during the UF procedure. This was thought to be due to hyponatremia, and the cramps resolved when the replacement fluid of lactated Ringer's solution was supplemented to raise the sodium concentration to 154 mEq/L and the calcium concentration to 3.5 mEq/L.

Catheter-related problems were the major complications

of UF therapy. Frequent catheter clotting required intracatheter instillation of streptokinase. Daily aspirin therapy was tried, without benefit. Patients later were given warfarin sodium, aimed at maintaining prothrombin time 50% greater than control, with resolution of catheter clotting. One patient developed catheter sepsis, requiring removal of the catheter. The same patient had a second catheter placed on the opposite side, with resulting ileofemoral thrombosis.

Serum levels of SIFs were measured by means of the HPLC technique in those patients undergoing UF therapy. This examination revealed the ability of UF to remove SIFs (Fig 2). Serum levels of SIFs were decreased by more than 90% after UF. Levels of SIFs would return to near pretreatment values between UF sessions. Periodic UF was able to reduce serum levels of SIFs over time. No patient in the treatment group demonstrated significant reduction of tumor size during the two-month period of UF therapy. Of the six patients in the trial, five were anergic. No change in response to skin test antigens occurred in these patients during the trial period.

COMMENT

The initial observation was that ultrafiltrate from normal volunteers suppressed lymphocyte blastogenesis. A portion of this effect may be due to the absence of lymphokines such as interleukin 1, interleukin 2, and interferon, all of which have molecular weights greater than 10 kd. An additional component of suppression may be the lack of osmotic buffers provided by macromolecules. The third component of ultrafiltrate-mediated suppression is that of SIFs. One third of patients with cancer had suppressive serum. The ultrafiltrate of serum from these patients was suppressive in 78% of patients. The finding of suppressor activity in the ultrafiltrate of normal individuals with increased amounts in patients with cancer suggests that SIFs are normal serum constituents and are significantly increased in advanced cancer. They may be offset by simultaneous elaboration of enhancing factors, accounting for lesser suppression of blastogenesis by intact serum from patients with cancer compared with ultrafiltrate from these same patients.

Next, efforts were aimed at providing additional evidence to support the presence of SIFs. This was accomplished by diluting ultrafiltrate with tissue culture medium. The reversal of suppression of lymphocyte blastogenesis noted in ten of 14 samples after dilution further supported the presence of increased amounts of SIF rather than lack of lymphocyte-enhancing factors. The presence of SIFs was assured with the HPLC technique, which demonstrated increased levels of SIFs correlating closely with suppression in the blastogenesis assay. The ease and reliability of the HPLC method has supplanted the bioassay to detect SIFs in our laboratory.

The phase I trial of continuous plasma UF was successful in terms of feasibility and toxic effects. The UF controller we used functioned well, handled blood at adequate rates, and provided sufficient control over flow rates, transmembrane pressures, and line pressures to optimize plasma UF. Adequate safeguards were supplied in the form of automatic line clamps and bubble detectors. The filter (Diafilter 30) functioned well, without failure at transmembrane pressures as high as 350 mm Hg. The limiting factor in terms of UF rate was the lumen size of the dialysis catheter. With catheter-related problems representing the major obstacle to continuous UF, it is difficult to envision the use of larger catheters.

None of the six patients in the UF trial manifested significant clinical benefit from UF. Of the five patients with anergy before therapy, all were unresponsive to skin testing after treatment. When the analogy to the animal model is considered, this result is not unexpected. We currently view the suppressor effect of cancer serum as the net result of lack of enhancing factors combined with increased levels of SIFs. In the population studied, only SIFs would be expected to be present. The ability to remove SIFs by continuous UF was clearly demonstrated. What is likely required for successful immunotherapy with UF is earlier intervention when endogenous lymphokine levels remain high or the simultaneous administration of exogenous lymphokine.

Despite the vast increase in knowledge relating to cellular immunology, only recently have significant results been achieved with the use of biologic agents as cancer therapy.[13,14] Responses have been brief, occurring only in a small portion of patients. The general lack of benefit of biologic response modifiers may be a failure to address adequately the suppression side of the immune response to cancer. It is overly simplistic to view cancer-related immunosuppression solely as the result of the presence of low-molecular-weight SIFs. Yet, in our animal models, these factors appear to exert a major biologic influence. The use of continuous UF combined with interleukin 2 may augment response to interleukin 2 with lower doses and less toxic reaction. This combined approach, simultaneously removing suppressor molecules and adding enhancing factors, may be required for effective cancer immunotherapy.

I am grateful for the support of COBE Laboratories, Lakewood, Colo, and Amicon Corp, Danvers, Mass, for furnishing essential devices and supplies. I greatly appreciate the superb nursing assistance provided by Kelly Gullixson.

References

1. Keller SE, Ioachim HL, Pearse T, et al: Decreased T-lymphocytes in patients with mammary cancer. *Am J Clin Pathol* 1976;65:445-449.
2. Papatestas AE, Lesnick GJ, Genkins G, et al: The prognostic significance of peripheral lymphocyte counts in patients with breast carcinoma. *Cancer* 1976;37:164-168.
3. Eilber FR, Morton DL: Impaired immunologic reactivity and recurrence following cancer surgery. *Cancer* 1970;25:362-367.
4. Roth JA: Tumor induced immunosuppression. *Surg Gynecol Obstet* 1983;156:233-240.
5. Rangel DM, Golub SH, Morton DL: Demonstration of lymphocyte blastogenesis-inhibiting factors in sera of melanoma patients. *Surgery* 1977; 82:224-232.
6. Giuliano AE, Rangel D, Golub SH, et al: Serum mediated immunosuppression in lung cancer. *Cancer* 1979;43:917-924.
7. Sugden PJ, Lilleyman JS: Impairment of lymphocyte transformation by plasma from patients with advanced Hodgkin's disease. *Cancer* 1980; 45:899-906.
8. Hadjipetrou-Kourounakis L, Manikou H, Tsougranis A: Restoration of immunosuppression in lung cancer by normal sera. *J Clin Lab Immunol* 1985;16:149-153.
9. Wile AG, Henson D, Nahabedian M, et al: Soluble suppressor factors elaborated in experimental malignant ascites. *Cell Immunol* 1984;86:347-353.
10. Cohen R, Contino M, Henson D, et al: Heterogeneity of soluble suppressor factors in rat malignant ascites. *Oncology* 1988;45:230-235.
11. Wile AG, Cohen RA, Terem TM, et al: Sequential elaboration of lymphocyte enhancing and suppressing factors in the sera of tumor bearing animals. *J Surg Oncol* 1987;35:207-212.
12. Snyder L, Kar R, Wile A: Plasma ultrafiltration as successful therapy of the rabbit VX-2 carcinoma. *J Surg Oncol*, in press.
13. Rosenberg SA, Lotze MT, Muul LM, et al: A progress report on the treatment of 157 patients with advanced cancer using lymphokine activated killer cells and interleukin-2 or high dose interleukin-2 alone. *N Engl J Med* 1987;316:889-905.
14. West WH, Tauer KW, Yannelli JR, et al: Constant-infusion recombinant interleukin-2 in adoptive immunotherapy of advanced cancer. *N Engl J Med* 1987;316:898-905.

Discussion

Q Do you have any idea what these factors are? Have you done these studies on them?

A Yes and no. We have been working with the suppressor factors on a variety of different levels. We have extensively characterized these factors in the rat model, and a characterization actually appears in the *Journal of Oncology*.

Endoscopic Ablation of Esophageal Malignancies With the Neodymium-YAG Laser and Electrofulguration

Hector R. Nava, MD; Marlys E. Schuh, MD; Raman Nambisan, MD; John L. Clark, MD; Harold O. Douglass, Jr, MD

• The case reports of 40 patients with obstructive esophageal cancer treated with electrofulguration (EF) or neodymium (Nd)-YAG laser were reviewed. Surgery was contraindicated because of advanced carcinoma (17 patients), recurrence after resection (13 patients), recurrence after irradiation (four patients), and poor medical condition (four). Two patients refused surgery. There were 31 men and four women; mean age was 62 years. There were 31 adenocarcinomas, eight squamous cell carcinomas, and one metastatic breast carcinoma. Tumor locations were lower esophagus in 35 patients, middle esophagus in three, and cervical esophagus in two. Thirty-five patients had obstructions; two, bleeding, and three, both. None of the patients could swallow solids. A total of 255 treatments were given (mean, 6.6 per patient). The mean number of Nd-YAG treatments was 1.9; for EF, 1.3. All 40 patients tolerated solid food after treatment and the esophagus remained open from three to 14 weeks. Mean survival from first treatment was 11 months; from diagnosis, 17 months. Both techniques were safe and effective.

(*Arch Surg* 1989;149:225-228)

Since the five-year cure rate of esophageal carcinoma remains poor, palliation is often the main goal of treatment.[1] A number of modalities used in the past to achieve palliation resulted in varying degrees of efficacy. These include surgery, radiation therapy, dilatation, and intubation.[2-4] In recent years, however, endoscopic treatment of malignant esophageal obstructive lesions with the neodymium (Nd)-YAG laser has emerged as a promising therapeutic option.[5,6] This report is a retrospective review of the palliative treatment of esophageal carcinoma with endoscopic Nd-YAG laser and endoscopic monopolar electrofulguration (EF) in 40 patients treated at Roswell Park Memorial Institute, Buffalo, between May 1984 and December 1986.

Accepted for publication July 8, 1988.

From the Department of Surgery, Roswell Park Memorial Institute, Buffalo.

Read before the Annual Meeting of the Society of Surgical Oncology, New Orleans, May 23, 1988.

Reprint requests to Roswell Park Memorial Institute, 666 Elm St, Buffalo, NY 14263 (Dr Nava).

PATIENTS AND METHODS

The case histories of 40 patients who were seen consecutively at Roswell Park Memorial Institute between May 1984 and December 1986, and were diagnosed as having carcinoma of the esophagus for which palliative therapy was administered were reviewed. Surgical treatment was contraindicated in these patients for the following reasons: the presence of advanced carcinoma at the time of diagnosis, 17 patients; recurrent carcinoma following resection, 13 patients; recurrent carcinoma following radiation therapy, four patients; and unsatisfactory medical condition, four patients. Two patients refused surgery. Adenocarcinoma of the esophagus was diagnosed in 31 patients; eight patients were found to have squamous cell carcinoma; and one patient had adenocarcinoma of the breast with metastasis to the esophagus. The mean age of the patients in this series was 62 years, with a range of 32 to 86 years.

Thirty-six of the patients were men; four were women. The majority of the malignant esophageal lesions (35 of 40) were located at or distal to 35 cm. In one patient, the lesion was present in the upper part of the esophagus at 19 cm from the incisors, and in the remaining four patients, the lesion was located in the middle of the esophagus at 22 to 34 cm.

Obstruction was the predominant presenting symptom in 35 patients. Acute bleeding was the reason for referral in two patients, and three patients reported symptoms of both obstruction and hemorrhage. The degree of esophageal obstruction was such that all 40 patients were unable to tolerate solid food. Obstructive dysphagia was severe enough in several patients to preclude even passage of saliva. Although a few patients in this series were able to swallow liquids, at the time treatment was administered none was capable of oral intake sufficient to maintain energy requirements.

TREATMENT TECHNIQUE

Endoscopic laser therapy was performed using an Nd-YAG laser (Medilas-2) with a power output calibrated to deliver 80 to 100 W. Laser energy was applied via quartz fibers placed through the operating channel of the fiberoptic endoscope (Pentax-FG 36TA), with a white ceramic tip adapted for the laser, or through the smaller-diameter fiberoptic endoscope (Pentax-FG 34JH). Laser energy was applied under direct vision in short pulses, visually regulated not to exceed 2 s. Treatment was performed in a retrograde fashion whenever possible, but due to the degree of

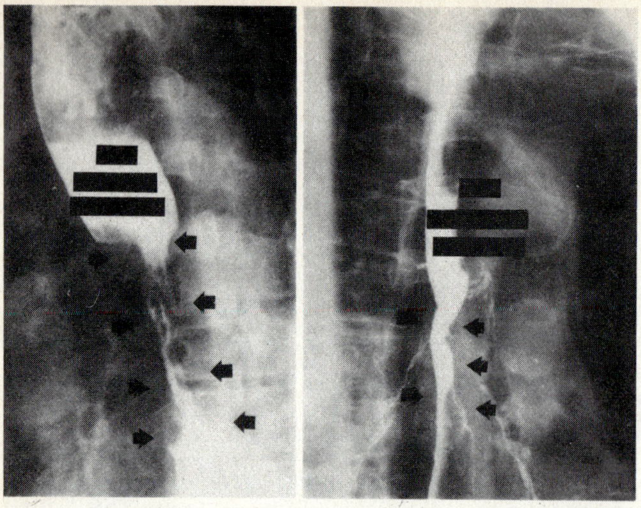

Fig 1.—Left, Adenocarcinoma with nearly complete obstruction. Notice dilatation proximal to tumor. Right, Eight weeks later, no tumor is seen in lumen: shouldering effect and proximal dilatation have disappeared. Arrows indicate location of tumor before and after electrofulguration.

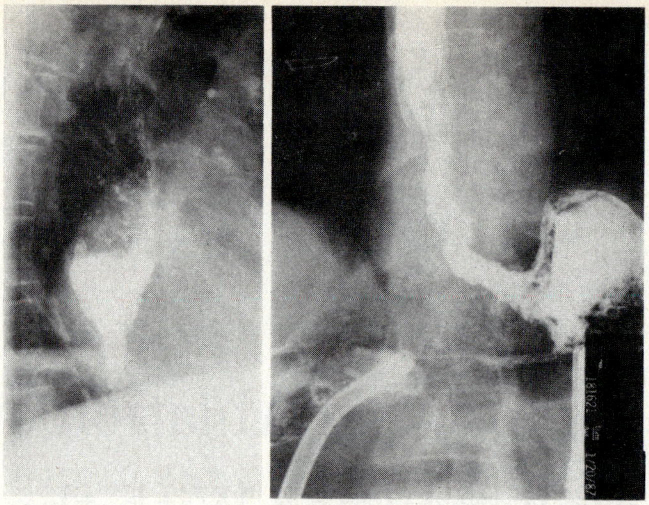

Fig 2.—Left, Complete obstruction by adenocarcinoma. Right, Final result after several neodymium-YAG laser treatments; raggedy edges outline channel created. Percutaneous endoscopic gastrostomy tube has been placed for nutritional supplementation.

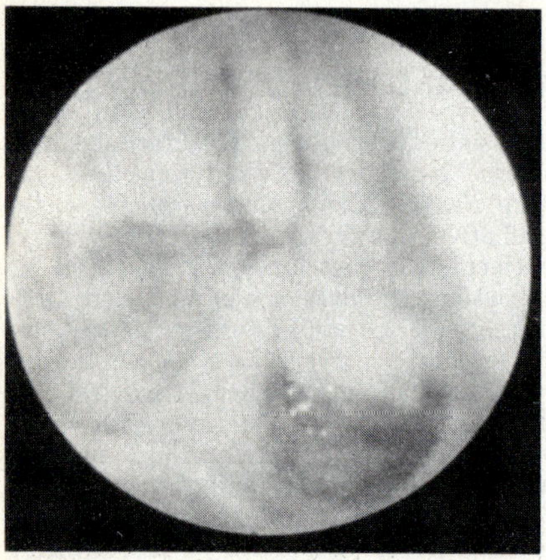

Fig 3.—Complete esophageal obstruction by adenocarcinoma. Lumen is not discernible at junction of folds.

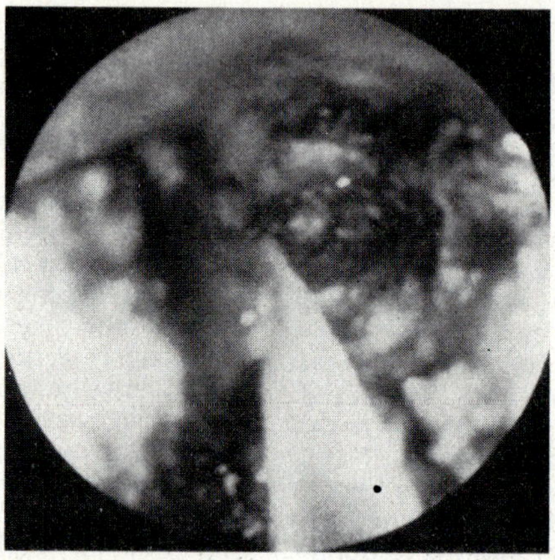

Fig 4.—Circumferential necrosis of esophageal tumor after endoscopic electrofulguration. Monopolar electrocautery probe inside of stricture.

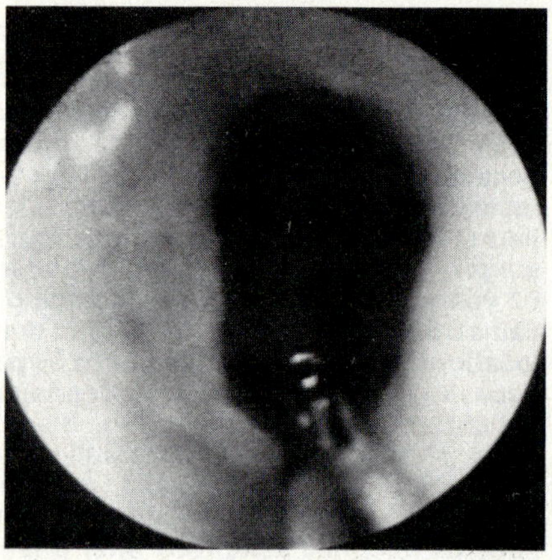

Fig 5.—Final result three weeks after endoscopic electrofulguration. Lumen wide open, biopsy forceps in place for comparison. Patient tolerating solid food.

obstruction present, this could be accomplished only if esophageal dilatation was first performed with Savary or balloon dilators. Thus, most treatments were administered in an antegrade fashion with the laser directed at the obstructed lumen (Figs 1 and 2).

Endoscopic EF therapy was performed using a monopolar unit (Valleylab SSE2-K) with the electrode (ACMI ball-tip) placed through the operating channel of the fiberoptic endoscope (Pentax-FG 34JH). The power setting on this instrument was 80 W. Treatment was administered in a retrograde fashion whenever possible, but unlike the Nd-YAG laser, the smaller diameter of the electrocautery EF probe permitted passage distal to the strictured lumen (Figs 3 through 5).

In the earlier years of the period under review, most patients were treated by EF, with treatment using the Nd-YAG laser becoming more frequent in the later years of the study. It was observed that a number of patients underwent both therapeutic modalities during different treatment courses.

For each type of therapy, treatments were repeated at 48- to 72-hour intervals until luminal patency was sufficiently established to allow the passage of the 11-mm-diameter endoscope into the stomach and to allow oral intake of solid food. During the period under review, a total of 12 percutaneous endoscopic gastrostomy tubes and one nasogastric feeding tube were placed.

RESULTS

The 40 patients examined in this study received a total of 255 treatments. The average number of treatments per patient was 6.6 (range, one to 32 treatments). It was determined that it required an average of 1.8 treatments (range, one to six treatments) with the Nd-YAG laser to establish luminal patency as compared with 1.3 treatments (range, one to four treatments) when employing the electrocautery EF probe. This result was independent of whether or not the patient was receiving chemotherapy in addition to endoscopic therapy.

The duration of response was variable. It was found that courses of treatment to reestablish adequate luminal patency were required on average every four weeks. In several patients, re-treatment was necessary in as little as three weeks, whereas other patients did not develop severe

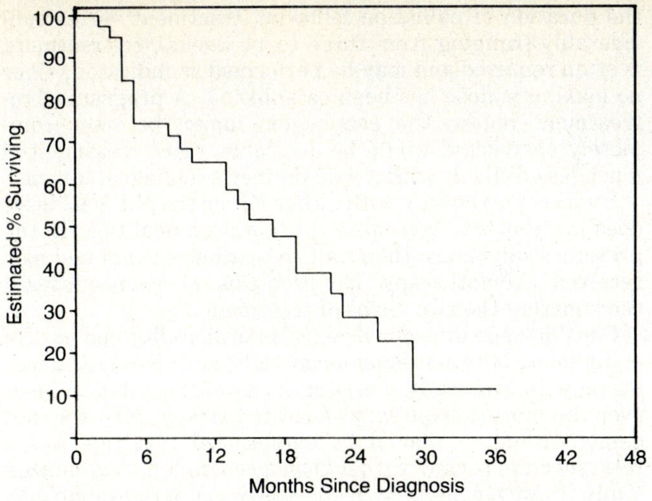

Fig 6.—Estimated survival time since diagnosis of 40 patients with esophageal malignant obstruction treated endoscopically.

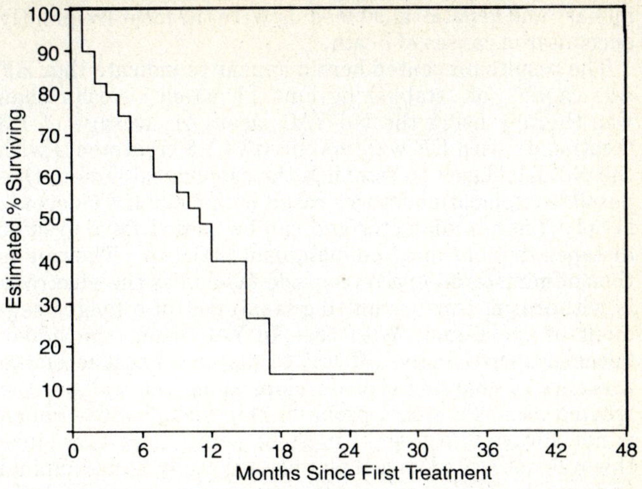

Fig 7.—Estimated survival time since first endoscopic treatment.

obstruction for approximately eight to ten weeks.

Of the five patients with symptoms of hemorrhage, bleeding was controlled with EF in three of them. In the remaining two patients, hemostasis could not be achieved with either the Nd-YAG laser or EF. Angiographic embolization of the left gastric artery was attempted in both patients, but treatment was unsuccessful and these two patients subsequently died of exsanguination.

The median survival time in all 40 patients from the time of the first endoscopic treatment was 11 months. The estimated one-year survival was 40%. In this patient population, median survival time from diagnosis was 17 months, with an estimated one-year survival of 65% (Figs 6 and 7).

At the time this review was carried out, 24 patients had died. The cause of death was progressive metastatic disease in nine patients, respiratory failure (eg, tracheoesophageal fistula, from tumor breakdown, aspiration pneumonia, or tumor involvement) in five patients, bleeding in five patients, sepsis in three patients, and myocardial infarction in two patients.

COMPLICATIONS OF THERAPY

Transient febrile (temperature >38.5°C) episodes occurred in three patients. Blood cultures did not yield the causative organism and the fevers resolved without antibiotic therapy. Antibiotics were required to treat two patients who developed fever and had positive blood cultures (*Escherichia coli*) subsequent to endoscopic therapy. Both patients recovered without further sequelae. One patient with diffuse abdominal carcinomatosis developed abdominal distention and crampy pains following endoscopic treatment. This was attributed to air insufflation and resolved without other therapy. Significant posttreatment pain, requiring parenteral narcotics for several days, occurred in one patient.

In addition to the five patients treated initially for bleeding, another 13 patients developed acute or chronic bleeding during the treatment period. None of the patients whose tumors were located in the middle or upper parts of the esophagus experienced significant bleeding. Hemorrhage from the tumor in the distal part of the esophagus appeared to increase in frequency and severity with repeated treatment courses, with most bleeding occurring as chronic oozing from the tumor surface. Several patients, however, developed acute massive bleeding. In one patient, angiographic embolization of the left gastric artery was successfully carried out. In the other patients, hemostasis was achieved endoscopically. Exsanguination was a direct cause of death in five patients. Hemorrhage seemed to occur with equal frequency whether treatment was performed with the laser or EF. However, all patients with massive hemorrhage were treated using the Nd-YAG laser.

COMMENT

It was found that endoscopic treatment with either the Nd-YAG laser or monopolar EF was well tolerated by all the patients in this series. No esophageal perforations or cases of aspiration pneumonia attributable to treatment were encountered. Treatment resulted in some transient febrile episodes (2%), with occasional bacteremia requiring antibiotic therapy (0.8%).

Symptomatic relief of the mechanical obstruction was achieved in all 40 patients, since ability to tolerate solid food was improved after treatment. Despite this, it was observed that in a number of patients, energy intake did not improve significantly after treatment. Whenever possible and acceptable to the patient, placement of a percutaneous endoscopic gastrostomy tube was carried out to enhance the nutritional status of these anorexic patients. It was also found that opening the percutaneous endoscopic gastrostomy tube during treatment aided in smoke evacuation and prevented any gastric dilatation as a result of insufflation.

It appeared that extensive tumor involvement with vascular encasement occurred in patients having the type of malignant stricture evaluated in this study. Endoscopic treatment with either the Nd-YAG laser or EF resulted in tumor ablation, with erosion of the involved vessels. Although the small bleeding points could be readily controlled endoscopically, as larger vessels were encountered, the resulting hemorrhage could become massive and life threatening.

Aspiration pneumonia and malnutrition are generally considered to be the usual causes of death from esophageal carcinoma. However, this was not true for the patients in this series. Aspiration pneumonia accounted for only one death. Progressive metastatic disease (particularly pulmonary and hepatic) and bleeding were the most frequently encountered causes of death.

The results presented herein appear to indicate that EF was capable of establishing luminal patency earlier than was therapy using the Nd-YAG laser. An average of 1.3 treatments with EF were required vs 1.8 treatments with the Nd-YAG laser, to establish the esophageal lumen. One possible explanation for this result is that the EF electrode is only 2 mm in diameter and can be passed for a greater distance distally into the malignant stricture. Therapy is thus administered in a retrograde fashion as the electrode is withdrawn, thus permitting treatment of a longer segment of the tumor. With the Nd-YAG laser, the lumen becomes increasingly difficult to discern, because of the presence of charring that develops along the walls of the treated area. Passing a probe to help visualize the lumen is not always effective. It must be pointed out that since this was not a randomized prospective study, exact luminal measurements before and after treatment were not available. Therefore, differences in treatment efficacy between the Nd-YAG laser and EF must be interpreted in that context.

The survival data in this series indicate that adequate palliation was maintained for prolonged periods. Because the duration of palliation following treatment varies considerably (ranging from three to 14 weeks), re-treatment is often required and may be performed as indicated, since no maximum dose has been established. A program of re-treatment before the esophageal lumen becomes completely obstructed would be desirable, since treatment is much less difficult with a well-defined esophageal lumen.

Endoscopic therapy with either EF or the Nd-YAG laser does not preclude treatment with other modalities. In the present study, more than half the patients examined also received chemotherapy. No problems were encountered coordinating the two forms of treatment.

Considerable differences exist in availability and cost of equipment between monopolar EF and Nd-YAG laser therapy. In this study, the superiority of the Nd-YAG laser over the more conventional form of therapy (EF) was not demonstrated. It should be emphasized that this was a retrospective review, rather than a controlled, randomized study. However, in view of the equivocal data available to date and given the cost factors involved, we would recommend that a randomized, controlled study be carried out as soon as possible to objectively evaluate these two modalities in the palliative treatment of malignant stricture resulting from the presence of esophageal carcinoma.

References

1. Ellis FH: Carcinoma of the esophagus. *CA* 1983;33:264-281.
2. Cukingnam RA, Carey JS: Carcinoma of the esophagus. *Ann Thorac Surg* 1978;26:274.
3. Gunnlangsson GH, Wychulis AR, Roland C, et al: Analysis of the records of 1657 patients with carcinoma of the esophagus and cardia of the stomach. *Surg Gynecol Obstet* 1970;130:997.
4. Cassidy DE, Nord HJ, Boyce HW Jr: Management of malignant esophageal strictures: Role of esophageal dilation and peroral prosthesis. *Am J Gastroenterol* 1981;76:173.
5. Fleischer D, Kessler F: Endoscopic Nd:YAG laser therapy for carcinoma of the esophagus: A new form of palliative treatment. *Gastroenterology* 1983;85:600-606.
6. Mellow MH, Pinkas H: Endoscopic therapy for esophageal carcinoma with Nd:YAG laser. *Gastrointest Endosc* 1984;30:334-339.

Discussion

Q What specific laser settings did you use?

A In reference to the YAG laser, the laser was set between 60 and 100 W. I usually prefer to use maximum power; the higher the power, the quicker the effect, and the less the penetration; this has been documented by others as the better way to use the laser.

Q What was the origin of the bleeding?

A In two patients the origin of the bleeding was documented arising in branches of the left gastric artery. Both of those patients had adenocarcinomas of the gastroesophageal junction and they did not bleed at the time of treatment. Subsequently, they experienced massive bleeding and it was very hard to determine whether it was the effect of the laser or just the natural course of the disease.

Q Can you use these techniques on benign structures?

A Actually, what prompted us to use these techniques, especially electrocautery, were reports from Germany using monopolar electrocautery to open benign postsurgical strictures. Definitely, both techniques can be used for benign strictures and we have done so on patients who developed benign strictures following esophagogastrectomies.

Q Did it work?

A Very well.

Q How about the contact laser?

A We had tried the contact laser with tips. The advantage of the contact method is that it reduces the depth of penetration of the laser; however, because of that it takes more time to debulk large amounts of tumor.

Q Which of the techniques is the best?

A Obviously a prospective randomized study needs to be done, not only between these two techniques, but with photodynamic therapy, bipolar therapy, and the heater probe, which are also techniques reported as being useful in this type of problem. We have continued to accumulate experience with the YAG laser. Since we have a lot of experience with monopolar EF, we are now in a position where we should be able to run a prospective randomized study between these two techniques. The recommendation to the group is that if the YAG laser is available it is perhaps the treatment of choice as long as there is someone who can use it. But, if it is not available, then you have the alternative, less expensive, form of therapy, which is monopolar EF.

Are Complications in Intraoperative Radiation Therapy More Frequent Than in Conventional Treatment?

Douglas T. Cromack, MD; Michelle M. Maher, RN; Harald Hoekstra, MD, PhD;
Timothy J. Kinsella, MD; William F. Sindelar, MD, PhD

• To evaluate whether intraoperative radiation therapy (IORT) results in higher complication rates than conventional radiotherapy, 119 patients were studied who entered four prospectively randomized clinical trials that compared IORT with conventional therapy. Malignant neoplasms included 33 gastric carcinomas, 35 retroperitoneal sarcomas, 22 resectable pancreatic cancers, and 29 unresectable pancreatic cancers. One hundred thirty-six complications developed among 66 patients who received conventional therapy, and 108 complications developed among 53 patients who received IORT. There was no statistical significance between treatment groups with respect to the overall incidence of complications. Analysis of types of complications by tumor type using Fisher's exact test revealed only one significant complication: an increased rate of sepsis among the patients with retroperitoneal sarcoma who received conventional therapy compared with their IORT cohorts. The overall complication rate associated with IORT was equivalent to conventional radiotherapy in the treatment of these malignant neoplasms and supported the use of IORT where clinically indicated.

(*Arch Surg* 1989;124:229-234)

Achieving local and regional control of many intra-abdominal malignant neoplasms remains a difficult and unrewarding task for the surgical oncologist despite the current availability and use of multimodality therapy. During the past decade, increasing enthusiasm for the use of intraoperative radiation therapy (IORT) has developed in some oncology centers.[1] Intraoperative radiation therapy allows the delivery of a single radiation dose directly to a tumor mass or to a resected tumor bed during a surgical procedure. Intraoperative radiation therapy potentially spares normal tissue in the vicinity of the treatment volume by operative displacement of tissues out of the treatment field. Intraoperative radiation therapy allows the delivery of large tumoricidal radiation doses to a malignant neoplasm with a low risk of radiation damage to normal tissues.

While complications associated with the use of IORT have been recognized, there have been no systematic reports comparing the types of IORT-related complications, their frequency, and their time course with the types of complications associated with conventional external-beam radiation therapy. In light of the theoretical treatment advantages of IORT in cancer therapy, objective analyses of the complications associated with the use of IORT are needed. For several years, the National Cancer Institute (NCI) has conducted randomized trials evaluating surgery in combination with IORT compared with surgery in combination with conventional radiotherapy for the treatment of retroperitoneal sarcomas, gastric adenocarcinomas, and both resected and unresected pancreatic cancers.[1-4] These trials have suggested a benefit in local disease control but not in overall survival. The trials have not yet, however, sufficiently matured to draw firm conclusions on the efficacy of IORT compared with conventional radiotherapy. The present study analyzes both IORT and control groups to address whether the complications of IORT differ from those of conventional treatment.

PATIENTS AND METHODS

Patients and Characteristics

The clinical courses of 119 patients were analyzed for complications secondary to therapy, representing all patients who were prospectively randomized to approved NCI treatment protocols that involved retroperitoneal sarcomas, gastric cancers, or pancreatic cancers. In all protocols, patients received either surgery with IORT or surgery with conventional radiotherapy (Table 1). The IORT and control patient populations had similar surgical procedures performed and were comparable with respect to sex, age, and disease state (Table 2). Three reviewers classified every clinical complication in each patient as to the probable underlying cause: radiation therapy (IORT or conventional), surgery, chemo-

Accepted for publication Nov 29, 1988.

From the Surgery (Drs Cromack, Hoekstra, and Sindelar and Ms Maher) and Radiation Oncology (Dr Kinsella) Branches, National Cancer Institute, National Institutes of Health, Bethesda, Md.

Read before the Annual Meeting of the Society of Surgical Oncology, New Orleans, May 23, 1988.

Reprint requests to Surgery Branch, National Cancer Institute, National Institutes of Health, Bethesda, MD 20892 (Dr Sindelar).

Table 1.—Randomized Treatment Protocols*

Disease Type	Experimental Therapy Arm	Conventional Therapy Arm
Retroperitoneal sarcoma	Surgical excision of lesion + IORT (2000 cGy) to resection bed + EBRT (4500 cGy) to wide field postoperatively	Surgical excision of lesion + EBRT (6000 cGy) to wide field postoperatively
Gastric carcinoma	Gastrectomy + IORT (2000 cGy) to resected bed (all stages)	Gastrectomy (stage I), gastrectomy + EBRT (5000 cGy) postoperatively (stages II-IV)
Pancreatic carcinoma (resected)	Pancreatectomy + IORT (2000 cGy) to resected bed (all stages)	Pancreatectomy (stage I), pancreatectomy + EBRT (5000 cGy) postoperatively (stages II-IV)
Pancreatic carcinoma (unresected)	Gastric + biliary diversion + IORT (2500 cGy) to primary + EBRT (5000 cGy) postoperatively + fluorouracil (500 mg/m²) daily for 3 days in twelve 4-wk cycles	Gastric + biliary diversion + EBRT (6000 cGy) postoperatively in three 2-wk cycles of 2000 cGy + fluorouracil (500 mg/m²) daily for 3 days in twelve 4-wk cycles

*IORT indicates intraoperative radiation therapy; EBRT, external-beam radiotherapy.

Table 2.—Patient Characteristics*

Category	Treatment Group	Pancreas Resected	Retroperitoneal Sarcoma	Gastric Carcinoma	Pancreas Unresected
No. of patients	Control	12	20	21	13
	IORT	10	15	12	16
Sex, M/F	Control	6/6	9/11	15/6	8/5
	IORT	4/6	9/6	2/10	8/8
Age range (median), y	Control	48-76 (57)	22-66 (55)	33-67 (55)	42-66 (58)
	IORT	44-76 (57)	27-62 (45)	35-75 (65)	28-66 (57)
Disease stage†					
I	Control	3	0	3	3
	IORT	0	0	1	0
II	Control	1	4	0	0
	IORT	1	1	0	0
III	Control	4	8	11	4
	IORT	7	4	6	6
IV	Control	4	8	7	6
	IORT	2	10	5	10

*IORT indicates intraoperative radiation therapy.
†Number of patients is given throughout for each disease stage.

therapy, progressive malignant neoplasm, or other factors. The complications due to surgery or radiation therapy are considered in this analysis. Complications were graded by type, severity, frequency, and chronologic occurrence. Every complication episode was recorded throughout the entire clinical course of every patient, so that some patients were scored as having multiple episodes of the same type of complication. Twenty-nine separate types of complications were identified within seven general categories: gastrointestinal, urologic, vascular, neurologic, cardiorespiratory, infectious, and miscellaneous (Table 3). Early complications were defined as those that occurred within 30 days of surgery. Late complications were defined as those that occurred more than 30 days after surgery. Complications that resolved spontaneously or with little medical intervention were assessed as minor. Complications that required active therapy, invasive intervention, or surgery, and those that were life threatening were considered major. Treatment-related mortality was defined as any death that occurred within 65 days of surgery during the initial hospital admission. The lengths of the hospital stays that were required due to primary treatment and radiation-related complications were recorded for all patients, and the percentage of overall survival time spent in the hospital was calculated.

Statistical Methods

Statistical analysis by the χ^2 test was used to compare IORT and control patient populations for the frequency of complications, the overall incidence of complications, treatment-related mortality, and the frequency and incidence of specific types of complications. Fisher's exact test was utilized to compare the incidence of early and late complications and to evaluate complication subgroups by tumor type and method of radiation. Student's t test was used to compare the frequency of complications per patient among the various tumor types and treatment arms. Hospitalization durations were compared using the Wilcoxon rank-sum test.

RESULTS

Patient Groups

One hundred nineteen patients in four randomized studies at the NCI were evaluated for complications that resulted from therapy. Sixty-six patients received conventional therapy and were considered to form the control group. Fifty-three patients received IORT and constituted the experimental group. Tumor types and the distribution of disease stages were similar (Table 2). The median follow-up time was 53 months for the control group and 54 months for the experimental group.

Incidence of Complications

A total of 136 complications developed among 66 patients who received conventional therapy, and 108 complications developed among 53 patients who received IORT (Table 3). No statistically significant differences were present between the control and IORT groups with respect to the overall incidence of complications. No differences in complication incidence were present when each specific tumor type was analyzed independently.

The majority of complications occurred within the gastrointestinal category and included enteritis, bowel obstruction, and hemorrhage (Table 3). Analysis within the

Table 3.—Complications by Tumor Type and Treatment*

	Tumor Type									
	Resected Pancreatic		Retro-peritoneal Sarcoma		Gastric		Unresected Pancreatic		Total	
Complications	**C**	**I**	**C**	**I**	**C**	**I**	**C**	**I**	**C**	**I**
GI										
Fistula	0	1	2	0	4	5	1	0	**7**	**6**
Hemorrhage, GI	2	2	1	0	0	1	2	6	**5**	**9**
Hemorrhage, intra-abdominal	0	1	1	0	1	1	1	0	**3**	**2**
Enteritis-obstruction, mild†	2	0	1	3	1	0	0	3	**4**	**6**
Enteritis-obstruction, surgery‡	0	0	7	2	5	0	2	1	**14**	**3**
Nutritional	2	1	0	0	3	1	0	1	**5**	**3**
Stricture	0	0	0	1	2	4	0	0	**2**	**5**
Other major	4	0	2	3	3	4	1	3	**10**	**10**
Other minor	4	4	1	0	4	1	4	2	**13**	**7**
Subtotal	**14**	**9**	**15**	**9**	**23**	**17**	**11**	**16**	**63**	**51**
Infectious										
Wound infection	1	0	3	0	1	0	0	0	**5**	**0**
Intra-abdominal abscess	4	4	4	0	5	5	1	2	**14**	**11**
Sepsis	2	5	6	0	4	5	2	2	**14**	**12**
Subtotal	**7**	**9**	**13**	**0**	**10**	**10**	**3**	**4**	**33**	**23**
Urologic										
Ureteral obstruction	0	1	1	2	2	0	0	0	**3**	**3**
Other	0	1	1	1	2	0	0	0	**3**	**2**
Subtotal	**0**	**2**	**2**	**3**	**4**	**0**	**0**	**0**	**6**	**5**
Vascular										
Ischemia, occlusion	1	1	2	1	0	0	2	0	**5**	**2**
Coagulopathy	1	2	0	0	0	0	0	0	**1**	**2**
Pericarditis	0	0	0	0	2	0	0	0	**2**	**0**
Other	0	0	0	1	2	3	0	0	**2**	**4**
Subtotal	**2**	**3**	**2**	**2**	**4**	**3**	**2**	**0**	**10**	**8**
Neurologic										
Neuropathy, early	1	0	4	4	0	0	1	0	**6**	**4**
Neuropathy, late	0	0	5	8	0	0	0	0	**5**	**8**
Stroke	0	0	0	1	0	0	0	0	**0**	**1**
Subtotal	**1**	**0**	**9**	**13**	**0**	**0**	**1**	**0**	**11**	**13**
Cardiorespiratory										
Myocardial infarction	0	0	0	0	0	1	0	0	**0**	**1**
Pulmonary embolus	0	1	1	1	1	0	1	1	**3**	**3**
T-E fistula	0	0	0	0	2	0	0	0	**2**	**0**
Pneumonia	1	0	0	0	2	0	0	1	**3**	**1**
Subtotal	**1**	**1**	**1**	**1**	**5**	**1**	**1**	**2**	**8**	**5**
Miscellaneous										
Technical problem	0	1	1	0	1	0	0	0	**2**	**1**
Osteoradionecrosis	0	0	0	1	0	0	0	0	**0**	**1**
Radiation dermatitis	0	0	0	1	0	0	0	0	**0**	**1**
Other	0	0	3	0	0	0	0	0	**3**	**0**
Subtotal	**0**	**1**	**4**	**2**	**1**	**0**	**0**	**0**	**5**	**3**
Cumulative total	**25**	**25**	**46**	**30**	**47**	**31**	**18**	**22**	**136**	**108**

*C indicates control; I, intraoperative radiation therapy; GI, gastrointestinal; and T-E, tracheoesophageal.
†Resolved by conservative therapy.
‡Required surgical intervention.

categories of gastrointestinal, urologic, vascular, neurologic, cardiorespiratory, infectious, and miscellaneous revealed no overall differences in the incidence of complications between the control and IORT patient groups (Table 3 and Figure). However, analysis of complications within each tumor type revealed one area of significant difference (Figure): There was a greater incidence of sepsis among patients with retroperitoneal sarcomas who received conventional therapy compared with patients with retroperitoneal sarcoma patients who received IORT.

Complication Episodes

Nine patients (17%) who received IORT and 15 patients (23%) who received conventional therapy had no compli-

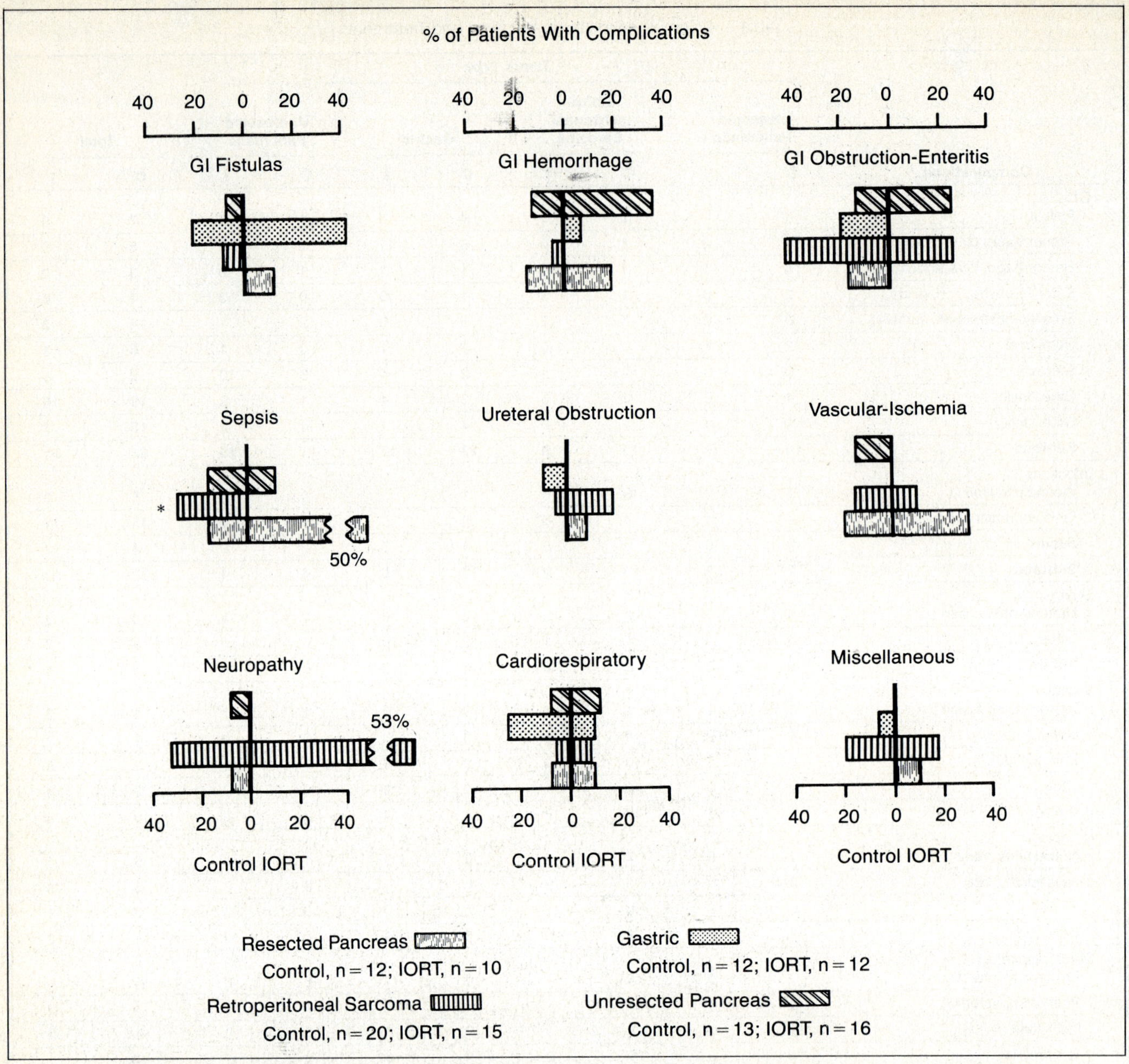

Incidence is reported as percentage of patients developing indicated complication in each tumor type. Statistical comparison of controls and patients who received intraoperative radiation therapy (IORT) by Fisher's exact test is shown. Significant values ($P<.05$) are indicated by asterisk. GI denotes gastrointestinal.

cation episodes at any time, while 44 IORT patients and 51 control patients suffered one or more complication episodes after therapy. The maximum episodes in a single patient was 17 for the control group and 12 for the IORT cohort. Repeated episodes of intra-abdominal or gastrointestinal bleeding and life-threatening sepsis in the immediate postoperative period accounted for more than 50% of the complication episodes, resulting in 54 operative interventions for the treatment of complications and, ultimately, in ten of the 11 postoperative deaths.

Comparison of IORT and control patient groups revealed no significant differences in the overall numbers of complication episodes and no differences in the numbers of episodes grouped according to complication category. Analysis by tumor type revealed no area of significant difference between IORT and control patients.

Mortality

Overall treatment-related mortality among the treatment groups and tumor types did not differ significantly. There were five deaths among the control patients and seven deaths among the IORT patients (Table 4).

Early and Late Complications

Early and late complications occurred in similar overall frequency in both the IORT and control treatment groups. Early complications comprised 58% of the total control group complication episodes and 47% for the IORT group episodes. Late complications comprised 42% of all control group complication episodes and 53% of all IORT episodes.

Table 4.—Mortality by Treatment Group and Tumor Type*						
Tumor Type	**Pancreas Resected**	**Retroperitoneal Sarcoma**	**Gastric Carcinoma**	**Pancreas Unresected**	**Total**	***P***
Control	1	2	0	2	5	NS
IORT	4	1	1	1	7	NS

*NS indicates not significant; IORT, intraoperative radiation therapy.

Table 5.—Proportion of Overall Survival Time Spent in Hospital*			
Overall Survival Time, mo	**Overall Survival, %**		
	Control	**IORT**	***P***
<6	15.4	39.7	NS
6-12	16.7	24.5	NS
12-24	10.7	13.8	NS
>24	5.5	4.8	NS
Total	11.0	17.7	NS

*Postoperative deaths are excluded. IORT indicates intraoperative radiation therapy; NS, not significant.

Hospitalization due to Complications

The total durations of hospitalization time due to complications or related treatment were similar for both IORT and control treatments, as measured by the percentage of time spent in the hospital adjusted for overall survival (Table 5). Hospitalization time for all control patients averaged 11% of overall survival and averaged 18% for IORT patients.

COMMENT

Intraoperative radiation therapy, while first utilized as early as 1909, gained increased acceptance during the late 1970s after the development of high-energy linear accelerators and initial clinical trials.[1,5] Presently, IORT remains an experimental therapy utilized at several cancer centers to achieve local-regional control of various intra-abdominal malignant neoplasms. Limited information is available for an accurate assessment of the risk of complications due to IORT. Published results of IORT trials have recognized certain treatment-related complications. A report from the Massachusetts General Hospital, Boston, compared historical controls who had colorectal cancer with IORT-treated patients and found no increase in complication rates resulting from the experimental therapy.[6] However, no prospective comparisons of complications between conventional radiotherapy and IORT have been published.

The IORT-related complications recognized by previous authors have included gastrointestinal bleeding,[7,8] intestinal obstruction,[9] infectious complications,[10] and peripheral neuropathies.[11] Similar types of complications occurred in the prospective randomized NCI trials, reviewed here, that compared IORT with conventional radiotherapy in the treatment of retroperitoneal sarcomas, gastric adenocarcinomas, and resected and unresected pancreatic cancers. Importantly, no significant differences in complication rates emerged between IORT and control groups when analyzed by type of radiation therapy, functional category, or type of tumor. Consequently, an equivalent complication risk exists between IORT and conventional radiotherapy in the treatment of intra-abdominal malignant neoplasms. Oncologists can recommend experimental IORT when clinically indicated without subjecting patients to an increased risk of complication, compared with conventional radiotherapy.

Early in the development of IORT, there were theoretical concerns of the possibility of increased infectious complications in IORT due to technical manipulations (transportation of patients under anesthesia between operating and radiotherapy suites) and the temporary placement of foreign bodies within the abdominal cavity (IORT applicators, shielding, and tissue retractors). Such concerns have been proved to be unfounded based on the data in the current study. The incidence of infectious complications was similar in both IORT and conventional radiotherapy groups. Separate analysis by tumor type actually revealed an excess of infectious complications among the conventional-treated patients with retroperitoneal sarcomas.

Analysis of specific tumor types revealed findings that appeared to correlate with previously described IORT-associated complications. Kinsella et al[11] reported late-appearing peripheral neuropathies both in an experimental IORT model in dogs and in patients who received IORT for retroperitoneal or pelvic tumors. While the current results failed to show a statistically significant overall difference between conventional radiotherapy and IORT, there was a tendency toward increased late peripheral neuropathies in patients with retroperitoneal sarcomas who received IORT. As was demonstrated in experimental animal models, IORT applied to the area of lumbar or sacral plexus can produce demyelination and peripheral neuropathy, a phenomenon that was dose related.[11] Limited patient survival due to tumor recurrence may have prevented the appearance of a higher rate of late peripheral neuropathy among the patient group with retroperitoneal sarcomas at the NCI.

Upper gastrointestinal tract bleeding associated with IORT for pancreatic cancers has been reported.[7] Current NCI results have demonstrated a tendency toward an increased gastrointestinal bleeding after IORT in patients with unresectable pancreatic carcinoma. Hemorrhage typically occurred four to six months after treatment and was due to ischemic necrosis of the mucosa on the medial duodenal wall, an area routinely included in IORT portals to encompass tumor masses in the head of the pancreas.[8,12] In all patients who experienced duodenal hemorrhage, the bleeding episodes were self-limiting and ceased after the denuded duodenal wall healed with scar formation six or more months after therapy. This complication may be an expected complication of IORT applied to unresected pancreatic cancer and appears to occur in 20% to 30% of treated patients who survive six or more months.

Enteritis and associated bowel obstruction are recognized complications of wide-field, high-dose, external-beam abdominal radiation therapy, occurring in up to 25% of patients.[13] A theoretical advantage to IORT is a lessening of intestinal exposure to radiation dose and a consequent reduction of the risk of late radiation-related enteritis and associated bowel obstruction. This theoretical advantage for IORT may be validated by the current study, since a lower incidence of enteritis was observed in those patients who received IORT for resected pancreatic cancer and for gastric carcinoma (both trends bordering on significance).

Intraoperative radiation therapy did not increase the overall risk of complications or overall mortality among patients in the NCI prospectively randomized trials. Therefore, it appears that IORT can be used for treatment, where clinically indicated, without exposing patients to an increased risk of treatment-related complications. The small number of patients and the high overall complication rate could mask small differences between control and experimental groups. Comparison of radiated and nonradiated patients in a prospective trial would be of interest in determining the risk added to surgery by radiotherapy in general.

Although IORT may increase the risk of duodenal hemorrhage and peripheral neuropathy in certain circumstances, IORT does appear to enable the delivery of high radiation doses to large abdominal fields with a lower incidence of long-term intestinal complications. This report of complications developing during randomized clinical trials demonstrates the relative safety of IORT and supports continued investigation into its clinical role as a cancer treament.

The authors thank Seth Steinberg, PhD, Rosalie Smith, RN, and Donald White, MS, for their help in the preparation of this manuscript.

References

1. Kinsella TJ, Glatstein E, Sindelar WF: Intraoperative radiotherapy. *Hosp Pract Off* 1985;20:125-141.

2. Kinsella T, Sindelar W, Glatstein E, et al: Preliminary results of a prospective randomized trial of intraoperative (IORT) and low dose external beam radiotherapy vs high dose external beam radiotherapy as adjunctive therapy in resectable soft tissue sarcomas of the retroperitoneum, abstracted. *Int J Radiat Oncol Biol Phys* 1986;12(suppl 1):183.

3. Sindelar WF, Kinsella TJ: Randomized trial of intraoperative radiotherapy in unresected carcinoma of the pancreas, abstracted. *Int J Radiat Oncol Biol Phys* 1986;12(suppl 1):148.

4. Sindelar WF, Kinsella TJ: Randomized trial of intraoperative radiotherapy in unresected carcinoma of the pancreas, abstracted. *Int J Radiat Oncol Biol Phys* 1986;12(suppl 1):148-149.

5. Gunderson LL, Tepper JE, Briggs PJ, et al: Intraoperative ± external beam irradiation. *Curr Probl Cancer* 1983;7:1-69.

6. Tepper JE, Gunderson LL, Orlow EL, et al: Complications of intraoperative radiation therapy. *Int J Radiat Oncol Biol Phys* 1984;10:1831-1839.

7. Goldson AL, Ashaveri E, Espinoza MC, et al: Single dose electrons for advance stage pancreatic cancer: Phase 1 pilot study. *Int J Radiat Oncol Biol Phys* 1981;7:869-874.

8. Sindelar WF, Kinsella TJ, Hoekstra H, et al: Duodenal hemorrhage as a complication of intraoperative radiotherapy for unresectable carcinoma of the pancreas, abstracted. *Proc Am Soc Clin Oncol* 1985;4:277.

9. Sindelar WF, Kinsella TJ, Tepper JE, et al: Experimental and clinical studies with intraoperative radiotherapy. *Surg Gynecol Obstet* 1983;157:205-219.

10. Shipley WU, Wood WC, Tepper JE, et al: Intraoperative electron beam irradiation for patients with unresectable pancreatic carcinoma. *Ann Surg* 1984;200:289-296.

11. Kinsella TJ, Sindelar WF, DeLuca AM, et al: Tolerance of peripheral nerve to intraoperative radiotherapy (IORT): Clinical and experimental studies. *Int J Radiat Oncol Biol Phys* 1985;11:1579-1585.

12. Sindelar WF, Hoekstra H, Kinsella TJ: Surgical approaches and techniques in intraoperative radiotherapy for intra-abdominal, retroperitoneal, and pelvic neoplasms. *Surgery* 1988;103:247-256.

13. Glenn J, Sindelar WF, Kinsella TJ, et al: Results of multimodality therapy of resectable soft-tissue sarcomas of the retroperitoneum. *Surgery* 1985;97:316-325.

Discussion

Q I recently reviewed the series of the radiation therapy oncology group. We have almost 200 cases, and our data are very similar to what you presented with regard to the complication rate. Most of the institutions that are participating are transporting patients. I know you transported patients early on in your studies. How many of your patients were transferred vs how many were treated in your dedicated unit?

A The breakdown is approximately 40% of patients were transported, and approximately 55% to 60% of patients were treated in the dedicated unit. We found that the actual incidence of complications, which were all wound infections, between the two groups were virtually identical. We are not sure whether we can attribute that to the transport problem or just to the overall technique and attention to detail.

Q Are there ongoing controlled trials of IORT? Can you separate radiation from surgical complications?

A Initially, there were four separate clinical trials, looking at IORT vs the external-beam radiation therapy arm. Several of the trials are ongoing and continue to accumulate patients. Regarding the second point of your question, we felt that it would be very difficult to try to distinguish between those complications that were solely related to the surgical treatment and those related to radiation. Some would be very easy to break out, and some were in the overlap area. We felt that since radiation therapy, given at the time of surgery, involves additional manipulation of the surgically exposed tumors, we should examine the complications of both the surgery and the radiation treatment. As far as the overall incidence of complications, as compared with that reported in the literature, again we tried to be very meticulous about those complications that we classified as complications vs what we would routinely expect in a normal patient. I believe our data correlate well with other reported literature, as far as the incidence of complications in treated patients who did not receive radiation therapy.

The Influence of Natural Killer Cells in Neuroblastoma

John V. Reynolds, FRCS(I); Jian Shou, MD; Hoon Choi, MD; Robert Sigal, MD; Moritz M. Ziegler, MD; John M. Daly, MD

• Human neuroblastoma (NRB) cell lines are markedly sensitive to natural killer (NK) cell lysis in vitro, but patients with NRBs have low or absent NK activity. This study evaluated the NK sensitivity of murine NRBs (C1300 and TBJ) in the regulation of NRB growth and determined the effects of recombinant (r) interferon gamma and recombinant interleukin 2 (rIL-2). Both basal (8% ± 3% specific cytotoxicity) and induced (20% ± 3%) NK lyses of C1300-NRB were observed. In vivo depletion of NK cells with anti–asialo GM-1 significantly enhanced growth of C1300-NRB and deceased survival. Treatment wth r–interferon gamma or rIL-2 on days 1 through 3 after C1300-NRB inoculation significantly prolonged the mean tumor latency period, decreased the tumor growth rate, and enhanced in vitro NK killing of C1300-NRB and YAC-1. The effects of r–interferon gamma and IL-2 were abrogated by pretreatment with anti–asialo GM-1. These results demonstrated that NK cells form one important component of regulation of a murine NRB, but immunomodulation with potent lymphokines requires cooperation of more than one cell type.

(*Arch Surg* 1989;124:235-239)

Neuroblastoma (NRB), first described by Virchow[1] in 1865, represents the most common extracranial solid tumor seen in childhood. Despite multimodality therapy, including surgery, radiotherapy, chemotherapy, and bone marrow transplantation, the overall three-year survival remains at 35%.[2]

Neuroblastoma may be influenced by immunologic mechanisms since spontaneous regression of tumor has been observed.[3-5] Cytotoxic lymphocytes, humoral responses, and tumor-induced "blocking" antibodies have also been demonstrated in patients with NRB, although their prognostic significance is unclear.[6]

Recently, Lampson et al[7] and Main et al[8] characterized human NRB cell lines in terms of both HLA-A, HLA-B, and HLA-C (class 1 major histocompatibility complex [MHC]–encoded antigens) expression and sensitivity to cytotoxic effector mechanisms. Human NRB cell lines lack significant class 1 antigens, but these can be readily induced by interferon gamma.[9] This implies that class 1 MHC-restricted cytotoxic T-cell (CTL) killing of NRB is unlikely to be significant in vivo unless class 1 antigens are upregulated by endogenous or exogenous interferon gamma. Immunologic manipulation, based on upregulating natural killer (NK) function, modulating class 1 MHC expression, or combinations of both, may have therapeutic application. Recombinant interleukin 2 (rIL-2) and recombinant (r) interferon gamma are potent activators of NK cells that have the capacity to modulate class 1 expression.[10-12]

Natural killer cells represent a subpopulation of lymphocytes that mediate non-MHC-restricted killing of certain target and tumor cells.[13,14] Natural killer cells have been demonstrated to modulate the development of primary tumors and to control the development of metastases.[15,16] Phenotypically, NK cells are Thy-1.2$^-$ and Lyt-2$^-$ but express the surface antigen, asialo GM-1.[17] The CTLs are phenotypically Thy-1.2$^+$ and Lyt-2$^+$ and may express asialo GM-1 to a variable degree.[18] In vivo depletion of NK cells by treatment with antiserum to asialo GM-1 has been demonstrated to facilitate local tumor growth and metastases.[19,20]

This study was designed to determine whether NK cells have a regulatory role in murine NRBs. Both in vivo depletion and in vivo activation experimental regimens were used to modulate NK function at a period when NK resistance to tumor growth might be most critical.[21] The overall objective of the study was to determine whether a suitable animal model of NRB exists, comparable with human NRB, so that immunotherapeutic modalities of treatment with potential clinical application may be fully evaluated.

MATERIALS AND METHODS

Mice

Six-week-old male A/J (H-2^a), CBA/J (H-2^h), CFW (H-2^k), and DBA/2 (H-2^d) strain mice were obtained from the Jackson Laboratory, Bar Harbor, Me.

Tumors

The C1300-NRB arose from the spinal cord region of A strain mice in 1940, and it has been maintained by serial in vivo and in vitro passage ever since. The TBJ-NRB is a clonal variant of C1300-NRB with markedly reduced immunogenicity. The antigenic characteristics of both tumors have been previously described.[22] The P815, syngeneic to strain DBA/2, and the YAC-1 lymphoma of A/Sn origin were maintained in continuous in vitro culture.

Medium

Unless otherwise stated, all assays were performed in complete medium (CM), which consisted of RPMI 1640 supplemented with 10% heat-inactivated fetal calf serum, antibiotics (100 mg/L of penicillin and 100 U/mL of streptomycin), 2-mmol/L L-glutamine, and 5×10^{-5} 2-mercaptoethanol.

Reagents

Human rIL-2 was generously provided by a commercial manufacturer (Hoffmann-LaRoche Inc, Nutley, NJ). Murine interferon gamma was used. Polyriboinosinic:polyribocytidylic acid (Poly IC) was purchased commercially (Sigma Chemical Co, St Louis).

Preparation of Single Cell Suspensions

Single cell suspensions of spleen were prepared by mechanical disruption, followed by filtration through nylon mesh (Nytex, Tetko, Elmsford, NY). Cells were washed twice in RPMI 1640 and resuspended in CM.

Cytotoxicity Assays

Cytotoxicity to tumor targets was assessed using chromium 51–release assays. Labeling was performed by incubation of a $\times 10^7$ viable target (C1300, TBJ, YAC, and P815) cells with 150-µL of sodium chromate 51 (2 mCi/mL, New England Nuclear, Boston) for 90 minutes. The assay was performed in V-bottomed microwells by adding serial dilutions of effector cells to 1×10^4 ^{51}Cr-labeled target cells in a total volume of 200-µL CM. The plates were centrifuged (800 revolutions per minute for five minutes) at the beginning of the assay, incubated at 37°C for four or 18 hours, and centrifuged again (1200 revolutions per minute for ten minutes). A volume of 100 µL was removed from each well for gamma counting. Percent-specific ^{51}Cr release was computed according to the formula: $(E - S)/(M - S) \times 100\%$, where E is the ^{51}Cr release in the presence of effector cells, S is the spontaneous ^{51}Cr release in the presence of the medium, and M is the maximum

Accepted for publication Oct 12, 1988.

From the Departments of Surgery, The Harrison Department of Surgical Research (Drs Reynolds, Shou, Sigal, and Daly) and the University of Pennsylvania School of Medicine, Philadelphia, and the Joseph Stokes, Jr, Research Institute, The Children's Hospital of Philadelphia (Drs Choi and Ziegler).

Read before the Annual Meeting of the Society of Surgical Oncology, New Orleans, May 24, 1988.

Reprint requests to Division of Surgical Oncology, Department of Surgery, Hospital of the University of Pennsylvania, 3400 Spruce St, Philadelphia, PA 19104 (Dr Daly).

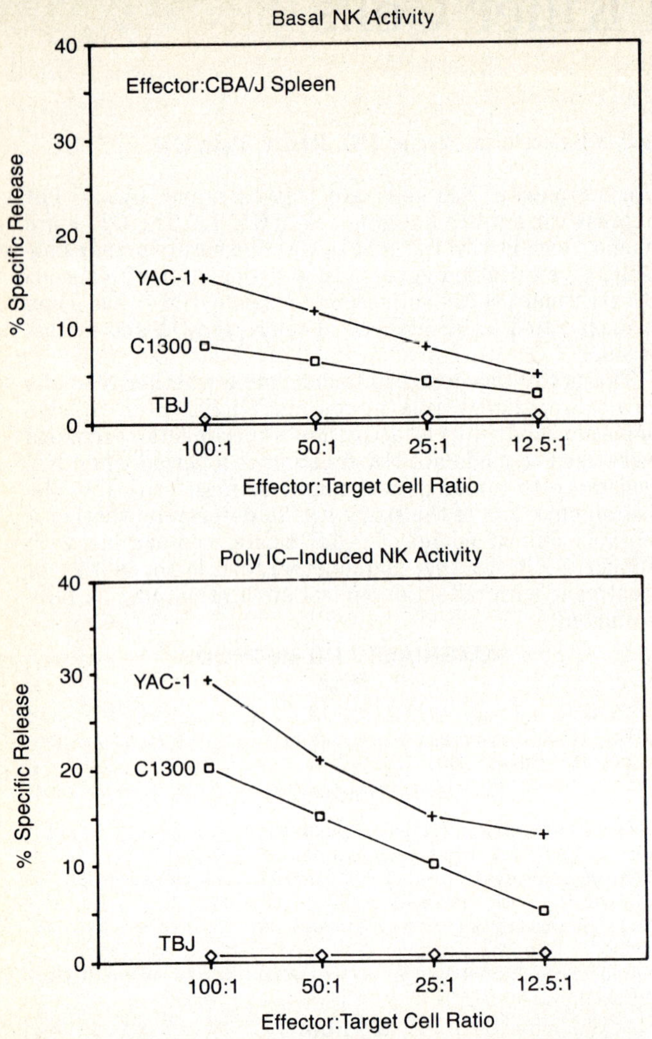

Fig 1.—Ability of strain CBA/J spleen cells to lyse C1300-neuroblastoma (NRB), TBJ-NRB, and YAC-1 in standard four-hour chromium 51–release assay using either fresh spleen cells or spleen cells from mice injected with polyriboinosinic:polyribocytidylic acid (Poly IC) (100 μg intraperitoneally) 16 to 24 hours previously. Results represent mean of eight experiments; SDs ranged from 2% to 5%. NK indicates natural killer.

release obtained by the addition of the targets to an equal volume of 1% Triton X-100. The results are expressed as the mean percent lysis of triplicate experiments.

Generation of Lymphokine-Activated Killer (LAK) Cells

The LAK cells were prepared by incubating erythrocyte-free spleen cells at a concentration of 5×10^6/mL in 8-mL CM that contained 200 U/mL of rIL-2 in 25-cm^3 tissue culture flasks. After three days of incubation at 37°C with 5% carbon dioxide, cells were harvested and were tested for lytic activity against P815, YAC, and C1300-NRB in four-hour ^{51}Cr-release assays as described above.

Generation of Allogeneic CTL

The CTLs were generated by coincubating responder strain A/J splenocytes (4×10^6/mL) with x-irradiated (20 Gy) strain DBA/2 stimulator spleen cells (2×10^6/mL) in a total volume of 8 mL. The resultant CTLs were tested against P815 in a four-hour ^{51}Cr-release assay as described above.

In Vivo Treatment With Monoclonal Antibodies or Antiserum

Anti–asialo GM-1 (Wako Chemicals, Dallas) was diluted 1/20 in phosphate-buffered saline (PBS) and filtered through a 0.22 μm filter (Millipore) (0.22 μm) before intravenous (IV) injection (0.4 mL per mouse). Injection of pooled normal rat serum served as a control. Purified anti–Lyt-2 (derived from hybridoma 2.43) was obtained commercially (Becton Dickinson, Sunnyvale, Calif), and 50 μg was injected IV in a total volume of 0.4 mL. Injection of rat IgG served as a control. These doses of antibody have previously been demonstrated to deplete specific target cells in vivo.[23,24]

Fluoresence-Activated Cell Sorter Analysis

The fluorescein isothiocyanate (FITC)–labeled anti–Lyt-2 and phycoerythrocin-labeled anti-L3T4 were purchased commercially (Becton Dickinson). The corresponding second reagent to anti–asialo GM-1, FITC goat anti–rabbit IgG (ab′)2, was a gift. For staining, 10^6 cells were incubated with an appropriate concentration of primary antibody diluted in PBS that contained 2% fetal bovine serum and 0.1% sodium azide for 45 minutes at 4°C. They were then washed thoroughly and incubated with an excess of FITC-labeled second antibody for 30 minutes. Analysis of 50 000 cells per sample was performed on fluorescence-activated cell sorter microfluorometer (Ortho Cytofluorograf, Ortho Diagnostic Systems Inc, Raritan, NJ).

Experimental Protocol

Tumor (C1300-NRB or TBJ-NRB) was injected subcutaneously (1×10^6) on day 0. For in vivo depletion, ASGM-1 or Lyt-2 was injected on day 1 (in some experiments, injections were repeated every five days). On days 1 through 3, mice received rIL-2 (10^5 U intraperitoneally [ip] three times per day), r-interferon gamma (10^5 U/ip), Poly IC (100 μg ip), or PBS; all injections were administered in a total volume of 0.4 mL. The tumor incidence and latency period were recorded, and the tumor volume (major axis × minor axis) was measured every three days. On day 21, mice were killed by carbon dioxide insufflation, and the tumor weight was measured. In representative mice in each group, the liver and lung were examined for metastases as described by Wexler.[25]

Statistics

Statistical significance was determined by a two-tailed Student's t test.

RESULTS

Susceptibility to Lysis by NK Cells

As shown in Fig 1, the sensitivity of C1300-NRB, TBJ-NRB, and YAC-1 (positive control) to lysis by fresh and Poly IC (100 μg ip, 16 to 24 hours before the mice were killed) induced spleen cells from a number of strains of mice was determined. Natural cytotoxicity was manifest against C1300-NRB, which was enhanced with Poly IC pretreatment. However, no cytotoxicity, basal or induced, was manifest against TBJ-NRB.

Efficacy of In Vivo Depletion of NK (Anti–Asialo GM-1) and CTL (Lyt-2) Cells

Strain A mice (n = 6 per group) were injected IV with anti–asialo GM-1, anti–Lyt-2, or control normal rabbit serum and rat IgG, respectively. Three days after injection, fresh spleen cells were phenotypically analyzed for Thy-1.2, L3T4, Lyt-2, and asialo GM-1 and assessed for NK activity, CTL activity, and the potential to generate LAK cells. As shown in Table 1, anti–asialo GM-1 treatment markedly abrogated NK killing and significantly reduced LAK generation but did not alter CTL development. Anti–Lyt-2 treatment did not affect NK or LAK mechanisms but significantly decreased CTL development.

Effect of In Vivo Depletion of NK Cells or CTLs

Mice were pretreated before tumor inoculation (10^6 cells subcutaneously), and depletion was maintained by repeated IV injections (anti–asialo GM-1 every five days and anti–Lyt-2 every seven days). As shown in Table 2, in mice bearing C1300-NRB, the mean tumor weight was significantly (P<.001) increased by in vivo depletion with either anti–asialo GM-1 or anti–Lyt-2, compared with controls. The percentage mortality by day 21 was 4.5% for control mice, 45% for anti–asialo GM-1–treated mice, and 37.5% for anti–Lyt-2–treated mice. The effects of in vivo depletion with these antibodies in mice bearing TBJ-NRB were less

Table 1.—Anti–Asialo GM-1 and Anti–Lyt-2 Treatment Efficacy*

Treatment	Lysis (Effector-Target Ratio 100:1): NK† Cells	LAK‡ Cells	CTLs§	Spleen Cell Phenotype: Thy-1.2‖ Cells	Anti–Asialo GM-1‖ Cells	Lyt-2‖ Cells
NRS¶	12	68	52	53	9.7	17.3
Anti–Asialo GM-1¶	0	29	50	51	2.5	15.5
Anti–Lyt-2¶	10	63	24	53	8.7	5.1

*Data represents the mean of three separate experiments; SD range, 2% to 10%. NK indicates natural killer; LAK, lymphokine-activated killer; CTLs, cytotoxic T lymphocytes; and NRS, normal rabbit serum.
†Percent lysis of YAC-1 by fresh spleen cells in a four-hour chromium 51–release assay.
‡LAK cells were generated by three-day culture in complete medium containing 200 U/mL of recombinant interleukin 2, and cytotoxicity to P815 was determined in a four-hour ^{51}Cr-release assay.
§CTLs were generated by coincubation of spleen cells from treated animals with x-irradiated DBA/2 spleen cells for five days, and cytotoxicity was determined in a four-hour chromium 51–release assay.
‖Percentage-positive antibody staining determined by fluorescein isothiocyanate–indirect immunofluorescence and quantitated by fluorescence-activated cell sorter analysis.
¶Anti–asialo GM-1 (0.4 mL) (diluted 1:20), anti–Lyt-2 (50 μg), or normal rabbit serum was injected intravenously in strain A/J mice (n = 8 per group), and assays were performed three days after the injection.

Table 2.—Incidence, Mortality, and Tumor WT Effects on Day 21 in Mice Bearing C1300-NRB and TBJ-NRB*

	C1300-NRB: Incidence	Mortality	Tumor WT	TBJ-NRB: Incidence	Mortality	Tumor WT
NRS†	22/22	1/22	2.4 ± 1.3‡	12/12	6/12	4.2 ± 1.3
Anti-asialo GM-1†	22/22	10/22	4.8 ± 0.9	12/12	7/12	4.9 ± 1.6
Anti–Lyt-2†	16/16	6/16	4.0 ± 0.2	12/12	7/12	4.8 ± 0.6

*NRB indicates neuroblastoma; WT, weight; and NRS, normal rabbit serum. Weight is given in grams as mean ± SD.
†Anti–asialo GM-1, anti–Lyt-1, anti–Lyt-2, or NRS was injected (0.4 mL) before tumor inoculation and repeated every five days (anti–asialo GM-1 and NRS) and every seven days (anti–Lyt-2).
‡$P < .001$, compared with both treatment groups.

dramatic, with a 14% increase in tumor weight in both treatment groups observed on day 21.

Efficacy of In Vivo Activation of NK With rIL-2 and Recombinant (r)–Interferon Gamma

Mice (strains CFW and A/J, n = 6 per group) were treated for three days with PBS (control), rIL-2 (10^5 U three times per day), or r-interferon gamma (10^5 U daily). On day 4, cytotoxicity of fresh spleen cells was tested against YAC-1, C1300-NRB, and P815 (NK-insensitive but LAK-sensitive control). As shown in Fig 2, the enhanced cytotoxic effect was more marked in rIL-2–treated mice than with r–interferon gamma treatment. These results were similar using YAC-1. No lysis of P815 was observed in any group. Basal NK killing was greater in strain CFW mice than in strain A/J mice, but r–interferon gamma– and rIL-2–induced killing was comparable in both groups (data not shown).

Antitumor Effect of rIL-2 and r–Interferon Gamma

The strain A/J mice (n = 10 per group) were injected with 10^6 cells subcutaneously on day 0 and received either PBS, r–interferon gamma, or rIL-2 from days 1 through 3. As shown in Fig 3, the tumor incidence on day 21 decreased from 100% in control mice to 80% in rIL-2–treated mice and to 50% in mice treated with r–interferon gamma. The mean latency period increased from seven days in control mice to 11 days in rIL-2–treated mice and to 14 days in r–interferon gamma–treated mice. There was a 64% reduction in the mean tumor weight on day 21 in rIL-2–treated mice (1.5 g) and a 78% reduction in tumor weight in r–interferon gamma–treated mice (1.2 g), compared with control mice (3.9 g).

Effect of In Vivo Depletion With Anti–Asialo GM-1

The strain A/J mice (n = 6 per group) were injected IV with anti–asialo GM-1, anti–Lyt-2, or normal rabbit serum one day before commencing on a three-day course of treatment with rIL-2, r–interferon gamma, or control PBS

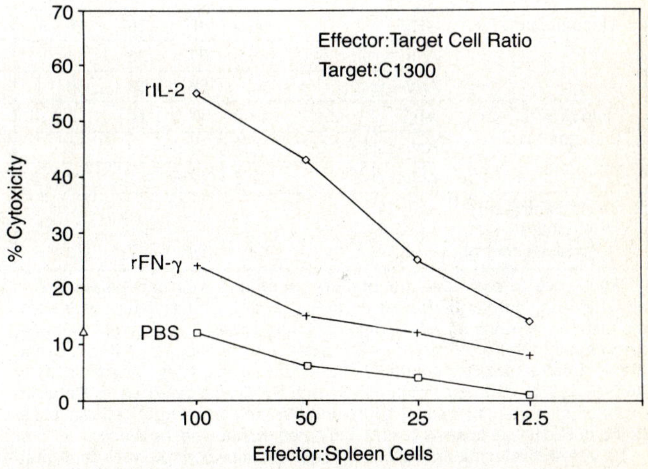

Fig 2.—Augmentation of cytotoxicity to C1300-neuroblastoma (NRB) in treated mice. Strain A/J mice (n = 6 per group) were injected intraperitoneally with either recombinant interleukin 2 (rIL-2) (10^5 U three times per day) recombinant interferon gamma (rIFN-γ) (10^5 U daily), or phosphate-buffered saline (PBS) in volume of 0.4 mL for three days. On day 4, lysis of C1300-NRB was measured in a four-hour chromium 51–release assay. Similar observations were made using YAC-1 as targets. No killing of P815 was observed.

in doses utilized above. Cytotoxicity of fresh spleen cells was determined on day 4 against YAC-1, C1300-NRB, and P815 as before. The results are shown in Table 3. Pretreatment with anti–asialo GM-1 completely abrogated the effect of r–interferon gamma on NK activity. Surprisingly, however, anti–asialo GM-1 pretreatment did not abrogate the marked cytotoxic activity of spleen cells of rIL-2–treated mice.

In a subsequent experiment, the strain A/J mice were pretreated with specific monoclonal antibody one day before inoculation with C1300 and were randomized to

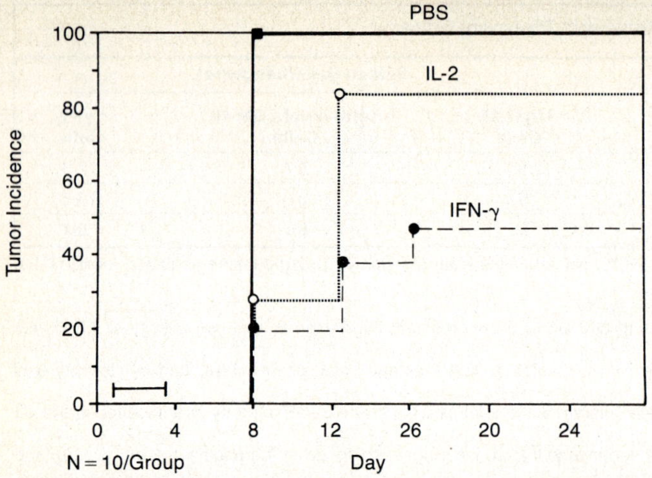

Fig 3.—Tumor incidence at day 21 decreased from 100% in phosphate-buffered saline (PBS)–treated animals to 50% in animals treated with recombinant interferon gamma (IFN-γ) IL-2 indicates interleukin 2.

Table 4.—Tumor Incidence and Weight Results on Day 21 in Strain A/J Mice*

Treatment	mAb	n	Tumor Incidence, %	Tumor Weight, g†
PBS	NRS	8	100	3.9 ± 0.5
	Anti–asialo GM-1	6	100	4.8 ± 1.3
	Anti–Lyt-2	5	100	4.7 ± 2.2
Recombinant IL-2	NRS	8	80	1.5 ± 0.8
	Anti–asialo GM-1	14	100	4.5 ± 1.8
	Anti–Lyt-2	8	100	5.0 ± 1.3
Interferon gamma	NRS	10	50	1.2 ± 1.1
	Anti–asialo GM-1	6	100	5.2 ± 3.7
	Anti–Lyt-2	7	58	6.8 ± 2.7

*Strain A/J mice were injected intravenously with anti–asialo GM-1, anti–Lyt-2, or normal rabbit serum (NRS) one day before subcutaneous inoculation with C1300–neuroblastoma (day 0). Mice were treated with recombinant interleukin 2 (IL-2) (10^5 U three times per day), recombinant interferon gamma (10^5 U daily), or phosphate-buffered saline (PBS) from days 1 through 3.

†Mean ± SD tumor weight.

Table 3.—Cytotoxic Results With mAb, YAC-1, and C1300-NRB*

		YAC-1		C1300-NRB	
Treatment	mAb	100:1	50:1	100:1	50:1
PBS	NRS	7.5	2.3	4.5	1.5
	Anti–asialo GM-1	1.5	0	0	0
	Anti–Lyt-2	7.9	4.5	5.5	2.5
Recombinant IL-2	NRS	55.3	48	28	16
	Anti–asialo GM-1	50.5	37	25	14
	Anti–Lyt-2	81.1	64	59	55
Interferon gamma	NRS	27.2	17	14	8
	Anti–asialo GM-1	2.2	0.5	0	0
	Anti–Lyt-2	26.3	17.5	12	7.5
In vitro activated NK cells† (positive control)	. . .	69	59	57	30

*Mice (five to eight per group) were pretreated with anti–asialo GM-1, anti–Lyt-2, or normal rabbit serum (NRS) and, 24 hours later, were commenced on a regimen of recombinant interleukin 2 (IL-2) (10^5 U tds), recombinant interferon gamma (10^5 U daily), or phosphate-buffered saline (PBS). Treatment was continued for three days, and on day 4, cytotoxicity to YAC-1, C1300–neuroblastoma (NRB), and P815 was determined. Data are expressed as percent lysis at 100:1 and 50:1 effector–target cell ratios. No killing of P815 was observed. mAb indicates monoclonal antibody.

†In vitro activated natural killer (NK) cells (positive control) were generated by incubating spleen cells in complete medium containing 200 U/mL of recombinant IL-2 for 48 hours.

regimens with rIL-2 or r–interferon gamma. Table 4 indicates the results in terms of tumor incidence and tumor weight on day 21. Either anti–asialo GM-1 or anti–Lyt-2 pretreatment completely abrogated the antitumor effect of rIL-2 and r–interferon gamma.

COMMENT

The challenge in improving the responsiveness of tumors to immunotherapeutic modalities of treatment involves (1) an understanding of the cellular effector mechanisms involved in vivo during the regression of tumors that respond and (2) an understanding of the interaction of tumor components (MHC-regulated or otherwise) with effector cells, such as CTL and NK, and the potential for modulation of this interaction. For human NRB, Main et al[8] demonstrated that human NRB cell lines lacked class 1 antigen and were not susceptible to killing by CTLs but were highly sensitive to NK cell killing. This is consistent with evidence that NK cell killing varies inversely with class 1 expression.[26] The clinical implications of their findings is that the aggressiveness of human NRB may relate to a lack of CTL development by the host, or alternatively, it may relate to impaired NK activity. From a therapeutic viewpoint, tumors, such as NRB with low but inducible class 1 MHC levels, may be suitable for therapies that modulate class 1 MHC levels or for therapies that augment NK activity.

This study demonstrated the immunologic relevance of murine C1300-NRB to human NRB. The NK sensitivity was demonstrated using both basal and Poly IC–induced splenic effector cells from strain CBA/J mice. The C1300-NRB, however, is syngeneic to strain A mice, which is a relatively low-responder strain for expression of natural cytotoxic reactivity to YAC-1, with minimal killing observed in short-term ^{51}Cr-release assays. Herberman et al[27] demonstrated that strain A mice are not generally low reactors in natural cytotoxicity, but are only low in their reactivity against some of the antigens recognized by NK cell mechanisms, including YAC-1. In support of this, we have observed no differences in basal anti–asialo GM-1 receptor expression in strain A/J spleen cells, compared with strain CFW spleen cells, which have a higher basal reactivity against YAC-1. Furthermore, activated NK from strain A mice lyse YAC-1 efficiently in short-term assays.

In vivo depletion with anti–asialo GM-1 resulted in rapid tumor growth and significantly increased mortality by day 21 after inoculation, compared with control mice. These effects were relatively more pronounced than depletion of Lyt-2–positive cells, suggesting that NK cells may have a greater regulatory role than CTLs in untreated animals.

The biologic effects of r–interferon gamma were more marked than high-dose rIL-2 in this study, where treatment was instituted at an early period of tumor development. This was not explained by differences in NK activity as the enhancement of NK cytotoxicity by r–interferon gamma was considerably less than that observed with rIL-2. An immunologic explanation for this effect, rather than an explanation based on a potential antiviral and antiproliferative effect, is likely in view of the fact that pretreatment with anti–asialo GM-1 or anti–Lyt-2 abolished the antitumor effect. This indicates that both cells of the NK and CTL phenotype are required for r–interferon gamma to be effective in this model. There are two likely mechanisms to explain the influence of CTLs in this phenomenon: (1) r–interferon gamma is a potent modulator of class 2 (Ia) on antigen-presenting cells, such as macrophages and dendritic cells, such that the host capacity to present C1300 and to sensitize host lymphocytes may be enhanced[12]; and (2) r–interferon gamma may directly enhance class 1 and class 2 expression on the tumor in vivo, resulting in enhanced generation of CTLs. In this respect, we have demonstrated that r–interferon gamma at a concentration of 500 U/mL induces class 1 expression on C1300-NRB cells in vitro, with the effect being observed at 24 hours and maximal after 72 hours.[28]

The effectiveness of high-dose rIL-2 in this model was also abrogated by selective depletion of anti–asialo GM-1–positive or Lyt-2–positive cells. Pretreatment with anti–asialo GM-1 did not significantly reduce the enhanced cytotoxic activity against YAC-1 or C1300-NRB. This phenomenon may have involved facilitated non-MHC-restricted lysis of these targets by Lyt-2+ T cells, as has been observed in CTL clones stimulated with rIL-2.[29] The influence of in vivo LAK cell generation in this study is unclear, although we observed no significant killing of the LAK-sensitive P815 cell line by spleen cells from treated mice.

Phase I/II studies evaluating r–interferon gamma in advanced human NRB have been initiated, and augmented NK killing and tumor class 1 expression have been observed in a small study.[30] No clinical response has been observed to date. Perhaps the greatest application of r–interferon gamma will be in low-volume disease, such as following cytoreductive surgery or after multimodality treatment and bone marrow transplantation, since experimental evidence suggests that NK mechanisms and MHC modulation are of greater benefit with smaller tumor burdens. Clearly, future experimental and clinical studies will evaluate r–interferon gamma in combination treatment modalities, with cytokines, such as tumor necrosis factor and rIL-2, and in combination with LAK cell or tumor-infiltrating lymphocytes. Based on the evidence from this study, murine C1300-NRB can be a suitable model for evaluation of such immunotherapeutic modalities.

This study was supported in part by the Georgene S. Harmelin Surgical Oncology Research Fund, Philadelphia.

James Markmann, University of Pennsylvania, Philadelphia, provided the murine interferon gamma and the fluorescein isothiocyanate goat anti-rabbit IgG (ab')2 used in this study.

References

1. Virchow R: *Die Krankaften Geschwultse.* Berlin, August Herschwald, 1865, vol 2, p 78.
2. Simone JV, Cassady RJ, Filler RM: Cancers of childhood, in De Vita VT, Hellman S, Rosenberg SA (eds): *Cancers: Principles and Practice of Oncology.* Philadelphia, JB Lippincott, 1982, pp 1254-1330.
3. Bill AH: Immune aspects of neuroblastoma. *Am J Surg* 1971;122:142-147.
4. Everson TC, Cole WH: *Spontaneous Regression of Cancer.* Philadelphia, WB Saunders Co, 1966, pp 88-163.
5. D'Angio GJ, Evans EA, Koop CE: Special pattern of widespread neuroblastoma with a favourable prognosis. *Lancet* 1976;1:1046-1049.
6. Hellstrom I, Hellstrom KE, Bill AH, et al: Studies on cellular immunity to human neuroblastoma cells. *Int J Cancer* 1970;6:172-188.
7. Lampson LA, Fischer CA, Whelan JP: Striking paucity of HLA-A, B, C and B2 microglobulin on human neuroblastoma cell lines. *J Immunol* 1983;130:2471-2478.
8. Main EK, Lampson LA, Hart MK, et al: Human neuroblastoma cell lines are susceptible to lysis by natural killer cells but not by cytotoxic T lymphocytes. *J Immunol* 1985;135:242-246.
9. Lampson LA, Fisher CA: Weak HLA and beta$_2$-microglobulin expression of neuronal cell lines can be modulated by interferon. *PNAS* 1984;81:6476-6480.
10. Henney CS, Kuribayashi K, Kern DE, et al: Interleukin-2 augments natural killer cell activity. *Nature* 1981;291:335-338.
11. Gidlund M, Orn A, Wigzell H, et al: Enhanced NK activity in mice injected with interferon and interferon inducers. *Nature* 1978;273:759-761.
12. Bonnen EM, Oldham RK: Gamma-interferon: Physiology and speculation on its role in medicine. *J Biol Response Mod* 1987;6:275-301.
13. Reynolds CW, Ortaldo JR: Natural killer activity: The definition of a function rather than cell type. *Immunol Today* 1987;8:172-176.
14. Zingernagel RM, Doherty PC: H-2 compatibility requirement for T-cell mediated lysis of target cells infected with lymphocytic choriomeningitis virus: Different cytotoxic T cell specificities are associated with structures coded from in H-2K or H-2D. *J Exp Med* 1975;141:1427-1436.
15. Hanna N, Burton RC: Definitive evidence that natural killer (NK) cells inhibit experimental tumor metastasis in vivo. *J Immunol* 1981;127:1754-1758.
16. Gorelik E, Wiltrout RH, Okumura K, et al: Role of NK cells in the control of metastatic spread and growth of tumor cells in mice. *Int J Cancer* 1982;20:107-112.
17. Kasai M, Iwamori M, Nagai Y, et al: A glycolipid on the surface on mouse natural killer cells. *Eur J Immunol* 1980;10:175-180.
18. Suttles J, Schwarting GA, Stout RD: Flow cytometric analysis reveals the presence of asialo-GMi on the surface membrane of alloimmune cytotoxic T cells. *J Immunol* 1986;136:1586-1592.
19. Habu S, Fukui H, Shimamura K, et al: In vivo effects of anti-asialo GM1: I. Reduction of NJ activity and enhancement of transplanted tumor growth in nude mice. *J Immunol* 1981;127:34-38.
20. Barlozzari T, Leonhardt J, Wiltrout R: Direct evidence for the role of LGL in the inhibition of experimental tumor metastases. *J Immunol* 1985;134:2783-2789.
21. Karre KG, Klein R, Kiessling G, et al: Low natural in vivo resistance to syngeneic leukaemias in natural killer-deficient mice. *Nature* 1980;284:624-627.
22. Karpeh MS, Kehne JA, Choi SH, et al: Tumor immunogenicity, nutritional repletion and cancer. *Surgery* 1987;102:283-290.
23. Kasai M, Yoneda T, Habu S, et al: In vivo effect of anti-asialo GM1 on natural killer cell activity. *Nature* 1981;291:334-335.
24. Cobbold SP, Jayasuriya A, Nash A, et al: Therapy with monoclonal antibodies by elimination of T cell subsets in vivo. *Nature* 1984;312:548-551.
25. Wexler H: Accurate identification of experimental pulmonary metastases. *JNCI* 1966;36:641-647.
26. Storkus WJ, Howell DN, Slater RD, et al: NK susceptibility varies inversely with target class 1 HLA antigen expression. *J Immunol* 1987;138:1657-1659.
27. Herberman RB, Nunn ME, Holden HT, et al: Augmentation of natural cytotoxic reactivity of mouse lymphoid cells against syngeneic and allogeneic target cells. *Int J Cancer* 1977;19:555-564.
28. Sigal RK, Reynolds JV, Markmann J, et al: Upregulation of MHC class 1: Effect on growth and LAK sensitivity of neuroblastoma. *Surg Forum* 1988;39:572-574.
29. Farrar JJ, Benjamin WR, Hilfiker ML: The biochemistry, biology and role of interleukin 2 in the induction of cytotoxic T cell and antibody-forming B cell responses. *Immunol Rev* 1982;62:129-166.
30. Evans A, Lampson L, Main E, et al: Effects of gamma interferon on the NK and tumor cells of children with neuroblastoma, abstract 1656. *Proceedings of the American Association for Cancer Research,* 1988, vol 29, 1656 p 416.

Discussion

Q Dr Reynolds, I know you mentioned in the beginning that NRB may be an immunogenic tumor; however, this model is a sub-Q model, and what effect do you think the blood-brain barrier would have on the immune response? How do you think that you could translate a model like this from a mouse system to a human condition?

A This NRB was originally a metastatic tumor, but by years of serial and in vivo transplantation and keeping it in vitro, it lost a capacity to metastasize. In terms of the blood-brain barrier, I am really unsure as to how we could influence that. The only suggestion is, and this is based on work done with human NRB cell lines at The Children's Hospital of Philadelphia, that interferon very potently induces class 1 induction of the human NRB, and specific cytotoxic responses can develop to the tumor in the class 1–induced state. They feel, though they have not proved it experimentally, nor have we, that this may be an important modality for future treatment. Local-sensitized CTLs may exert an antitumor effect on class 1–upregulated NRBs.

Q After the anti–asialo GM-1 therapy, did the NK cell count decrease?

A Yes, it did. It decreased from a mean of about 15% in the untreated state to a mean of about 4% positivity in the treated animals after three days.

Q Now that you have established with this sub-Q model that you can boost the immune response, increase NK activity, and essentially show a difference, where are you going to take this? Is this model something you are going to continue with; what is your next experiment?

A I think the most exciting feature of working with neurotumors, in the experimental system, is that they do not express class 1 antigens. So early treatment with interferon and tumor necrosis factor, which induces class 1 induction on the tumors, followed later on by treatment with potent adaptive immunotherapy, such as LAK cells or tumor-infiltrating lymphocytes, may, I feel, give the best results.

Pseudocysts in Chronic Pancreatitis

Surgical Results in 102 Consecutive Patients

Tuula Kiviluoto, MD; Leena Kivisaari, MD; Eero Kivilaakso, MD; Matti Lempinen, MD

• Preoperative symptoms, diagnoses, and postoperative outcomes in 102 consecutive patients with pancreatic pseudocysts were analyzed. Upper epigastric pain, loss of weight, obstructive jaundice, and sudden arterial bleeding from the pseudocyst were the most common preoperative symptoms. Ultrasonography, computed tomography, and endoscopic retrograde cholangiopancreatography were the most useful diagnostic tools in the evaluation of the presence, size, location, and possible pancreatic ductal communications of the pseudocyst. In a single thick-walled pseudocyst, the best long-term results were achieved by internal drainage. Pancreatic resection is justified if the patient already has diabetes or multiple pseudocysts or if the pseudocyst is not amenable to internal drainage. The most fatal preoperative complication was a sudden arterial bleeding from a pseudocyst. In treating this complication, hemostasis with transcystic arterial ligation and external drainage of the pseudocyst gave the best results.
(*Arch Surg* 1989;124:240-243)

Several unsettled questions still exist with regard to the optimal timing and different methods of surgery for pancreatic pseudocysts. Nowadays, ultrasonography (US), computed tomography (CT), and endoscopic retrograde cholangiopancreatography (ERCP) can possibly make the exact preoperative determination of the wall thickness, diameter, number, and size of pseudocysts. Thus, there are improved premises for exact planning of the treatment, as well as for comparing the surgical results. In 1981, Crass and Way[1] emphasized the importance of distinguishing between acute pseudocysts following an attack of acute pancreatitis and pseudocysts associated with chronic pancreatitis. Obviously, the pathophysiology, natural history, and treatment are different in these two conditions.

With regard to the operative treatment of uncomplicated pseudocysts, one should choose between several different operative techniques, including external and internal drainage of the pseudocyst, as well as pancreatic resections.

This study reviews 102 consecutive patients who underwent operations for pancreatic pseudocysts. All patients had chronic pancreatitis. Preoperative symptoms, diagnoses, timing of the operation, and postoperative outcomes after different operations were analyzed.

Accepted for publication April 12, 1988.
From the Second Department of Surgery (Drs Kiviluoto, Kivilaakso, and Lempinen) and Department of Diagnostic Radiology (Dr Kivisaari), Helsinki University Central Hospital.

Reprint requests to Second Department of Surgery, Helsinki University Central Hospital, Haartmanink 4 00290 Helsinki, SF-Finland (Dr Kiviluoto).

PATIENTS AND METHODS

Between 1971 and 1984, 102 patients underwent operations for pancreatic pseudocysts caused by chronic pancreatitis at the Second Department of Surgery, Helsinki University Central Hospital. The mean age of the patients was 39 years (age range, 20 through 71 years). There were 81 men and 21 women. Alcohol was the principal causal factor for chronic pancreatitis in 87 (85%) of the patients. The first pancreatic attack was diagnosed, on an average, four years (range, one to 12 years) before the operation for a pseudocyst. Cholelithiasis was diagnosed in four patients, but none of them had concrements in the common bile duct. In four patients, the pseudocyst was secondary to blunt abdominal trauma. Hyperparathyreosis was detected in two patients, and in five patients, the origin of chronic pancreatitis remained unknown.

The preoperative symptoms are listed in Table 1. More than half (68%) of the patients had upper epigastric abdominal pains that often radiated to the back. A palpable intra-abdominal mass and loss of weight (>5 kg) were other common signs (32% and 27%, respectively). Permanent or intermittent obstructive jaundice (18%) was a sign that suggested compression of the common bile duct by a pancreatic mass. Vomiting (8%) was often evoked by compression of the pyloric outlet or duodenum. Acute bleeding originating from an arterial pseudoaneurysm, secondary to a pseudocyst, occurred in 18 patients (17%). Left pleural effusion, caused by a spontaneous pancreatic fistula, was detected in three patients. Fifteen patients had previously undergone some kind of abdominal operation as follows:

Type of Operation	No. of Patients
Cholecystectomy	4
External drainage of pseudocyst	5
Pancreatic caudal resection	4
Longitudinal wirsungo-jejunostomy	1
Antrectomy and vagotomy	1
Total	**15**

Preoperative Findings

Considerable hemorrhagic anemia with a hematocrit less than 0.34 was present in 24 patients, and in 18 patients (18%), the anemia was attributable to sudden blood loss into the gastrointestinal tract, peritoneal cavity, or retroperitoneal space. Leukocytosis ($>10^9$/L) was present in ten patients (10%) during the first few days of admission. Usually, the leukocyte count fell to normal

Table 1.—Preoperative Symptoms and Findings in 102 Patients Operated on for Chronic Pseudocysts

Symptom/Finding	External Drainage (n=39)	Internal Drainage (n=22)	Excision/Pancreatic Resection (n=41)	Total
Intra-abdominal pain	31	15	23	**69**
Loss of weight (>5 kg)	9	8	11	**28**
Fever	5	1	5	**11**
Nausea/vomiting	2	4	2	**8**
Icterus	2	1	16	**19**
Gastric outlet symptoms	3	5	3	**11**
Diabetes mellitus	5	4	2	**11**
Palpable abdominal resistance	20	5	8	**33**
Diarrhea	2	1	0	**3**
Cardiac insufficiency	1	1	1	**3**
Essential hypertony	3	0	3	**6**
Sudden loss of hemoglobin	11	0	7	**18**
Pleural effusion	0	0	3	**3**

Table 2.—Postoperative Complications and Outcome of 102 Patients Operated on for Pseudocysts

	External Drainage (n=39)	Internal Drainage (n=22)	Excision/ Resection (n=35)	Whipple's Procedure or Total Pancreatectomy (n=6)	Total
Hospital mortality	2	0	4	1	**7**
Wound infection/dehiscence	1	0	1	0	**2**
Postoperative pneumonia	1	3	9	1	**14**
Recidivistic pseudocyst	3	0	4	0	**7**
Reoperation	11	5	8	0	**24**
Postoperative diabetes*	10 (5)	6 (4)	9 (2)	3	**28**
Postoperative abdominal pains	9	7	13	0	**29**
Late mortality	1	1	4	0	**6**
Unable to work	4	3	4	3	**14**

*Numbers in parentheses are counts of preoperative diabetes.

before the surgical therapy. The urine serum amylase values were elevated during the hospital stay in 36 patients (35%) and often showed marked fluctuations. Evidence of extrahepatic biliary tract obstruction with elevation of the serum alkaline phosphatase and/or serum bilirubin levels was noted in 19 patients (19%). In three patients with left pleural effusion, due to a pancreatopleural fistula, the amylase level in the pleural fluid was above 10 000 U/L (Table 1).

In 73 patients (72%), the preoperative diagnosis was confirmed by US, ERCP, and/or CT. In 35 patients, the pseudocyst was localized in the head or uncinate process, in 31, in the body, and in 36, in the tail of the pancreas.

Operations

External Drainage.—Thirty-nine patients (38%) underwent an external drainage of the pseudocyst. This operation was usually chosen in the case of a relatively thin-walled pseudocyst with potentially infected cystic fluid. However, 11 of these patients were operated on by transcystic ligatures for a sudden hemorrhage, originating from a pseudoaneurysm that was generated by an arterial erosion by the pseudocyst.

Internal Drainage.—Single pseudocysts with a thick wall were candidates for internal drainage. In 18 patients (18%), a cystojejunostomy using Roux-en-Y reconstruction with a 35- to 40-cm jejunal blind loop was performed. In one patient, the cystic wall was adherent to the gastric wall, and a cystogastrostomy was performed. In addition, in two patients (2%), multiple intrapancreatic pseudocysts were in connection with the dilated main pancreatic duct, and a lateral wirsungojejunostomy was performed.

Pancreatic Resection.—Pseudocysts, especially multiple ones, destroying pancreatic parenchyma without a dilated main pancreatic duct, were usually treated with resection. Resection of the pseudocyst, only without removal of pancreatic parenchyma, was possible in three patients (3%), whereas in 38 patients (38%), pancreatic resection also was necessary. In four of them, multiple pseudocysts were localized in the head of the pancreas, causing intrapancreatic obstruction of the main biliary tract, and a pancreaticoduodenectomy was performed. In five patients, a distal pseudocyst was removed by caudal pancreatic resection. Because of the dilated pancreatic duct, these patients also underwent distal pancreaticojejunostomy (Table 2).

Follow-up

Seventy-five (74%) of the 102 patients had a checkup examination, on average, 6.5 years after the operation (range, two to 12 years). Thirteen patients had died, and 14 patients could not be traced. In addition to the routine clinical examination and laboratory tests, ERCP was performed in 27 patients, US in 49 patients, and CT in eight patients.

RESULTS

Hospital Mortality

Seven patients died within 30 days after the operation, giving a hospital mortality of 7%. One patient died of cardiac insufficiency after an elective pancreatic resection with distal pancreaticojejunostomy (DuVal). The other six patients died after an emergency operation due to a massive hemorrhage from the pancreatic pseudocyst. Two

Table 3.—Surgical Procedures and Clinical Outcome of 18 Patients Operated on for Pancreatic Pseudocyst and Hemorrhage

	No. (%)		
	Transcystic Arterial Ligation (n=11)	Distal Pancreatic Resection (n=5)	Whipple's Procedure or Total Pancreatectomy (n=2)
Reoperation	4 (36)	1 (20)	0
Hospital mortality	2 (18)	3 (60)	1 (50)
Late mortality	2 (18)	0	0
Good postoperative outcome	4 (36)	1 (20)	1 (50)

of these patients had primarily undergone transcystic arterial ligation and external drainage of the pseudocyst. After the operation, one patient had massive bleeding from the gastroduodenal artery during the primary operation, and the other patient died of a rebleeding from the superior pancreatoduodenal artery 22 days after the operation. Four patients died after a left-sided pancreatic resection or total pancreatectomy. The reasons for death were postoperative bacterial sepsis with diffuse intra-abdominal and/or gastrointestinal bleeding in two of these patients, and general sepsis and wound dehiscence in the remaining two patients.

Postoperative Complications

External Drainage.—Six patients underwent reoperations for recurrent pseudocysts after primary external drainage, and pancreatic resection was performed. Three patients developed a persistent pancreatocutaneous fistula after an operative external drainage of a pseudocyst; the treatment in these patients was a sparing distal pancreatic resection. Similarly, two patients were operated on for massive pseudoaneurysmal hemorrhage by hemostatic transcystic ligature and external drainage; they developed a new bleeding episode, and a pancreatic resection was performed.

Internal Drainage.—There was no hospital mortality in this group. Postoperatively, three patients developed pneumonia. Later on, four patients underwent pancreatic resection for abdominal pains and recurrent attacks of pancreatitis. In addition, one patient had sudden bleeding from a pseudoaneurysm in the wall of the pancreaticoduodenal artery. This patient underwent a total pancreatectomy, and died a few days later for a disseminated intravascular coagulation–like diffuse bleeding and sepsis.

Pancreatic Resection.—Recurrent pseudocysts developed in four (13%) of the 32 patients who were primarily treated by a distal pancreatic resection. Three of these patients were treated by an additional pancreatic resection, and internal drainage of the pseudocyst by a jejunal Roux-en-Y procedure was performed in the remaining patient. In addition, four other patients needed an extensive pancreatic resection due to progression of chronic pancreatitis. One patient had signs of biliary tract obstruction with elevated serum alkaline phosphatase and bilirubin levels, but without subjective symptoms. The patient had these symptoms one year after near-total pancreatectomy (leaving a rim of pancreas along the duodenal loop).

In three asymptomatic patients, a silent pseudocyst was revealed by using US, CT, and/or ERCP in the checkup examination. In addition, ERCP and CT showed a noticeable progression of chronic pancreatitis in 15 of the patients.

Fourteen (19%) of the 75 reexamined patients were unable to work because of symptoms attributable to chronic pancreatitis.

COMMENT

Several factors should be considered in the choice of a suitable surgical method for the treatment of pancreatic pseudocysts in chronic pancreatitis. Important factors include the general condition of the patient, pancreatic endocrine and exocrine functional capacity, as well as the site, number, and possible complications of the pseudocysts. Mechanical obstruction of the biliary tract and gastric outlet is clinically important. The differential diagnosis between pseudocysts and other inflammatory masses and neoplasms is also necessary. Ultrasonography combined with fine-needle biopsies, CT, and ERCP are the most important diagnostic tools in the evaluation of these patients.

Most authors agree that resection of the pancreas with a pseudocyst is, in certain cases, indicated.[2-7] Without dilatation of the main pancreatic duct, multiple pseudocysts that constitute the head of the pancreas are not appropriate for the internal drainage procedure, and resection of the proximal portion of the pancreas is often the only possibility. In such situations, our method of choice is usually pancreaticoduodenectomy (Whipple's procedure) or duodenum-saving near-to-total pancreatectomy. Resection is also often indicated, when the patient already has severe pancreatic endocrine insufficiency. However, diabetes and steatorrhea, often combined with continual alcohol consumption, impaired the late results in these patients.

Internal drainage of the pseudocyst with a Roux-en-Y cystojejunostomy proved to yield the best short- and long-term results. In this respect, our results are in accordance with those found by several other authors.[5,8,9] Also, when the pseudocysts are in connection with the dilated main pancreatic duct, lateral wirsungojejunostomy with Roux-en-Y reconstruction often seems to yield satisfying results.[8]

In our series, only one patient had undergone cystogastrostomy, and he needed a new operation because of recurrence of the pseudocyst. However, this procedure is often advocated in cases when a mature pseudocyst extends out from the lesser sac and is intimately adherent to the posterior wall of the stomach; this procedure seems to yield satisfactory results in these cases.[5-8,10]

The complication rate was clearly highest (24%) after external drainage of the pseudocysts. Also, in the literature, the complication rate ranges from 25% to 50%.[11] Furthermore, the recurrence rate after this procedure is high, ranging from 20% and 30%.[12] These results strongly suggest that this procedure is rarely warranted in elective surgery.

The most serious complication of a pseudocyst was acute bleeding due to erosion and aneurysmal degeneration of the splanchnic arteries on the wall of the pseudocyst (Table 3). These patients had a very high postoperative mortality (33%). In our series, seven patients of the total 18 patients with pseudoaneurysmal bleeding underwent pancreatic resection as the primary intervention.[13] Four of these patients died during the first month after the operation. The general condition of these patients was often poor due to massive bleeding, and resectional surgery as an emergency intervention therefore carries a very high complication risk. Our results favor a more "conservative" surgical approach, such as hemostasis with transcystic ligatures with external drainage, for the treatment of this complication, yielding clearly a better outcome. However, in selected cases, good results seem to be achieved also by angiographic arterial embolization,[14,15] but we do not have any personal experience with this method in the management of this complication. Obviously, transcystic ligature and other pancreatic parenchyma–sparing procedures are not always successful, and more extensive surgical interventions, such as pancreatic resection, become mandatory.

The diagnosis of a pseudocyst may be difficult, particularly in situations where pleural effusion is the first sign of pancreatic disease. One of our patients had undergone a left pleural decortication before the correct diagnosis. A high amylase concentration in the pleural fluid is characteristic of this condition. In our series, three patients had a distal pancreatic pseudocyst and pleural fistula. A sparing distal pancreatic resection and removal of the cyst yielded good short- and long-term results.

Unexpectedly, a high frequency of preoperative complications were encountered in the patients with chronic pancreatitis and pseudocysts. Also, improved preoperative diagnostic methods have revealed that the frequency of silent pseudocysts is much higher than was earlier presumed. Prolonged waiting before the operation carries a high morbidity and mortality risk.[2,6,16,17] Thus, early and elective surgery in this disease is recommended.

References

1. Crass RA, Way LW: Acute and chronic pseudocysts are different. *Am J Surg* 1981;142:660-663.
2. Sankaran S, Walt A: The natural and unnatural history of pancreatic pseudocysts. *Br J Surg* 1975;62:37-44.
3. Van Heerden JA, ReMine WH: Pseudocyst of the pancreas. *Arch Surg* 1975;110:500-505.
4. Frey CF: Pancreatic pseudocyst: Operative strategy. *Ann Surg* 1978;188:652-662.
5. Sandy JT, Taylor RH, Christensen RM, et al: Pancreatic pseudocysts: Changing concepts in management. *Am J Surg* 1981;141:574-576.
6. Brooks JR: Pseudocysts of the pancreas, in Brooks JR (ed): *Surgery of the Pancreas.* Philadelphia, WB Saunders Co, 1983, pp 212-229.
7. Alrabeeah AA, Cattral M, Siegenberg J: Unusual presentation of a pancreatic pseudocyst: A case report. *Can J Surg* 1987;30:281-282.
8. Munn JS, Aranha GV, Greenlee HB, et al: Simultaneous treatment of chronic pancreatitis and pancreatic pseudocyst. *Arch Surg* 1987;122:662-667.
9. Kohler H, Schafmayer A, Lundtke FE, et al: Surgical treatment of pancreatic pseudocyst. *Br J Surg* 1987;74:813-815.
10. Frick S, Ebert M, Ruckert K: Surgery in chronic pancreatitis: II. Late results following nonresection operations. *Dtsch Med Wochenschr* 1987;112:832-837.
11. Elechi EN, Callender CO, Leffal LD, et al: The treatment of pancreatic pseudocysts by external drainage. *Surg Gynecol Obstet* 1979; 148:707-710.
12. Martin EW Jr, Catalano P, Cooperman M, et al: Surgical decision making in the treatment of pancreatic pseudocysts: Internal versus external drainage. *Am J Surg* 1979;138:821-824.
13. Kiviluoto T, Schröder T, Kivilaakso E, et al: Acute haemorrhage associated with pancreatic pseudocyst and chronic pancreatitis. *Ann Chir Gynaecol* 1984;73:214-218.
14. Freeny PC, Lawson TL: Complications in pancreatitis, in Freeny PC, Lawson TL (eds): *Radiology of the Pancreas.* New York, Springer-Verlag NY Inc, 1982; pp 306-386.
15. Reuter SR, Chuang VP, Bree RL: Selective embolization for control of massive upper gastrointestinal bleeding. *AJR* 1975;125:119-126.
16. Pollak EW, Michas CA, Wolfman EF: Pancreatic pseudocyst: Management of 54 patients. *Am J Surg* 1978;135:199-201.
17. Hanna W: Rupture of pancreatic cysts: Report of a case and a review of the literature. *Br J Surg* 1960;47:495-498.

Editorial Comment

There appears to be less uniformity to pancreatitis and its complications from country to country than exists for many other surgical diseases. This large series of pancreatic pseudocysts from Finland, whose citizens appear to be no less vigorous in their alcoholic consumption than our own, reflects some clear differences. Fewer had pain, and none had pancreatic abdominal ascites, which is surprising. In contrast, the incidence of jaundice (18%) is unusually high. No less than 17% had the dreaded complication of acute bleeding from a pseudoaneurysm in the pseudocyst wall, and these had a 33% mortality rate. The authors note that arterial embolization was not available for these patients, but it may also be significant that recurrent bleeding caused death in some patients in whom transcystic ligation of the aneurysm was performed rather than resection. In our experience, resection, whenever feasible, is the more desirable and, ultimately, safer approach.

Considering that all the operations were done for well-established pseudocysts associated with chronic pancreatitis, the frequency of external drainage (38%) is surprisingly high. Paradoxically, the resection rate of 40% was also unusually high when compared with most series, but the authors may have been ahead of their time in that there is an increasing use of resection in many institutions today. The ratio of 21:1 for cystojejunostomy/cystgastrostomy is unusual although essentially unimportant, and a concomitant lateral pancreaticojejunostomy (modified Puestow) for pain was infrequently added.

Finally, no mention is made of percutaneous or transgastric drainage of pseudocysts. Although not introduced until recent years, consideration of the role of these approaches, desirably based on a preliminary endoscopic retrograde cholangiopancreatography road map, is increasing.

Alexander J. Walt, MB, ChB
Detroit

Single-Dose Antibiotic Prophylaxis in Contaminated Abdominal Surgery

John C. Hall, FRACS; J. McK. Watts, FRACS; Lexi Press, RN; P. O'Brien, FRACS; J. Turnidge, FRACP; P. McDonald, FRACP

• Although perioperative antibiotic cover reduces the incidence of septic complications associated with abdominal surgery, the optimum duration of antibiotic exposure is open to question. This clinical trial compared the efficacy of a single dose of moxalactam (1 g intravenously) with an extended course of moxalactam (1 g intravenously for eight doses) in 1027 patients undergoing contaminated abdominal surgery. The wound infection rate was 5.4% (28/519) for the single-dose schedule and 6.1% (31/508) for the extended-cover regimen (the respective 95% confidence intervals being 3.6% to 7.7% and 4.2% to 8.6%). Over 80% of all patients undergoing abdominal surgery during the period of study were entered into the trial. There was no significant difference in the incidence of other complications between the two groups under study. It is concluded that a single dose of moxalactam is as effective as a 48-hour course when attempting to prevent infection after contaminated abdominal surgery.

(*Arch Surg* 1989;124:244-247)

It has been suggested that a single dose of an appropriate antibiotic will provide adequate prophylaxis against infection in patients undergoing contaminated abdominal surgery. Single-dose prophylaxis is attractive because it minimizes the development of bacterial resistance, reduces the risk of morbidity associated with the use of antibiotics, and is cheaper than more prolonged regimens.

However, the evidence in support of this concept contains major deficiencies. Most of the studies addressing this question have either compared a single-dose regimen with a placebo or have compared a single dose of one agent with the prolonged administration of other agents.[1] Only a small number of studies[2-4] have used the same antibiotic to compare a single-dose regimen with an extended course (Table 1). Furthermore, the methodological standards of such studies have recently come under close scrutiny.[5,6] In particular, there has been discussion about the dangers of drawing conclusions from studies that have evaluated relatively small numbers of patients (studies that contain a high probability of a type II error). The small sample sizes used in the studies detailed in Table 1 detract from the reliability of the observed results. Another consideration is the evaluation of an adequate spectrum of patients. At the present time, there is a lack of information concerning the relative value of prophylactic antibiotics across a range of contaminated abdominal operations. Most published studies have concentrated on either biliary or colorectal surgery. Far less information is available concerning gastric and small-bowel surgery.

This clinical trial evaluates the efficacy of moxalactam, a semisynthetic, broad-spectrum, β-lactam antibiotic, given as a single dose or as a 48-hour regimen for a range of potentially contaminated abdominal operations. All patients undergoing abdominal surgery during the period of study were considered for entry into this trial, and the number of patients required to substantiate a claim of "no significant difference" has been predetermined using strict statistical criteria.

METHODS

Consecutive patients over 14 years of age undergoing potentially contaminated abdominal surgery at Flinders Medical Centre, Bedford Park, Australia, or the Repatriation General Hospital, Daw Park, Australia, were considered for entry into the study. It was prospectively decided that an absolute difference of 5% in wound infection rates between the groups (ie, 5% vs 10%) would be of clinical significance. A sample size that could reliably detect or reject such a difference using a two-tailed test with a confidence of 95% ($P=.05$) and a power of 80% was estimated to be 1022.[7]

Patients being considered for entry into the trial received 1 g of moxalactam in 10 mL of water intravenously at the time of induction of anesthesia. Because of reports of coagulopathy associated with the administration of moxalactam,[8,9] patients were given 10 mg of vitamin K intramuscularly prior to operation. Informed consent was obtained from all of the patients investigated in this study, and the protocol was approved by the human ethics committees of the participating hospitals.

The following operative procedures were standardized for all patients within the study. Povidone iodine was used to prepare the skin prior to surgery. Nylon suture was used for the closure of the aponeurotic layer of all vertical incisions. Oblique or transverse incisions were closed using an absorbable synthetic suture. Intra-abdominal drain tubes were passed not through the wound but through a separate stab incision. Wound drains, subcutaneous fat sutures, or tension sutures were not used. The maximum depth of subcutaneous fat in the wound was measured in millimeters using a steel ruler. The skin was closed using stainless-steel staples. No local antibiotic or antiseptic preparation was used in the wound. All patients undergoing elective colorectal surgery had a two-day mechanical bowel preparation (no oral antibiotics were administered).

Patients were entered into the study at the completion of their operation using a stratified randomization technique. Envelopes were grouped according to stratification and placed in a box within

Table 1.—Studies Comparing Single Dose With Extended Course of Same Antibiotic(s)

Source	Patients Studied	Rate of Wound Sepsis, %
Strachan et al[2]	Routine cholecystectomy (N=201)	Control, 16.9; single-dose cefazolin, 3.2; 5-d cefazolin, 5.5
Higgins et al[3]	Colorectal surgery (N=60)	Single-dose co-trimoxazole and metronidazole, 7.0; 5-d co-trimoxazole and metronidazole, 9.6
Tornqvist et al[4]	Elective colorectal surgery (N=196)	Single-dose doxycycline (200 mg preoperative), 13; single-dose doxycycline (600 mg preoperative), 7; single-dose doxycycline (600 mg postoperative), 20; doxycycline (200 mg preoperative plus 3-d postoperative course), 19

Accepted for publication Dec 7, 1987.

From the Department of Surgery, Royal Perth Hospital, Perth, Western Australia (Dr Hall); the Departments of Surgery (Dr Watts and Ms Press) and Clinical Microbiology (Drs Turnidge and McDonald), Flinders Medical Centre, Bedford Park, South Australia; and the Department of Surgery, Alfred Hospital, Melbourne (Dr O'Brien).

Reprint requests to Department of Surgery, Royal Perth Hospital, Wellington Street, Perth, Western Australia 6000, (Dr Hall).

the operating suite of each hospital. These envelopes were sequentially numbered, opaque, and sealed. They contained the drug regimen to be used (previously determined on the toss of a coin) and a perioperative data sheet. The clinical details of patients who were not entered into the study by completion of the randomization procedure and were thereby excluded from study were documented.

The stratification groups were as follows: appendectomy; cholecystectomy; bile duct surgery (including exploration of the common bile duct); elective colorectal surgery; emergency colorectal surgery; gastroduodenal surgery (excluding closed procedures, such as highly selective vagotomy, gastroplasty, and fundoplication); and small-bowel surgery. In addition, there was a set of envelopes present to document patients who were excluded from study. The reasons for exclusion from the study were as follows:

Reason for Exclusion	No.
Postoperative antibiotics for residual infection	75
Antibiotics within 48 h prior to operation	74
Viscus not opened at operation	46
Failure to give informed consent	15
Failure to give initial dose of moxalactam	14
History of cephalosporin sensitivity or penicillin anaphylaxis	11
Established renal or liver failure	3
Reaction to initial dose of moxalactam	2
Total	**240**

The major reasons for exclusion were the preoperative or postoperative use of other antibiotics. Preoperative antibiotics were used to treat the primary disease (61), for the management of concurrent disease (eight), and as preventative measures in patients with prostheses (five). Antibiotics were administered in the postoperative period if residual infection was present at the completion of surgery. This clinical decision was made by the attending surgeon and resulted in a minimum of five days of antibiotic therapy. The wound infection rate for these patients while they were in the hospital was 13.3% (10/75). The end result was that 81.3% of all patients undergoing abdominal surgery during the period of study entered the trial, ie, 1034 of 1272.

Patients assigned to the single-dose regimen received no further antibiotic. Patients assigned to an extended-course regimen received 1 g of moxalactam intravenously at six-hour intervals for a further seven doses. This provided a total of 8 g of moxalactam administered within 48 hours. The dosages of moxalactam were chosen to exceed the minimum inhibitory concentration of 90% of strains of *Bacteroides fragilis* (10 mg/L) for six and 48 hours, respectively.

Each patient was evaluated daily while in the hospital by a nurse epidemiologist. The state of the wound and evidence of postoperative morbidity were noted and recorded. *Wound infection* was defined as a purulent wound discharge or a serous wound discharge with culture of pathogenic organisms. A wound infection was classified as *major* if it resulted in an extension of the hospital stay or required dressings at home for more than seven days and as *minor* if neither of these features occurred. Peritoneal infection was declared if pus or peritoneal fluid containing pathogenic organisms was found at operation, if there was spontaneous discharge or needle aspiration of pus from the peritoneal cavity, or if there was a collection of pus present at autopsy. All patients were reviewed during the fifth postoperative week for evidence of wound infection and the final pro forma was completed by the nurse epidemiologist at this time.

Confidential monitoring of the trial was performed using a group sequential analysis technique.[10] This allowed for an assessment of the trial results, after each consecutive group of 100 patients had been assessed, with the use of an appropriately modified level of statistical significance ($P=.011$). All comparisons of differences between groups were performed using a two-tailed χ^2 test or Fisher's exact test with declaration of the 95% confidence limits.[11]

RESULTS

Five patients were withdrawn from the study because of an inadequate randomization procedure, and two patients were unavailable for follow-up after discharge from the hospital. The equivalence of the stratification procedure for the remaining 1027 patients who completed the study is demonstrated in Table 2. The proportion of patients undergoing emergency surgery varied between the stratification groups, ie, 16.5% (41/248) for colorectal surgery, 27.0% (27/100) for bile duct surgery, 32.2% (91/283) for cholecystectomy, 53.3% (64/120) for gastroduodenal surgery, 87.9% (27/33) for small-bowel surgery, and 99.2% (244/246) for appendectomy.

Table 2.—Distribution of Randomized Patients According to Sex

	Single Dose		48-h Schedule	
Stratum	**M**	**F**	**M**	**F**
Appendectomy	68	59	64	55
Cholecystectomy	57	89	49	91
Bile duct surgery	25	26	26	20
Elective colorectal	73	28	68	39
Emergency colorectal	8	9	11	9
Gastroduodenal	24	34	32	27
Small-bowel surgery	9	7	9	8
Total	**264**	**255**	**259**	**249**

Table 3.—Wound Infections

	No. (%) of Patients		
Stratum	**Single Dose**	**48-h Schedule**	**Total %**
Cholecystectomy	3/145 (2.0)	3/138 (2.1)	2.0
Bile duct surgery	3/52 (5.8)	2/48 (4.1)	5.1
Appendectomy	3/127 (2.3)	10/119 (8.4)	5.2
Colorectal elective	11/102 (10.7)	6/105 (5.6)	8.2
Gastroduodenal	6/60 (10.0)	4/60 (6.7)	8.4
Small-bowel surgery	1/16 (6.2)	2/17 (11.7)	9.0
Colorectal emergency	1/17 (5.8)	4/21 (20.0)	13.5
Total	**28/519** (5.3)	**31/508** (6.1)	5.7

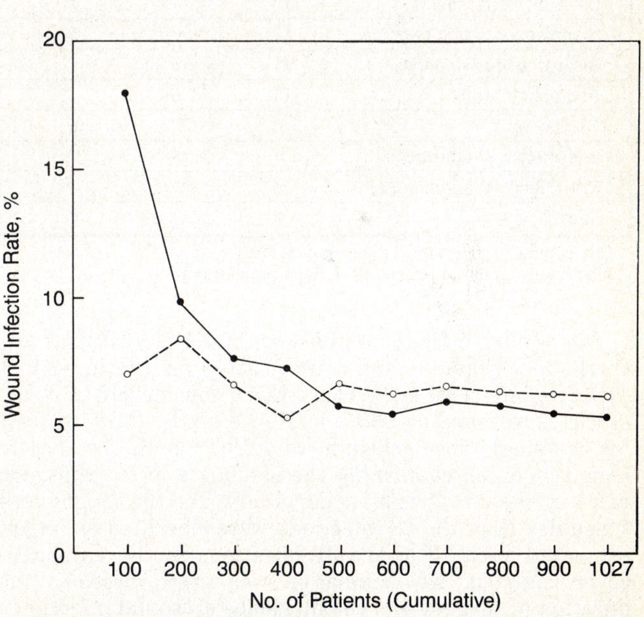

Comparison of cumulative infection rate for two groups under study: single-dose schedule, straight line; 48-hour course, broken line.

Table 4.—Other Infective and Noninfective Complications

	Single Dose	48-h Schedule
Perineal wound infection	6/11	6/11
Intra-abdominal sepsis	10	6
Anastomotic leak	8	9
Superficial wound dehiscence	8	7
Incisional hernia	4	3

Table 5.—Depth of Subcutaneous Abdominal Fat

Treatment Schedule	N	Median Depth, mm	Interquartile Range, mm	Absolute Range, mm
Single dose (no wound infection)	491	21	12-38	1-100
48-h regimen (no wound infection)	477	20	14-36	1-90
All patients with wound infection	59	21	15-40	1-72

Table 6.—Culture Isolates From Abdominal Wound Infections*

Organisms	Total No.	Single Dose	48-h Schedule
Staphylococcus aureus†	20	12	8
Enterococcus	13	5	8
Enterobacteriaceae	13	4	7
Staphylococcus epidermidis	11	6	5
Streptococcus viridans	11	6	5
Bacteroides spp	10	6	4
Coryneforms	8	2	6
β-Hemolytic streptococcus	4	2	2
Pseudomonas aeruginosa	4	1	3
Yeast	2	1	1

*No culture obtained in 13 infected wounds.
†Includes methicillin-resistant *S aureus* (one strain).

The wound infection rates were 5.4% (28/519) for the single-dose schedule and 6.1% (31/508) for the extended-cover regimen (Table 3). There was a considerable overlap of the corresponding 95% confidence limits (3.6% to 7.7% for the single-dose schedule vs 4.2% to 8.6% for the 48-hour schedule), confirming the similarity of the infection rates in the two groups under study. For the single-dose schedule, 12 of the 28 infections were classified as major, compared with 13 of the 31 infections in the extended-cover regimen. No correlation was found between the duration of surgery and the incidence of wound infections. No deaths were attributable to the choice of moxalactam as the prophylactic agent.

The infection rates of each group were monitored using a group sequential technique and began to stabilize after 500 patients had been studied (Figure). Comparison of infection rates within each of the stratification groups also failed to achieve statistical significance, but the relative number of patients in each of these groups is small.

The time of presentation of the wound infections after operation was at a median of eight days, with a range of three to 28 days. No differences in time of presentation of infection was evident between the two treatment groups under study. The median duration of hospital stay was 11 days (range, three to 37 days) for patients having the single-dose regimen and 12 days (range, three to 48 days) for those patients having the extended-cover regimen. Table 4 lists the incidence of other infective or noninfective complications for the two groups. No significant differences between the two dosage regimens was evident for these various complications. The depth of subcutaneous fat, as measured at the time of surgery, was unrelated to the risk of developing an infected wound (Table 5).

Two patients were withdrawn because of possible allergic reactions to moxalactam. Both patients developed a rash soon after administration of the initial dose, and one of the patients had transient respiratory distress that settled without specific therapy. Postoperative bleeding led to reoperation in five patients and to transfusion alone in two patients. A hematologist was consulted on each occasion; however, moxalactam was not implicated in any of these episodes.

Twenty-one (2%) of the 1027 patients died during the course of the study. This mortality reflects the type of patients who were included in this study. The mortalities were as follows: 0% for cholecystectomy (0/283) and appendectomy (0/246); 1.0% (1/100) after bile duct surgery; 3.4% (7/207) after elective colorectal surgery; and 19.4% (13/67) after an emergency resection of the large or small bowel. Information concerning the patients who died during the postoperative period was included in the results (the study was analyzed on an intention-to-treat basis).

The microbiologic features of the wound infections are shown in Table 6. Multiple organisms were cultured in 26 patients or 58% of wound cultures. Nonenteric organisms, most commonly *Staphylococcus aureus*, were cultured as a single or mixed growth in 36 patients (80%). An analysis of the sensitivity patterns of the bacteria confirmed that prophylaxis did not promote the emergence of strains that were resistant to moxalactam.

COMMENT

This study demonstrates that a single dose of moxalactam is as effective as a two-day course of the same antibiotic when trying to prevent infection after contaminated abdominal surgery. No significant differences were noted within the stratification groups. However, two groups with moderate numbers of patients, the appendectomy and elective colorectal surgery groups, both showed trends, but interestingly, in opposite directions.

When the patients who had colorectal surgery (both elective and emergency) were considered as a group, the patients receiving a single dose of moxalactam had a wound infection rate of 10.1% (12/119), compared with 7.9% (10/126) for the 48-hour schedule. While it does not appear that patients were disadvantaged by the use of a single-dose regimen, the overall wound infection rate was still considerable. The same comment can be made for the wound infection rate after gastroduodenal (8.4%) and small-bowel surgery (9.0%).

One factor that might have influenced the wound infection rate relates to the selection of patients. The decision as to whether a patient should be included in this prophylactic study, or receive a full course of antibiotics, was made by the attending surgeon at the completion of each operation. The desire by surgeons to cooperate and enter patients into the trial resulted in the accrual of over 80% of all patients undergoing abdominal surgery during the period of study, but may also have led to the inappropriate inclusion of some patients who had a high risk of developing a septic complication. Against this is the report by Sauvens et al[12] of a wound infection rate of 19.6% (9/46) after ileocolorectal surgery preceded by a similar single prophylactic dose of moxalactam, the report by Hinchey et al[13] of a 7.8% wound infection rate for elective colon surgery after a three-dose schedule of prophylaxis with moxalactam, and the fact that the rate of wound sepsis observed in this trial compares favorably with that found in other studies.[14]

When designing the protocol for this study, we decided to include all patients undergoing elective cholecystectomy. Many of these patients have a low probability of developing a septic complication; however, it is impossible to identify all of the high-risk patients prior to surgery. In particular, the need for exploration of the common bile duct may only become evident during the course of an operation.

A number of previous studies have demonstrated that the use of perioperative cover alone is at least as good as a "treatment course." Stone and coworkers[15] randomly allocated 220 patients undergoing elective gastric, biliary, or colonic surgery into one group having a three-dose perioperative administration of cefamandole and a further group having this same antibiotic continued beyond the perioperative period for a further five days. No significant differences were found between the groups in the rate of wound infection or other septic complications. In a smaller study Kling et al[16] compared the efficacy of metronidazole and doxycycline in patients having colorectal surgery. Some patients were given a single dose of the agents and some had the antibiotics continued for between two and seven days. Metronidazole was seen to provide more effective prophylaxis than doxycycline. Two of 41 patients having a single dose of metronidazole developed a wound infection and none of the nine patients having prolonged prophylaxis developed wound infection.

Other studies have compared a single-dose schedule with an extended course of the same antibiotic. A study by Strachan and others[2] evaluated cefazolin in 201 patients undergoing routine cholecystectomy. A high rate of wound sepsis occurred in patients used as controls (16.9%), but much lower figures were recorded in patients receiving either a single dose or a five-day course (3.2% and 5.5%, respectively). The investigators concluded that cefazolin "is effective when given as a single dose, which reduces cost, saves nursing time, and is less likely to produce bacterial resistance." Higgins et al[3] reported a small study in which a single dose of co-trimoxazole and metronidazole, given at the onset of colorectal operations, was compared with the use of these same antibiotics for five days. No difference between the treatments was evident (7.0% vs 9.6%, respectively).

A study by Tornqvist et al[4] evaluated the prophylactic effect of doxycycline in elective colorectal surgery. The 196 patients were randomized into four groups. The lowest incidence of wound infection (7%) occurred when 600 mg of doxycycline was administered in the preoperative period, while the highest incidence of wound infection (20%) was associated with the postoperative administration of that antibiotic (the first dose was given in the recovery room).

The results of our study are consistent with the view that it is only necessary to have adequate tissue concentrations of an appropriate antibiotic during the period of contamination. It takes several hours for contaminating bacteria to become localized, and antibiotic drugs administered after this period cannot prevent the development of a septic process.[17] At the present time, the use of cephalosporins with activity against anaerobic bacteria is appropriate when trying to prevent sepsis after contaminated abdominal surgery.[18] Most cephalosporins achieve maximal tissue concentrations within two hours after their intravenous injection and persist at a concentration higher than in the blood for several hours. The administration of a second dose of a prophylactic antibiotic is probably only appropriate when surgery is prolonged. Fry[19] recommended that prophylactic antibiotics should be given twice as often as therapeutic regimens. For example, a second dose of moxalactam would only be necessary if an operation was still in progress three hours after the initial dose was given.

Cephalosporins, such as moxalactam, that contain a methylthiotetrazole side-chain are capable of inhibiting vitamin K utilization by the liver.[8] The hypoprothrombinemia can be prevented or reversed by vitamin K therapy. Although this is more likely to occur in patients with renal failure who are receiving prolonged courses of therapy, it has also been reported after short-term therapy in healthy patients.[9] Prophylactic vitamin K was administered during this study, and there was no clinical evidence of an increased tendency for the patients to bleed. This contrasts with the findings of Morris et al,[20] who found that the administration of vitamin K failed to prevent excessive bleeding in five patients after colorectal surgery. Salem et al[21] refrained from using vitamin K prophylaxis in a careful study of 40 patients and concluded that there was no difference between moxalactam and piperacillin in their ability to produce clinical disturbances of hemostasis.

Although the search for the "best" prophylactic antibiotic for patients submitted to contaminated abdominal surgery will continue, the results of this clinical trial confirm that a single preoperative dose of an appropriate antibiotic provides optimal prophylaxis against infection.

References

1. DiPiro JT, Cheung RPF, Bowden TA Jr, et al: Single dose systemic antibiotic prophylaxis of surgical wound infections. *Am J Surg* 1986;152:552-559.

2. Strachan CJL, Black J, Powis SJA, et al: Prophylactic use of cephazolin against wound sepsis after cholecystectomy. *Br Med J* 1977;1:1254-1256.

3. Higgins AF, Lewis A, Noone P, et al: Single and multiple dose cotrimoxazole and metronidazole in colorectal surgery. *Br J Surg* 1980;67:90-92.

4. Tornqvist A, Ekelund G, Forsgren A, et al: Single dose doxycycline prophylaxis and peroperative bacteriological culture in elective colorectal surgery. *Br J Surg* 1981;68:565-568.

5. Watts JMcK, McDonald PJ, Woods PJ: Clinical trials of antimicrobials in surgery. *World J Surg* 1982;6:321-326.

6. Evans M, Pollock AV: Trials on trial: A review of trials of antibiotic prophylaxis. *Arch Surg* 1984;119:109-113.

7. Fleiss JL: *Statistical Methods for Rates and Proportions,* ed 2. New York, John Wiley & Sons Inc, 1981.

8. Neu HC: Adverse effects of new cephalosporins. *Ann Intern Med* 1983;98:415-416.

9. Jones SR, Kimbrough RC: Moxalactam and haemorrhage. *Ann Intern Med* 1983;99:126.

10. Pocock SJ: Size of cancer clinical trials and stopping rules. *Br J Cancer* 1978;38:757-766.

11. Gardner MJ, Altman DG: Confidence intervals rather than p values: Estimation rather than hypothesis testing. *Br Med J* 1986;292:746-750.

12. Sauvens P, Playforth MJ, Smith GMR, et al: Single dose antibiotic prophylaxis of abdominal surgical wound infection: A trial of preoperative latamoxef against peroperative tetracycline lavage. *J R Soc Med* 1986; 79:137-141.

13. Hinchey EJ, Richards GK, Lewis R, et al: Moxalactam as single agent prophylaxis in the prevention of wound infection following colon surgery. *Surgery* 1987;101:15-19.

14. Guglielmo BJ, Hohn DC, Koo PJ, et al: Antibiotic prophylaxis in surgical procedures: A critical analysis of the literature. *Arch Surg* 1983;118:943-955.

15. Stone HH, Haney BB, Kolb LD, et al: Prophylactic and preventative antibiotic therapy. *Ann Surg* 1979;189:691-699.

16. Kling P, Holmund D, Burman LG: Single dose intravenous metronidazole v doxycycline prophylaxis in colorectal surgery. *Acta Chir Scand* 1985;151:163-168.

17. O'Brien P, McDonald P: Preventative antibiotics in surgical practice. *Med J Aust* 1985;143:149-152.

18. Jones RC: Newer antibiotics for the surgeon. *Am J Surg* 1986;152:577-582.

19. Fry DE: Third generation cephalosporin antibiotics in surgical practice. *Am J Surg* 1986;151:306-313.

20. Morris DL, Fabricius PJ, Ambrose NS, et al: A high incidence of bleeding is observed in a trial to determine whether addition of metronidazole is needed with lactamoxef for prophylaxis in colorectal surgery. *J Hosp Infect* 1984;5:398-408.

21. Salem RR, McIndoe A, Matkin JA, et al: The hematologic effects of latamoxef sodium when used as a prophylaxis during surgical treatment. *Surg Gynecol Obstet* 1987;164:525-529.

Long-term Survival in Carcinoma of the Biliary Tract

Analysis of Prognostic Factors in 146 Resections

Kiyoaki Ouchi, MD; Seiki Matsuno, MD; Toshio Sato, MD

• In 146 consecutive patients undergoing resection for carcinoma of the biliary tract, various tumor characteristics that affected long-term survival of the patients were studied. Patients with gallbladder carcinoma whose tumors had no serosal infiltration or vessel invasion were grossly papillary, or were papillary or well-differentiated adenocarcinoma histologically survived longer than those without these tumor characteristics. In upper-third lesions, patients whose tumors showed no serosal infiltration or vessel invasion, were grossly papillary, were papillary or well-differentiated adenocarcinoma histologically, or were treated with hepatic lobectomy had a higher chance of long-term survival. Patients with the middle-third lesions, whose tumors were grossly papillary or nodular or whose margins were tumor-free, were apt to survive longer. Long-term survival for patients with lower-third lesions was obtained most often in patients without lymph node metastasis or vessel invasion.

(*Arch Surg* 1989;124:248-252)

Carcinomas of the extrahepatic biliary tract, including the gallbladder, are almost always accompanied by an unfavorable prognosis. In most cases the resectability rate is low because of the direct extension of tumor to adjacent vital organs. Even though the diagnostic methods, surgical techniques, and appropriate chemotherapy or radiotherapy or both have improved, the management of these patients has been extremely difficult. Conversely, there have been reports of long-term survival following resection.[1,2] The published studies have concluded that, whenever possible, aggressive resection is the best approach to these diseases.[3,4]

In an effort to identify various factors that might have prognostic value, the records of patients treated for resection of these carcinomas at the First Department of Surgery, Tohoku University Hospital, Sendai, Japan, were reviewed.

Accepted for publication May 15, 1987.

From the First Department of Surgery, Tohoku University School of Medicine, Sendai, Japan.

Reprint requests to First Department of Surgery, Tohoku University School of Medicine, 1-1 Seiryo-cho, Sendai 980, Japan (Dr Ouchi).

MATERIALS AND METHODS

The complete clinical records of all patients with histologically proved carcinomas of the biliary tract treated between April 1960 and September 1986 were reviewed retrospectively. Carcinomas of the gallbladder were included, while those of the intrahepatic bile ducts and ampulla of Vater were excluded.

Of 146 patients with carcinoma of the biliary tract who underwent resection, carcinoma of the gallbladder was found in 43 patients and carcinoma of the bile duct was found in 103 patients. The upper third was involved in 36 patients, the middle third was involved in 21 patients, and the lower third was involved in 46 patients.

Of the 43 patients with carcinoma of the gallbladder, 16 were treated with simple cholecystectomy, 25 were treated with cholecystectomy (including wedged resection of the gallbladder bed of the liver and regional lymphadenectomy, namely, extended cholecystectomy), and two were treated with right hepatic lobectomy. Of the 36 patients with carcinoma of the upper bile duct, ten underwent hepatic resection associated with bile duct resection with hepaticojejunostomy and 26 underwent bile duct resection with hepaticojejunostomy. Of the 21 patients with carcinoma of the middle bile duct, six received pancreaticoduodenectomy and 15 received bile duct resection with hepaticojejunostomy. All patients with carcinoma of the lower bile duct were treated with pancreaticoduodenectomy except for one, who underwent total pancreatectomy.

Resection was not indicated when the common or proper hepatic artery or portal trunk or both were involved and when liver metastasis, distant metastasis, or peritoneal seeding was observed.

The patients were divided into two groups. Patients with carcinoma of the gallbladder who survived more than five years and those with carcinoma of the bile duct who survived more than three years constituted group 1 (long-term survivors). The patients with carcinoma of the gallbladder and bile duct who died within five and three years, respectively, constituted group 2 (short-term survivors). Patients who died within one month after surgery and those with carcinoma of the gallbladder and bile duct alive less than five and three years, respectively (ten cases of gallbladder cancer and four of upper, four of middle, and eight of lower bile duct cancer), were excluded from the analysis of prognostic factors. Among the long-term survivors with carcinoma of the bile duct, only three patients with upper-third lesions, three with middle-third lesions, and nine with lower-third lesions survived five or more years after operation. Therefore, the analysis of prognostic factors for cancer of the bile duct was undertaken between three-

Table 1.—Patients Undergoing Resection

	Cancer of Gallbladder	Cancer of Bile Duct: Upper Third	Middle Third	Lower Third
No. of patients resected	43	36	21	46
No. of long-term survivors	10	4	5	14
No. of short-term survivors	19	23	9	20

Table 2.—Resectability Rate

Location	No. of Patients Admitted	No. of Patients Resected	Resectability Rate, %
Gallbladder	144	43	30
Bile duct			
Upper third	117	36	31
Middle third	47	21	45
Lower third	77	46	60

Table 3.—Operative Mortality

Location	No. of Patients	No. of Operative Deaths	Mortality, %
Gallbladder	43	4	9
Bile duct			
Upper third	36	5	14
Middle third	21	3	14
Lower third	46	4	9

year survivors and the patients who died within three years. Group 1 consisted of ten patients with carcinoma of the gallbladder, four with carcinoma of the upper bile duct, five with carcinoma of the middle bile duct, and 14 with carcinoma of the lower bile duct (Table 1). In group 2 there were 19 patients with carcinoma of the gallbladder, 23 with carcinoma of the upper bile duct, nine with carcinoma of the middle bile duct, and 20 with carcinoma of the lower bile duct.

Retrospective studies were made to search for statistically significant prognostic indicators between both groups for each location of lesion. The indicators studied were as follows: the gross and microscopic features of tumors; depth of invasion; lymph node metastasis; infiltration to the liver, the duodenum, or the pancreas; involvement of major vessels; histologic venous, lymphatic, or perineural invasion (vessel invasion); resected margin; and types of operative procedures. All statistical analyses were done by the χ^2 method. Cumulative survival rates for patients with each type of lesion of the biliary tract system were obtained by the Kaplan-Meier method.

RESULTS

Operations

The resectability rate for gallbladder carcinoma was 30% (43/144), with a mortality of 9% (4/43) (Tables 2 and 3). Lesions in the upper, middle, and lower third of the bile duct were resectable in 31% (36/117), 45% (21/47), and 60% (46/77) of the patients admitted, respectively. Resection was associated with 14% operative mortality in carcinomas of the upper (5/36) and middle bile ducts (3/21) and with 9% (4/46) in carcinoma of the lower bile duct.

When the cumulative postoperative survival rates, including operative mortality, were analyzed according to the location of the lesion, the five-year survival rates were as follows: gallbladder carcinomas, 41%; upper-third lesions of the bile duct, 17%; middle-third lesions, 20%; lower-third lesions, 29% (Fig 1). The exact cause of late death was often difficult to ascertain, but, in the majority of patients in group 2, death was directly related to the biliary tract, ie, progressive or recurrent tumor or liver failure.

Prognostic Factors

Cancer of the Gallbladder.—Eight of ten patients in group 1 were alive with disease-free conditions. All patients in group 1 had tumors superficial to the subserosa; three showed only mucosal, four showed muscular, and three showed subserosal involvements. Conversely, there was spread of tumors beyond the gallbladder serosa in 14 (74%) of 19 patients in group 2 ($P<.01$ compared with group 1, Fig 2). Hepatic infiltration of carcinoma was found in one of the ten patients in group 1 and 11 (58%) of the 19 patients in group 2, and there was a statistically significant difference in the presence of hepatic infiltration between groups 1 and 2 ($P<.05$). The gross pathologic findings revealed that in group 1 seven of ten patients had tumors associated with the papillary form, while in group 2 thirteen (68%) of 19 patients had tumors of the infiltrative or nodular form; this difference was statistically significant ($P<.05$). With respect to the microscopic findings, group 1

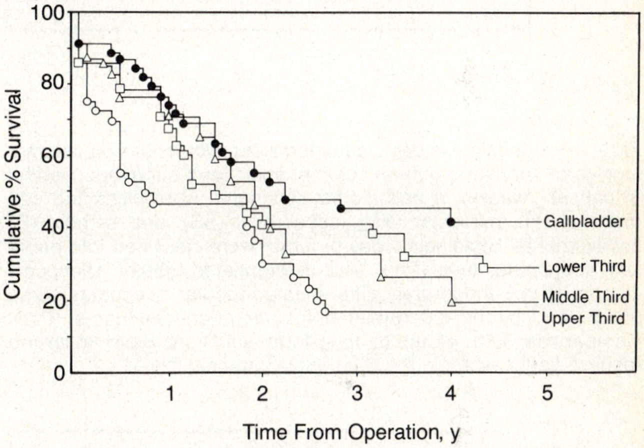

Fig 1.—Survival curves after resection according to location of lesion within biliary system (Kaplan-Meier method).

consisted of nine papillary and one well-differentiated tubular adenocarcinomas, while eight patients in group 2 (42%) had moderately or poorly differentiated tubular adenocarcinomas. This difference was significant ($P<.05$). Venous, lymphatic, or perineural invasion or a combination thereof was found by histopathologic examination in three (30%) of ten patients in group 1 and in 16 (84%) of 19 patients in group 2. Thus, the presence of vessel invasion differed significantly between groups 1 and 2 ($P<.01$). In group 1, five patients survived five or more years after simple cholecystectomy; three had tumors limited to the gallbladder mucosa and two had tumors limited to the muscular layer. The remaining five patients in group 1 underwent extended cholecystectomy; two had tumors limited to the muscular layer and three had tumors limited to the subserosal layer. Conversely, in group 2, nine died after simple cholecystectomy and ten died after extended cholecystectomy. The former included patients with involvement of the mucosa (one), the muscular layer (three), the subserosal layer (one), and the serosal layer (four). All of the latter ten patients had tumors exposed to the serosa.

Cancer of the Upper Bile Duct.—Three (75%) of four

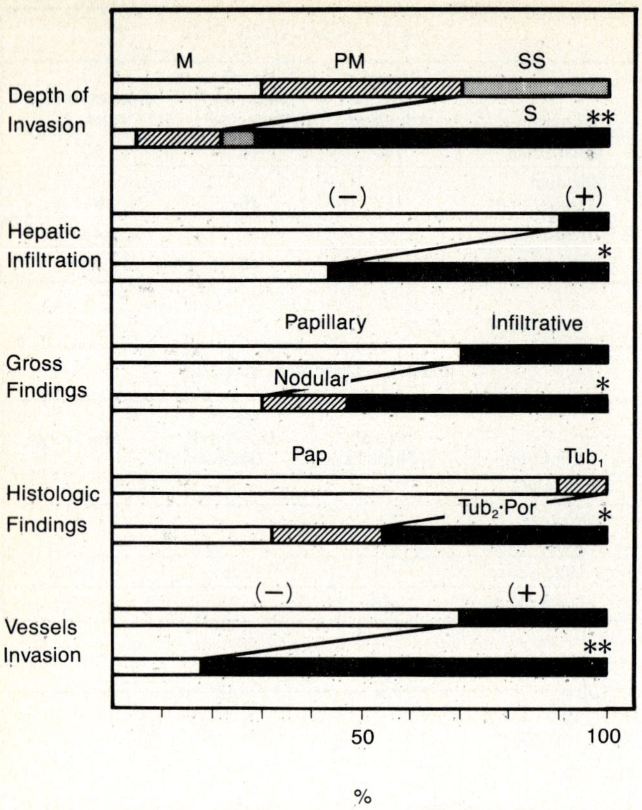

Fig 2.—Prognostic factors in carcinoma of gallbladder. Top column, long-term survivors; bottom column, short-term survivors. Depths of cancer invasion in gallbladder carcinoma were classified into mucosal (M), muscular (PM), subserosal (SS), and serosal (S) involvements. Histologic types of tumor were classified into papillary adenocarcinoma (Pap), well-differentiated tubular adenocarcinoma (Tub_1), moderately differentiated tubular adenocarcinoma (Tub_2), and poorly differentiated tubular adenocarcinoma (Por). Comparison with group of long-term survivors gave following results: single asterisk, $P<.05$; double asterisk, $P<.01$.

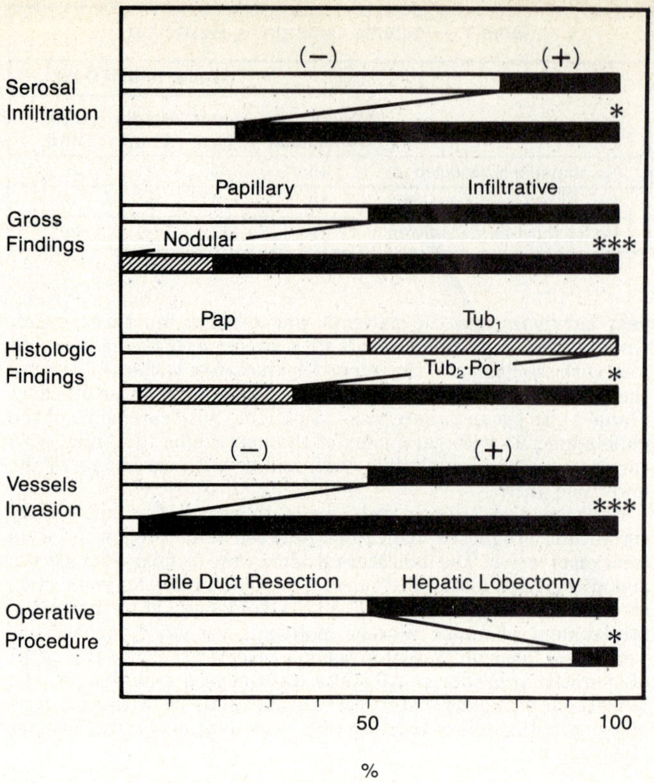

Fig 3.—Prognostic factors in carcinoma of upper bile duct. Top column, long-term survivors; bottom column, short-term survivors. Comparison with group of long-term survivors gave following results: single asterisk, $P<.05$; triple asterisk, $P<.001$.

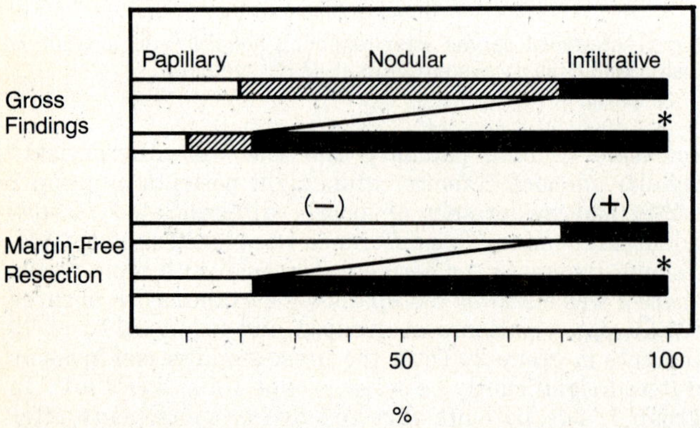

Fig 4.—Prognostic factors in carcinoma of middle bile duct. Top column, long-term survivors; bottom column, short-term survivors. Asterisk indicates comparison with group of long-term survivors, $P<.05$.

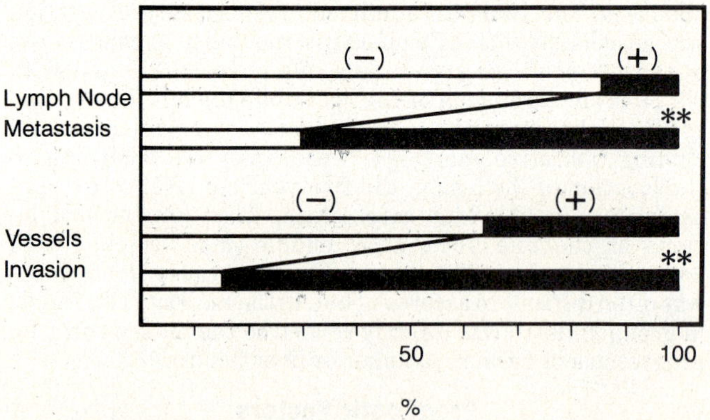

Fig 5.—Prognostic factors in carcinoma of lower bile duct. Top column, long-term survivors; bottom column, short-term survivors. Double asterisk indicates comparison with group of long-term survivors; $P<.01$.

patients in group 1 had no cancer infiltration of the serosa of the bile duct, and two of them had involvement limited only to the fibromuscular layer of the bile duct. In contrast, 18 (78%) of 23 patients in group 2 showed cancer infiltration of the serosa and only five did not (Fig 3). Therefore, in group 2 the presence of serosal infiltration was higher than in group 1 ($P<.05$). With respect to the gross findings, the papillary form was seen in three patients. Two of them, belonging to group 1, survived three or more years and died of diseases not related to the carcinoma; their survival periods after operation were 13 and 5.5 years, respectively. The remaining patient with the papillary tumor was still alive without any sign of recurrence 2.7 years after operation. None of the group 2 patients, in contrast, had papillary-type tumors. Group 2 included 19 patients with infiltrative tumors and four with nodular tumors, and this incidence was significantly different from group 1

($P<.001$). Histologic examination revealed there were two papillary adenocarcinomas and two well-differentiated tubular adenocarcinomas in patients in group 1, whereas 15 patients (65%) in group 2 had moderately or poorly differentiated tubular adenocarcinomas. This difference was statistically significant ($P<.05$). Venous, lymphatic, or perineural invasion or a combination thereof was found in two of four patients from group 1 and in 22 (96%) of 23 patients from group 2 ($P<.001$). Margin-free resection could be achieved in all four group 1 patients; two underwent hepatic lobectomy with bile duct resection and two had bile duct resection alone. Although specimens from ten patients in group 2 showed tumor in their margins, the incidence of tumor-free margins was not significantly different from group 1. However, the use of hepatic lobectomy with bile duct resection was significantly more frequent in group 1 than in group 2, in which 22 (96%) of 23 patients underwent bile duct resection alone ($P<.05$).

Cancer of the Middle Bile Duct.—The gross findings indicated that group 1 consisted of one papillary and three nodular carcinomas (Fig 4). In contrast, seven (78%) of nine tumors in group 2 patients were of the infiltrative type. This incidence was significantly higher in group 2 ($P<.05$). The histologic findings revealed that in all cases, carcinoma of the middle bile duct was either papillary or well-differentiated tubular adenocarcinoma, and no difference in the type of histologic shape could be found between groups 1 and 2. Venous, lymphatic, or perineural invasion or a combination thereof was frequently recognized in both groups: four of five patients in group 1 and seven of nine patients in group 2. A tumor-free margin was achieved in four patients (80%) in group 1, which was a significantly better result than in group 2, in which only two patients (22%) had tumor-free margins ($P<.05$). Four of five patients in group 1 and all patients in group 2 underwent bile duct resection alone. One among the group 1 patients underwent pancreaticoduodenectomy.

Cancer of the Lower Bile Duct.—In cases of lower bile duct cancer, there was a higher incidence of pancreatic, duodenal, and major vessel invasion in 20 patients who died within three years after operation (group 2) than in 14 patients who survived three or more years (group 1), but the difference was not significant. Lymph node metastasis was found in 14 (70%) of 20 patients in group 2 but was found in only two (14%) of 14 patients in group 1 ($P<.01$, Fig 5). Venous, lymphatic, or perineural invasion was significantly less frequent in group 1 than in group 2 (36% [5/14] vs 85% [17/20], respectively; $P<.01$). No significant difference could be demonstrated for various forms of gross and histologic characteristics of tumors between groups 1 and 2.

COMMENT

Cancers of the gallbladder were associated with a poor resectability rate due to extensive local extension to the adjacent vital organs, which precludes curative resection. Many of the cases were far advanced and extensive when diagnosed because the disease does not cause specific symptoms in its early stage. The disease that is often indicated for curative resection is rarely diagnosed preoperatively. Correct preoperative diagnosis of gallbladder carcinoma was made in 15 of 43 patients who underwent resection and in only two who survived five or more years after operation. The conditions of the remaining eight long-term survivors were diagnosed intraoperatively or after the histologic examination of the resected specimens. Bergdahl[5] found that the majority of patients who lived longer than five years were usually those whose carcinoma was diagnosed during microscopic examination of gallbladders removed for presumed benign disease. Our experience suggests that only when carcinoma is localized inside the gallbladder is there a reasonable chance of long-term survival. Among the ten long-term survivors, macroscopically seven had papillary tumors and, histologically, all except one had papillary adenocarcinoma. No patient with moderately or poorly differentiated carcinoma survived longer than five years. All the tumors limited to the mucosa and six of seven tumors limited to the muscularis layer were of the papillary form. In contrast, 11 of 17 tumors spread beyond the serosa were of the infiltrative type. Papillary adenocarcinoma was found in five of seven tumors with mucosal involvement and in six of seven with muscular involvement. Conversely, of 17 tumors spread beyond the gallbladder serosa, seven had moderately or poorly differentiated tubular adenocarcinoma, which was not found in tumors superficial to the subserosa. Appleman et al[6] reported that in 21 patients who lived five or more years, the gross appearance of tumors was papillary in 12, and ten were histologically well-differentiated carcinoma. It can be said that the prognosis of gallbladder carcinoma is highly influenced not only by the depth of invasion but also by the biologic nature of the tumor, ie, gross and histologic characteristics of tumor. Tumors characterized as infiltrative are frequently associated with venous, lymphatic, or perineural invasion. Eighty-four percent of the patients who died less than five years after operation had venous, lymphatic, or perineural invasion. One patient with a mucosa-limited, well-differentiated, tubular adenocarcinoma and three patients with muscular tumor died of recurrence within five years after performance of simple cholecystectomy. Fahim et al[7,8] reported that the only place for simple cholecystectomy is for noninfiltrative, grade 1 papillary adenocarcinoma. An adequate operation for carcinomas superficial to the gallbladder subserosa should be extended cholecystectomy. Ten patients with tumors spread beyond the serosa died within five years after performance of extended cholecystectomy. Thus, for advanced disease that involves the gallbladder serosa, more than extended cholecystectomy should be performed.

The outcome for patients with carcinoma of the upper bile duct is poor because of the low frequency of curative resection owing to the technical difficulties associated with resection and extension of tumor to the liver or to the main vessels. Resectability rates in recent years have ranged from 25% to 47%.[1,3,9,10] The resectability rates in our series were 31% for all admitted patients and 41% for all operated-on patients. Histologically curative resection (tumor-free resection) was obtained in only 16 of 36 patients who underwent resection. In the series of Beazley et al,[9] only four of 16 patients obtained curative resection. As similarly shown in carcinoma of the gallbladder, morphologic features in carcinoma of the upper bile duct are intimately related to the prognosis of the patients. Macroscopically papillary tumors were seen in half of the three-year survivors and papillary or well-differentiated adenocarcinomas were seen in all of the three-year survivors. Two of three papillary carcinomas were limited to the fibromuscular layer of the bile duct and one was limited to the subserosal layer. Kozuka et al[11] reported that of eight patients with papillary carcinoma, seven with carcinoma limited to the fibromuscular layer showed better prognosis than those having carcinoma of other types. They also mentioned that all the noninfiltrating cancers were papillary adenocarcinomas and all the poorly differentiated cancers had spread beyond the fibromuscular layer. No patients with poorly differentiated carcinoma in our series survived two or more years. Thirteen of 14 cases of moderately or poorly differentiated carcinoma were associated with venous, lymphatic, or perineural invasion. In our series of patients undergoing resection, two long-term survivors received hepatic lobectomy combined with resection of the bile duct, while a majority of short-term survivors received bile duct resection alone. Excluding hospital deaths, five patients who underwent hepatic lobectomy showed a two-year survival rate of 75% and 20 patients who underwent bile duct resection alone showed a two-year rate of 30%. If the tumor is infiltrative and localized to the confluence of the hepatic ducts, a hepatic lobectomy along with bile duct resection and hepaticojejunostomy should be chosen. Bile duct resection is preferentially indicated only when the papillary tumor is localized to the common hepatic duct. The longest survivor alive and well 13 years after bile duct resection had papillary tumor limited to the fibromuscular layer.

In cancer of the middle bile duct, both gross findings of tumor and resection margins influenced the prognosis of the patients. Most long-term survivors had papillary or nodular tumors, while most short-term survivors had infiltrative tumors. There are considerable difficulties associated with macroscopic evaluation of the resected margins. In our four patients undergoing resections of the bile duct along with Roux-en-Y hepaticojejunostomy, duodenal margins that seemed to be tumor-free during surgery proved to show tumor invasion on histologic examination. As perineural invasion was highly associated with cancer of the middle bile duct, exposed connective tissues around the major vessels in the hepatoduodenal ligament were apt to show cancer invasion. To eliminate cancerous duodenal margins and to dissect pericholedochal and pancreaticoduodenal lymph nodes completely, pancreaticoduodenectomy is highly recommended except for patients with localized and papillary or nodular tumors.

The lesions of the lower third were associated with the best results of resection among lesions of the bile duct, mostly because of the highest resectability rate. Gibby et al[4] failed to demonstrate an increased survival rate with pancreaticoduodenectomy in their nine patients with cancer of the lower bile duct, while Tompkins et al[1] reported the most significant improvement in survival rate with pancreaticoduodenectomy. It is clear that resection carries the best hope of cure. Fourteen patients who had resections survived three or more years, and the longest survivor in our series was alive 12 years after surgery. The results of the present study revealed that prognosis of the patients undergoing resection of carcinoma of the lower bile duct depends on the presence or abscence of lymph node metastasis and venous, lymphatic, or perineural invasion, prognostic factors that are similar to those of cancer of the head of the pancreas.[12] Neither gross nor histologic features of tumors of the lower bile duct were important factors for long-term prognosis, and this evidence was different from other lesions of the biliary tract system. It can be said that in cancer of the lower bile duct, the infiltration to the surrounding tissues is more important than the biologic characteristics of tumor for defining prognosis. The long-term prognosis for patients who had lymph node metastasis and vessel invasions has not been satisfactory even after pancreaticoduodenectomy.

References

1. Tompkins RK, Thomas D, Wile A, et al: Prognostic factors in bile duct carcinoma: Analysis of 96 cases. *Ann Surg* 1981;194:447-455.
2. Launois B, Campion J-P, Brissot P, et al: Carcinoma of the hepatic hilus: Surgical management and the case for resection. *Ann Surg* 1979;190:151-157.
3. Evander A, Fredlund P, Hoevels J, et al: Evaluation of aggressive surgery for carcinoma of the extrahepatic bile ducts. *Ann Surg* 1980;191:23-29.
4. Gibby DG, Hanks JB, Wanebo HJ, et al: Bile duct carcinoma: Diagnosis and treatment. *Ann Surg* 1985;202:139-144.
5. Bergdahl L: Gallbladder carcinoma first diagnosed at microscopic examination of gallbladders removed for presumed benign disease. *Ann Surg* 1980;191:19-22.
6. Appleman RM, Morlock CG, Dahlin DC, et al: Long-term survival in carcinoma of the gallbladder. *Surg Gynecol Obstet* 1963;117:459-464.
7. Fahim RB, McDonald JR, Richards JC, et al: Carcinoma of the gallbladder: A study of its modes of spread. *Ann Surg* 1962;156:114-124.
8. Fahim RB, Ferris DO, McDonald JR: Carcinoma of the gallbladder: An appraisal of its surgical treatment. *Arch Surg* 1963;86:334-341.
9. Beazley RM, Hadjis N, Benjamin IS, et al: Clinicopathological aspects of high bile duct cancer: Experience with resection and bypass surgical treatment. *Ann Surg* 1984;199:623-634.
10. Cameron JL, Broe P, Zuidema GD: Proximal bile duct tumors: Surgical management with Silastic transhepatic biliary system. *Ann Surg* 1982;196:412-417.
11. Kozuka S, Tsubone M, Hachisuka K: Evolution of carcinoma in the extrahepatic bile ducts. *Cancer* 1984;54:65-72.
12. Matsuno S, Sato T: Surgical treatment for carcinoma of the pancreas: Experience in 272 patients. *Am J Surg* 1986;152:499-503.

Follow-up of Patients With Aspirated Breast Cysts Is Necessary

Hisham Hamed, MD; Andrew Coady, MS; Murid A. Chaudary; Ian S. Fentiman, MD

• A review was conducted of 401 women who presented with breast lumps that proved to be cysts by yielding fluid on aspiration. The aim was to determine the proportion of patients with cancers that masqueraded as cysts and to establish whether short-term follow-up was necessary. After the first visit, six patients had biopsies because of a residual mass or a bloodstained aspirate. Of these patients, two were found to have cancer. After the follow-up visit, 20 further biopsies were carried out for presence of a mass, bloodstained fluid, or recurrent fluid, and two more cancers were diagnosed. Of the four patients with malignancy, only one had an intracystic carcinoma, two had necrotic grade 3 ductal carcinomas, and one had a malignant phyllode tumor. These findings underline the value of a single return visit after cyst aspiration.

(*Arch Surg* 1989;124:253-255)

The appearance of a breast lump may provoke great anxiety in a woman, particularly if the mass appears suddenly. Fortunately, many of these lumps prove to be cysts that disappear after aspiration. Gross cystic disease of the breast was first described by Sir Astley Cooper[1] in 1840, and this condition is the most frequent cause of benign breast lumps. At Guy's Hospital Breast Unit, London, approximately 7% of all new patients are found to have gross breast cysts. Such patients are treated by needle aspiration. Provided that the aspirate is not bloodstained, there is complete resolution of the lump following aspiration, and there are no signs to indicate an underlying malignant neoplasm, they are asked to return to the clinic in six to eight weeks for reexamination. The reason for follow-up is to exclude cyst recurrence and a malignant neoplasm that masquerades as a cyst. This routine review, apart from putting the patient to the inconvenience of another hospital visit, often takes up a considerable amount of the physician's time in a busy clinic. However, with the advent of mammography and its use in symptomatic women aged over 35 years, it is possible that return visits are unnecessary provided that the malignant neoplasm is excluded roentgenographically. Against this, it has been claimed that gross cystic disease of the breast carries a twofold to threefold increase in risk of subsequent carcinoma,[2] and therefore, these patients should be closely monitored. This apparently increased risk was derived from studies in which benign breast disease was considered collectively without detailed histological description. However, recent long-term follow-up studies of patients with histologically characterized benign breast lesions have shown that the risk is only carried by a small proportion of such patients who have atypical epithelial hyperplasia, and this risk is further increased by a positive family history.[3] Attempts have been made to subdivide cysts into flattened and apocrine, based on the biochemical content.[4,5] Dixon et al[6] showed in a retrospective study that 11 of 80 patients with apocrine cysts developed a subsequent malignant neoplasm, as compared with only one of 30 of those patients with flattened cysts. To our knowledge, no prospective study has yet been carried out to assess the significance of cyst type and cancer risk. The aim of this study was to review the experience of a busy breast clinic to determine first the number of cancers that presented as cysts and second whether routine short-term follow-up of those patients with benign cysts was necessary.

PATIENTS AND METHODS

The case records of 401 women with gross cystic disease who attended the Guy's Hospital Breast Unit between 1978 and 1980 were reviewed. The diagnosis of a cyst was made clinically on the basis of a lump that resolved after aspiration. At the time of first presentation, provided that aspiration was successful, bilateral mammography was arranged for those patients aged 35 years or older. The cyst aspirate was not subjected to any routine cytological or biochemical examination. All patients were reviewed six to eight weeks after first attending.

Patients were considered to have had recurrence of a cyst if, at their second visit, there was reaccumulation of fluid at the site of previous aspiration. Those cysts in a different quadrant of the same breast, or in the contralateral breast, were not regarded as recurrences. Repeated aspiration was performed, but a biopsy was carried out if there was a residual palpable mass, if a bloodstained aspirate was obtained, or if there was a recurrence of the cyst at the same site on more than two occasions. Usually, those patients without a recurrence and with normal mammograms were then discharged.

Accepted for publication Dec 3, 1987.

From the Clinical Oncology Unit (Drs Hamed and Fentiman and Mr Chaudary) and Department of Clinical Microscopy (Mr Coady), Guy's Hospital, London.

Reprint requests to Clinical Oncology Unit, Guy's Hospital, London SE1 9RT, England (Dr Fentiman).

Table 1.—Features at First Presentation With Breast Cyst	
Feature	**Mean**
Age, y	
Mean	45.7
Range	14-72
No. of patients	
Premenopausal	344
Postmenopausal	19
Previous hysterectomy	38
Side of cyst appearance	
R	153
L	215
Bilateral	33
Site of cyst	
Medial	64
Central	95
Lateral	181
Multiple	61

RESULTS

Clinical Features

The clinical features of the patients are shown in Table 1. Three hundred forty-four women (86%) were premenopausal. Thirty-eight women (9.5%) had had a previous hysterectomy, and 19 (4.5%) were postmenopausal (last period more than six months before the visit). It is interesting that of those patients with unilateral cysts, 153 (42%) were right sided, and 215 (58%) were left sided which mirrors the left-sided predilection of breast cancers. Cysts were single in 340 patients (85%) and multiple in 61 patients (15%). The clinical findings after aspiration were as follows:

Finding	No. of Patients
Complete resolution	395
Residual mass and bloodstained aspirate	2
Residual mass	3
Bloodstained aspirate	1

One patient had bloodstained fluid aspirated but without a residual mass. Five patients had a residual mass, and two of these patients also had bloodstained aspirates. A biopsy was performed in all six of these patients with signs that were suggestive of a malignant neoplasm, and a histological diagnosis of carcinoma was made in two patients, both of whom had a residual mass and bloody aspirate. The clinical findings on review six to eight weeks later are shown as follows:

Finding	No. of Patients
No abnormality	315
Mass at site of previous cyst	20
Recurrent cyst	44
New cyst	22

Patients with a mass at the original site of cyst aspiration that did not disappear on the second attempted aspiration are given separately in the above tabulation. Those patients with a mass that was at the site of the original cyst and disappeared after a second aspiration were described as having recurrent cysts. As a result of the finding of recurrence of the cyst on one or more occasions or aspiration of bloodstained fluid or a mass at the site of aspiration, 20 further biopsies were performed. Among these, carcinoma was diagnosed histologically in a further two patients, in both of whom there was a mass at the site of the aspiration. One hundred fifty-five patients had mammography. No biopsies were performed because of mammographic abnormalities alone. A possible explanation was because the majority of these patients were premenopausal with dense breast tissue that could have masked a mass, microcalcification, or trabecular distortion.

Table 2.—Clinical Features of Patients With Breast Cancer Presenting With Cysts			
Patient/ Age, y	Clinical Finding: 1st Visit	Clinical Finding: 2nd Visit	Histological Finding
1/23	Lump and bloody aspirate	...	Necrotic ductal grade 3
2/66	Lump and bloody aspirate	...	Phyllode tumor
3/72	Straw-colored fluid, no residual lump	3-cm-diameter mass	Intracystic papillary carcinoma
4/69	Clear fluid, no residual mass	7-cm-diameter mass	Necrotic grade 3

Table 3.—Histological Findings in 21 Benign Breast Biopsy Specimens	
Histological Finding	**No. of Specimens**
Large Cyst, Total	**18**
Cyst lining	
Apocrine	5
Flat	7
None	6
Small cysts	17
Apocrine metaplasia	18
Sclerosing adenosis	5
Radial scar	1
Ductal Epithelial Hyperplasia, Total	**12**
Mild	6
Moderate	5
Marked	1
Fibroadenoma	1

Histological Findings

The histological sections from 25 of the 26 patients in whom biopsy specimens were obtained were reviewed, but the slides could not be traced for one patient. (A median of two blocks was taken per case, with a range of one to eight blocks.) Four patients had malignant lesions, and three of these lesions were grossly cystic. One lesion was an intracystic papillary carcinoma, the second lesion was a centrally necrotic grade 3 infiltrating ductal carcinoma, and the third lesion was a malignant phyllode tumor with areas of cystic degeneration. The remaining patient had a grade 3 infiltrating ductal carcinoma that showed extensive necrosis on histological examination, although it was not described as being cystic on gross examination. The clinical features of the patients with biopsy-proved carcinoma are given in Table 2.

The histological features of the 21 benign breast biopsy specimens are shown in Table 3. A large cyst was noted in 13 biopsy specimens, and in five further specimens, three of which had no gross description, an obvious large cyst was identified in the section. Five of the cysts were lined by apocrine epithelium and seven with a flattened epithelium. In many cases, only a small fragment of the epithelium was identified, with the remaining cysts being lined by fibrous tissue without an epithelial lining. In six cases, no lining was demonstrable. There was increased fibrous tissue in the wall of eight of the large cysts, and this was usually accompanied by a chronic inflammatory cell reaction. Two of the three cases in which large cysts were absent contained microcysts on histological examination. The remaining case showed occasional mildly dilated cuts but no true cyst. Microscopic cysts were present in all but three of the cases in which a macroscopic cyst was identified, and apocrine metaplasia was present in surrounding tissue in all but two of the cases with a large cyst. Ductal epithelial hyperplasia was present in 12 cases, but no examples of atypical hyperplasia of either the ductal or lobular type were seen.

COMMENT

In this study, only 1% of patients presenting with a cystic lump were found eventually to have an underlying malignant neoplasm, and this is consistent with the incidence reported by others.[7-9] Of the entire group of patients, 147 (37%) were followed up for more than one year, 129 (32%) were followed up for more than three years, and 55 (14%) were followed up for more than five years; none of these patients were known to have developed breast cancer. Although a small group of these women were regularly followed up during a long period of time, most return visits were self-referrals as a result of the development of new problems.

A bloody aspirate is not diagnostic of malignant neoplasm as it may be the result of an inadvertent puncture of a blood vessel at the time of aspiration. Similarly, cyst recurrence does not usually imply that there is any underlying carcinoma and is usually due to incomplete aspiration at the first visit. When clinical signs that are thought to be suggestive of a malignant neoplasm were examined in the present study, it was found that the combination of a residual mass and a bloody aspirate were the strongest indicators of underlying cancers. It is of interest that three of the four patients with cystic carcinomas were aged over 60 years.

The main reason for conducting this study was to determine the necessity for short-term follow-up. The results indicate that a review of these patients after six to eight weeks was necessary to detect an underlying malignant neoplasm that was not apparent at the first visit, with one half of the cancers being diagnosed after a biopsy resulting from the second examination.

Provided that the previously mentioned criteria for biopsy are adhered to, a policy of cyst aspiration is safe. However, to reduce the likelihood of overlooking a cystic cancer at the first visit, at least one subsequent reexamination of the breast is recommended after six to eight weeks. Any routine follow-up after this period would appear not to be essential in those patients without recurrence and with normal mammograms. Such a policy would certainly reduce the cost of health care and its burden to the patient. On the second visit to the clinic, the patient can be instructed in self-examination and told to come back if a lump should develop. To minimize patient anxiety, it is helpful to have an open-door policy that affords the patient ready access to the surgeon.

References

1. Cooper AP: *Illustrations of the Diseases of the Breast: I.* New York, Longman Inc, 1829.
2. Haagensen CD: *Diseases of the Breast.* Philadelphia, WB Saunders Co, 1971.
3. Dupont WD, Page DC: Risk factors for breast cancer in women with proliferative breast disease. *N Engl J Med* 1983;312:146-151.
4. Dixon JM, Scott WN, Miller WR: Natural history of cystic disease: The importance of cyst type. *Br J Surg* 1985;72:190-192.
5. Dixon JM, Miller WR, Scott WN, et al: The morphological basis of human breast cyst populations. *Br J Surg* 1983;70:604-606.
6. Dixon JM, Lunsden AD, Miller WR: The relationship of cyst type to risk factors of breast cancer and the subsequent development of breast cancer in patients with breast cystic disease. *Eur J Cancer Clin Oncol* 1985;21:1047-1050.
7. Devitt JE, Barr JR: The clinical recognition of cystic carcinoma of the breast. *Surg Gynecol Obstet* 1984;159:130-132.
8. Pain RA, Jackson DB: Cystic tumours of the breast. *Ann R Coll Surg Engl* 1980;62:228-229.
9. Czernobilsky B: Intracystic carcinoma of the female breast. *Surg Gynecol Obstet* 1967;124:93-98.

Editorial Comment

This report from a well-recognized breast clinic in England asks if all patients with successfully aspirated, nonsuspicious breast cysts should be *routinely* reexamined in six to eight weeks, and it concludes that they should be. This conclusion is based on the fact that of the 401 patients in the series, one woman aged 72 years had a 3-cm intracystic papillary carcinoma, and another woman aged 69 years had a 7-cm necrotic grade 3 carcinoma that was undiscovered at the first aspiration. The mammographic status of these patients is not known, but their age is highly significant as any distinct cystic (or solid) mass must be viewed with substantial suspicion in all women older than 60 years. It can be conjectured, however, that a combination of self-examination, more accurate initial aspiration, and detailed mammography may well have obviated the subsequent unpleasant surprises experienced by these two patients. Consequently, the data provided do not make an unequivocal case for the hypothesis advanced.

A second visit by the patient three to eight weeks after aspiration is certainly the conventional wisdom and perhaps the safest course to follow as long as the medicolegal atmosphere is as highly charged as it is in the United States. It is a sad fact that lawyers increasingly drive clinical decisions. When the clinical problem is viewed more objectively, however, the concept that routine reexamination is the standard of practice may be vigorously challenged, particularly in a "resource-sensitive" society. Time lost from work, the need often to travel long distances, the high sensitivity of the modern mammogram, the cost of the second visit, and the medical intelligence of many of our patients who are well able to determine the status of their own breasts may justify a telephonic report that confirms the complete regression of the cystic area in question when clear nonsanguineous fluid has been aspirated initially. This is especially true in those patients under the age of 50 years who constitute the significant majority of patients with cysts.

Two or three decades ago, depending on the region of the world, the concept of aspiration of cysts in the breast was an anathema to a great segment of surgeons. Today, the technique and the principles that underpin aspiration are universally accepted. As confidence increased, routine cytological examination of the cyst fluid was advocated as a safety net. The value of this approach has now been disproved. Attitudes change and given the new technology, the increased sophistication of our patients with their desire to share in their own care, and the drive to reduce the cost of medical care, routine reexamination at six weeks of premenopausal patients with successfully aspirated, nonsanguineous cysts and nonsuspicious mammograms is probably unnecessary *as a routine* in this large group of patients.

Alexander J. Walt, MB, ChB
Detroit

Treatment of Peritoneal Mesothelioma

To the Editor.—The discussion of management of peritoneal mesothelioma by Plaus[1] is good but incomplete. The behavior of these neoplasms is highly variable in the degree of aggressiveness and the physician risks adding to morbidity by overtreating. The use of a peritoneovenous shunt is not without risk, and with it or without it other approaches may be useful.

In the presence of malignant ascites, copious irrigation of the peritoneal cavity with 5% dextrose in water (DW) at laparotomy is essential. The mucopolysaccharide responsible for the viscosity of malignant ascites (as with pseudomyxoma peritonei) is miscible in 5% DW. Viable tumor cells persist in a third-space haven when this is not done. Pulmonary capillary occlusion and coagulopathies have been reported with peritoneovenous shunts.

The mesothelium is also particularly sensitive to hyperthermia. (We use 5% DW heated to 50°C for a three-minute wash after the wash with 5% DW at body temperature and just before closure.) Finally, whenever intracavitary chemotherapy is administered, each administration must be given diluted to 2000 mL (preferably, 5% DW). This volume is necessary to ensure uniform exposure of the peritoneum to the drug, avoiding streaming and pooling.[2]

JOHN S. SPRATT, MD
Louisville

1. Plaus WJ: Peritoneal mesothelioma. *Arch Surg* 1988;123:763-766.
2. Spratt JS, Edwards M, Kubota T, et al: Peritoneal carcinomatosis: Anatomy, physiology, diagnosis, management. *Curr Probl Cancer* 1986;10:555-584.

Breast Cancer Diagnosis in the Augmented Patient

To the Editor.—Silverstein et al[1] report that in their clinic, breast cancers diagnosed in women with augmentation mammoplasties were more advanced than in nonaugmented patients. They imply that the delay in diagnosis is due to the implant obscuring and compressing the breast, thus reducing the effectiveness of mammography. In light of published evidence that they did not discuss, and in light of potentially serious design flaws in their study, their data do not support their conclusions and should be considered with great skepticism.

Specialty clinics in large urban areas are exceptionally vulnerable to referral bias that can produce overestimations or underestimations of associations. No referral information is provided, and the fact that none of the augmented patients presented until their masses had been palpable for up to two years (mean, 123 days) suggests that the behavior of these patients may be much different from that of the nonaugmented patients.

The ages of the two groups differ substantially, and both the rate of disease progression and screening behavior are likely to be associated with age. While the authors eliminated the nonaugmented patients over age 58 years as an *age adjustment* (an uncustomary usage of the term), they offer no evidence that the age distributions are similar other than comparing means.

We have published a retrospective cohort study[2] of the relationship between breast cancer and augmentation mammoplasty in 3111 patients. Although the authors cite our reference as evidence that implants do not increase cancer risk, they ignore our findings in the relatively early stage of diagnosis when compared with population-based Los Angeles County data. We are now in the process of adding five more years of information and, thus far, have identified 17 breast cancers in this cohort. The stages at detection are as follows: in situ, two; local, eight; regional spread, four; distant spread, two; and unknown, one. The following tabulation illustrates that the breast cancer stage distribution at diagnosis was not different for patients with implants when compared with 5876 women with breast cancer, aged 45 to 54 years and diagnosed between 1972 and 1985:

	All Patients in Los Angeles County, %	Implant Patients in Los Angeles County, %
In situ	7.1	12.5
Local	50.2	50.0
Nonlocal	42.7	37.5

Of the nine cancers detected in patients in the published report (1972-1981), seven were self-discovered as a mass. No detection information is available for the other two. Of the eight cancers diagnosed in patients between 1982 and 1986, three were discovered by routine mammography, and five presented as a mass. Thus, we conclude that breast cancer diagnosis in augmented patients is comparable with the nonaugmented population.

Modern mammography offers the best opportunity for early detection of breast cancer. Film quality in the augmented patient can be comparable with that of the normal breast if one uses the adjustment in technique described by Eklund,[3] supplemented on occasion by some extra tangential views. The pictured mammograms (Figure) were taken by the same tech-

Left, Mammogram taken utilizing conventional technique. Right, Mammogram taken utilizing Eklund's modification (reversed for contrast).

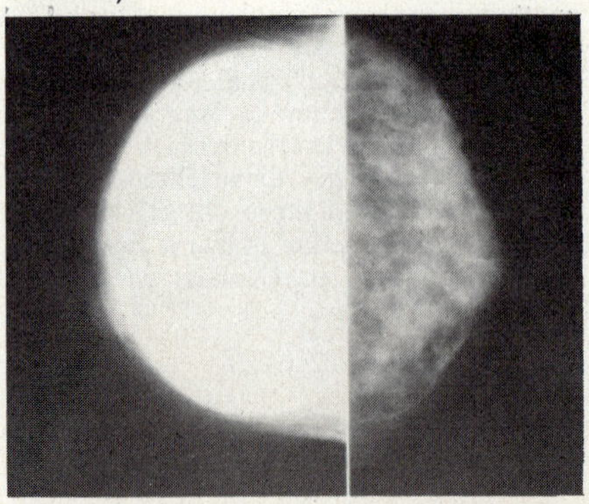

nician on the same patient with the same equipment five minutes apart. The picture on the left utilized conventional technique, and the one on the right (reversed for contrast), Eklund's modification. One should not ignore, of course, the additional detection modalities of self-inspection and regular physical examination by a physician familiar with the implanted breast.

Considering the available evidence to date, we are concerned that this report may foster undue concern among women with breast implants, and fear that it could in fact lead these patients to the unfortunate belief that mammography is of no value. The major cause of delayed detection of cancer in all patients remains ignorance, neglect, denial, and complacency. In an article making several procedural recommendations, we believe a balanced and critical discussion of the evidence should have been presented.

Garry S. Brody, MD
Dennis M. Deapen, DrPH
Downey, Calif

The mammograms were provided through the courtesy of Tom W. Staple, MD, Memorial Breast Evaluation Center, Long Beach, Calif.

1. Silverstein MJ, Handel N, Gamagami P, et al: Breast cancer in women after augmentation mammoplasty. *Arch Surg* 1988;123:681-685.
2. Deapen DM, Pike MC, Casagrande JT, et al: The relationship between breast cancer and augmentation mammoplasty: An epidemiologic study. *Plast Reconstr Surg* 1986;77:361-367.
3. Eklund GW, Busby RC, Miller SH, et al: Improved imaging of the augmented breast. *AJR* 1988;151:469-473.

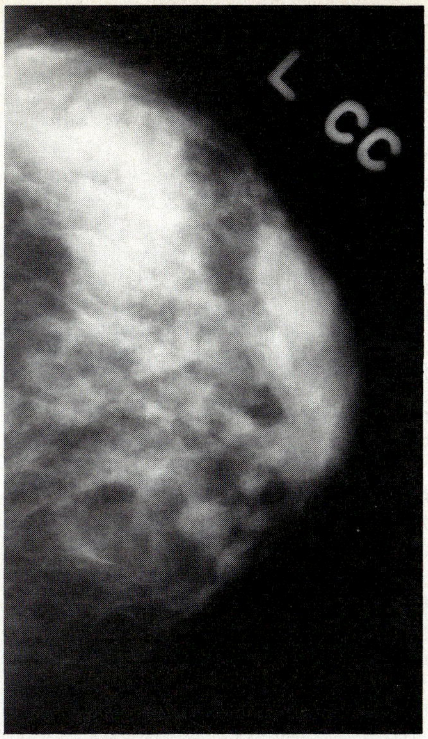

Fig 1.—Preaugmentation mammogram (craniocaudal view) in 30-year-old woman with average-sized breasts reveals 166 cm² of visualizable breast tissue.

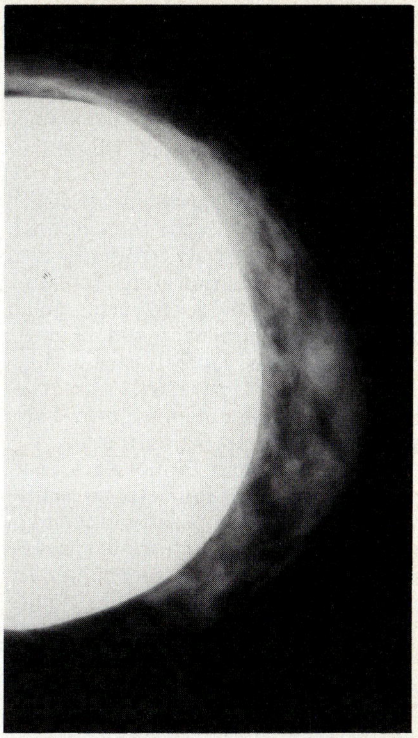

Fig 2.—Postaugmentation mammogram using standard (implant compression) technique reveals 61 cm² of visualizable breast tissue, a 63% reduction. The silicone-gel–filled implant is in subglandular (prepectoral) position.

In Reply.—My colleagues and I wish to thank Drs Brody and Deapen for their letter and continued interest in our article.

The typical American woman with breast cancer presents with a palpable lesion with an average diameter of 2.7 cm, with symptoms that have persisted approximately one to three months, and with metastases to axillary nodes 40% of the time. Our group of previously augmented patients with breast cancer and their group both have patients who are quite similar to this average patient with breast cancer. Neither of the groups' patients have early breast cancer by current standards.

Drs Brody and Deapen have 17 previously augmented patients, 38% of whom had positive nodes; our article presented 20 patients, 65% of whom had positive nodes (we currently have 27 patients, 56% of whom had metastases to axillary nodes at the time of presentation). The Los Angeles County registry has 5876 similarly aged, nonaugmented patients, 43% of whom had positive nodes. All of these patients are representative of average breast cancer; therein lies the problem: we should not be satisfied finding average breast cancer.

Early and more curable breast cancers are found by mammography alone. Microcalcifications, asymmetries, architectural distortions, tiny stellate masses, etc, are the only findings, and they are roentgenographic findings. There are no physical findings. There is no palpable lesion. Biopsy must be done using needle, dye, or hooked-wire–directed techniques. Breast cancer diagnosed this way represents the state of the art. Five-year survival rates for this type of patient are in excess of 90% to 95%, compared with 50% to 70% for patients presenting with palpable lesions. Nodal positivity using state-of-the-art screening mammography has been reported to be as low as 4%.[1] Any procedure that interferes with our ability to radiographically visualize breast tissue interferes with our ability to find and diagnose these early nonpalpable lesions. Such a procedure should be challenged.

Hayes and colleagues[2] have published a warning for plastic surgeons and their augmented patients. They

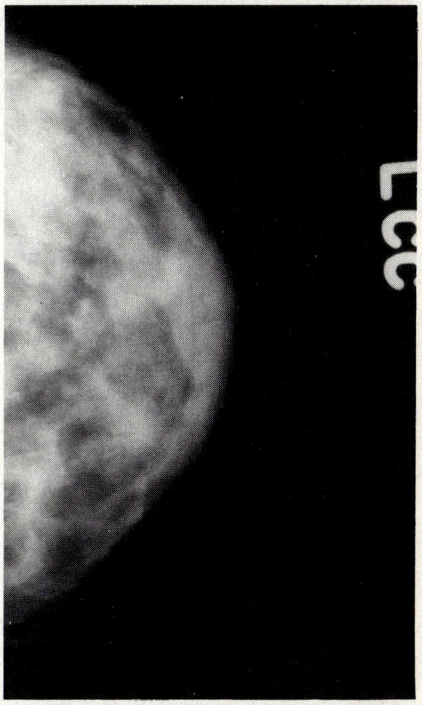

Fig 3.—Postaugmentation mammogram using Eklund (implant displacement) technique reveals 90 cm² of visualizable breast tissue, an improvement when compared with implant compression technique, but more importantly, a continued reduction of 46% when compared with preaugmentation view.

report that 22% to 83% of visualizable breast tissue is obscured by augmentation mammoplasty. Hayes et al state that "this wide variation casts serious doubt on the reliability of routine film-screen mammography in these patients."

Drs Brody and Deapen submit mammograms taken with the conventional (implant compression) technique and Eklund's modification (implant displacement) as evidence that good mammograms can be taken in augmented patients. Unfortunately, they omit the most important film: the preaugmentation mammogram. We are currently completing a study involving more than 50 patients that compares the preaugmentation mammogram with postoperative mammograms done using both the compression and displacement technique. In subglandular (prepectoral) augmented patients, the compression technique obscures an average of 47% (range, 15% to 87%) of visualizable breast tissue. The displacement technique, while better, continues to obscure an average of 31% of visualizable breast tissue (Figs 1 through 3). In addition, as the capsular scar increases, the displacement technique becomes less effective.

When the implant is placed submuscularly and the displacement technique is used, there is no significant loss in visualized square surface area. However, all augmented patients, regardless of the position of the implant, develop some degree of postoperative scarring, which results in various degrees of parenchymal distortion and makes mammographic interpretation more difficult. We caution plastic surgeons not to delude themselves into believing that postaugmentation mammography is as accurate as preaugmentation mammography.

There is nothing wrong with augmentation mammoplasty for properly informed patients. It is, however, the plastic surgeon's duty to inform patients that state-of-the-art mammography, which is the current "gold standard" for early breast cancer diagnosis, will no longer be possible after augmentation. Patients who are at high risk for the development of breast cancer should be discouraged from undergoing augmentation mammoplasty.

We must confront one additional criticism, that is, the mean delay of 123 days in our patients between the first onset of symptoms and diagnosis. We should have reported the median delay, which was 21 days. The elongated average delays occurred because of four patients whose symptoms persisted one to two years. Three of these patients had been reassured by their plastic surgeons that the lump they were feeling was capsular scarring.

Melvin J. Silverstein, MD
Van Nuys, Calif

1. Silverstein MJ, Gamagami P, Rosser RJ, et al: Hooked-wire–directed breast biopsy and overpenetrated mammography. *Cancer* 1987;59:715-722.

2. Hayes H, Vandergrift J, Diner WC: Mammography and breast implants. *Plast Reconstr Surg* 1988;82:1-8.

Books

Medicine: Preserving the Passion, by Phil R. Manning and Lois DeBakey, New York, Springer-Verlag NY Inc, 1987.

There is some obfuscation associated with the title of this monograph, and the authors use a somewhat compromising approach to data procurement. The title suggests that here is an evangelistic presentation intended to get the juices flowing and rekindle our excitement for our chosen profession. There is also the anticipation that Dr Manning will teach us how to continue learning and Dr DeBakey will focus on how to improve our writing skills.

The book is a well-constructed collection of anecdotal observations obtained by interviews from recognized leaders in medicine. These are supplemented by quotations from notables such as Samuel Johnson ("Curiosity is, in great and generous minds, the first passion and the last") and Seneca ("Men learn while they teach").

There is a collection of "personal essays" produced by 11 accomplished physicians and educators directed at describing the various techniques of continued learning these individuals have developed over the years that have contributed to their success. While some of the methods are general, such as working hard and using time efficiently, others are very specific. As an editor of the *Year Book of Medicine*, for example, Dr Greenberger at the Kansas University School of Medicine, Kansas City, receives 10 000 articles a year to review for possible inclusion in the *Year Book*, providing an obvious continuing education. Accompanying each personal commentary are laudatory phrases and statements concerning the commentators from recognizable peers, indicating the strength of the commentators' credentials.

There is a serious imbalance between information and photographs in this book. The value or purpose of the plethora of photographs of the people being quoted is unclear. Several individuals are quoted in a single brief phrase or sentence, yet there is a full-page photograph. One feels as if one has purchased a photo album.

The book is replete with useful information directed at stimulating and helping physicians improve their self-education patterns. Two chapters deal with the educational characteristics of female physicians and the role of physicians' families. Both chapters are directed at the overall aspects of women as physicians and at the interactions of the physicians with their families and, of course, provide useful information.

The final chapter, which discusses computers in continuing medical education, is excellent and should stimulate all of us to dust off our personal computers and get going.

I hope that Drs Manning and DeBakey will now write about their ideas on continuing to learn and write.

Donald L. Kaminski, MD
St Louis

Abdominal Wound Dehiscence, by Galen V. Poole, Jr, 129 pp, Potts Point, Australia, MacDonald Futura, 1987.

Few complications in general surgery are as distressing for the patient or as embarrassing for the surgeon as an abdominal wound dehiscence. The responsibility for most of these mishaps rests with the surgeon, as dehiscence usually occurs before significant fascial healing has begun. The patient pays the price when meticulous technique is exercised during the intra-abdominal portion of the operation but forgotten when the abdominal wall is closed.

In this monograph, Poole discusses the various methods of wound closure, the process of wound healing, and the causes of wound failure.

The author begins with a brief introduction on wound healing. The detail of this preface is sufficient only to make a valid point: delayed or failed wound healing has very little to do with most dehiscences, and faulty surgical technique is usually the culprit.

Additional insights are then provided by a short review of the epidemiology of dehiscence. Despite innumerable studies on wound closure, the rate of dehiscence following abdominal surgery and its associated mortality remain stable at 0.65% and 20%, respectively. The author points out that the incidence of dehiscence is often underestimated by clinicians because they do not follow up their patients long enough; an early, small fascial separation may not be detected until the later appearance of an incisional hernia.

The monograph then covers the various factors that have been associated with retarded wound healing. Despite the evidence that malnutrition, age, corticosteroid and chemotherapeutic therapies, and other factors do delay wound healing, there is little evidence that any of them promote dehiscence. This is to be expected, as most dehiscences occur early after surgery when little wound healing has taken place.

The factors that most directly affect a wound, ie, surgical technique and suture material, are then discussed in some detail. Experienced surgeons will be familiar with the highlights of this chapter. For example, wound length, position, and direction have little effect on dehiscence as long as the fascial closure is accomplished with adequate bites, minimal tension, and stout suture (interrupted, running, slowly absorbable, or nonabsorbable).

The text then closes with a chapter on the clinical diagnosis of dehiscence and its management.

The serious student of wound healing will be disappointed with this monograph's brevity, the less-than-exhaustive bibliography, and the omission of topics such as the use of prosthetic materials in wound closure. However, the book will provide the medical student and surgical house officer with a sound understanding of dehiscence and its prevention. It will also be an enjoyable review for the experienced surgeon. We as surgeons can all benefit from an occasional reminder that the abdominal wall should be treated with all the respect we show the intra-abdominal organs.

William J. Plaus, MD
Denver

The Art of Surgical Technique, by Milton T. Edgerton, 218 pp, with illus, $41.50, Baltimore, Williams & Wilkins, 1988.

Despite two forewords, a preface, and an introduction, the objective of this book is unclear. The author is a highly respected elder statesman of plastic surgery, and this summary of principles of technique is clearly a labor of love by a thoughtful scholar and gentleman.

The book is comparable in several ways with Dr Ralph Millard's books on plastic surgery, which also contain a mixture of anecdotes, tradition, scientific data, pearls of wisdom, and personal opinions. *The Art of Surgical Technique* is a book to be enjoyed by all of us and one to be studied by medical students considering surgery, surgical residents, surgical assistants, scrub nurses, and technicians. Practicing surgeons, and specifically plastic surgeons, will profit by seeing much of what they do instinctively spelled out, as well as by learning a few new things.

Although it is worth understanding one's professional roots, in this book there is perhaps too much emphasis on outdated instruments and techniques such as freehand skin grafting knives and drum dermatomes. Even Barton dressings for jaw fractures are mentioned. Some modern techniques and materials, such as skin staples, lasers, and monofilament absorbable suture, are omitted. Surgical dogma inserted without scientific support is at least worthy of an opposing viewpoint. Use of antibiotic irrigation and topical thrombotic agents are two examples. Holding suture needles at the end and using drains to prevent hematomas are two other controversial techniques.

Dr Edgerton admits his biases, and I could imagine my knuckles being rapped if I violated them as a surgical resident. The "suction cannula . . . is an instrument of the devil"; "a quiet operating room improves the quality of surgery"; "sponging . . . is often done badly by surgeons or their assistants." Such aphorisms are instructive and add charm.

I applaud the emphasis on the nearly lost arts of surgical assisting and scrub nursing. Hand signals for silent passing of instruments are described in detail. Such gentlemanly concern with the technique of dignified and efficient interaction between the surgeon and his or her assistants makes this a unique contribution. There is also an excellent section on the art (and underlying science) of dressings and wound care. As anticipated from a surgeon nurtured in the halstedian tradition, atraumatic handling of tissues is repeatedly emphasized.

This is not a long book and, in common with many modern surgical texts, it contains much blank space and repeated figures, although the illustrations are very nicely done. *The Art of Surgical Technique* can be read and enjoyed in a night or two and will make a valued gift to a special resident or assistant, as well as contributing to the body of surgical literature.

Scott L. Replogle, MD
Denver

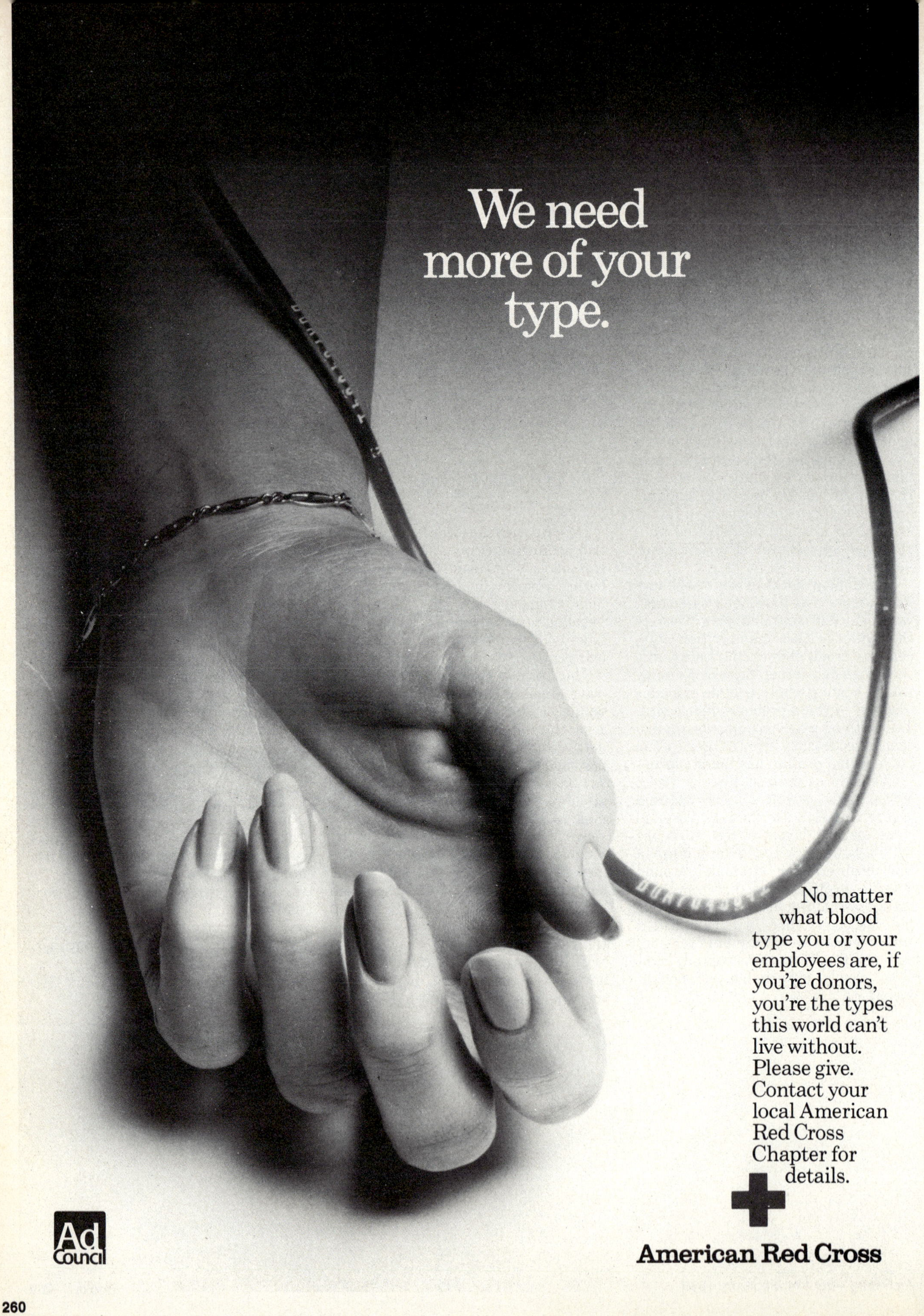
We need more of your type.
No matter what blood type you or your employees are, if you're donors, you're the types this world can't live without. Please give. Contact your local American Red Cross Chapter for details.
Ad Council
American Red Cross

Evaluation of Prostacyclin Production by Human Gallbladder

Donald L. Kaminski, MD; Y. G. Deshpande, MS; Scott Westfall, MD; David Herbold, MD

• The prostanoids have been demonstrated to be involved in gallbladder physiology and disease. In previous reports, prostaglandin E (PGE) compounds were found to be increased in inflamed human gallbladders. Prostaglandin synthetase inhibition decreased PGE formation by human gallbladders; however, the relief of symptoms of cholecystitis did not correlate well with the decrease in PGE formation. This suggested that other prostanoids may be involved in cholecystitis. The purpose of this study was to evaluate the production of the proinflammatory arachidonic acid metabolite prostacyclin by gallbladders from patients with calculous cholecystitis. The formation of PGE and 6-ketoprostaglandin $F_{1\alpha}$ (6-keto-$PGF_{1\alpha}$), the stable metabolite of prostacyclin, in normal human gallbladder mucosal cells and muscle tissue was compared with that produced by diseased mucosal cells and muscle tissue. Normal human gallbladders produced small amounts of 6-keto-$PGF_{1\alpha}$, and no differences in formation rates were evident when muscle tissue was compared with mucosal cells. Diseased gallbladders produced significantly greater amounts of 6-keto-$PGF_{1\alpha}$ than did normal gallbladders, and diseased gallbladder muscle produced approximately four times greater amounts of 6-keto-$PGF_{1\alpha}$ than did diseased gallbladder mucosa. Prostacyclin formation is increased in diseased human gallbladders and may be an important mediator of the inflammatory changes of cholecystitis.

(*Arch Surg* 1989;124:277-280)

Arachidonic acid metabolites are recognized as having an important role in inflammatory processes involving the liver[1] and biliary tract[2] and possibly as being involved in gallstone formation.[3] Prostaglandin synthetase inhibitors have been found to be effective in the treatment of the pain of cholecystitis.[4]

In a previous report, the cyclo-oxygenase inhibitor ibuprofen relieved the pain of gallbladder disease. However, the inhibition of prostaglandin E (PGE) production did not correlate well with relief of pain.[4] This suggested that other prostanoids may be involved in the production of the pain and the inflammatory response associated with cholecystitis. Prostacyclin is an arachidonic acid derivative present in most tissues that inhibits platelet aggregation and is a vasodilator substance. Prostacyclin has considerable proinflammatory effects and, in most systems, is more potent than are the PGE compounds.[5]

The purpose of the present study was to evaluate prostacyclin production by human gallbladder tissue, by measuring the stable metabolite of prostacyclin, 6-keto-prostaglandin ($PGF_{1\alpha}$).[6] We intended to compare 6-keto-$PGF_{1\alpha}$ levels in normal gallbladders with those found in diseased gallbladders with various degrees of inflammation.

SUBJECTS AND METHODS

Twenty-four patients underwent cholecystectomy, with measurement of the amount of PGE and 6-keto-$PGF_{1\alpha}$ formed by gallbladder tissue. Four male and two female patients (54 ± 7 years of age [mean ± SD]) had no gallbladder symptoms or known biliary tract disease and underwent incidental cholecystectomy at the time of hepatic resection or insertion of hepatic artery catheters for regional chemotherapy to treat hepatic colorectal cancer metastases. These gallbladders were used to determine normal values.

Eighteen patients, six men and 12 women (47 ± 5 years of age), had acute or chronic calculous cholecystitis and underwent cholecystectomy for gallbladder disease.

Informed consent to perform the experiment was obtained from the patients, and the study was approved by the Institutional Review Board for Human Experimentation, St Louis University Medical Center. None of the patients had used cyclo-oxygenase or lipo-oxygenase inhibitors, including aspirin, before the operation.

Immediately following removal of the gallbladder, it was opened and the fluid contained collected on ice for measurement of its protein content by the method of Bradford.[7] The gallbladder was then washed in iced saline solution and the mucosal surface inspected by a pathologist. If no mucosal tumors were present, two 1 × 2-cm full-thickness strips were excised. One was placed in 4% formaldehyde solution for histologic evaluation. The other strip was placed in ice-cold 50-mmol/L TRIS hydrochloride buffer, pH 7.0, containing 2.5 mmol/L of edetic acid, homogenized and used for measurement of β-glucuronidase activity.[8] The activity of the enzyme is reported as units per milligram of homogenate protein. The remainder of the gallbladder was placed in iced tissue culture medium. Utilizing techniques described previously,[4] the gallbladders underwent immediate separation of mucosal cells from muscle tissue. An ice-cold solution of 0.25 mol/L of sodium chloride and 2.5 mmol/L of edetic acid, pH 7.5, was injected into the submucosa with a 25-gauge needle. The gallbladder was soaked in the same ice-cold medium for five minutes and shaken to release

Accepted for publication March 15, 1988.

From the Department of Surgery, St Louis University Medical Center.

Reprint requests to Department of Surgery, St Louis University Medical Center, 1325 S Grand Blvd, St Louis, MO 63104 (Dr Kaminski).

Table 1.—Comparison of Levels of 6-Keto-PGF$_{1\alpha}$ and PGE in Gallbladder Muscle Tissue and Mucosal Cells in Tissue Culture Medium and Homogenates*

	6-Keto-PGF$_{1\alpha}$, pg/mg of Protein	PGE, pg/mg of Protein
Mucosal cells		
Medium	128±39	733±317
Homogenate	198±61	1594±469
Muscle tissue		
Medium	661±316	1599±377
Homogenate	1009±453	1957±507

*6-Keto-PGF$_{1\alpha}$ indicates 6-ketoprostaglandin F$_{1\alpha}$; PGE, prostaglandin E. Each tissue culture medium value is the mean±SEM of 24 values obtained from the mean of three hourly samples from 24 gallbladders. Each homogenate value is the mean±SEM of 24 values.

Table 2.—6-Keto-PGF$_{1\alpha}$ and PGE Production by Normal and Diseased Human Gallbladders*

	Normal (n=6)	Diseased (n=18)
β-Glucuronidase, U/mg of protein	49±5	189±35†
Histologic score of inflammation	8.6±1.1	15.8±1.5†
Gallbladder fluid protein content, mg/mL	16.6±3.3	12.0±1.2
6-Keto-PGF$_{1\alpha}$ mucosal cells		
Medium	19±9	168±49†
Homogenate	16±7	259±77†
6-Keto-PGF$_{1\alpha}$ muscle tissue		
Medium	24±6	490±108†
Homogenate	17±7	530±164†
PGE mucosal cells		
Medium	265±63	898±418
Homogenate	481±83	1987±621†
PGE muscle tissue		
Medium	729±157	1990±484†
Homogenate	508±144	2440±637†

*6-Keto-PGF$_{1\alpha}$ indicates 6-ketoprostaglandin F$_{1\alpha}$; PGE, prostaglandin E. These values are expressed in picograms per milligram of protein. Each tissue culture medium value is the mean±SEM of the number of values indicated obtained from the mean of three hourly samples. Each homogenate value is the mean±SEM of the number of values indicated.

†Diseased gallbladder value is significantly different from normal gallbladder value.

the mucosal cells. The gallbladders were again soaked for five minutes in fresh edetic acid medium and shaken. The solutions were pooled and the mucosal cells collected by centrifugation for five minutes at 2500 g. The pellet was washed twice in iced Krebs-Ringer phosphate solution, pH 7.5, to remove white and red blood cells[4] and the sample pooled by centrifugation at 200 g for one minute. The separation techniques yielded 200 to 500 mg of mucosal cells.

The remaining gallbladder mucosal surface was scraped by a glass slide and the gallbladder wall washed with Krebs-Ringer phosphate solution, pH 7.5. A 200- to 300-mg piece was minced with scissors and knife to the smallest pieces possible and the resulting tissue washed twice with Krebs-Ringer phosphate solution and the samples were pooled by centrifugation at 200 g for one minute.

Mucosal cells and muscle tissue cultures were performed as described previously in 15 mL of medium.[4] Mucosal cells and muscle tissue were viable as estimated by trypan blue exclusion before and at the end of three hours of culture (>80% viable). Hourly 1-mL samples of culture medium were withdrawn and replaced with fresh medium. At the end of three hours, the medium containing mucosal cells and muscle tissue was removed from the incubator and centrifuged for five minutes at 2500 g. One milliliter of medium was removed, and the mucosal cells and muscle tissue were processed for determination of PGE and 6-keto-PGF$_{1\alpha}$ concentrations by homogenization in 1 mL of ice-cold 50-mmol/L TRIS hydrochloride buffer, pH 7.0, containing edetic acid. The amount of protein present in the mucosal cell or muscle tissue pellet was determined by the method of Bradford.[7]

Prostaglandins in the tissue culture media and homogenates were extracted, purified, and measured by radioimmunoassay according to the method reported by Powell,[9] as modified by Stephenson et al[10] and Suzuki et al.[11] To determine recovery, 2000 to 3000 cpm of tritiated PGE$_2$ or 6-keto-PGF$_{1\alpha}$ was added. One milliliter of tissue culture medium or tissue homogenate was adjusted to a pH of 3.0 with 0.1N hydrochloric acid, and then 4 mL of 1:1 mixture of ethylacetate-cyclohexane was added. The mixtures were vortexed and then centrifuged at 1500 g for ten minutes. The organic layer was separated and the extraction was repeated again. The organic layers were dried under nitrogen at 4°C.

The dried samples were mixed with 2.25 mL of water and 0.75 mL of alcohol, then vortexed, and 0.14 mL of 1N hydrochloric acid was added. The samples were applied to octadecylsilane packed (Sep-Pack C$_{18}$) columns that had been previously washed with 20 mL of alcohol, 20 mL of high-performance liquid chromatography water, and 20 mL of 15% alcohol to remove polar lipids and then with 20 mL of petroleum ether. The columns were eluted with 10 mL of methyl formate, which removed the prostaglandins. The methyl formate fractions were collected, evaporated to dryness under nitrogen, and then dissolved in 1 mL of 0.05 mol/L of phosphate buffer, pH 6.8, containing 0.9% sodium chloride, 0.01% edetic acid, 0.3% bovine gamma globulin, 0.005% (octy)phenoxy polyethoxyethanol (Triton-X-100), and 0.05% sodium azide. Recovery was determined by counting 100 μL. Prostaglandin E level was measured by radioimmunoassay as described previously.[4]

For radioimmunoassay of 6-keto-PGF$_{1\alpha}$, the tracer iodine 125–labeled 6-keto-PGF$_{1\alpha}$ was diluted with 50 mmol/L of phosphate buffer, pH 6.8, to a specific activity of 10 000 cpm/dL. The antibody was similarly diluted to provide binding of 50% to 60%. The assay was carried out in 12×7.5-mm siliconized glass tubes with standard 6-keto-PGF$_{1\alpha}$ from 2.0 to 500 pg/100 μL per tube. To all the tubes, including the samples, 100 μL of diluted ^{125}I–6-keto-PGF$_{1\alpha}$ was added. This was followed by adding 100 μL of diluted antibody except for the total count and nonspecific binding tubes. The tubes were vortexed and incubated overnight at 2°C. Following incubation, the tubes were placed in an ice-water bath. One milliliter of polyethylene glycol (16%; molecular weight, 6000) as a precipitating agent was added to all the tubes except the total count tubes. The tubes were vortexed and then centrifuged at 1500 g for 30 minutes. The supernatant was decanted, and the pellet was counted in a gamma counter.

The amount of cross-reaction between the antibody for 6-keto-PGF$_{1\alpha}$ was 2.6% with PGF$_{2\alpha}$, 1.9% with PGE, 1.4% with thromboxane B$_2$, and less than 1% with all other prostanoids. Recovery of 6-keto-PGF$_{1\alpha}$ ranged from 60% to 65%. The intra-assay coefficient of variation was 2%, and the interassay coefficient of variation was 5%.

Each section of gallbladder wall was evaluated histologically after hematoxylin-eosin staining. The histologic evaluation of the amount of inflammation present was performed by a pathologist using a scoring system estimating the amount of inflammatory cell infiltrate, edema, tissue necrosis, muscle thickening, and fibrosis, with 0 being none and 3 being severe.[12] The histologic slides were coded to "blind" the pathologist.

Statistical analysis of the difference between mean (±SEM) values was performed by analysis of variance or Student's *t* test. Determination of correlation coefficients by the method of least squares was used to determine the relationship between prostaglandin levels and β-glucuronidase activity. Spearman rank correlation and Wilcoxon rank-sum test were used to evaluate the histologic scores of inflammation and prostaglandin levels. As used throughout the manuscript, significant indicates $P<.05$.

RESULTS

Normal and diseased human gallbladder mucosal cells and muscle tissue released PGE and 6-keto-PGF$_{1\alpha}$ into tissue culture medium, and cell and tissue homogenates were found to contain both prostanoids. Both 6-keto-$PGF_{1\alpha}$ and PGE were identifiable in all gallbladders evaluated. Muscle tissue produced significantly more 6-keto-$PGF_{1\alpha}$ than did mucosal cells (Table 1). Human gallbladders produced more PGE than 6-keto-$PGF_{1\alpha}$. Mucosal cells and muscle tissue appeared to produce similar amounts of PGE, as evaluated in tissue culture medium and in muscle tissue homogenates (Table 1).

It has been difficult previously to obtain normal gallbladders, and we previously compared gallbladders with minimal inflammation with those with severe inflammation.[4,12] In the present study, access to an adequate-sized sample of normal gallbladders enabled us to compare normal with diseased tissue (Table 2).

We have been attempting to identify an objective, quantitative index of the degree of cholecystitis present. The lysosomal enzyme, β-glucuronidase, is derived from invading inflammatory cells, and the activity of the lysosomal enzyme parallels the severity of the inflammatory response.[13,14]

Both β-glucuronidase activity and the histologic score of inflammation were significantly greater in diseased gallbladders than in normal gallbladders (Table 2). A significant correlation existed ($r=.637$, $P<.001$) between the histologic score of inflammation and β-glucuronidase activity.

Protein concentration in gallbladder fluid has been implicated in gallstone formation and has been demonstrated to increase in experimental cholecystitis.[15,16] Comparison of the protein concentration of the luminal contents of normal gallbladders with that present in diseased gallbladders revealed no significant differences (Table 2).

Normal gallbladder mucosal cells and muscle tissue produced relatively small and similar amounts of 6-keto-$PGF_{1\alpha}$ in culture media and homogenates. Significantly greater 6-keto-$PGF_{1\alpha}$ was produced by diseased gallbladders than normal gallbladders (Table 2).

Greater amounts of PGE than 6-keto-$PGF_{1\alpha}$ were produced by normal and diseased gallbladders. Diseased gallbladders produced greater amounts of PGE than did control gallbladders for all factors evaluated except when mucosal cells in tissue culture media were evaluated (Table 2).

Attempts to evaluate the degree of correlation between β-glucuronidase activity levels or the histologic score of inflammation with 6-keto-$PGF_{1\alpha}$ levels revealed no significant correlations. When normal values were included in the analysis and when they were not, such significant correlations were able to be demonstrated when comparing β-glucuronidase and histologic inflammation with PGE production. As has been found previously,[4,12] when histologic score was compared with mucosal cell homogenate PGE values, the correlation coefficient was $r=.541$ ($P<.05$). Prostaglandin E production appeared to be more positively correlated with inflammation than was 6-keto-$PGF_{1\alpha}$.

COMMENT

Prostacyclin is formed by human gallbladder muscle and mucosa. In the canine intestinal tract, prostacyclin is formed by both muscularis and mucosal tissues.[17] As is true in human gallbladder muscle tissue (Table 2), the intestinal tract and stomach muscle tissue produce more prostacyclin than is formed by mucosal cells.[17]

Others have demonstrated prostacyclin production by guinea pig[18] and prairie dog[3] gallbladders, unspiked by arachidonic acid, with 6-keto-$PGF_{1\alpha}$ levels quantitatively similar to those produced by human gallbladders. Prostaglandin E compounds may play a role in gallbladder muscle contraction[19] and mucosal water transport,[20] as well as gallbladder inflammation.[2] We are unaware of any studies having been performed to ascertain if prostacyclin alters any physiologic gallbladder function. The prostacyclin in gallbladder muscle and mucosa may be formed by blood vessels[17] and may function in the vasodilation associated with inflammation.

In an experimental model of gallstone formation, produced by feeding prairie dogs a high-cholesterol diet, prostaglandins have been shown to be involved in gallstone formation. Prostaglandin formation is stimulated by increased bile cholesterol.[21] Prostaglandins stimulate secretion of mucin, which acts as a nidus for gallstone formation.[3] Mucin secretion and experimental gallstone formation are inhibited by prostaglandin synthetase inhibitors.[22,23] In experimental cholelithiasis, mucin secretion appears to be regulated by endogenous prostacyclin levels.[22] The data in the present report demonstrate significantly greater prostacyclin levels produced by gallbladders from patients with gallstones than from patients with normal gallbladders. The increased prostanoid levels may be contributing to stone formation as well as subsequent inflammation.

We have previously demonstrated that systemic infusion of prostacyclin increases hepatic bile flow, producing a bicarbonate-rich choleresis mediated by cyclic adenosine monophosphate.[24] The response produced was not due to regional blood flow changes.[24] It will be important for improved understanding of the results in the present study to determine if prostacyclin has any effect on gallbladder contraction or absorption.

Our previous studies of prostaglandin formation by diseased human gallbladder was inhibited by the relative difficulty in obtaining normal gallbladders for comparison. Organ donors are not a suitable source for normal gallbladders for prostanoid evaluation because of the steroid therapy used for immunosuppression. Currently, a variety of operative procedures are performed that require incidental cholecystectomy, such as regional hepatic chemotherapy and hepatic resection, providing access to disease-free gallbladders. As these gallbladders require operative removal, with the associated tissue trauma[25] and hypoxia,[26] the prostanoid levels present may not be absolutely normal. The ability in this study to compare similarly procured normal and diseased gallbladders enhanced our understanding of the changes in arachidonic acid metabolism that was occurring.

Measurement of the lysosomal enzyme β-glucuronidase as a marker of white blood cell invasion correlated well with the severity of inflammation present, as evaluated histologically. It is likely that measurement of other lysosomal enzymes[27] would produce similar information, and perhaps lysosomal enzymes even more specific for gallbladder inflammation will be identified. β-Glucuronidase measurements clearly allowed the separation of normal from diseased gallbladders.

In acute experimental models of cholecystitis, diseased gallbladders secrete a protein-rich fluid into the lumen of the gallbladder.[16] This process is believed to be mediated by prostaglandins, as it is inhibited by prostaglandin synthetase inhibition.[28] In the present study, the protein content of fluid obtained from the gallbladders at the time of cholecystectomy in normal gallbladders was not significantly different from that found in diseased gallbladders. All of the diseased gallbladders contained gallstones, and perhaps intraluminal fluid protein content may only be important in acalculous cholecystitis.[16]

Though previous studies have demonstrated that PGE production by human gallbladder muscle tissue and mucosal cells increased with increasing severity of the inflammatory process,[4,12] the present study indicates that gallbladders from patients with calculous cholecystitis have increased PGE production compared with normal gallbladders (Table 2). The increased PGE levels may contribute to the inflammatory response,[4,12] pain,[19] and gallbladder fluid accumulation[20] and indeed may be involved in gallstone formation related to prostaglandin-mediated production of mucin, which acts as a nidus for nucleation of cholesterol crystals.[3] Prostanoid formation appears to be an important factor in human gallbladder disease.

This study was supported by grant DK 27695 from the US Public Health Service.

References

1. Hagman W, Steffan AM, Kirn A, et al: Leukotrienes as mediators in frog virus 3–induced hepatitis in rats. *Hepatology* 1987;7:732-736.
2. Kaminski DL, Deshpande YG, Qualy J, et al: The role of prostaglandins in feline experimental cholecystitis. *Surgery* 1985;98:760-786.
3. LaMorte WW, Lamon JT, Hale W, et al: Gallbladder prostaglandins and lysophospholipids as mediators of mucin secretion during cholelithiasis. *Am J Physiol* 1986;251:G701-G707.
4. Kaminski DL, Deshpande YG, Thomas L, et al: The effect of oral ibuprofen on the formation of prostaglandins E and F by human gallbladder muscle and mucosa. *Dig Dis Sci* 1985;30:933-940.
5. Samuelsson B: Leukotrienes: Mediators of immediate hypersensitivity reactions and inflammation. *Science* 1983;220:568-575.
6. Moncada SR, Gryglewski R, Bunting S, et al: An enzyme isolated from arteries transforms prostaglandin endoperoxides to an unstable substance that inhibits platelet aggregation. *Nature* 1976;263:603-609.
7. Bradford MM: A rapid and sensitive method for the quantitation of microgram quantities of protein utilizing the principle of protein-dye binding. *Anal Biochem* 1976;72:248-254.
8. Talalay P, Fishman WH, Huggins C: Chromagenic substrates: II. Phenolphthalein glucuronic acid as substrate for the assay of glucuronidase activity. *J Biol Chem* 1946;166:757-772.
9. Powell WS: Rapid extraction of arachidonic acid metabolites from biological samples using octadecysilyl silica. *Methods Enzymol* 1982;86:467-470.
10. Stephenson AH, Sprague RS, Dahms TE, et al: Unilateral acute lung injury induced by ethchlorvynol in anesthetized dogs. *J Appl Physiol* 1984;56:1252-1258.
11. Suzuki Y, Harada Y, Veno A, et al: Release of endogenous prostaglandins by mild hyperosmotic saline inhibits tetra-gastrin–stimulated gastric acid secretion in rats. *Prostaglandins* 1986;32:201-211.
12. Kaminski DL, Deshpande YG, Thomas L, et al: Evaluation of the role of prostaglandins E and F in human cholecystitis. *Prostaglandins Leukotrienes Med* 1984;16:109-120.
13. Ammendola G, DiRosa M, Sorrentino L: Leucocyte migration and lysosomal enzyme release in rat carrageenin pleurisy. *Agents Actions* 1975;5:250-254.
14. Doherty NS, Robinson BV: Some biological and pharmacological properties of inflammatory exudates. *J Pharm Pharmacol* 1976;28:859-864.
15. Burnstein MJ, Ilson RG, Petrunka CN, et al: Evidence for a potent nucleating factor in the gallbladder bile of patients with cholesterol gallstones. *Gastroenterology* 1983;85:801-807.
16. Neiderhiser DH: Animal model of human disease: Acute acalculous cholecystitis induced by lysophosphatidylcholine. *Am J Pathol* 1986;124:559-563.
17. LeDuc LE, Needleman P: Regional localization of prostacyclin and thromboxane synthesis in dog stomach and intestinal tract. *J Pharm Exp Ther* 1979;211:181-188.
18. Booker ML, LaMorte WW: Prostaglandin release from in vitro guinea-pig gallbladder. *Prostaglandins* 1983;25:143-153.
19. Nakano J, McCloy RF, Gin AC, et al: Effects of prostaglandins E, E_1, E_2 and F_2 and pentagastrin on gallbladder pressure in dogs. *Eur J Pharmacol* 1975;30:107-112.
20. Heinze K, Leinesser W, Peterson KU, et al: Triphasic effect of prostaglandins E_1, E_2, and $F_{2\alpha}$ on the fluid transport of isolated gallbladder of guinea pigs. *Prostaglandins* 1975;9:209-322.
21. LaMorte WW, Booker ML, Scott TE, et al: Increases in gallbladder prostaglandin synthesis before the formation of cholesterol gallstones. *Surgery* 1985;98:445-451.
22. LaMont JT, Turner BS, DiBenedetto D, et al: Arachidonic acid stimulates mucin secretion in prairie dog gallbladder. *Am J Physiol* 1983;245:G92-G98.
23. Lee SP, Carey ML, LaMont JT: Aspirin prevention of cholesterol gallstone formation in prairie dogs. *Science* 1981;211:1429-1431.
24. Kaminski DL, Deshpande YG: The effects of prostacyclin on canine hepatic bile flow. *Hepatology* 1984;4:644-650.
25. Ferreira SH: Prostaglandins, in Houck JC (ed): *Chemical Messengers of the Inflammatory Response.* Amsterdam, Elsevier Science Publishers, 1979, p 113.
26. Jelkmann W, Kurtz A, Forstermann U, et al: Hypoxia enhances prostaglandin synthesis in renal mesangial cell cultures. *Prostaglandins* 1985;30:109-118.
27. Bonney BJ, Wightman PD, Davies P, et al: Regulation of prostaglandin synthesis and of the selective release of lysosomal hydrolases by mouse peritoneal macrophages. *Biochem J* 1978;176:433-442.
28. Svanik JE, Thornell L, Zettergren L: Gallbladder function in experimental cholecystitis: Reversal of the inflammatory net fluid secretion into the gallbladder by indomethacin. *Surgery* 1981;89:500-506.

The Efficacy of Oral Antimicrobials in Reducing Aerobic and Anaerobic Colonic Mucosal Flora

Jonathan I. Groner, MD; Charles E. Edmiston, Jr, PhD; Candace J. Krepel;
Gordon L. Telford, MD; Robert E. Condon, MD, MS

• We investigated the impact of intestinal antisepsis on the colonic mucosa-associated flora. Four groups of dogs were studied: group A received no bowel preparation, group B received a three-day clear-liquid diet, group C underwent mechanical cleansing of the bowel, and group D had mechanical cleansing followed by oral neomycin and erythromycin. Mucosal biopsy specimens were obtained for bacteriologic and scanning electron microscopic (SEM) studies. No significant difference in recovery of mucosal bacteria was observed between groups A and B. A significant decrease in recovery of aerobes was observed in group C, and a significant decrease in both aerobes and anaerobes was observed in group D compared with group A; Enterobacteriaceae and *Bacteroides* were either eliminated or greatly reduced. The SEM analysis of group D revealed a marked decrease in mucosa-associated microflora compared with groups B and C. Oral neomycin-erythromycin produced a significant quantitative reduction in the colonic mucosa-associated bacterial population, including the potentially pathogenic *Escherichia coli* and *Bacteroides fragilis* group isolates. These mucosa-associated bacteria are a likely source of contamination of the abdominal cavity and wound at the time of colon surgery.

(*Arch Surg* 1989;124:281-284)

The use of prophylactic antimicrobials in patients undergoing elective colon surgery has been extensively studied, clinically and experimentally, for over 30 years.[1] In current clinical practice, prophylaxis is administered by parenteral, oral, or combination regimens.[2] The strategy behind parenteral preoperative antimicrobial administration is to assure that adequate microbicidal levels of the drug are present in the wound at the time of initial tissue contamination.[3] In comparison, the strategy behind the administration of the oral combination of erythromycin and neomycin is to reduce the microbial flora in the colonic lumen. This combination has been demonstrated to reduce the incidence of septic complications in a blinded, randomized, controlled clinical trial.[4] Erythromycin, a macrolide antibiotic, exhibits activity against anaerobes as well as gram-positive aerobic (including facultatively aerobic) microorganisms. Bactericidal levels of erythromycin can be found in the serum and stool of patients after oral doses of this drug.[5] Neomycin, an aminoglycoside, is active against aerobic and facultative coliforms; it is poorly absorbed and acts within the bowel lumen.

Intraluminal sampling has demonstrated that oral administration of neomycin and erythromycin reduces bacterial counts in the residual colonic contents.[6] However, the impact of oral prophylaxis on the bacteriology of the colonic mucosal surface has not been previously examined. Previous studies in man have demonstrated that the mucosa-associated colonic bacteria are a discrete subpopulation of the luminal flora exhibiting strong adherence to the brush-border surface. This adherent microflora includes *Bacteroides*, fusobacteria, peptostreptococci, and some members of the Enterobacteriaceae that are resistant to removal by mechanical cleansing or mucosal washes.[7]

Subinhibitory levels of antimicrobials have been documented to alter microbial adhesion in vitro.[8] The administration of oral antibiotics may be effective in reducing the concentration of mucosa-associated bacteria, theoretically leading to a reduction in wound contamination and infection risk. The purpose of the present investigation was to determine whether mechanical bowel preparation, followed by oral administration of neomycin and erythromycin, is effective in reducing the numbers of aerobic (facultative) and anaerobic (obligate) mucosa-associated colonic bacteria.

MATERIALS AND METHODS

Animals

This study was approved by the animal experimentation institutional review board. Twenty-eight dogs were randomly assigned to four different groups. In group A (n=6), six dogs received food

Accepted for publication April 29, 1988.

From the Surgical Microbiology Research Laboratory, Department of Surgery (Drs Groner, Edmiston, Telford, and Condon and Ms Krepel); and the Vince Lombardi Cancer Center (Drs Telford and Condon), Medical College of Wisconsin, and Zablocki Veterans Administration Medical Center (Drs Groner, Telford, and Condon), Milwaukee.

Reprint requests to Department of Surgery, Medical College of Wisconsin, 8700 W Wisconsin Ave, Milwaukee, WI 53226 (Dr Edmiston).

Table 1.—Quantitative Recovery of Aerobic and Anaerobic Mucosa-Associated Bacteria From Canine Colonic Segments*

Group	Microbial Recovery		
	Proximal	Midcolon	Distal
Aerobes			
A	8.6±0.5	8.3±0.6	8.7±0.5
B	7.4±1.6	6.7±2.0	7.2±1.7
C	5.5±0.6	5.4±0.8	5.7±1.0
D	2.4±0.7	3.1±0.2	2.5±1.2
Anaerobes			
A	9.5±0.4	9.7±0.4	9.8±0.9
B	9.0±0.9	8.6±2.1	8.6±1.6
C	8.2±0.9	7.4±0.7	7.4±1.0
D	2.6±1.0	3.0±1.4	2.6±1.1

*Expressed as log_{10} colony-forming units per milligram (wet weight) of tissue, mean±SD. Group A (n=6) received no bowel preparation; group B (n=7), clear-liquid diet; group C (n=8), mechanical preparation; and group D (n=7), oral antimicrobial prophylaxis.

Table 2.—Relative Prevalence of Bacteria From Mucosa of Canine Colonic Segments*

	Group			
	A	B	C	D
Aerobes				
Enterobacteriaceae†	16	15	14	0
Enterococcus	6	8	9	0
Streptococcus	4	2	6	9
Miscellaneous‡	2	5	9	1
Anaerobes				
Bacteroides	17	15	20	4
Fusobacterium	14	12	5	4
Clostridium	9	5	15	0
Eubacterium	5	1	9	12
Lactobacillus	4	2	4	11
Peptostreptococcus	11	7	12	5
Miscellaneous§	3	4	7	3

*Counts reflect number of biopsy specimens harboring each isolate. Total number of biopsy specimens per study group: A, 18; B, 21; C, 24; and D, 21.

†Recovered Enterobacteriaceae included *Escherichia coli, Klebsiella, Enterobacter, Citrobacter, Proteus,* and *Morganella; E coli* was the most predominant isolate in groups A, B, and C.

‡Aerobic miscellaneous isolates included corynebacteria, facultative lactobacilli, and staphylococci.

§Anaerobic miscellaneous isolates included bifidobacteria, *Megasphaera,* propionibacteria, and *Veillonella.*

and water ad libitum without any bowel preparation. Group B (n=7) dogs were placed on a 72-hour clear-liquid diet. The third group of dogs, group C (n=8), was given a 72-hour clear-liquid diet, and then 280 g of magnesium citrate orally, followed by a tap water enema. Group D dogs (n=7) underwent a similar mechanical bowel preparation and, in addition, received oral neomycin sulfate (500 mg) and erythromycin base (500 mg) at noon, 1, and 6 PM on the day before study.

In groups A, B, and D, mucosal biopsy specimens were obtained at laparotomy. In group C, the specimens were obtained by colonoscopy (Olympus Model CF-1B). To obtain a mucosal biopsy sample free of contamination by flora foreign to the immediate sample site, a sealed polyethylene catheter (Clay Adams PE 160) containing a gas-sterilized biopsy instrument was introduced through the biopsy channel of the colonoscope. At the biopsy site, the instrument was pushed through a paraffin seal at the catheter tip, and the mucosa underwent biopsy. The biopsy instrument was drawn back into the catheter and the biopsy probe and catheter were removed together from the colonoscope. The process was repeated for each biopsy in the proximal, middle, and distal colon using a fresh catheter-sheath instrument.

Dogs undergoing laparotomy (groups A, B, and D) had a ventral midline incision performed using general endotracheal anesthesia after skin preparation with povidone-iodine scrub solution and sterile draping. The colon from just distal to the cecum to just proximal to the rectum was isolated and divided. Using separate sterile scissors for each biopsy, a sample of mucosa was obtained from proximal, middle, and distal colon sites. All samples were immediately placed in gassed-out vials and transported to the laboratory.

Bacteriology

After wet-weight determination (tissue weight range, 2.1 to 12.9 mg), the biopsy specimens were placed inside an anaerobic chamber where all tissue homogenization, serial dilution with buffered gelatin diluent, and plating was carried out. The following media for aerobic and anaerobic isolation were inoculated using a 0.01-mL calibrated loop: trypticase-soy blood agar, colistin-nalidixic acid blood agar, *Enterococcus*-selective agar, Sabouraud dextrose agar, Centers for Disease Control (CDC formulation) anaerobic blood agar, kanamycin-vancomycin blood agar, egg yolk agar, phenylethyl alcohol agar, *Lactobacillus*-selective agar, modified *Fusobacterium* medium, and *Bifidobacterium* medium. Aerobic media were incubated at 36.5°C and examined at 24 and 48 hours. All aerobic bacterial isolates were characterized by standard methods.[9]

Anaerobic bacteria initially were characterized on the basis of macroscopic and microscopic criteria. The isolates were tested for oxygen tolerance in an atmosphere supplemented with 5% carbon dioxide. Strict anaerobes were inoculated into prereduced, anaerobically sterilized, carbohydrate media. Volatile and nonvolatile metabolic by-products were analyzed by gas-liquid chromatography. Biochemical evaluations were carried out using standard techniques.[10] Microbial quantitation was expressed as log_{10} colony-forming units (CFUs) per milligram (wet weight) of mucosal tissue.

Scanning Electron Microscopy

Specimens for scanning electron microscopy (SEM) were immediately prefixed for eight hours in 2% glutaraldehyde, buffered with 0.15 mmol/L of sodium cacodylate (pH, 7.4). After several buffered washes, the specimens were postfixed in 1% osmium tetroxide. Following serial dehydration, the specimens were critical point dried from liquid CO_2 and then coated with gold-palladium in an evaporator. The processed specimens were viewed in an SEM at 20 kV with a spot size of 8 nm.

Statistical Analysis

The quantitative data were analyzed by the paired t test to compare biopsy sites within a given treatment group. Comparisons of bacterial recovery for different treatment groups at a given site were performed using analysis of variance and the nonpaired t test.

RESULTS

Eighty-four colonic mucosal biopsy specimens were obtained from 28 dogs. The mean biopsy weight was 9.2 mg in group A (no preparation), 8.7 mg in group B (clear-liquid diet), 7.1 mg in group C (mechanical preparation), and 10.8 mg in group D (antibiotic preparation group). No significant differences in quantitative aerobic or anaerobic recovery were observed between biopsy sites within a study group (Table 1) or between groups A and B. There was a significant difference in recovery of aerobes between groups B and C ($P<.05$) but no difference in obligate anaerobe recovery. Both aerobes and anaerobes were significantly decreased in group D dogs ($P<.01$) compared with controls (group A).

A broad and complex microbial flora was recovered in

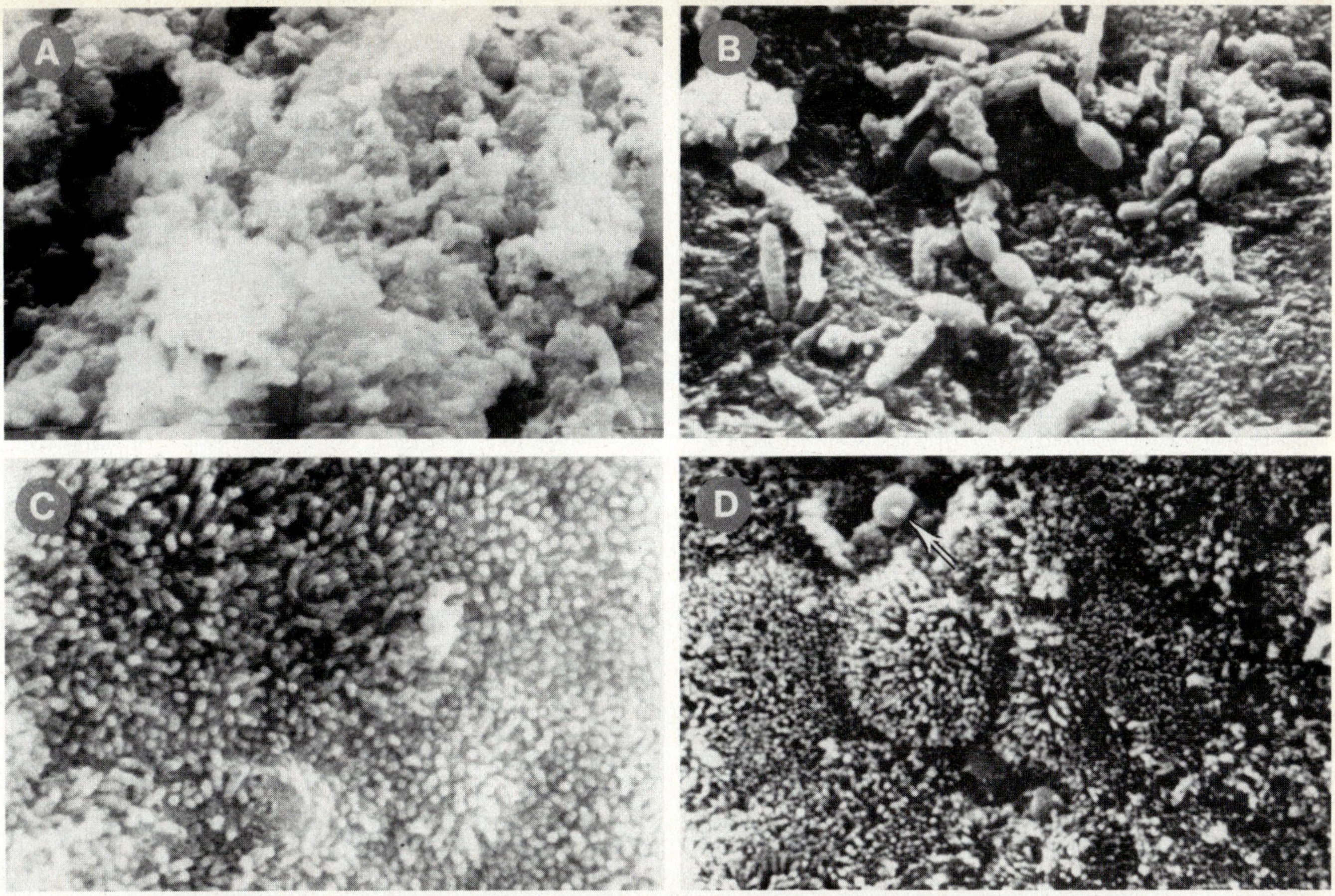

A, Scanning electron micrograph of colonic mucosal surface in group B dog (clear-liquid diet regimen) demonstrating intact mucin sheath in which rods and cocci are embedded (×2400). B, Colonic mucosal surface in group C dog (mechanical preparation) demonstrates some mucus debris along with heterogeneous mucosa-associated bacteria (×3000). C, Mucosal surface in group D dog (given oral antibiotics) showing no microorganisms present in proximal colonic biopsy specimen (×4000). D, Arrow points to single coccilike organism residing on brush-border surface in another group D biopsy specimen (×3200).

group A (Table 2). *Bacteroides*, Enterobacteriaceae, fusobacteria, peptostreptococci, and clostridia were the predominant mucosa-associated flora in the control (group A) dogs as well as in groups B and C. In group D, no Enterobacteriaceae or clostridia were recovered from any of the 21 biopsy samples. *Bacteroides*, *Fusobacterium*, and peptostreptococci were recovered from less than one quarter of the group D specimens.

In group B, SEM revealed a mucosal surface with a dense mucin layer. Numerous rods and cocci were observed residing within the gel-like matrix (Figure, part A). Mechanical preparation removed much of the mucin from the mucosal surface, revealing a luxurious mucosa-associated microflora (Figure, part B). Treatment with oral neomycin and erythromycin removed most of the mucosa-associated microorganisms (Figure, parts C and D).

COMMENT

Postoperative septic complications following elective colon surgery are usually the result of contamination by endogenous microorganisms.[11] The predominant bacteria in the large bowel are the anaerobic gram-negative, non-spore-forming bacilli. These organisms are present in the colon lumen at concentrations of 10^9 to 10^{11} organisms per gram of stool.[4] Aerobic (facultative) gram-negative bacilli represent only 1% to 10% of the total endogenous colonic flora; however Enterobacteriaceae are a significant cause of morbidity and mortality following elective abdominal surgery.[12,13] A variety of other aerobes and anaerobes, including clostridia and enterococci, also can be cultured from the stool, while fungi in large numbers are rarely cultured from the stool of young, healthy individuals.[14,15] Bartlett et al[16] and Edmondson and Rissing[17] have shown that the predominant isolates recovered from infected sites following elective colon operations were *Bacteroides fragilis* and *Escherichia coli*.

Previous reports have documented the failure of mechanical preparation alone to reduce significantly the intraluminal microbial population of the colon.[6,12] Furthermore, the use of mechanical preparation by itself has been shown to be associated with a higher incidence of septic complications.[4,11] Using tissue biopsy, we have demonstrated that vigorous mechanical preparation appears to eliminate mucin-bound bacteria but does not significantly reduce mucosa-associated aerobes or anaerobes compared with a nonmechanically (liquid diet) prepared group of dogs.

In dogs receiving both mechanical preparation and oral antimicrobials, there was a significant reduction in both aerobes and anaerobes compared with the control group (aerobic-facultative reduction, 5.2 to 6.2 $\log_{10}$ CFUs/mg of tissue vs group A; anaerobic reduction, 6.7 to 7.2 $\log_{10}$ CFUs/mg of tissue vs group A). The concentration of residual mucosa-associated bacteria in group D following oral administration of neomycin-erythromycin (Table 1) was below the microbial density often present in a wound following a clean-contaminated procedure, and below the concentration (10^5) at which wound infection may occur. Furthermore, qualitative analysis demonstrated that Enterobacteriaceae and *Bacteroides* were either eliminated or significantly decreased in the oral antimicrobial–treated group (Table 2). The predominant organisms isolated after oral prophylaxis were of low inherent virulence (eubacteria, lactobacilli, and facultative streptococci) and, therefore, unlikely to cause postoperative septic complications.

In conclusion, a regimen of mechanical bowel cleansing followed by oral administration of neomycin and erythromycin significantly decreases the mucosa-associated facultative and obligate microbial populations of the colon and, in so doing, eliminates or reduces those bacteria often responsible for postoperative intra-abdominal and wound infections. Without the addition of oral antimicrobials, such as neomycin and erythromycin, the mucosa-associated bacteria remain unchanged and are a potential source of contamination of the wound and abdominal cavity at the time of operation.

We wish to thank Marcey Jaskulski for her technical assistance in preparing the manuscript.

References

1. Baum ML, Anish DS, Chalmers TC, et al: A survey of trials of antibiotic prophylaxis in colon surgery: Evidence against further use of no-treatment controls. *N Engl J Med* 1981;305:795-799.
2. Condon RE, Bartlett JG, Greenlee H, et al: Efficacy of oral and systemic antibiotic prophylaxis in colorectal operations. *Arch Surg* 1983;118:496-502.
3. MilesAA, Miles EM, Burke JF: The value and duration of defense reaction of the skin to the primary lodgement of bacteria. *Br J Exp Pathol* 1957;38:79-96.
4. Clarke JS, Condon RE, Bartlett JG, et al: Preoperative oral antibiotics reduce septic complications of colon operations: Results of a randomized, double-blind clinical study. *Ann Surg* 1977;186:251-259.
5. Nichols RL, Condon RE, DiSanto AR: Preoperative bowel preparation. *Arch Surg* 1977;112:1493-1496.
6. Nichols RL, Condon RE, Gorbach SL, et al: Efficacy of preoperative antimicrobial preparation of the bowel. *Ann Surg* 1972;176:227-313.
7. Edmiston CE, Avant GR, Wilson FA: Anaerobic bacterial populations on normal and diseased human biopsy tissue obtained at colonoscopy. *Appl Environ Microbiol* 1982;43:1173-1181.
8. Vosbeck K, Handschin H, Menge E, et al: Effects of subminimal inhibitory concentrations of antibiotics on adhesiveness of *Escherichia coli* in vitro. *Rev Infect Dis* 1979;1:845-851.
9. Lennette FH, Spaulding EH, Truant JP (eds): *Manual of Clinical Microbiology*, ed 3. Washington, DC, American Society for Microbiology, 1985.
10. Holdeman LV, Moore WE: *Anaerobic Laboratory Manual*, ed 4. Blacksburg, Va, Virginia Polytechnical Institute and State University, 1977.
11. Nichols RL, Broido P, Condon RE, et al: Effect of preoperative neomycin-erythromycin intestinal preparation on the incidence of infectious complications following colon surgery. *Ann Surg* 1973;178:453-462.
12. Nichols RL, Condon RE: Antibiotic preparation of the colon: Failure of commonly used regimens. *Surg Clin North Am* 1971;51:223-231.
13. Kleighley MRB, Drysdale RB, Quoralshi AH, et al: Antibiotic treatment of biliary sepsis. *Surg Clin North Am* 1975;55:1379-1390.
14. Jones FE, Malangoni MA, Spiegel C, et al: Antibiotic management of intra-abdominal sepsis. *Infect Surg* 1987;65:15-24.
15. Finegold SM, Flora DJ, Attebery HR, et al: Fecal bacteriology of colonic polyp patients and control patients. *Cancer Res* 1975;35:3407-3417.
16. Bartlett JG, Condon RE, Gorbach SL, et al: Veterans Administration cooperative study on bowel preparation for elective colorectal operations. *Ann Surg* 1978;188:249-254.
17. Edmondson HT, Rissing JP: Prophylactic antibiotics in colon surgery. *Arch Surg* 1983;118:227-231.

In Other AMA Journals

ARCHIVES OF INTERNAL MEDICINE

Factors Predictive of Acute Renal Failure in Rhabdomyolysis

Michael M. Ward, MD, MPH

In a historical cohort study, acute renal failure developed in 16.5% of 157 patients with rhabdomyolysis over a two-year study period. Underlying clinical, laboratory, and causative factors associated with the development of acute renal failure were examined. Factors predictive of renal failure in this setting, determined by multiple logistic regression analysis, included the degree of serum creatine kinase, serum potassium, and serum phosphorus level elevation; the degree of depression of serum albumin level; and the presence of dehydration at presentation or sepsis as the underlying cause. The predictive model that was developed correctly classified 93% of subjects and was statistically validated (*Arch Intern Med* 1988;148:1553-1557).

Reprints not available.

Emergency Abdominal Operations in the Patient With Acquired Immunodeficiency Syndrome

Joshua H. Burack, MD; Marc S. Mandel, MD; Lawrence S. Bizer, MD

• We have reviewed the medical records of ten patients with acquired immunodeficiency syndrome who required emergency celiotomy in a three-year period. These operations are characterized by a high morbidity and mortality. Careful attention to the support of these immunosuppressed, malnourished patients if emergency operation is necessary may improve the poor results reported herein.

(*Arch Surg* 1989;124:285-286)

Acquired immunodeficiency syndrome (AIDS) has become a recognized disease entity to most physicians. The protean infectious and malignant complications of AIDS and its causative agent(s) have been identified. The diagnosis and treatment of intra-abdominal pathologic conditions in patients with AIDS represent a formidable challenge to surgeons. Furthermore, as would be expected, major surgical procedures result in high morbidity and mortality in a group of patients with marked immunosuppression abetted by frequent protein calorie malnutrition. The following report documents our experience with emergency celiotomy in patients with AIDS.

PATIENTS AND METHODS

A medical record review at Montefiore Medical Center, Bronx, NY, and its two affiliated municipal hospitals over a three-year period (June 1984 to July 1987) revealed ten patients with AIDS who underwent emergency celiotomy for acute intra-abdominal disease. All ten patients met Centers for Disease Control criteria for the diagnosis of AIDS.[1] All patients were followed up until their deaths or the time of this writing. Particular attention was paid to the preoperative opportunistic infections the patients had acquired as well as the likely cause of human immunodeficiency virus transmission and the nutritional status of the patients. Presenting signs and symptoms of intra-abdominal pathologic conditions, preoperative and postoperative diagnosis, surgical procedures performed, and pathologic examination of the tissue removed at operation were all examined. In addition, close attention was paid to postoperative complications and mortality.

RESULTS

Nine of the ten patients were men. The average age was 36.7 years (range, 27 to 44). Eight (80%) of the ten patients were intravenous drug abusers, one was a homosexual, and the tenth patient was a heterosexual with prostitute contacts. All of the patients appeared malnourished, and, although nutritional profiles had not been done, the mean serum albumin level was 26 g/L (range, 18 to 35 g/L), with 70% having a level below 30 g/L. The diagnosis of AIDS had been established an average of 5.5 months before operation. Five patients had *Pneumocystis carinii* pneumonia and one each had disseminated histoplasmosis, cryptococcal meningitis, and Kaposi's sarcoma. The remaining two patients had documented *Candida* esophagitis. Six of the infections were active at the time abdominal symptoms began.

In every case, the patient initially complained of abdominal pain. The average rectal temperature was 38.2°C, with a range from 36.7°C to 38.9°C. Two patients were afebrile (temperature, <37.8°C). Seven of the ten patients had involuntary guarding and rebound tenderness, whereas in three patients there was only mild abdominal tenderness. Interestingly, the average white blood cell count was only 6.8×10^9/L, with a range from 2.1 to 15×10^9/L. Nine of the ten patients had a white blood cell count of less than 10×10^9/L, but 50% of patients had 10% or more band forms seen on differential count.

In five patients, clinical presentation alone mandated an operation. In the other five patients, the decision to operate was based on additional radiographic findings: a radionuclide biliary scan showing acute cholecystitis (two), pneumoperitoneum on upright chest roentgenography (two), and progressive small-bowel obstruction on abdominal roentgenograms (one).

In 40% of the patients, the preoperative and operative diagnosis differed, but all abdominal explorations were indicated (Table). Postoperative complications were frequent. They included three wound infections, three wound dehiscences, one intestinal anastomotic leak, one ostomy revision required because of bowel necrosis, two postoperative small-bowel obstructions (both requiring reoperation), and four patients with ventilator-dependent respiratory failure postoperatively.

Seven of the ten patients died postoperatively; six never left the hospital, and the seventh patient was readmitted soon after hospital discharge for an anastomotic leak and abdominal wound dehiscence and died five weeks later. Three patients survived their postoperative course; two died five and 24 months postoperatively of AIDS-related diseases, and one patient is still alive six months postoperatively.

COMMENT

In 1984, Potter et al[2] described five patients with AIDS with abdominal pain, four of whom underwent celiotomy. Two of the four patients died within one month of operation. Subsequent reports in the English-language literature

Accepted for publication Jan 20, 1988.
From the Department of Surgery, Montefiore Medical Center–Albert Einstein College of Medicine, Bronx, NY.
Reprints not available.

Operative Results in Ten Patients With AIDS*

Patient No.	Preoperative Diagnosis	Findings	Surgical Procedure	Outcome/Cause
1	Appendicitis	Acute appendicitis	Appendectomy	Death/sepsis
2	Appendicitis	Acute appendicitis	Appendectomy	Death/sepsis
3	Appendicitis	Strangulated ileocecal intussusception	Right hemicolectomy	Death/multisystem organ failure
4	Cholecystitis	Acute cholecystitis	Cholecystectomy	Survival†
5	Cholecystitis	Acute cholecystitis	Tube cholecystostomy	Survival†
6	Perforated duodenal ulcer	Perforated duodenal ulcer	Omental patch	Death/sepsis
7	Perforated duodenal ulcer	Perforated cecum	Ileostomy and mucous fistula	Death/sepsis
8	Perforated duodenal ulcer	Jejunal perforation	Plication of perforation	Death/multisystem organ failure
9	Perforated sigmoid	Unresectable perforated sigmoid cancer	Diverting colostomy and plication of perforation	Survival†
10	Adhesive small-bowel obstruction	Small-bowel stricture	Small-bowel resection and anastomosis	Death/sepsis

*AIDS indicates acquired immunodeficiency syndrome.
†Greater than two months.

document a total of at least 11 cases of emergency celiotomy in patients with AIDS. Six died within one month of operation. An unusual spectrum of pathologic conditions was found in these cases. Cytomegalovirus was responsible for four colon perforations, one small-bowel perforation, and a megacolon in one patient. In addition, cases of disseminated intra-abdominal cryptococcosis, atypical Kaposi's sarcoma, and lymphoma are described.[3-6] The majority of our patients had intra-abdominal surgical problems commonly seen in patients without AIDS, but we did treat one patient with a cecal perforation due to cytomegalovirus, a small-bowel stricture due to *Strongyloides* infestation, and an ileocecal intussusception due to atypical mycobacteria infection (Table).

Fever and leukocytosis are variably present in these individuals, as is typical of immunosuppressed patients. Hubbard et al[7] reported a series of seven renal transplant patients who developed peritonitis. Only two were febrile, and another two patients had leukocytosis.

The atypical histories in these patients with previous or ongoing infections in other organ systems and immunosuppression all contribute to the difficulty of establishing a diagnosis requiring operative intervention. In addition, patients with AIDS are poor surgical risks. Typically, the postoperative course is punctuated by complications directly related to the surgical procedure and a high incidence of ventilatory failure. The patients commonly spend a protracted postoperative period in the intensive care unit, only to succumb to sepsis and multiple organ failure (Table).

In the United Kingdom, the patient with AIDS has an average life expectancy of 13.5 months from the time of diagnosis.[8] In our small series of patients, the average survival from the time of a diagnosis of AIDS was only ten months, suggesting that emergency abdominal operations (and the disease that necessitated operation) hasten the patient's demise. Others have questioned whether emergency surgical procedures should be performed in these patients, particularly if they appear near death before the development of a surgical catastrophe.[9] Our limited data cannot answer this question.

It is also important to remember that this series of patients represents the high morbidity and mortality of emergency celiotomy in the patient with AIDS, and the results do not necessarily pertain to elective surgical procedures in patients with AIDS. Furthermore, the results do not necessarily pertain to elective or emergency surgical procedures in patients who are human immunodeficiency virus antibody positive or who have AIDS-related complex (ARC). There is, however, evidence that elective anorectal surgical procedures in patients with AIDS or ARC are fraught with a high incidence of complications and poor wound healing.[10] Thus, one would expect that subsequent reports in the medical literature will document great difficulties in successfully operating on patients with AIDS or ARC electively and for surgical emergencies.[4]

References

1. Centers for Disease Control: Revision of case definition of acquired immunodeficiency syndrome (AIDS)–United States. *MMWR* 1985;34:373-375.
2. Potter DA, Danforth DN, Macher AM, et al: Evaluation of abdominal pain in the AIDS patient. *Ann Surg* 1984;199:332-339.
3. Barone JE, Gingold BS, Arvantis ML, et al: Abdominal pain in patients with acquired immune deficiency syndrome. *Ann Surg* 1986;204:619-623.
4. Frank D, Raicht RF: Intestinal perforation associated with cytomegalovirus infection in patients with acquired immune deficiency syndrome. *Am J Gastroenterol* 1984;79:201-205.
5. Kram HB, Stanley HT, Cohen RE, et al: Spontaneous colonic perforation secondary to cytomegalovirus in a patient with acquired immune deficiency syndrome. *Crit Care Med* 1984;12:469-471.
6. Robinson G, Wilson SE, Williams RA: Surgery in patients with acquired immunodeficiency syndrome. *Arch Surg* 1987;122:170-175.
7. Hubbard SG, Brack BA, Litvak AS: Acute abdomen in the transplant patient. *Am Surg* 1980;46:116-120.
8. Marasca G, McEvory M: Length of survival of patients with acquired immune deficiency syndrome in the United Kingdom. *Br Med J* 1986;292:1727-1729.
9. Miller JI: The thoracic surgical spectrum of acquired immune deficiency syndrome. *J Thorac Cardiovasc Surg* 1986;92:977-980.
10. Wexner SD, Smithy WB, Wilson JW, et al: The surgical management of anorectal diseases in AIDS and pre-AIDS patients. *Dis Colon Rectum* 1986;29:719-723.

Errors in Estimating Energy Expenditure in Critically Ill Surgical Patients

Vincente Cortes, MD, Loren D. Nelson, MD

• Thirty-one critically ill surgical patients were receiving central parenteral nutrition. All were intubated, and 29 were receiving mechanical ventilatory support. Nutritional and metabolic data were recorded at the time of indirect calorimetry. Measured energy expenditure (MEE) was compared with predictions of basal energy expenditure (BEE) and *calculated energy expenditure,* defined as the product of BEE and a stress factor estimated by the nutrition support service to account for severity of illness and activity. The MEE was significantly greater than the BEE and significantly less than the calculated energy expenditure. The estimated stress factor was significantly greater than the actual MEE/BEE ratio, and the correlation between these values was poor. Clinical assessment may overestimate energy expenditure in critically ill patients because of the apparent degree of illness used to determine the stress factor. Bedside indirect calorimetry may be useful to assess more accurately energy expenditure and optimize nutritional support.

(*Arch Surg* 1989;124:287-290)

Central parenteral nutrition (CPN) regimens are formulated to optimize total energy intake and fractional requirements of protein, carbohydrate, and fat. Total energy requirement is frequently calculated using the Harris-Benedict equations to estimate basal energy expenditure (BEE).[1] The clinical estimate of a patient's actual energy expenditure (calculated energy expenditure [CEE]) is the product of BEE times a stress factor to estimate the fraction by which actual energy expenditure exceeds the basal value.[2-4] Energy expenditure can also be measured by direct or indirect calorimetry.

Increased interest in nutritional support of hospitalized patients brought about the rebirth of indirect calorimetry.[5-8] Technical considerations have limited the application in intubated patients receiving supplemental oxygen and mechanical ventilatory support. The development of an adequate interface between ventilator and patient and the refinement of precise measuring instruments have made indirect calorimetry a reality in these cases.[9,10]

We used indirect calorimetry to assess clinical estimates of energy expenditure as a reflection of actual energy expenditure in a group of critically ill surgical patients.

SUBJECTS AND METHODS

Patient Population

The records of 100 consecutive patients studied by indirect calorimetry in the Surgical Intensive Care Unit at Jackson Memorial Hospital, Miami, were reviewed. Indications for metabolic measurements included carbon dioxide retention, difficulty in ventilator weaning, shock, sepsis, acute respiratory failure, and monitoring of CPN. Thirty-one of these patients who were receiving CPN at the time of measurement were selected for this study. Twenty-five patients had undergone major surgery, and six had sustained thoracoabdominal trauma. All patients were intubated and were receiving supplemental ventilatory support sufficient to produce a comfortable breathing pattern and respiratory rate.

All the patients had been evaluated by the Nutritional Support Service, and recommendations for specific CPN regimens, including total energy requirement and percentages of each major component (protein, carbohydrate, and lipid), had been made. The consultation forms entered in the patient's chart by the Nutritional Support Service were reviewed, and information regarding height, weight, BEE calculated according to the Harris-Benedict equations, stress factor, CEE, and nutritional recommendations were obtained for each patient. Nitrogen balance was calculated as protein intake divided by 6.25 minus the 24-hour urinary urea nitrogen excretion plus 3 g for insensible losses.

Other information recorded included level of mechanical ventilatory support, arterial blood gas results, actual nutritional components being infused, and the estimated activity level of the patient at the time of measurements. All patients were intubated, and all but two were receiving mechanical ventilatory support (fractional inspired oxygen concentration, 0.21; intermittent mandatory ventilation rate, two or more breaths per minute; positive end-expiratory pressure, ≥5 cm H_2O).

Indirect Calorimetry

Oxygen consumption and carbon dioxide production were measured using a portable bedside indirect calorimeter (Metabolic Gas Monitor—MGM/Two, Utah Medical Products, Midvale). The device measures differences in the concentration of oxygen and carbon dioxide between inspired gas and expired gas, as well as the minute expired volume. It has previously been subjected to bench testing[9] and clinical validation in similar critically ill patients using the same interface between the device and the ventilatory

Accepted for publication July 15, 1988.
From the Departments of Surgery, University of Miami School of Medicine (Dr Cortes) and Vanderbilt University School of Medicine, Nashville, Tenn (Dr Nelson).

Reprints not available.

Variable*	n	Mean ± SD	Range
pH	31	7.36 ± 1.30	7.14-7.49
Pa_{O_2}, mm Hg	31	98 ± 32	50-152
Pa_{CO_2}, mm Hg	31	46 ± 14	28-79
Sa_{O_2}, %	31	95 ± 17	85-99
BEE, kJ/d	29	5910 ± 1310†	4140-8820
SF	29	1.47 ± 0.13	1.2-1.7
CEE, kJ/d	30	8590 ± 1690‡	6300-13 240
MEE, kJ/d	29	7730 ± 2050	3300-11 860
MEE/BEE	29	1.32 ± 0.36§	0.78-2.02
V_{O_2}, mL/min	31	252 ± 83	107-412
V_{CO_2}, mL/min	31	258 ± 76	126 ± 387
RQ	31	1.03 ± 0.22	0.79-1.29

Table 1.—Blood Gas and Energy Expenditure Data

*Pa_{O_2} indicates arterial oxygen tension; Pa_{CO_2}, arterial carbon dioxide tension; Sa_{O_2}, arterial oxygen saturation; BEE, basal energy expenditure; SF, stress factor; CEE, calculated energy expenditure; MEE, measured energy expenditure; V_{O_2}, oxygen consumption; V_{CO_2}, carbon dioxide production; RQ, respiratory quotient.

†Significantly less than MEE ($P<.001$).

‡Significantly greater than MEE ($P<.01$).

§Significantly less than SF ($P<.025$).

circuit.[10] The measurements were made over periods ranging from 30 minutes to two hours. When steady-state values were obtained, measured energy expenditure (MEE), oxygen consumption, carbon dioxide production, and respiratory quotient were recorded.

Statistical Analysis

Measurements of various parameters are expressed as mean ± SD. The Student's t test for paired data was used for determinations of differences between variables. Correlation between values was assessed by linear regression analysis. Probability values less than .05 were considered statistically significant.

RESULTS

The group included 15 male and 16 female patients, with a mean age of 56 ± 20.6 years (range, 15 to 82 years) and a mean body surface area of 1.78 ± 0.41 m^2 (range, 1.4 to 2.3 m^2). The mean mechanical ventilatory support levels were as follows: fractional inspired oxygen concentration, 0.40 ± 0.11 (range, 0.21 to 0.47); intermittent mandatory ventilation rate, 3.2 + 2.1 breaths per minute (range, zero to eight breaths per minute); and positive end-expiratory pressure, 5.5 ± 2.2 cm H_2O (range, 5 to 15 cm H_2O). Arterial

Table 2.—Diagnoses, Energy Expenditure, and Nitrogen Excretion*

Case	Primary Diagnosis	MEE, kJ/d	BEE, kJ/D	Stress Factor	CEE, kJ/d	UUN, mmol/d	MEE/BEE
1	Tongue carcinoma	7250	5330	1.4	7470	640	1.36
2	Pelvic inflammatory disease	9420	5940	1.5	8910	110	1.58
3	Colon AV malformation	6500	4630	1.4	6480	240	1.40
4	Perforated ulcer	11 860	7170	1.4	10 040	...	1.65
5	Abdominal trauma	8080	6750	1.5	10 120	660	1.20
6	Toxic megacolon	5040	4910	1.5	7860	160	1.02
7	Perforated diverticulum	10 390	5130	1.5	7700	150	1.02
8	Multiple gunshot wounds	11 840	7990	1.3	10 390	430	1.48
9	Pancreatitis	8870	5120	1.4	7170	450	1.73
10	Pancreatitis	7750	8600	1.2	10 330	560	0.90
11	Liver cystic disease	7360	6190	1.3	8050	220	1.19
12	Pancreatitis	5800	4137	1.7	7030	...	1.40
13	Perforated appendicitis	7390	4200	1.5	6300	400	1.76
14	Lye ingestion	6590	5300	1.65	8740	410	1.24
15	Rectal carcinoma	6720	4780	1.5	7170	230	1.40
16	Carcinoid	6700	5450	1.5	8170	90	1.23
17	Pancreatitis	10 270	7000	1.35	9450	210	1.47
18	Perforated gastric lymphoma	3710	4390	1.6	7030	140	0.84
19	Ovarian carcinoma	6790	5190	1.5	7780	220	1.31
20	Multiple trauma	8359	6750	1.5	10 120	820	1.24
21	Diabetic foot ulcer	3310	4230	1.65	6980	250	0.78
22	Hypothyroid obesity	6160	...	...	7680	370	...
23	Bladder carcinoma	6270	5250	1.3	6820	200	1.20
24	Cervical fracture	7850	5440	1.5	8160	260	1.44
25	Cholangitis	5480	...	...	8500	610	...
26	Laryngeal carcinoma	9000	6510	1.6	10 420	320	1.38
27	Multiple gunshot wounds	7710	7790	1.7	13 240	160	0.99
28	Rectal carcinoma	6330	5080	1.5	7620	250	1.25
29	Multiple trauma	10 130	8820	1.4	12 570	600	1.15
30	Tongue carcinoma	8440	6770	1.4	9470	480	1.25
31	Esophageal carcinoma	8520	6630	1.3	8620	170	1.28

*MEE indicates measured energy expenditure; BEE, basal energy expenditure; CEE, calculated energy expenditure; UUN, urinary urea nitrogen excretion; AV, arteriovenous.

blood gas results and metabolic measurements are shown in Table 1.

The patient's diagnosis, MEE and estimated energy expenditure, stress factor, ratio of MEE to BEE, and 24-hour urinary urea nitrogen excretion are listed in Table 2. Nitrogen balance varied widely in these patients; mean nitrogen balance was a positive 1.0 ± 6.9 g/d.

Measured energy expenditure (7730 ± 2050 kJ/d) was significantly greater than BEE (5910 ± 1310 kJ/d) ($P<.001$), and there was a significant correlation between the two values ($r=.67$, $P<.001$) (Fig 1). Measured energy expenditure (7670 ± 2040 kJ/d) was significantly less than CEE (8590 ± 1700 kJ/d) ($P<.01$), and there was a significant correlation between the two values ($r=.56$, $P<.005$, Fig 2).

The estimated stress factor (1.47 ± 0.13) was significantly greater than the actual ratio between MEE and BEE (1.32 ± 0.36) ($P<.025$), and the correlation between those two values was poor ($r=-.13$, $P>.05$, Fig 3).

Neither the estimated stress factor nor the ratio of MEE to BEE correlated with the 24-hour urinary urea nitrogen value ($r=-.01$, $P>.05$).

COMMENT

Frequent use of nutritional support has increased the desire to appraise energy requirements of critically ill patients. Calculation of BEE and measurement of actual energy expenditure have been used clinically.[11,12] Basal energy expenditure is the energy requirement of a normal individual at rest in the fasting state, ten to 18 hours after a meal, and physically relaxed in a neutral-thermal environment and is also called *basal metabolic rate*. The clinical estimate of a patient's actual energy expenditure (CEE) is the product of BEE times a stress factor to estimate the fraction by which actual energy expenditure exceeds that basal value.[2-4]

One of the most common methods to estimate BEE uses multiple regression equations developed by Harris and Benedict in 1919. These calorimetric studies, performed on awake, resting, normal subjects, indicated that sex, height, weight, and age are the primary determinants of BEE.[1]

Since BEE estimates "basal" energy expenditure, it is multiplied by a stress factor to estimate the energy requirements for a specific individual and circumstance.[3] The stress factor accounts for the increased expenditure related to specific dynamic action of the nutrients, activity, illness, fever, trauma, and surgery. Cerra[13] suggested a simple system for the estimation of the stress: low, 1.3; moderate, 1.5; severe, 2.0.

Indirect calorimetry has been reintroduced for the bedside measurement of energy expenditure, but technical difficulties have limited application in critically ill patients receiving supplemental oxygen and mechanical ventilatory support.[7,8,12] These same patients are often highly stressed, and the correction factors used to calculate energy expenditure vary widely. Overfeeding of carbohydrate substrate may result in hyperglycemia, hyperosmolar states, osmotic diuresis, fatty infiltration of the liver, increased carbon dioxide production, and worsening of respiratory failure.[14-22]

With the use of indirect calorimetry, we detected errors in the estimation of energy expenditure in patients in the surgical intensive care unit. While BEE, CEE, and MEE correlated statistically, MEE was significantly greater than BEE, calculated using the Harris-Benedict equations, and significantly less than the CEE, calculated using an estimated stress factor. The stress factor used for the CEE

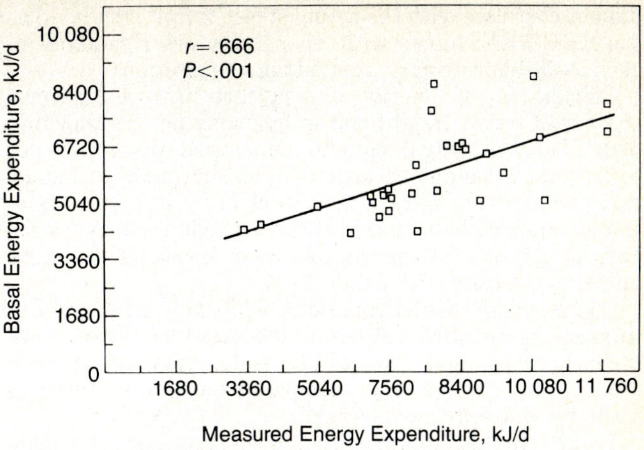

Fig 1.—Correlation between measured and basal energy expenditure ($r=.67$, $P<.001$) ($y=620+0.43x$).

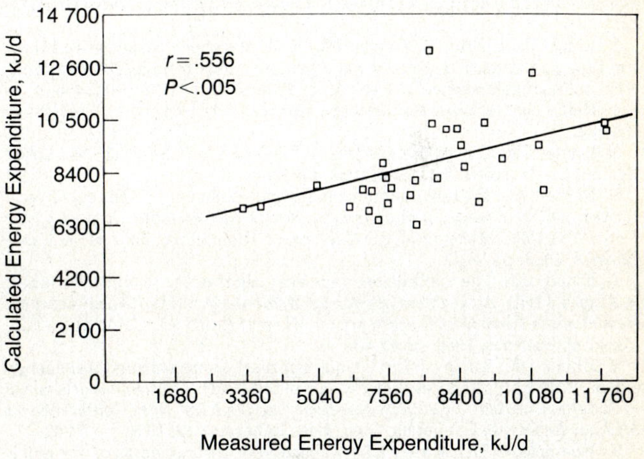

Fig 2.—Correlation between measured and calculated energy expenditure ($r=.56$, $P<.005$) ($y=1199+0.46x$).

Fig 3.—Correlation between ratio of measured to basal energy expenditure (MEE/BEE) and estimated stress factor ($r=-0.13$, $P<.05$) ($y=1.72-0.27x$).

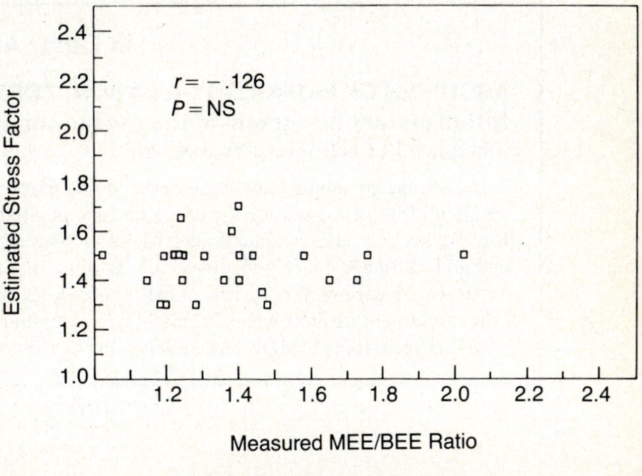

did not correlate with the actual stress factor calculated as the MEE/BEE ratio or with other indicators of catabolism, such as 24-hour urinary urea nitrogen excretion.[3]

Calculation of energy expenditure involves several sources of error. Height and weight may not be known in bedridden, critically ill patients. Measured weight may not reflect usual weight because of prehospitalization losses, water volume changes related to primary illness or associated complications, and intravenous fluid resuscitation.[23] Height may not be known, and measurements of length may not correlate with height.[24]

The Harris-Benedict equations, while validated by other workers to within ±5% from 1936 to 1956, have more recently been shown to yield results varying between −14.1% to +19.1% when compared with measurements made by indirect calorimetry.[25]

It appears that clinical estimation of stress is responsible for the observed divergence between CEE and MEE. Clinical impressions may overestimate actual stress because support technology makes the patient appear to be sicker than he is. Our results support this contention and point to the estimation of the stress factor as the primary source of error.

While it is possible that this overestimate of metabolic needs is specific to our institution, it is our impression that it is more widespread. Physician awareness of this problem will be important to avoid overfeeding of critically ill patients. More frequent use of indirect calorimetry in the critical care setting may facilitate the administration of nutritional support by providing objective measurements of actual energy expenditure and substrate use.

Hans Anderson, RRT, assisted in the development of the interface techniques and validation of the metabolic monitor. Cliff Reistler and the Nutritional Support Service at Jackson Memorial Hospital performed the metabolic assessments.

References

1. Harris JA, Benedict FG: *Biometric Studies of Basal Metabolism in Man,* publication 279. Carnegie Institute of Washington, 1919.
2. Blackburn GL, Bistrian BR, Maini BS, et al: Nutritional and metabolic assessment of the hospitalized patient. *J Parenteral Enteral Nutr* 1977;1:11-22.
3. Long CL, Shaffel N, Geiger JW, et al: Metabolic response to injury and illness: Estimation of energy and protein needs from indirect calorimetry and nitrogen balance. *J Parenteral Enteral Nutr* 1979;3:452-456.
4. Reilly JJ, Gerhardt AL: Modern surgical nutrition. *Curr Probl Surg* 1985;22.
5. Kinney JM: Energy metabolism, in Fisher JR (ed): *Surgical Nutrition.* Boston, Little Brown & Co Inc, 1983, pp 42-48.
6. Norton AC: Portable equipment for gas exchange, in Kinney J (ed): *Assessment of Energy Metabolism in Health and Disease: Report of the First Ross Conference on Medical Research.* Columbus, Ohio, Ross Laboratories, 1980, pp 36-41.
7. Kinney JM: The application of indirect calorimetry to clinical studies, in Kinney J (ed): *Assessment of Energy Metabolism in Health and Disease: Report of the First Ross Conference on Medical Research.* Columbus, Ohio, Ross Laboratories, 1980, pp 42-48.
8. Elwyn DH, Kinney JM: A unique approach to measuring total energy expenditure by indirect calorimetry, in Kinney J (ed): *Assessment of Energy Metabolism in Health and Disease: Report of the First Ross Conference on Medical Research.* Columbus, Ohio, Ross Laboratories, 1980, pp 54-62.
9. Westenskow DR, Cutler CA, Wallace WD: Instrumentation for monitoring gas exchange and metabolic rate in critically ill patients. *Crit Care Med* 1984;12:183-187.
10. Nelson LD, Anderson HB, Garcia H: Clinical validation of a new metabolic monitor suitable for use in critically ill patients. *Crit Care Med* 1987;15:951-957.
11. Rutten P, Blackburn GL, Flatt JP, et al: Determination of optimal hyperalimentation infusion rate. *J Surg Res* 1975;18:477.
12. Long CL, Carlo MA, Schaffel NA, et al: A continuous analyzer for monitoring respiratory gases and expired radioactivity in clinical studies. *Metabolism* 1979;28:320-332.
13. Cerra FB: *Pocket Manual of Surgical Nutrition.* St Louis, CV Mosby Co, 1984.
14. Wolfe RR, Allsop JR, Burke JF: Glucose metabolism in man: Response to intravenous glucose infusion. *Metabolism* 1979;28:210-220.
15. MacFie J, Smith RC, Hill GL: Glucose or fat as a nonprotein energy source? *Gastroenterology* 1981;80:103-107.
16. Ausman RK, Hardy G: Metabolic complications of parenteral nutrition, in Jonston LDA (ed): *Advances in Parenteral Nutrition.* Lancaster, England, MTP Press Ltd, 1977, pp 111-117.
17. Burke JF, Wolfe RR, Mullany CJ, et al: Glucose requirements following burn injury: Parameters of optimal glucose infusion and possible hepatic and respiratory abnormalities following excessive glucose intake. *Ann Surg* 1979;190:274-285.
18. Saltzman HA, Salzano JV: Effects of carbohydrate metabolism upon respiratory gas exchange in normal men. *J Appl Physiol* 1971;30:228-231.
19. Gieseke T, Gurushanthaiah G, Glauser FL: Effects of carbohydrates on carbon dioxide excretion in patients with airway disease. *Chest* 1977;71:55-58.
20. Askanazi J, Elwin DH, Silverberg PA, et al: Respiratory distress secondary to a high carbohydrate load: A case report. *Surgery* 1980;87:596-598.
21. Askanazi J, Rosenbaum SH, Hyman AI, et al: Respiratory changes induced by the large glucose loads of total parenteral nutrition. *JAMA* 1980;243:1444-1447.
22. Covelli HD, Black JW, Olsen MS, et al: Respiratory failure precipitated by high carbohydrate loads. *Ann Intern Med* 1981;95:579-581.
23. Gump FE, Kinney JM, Iles M, et al: Duration and significance of large fluid loads administered for circulatory support. *J Trauma* 1970;10:431-439.
24. Mitchell CO, Lipschitz DA: Arm length measurement as an alternative to height in nutritional assessments of the elderly. *J Parenteral Enteral Nutr* 1982;6:226.
25. Daly JM, Heymsfield SB, Head CA, et al: Human energy requirements: Over estimation by widely used prediction equation. *Am J Clin Nutr* 1985;42:1170-1174.

In Other AMA Journals

ARCHIVES OF PATHOLOGY & LABORATORY MEDICINE

Inflammatory Aneurysm of the Aorta, Aortitis, and Coronary Arteritis

Stephen D. Cohle, MD, J. T. Lie, MD

Inflammatory aneurysm of the aorta is not merely a variant of atherosclerosis, but more probably it is a manifestation of a peculiar systemic disease related to idiopathic retroperitoneal and mediastinal fibrosis. Rarely, aortitis and coronary arteritis may coexist with the inflammatory aneurysm; one of each of such unusual cases are described. Because inflammatory aneurysms of the aorta tend to occur in elderly persons, aortitis and coronary arteritis, when present, cannot be distinguished from the concomitant age-related atherosclerosis without a careful histologic examination (*Arch Pathol Lab Med* 1988;112:1121-1125).

Reprint requests to Blodgett Memorial Medical Center, 1840 Wealthy St SE, Grand Rapids, MI 49506 (Dr Cohle).

Hemostasis of Solid Viscus Trauma by Intraparenchymal Injection of Fibrin Glue

Carl J. Hauser, MD

• Fibrin glue (FG) is an effective hemostatic agent applied topically to the spleen. In this study, FG was found to be an effective hemostatic agent when applied topically in standardized wounds of the canine liver, spleen, and pancreas. It was markedly more effective, however, when injected intraparenchymally. In a case of severe blunt trauma in a patient with acute alcoholic hepatitis, intraparenchymal FG was lifesaving. Fibrin glue is a useful adjunct in the management of trauma to all the abdominal solid viscera. Intraparenchymal injection is the preferred mode of FG application.

(*Arch Surg* 1989;124:291-293)

Hemorrhage from injured solid organs may be difficult to control. Solid viscera hold sutures poorly, injured vessels may be deep within the organ, and bleeding from the parenchyma itself may be life-threatening, especially when coagulopathy occurs. On occasion, the surgeon must perform undesirable resective procedures,[1,2] pack the abdomen,[3-5] or accept incomplete hemostasis at the time of closure. Such situations might be avoided if more effective methods of solid organ hemostasis were available.

Fibrin glue (FG) is formed by mixing a source of concentrated fibrinogen with thrombin and is hemostatic in mild to moderate splenic trauma.[6-8] When splenic trauma is severe, however, FG is less effective.[7] In these cases, FG tends to be washed off by the stream of blood prior to polymerization or to be lifted off of the treated surface soon afterward by bleeding beneath the coagulum. Thus, a method of application appropriate to the parenchymal injuries seen in hepatic and severe splenic trauma has not been described. This communication reports my experience using intraparenchymal FG (IPFG) to avoid such displacement of the FG coagulum.

METHODS

Experimental Injuries

Twenty-four hepatic injuries were produced in 12 mongrel dogs. General anesthesia was induced by ketamine hydrochloride and pentobarbital sodium (Nembutal). The liver was exposed at laparotomy. Injuries were produced in a random sequence. In each dog, a slash incision 8 cm in length and 1.5 cm deep was made in the right lobe of the liver, and a stab incision was made in the left lobe by plunging a No. 10 scalpel into the liver to a depth of 5 cm. All wounds bled freely (>50 mL/min). Twelve wounds were fashioned in the spleens of six of the above dogs. One slash wound 4 cm long and 1 cm deep and one stab wound formed by plunging a No. 10 scalpel blade to a depth of 2.5 cm were created in each animal's spleen. In six dogs, the distal 2.5 cm of the descending limb of the pancreas was dissected free from the duodenal mesentery and amputated.

Administration of FG

Fibrin glue was prepared from a kit containing concentrated fibrinogen and bovine thrombin. The two substrates are mixed as the glue is delivered through a needle. By using concentrated thrombin solution, polymerization was effected within 10 to 15 s. Wounded areas were first compressed to obtain hemostasis until the glue had polymerized. Fibrin glue was applied topically (TFG) by allowing it to flow freely onto the cut surface until a polymerized seal had formed. Injection into the wound (IPFG) was performed using a sharp 18-gauge needle advanced 1 cm into the parenchyma via the capsular wound and then moved back and forth during injection as for the creation of a field block with a local anesthetic. Injections were done such that FG oozed out of tissue and polymerized on the surface of the wound. The temporary compression of the organ was then released.

Half of the wounds of each type were treated, respectively, with TFG and IPFG as the initial hemostatic modality. In all cases, each treatment used 4 to 6 mL of glue. As an internal control to test for the effects of the wound compression on hemostasis in these wounds, four hepatic stab and four hepatic slash wounds were each initially compressed for a period of one minute and then released. In all cases, free bleeding recurred immediately, and these wounds were subsequently treated with TFG or IPFG. In subsequent dogs, this test was omitted. After release of compression, the wounds were inspected for one minute and then were judged hemostatic (no assessable bleeding) or nonhemostatic (showing continued free bleeding or hematoma formation). Nonhemostatic wounds were treated with a second application of TFG or IPFG. If two applications of FG failed, that wound was "crossed over" to the other method of FG administration.

Statistical Analysis

Dogs were reoperated on and killed at one week to three months to assess any possible complications of therapy and to determine the fate of the wound repairs. The abilities of TFG, IPFG, and

Accepted for publication June 20, 1988.
From the Division of Trauma, Hollywood Presbyterian Medical Center, Los Angeles.
Reprint requests to Department of Medical Education, Hollywood Presbyterian Medical Center, 1300 N Vermont Ave, Los Angeles, CA 90027 (Ms Kay Biggs).

Table 1.—Hemostasis in Hepatic Slash Wounds*

	Control Achieved		Control Not Achieved
	1 Application	2 Applications	
Tamponade	0	0	4
TFG	3	3	0
IPFG	6	0	0

*TFG indicates topical fibrin glue; IPFG, intraparenchymal fibrin glue. Both TFG and IPFG were significantly more effective hemostatic modalities than simple tamponade of the wound ($\chi^2=14.6$, $P<.001$ for both modes of administration). Intraparenchymal FG was successful after the first application significantly more frequently than was TFG ($\chi^2=5.45$, $P<.02$).

Table 2.—Hemostasis in Hepatic Stab Wounds*

	Control Achieved		Control Not Achieved
	1 Application	2 Applications	
Tamponade	0	0	4
TFG	0	3	3
IPFG	6	0	0

*TFG indicates topical fibrin glue; IPFG, intraparenchymal fibrin glue. Both TFG and IPFG were significantly more effective hemostatic modalities than simple tamponade of the wound ($\chi^2=5.73$ [$P<.02$] and $\chi^2=14.6$ [$P<.001$], respectively). One application of IPFG was significantly more likely to effect hemostasis in a deep hepatic stab wound than either one or two applications of TFG ($\chi^2=16.33$ [$P<.001$] and $\chi^2=7.11$ [$P<.01$], respectively).

compression alone to produce hemostasis were compared by χ^2 analysis, with statistical significance assumed at the $P<.05$ level.

RESULTS

Of the six hepatic slash wounds treated with TFG, all showed marked initial diminution of bleeding, but in three of six the bleeding recurred. A second TFG application achieved complete hemostasis in all six. Of the six slash wounds treated primarily with IPFG, all achieved complete hemostasis on the first application (Table 1).

Six hepatic stab wounds were treated initially with TFG. Three achieved hemostasis, in each case after two applications. Two stab wounds continued to bleed, and one formed a hematoma despite two TFG applications. These three wounds were treated with IPFG and were hemostatic after one IPFG application. Of six hepatic stab wounds treated primarily with IPFG, all became hemostatic after the first application (Table 2).

The six superficial lacerations of the spleen were all treated successfully with either one (four of six) or two (two of six) applications of TFG. Intraparenchymal FG was not tested in these injuries. Of the deep splenic lacerations, three of six were successfully treated with a single application of TFG. The other three injuries bled despite two applications of TFG, but were then controlled by a single application of IPFG.

Topical FG did not achieve hemostasis in any pancreatic injuries. Hemorrhage from arteries in the pancreatic substance easily lifted the FG seal off of the pancreas. Intraparenchymal FG was used subsequently and achieved somewhat better success. Hemostasis was achieved in all cases; however, two applications of IPFG were required in four of the six injuries, and in three of these four cases hematomas formed beneath the FG seal.

Except for one dog who died intraoperatively of an anesthetic complication, all dogs recovered in a routine fashion. No dog developed clinical peritonitis, jaundice, or sepsis. At reexploration, no dog was found to have bile leakage, pancreatitis, ascites, or hemoperitoneum. No hepatic parenchymal hematomas were noted. In pathologic specimens obtained during the first postoperative week, IPFG administration sites were noted to form a continuous gel that traversed the wounds, filling the parenchyma as well as the wound itself. Intraparenchymal FG caused a slight space-occupying effect, with bulging of the specimen's cut surface at the IPFG injection site. Topical FG and IPFG sites disappeared over the course of three to four weeks, leaving a fibrous capsular scar.

REPORT OF A CASE

A 32-year-old man was found lying in the street and was brought to Hollywood Presbyterian Trauma Center, Los Angeles. He was hypotensive, agitated, and jaundiced. A thoracoabdominal tire-track mark was noted. The hematocrit reading was 0.23; the blood alcohol level was 428 mg/dL. After resuscitation, the patient was taken to the operating room. Laparotomy revealed an enormously enlarged, fatty liver. The posterior lateral left hepatic lobe was severely fractured, as was the spleen. Acute pancreatitis with saponification was noted. Rapid splenectomy was performed. Attempts at suture of the friable liver exacerbated the bleeding. Hepatic artery ligation and lobar resection were thought contraindicated by hepatitis and saponification in the porta hepatis. The liver was packed, and the abdomen was closed. Over the next 48 hours, the patient required 6 U of packed red blood cells. He was treated for cardiac and pulmonary contusions, acute respiratory distress syndrome, delirium tremens, Wernicke's encephalopathy, and coagulopathy. On the third hospital day, the patient developed polymicrobial sepsis. After Food and Drug Administration approval of possible use of FG on humanitarian grounds, the patient underwent another laparotomy. The left upper quadrant was exposed by division of the costal margin. Packs were gently dissected off the liver using a water pick. Nonetheless, life-threatening hemorrhage recurred. The liver was compressed medial to the injuries, and FG was injected into the liver parenchyma around the fracture sites until it ran into the fractures and filled them up. Compression was maintained for two minutes and then released. Hemostasis was complete. A subcapsular hematoma due to retraction of the liver was noted. The hematoma was unroofed, revealing diffuse bleeding but no fracture. This was controlled by TFG. Multiple soft silicone sump drains were placed, and the abdomen was closed. The drains were nonproductive and were removed at one week. The patient was discharged one month after his injury. Computed tomographic scan performed three weeks after injury showed continued fatty replacement but no residual injuries.

COMMENT

The efficacy of TFG in human splenic salvage has been established in European studies,[6,7] but to my knowledge the use of FG in hepatic trauma has not been reported. Topical FG seems to be quite adequate to obtain hemostasis in the mildly to moderately injured spleen. In the deeply lacerated spleen and in the injured liver, however, IPFG seems to be more effective. In these experimental injuries, immediate hemostasis was achieved more frequently by IPFG than TFG, in both the slash ($\chi^2=5.45$, $P<.02$) and the stab ($\chi^2=16.33$, $P<.001$) wounds. This seems to be related to three factors. First, the fibrin is anchored to the wound by extension of the polymer into the adjoining parenchyma. Second, causing the FG to "percolate" through the parenchyma seals the parenchymal sites, which may persist in bleeding after discrete bleeding sites have been controlled. Third, injection of FG directly into the parenchyma seems to cause a "mass effect," with tamponade of bleeding from surrounding tissues.

In bleeding pancreatic injuries, FG was less effective.

Topical FG was easily lifted off of the organ capsule by the bleeding. Also, IPFG did not spread through pancreatic parenchyma as readily as through liver or spleen. Thus, arterial bleeding from the pancreas was only controlled by repeated application of IPFG. Venous bleeding, however, and leakage of pancreatic juices were controlled by IPFG.

The case study demonstrates that use of FG can effect hemostasis where bleeding might not be controllable by conventional methods. The lack of bile leakage seen in this patient, as well as in the canine model, suggests that FG prevents leakage of bile from hepatic injuries. The absence of residual computed tomographic evidence of injury at three weeks suggests that the human liver heals rapidly in the presence of FG, with total reabsorption at three to four weeks, as reported in canine spleen.[8]

Fibrin glue is an effective hemostatic agent in solid organ trauma. It should not be expected to control bleeding from major vessels, but it is extremely effective in the control of parenchymal bleeding persisting after major vascular sources have been controlled. The degree of effectiveness varies, depending on the organ and injury in question and on the mode of administration. This study suggests that IPFG is preferred in deep injuries, especially injuries of the liver. Compression of the parenchyma to be injected until the FG polymerizes is useful to maximize local adherence, as well as to eliminate the theoretical danger of embolism to the lungs.

When FG is produced from pooled plasma, its use carries a high risk of hepatitis transmission and thus Food and Drug Administration approval has been limited to individual cases of compassionate need. However, as manufacture of FG from individual donors or synthesized fibrinogen becomes practical,[9] FG will become an important therapeutic modality in solid organ hemorrhage.

References

1. Donovan AJ, Michaelian MJ, Yellin AE: Anatomic hepatic lobectomy in trauma to the liver. *Surgery* 1973;73:833-847.
2. Pachter HL, Spencer FC, Hofstetter SR, et al: Experience with the finger fracture technique to achieve intrahepatic hemostasis in 75 patients with severe trauma to the liver. *Ann Surg* 1983;179:771-777.
3. Stone HH, Lamb JM: Use of pedicled omentum as an autogenous pack for control of hemorrhage in major injuries of the liver. *Ann Surg* 1975; 141:92-94.
4. Feliciano DV, Mattox KL, Jordan GL Jr: Intraabdominal packing for control of hepatic hemorrhage: A reappraisal. *J Trauma* 1981;21:285-289.
5. Carmona RH, Peck DZ, Lim RC Jr: The role of packing and planned reoperation in severe hepatic trauma. *J Trauma* 1984;24:779-782.
6. Brands W, Menniken C, Beck M: Preservation of the ruptured spleen with highly concentrated human fibrinogen: Experimental and clinical results. *World J Surg* 1982;6:366-368.
7. Scheele J, Gentche HH, Matteson E: Splenic repair by fibrin tissue adhesive and collagen fleece. *Surgery* 1984;95:6-13.
8. Kram HB, Shoemaker WC, Hino ST, et al: Splenic salvage using biologic glue. *Arch Surg* 1984;119:1309-1311.
9. Dresdale A, Rose EA, Jevanandam V, et al: Preparation of fibrin glue from single donor fresh frozen plasma. *Surgery* 1985;97:750-755.

In Other AMA Journals

ARCHIVES OF OTOLARYNGOLOGY–HEAD & NECK SURGERY

Sinusitis in the Nasotracheally Intubated Patient

Barry E. Linden, MD; Eugenio A. Aguilar, MD; Steven J. Allen, MD

Maxillary sinusitis as a complication of nasotracheal intubation has long been recognized as difficult to diagnose and equally difficult to treat. To better define this problem from a diagnostic and therapeutic standpoint, we studied patients admitted to the surgical intensive care unit at the University of Texas Health Science Center at Houston-Hermann Hospital over a six-month period. During this time, we identified 19 cases of maxillary sinusitis. Diagnostic criteria included fever, leukocytosis, purulent rhinorrhea, and maxillary sinus opacification or air fluid level noted on sinus roentgenograms. Patients who met these criteria underwent maxillary sinus aspiration. Sixteen patients were receiving antibiotic therapy when sinusitis was diagnosed. All patients had their endotracheal tubes replaced orally, had diseased maxillary antra lavaged, and underwent appropriate antibiotic therapy guided by culture and sensitivity studies. Four of 19 patients required more than one sinus lavage, but all patients had their sinus disease resolve. These data suggest an aggressive approach to diagnosing sinusitis in the nasotracheally intubated patient is needed. A maxillary sinus aspiration and lavage should be an integral part of the diagnosis and treatment of these patients (*Arch Otolaryngol Head Neck Surg* 1988;114:860-861).

Reprint requests to the Department of Otolaryngology-Head and Neck Surgery, The University of Texas Health Science Center at Houston, 6431 Fannin, MSMB 6.132, Houston, TX 77030 (Dr Linden).

Neutron Therapy for Nonresectable Radioresistant Tumors

Lionel Cohen, MD, Frank R. Hendrickson, MD

• Locally advanced, nonresectable, radioresistant tumors can often be ablated by external irradiation using high-energy fast neutron beams. Long-term local control has been achieved in a wide range of malignant tumors, notably sarcomas of bone and soft tissue and adenocarcinomas in various sites. Complete response and long-term remission, with local control rates between 50% and 70%, have been reported in a number of very large osteogenic sarcomas, soft-tissue sarcomas (particularly neurogenic tumors), melanomas, and adenocarcinomas of the alimentary tract. Malignant salivary gland tumors and carcinoma of the prostate appear to be the most responsive to neutrons, with a high frequency (70% to 90%) of successful remission and significantly improved survival even in advanced stages of disease. The biological mechanisms underlying radioresistance of tumor cells and the rationale for using heavily ionizing particles are described. Neutrons are shown to be a valuable adjunct in managing nonresectable malignant tumors that resist conventional therapy.

(*Arch Surg* 1989;124:294-300)

Surgery, radiotherapy, and chemotherapy are the only modalities, used singly or in combination, that can provide long-term local control of nonmetastatic cancer. In suitably responsive tumors (lymphomas or small epidermoid carcinomas, for example), radiotherapy and/or chemotherapy may be the preferred treatment. In most other situations, complete surgical resection, with or without preoperative or postoperative adjuvant therapy, is the only potentially curative option. However, a real dilemma is posed when a nonresectable tumor, which is also resistant to radiotherapy and chemotherapy, is encountered. Under these circumstances it would be reasonable to explore other modalities that are theoretically able to control such tumors.

MATERIALS AND METHODS

Radioresistant Tumors

Commonly encountered radioresistant tumors include melanoma, sarcoma of the bone and soft tissue, adenocarcinoma of the thyroid, respiratory, and alimentary systems, and peripheral nerve tumors (Table 1). In all these tumor types, permanent ablation can be achieved by radiation, but only with exceptionally large doses, often beyond safe normal tissue tolerance limits.

The resistance of these tumors to conventional radiotherapy has been attributed to (1) the presence, in many tissues and tumors, of repair enzymes that confer on the associated tumor cells an unusually high capacity to sustain and recover from radiation injury; (2) the existence in large necrotic tumors of ischemic (hypoxic) zones in which tumor cells are protected from the lethal effects of the oxidizing radicals normally produced by ionizing radiation in well-oxygenated tissues; (3) production of intracellular reducing substances (such as melanin) that can intercept oxidizing radicals before they can react irreversibly with chromosomal DNA; and (4) variation in the response of cells in different phases of the cell cycle, with the result that slow-growing tumors, having a large proportion of noncycling, relatively insensitive cells, can survive doses of radiation that would be lethal in more rapidly cycling tumors.

These mechanisms are known to be responsible for repair and recovery from sparsely ionizing (low–linear energy transfer [LET]) radiations, which include electrons, x-rays, and gamma rays generally used for radiotherapy. By contrast, irradiation with high-LET particles such as neutrons produces irreversible chromosomal disruption (double-strand breaks), which kills or sterilizes cells independently of the cell cycle, biochemical environment, or treatment time. For this reason, tumors that are resistant to conventional radiotherapy are expected to be markedly more responsive to neutron beam therapy.[1] A number of clinical studies have also confirmed this expectation.[2-4]

Previous Clinical Studies

An active "historical" phase in neutron therapy research was pursued from 1970 to 1985 following reports by Catterall[3] in London on the striking results of neutron therapy for locally advanced cancer of the upper aerodigestive tract. During that period, some 9000 patients were treated in 20 centers throughout the world using relatively low-energy (15- to 30-MeV) cyclotrons designed for research in nuclear physics and adapted for clinical use. Although these beams were not well suited for treatment of deep-seated cancers, some impressive results were reported in a variety of nonresectable radioresistant tumors (Table 2). The current phase of this work commenced at Fermilab in Chicago in 1976 with the development of a high-energy (66-MeV) neutron beam suitable for cross-firing, deep-seated tumors in an isocentric mode analogous to a modern linear accelerator. Hospital-based high-energy cyclotrons now exist in several other centers: Houston, Los Angeles, Seattle, Cleveland, and Detroit in the United States and Louvain, Belgium, Liverpool, England, and Cape Town, South Africa, abroad. Results of current studies, using high-

Accepted for publication March 15, 1988.
From the Midwest Institute for Neutron Therapy at Fermilab, Batavia, Ill.

Reprint requests to Midwest Institute for Neutron Therapy at Fermilab, PO Box 5004, MS-301, Batavia, IL 60510 (Dr Cohen).

energy equipment, in selected groups of patients with unresectable, radioresistant tumors, will be described below.

RESULTS

With the exception of the gliomas, in which intensive investigation has so far not shown any advantage of neutron therapy over standard treatment, most radioresistant tumors appear to respond well to high-LET radiations.

Head and Neck

In cancer of the head and neck, stage and histological nature are major determinants of the response to irradiation. In general, locally advanced epidermoid carcinomas and most adenocarcinomas were found to be relatively resistant to conventional radiotherapy and significantly more responsive to neutrons (Color Fig 1).[4,5] Although no survival advantage could be demonstrated in epidermoid carcinomas, neutron therapy did yield a high rate of local control in large tumors and a low incidence of bone necrosis with repair of some bones eroded by tumor, which correlates well with their known physical and biological attributes.[4]

Seventy-six patients with locally advanced cancers of the head and neck have been treated with neutrons at Fermilab.[5] Results were analyzed to study the influence of stage, previous management, site of origin, and tumor histological type on local control of the disease. The most significant factor determining the outcome was the histological type. Long-term local control was achieved in 17 (49%) of 35 patients with epidermoid carcinoma and in 28 (72%) of 39 with nonepidermoid neoplasms (adenocarcinoma, cylindroma, mucoepidermoid carcinoma, and salivary-type tumor). The analysis also showed a survival advantage in nonepidermoid tumors treated with neutrons. It was concluded that neutron beam therapy was probably the treatment of choice for nonresectable or recurrent nonepidermoid cancers of the head and neck. Typical response of a large nonepidermoid oropharyngeal tumor is illustrated in Color Fig 2.

Salivary Gland Tumors

Tumors of the major and minor salivary glands, as well as salivary-type tumors in ectopic sites, have proved particularly responsive to neutron beam therapy, which has now become accepted as the treatment of choice in nonresectable salivary tumors.[6] Locally advanced salivary tumors with commencing facial nerve encroachment have been well controlled, often with full restoration of facial nerve function.[7] Color Fig 3 illustrates a typical result of neutron irradiation for nonresectable carcinoma of the parotid gland.

One hundred thirteen patients with recurrent and/or unresectable malignant salivary-type tumors treated with fast neutron therapy at Fermilab were analyzed for local control, sites of failure, and treatment-related morbidity.[6] Local control was achieved in 42 (67%) of 63 with major, and 29 (58%) of 50 patients with minor, salivary gland tumors. In a subset of patients with oropharyngeal and oral cavity salivary-type tumors, 19 (79%) of 24 were controlled. When the tumor was less than 6 cm in diameter, 74% were controlled; with larger lesions the control rate was 30%. Median survival times were three years for patients with major salivary gland tumors and four years for those with minor salivary gland tumors. In the usual dose range, the complication rate was 16%; these were all successfully managed with minimal residual disability. Results are summarized in Table 3. Neutron irradiation of nonresectable thyroid tumors has yielded essentially similar results.[8]

Table 1.—Radioresistant and Unresponsive Tumors

Organ or System	Tumors
Skin	Melanoma*
Musculoskeletal	Osteosarcoma*
	Chondrosarcoma*
	Soft-tissue sarcoma*
Respiratory	Adenocarcinoma (trachea, bronchus, lung)
	Mesothelioma
Vascular	Hemangioendothelioma
Alimentary	Salivary tumors (major and minor salivary glands)*
	Adenocarcinoma of stomach, intestine, colon
	Carcinoma of rectum
	Carcinoma of pancreas, bile duct*
Urinary	Renal cell carcinoma
	Carcinoma of prostate†
Endocrine	Adenocarcinoma of thyroid*
	Adrenal gland tumors
Nervous	Peripheral nerve tumors (neurofibroma, schwannoma)*
	Glioma

*Proved sensitivity to high–linear energy transfer radiation.[2,4,8]
†Prostatic cancer can be ablated with conventional radiotherapy; however, neutrons have been shown to be significantly more effective in this regard.[12]

Sarcoma of Bone and Soft Tissue

Osteosarcoma and chondrosarcoma are traditionally treated by radical or conservative surgery, with or without chemotherapy. When total tumor ablation is achieved, this method yields a high rate of local control, the major cause of failure being distant metastases. When adequate surgery is not feasible, radical radiotherapy may be the only option, but the very high doses required for cure are not well tolerated by the normal tissues, and the consequences are often destructive. In the axial skeleton, where the target volume may impinge on vital organs, it may be impossible to deliver adequate doses for these relatively radioresistant tumors.

The accepted treatment for soft-tissue sarcomas is resection and postoperative irradiation for ablation of residual microscopic disease. However, surgery may not always be feasible when these tumors occur in the neck or trunk and may be undesirable when a nerve sheath is involved. In these nonresectable soft-tissue sarcomas, conventional radiotherapy has been effective in only a small proportion of patients treated, and for this reason a number of trials with neutron beam irradiation have been instituted in various countries. These trials have generally yielded local control rates between 50% and 70% (Table 2). International experience of 286 soft-tissue sarcomas treated with neutrons yielded 144 (50%) with local control. Similarly, of 118 sarcomas of bone so treated, 74 (63%) were controlled.

A total of 51 patients with exceptionally large tumors were treated at Fermilab[10] for sarcoma of bone (25 patients) and soft tissue (26 patients). Chondrosarcoma was particularly responsive, with a 56% (9/16) control rate. Among the soft-tissue tumors, liposarcoma and neurogenic sarcoma were most responsive. The overall five-year survival rate was 40% in the entire series. Response of a typical nonresectable malignant bone tumor (chondrosarcoma of the chest wall) is shown in Color Fig 4. Responses of irradiated soft-tissue sarcomas (neurogenic sarcoma of the neck and fibrosarcoma of the maxillary antrum) are illustrated in Color Fig 5 and Fig 1.

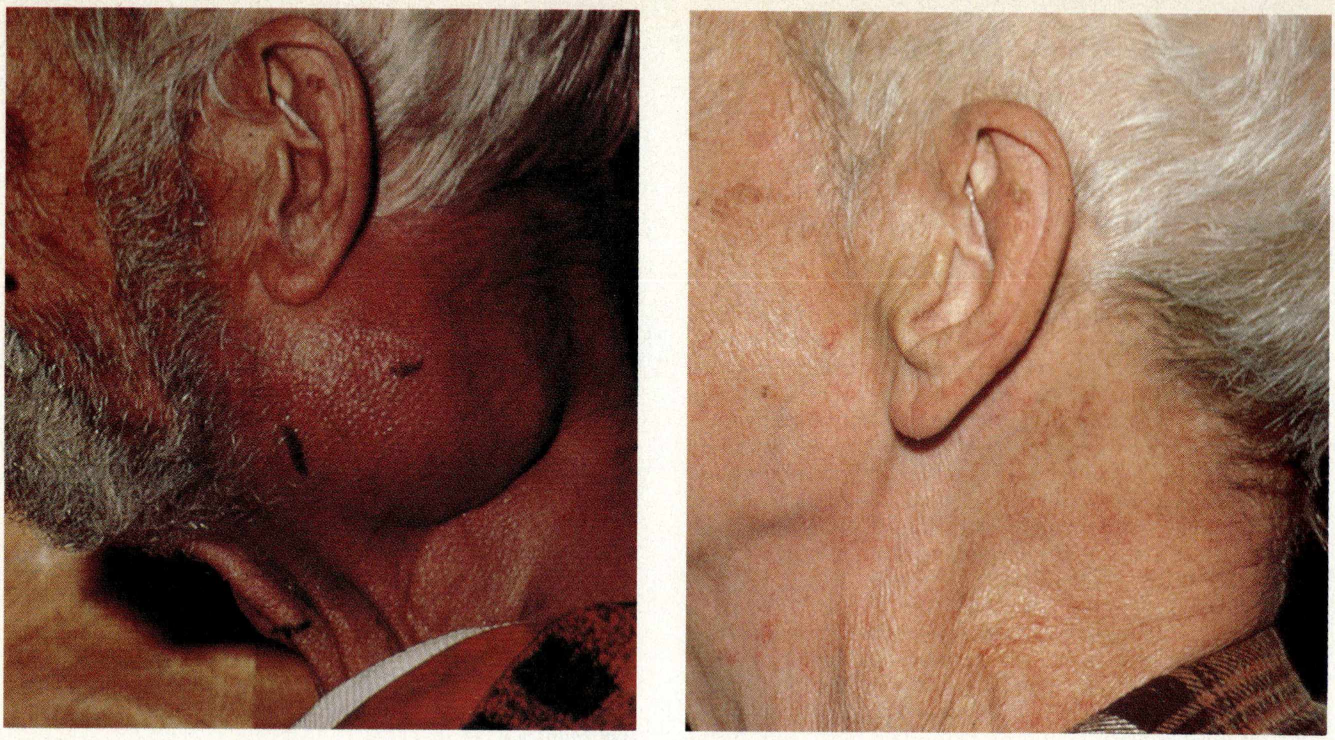

Color Fig 1.

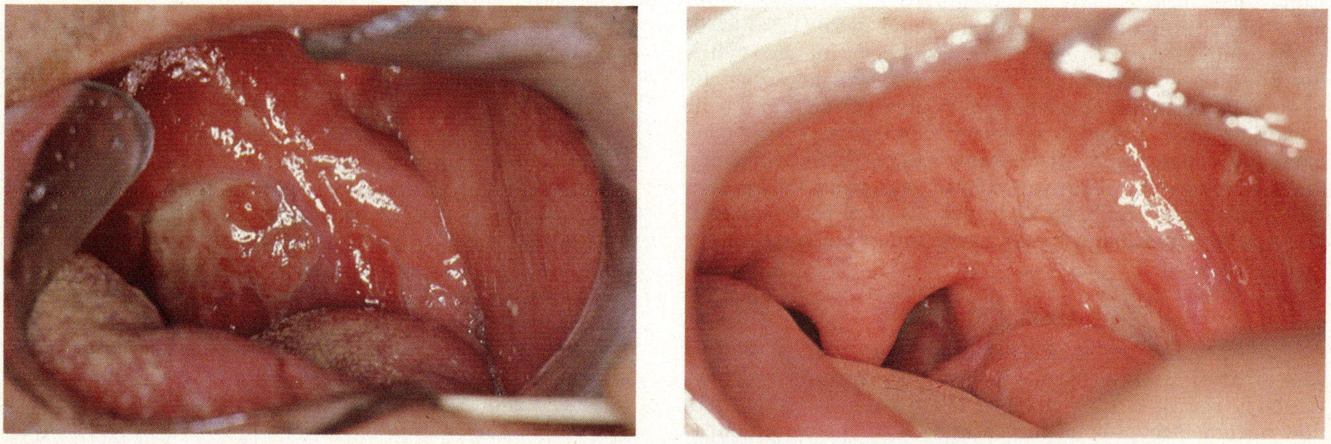

Color Fig 2.

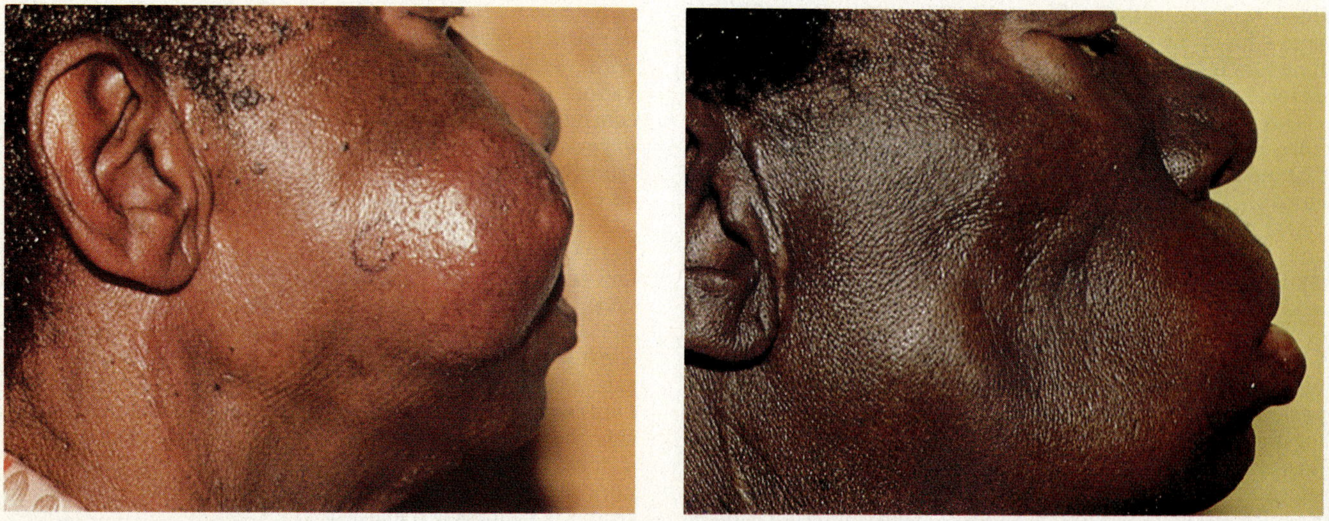

Color Fig 3.

Table 2.—Long-term Local Control in Nonresectable Radioresistant Tumors Treated by Neutrons: International Experience to 1987*			
Tumor Type	**Facility**	**Treated**	**Controlled (%)**
Salivary tumors	Hammersmith	65	50
	Amsterdam	30	22
	Seattle	32	26
	Houston	9	6
	Edinburgh	14	12
	Fermilab	113	71
	Total	**263**	**187** (71)
Sarcoma of bone	MANTA	10	8
	NIRS	42	34
	Essen	24	12
	Seattle	13	9
	Houston	5	4
	Fermilab	25	11
	Total	**118**	**78** (66)
Soft-tissue sarcoma	Houston	29	18
	MANTA	10	4
	NIRS	12	7
	EORTC	199	97
	Seattle	10	5
	Fermilab	26	13
	Total	**286**	**144** (50)
Melanoma	NIRS	14	12
	Fermilab	7	3
	Total	**21**	**15** (71)
Rectosigmoid cancer	Amsterdam	25	13
	Edinburgh	35	7
	Total	**60**	**20** (33)
Bladder cancer	Amsterdam	22	10
	Edinburgh	53	23
	Fermilab	18	12
	Total	**93**	**45** (48)

*Report on patients receiving neutron doses over 16 Gy. Facilities include the following: Hammersmith: MRC Cyclotron Unit, Hammersmith Hospital, London[3,7]; MANTA: Mid-Atlantic Neutron Therapy Association, Naval Research Laboratory, Washington, DC (facility closed)[2]; NIRS: National Institute of Radiological Science, Chiba-Shi, Japan[9]; EORTC: European Organization for Research and Treatment of Cancer, Louvaire, Belgium[8,9]; and Fermilab: Midwest Institute for Neutron Therapy, Fermi National Accelerator Laboratory, Batavia, Ill.[5,8,10]

Color Fig 1.—Typical response of neutron-irradiated T2, N3 carcinoma of head and neck. Left, Primary of piriform fossa with associated large neck node before treatment; right, follow-up two years after treatment with neutrons (20 Gy).

Color Fig 2.—Adenocystic carcinoma of soft palate (T3). Left, Before treatment; right, follow-up two years after treatment (20 Gy).

Color Fig 3.—Nonresectable mucoepidermoid carcinoma of parotid gland. Left, Before treatment; right, follow-up appearance after neutron therapy (20 Gy).

Table 3.—Unresectable Nonepidermoid Carcinomas: Response to Neutrons			
Site of Origin	**No. of Patients**	**No. Controlled**	**Control Rate, %**
Major salivary glands			
Parotid	51	33	...
Submaxillary	12	8	...
Subtotal	63	41	65
Ectopic and minor salivary gland tumors			
Oropharynx	14	13	...
Oral cavity	10	6	...
Maxillary antrum	14	4	...
Nasopharynx	6	4	...
Trachea	5	3	...
Larynx	1	0	...
Subtotal	50	30	60
Total	**113**	**71**	63

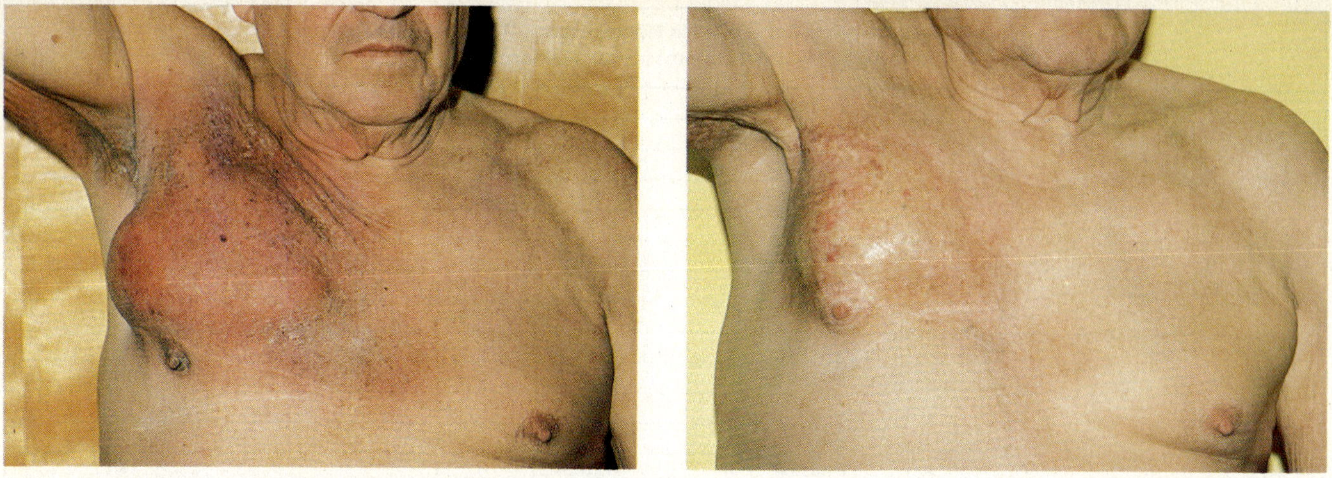

Color Fig 4.—Nonresectable chondrosarcoma of chest wall. Left, At commencement of neutron irradiation; right, follow-up three years after treatment.

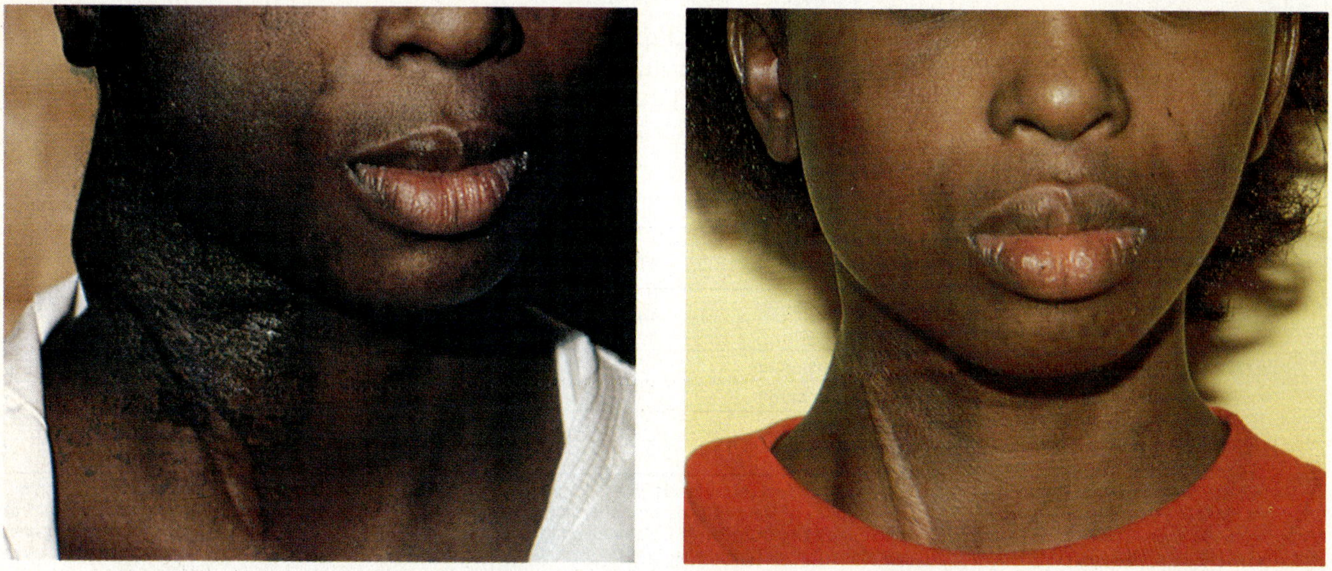

Color Fig 5.—Massive neurogenic sarcoma of neck recurrent after excision. Left, During course of neutron therapy; right, follow-up two years after irradiation.

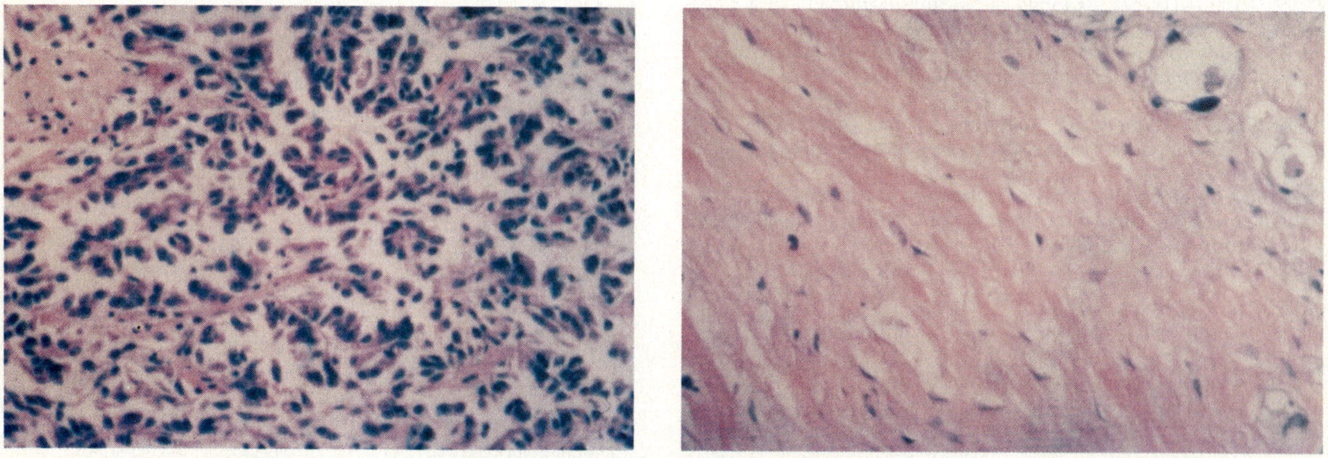

Color Fig 6.—Response of carcinoma of pancreas to neutrons. Left, Original biopsy specimen of pancreatic adenocarcinoma; right, autopsy specimen of tumor site showing local control with extensive fibrosis one year after irradiation with neutrons (21 Gy). Death was due to metastases (Masson's trichrome, original magnification × 100).

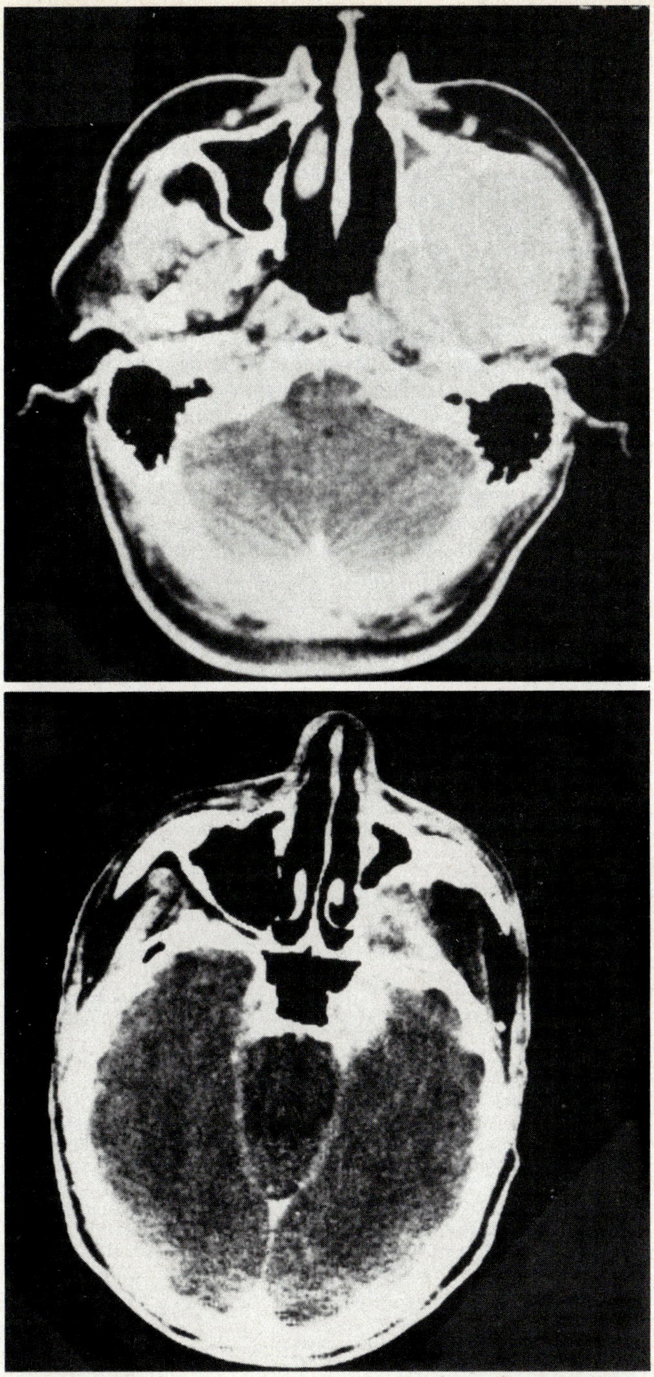

Fig 1.—Computed tomographic scans of large fibrosarcoma of left maxillary antrum. Top, Before treatment; bottom, follow-up after irradiation with neutrons (22 Gy).

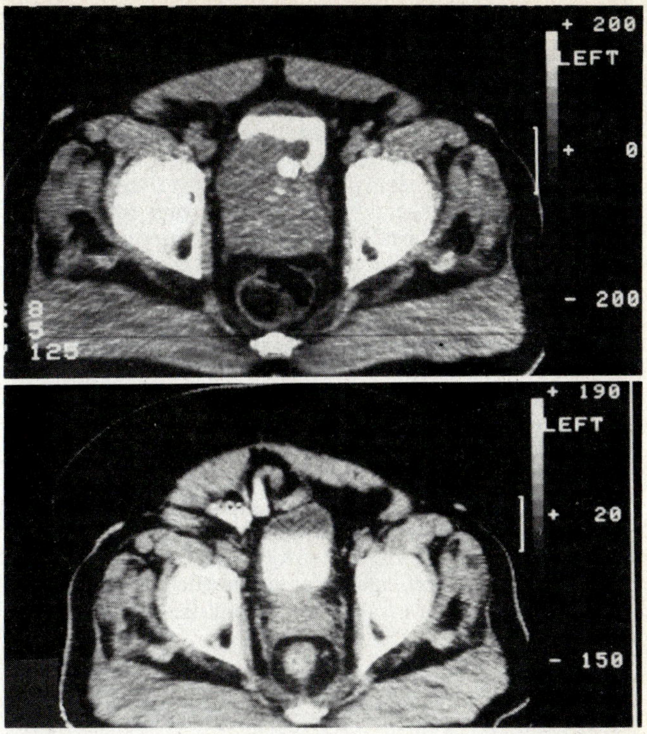

Fig 2.—Adenocarcinoma of prostate, stage D1. Top, Pretreatment computed tomographic scan showing massive tumor with bladder invasion; bottom, first six-month follow-up showing initial response. Patient remains well at last checkup (May 1987).

Colorectal and Pancreatic Adenocarcinoma

Unresectable, residual, or recurrent adenocarcinomas of the gastrointestinal tract (stomach, bowel, rectum) are relatively resistant to irradiation. Initial studies suggest that these tumors may respond better to neutron irradiation,[3] but this has not been confirmed in controlled trials. The response of pancreatic cancer to local irradiation with high-energy neutrons has been thoroughly evaluated at Fermilab.[11] Seventy-seven patients with locally advanced, nonresectable, biopsy-proved adenocarcinoma of the pancreas have been treated with bypass surgery followed by intensive neutron beam irradiation of the primary tumor site. No improvement in overall survival was observed. As with most treatments for pancreatic cancer, the median survival time was only six months, but symptomatic palliation was achieved in the majority of patients. With "second look" surgery and at autopsy (19 subjects), complete tumor regression, with reactive fibrosis and minimal residual microscopic tumor, was observed in all cases (Color Fig 6). The major cause of death was metastatic dissemination. Neutron irradiation apparently provides effective local control coupled with many deaths due to metastases, suggesting that better forms of systemic chemotherapy, possibly combined with local high-LET irradiation, would be worth exploring.

Prostate

Carcinoma of the prostate has proved to be exceptionally sensitive to neutron irradiation. Typically, even very large stage C and D1 prostatic tumors have regressed completely following treatment (Fig 2). In a recently completed randomized trial comparing conventional photon irradiation with mixed-beam (photon plus neutron) treatment,[12] the latter was shown to yield significantly better results in regard to both local control and survival.

Lung Cancer

A trial of high-LET radiations in the treatment of non–small-cell lung cancer is currently under way. Of 40 patients treated with neutrons[13] and followed up for two or more years, nine (23%) were locally controlled (seven alive without evident disease), four were alive with local residual disease, 24 (60%) had clinically evident metastases, and only three patients have died of local extension without metastases. These results are not greatly different from those with conventional radiotherapy.

Salvage of Radiation Failures

Few therapeutic options are available for a patient whose tumor has recurred within a field previously treated with a full radical dose of radiation. Neutrons have been used to re-treat patients with advanced recurrent tumors of the head and neck both at Hammersmith Hospital (London) and at Fermilab.[14,15] Forty-six patients who had received prior radical radiotherapy with photons were reirradiated with neutrons at Fermilab for locally recurrent disease. Overall, 21 (46%) of the 46 patients had a complete local response. The tumor regressed completely in eight (80%) of ten recurrent salivary tumors, in nine (39%) of 23 recurrent primary squamous cancers, and in four (67%) of six patients with neck node recurrences. Partial regression and/or palliation of symptoms occurred in a further 22 patients (48%). Only three of the 46 patients showed no response. Significant morbidity was seen in ten patients. It was concluded that neutron therapy can be tolerated by previously irradiated tissues and could be an effective treatment for patients with locally recurrent tumors. Though not without risk of severe side effects, neutron beam therapy is particularly recommended for recurrent salivary gland tumors and for recurrent disease in cervical lymph nodes.

Palliation of Radioresistant Metastatic Disease

Neutrons have generally been used for radical treatment of locally advanced but potentially curable tumors without overt metastases. However, because of the rapid response observed in many tumors that are relatively resistant to conventional radiotherapy, it seemed probable that metastases arising from such radioresistant tumors would also be more amenable to neutron therapy. Patients are currently being treated with neutrons for isolated metastases from adenocarcinomas (salivary gland, prostate, lung, kidney, and bowel) and sarcomas of all types. Although no survival statistics are available, palliation has generally been excellent and exceptionally rapid, often within a few days after starting treatment. Another advantage of neutron palliation is the very short course of treatment required. One to three fractions are usually sufficient to provide complete symptomatic relief.

CONCLUSIONS

Though neutron beam therapy is clearly not a panacea for all advanced cancer, there does appear to be a distinct subset of patients who can benefit substantially from this treatment. In particular, adenocarcinomas (all sites of origin) and sarcomas (soft tissue and bone) are usually amenable to neutron irradiation. The superiority of neutrons over conventional irradiation has been demonstrated unequivocally in the case of salivary gland tumors[6,7] and carcinoma of the prostate.[12] Neutrons are probably indicated in most locally advanced, nonresectable tumors that are classified histologically as radioresistant.

This investigation was supported in part by US Public Health Service grant CA18081 from the National Cancer Institute, Bethesda, Md.

This material was prepared as an account of work performed by Universities Research Association, Inc, Washington, DC, using facilities owned by the US Department of Energy.

The authors acknowledge Laurie Hanabarger for typing the manuscript. Bonnie Deke provided skillful color photograph production.

References

1. Batterman JJ, Breur K, Hart GAM: Observations on pulmonary metastases in patients after single doses and multiple fractions of fast neutrons and cobalt-60 gamma rays. *Eur J Cancer* 1981;17:539-548.

2. Cohen L, Hendrickson FR, Kurup P, et al: Clinical evaluation of neutron beam therapy: Current results and prospects. *Cancer* 1985;55: 10-17.

3. Catterall M: The treatment of advanced cancer by fast neutrons from the Medical Research Council's cyclotron at Hammersmith Hospital, London. *Eur J Cancer* 1974;10:343-347.

4. Catterall M, Errington RD, Bewley DK: A comparison of clinical and laboratory data on neutron therapy for locally advanced tumors. *Int J Radiat Oncol* 1987;13:1783-1791.

5. Kurup PD, Mansell J, TenHaken RK, et al: Response of epidermoid and non-epidermoid cancers of the head and neck to fast neutron irradiation: The Fermilab experience. *Int J Radiat Oncol* 1984;10:473-479.

6. Saroja KR, Mansell J, Hendrickson FR, et al: An update on malignant salivary gland tumors treated with neutrons at Fermilab. *Int J Radiat Oncol* 1987;13:1319-1325.

7. Catterall M: The treatment of malignant salivary gland tumors with fast neutrons. *Int J Radiat Oncol* 1981;7:1730-1738.

8. Franke HH, Schmidt R: Clinical results with fast neutrons (DT, 14 MeV). *Radiat Med* 1985;3:151-160.

9. Wambersie A: The European experience in neutron therapy at the end of 1981. *Int J Radiat Oncol* 1982;8:2145-2152.

10. Cohen L, Hendrickson FR, Mansell J, et al: Response of sarcomas of bone and of soft tissue to neutron beam therapy. *Int J Radiat Oncol* 1981;10:821-824.

11. Cohen L, Woodruff KH, Hendrickson FR, et al: Response of pancreatic cancer to local irradiation with high-energy neutrons. *Cancer* 1985;56:1235-1241.

12. Laramore GE, Krall JM, Thomas TJ, et al: Fast neutron radiotherapy for locally advanced prostate cancer. *Int J Radiat Oncol* 1985;11:1621-1627.

13. Cohen L: New modalities in radiation therapy of lung cancer. *Chest* 1986;89:3495.

14. Errington RD, Catterall M: Re-irradiation of advanced tumors of the head and neck with fast neutrons. *Int J Radiat Oncol* 1986;12:191-195.

15. Saroja KR, Hendrickson FR, Cohen L, et al: Re-irradiation of locally recurrent tumors with fast neutrons: Fermilab experience. *Int J Radiat Oncol* 1988;15:115-121.

In Other AMA Journals

ARCHIVES OF OTOLARYNGOLOGY–HEAD & NECK SURGERY

Ethical Use of Yellow Pages Listings by Physicians

Steven M. Denenberg, MD, Howard W. Smith, MD, DMD

A recent article in the *New England Journal of Medicine* examined the percentage of physicians listed under specialty headings in a Yellow Pages publication who were board certified. The authors presented findings that many of the physicians listed in the Yellow Pages, particularly under the heading of "Plastic Surgery," were not board certified. The source data employed in that article were obtained and reexamined, and it was found that the assumptions used were inaccurate and the methodology flawed. Almost every physician listed under "Plastic Surgery" in the Yellow Pages is board certified. We discuss the conclusions of the original article and its recommendations for control of Yellow Pages listings. We believe that these recommendations are not in the public's best interests and may be illegal as well (*Arch Otolaryngol Head Neck Surg* 1988;114:1392-1394).

Reprint requests to 7640 Pacific St, Omaha, NE 68114 (Dr Denenberg).

Gallbladder Response to Enteral Lipids in Injured Patients

Ronald C. Merrell, MD; Priscilla Miller-Crotchett, RN; Patricia Lowry, MD

• Severely injured patients are at risk for complications of gallbladder stasis in a spectrum from sludge formation and cystic duct occlusion by inspissation and, subsequently, acalculous cholecystitis. In a double-blind randomized trial, the effect of enteral lipids on the ability of the gallbladder to clear itself was tested. The gallbladder was assessed by ultrasonography for acute contractions, sludge, and dilatation on days 1, 3, and 7 after injury. There were no significant differences between patients who received enteral lipids and controls. Both groups showed modest enlargement of the gallbladder and failure of contraction. In a population at risk for biliary stasis following severe trauma, standard enteral lipids did not elicit, acutely or chronically, an appropriate reflexive evacuation of the gallbladder.

(*Arch Surg* 1989;124:301-302)

Although the cause of acalculous cholecystitis[1,2] is unknown, well-described groups of patients are at exceptional risk for this condition. These include diabetic patients, patients who receive total parenteral nutrition (TPN) for long periods, and critically ill patients in either a surgical or medical intensive care environment. Factors implicated in acalculous cholecystitis include anesthesia,[2] narcotic analgesics, multiple transfusions,[3] sepsis,[4] and hypotension.[5] One common feature among these patients is a diminished response of the contractile elements of the gallbladder either due to a relative insensitivity to cholecystokinin in the case of diabetic patients[6] or due to failure to elicit cholecystokinin release from the duodenum by lipid secretagogues because the patients are not eating.[7] If the gallbladder is not stimulated to contract, there is a tendency to progressive dilatation, the formation of sludge, and inspissation of this sludge in the cystic duct with cystic duct obstruction.[8] This occlusion is permissive for the development of cholecystitis. In this study, a double-blind design was chosen to test the ability of lipids, instilled into the gastrointestinal tract via nasogastric tube, to promote evacuation of the gallbladder. The hypothesis declared that reflexive emptying would avoid dilatation of the gallbladder, with sludging of the gallbladder bile.

Accepted for publication May 24, 1988.

From the Departments of Surgery (Dr Merrell and Ms Miller-Crotchett) and Radiology (Dr Lowry), The University of Texas Medical School at Houston.

Reprint requests to Department of Surgery, The University of Texas Medical School, 6431 Fannin, Suite 4292, Houston, TX 77030 (Dr Merrell).

PATIENTS AND METHODS

Injured patients between the ages of 20 and 65 years who required at least a one-day admission to the surgical intensive care unit and who were, in all likelihood, to take nothing by mouth for seven days were considered for inclusion in the study. Patients with a previous cholecystectomy or direct biliary or duodenal trauma were excluded. All patients had a nasogastric tube that was advanced far into the stomach, and they had no gallstones demonstrable by ultrasound. The patients were randomized to receive, in a "blinded" fashion, either 40 mL of safflower oil (Lipomul)[9-11] or water at 8 AM each day into the very distal nasogastric tube. Ultrasound examination was done on the first day before and after receipt of the safflower oil and then repeated on days 3 and 7. Bedside ultrasonography was performed, and the characteristics for notation included gallbladder length and diameter and wall thickness.[12-14] The presence or abscence of pericholecystic edema and the presence or absence of sludge were also noted. The trauma characteristics of the patients are listed in Table 1. The majority of patients arrived by air ambulance from the scene of injury. The representative laboratory values of the study population are listed in Table 2. These were severely injured patients who fit the risk description for acalculus cholecystitis.

RESULTS

All patients survived the observation period, and none was excluded for technical or clinical reasons. All patients were studied under the informed consent provisions of the Committee for the Protection of Human Subjects of The University of Texas Medical School at Houston. Consent was obtained from relatives. There were no complications of the safflower oil administration. No patients developed acute cholecystitis during the course of the study. The results of the measurements are displayed in Table 3. The results of safflower oil instillation on acute gallbladder dimensional changes (mean ± SEM) are as follows: longitudinal diameter, 7.1 ± 0.9 vs 7.0 ± 0.9 cm; transverse diameter, 3.2 ± 0.6 vs 2.8 ± 0.6 cm. These dimensions do not reflect any significant contraction of the gallbladder in response to safflower oil instillation. Safflower oil administration to normal subjects in these circumstances leads to a dramatic response in gallbladder dimension, with at least a 50% reduction in the diameters, and is a tactic that is commonly employed for biliary kinetic analysis in this institution and others.[10] Furthermore, the dimensions of the gallbladder throughout the course of observation showed a modest increase in the longitudinal axis that was

Table 1.—Characteristics of Traumatized Patients

Group	n	Patient's Mean(±SEM) Age, y	% Male	% Air Transport
Control	6	40±8	83	67
Lipid fed	6	30±6	83	100

Table 2.—Laboratory Values in Control and Lipid-Fed Groups

Laboratory Level	Mean±SEM Day 1	Day 3	Day 7
Control Group			
Total protein, g/L	50±7	54±8	58±3
Albumin, g/L	32±5	32±5	30±3
Total bilirubin, μmol/L	24±9	15±5	56±75
Alkaline phosphatase, U/L	52±16	72±24	165±64
Lipid-Fed Group			
Total protein, g/L	34±6	45±2	49±7
Albumin, g/L	21±4	26±3	27±4
Total bilirubin, μmol/L	15±10	27±12	50±101
Alkaline phosphatase, U/L	39±10	55±11	73±18

not affected by the daily administration of the enteral fat. One patient in the safflower oil–treated group and two in the saline solution–treated control group developed gallbladder sludge. Both groups of patients showed modest increases in gallbladder wall thickness throughout the course of this study. The mean total bilirubin level was elevated by day 7 in both groups. This seemed to be a population at risk for biliary complications, but no impact of safflower oil on biliary dimensions could be detected.

Table 3.—Biliary Images by Ultrasound Examination in Control/Lipid-Fed Groups

Biliary Image	Mean±SEM, Control/Lipid-Fed Group Day 1	Day 2	Day 3
Gallbladder length, cm	6.8±0.7/ 6.8±1.2	7.8±0.5/ 7.4±2.9	7.4±0.9/ 7.6±1.4
Gallbladder diameter, cm	3.0±0.8/ 2.6±0.4	2.8±0.6/ 2.8±0.4	2.6±0.8/ 2.4±0.7
Wall thickness, cm	0.25±0.05/ 0.3±0.1	0.3±0.1/ 0.4±0.2	0.4±0.04/ 0.4±0.1

COMMENT

Acute acalculous cholecystitis represents a serious and potentially fatal complication among massively injured patients. Although the cause of the condition is unknown, there is good reason to implicate biliary sludge that theoretically can occlude the cystic duct and commence the process of infection in an undrained hollow viscus. Other factors implicated in acalculous cholecystitis include anesthetic effects,[2] narcotic analgesics,[2] multiple transfusions,[3] sepsis,[4] and hypotension.[5] Acalculous cholecystitis has been recognized in patients receiving long-term TPN who are unable to eat.[7,15] Patients who receive long-term TPN also develop bilirubinate stones in addition to their problem with acalculous cholecystitis.[16] Recent data have strongly suggested a salutary effect of cholecystokinin in TPN models to flush and drain the gallbladder periodically.[17] This drainage is effective in prairie dogs that receive long-term TPN to avoid the formation of sludge and has even been useful in reducing cholesterol stone formation in cholesterol-fed prairie dogs. Safflower oil, introduced orally, has been a standard for many years to induce contraction of the gallbladder because of the cholecystokinin released in the duodenum in the presence of lipids. This measure was used for many years with oral cholecystography and, more recently, has been useful in studying gallbladder dynamics with ultrasonography. The technique of ultrasonography to detect gallbladder motility problems, sludge, and signs indicative of incipient or established acalculous cholecystitis has become a matter of general agreement. In this double-blind study, ultrasonography certainly demonstrated changes in the gallbladder that declare the population studied as one at risk for acalculous cholecystitis. However, the ultrasonography failed to show proper response of the gallbladder to enteral safflower oil either acutely or chronically. There are two possible conclusions of the results reported here. The first is that as a consequence of bowel edema and motility changes, there is no stimulation or cholecystokinin released by the enteral lipid. The other possibility is that in severe injury, the gallbladder is not especially responsive to circulating cholecystokinin. In either case, enteral lipid is not effective for reflexive evacuation of the gallbladder in injured patients.

References

1. Glenn F, Wantz GE: Acute cholecystitis following the surgical treatment of unrelated disease. *Surg Gynecol Obstet* 1956;102:145-153.

2. Glenn F, Becker CG: Acute acalculous cholecystitis. *Ann Surg* 1982;196:131-136.

3. Lindberg EF, Grinnan GL, Smith L: Acalculous cholecystitis in Vietnam casualties. *Ann Surg* 1970;171:152-157.

4. Munster AM, Goodwin MN, Pruitt BA Jr: Acalculous cholecystitis in burn patients. *Am J Surg* 1971;122:591-593.

5. Golden GT, Sears HF II, Wangensteen SL: Post-traumatic cholecystitis. *Am Surg* 1973;39:275-278.

6. Shreiner DP, Sarva RP, Thiel DV, et al: Gallbladder function in diabetic patients. *J Nucl Med* 1986;27:357-360.

7. Roslyn JJ, DenBesten L, Pitt HA, et al: Effects of cholecystokinin on gallbladder stasis and cholesterol gallstone formation. *J Surg Res* 1981;30:200-204.

8. Messing B, Bories C, Kunstlinger F, et al: Does total parenteral nutrition induce gallbladder sludge formation and lithiasis? *Gastroenterology* 1983;84:1012-1019.

9. Hopman WPM, Rosenbusch G, Jansen JBMJ, et al: Gallbladder contraction: Effects of fatty meals and cholecystokinin. *Radiology* 1985;157:37-39.

10. Hopman WPM, Jansen JBMJ, Rosenbusch G, et al: Effect of equimolar amounts of long-chain triglycerides and medium-chain triglycerides on plasma cholecystokinin and gallbladder contraction. *Am J Clin Nutr* 1984;39:356-359.

11. Fried GM, Ogden WD, Fagan CJ, et al: Comparison of cholecystokinin release and gallbladder emptying in men and in women at estrogen and progesterone phases of the menstrual cycle. *Surgery* 1984;95:284-289.

12. Raghavendra BN, Feiner HD, Subramanyam BR, et al: Acute cholecystitis: Sonographic-pathologic analysis. *Am J Res* 1981;137:327-332.

13. Shlaer WJ, Leopold GR, Scheible FW: Sonography of the thickened gallbladder wall: A nonspecific finding. *Am J Res* 1981;136:337-339.

14. Sanders RC: The significance of sonographic gallbladder wall thickening. *J Clin Ultrasound* 1980;8:143-146.

15. Peterson SR, Sheldon GF: Acute acalculous cholecystitis: A complication of hyperalimentation. *Am J Surg* 1979;138:814-817.

16. Muller EL, Grace PA, Pitt HA: The effect of parenteral nutrition on biliary calcium and bilirubin. *J Surg Res* 1986;40:55-62.

17. Doty JE, Pitt HA, Porter-Fink V, et al: Cholecystokinin prophylaxis of parenteral nutrition-induced gallbladder disease. *Ann Surg* 1985;201:76-80.

Gastric Adenocarcinoma

A Disease in Transition

Blake Cady, MD; Ricardo L. Rossi, MD; Mark L. Silverman, MD; William Piccione, MD; Thomas A. Heck, MD

• Two hundred eleven gastric adenocarcinomas diagnosed from 1967 to 1982 were analyzed. Thirty-four percent had a proximal location, a proportionate increase from previous decades that suggested a distinctive epidemiology. Diffuse histology occurred in 49% of cases overall and in 55% of unresectable cases, which were also increases from previous decades. No deaths followed curative resections, two (4%) of 50 patients with palliative resections died, and three (6%) of 54 patients who underwent exploration without resection died, indicating improved operative management. Superficial gastric cancer constituted 6% of cases; 91% were cured. Seventeen percent of cases were linitis plastica and required total gastrectomy in 77% of resections; only 13% of patients had curative operations; none were cured. Seventy-nine percent of cases were polypoid or ulcerated focal cancers. Of operable focal cancers, 72% were resected; 27 (47%) of 57 patients who underwent resection for cure survived five years, a distinct improvement from previous reports, as was the overall survival of 21%.

(*Arch Surg* 1989;124:303-308)

Until 1975 the incidence and death rate of gastric adenocarcinoma had been falling dramatically, but in 1986 the number of deaths predicted from gastric cancer was the same as in 1976, indicating a plateau in the death rate, while the estimated number of new cases actually rose by 8%, from 22 900 in 1976 to 24 700 in 1986.[1,2] Gastric cancer is the sixth leading cause of death by cancer in men and the ninth leading cause in women,[2] and thus still represents a formidable problem in clinical cancer treatment. A ten-year survey of the pathology and the results of therapy at the Lahey Clinic Foundation, Burlington, Mass, that concluded in 1966, with a ten-year follow-up, was published in 1977.[3] The present report covers the subsequent 15 years, from 1967 through 1981, with a minimum five-year follow-up. In 1982 we reported[4] a longer-term survey of the presentation and anatomical location of gastric adenocarcinoma in patients at the Lahey Clinic that covered the 40-year span from 1940 to 1980, and for the first time described a marked increase in the rate of a proximal location for gastric cancer and a corresponding decrease in the rate of a distal location. The present study further substantiates the changes in histologic pattern, location in the stomach, and surgical therapy, and describes current results of operative treatment in gastric adenocarcinoma.

Accepted for publication Oct 23, 1987.

From the Department of Surgery, New England Deaconess Hospital, Boston (Dr Cady); Departments of General Surgery (Dr Rossi) and Pathology (Dr Silverman), Lahey Clinic Foundation, Burlington, Mass; Department of Thoracic Surgery, Presbyterian–St Luke's Hospital, Chicago (Dr Piccione); and Department of Surgery, Good Samaritan Hospital, Dayton, Ohio (Dr Heck).

Read before the Annual Meeting of the Society of Surgical Oncology, London, April 28, 1987.

Reprint requests to 110 Francis St, Boston, MA 02215 (Dr Cady).

PATIENTS AND METHODS

All 211 cases of gastric adenocarcinoma recorded at the Lahey Clinic Foundation from 1967 through 1981 were reviewed, histologic material was reevaluated, and current status was determined. Lauren's histologic classification,[5,6] which defines lesions histologically as being of the "diffuse," "intestinal," or "mixed" type, was used. A small "other" group was recorded in which only biopsy material was available, with the lesion type remaining undefinable.

Three types of gastric adenocarcinoma presented at diagnosis. *Superficial gastric adenocarcinoma* was defined when malignant cells failed to penetrate beneath the muscularis propria. *Infiltrative gastric adenocarcinoma* (linitis plastica) was defined by the presence of malignant cells diffusely spread through a thickened gastric wall with a desmoplastic reaction and a typical clinical pattern. *Focal gastric adenocarcinoma* with a polypoid, fungate, or ulcerative appearance was defined when there was no extensive thickening of the gastric wall, no desmoplastic reaction, no wide lateral spread beneath the mucosa, and the cancer invaded through the muscularis propria. These three distinctive types can also be readily identified clinically.

Distal gastrectomy was defined as any operation that preserved a proximal portion of stomach and did not construct a proximal anastomosis to the esophagus. *Total gastrectomy* was defined as an operative specimen that included duodenum distally and esophagus proximally. *Esophagogastrectomy* was defined by the presence of esophagus at the proximal margin and stomach at the distal margin of the specimen. These operative categories separated the inherently more dangerous esophageal anastomoses and allowed us to address the continuing conflict regarding total gastrectomy as a manifestation of the extensiveness of local cancer removal in the stomach.

Location within the stomach was defined as *distal* if it arose in the distal one third of the stomach by analysis of radiology and endoscopy reports as well as operative notes and pathology reports. *Proximal* gastric cancer occurred in the proximal one third of the stomach, which included the cardia, upper lesser curvature, and fundus. Adenocarcinomas of the *body* of the

Table 1.—Patient Survival by Clinical Type and Surgery

Surgery	Clinical Type: Superficial	Infiltrating	Focal-Polypoid or Ulcerating
Curative resection, No. (%)	11 (100)	4 (13)	57 (34)
Cure, No. (%)	10 (91)	0 (0)	27 (47)
Median survival of deaths, mo (range)	9	12 (6-123)	38 (8-83)
Palliative resection, No. (%)	...	9 (28)	41 (25)
Median survival of deaths, mo (range)	...	13 (1-74)	11 (1-63)
Laparotomy and biopsy, No. (%)	...	16 (55)	38 (23)
Median survival of deaths, mo (range)	...	4 (1-48)	5 (1-13)
Biopsy only, No. (%)	1 (8)	3 (9)	31 (19)
Median survival of deaths, mo (range)	...	9 (6-12)	4 (1-33)
Total, No. (%)	**12** (6)	**32** (15)	**167** (79)

Table 2.—Survival After Curative Resections for Focal Polypoid or Fungating Gastric Cancer, 1967-1981

	No. (%) of Patients			
	Dead of Disease			
Resection	Before 5 y	After 5 y*	Cure	Total
Distal gastrectomy	21 (44)	3 (6)	24 (50)	**48** (84)
Total gastrectomy	1 (50)	0 (0)	1 (50)	**2** (4)
Esophagogastrectomy	4 (57)	1 (14)	2 (29)	**7** (12)
Total	**26** (46)	**4** (7)	**27** (47)	**57** (100)

*Of 31 patients who survived five years, four (13%) later died of disease.

Table 3.—Location and Resectability of Focal Gastric Adenocarcinoma

Procedure	Location, No. (%) of Cases: Proximal	Body	Distal
Resection			
Curative	12 (21)	15 (38)	30 (44)
Palliative	12 (21)	10 (25)	19 (28)
Laparotomy and biopsy	18 (31)	10 (25)	10 (15)
Biopsy only	16 (28)	5 (13)	10 (15)
Total	**58 (100)**	**40 (100)**	**69 (100)**

Table 4.—Histologic Types of Gastric Adenocarcinoma (Lauren[5])

	No. (%) of Cases: Diffuse	Intestinal	Mixed	Other
Study years				
1956-1967 (n=317)	133 (42)	112 (35)	32 (10)	40 (13)
1967-1981 (n=211)	104 (49)	76 (36)	20 (9)	11 (5)
Clinical types				
Superficial	1 (9)	11 (91)	...	...
Infiltrating	27 (84)	1 (3)	2 (6)	2 (6)
Focal	76 (46)	64 (38)	18 (11)	9 (5)
Focal cases only				
Biopsy only	17 (55)	8 (26)	2 (9)	...
Laparotomy and biopsy	17 (45)	13 (34)	3 (8)	...
Palliative resection	18 (44)	17 (42)	6 (15)	...
Curative resection	24 (42)	26 (46)	7 (12)	...

Table 5.—Changing Patterns of Gastric Cancer, 1940-1981*

Location of Gastric Cancer	Study Years, No. (%) of Cases: 1940-1949	1950-1959	1960-1969	1967-1981
Distal	286 (64)	217 (56)	106 (46)	69 (39)
Body	70 (16)	61 (16)	48 (21)	49 (28)
Proximal	90 (20)	111 (29)	79 (34)	60 (34)

*Significant changes over four decades: $P<.05$. Data on linitis plastica have been omitted.

stomach were located in the middle one third of the stomach and were undoubtedly an admixture of the distinctive proximal and distal types.

Curative resections were defined as the absence of gross residual disease at the conclusion of the surgery, while *palliative* resections left gross residual disease at completion, as recorded by the surgeon. The presence of a microscopically positive margin in the final pathology report did not change the designation of curative resection.

Operative mortality occurred when a patient died without leaving the hospital after surgery.

Only one patient (0.5%) was unavailable for follow-up less than five years after surgery and was considered dead of disease. This 99.5% follow-up provides assurance that the conclusions represent true clinical results. Postoperative deaths (five, 2.8%) were recorded as patients dead of disease.

Results will be presented in a fashion similar to that of our previous reports to enable estimation of time trends and provide direct comparisons. Where results of our initial study were also well substantiated in these patients and by other articles in the literature, further data are not reported. Thus, symptomatology, clinical presentation, and survival in relation to size, gastric wall penetration, number of lymph node metastases, and stage do not differ from our previous[3] and other recent reports.[7]

RESULTS

Results are not presented in the tumor-nodule-metastases (TNM) staging system because cases for the most part were treated before the system for stomach cancer had been accepted; the TNM system would have been inaccurate if applied retrospectively, particularly when describing the location of lymph node metastases. Furthermore, the present series emphasizes several features of gastric cancer that are important to prognosis, yet are not recognized by the current TNM system, such as location within the stomach (proximal vs distal), number of lymph node metastases (rather than their location relative to the stomach), histologic type (Lauren's classification), pattern of growth (linitis plastica), whether all disease could be resected (curative vs palliative resection), and the type of resection (conservative vs total gastrectomy).

Two hundred eleven documented cases of gastric adenocarcinoma were histologically confirmed at the Lahey Clinic Foundation from 1967 through 1981. Thirty-five cases (17%) were not explored because endoscopic biopsy documented the histologic diagnosis and the patients had evidence of metastatic disease, extensive intraperitoneal

Table 6.—Gastric Cancer Location Changes in Time: Theoretical Model

	Year				
	1945		1985		
	Absolute Incidence, No. of Cases	Relative Proportion, %	Absolute Incidence, No. of Cases	Relative Proportion, %	Fractional Reduction of Absolute Incidence
Overall incidence per 100 000 persons per year	25	100	7	100	...
Location					
Distal	16	64	2.7	39	1/6
Body	4	16	2.0	28	1/2
Proximal	5	20	2.4	34	1/2

Table 7.—Gastric Cancer: Changing Patterns of Surgery and Survival at the Lahey Clinic Foundation

	Years				
	1932-1939	1940-1949	1949-1958	1957-1966	1967-1982
Total No. of cases	308	981	641	403	211
Laparotomy, %	...	...	83	94	84
Operative mortality, %	23	9	7	6	2.8
Palliative resections, %	7	11	18	14	24
Curative resections, %	39	37	41	44	34
Total resection rate, %	46	47	59	58	58
5-year survival as proportion, %					
All cases	3	7	11	11	21
All resections	7	15	19	19	36
All curative resections	11	24	25	23	58

spread, hopelessly advanced local growth, or linitis plastica without symptoms requiring surgery. One patient had a biopsy specimen that confirmed superficial gastric adenocarcinoma but he died of advanced prostate cancer one month later without surgery for the obviously operable gastric cancer. This rate of inoperability was three times that noted in our earlier study (17% vs 6%) and undoubtedly reflects wider use of flexible endoscopic techniques with biopsy confirmation, compared with the infrequently used rigid gastroscopic biopsy available before 1967.

Infiltrative gastric adenocarcinoma (linitis plastica) was defined in 32 cases (15%). Focal (polypoid, fungating, or ulcerated) gastric cancers occurred in 167 cases (79%) (Table 1). These types were essentially identical in incidence to the 16% and 81% reported between 1957 and 1966.[3] Superficial gastric cancers were diagnosed in 12 patients (6%), a substantial rise from 3% of cases previously noted.[3] Table 1 demonstrates the curative resection rate and the cure rate in these patients. For the remaining patients, rates of palliative resection and laparotomy and biopsy are shown, as well as the median survival duration in months for patients who *died*. All patients with superficial gastric cancer who were operated on underwent resection, and ten of the 11 were cured. One patient died nine months after resection in unusual circumstances and while he was officially declared dead of gastric cancer, no autopsy was performed and no clinical evidence on hospital chart review at the time of death indicated recurrent, metastatic, or persistent gastric cancer; serious doubt exists that such failure occurred.

In the cases categorized as infiltrative (linitis plastica) or focal gastric adenocarcinoma, only 13% and 34%, respectively, of patients operated on underwent curative resection, a marked decline from our previous report in which 43% and 46%, respectively, were so defined. The median survival of these patients who eventually died of disease was 12 months and 38 months, respectively, compared with 14 months and 19 months previously. Palliative resections were carried out in 28% and 25% of cases, respectively, of infiltrating and focal gastric cancers in patients taken to surgery, a sharp increase compared with the previous study. The combined resection rates of all patients taken to surgery for infiltrative cancers decreased from 51% in the earlier study to 45% in the present study, but rose from 63% to 72% for focal cancers, reflecting better understanding of the outcome in linitis plastica and elimination of some candidates for exploration by wider use of endoscopy.

No patients died postoperatively after the 72 curative resections performed, and only two deaths (4%) occurred following the 50 palliative resections, for an overall mortality rate for gastric resections of 1.6%. There were three deaths (6%) among 54 patients who underwent laparotomy, for an overall operative mortality rate of 2.8% in 176 patients who underwent exploration. The postoperative mortality rate for gastric resection of 10% between 1957 and 1966 was thus sharply improved, as was the overall operative mortality rate (6.4% vs 2.8%) in all patients undergoing exploration.

Table 2 describes the outcome in patients undergoing curative resection of focal gastric cancer. Patterns of disease progression and survival rates after resection are best portrayed in the focal cancer group undergoing curative resection, since all patients with superficial gastric cancers survived and all patients with infiltrative cancers or palliative resection died of disease. The proportion of patients undergoing either total gastrectomy (4%) or esophagogastrectomy (12%) declined from our earlier series (14% and 29%, respectively), reflecting a more conservative attitude toward the use of total gastrectomy and the more selective use of esophagogastrectomy. Almost three fourths of distal, but only 42% of proximal, cancers could be resected. Our previous study noted that 24% of patients surviving five years eventually died of disease, while in the present study 13% of patients who were alive at five years eventually died of disease. No patients free of disease at this writing were expected to later die of gastric cancer because all 27 such patients had been followed up for more than six years. Three of the four patients who did die of disease after five years died in the sixth year. Thus, with few exceptions, six-year disease-free survival is tantamount to cure.

The rate of patients with proximal cancers undergoing curative resection was one half that of patients with distal gastric cancers (Table 3), and cancers in nearly one half of all patients undergoing exploration but not resection had a proximal location.

Lymph node metastases are important prognostic indicators. Forty-six percent of patients with negative nodes were cured, while 30% of those with one to three nodes, 16% of those with four to ten nodes, but none of those patients with more than ten node metastases were cured. However, whether the resection was classified as curative or palliative was of far more importance, since 49% of the patients with curative resections but none of those with palliative resections were cured. The number of lymph node metastases in palliative resections may not have been accurate since nodes left at the conclusion of surgery may have been the criterion for incomplete resection.

Table 4 illustrates the continuing increase in "diffuse histology" associated with a worse prognosis, as illustrated by its decreasing relative proportion as resection is performed; disease in 55% of patients undergoing biopsy only showed diffuse histology, but only 42% of cases with curative resections did. In contrast, 26% of patients undergoing biopsy only, but 46% of cases with curative resections, are classified as showing intestinal histology. While diffuse histology generally presents in a more advanced fashion and stage-for-stage carries a worse prognosis, of the 24 patients undergoing curative resections for focal gastric cancer classified as showing diffuse histology, 12 (50%) were cured. Thus, given the appropriate clinical presentation, diffuse histology by itself in no way indicates incurability.

There is a unique male predominance (4:1) in the sex ratio of proximal location, in contrast with distal gastric adenocarcinomas (1.2:1). Among focal cancers, the same unique sex ratio can be demonstrated; proximal cancers predominate among male patients (4:1), while distal cancers are equally distributed (1:1). Table 5 shows the changing anatomical location of gastric adenocarcinoma within the stomach since 1940. The three decades presented in the first columns are taken from our previous report[3] and the last column represents the present series. The sharp decline in the rate of distally located gastric cancers has continued while proximally located gastric cancers now constitute more than one third of cases. Table 6 offers a hypothetical extrapolation from the record of changing gastric adenocarcinoma incidence overall coupled with the relative change in location within the stomach. This theoretical model illustrates the extraordinarily rapid disappearance of distal gastric adenocarcinoma, in contrast with the far more modest decline in the absolute incidence of proximal and body cancers.

Table 7 illustrates the time trends in the surgical approach to gastric adenocarcinoma over five decades at the Lahey Clinic. The significant trends noted are the recent decrease in the rate of exploration and curative resections and the increasing rate of palliative resections. For the first time, a significant increase in five-year survival rates is noted, with an approximate doubling of the previously low rates in all cases diagnosed, all cases resected, and all cases undergoing curative resection.

COMMENT

Gastric adenocarcinoma continues to represent an oncologic and surgical challenge; in a 1977 report we[3] noted no improvement in the five-year survival rate over four decades. Other reports documented similar discouraging results.[7-11] Because we noted[4] changes in clinical presentation previously unrecognized but subsequently documented by others,[12,13] we undertook the present study to substantiate the increasing proportion of proximal gastric adenocarcinoma and diffuse histology (Lauren). Both trends have continued and call attention to the fact that gastric adenocarcinoma is not a single pathologic, clinical, or epidemiologic entity. For instance, while seldom separately reported in the United States, superficial gastric adenocarcinoma (also termed "early gastric cancer," but implications of duration in that description should be avoided) represents a distinct clinical entity,[14] with virtually all cases cured by relatively conservative distal gastric resections.[15-17] In the TNM staging system, such cases are categorized as T1 and, since node metastases are seldom detected, N0, and therefore are in stage 1. However, these cases may represent a unique biologic situation and not just an early stage. Such cases occasionally recur in the mucosa and can frequently be cured by further excisions, as one of our patients illustrated; such patients should undergo yearly follow-up endoscopy. In Japan, gastric adenocarcinoma is common; population screening by endoscopic surveillance has resulted in superficial involvement only (T1) in as many as 30% of all cases diagnosed[18] and represents a successful public health strategy. Such screening probably could not be justified in the United States because of the low incidence and high cost.

The rise in the rate of superficial gastric adenocarcinoma from 3% to 6% in our series and in other American reports[9,11,19] may be a result of the wider use of endoscopy and biopsy. The clinical course, duration, and natural history of superficial gastric adenocarcinoma are not yet well described, but the period between superficial involvement and invasive focal adenocarcinoma can be speculated on.[20] In 12 cases of superficial gastric adenocarcinoma, all but one was of an intestinal histology, and these patients had a median age of 61 years, while the median age of the 64 patients with focal cancer of intestinal histology was 67 years. Such a six-year lag time is consistent with time periods from in situ presentation to presentation with invasive clinical cancers occurring in the colon, cervix, and breast, and in melanoma.

The Lauren classification of gastric adenocarcinoma histologic types has proved useful since the two major types represent groups of patients with differing ages, sex ratios, survivals, epidemiology, and apparent origin.[6] Other reports[6,21,22] have noted a rise in the relative proportion of cases with diffuse histology from approximately 35% in the 1940s, to 45% in the 1960s, to almost 60% in the 1970s, at a time when the overall number of cases is decreasing. Patients whose cases are of diffuse histology tend to be younger,[23-25] with a slight predominance among women, and these cases have a relatively stable absolute incidence over time that produces the proportional increase in incidence. These trends have been exhaustively researched and summarized by Correa.[6] While the most marked clinical manifestation of the diffuse histologic pattern is the linitis plastica clinical type, which is easily recognized radiologically or surgically, many focal cases also have diffuse histology; these patients too have a slightly worse overall prognosis,[3] but their disease is curable if completely resected. Linitis plastica occurred in exactly the same proportion of cases as in our earlier report,[3] despite the proportional increase in diffuse histology. These facts suggest that linitis plastica is a peculiar host response to the cancer cells rather than just a unique histologic entity. Patients with linitis plastica all die of disease, usually after a short survival, but a few patients live for prolonged periods. Thus, all treatment of linitis plastica must be viewed as palliative. Indeed, the median survival of the few patients (14%) undergoing curative resection is no longer than that of patients undergoing palliative resection (12 months and 13 months, respectively). If resection is possible and safe, it probably should be attempted, but surgery may be avoided if obstruction or bleeding are not present.

Intestinal histology is seen in patients who have diet-related distal adenocarcinoma; thus, this manifestation is gradually declining in absolute incidence and overall relative proportion, both in the United States and in Europe.[6] Intestinal histology is seen in almost all superficial and many focal gastric cancers, and is more heavily represented in earlier and resectable cases.

The changing anatomical location of gastric adenocarcinoma reflects a little-noted trend that has an impact on the diagnosis and management of the disease. First reported by us in 1982,[4] other authors have documented a similar trend toward proximal location.[7,11-13] Proximally located gastric adenocarcinoma is marked by a relatively stable absolute incidence over time (in contrast with distal lesions), by a marked male predominance,[26] and by a generally worse prognosis. Despite some similarity of trends in diffuse histology (stable absolute incidence, increasing relative proportion, and worse prognosis), there are substantial differences (male predominance). Proximally located cancers are largely of intestinal histology and arise frequently on a background of dysplastic mucosa, indicating prolonged antecedent changes. These antecedent mucosal dysplasias frequently have produced hypochlorhydria or achlorhydria and proximally located cancers are marked by significantly elevated levels of serum gastrin as a result, in contradistinction to distally located cancers in which gastric acid is produced and serum gastrin levels are normal.[27]

Gastric stump adenocarcinomas,[28,29] those cancers arising in stomachs previously partially resected distally for benign duodenal ulcer, by definition are of the proximal type, and display the characteristics of proximal gastric cancers arising in intact stomachs (striking male predominance, hypochlorhydria, dysplasia of gastric mucosa, elevated gastrin levels, and poor prognosis). Although gastric stump adenocarcinomas are considered to be caused by the bile gastritis occurring with jejunal anastomoses to the stomach, we postulate that their incidence is similar to what would be expected in the population of at-risk patients followed up over the long term after ulcer operations. The more modern surgical therapy of duodenal ulcer without gastric resection has been used frequently only during the past decade; since the average lag period between gastrectomy and stump carcinoma is prolonged, it will be many years before we learn whether the preservation of the distal stomach, and even the pylorus, with reduced acid production from vagotomy but without bile gastritis, will be associated with the formation of proximal gastric adenocarcinomas.

The rising relative incidence of proximal adenocarcinoma highlights the rapid disappearance of distally located gastric cancers, which are clearly diet related, as noted by Correa.[6] Distally located cancers are "epidemic" in nature, and are related to dietary variations, while the proximal location is "endemic," as is diffuse histology. Thus, the decline in the incidence of distally located tumors in the United States has unmasked the endemic varieties, bringing them under investigation. Since significant adjustments in basic surgical approaches must be made for the treatment of proximally located cancers, and esophagogastrectomy is inherently more difficult, it was encouraging to note the sharp reduction in operative mortality. Currently, proximal gastrectomy and total gastrectomy can be performed with negligible operative mortality. The use of the circular stapling device had nothing to do with the results reported herein, since it was not used. Because proximal cancers may be resected via a transthoracic approach, members of general surgical services may have even less gastric adenocarcinoma experience than would be expected from incidence data; however, nearly all such cancers can be as effectively approached from the abdomen, with only an occasional need to open the chest for resection of esophageal extension, and thus their treatment should be within the competence and experience of surgical oncologists.

The overall resection rate has remained remarkably stable since 1950, while shifts in the proportions labeled palliative or curative have changed, reflecting changed attitudes regarding extensive lymph node resections for nodal metastases at some distance from the stomach and attempts to remove all direct spread to adjacent structures. Generally more conservative surgical approaches have been practiced since 1970. Routine sacrifice of the spleen, omentum, pancreas, and celiac nodes was infrequently performed and was used only in a highly selective fashion. Surgeons were less likely to attempt removal of extensive local evidence of disease once the primary gastric cancer and stomach were removed by gastrectomy when the goal was only palliation. The total gastrectomy rate was 13% of all resections and only 4% of curative resections, in contrast with the 14% rate reported in the 1960s, and over 30% reported in the 1950s, thus indicating a continued decline in the routine use of this procedure. Total gastrectomy was used only when indicated by the local extent of the disease in the stomach itself. This was illustrated by the fact that 26% of all patients undergoing palliative resection and 72% of all patients undergoing resection for linitus plastica required total gastrectomy.

The principal palliative goal is to rid the patient of the infected, bleeding, obstructed, necrotic, or ulcerated polypoid gastric lesion. For this purpose a limited gastric resection may suffice. Extension of the resection to other organs only occasionally cures the patient and sometimes does not justify the morbidity for a palliative goal. That such a conservative operative policy is practical and important is reflected in the median survival values of palliative cases, the sharply decreased operative mortality, the improved five-year survival rates for patients who undergo resection for cure, and the survival durations of patients who undergo curative resections but who nevertheless die of disease. Compared with our previous report, palliative resections bring about an improved median survival, partly reflecting the decreased operative mortality, but also reflecting the decreased morbidity and mortality of more restricted operations. A conservative surgical philosophy has yielded similar therapeutic benefits with other cancers.

Our better five-year survival and cure rates indicate that

a policy of routine total gastrectomy, as advocated by some authors,[27,28] is unnecessary and dangerous. Vigorous attempts to remove the cancer itself, along with a modest amount of surrounding uninvolved gastric wall encompassing the gross tumor, should be performed to produce an intact gastrointestinal tract. Previously we noted that the resection margin of normal stomach was not the determining factor in outcome. Thus, a reasonable local gastric margin of 3 to 4 cm should be sought,[29] but compromises are frequently required. Carcinoma that is evident at a distance from the primary cancer need not be resected, since such diseased tissue is associated with a fatal outcome regardless of its resection. Maximum potential palliation is achieved by clearing the gastrointestinal tract of the primary cancer.

The present study documents significant changes in the clinical and pathologic presentations of gastric adenocarcinoma. It also documents the benefits of a generally conservative surgical philosophy and indicates a surprising improvement in outcome as measured by median and five-year survival rates. Surgeons need to recognize these changes and transitions in disease to tailor properly their surgical therapy.

References

1. Seidman H, Silverberg E, Holleb A: Cancer statistics 1976. *CA* 1976;1:2-29.
2. Silverberg E, Lubera J: Cancer statistics 1986. *CA* 1986;1:9-25.
3. Cady B, Ramsden DA, Stein A, et al: Gastric cancer: Contemporary aspects. *Am J Surg* 1977;133:423-429.
4. Cady B, Choes DS: Changing patterns in gastric cancer, in Nieburg HE (ed): *Prevention and Detection of Cancer II*. New York, Marcel Dekker, 1984, pp 2041-2049.
5. Lauren P: The two histologic main types of gastric carcinoma: Diffuse and so-called intestinal type carcinoma: An attempt at a histo-clinical classification. *Acta Pathol Microbiol Scand* 1965;64:31-49.
6. Correa P: Clinical implications of recent developments in gastric cancer pathology and epidemiology. *Semin Oncol* 1985;1:2-10.
7. Meyers WC, Damiano RJ Jr, Rotolo FS, et al: Adenocarcinoma of the stomach: Changing patterns over the last four decades. *Ann Surg* 1987;205:1-8.
8. Adashek K, Sanger J, Longmire W: Cancer of the stomach. *Ann Surg* 1979;189:6-10.
9. Weed T, Nuessle W, Ochsner A: Carcinoma of the stomach. *Ann Surg* 1981;193:407-413.
10. Diehl J, Hermann R, Cooperman A, et al: Gastric carcinoma. *Ann Surg* 1983;198:9-12.
11. Lundegardh G, Adami HO, Malker B: Gastric cancer survival in Sweden. *Ann Surg* 1986;204:546-551.
12. Antonioli DA, Goldman H: Changes in the location and type of gastric adenocarcinoma. *Cancer* 1982;50:775-781.
13. Sons H, Borchard F: Cancer of the distal esophagus and cardia. *Ann Surg* 1986;203:188-195.
14. Murakami T: Pathomorphological diagnosis: Definition and gross classification of early gastric cancer, in Murakami T (ed): *Early Gastric Cancer: Gann Monograph on Cancer Research*. Tokyo, University of Tokyo Press, 1971, vol 2, pp 53-55.
15. Bringaze W, Chappuis C, Cohn I, et al: Early gastric cancer. *Ann Surg* 1986;204:103-113.
16. Longo W, Zucker K, Zdon M, et al: Role of endoscopy in the diagnosis of early gastric cancer. *Arch Surg* 1987;122:292-295.
17. Kajitani K, Takagi K: cancer of the stomach at Cancer Institute Hospital, Tokyo. *Gann* 1979;22:77-87.
18. Tsukuma H, Mishima T, Oshima A: Prospective study of early gastric cancer. *Int J Cancer* 1983;31:421-426.
19. Bloss R, Miller T, Copeland E: Carcinoma of the stomach in the young adult. *Surg Gynecol Obstet* 1980;150:883-886.
20. Grabiec J, Owen D: Carcinoma of the stomach in young persons. *Cancer* 1985;56:388-396.
21. Ikossi-O'Connor MG, Douglass HO: Gastric cancer in young patients. *J Surg Oncol* 1984;26:219-224.
22. Kalish RJ, Clancy P, Orringer MB, et al: Clinical epidemiologic and morphologic comparison between adenocarcinomas arising in Barrett's esophageal mucosa and in the gastric cardia. *Gastroenterology* 1984;86:461-467.
23. MacDonald WC: Clinical and pathologic features of adenocarcinoma of the gastric cardia. *Cancer* 1972;29:724-732.
24. McGuigan J, Trudeau W: Serum and tissue gastrin concentrations in patients with carcinoma of the stomach. *Gastroenterology* 1973;64:22-25.
25. Helsinger N, Hillestad L: Cancer development in the gastric stump after partial gastrectomy for ulcer. *Ann Surg* 1956;143:173-176.
26. Orlando R, Welch J: Carcinoma of the stomach after gastric operation. *Am J Surg* 1981;141:487-491.
27. Shiu M, Papacristou D, Kosloff C, et al: Selection of operative procedure for adenocarcinoma of the mid-stomach. *Ann Surg* 1980;192:730-737.
28. Paolini I, Tosato F, Cassese M, et al: Total gastrectomy in the treatment of adenocarcinoma of the cardia. *Am J Surg* 1986;151:238-243.
29. Bozzetti F, Bonfanti G, Bufalino R, et al: Adequacy of margins of resection in gastrectomy for cancer. *Ann Surg* 1982;196:685-690.

In Other AMA Journals

ARCHIVES OF INTERNAL MEDICINE

Cardiopulmonary Resuscitation in Patients With the Acquired Immunodeficiency Syndrome: A Prospective Study

Mario C. Raviglione, MD; Ruggero Battan, MD; Angelo Taranta, MD

To study the outcome of cardiopulmonary resuscitation (CPR) in patients with acquired immunodeficiency syndrome (AIDS), data on CPR in hospitalized patients were collected prospectively during a one-year study period. Of 43 consecutive patients with AIDS who underwent CPR, 23% were revived in the initial attempt, whereas of 293 patients with other diseases 42% were revived. One (2.3%) of 43 patients with AIDS survived until hospital discharge, and his arrest was iatrogenic, as opposed to 19 (6.5%) of 293 patients with diseases other than AIDS. A respiratory mechanism for the arrest was significantly more common in patients with AIDS. The duration of the unsuccessful attempt did not vary significantly; a higher number of temporary pacemakers was used in patients with diseases other than AIDS indicating a more invasive approach. Survival until hospital discharge is minimal in our series of patients with AIDS, undergoing CPR. We recommend that informative discussions take place early in the course of the disease to provide patients with a better understanding of the available options in case of cardiorespiratory arrest (*Arch Intern Med* 1988;148:2602-2605).

Reprint requests to Department of Medicine, Cabrini Medical Center, 227 E 19th St, New York, NY 10003 (Dr Raviglione).

Is Extensive Lymphadenectomy Necessary for Surgical Treatment of Intramucosal Carcinoma of the Stomach?

Keiji Iriyama, MD; Toyomatsu Asakawa, MD; Hiroshi Koike, MD; Hiroshi Nishiwaki, MD; Hiroshi Suzuki, MD

• This study was undertaken to elucidate those histological and gross features associated with gastric carcinoma that can be adequately treated by gastrectomy with less aggressive lymphadenectomy. The frequency of metastasis to the lymph nodes was analyzed in 514 cases of resected, solitary, gastric carcinomas. The frequency of metastasis to the lymph nodes increased in proportion to the increase in the extent of penetration by the cancer into the gastric wall. Lymph nodes were not involved in cases of intramucosal carcinoma of the intestinal type, by Laurén's histological classification. By contrast, metastasis to the lymph nodes was observed in cases of intramucosal carcinoma of the diffuse type, by Laurén's classification. We conclude that extensive lymphadenectomy is not mandatory for patients with intramucosal carcinoma of the stomach of the protruded type, since the lymph nodes do not become involved in this type of gastric carcinoma.

(*Arch Surg* 1989;124:309-311)

Extensive lymph node dissection in the surgical treatment of patients with carcinoma of the stomach has been advocated by Japanese surgeons[1-3] and has been adopted by surgeons all over the world. Since the intraoperative decision of whether or not the lymph nodes are involved is often inaccurate, extensive prophylactic lymphadenectomy seems to be necessary for the surgical treatment of patients with gastric carcinoma. However, the frequency of metastasis to the lymph nodes in patients with intramucosal cancer is extremely low and has been reported as varying from 1.9% to 7%.[4-8] Thus, we need to reconsider whether extensive lymphadenectomy is necessary for all patients with adenocarcinoma of the stomach, regardless of the extent of cancer. The present study was undertaken to elucidate the specific types of gastric carcinoma in which lymph nodes are not involved.

PATIENTS AND METHODS

From July 1, 1973, through Dec 31, 1986, there were 684 patients with primary adenocarcinoma of the stomach admitted to our clinic. Of these 684 patients, 553 (80.8%) underwent gastric resections. Thirty-nine patients with synchronous multiple carcinomas in the stomach were eliminated, so that the present analysis is based on the remaining 514 cases of resected stomachs. The operative mortality was 1.1%. The gross appearance of the carcinomas was classified into two principal types: the protruded type and the depressed type (Figure). The protruded type includes types I and IIa in the Japanese classification for early gastric cancer, and type 1 in Borrmann's classification. The depressed type includes types IIb, IIc, and III in the Japanese classification for early gastric cancer, and types 2, 3, and 4 in Borrmann's classification.[9] Most importantly, even if the principal gross feature of the cancer corresponded to the protruded type, any cancer that included even a minute ulceration, erosion, or excavation in the lesion was classified as the depressed type in the present study. The histological type was determined according to the report of the Japanese Research Society Committee on Histological Classification of Gastric Cancer,[10] and was classified into Laurén's classification as shown in Table 1. Papillary, well-differentiated, and moderately differentiated adenocarcinomas were classified as the intestinal type in Laurén's classification.[11] Poorly differentiated adenocarcinomas and signet-ring cell carcinomas were classified as the diffuse type in Laurén's classification. Because mucinous carcinomas were found to have structural characteristics in common with both the intestinal and the diffuse type, they were classified as being of the intestinal and the diffuse type by their structural features. One type, classified as the intestinal type, had distinct, usually large glandular lumina that were dilated and split by a profuse pool of mucus in which they floated. The other type had mucous masses that accumulated around isolated cells or loose clusters of cells and was classified as the diffuse type. Adenosquamous carcinomas were found mostly to be of the intestinal type.

Accepted for publication Dec 7, 1987.

From the Second Department of Surgery, Mie University School of Medicine, Tsu, Japan.

Reprint requests to Second Department of Surgery, Mie University School of Medicine, 2-174 Edobashi, Tsu 514, Japan (Dr Iriyama).

Macroscopic classification of early gastric cancer and Borrmann's classification of advanced gastric cancer, and corresponding classification of present study. Shaded area represents malignant tissue.

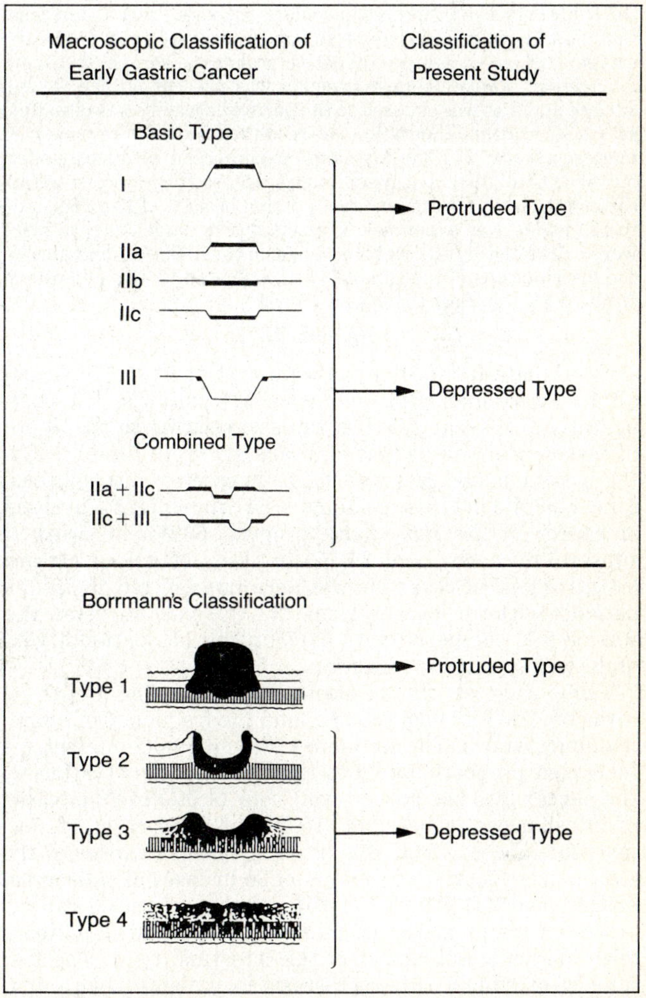

Table 1.—Histological Classification of Gastric Cancer

Japanese Research Society Committee on Histological Classification of Gastric Cancer	Laurén's Classification	General Structure
Papillary adenocarcinoma Tubular adenocarcinoma Well-differentiated type Moderately differentiated type	Intestinal type	Large glandular lumina; papillary fold formation; glandular structure is rarely completely absent
Poorly differentiated adenocarcinoma Signet-ring cell carcinoma	Diffuse type	Cells are found to be scattered; glandular lumina are rarely seen; cells seem to be only loosely attached to one another, forming no distinct epitheliumlike cords

Table 2.—Postoperative Five-Year Survival in Relation to Depth of Cancer Invasion*

Depth of Invasion	No. of Patients	Five-Year Survival Rate, %
ps(−)		
m	82	93.8
sm	84	86.4
pm	53	78.1
ss	36	66.9
ps(+)	259	31.0
Curative resection	146	52.9
Palliative resection	113	4.1

*ps(−) indicates negative prognostic serosal invasion; m, intramucosal; sm, submucosal; pm, muscularis propria; ss, subserosal; ps(+), cancer cells present on the serosal surface and exposed to the peritoneal cavity.

Cancers whose deepest layer of invasion into the gastric wall was the tunica mucosa including muscularis mucosae, tela submucosa, tela muscularis propria, and tela subserosa were included in the category of ps(−) cancers (negative prognostic serosal invasion). Any cancer whose deepest invasion was present on the serosal surface and that was exposed to the peritoneal cavity was classified as ps(+) cancer. Ulceration or resultant scars were analyzed microscopically. For the histologic examination of lymph nodes, one slice of all dissected lymph nodes, obtained by a cross section through the hilus at the central portion of each of the dissected lymph nodes, was examined. The cumulative crude survival rates were calculated by the Kaplan-Meier method. The significance of the distributions of the samples was evaluated by the χ^2 method. In the text, significant indicates $P<.05$.

RESULTS

Two hundred fifty-five patients with the ps(−) cancers (49.6%) were identified among the 514 patients. The postoperative five-year survival rates in relation to the depth of invasion of the gastric wall are given in Table 2. The five-year survival rate was 93.8% in cases of intramucosal cancer, 86.4% in cases of submucosal cancer, 78.1% in cases of cancer of the muscularis propria, 66.9% in cases of subserosal cancer, and 31.0% in cases of ps(+) cancer. Curative gastric resection was performed in 146 of the 259 patients with ps(+) cancer, and the five-year survival rate was 52.9%, compared with 4.1% in the 113 patients who underwent palliative resection.

Table 3 gives the relationship among the depth of invasion, the histological type, and the frequency of lymph node metastasis. The frequency of lymph node metastasis increased proportionately to the extent of penetration by the cancer into the gastric wall: four (4.9%) of 82 in cases of intramucosal cancer; 14 (16.7%) of 84 in cases of submucosal cancer; 21 (39.6%) of 53 in cases of cancer of the muscularis propria; 25 (69.4%) of 36 in cases of subserosal cancer; and 231 (89.2%) of 259 in cases of ps(+) cancer. However, lymph node metastasis was absent in all patients with intramucosal cancer of the intestinal type. The frequency of lymph node metastasis in patients with intramucosal cancer was significantly higher in cases of the diffuse type of cancer than in cases of the intestinal type ($P<.05$). The histological types did not influence the frequency of metastasis to the lymph nodes in cases with more extensive invasion by the cancer.

In the present series, four patients had intramucosal cancer with involvement of the regional lymph nodes, and their clinicopathological characteristics are given in Table 4. The common pathological features of their cancers were as follows. All were of the diffuse, depressed, superficially spreading type with maximum diameter more than 5 cm, and all had accompanying ulceration or resultant scars within the cancer. Metastasis was observed in the perigastric lymph node in these four patients.

Table 5 gives the relationship between the histological

Table 3.—Relationship Among Depth of Cancer Invasion, Histological Type, and Lymph Node Metastasis in Gastric Adenocarcinoma*

Depth	Histological Type, Lymph Node Metastasis	Negative	Positive	Subtotal	Total
ps(−)					
m	Intestinal	44 (100)	0 (0)	**44 (100)**	82 (16.0)
	Diffuse	34 (89.5)	4 (10.5)	**38 (100)**	
sm	Intestinal	35 (79.5)	9 (20.5)	**44 (100)**	84 (16.3)
	Diffuse	35 (87.5)	5 (12.5)	**40 (100)**	
pm	Intestinal	18 (64.3)	10 (35.7)	**28 (100)**	53 (10.3)
	Diffuse	14 (56.0)	11 (44.0)	**25 (100)**	
ss	Intestinal	7 (31.8)	15 (68.2)	**22 (100)**	36 (7.0)
	Diffuse	4 (28.6)	10 (71.4)	**14 (100)**	
ps(+)	Intestinal	11 (10.5)	94 (89.5)	**105 (100)**	259 (50.4)
	Diffuse	17 (11.0)	137 (89.0)	**154 (100)**	
Total	...	...	...	...	**514 (100)**

*Values are number (percent). ps(−) indicates negative prognostic serosal invasion; m, intramucosal; sm, submucosal; pm, muscularis propria; ss, subserosal; ps(+), cancer cells present on the serosal surface and exposed to the peritoneal cavity. Frequency of metastasis to lymph node in mucosal carcinoma is significantly low in the intestinal type as compared with the diffuse type ($P<.05$).

Table 4.—Clinicopathological Features of Mucosal Carcinoma of the Stomach With Lymph Node Metastasis*

Patient No./ Age, y/Sex	Maximum Diameter, cm	Lymph Node Involved
1/53/F	6.2	Infrapyloric
2/48/F	7.8	Lesser curvature
3/40/F	5.0	Lesser and greater curvature
4/41/F	7.5	Lesser curvature, infrapyloric

*In each case the cancer was the depressed, diffuse type, associated with ulceration.

Table 5.—Relationship Between Histological Type and Gross Appearance of Early Gastric Cancer*

	Depressed Type	Protruded Type
Intestinal type	71 (47.7)	17 (100)
Diffuse type	78 (52.3)	0 (0)
Total	**149 (100)**	**17 (100)**

*Values are number (percent).

Table 6.—Accuracy of Preoperative Assessment of Invasion in the Depressed Type of Early Gastric Carcinoma*

	Depth	
Assessment	**m**	**sm**
Preoperative	62	87
Histological		
m	50	19
sm	12	68
Accuracy, %	80.6	78.2

*m indicates intramucosal; sm, submucosal.

type and the gross appearance of early gastric cancer. The histological type of the protruded carcinomas was the intestinal type, without exception.

Table 6 gives the results of preoperative assessment of the depth of invasion by the cancer, in patients with the depressed type of early gastric cancer, by an upper gastrointestinal roentgenographic series and by endoscopic examination. We incorrectly assessed the depth of invasion in 20.8% of the patients with the depressed type of early gastric carcinoma. By contrast, we correctly assessed the depth of cancer invasion in all patients with the protruded type of early gastric carcinoma.

COMMENT

The prognosis of early gastric cancer is generally excellent, and the five-year survival rate has been reported to be greater than 90%. Certainly, the excellent five-year survival rate may be associated with treatment by gastrectomy with extensive lymphadenectomy.

Until two years ago, our surgical treatment for curatively resectable carcinoma of the stomach also included extensive lymphadenectomy with combined resection of the bursa omentalis, regardless of the extent of cancer. Since it is not unusual to observe metastasis to lymph nodes in cases of early gastric carcinoma, it seems reasonable to perform extensive lymphadenectomy uniformly in all patients with gastric carcinoma, regardless of the extent of cancer. The incidence of metastasis to lymph nodes in patients with early gastric cancer has been reported as varying from 1.9% to 7% in cases of intramucosal cancer, and from 7.4% to 20.9% in cases of submucosal cancer.[4-7,11] In the present study, the frequency of metastasis to lymph nodes was 4.8% in cases of intramucosal cancer, and 16.7% in cases of submucosal cancer. Because of these data, we do not criticize the performance of extensive lymphadenectomy in patients with gastric carcinoma that penetrates beyond the submucosal layer. However, in cases in which the gross and histological features of the intramucosal gastric carcinoma completely exclude the possibility of metastasis to lymph nodes, extensive lymphadenectomy with complete removal of the bursa omentalis is not necessary.

Korenaga et al[6] reported the clinicopathological features of 11 cases of intramucosal carcinoma with lymph node metastasis from a total of 568 patients with intramucosal carcinoma of the stomach. The histological classification of the tumor in nine of their 11 patients was the diffuse type, and ten patients had the depressed or flat type of tumor. They reported one case of a pure protruded type of intramucosal carcinoma of the intestinal type, in which the lymph node along the lesser curvature was involved. The size was 5.0×1.9 cm. This case is probably the first published case of metastasis to a lymph node seen in a case of a protruded type of intramucosal cancer of the intestinal type.

In the current study, the frequency of metastasis to the lymph nodes in cases of intramucosal cancer of the intestinal type was nil. However, we demonstrated that the differentiation, in terms of the depth of cancer invasion, between intramucosal and submucosal is often inaccurate in the depressed type of early gastric cancer. Consequently, four histological or gross features have ultimately emerged as the characteristics that eliminate the likelihood of metastasis to a lymph node: (1) intramucosal cancer, (2) the protruded type, (3) the intestinal type, and (4) a maximum size of less than 5 cm in diameter. An endoscopic feature of the cancer that satisfies the above-mentioned characteristics is a pure protruded type of cancer; in other words, the protruded type of cancer showing neither erosion nor excavation in the cancer, with a maximum diameter of less than 5 cm. The histological type of cancer demonstrating these characteristics is the intestinal type without exception, and the penetration of cancer into the gastric wall is probably confined to the mucosal layer. Lymph node is not involved in such a lesion. Thus, precise preoperative endoscopic evaluation is mandatory.

We conclude that gastrectomy with less aggressive lymphadenectomy may suffice as the curative surgical treatment for gastric cancer having the characteristics described above. The less aggressive lymphadenectomy that we emphasize in the current study is an operative procedure that includes dissections of the right cardial lymph node, the lymph nodes along the lesser and greater curvature, and the suprapyloric and infrapyloric lymph nodes, and preservation of the posterior portion of the bursa omentalis, ie, the capsule of the pancreas and the peritoneum around the common hepatic and splenic arteries. As the right and left omental arteries are resected, a combined removal of the greater omentum is therefore mandatory.

References

1. Jinnai D: Evaluation of extended radical operation for gastric cancer, with regard to lymph node metastasis and follow-up results. *Gann* 1968;3:225-231.
2. Soga J, Kobayashi K, Saito J, et al: The role of lymphadenectomy in curative surgery for gastric cancer. *World J Surg* 1979;3:701-708.
3. Kodama Y, Kano T, Tamada R, et al: Combined effect of prophylactic lymphadenectomy and long-term combination chemotherapy for curatively resected carcinoma of the stomach. *Jpn J Surg* 1982;12:244-248.
4. Abe S, Ogawa Y, Nagase N, et al: Early gastric cancer: Results in a general hospital in Japan. *World J Surg* 1984;8:308-314.
5. Ribichini P, Piccinini E, Perrucci A, et al: Early gastric cancer: Evaluation of diagnostic, clinicopathologic and therapeutic aspects in 60 cases. *Int Surg* 1984;69:325-329.
6. Korenaga D, Okamura T, Tamada R, et al: Clinicopathological features of mucosal carcinoma of the stomach with lymph node metastasis in 11 patients. *Br J Surg* 1986;73:431-433.
7. Iriyama K, Mori H, Suzuki H: Relationship between histological types and operative results in gastric carcinoma. *Cancer J* 1986;1:59-62.
8. Habu H, Takeshita K, Sunagawa M, et al: Lymph node metastasis in early gastric cancer. *Int Surg* 1986;71:244-247.
9. Japanese Research Society for Gastric Cancer: The general rules for the gastric cancer study in surgery and pathology: I. Clinical classification. *Jpn J Surg* 1981;11:127-139.
10. Japanese Research Society Committee on Histological Classification of Gastric Cancer: The general rules for the gastric cancer study in surgery and pathology: II. Histological classification of gastric cancer. *Jpn J Surg* 1981;11:140-145.
11. Laurén P: The two histological main types of gastric carcinoma: Diffuse and so-called intestinal-type carcinoma. *Acta Pathol Microbiol Immunol Scand* 1965;64:31-49.

THE NATURAL CHOICE

GORE-TEX®
SOFT TISSUE PATCH

In reconstructive surgery, a patient's own tissue is not always adequate. However, today surgeons do have alternatives. When a biomaterial is indicated, the GORE-TEX Soft Tissue Patch is the natural choice.

This remarkable sheet of GORE-TEX (expanded polytetrafluoroethylene) is engineered to provide improved performance in a wide range of applications. Since its introduction in 1982, the GORE-TEX Soft Tissue Patch has been used in more than 50,000 clinical cases worldwide.

The GORE-TEX Soft Tissue Patch combines high, balanced strength with softness and conformability. It is easy to shape and contour without fraying. Its microporous structure allows natural tissue ingrowth leading to potential treatability in the presence of infection. Next to delicate internal organs, the GORE-TEX Soft Tissue Patch has shown a significant reduction in adhesion formation and tissue erosion.

The exceptional versatility of the GORE-TEX Soft Tissue Patch makes it the natural choice in a wide range of applications.

- Abdominal Wall Reconstruction
- Hernia Repair
- Thoracic Wall Reconstruction
- Diaphragm Reconstruction
- Rectal and Vaginal Suspension
- Urethral Suspension
- Gastric Banding
- Facial Augmentation and Sling Procedures
- Related Pediatric Reconstructions

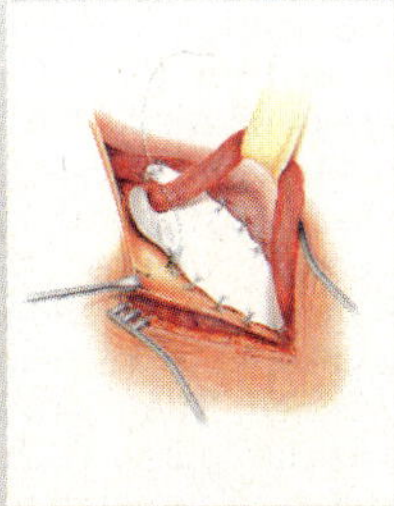
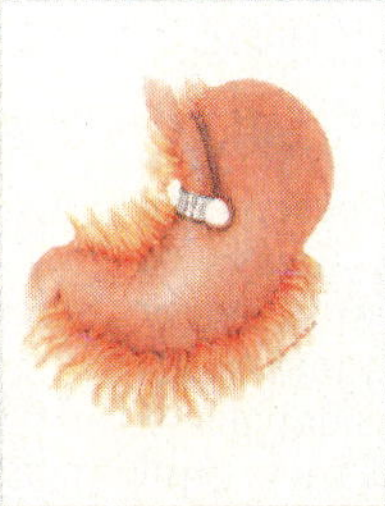
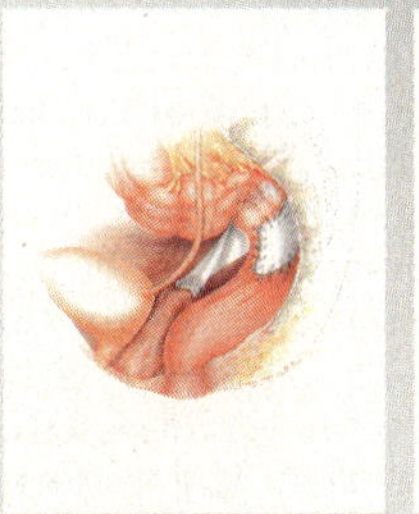
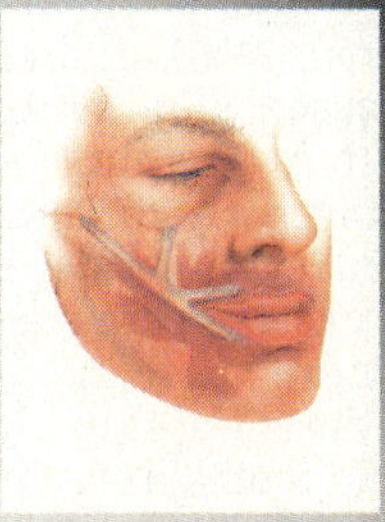

☐ Please send further information on the GORE-TEX Soft Tissue Patch.
☐ Please arrange for a free clinical sample.
☐ Please have your sales representative call for an appointment.

Name ______________________

Address ______________________

City ____________ State ________ Zip ________

Surgical Specialty ____________ Phone ____________

Hospital Affiliation ______________________

W.L. Gore & Associates, Inc.
P.O. Box 1220, Route 213 North Elkton, MD 21921

AOS-389

Everyday, more and more surgeons are coming to consider the GORE-TEX Soft Tissue Patch a superior alternative — the natural choice.

For specific clinical literature and information on the GORE-TEX Soft Tissue Patch, call 800-437-8181. In Arizona 800-528-1866.

GORE
CREATIVE TECHNOLOGIES WORLDWIDE

DNA Ploidy and Tumor Invasion in Human Gastric Cancer

Histopathologic Differentiation

Daisuke Korenaga, MD; Masaru Haraguchi, MD; Takeshi Okamura, MD; Hideo Baba, MD; Atsushi Saito, MD; Keizo Sugimachi, MD

• The relationship between DNA ploidy and tumor invasion in 254 patients with gastric carcinoma was studied, with particular emphasis on histopathologic features. In the differentiated type of adenocarcinoma, there were aneuploid lesions characterized by a relatively high incidence of lymph node metastasis and hematogenous recurrence, even when the invasion was limited to the submucosa. In the undifferentiated type, aneuploid lesions were rarely seen at the early stage, but the frequency remarkably increased with invasion into the deeper layers. Nodal involvement and disseminating metastasis were evident with serosal invasion. Analyzed by a multivariate Cox model, DNA ploidy significantly correlated with prognosis. Thus, DNA ploidy is a major determinant of survival, and the behavior of an aneuploid carcinoma is apparently controlled by individual histologic type.
(*Arch Surg* 1989;124:314-318)

Numerous DNA studies on human solid tumors revealed an association between the poor prognosis and abnormal DNA content.[1-3] This DNA abnormality corresponded to poorly differentiated tumors, as in carcinoma of the bladder, prostate, and breast,[3-5] but not always to cases of gastric carcinoma. Most recurrences in early carcinoma are those in which the lesion is well and moderately differentiated.[6,7] Cytophotometric DNA analysis of gastric carcinoma revealed that the differentiated type (DT), including well-differentiated and moderately differentiated adenocarcinomas, frequently had a dominant DNA distribution in the aneuploid range. The undifferentiated type (UT), consisting of poorly differentiated adenocarcinoma and signet-ring cell carcinoma, was predominantly of the diploid pattern.[8-10] While it is generally agreed that the UT has a favorable prognosis at the early stage of disease, some do become the highly malignant type of advanced carcinoma, characterized by rapid growth and by a poor prognosis.[11,12] This paradox suggested to us that the relationship between tumor progression and DNA abnormality, especially in cases of UT, had to be given attention.

The present study concerns progression of gastric carcinoma, with special focus on DNA abnormalities and histopathologic features.

Accepted for publication Feb 18, 1988.
From the Department of Surgery II, Kyushu University Faculty of Medicine, Fukuoka, Japan.

Reprint requests to Department of Surgery II, Kyushu University Faculty of Medicine, Fukuoka 812, Japan (Dr Korenaga).

PATIENTS AND METHODS

Patients

This study was based on 254 patients with gastric carcinoma treated in the Department of Surgery II, Kyushu University, Faculty of Medicine, Fukuoka, Japan, and affiliated hospitals, from 1965 to 1984.

Measurements of DNA Content

Cell nuclear DNA analysis of the resected specimens was performed on 10-μ-thick paraffin sections stained according to Feulgen's method.[13] The DNA content was measured with a microspectrophotometer (MMSP, Olympus Co, Japan) and the two-wavelength method.[14] Data processing was carried out using a personal computer (HP-85, Hewlett-Packard Co) combined with a microspectrophotometer. In each section, 100 cancer cells were measured, and the relative DNA content in each cancer cell was determined. The mean DNA value of 25 stromal lymphocytes was used as the control of the normal diploid chromosome complement (2c). The DNA distribution pattern was divided into low and high groups, according to the frequency of aneuploid cell population.[15-17] A carcinoma with a population of over 10% of cells beyond the hexaploid (6c) range was designated as *high ploidy* (aneuploid carcinoma) and that without such a population was classed as *low ploidy*.

Classifications of Clinicopathologic Factors

Clinicopathologic factors, including depth of invasion, tumor size, gross type, location, nodal involvement, and prognosis, were reviewed in relation to individual DNA ploidy and to the two main types of gastric carcinoma (DT and UT), according to the classification of Sugano et al.[12] Gross type of tumor was grouped into types 0 to 5, according to the general rules outlined by the Japanese Research Society for gastric cancer.[18] Type 0 indicates

Table 1.—DNA Ploidy and Clinicopathologic Characteristics			
	DNA Ploidy		
Pathologic Findings	Low Ploidy	High Ploidy	Significance, *P*
No. of cases	152	102	. . .
Mean age, y	53.6	57.4	NS*
Sex			
M	104	75	NS
F	48	27	
Tumor size, cm (mean ± SD)	4.4 ± 3.3	4.7 ± 3.6	NS
Depth of invasion			
Mucosa	57	18	<.01
Submucosa	43	36	
Muscularis propria	22	14	
Serosa	30	34	
Histology			
DT	61	71	<.01
UT	91	31	
Gross type			
0	100	54	<.01
1	1	0	
2	8	15	
3	10	20	
4	9	9	
5	24	4	
Location			
Upper	15	13	<.01
Middle	80	32	
Lower	52	49	
Whole stomach	5	8	
Nodal involvement			
Present	39	50	<.01
Absent	113	52	
Peritoneal dissemination			
Present	4	6	NS
Absent	148	96	
Liver metastasis			
Present	2	6	NS
Absent	150	96	
Curability			
Curative	141	85	<.05
Noncurative	11	17	
5-y survival rate, %	90.6	73.7	<.001

*NS indicates not significant.

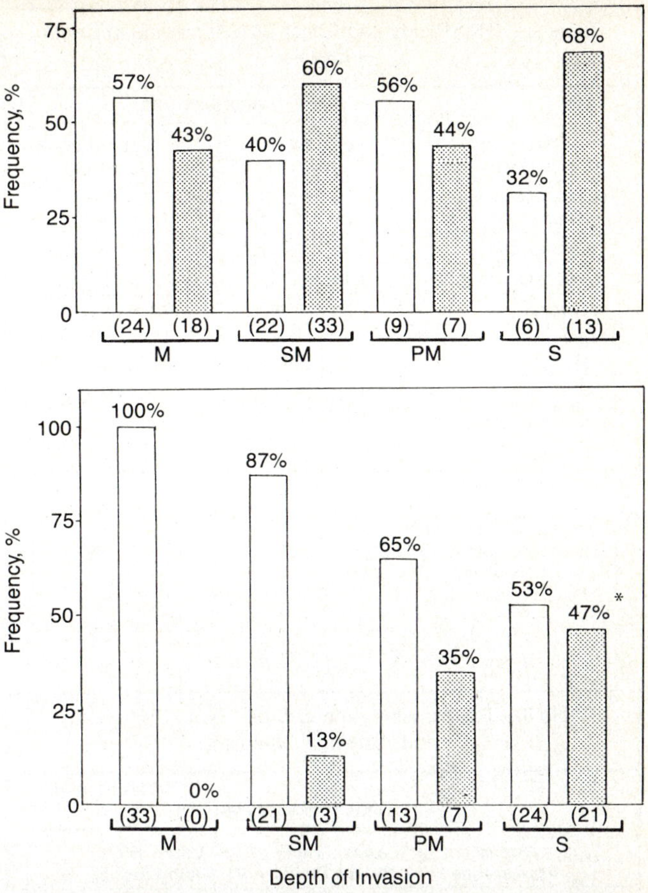

Fig 1.—Frequency of aneuploid carcinoma according to depth of invasion classified as differentiated (at top) or undifferentiated (at bottom). Number in parentheses indicates number of cases. Asterisk indicates significant difference compared with mucosa (M) ($P<.01$) and compared with submucosa (SM) ($P<.01$). PM indicates muscularis propria; S, subserosa and serosa. Shaded bars represent high ploidy; open bars, low ploidy.

early carcinoma confined to the mucosa or the submucosa, regardless of the presence of lymph node metastasis, and includes elevated, flat, and depressed types. Advanced carcinoma, with invasion extending into the muscularis propria or beyond it, was classified into types 1 to 5. Types 1 to 4 correspond to Borrmann's classification,[18] and type 5 is one that cannot be classified under any of the above types in which early cancer–simulating advanced carcinomas are involved.

Statistical Analysis

Statistical analysis for tumor size was made using Student's *t* test; other statistical analyses were performed using the χ^2 test. Survival rate was estimated on the basis of the method of Kaplan and Meier.[19] Statistical analyses of the survival rate were carried out using the generalized Wilcoxon test. In the multivariate analysis, Cox' proportional hazard's model[20] was used to determine the prognostic significance of the various factors discussed.

RESULTS

DNA Ploidy and Clinicopathologic Characteristics

Among the 254 patients were 102 (40.2%) cases of high ploidy, including 71 cases of the DT and 31 cases of the UT. Table 1 summarizes DNA ploidy and the clinicopathologic characteristics. There were statistically significant differences between low- and high-ploidy groups with regard to depth of invasion, histologic and gross types, tumor location, lymph node metastasis, curability in surgery, and the five-year survival rate. In cases of low ploidy, the carcinoma was confined to the mucosa, was UT in histologic type, was types 0 and 5 in gross appearance, involved the middle third of the stomach, showed no lymph node metastasis, and was resectable for potential cure. High ploidy was related to invasion into the serosal layer, was DT in histologic type, was types 2 and 3 in gross appearance, was located in the lower third of the stomach, showed nodal involvement, and was not resectable for potential cure. The five-year survival rate in the low-ploidy group was 90.6%, a value significantly higher than the five-year survival rate of 73.7% in the high-ploidy group ($P<.001$).

Frequency of Aneuploid Tumor Population According to Depth of Invasion

In DT cases, the rate of high ploidy was 42.9% at the mucosal stage and, at most, 68.4% at the serosal stage

Table 2.—DNA Ploidy and Tumor Size According to Depth of Invasion

Depth of Invasion	Tumor Size, cm*: Low Ploidy (n=152)	High Ploidy (n=102)
Differentiated type		
Mucosa	3.2±2.6 (24)	3.1±2.4 (18)
Submucosa	4.0±2.5 (22)	2.7±0.8 (33)
Muscularis propria	4.4±1.9 (9)	3.1±1.0 (7)†
Serosa	9.4±5.6 (6)	7.1±2.6 (13)†
Undifferentiated type		
Mucosa	3.6±2.0 (33)	. . .
Submucosa	3.6±1.8 (21)	3.1±1.5 (3)
Muscularis propria	4.1±2.5 (13)‡	4.4±1.2 (7)§
Serosa	6.7±5.0 (24)‡	8.8±4.7 (21)§

*Values are means±SDs. Number in parentheses indicates number of patients.
†Significantly different (*P*<.01).
‡Significantly different (*P*<.05).
§Significantly different (*P*<.01).

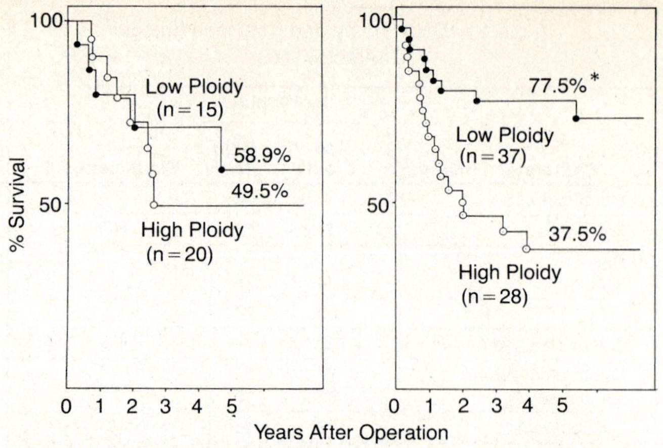

Fig 2.—Survival curves by DNA distribution pattern in patients with advanced carcinoma classified as differentiated (at left) or undifferentiated (at right). Asterisk indicates significant difference compared with high-ploidy group (*P*<.01).

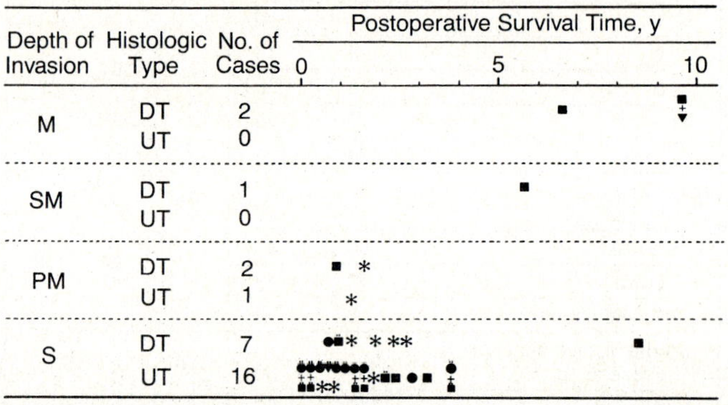

Fig 3.—Cause of death and postoperative survival time in patients with aneuploid carcinoma who died following recurrence. Squares indicate recurrence via hematogenous route; circles, recurrence via disseminating route; triangles, recurrence in remnant stomach; asterisk, unknown pattern of recurrence; double dots, origin of metastatic pattern was evident at surgery; M, mucosa; SM, submucosa; PM, muscularis propria; S, subserosa and serosa; DT, differentiated type; and UT, undifferentiated type.

Table 3.—Relationship Among Gross Type, DNA Ploidy, and Histologic Features

Gross Appearance	Differentiated Type: Low Ploidy	High Ploidy	*P*	Undifferentiated Type: Low Ploidy	High Ploidy	*P*
Early carcinoma (type 0)						
Elevated	15	33	<.01	2	1	. . .
Flat	2	1	. . .	2	0	. . .
Depressed	29	17	<.01	50	2	. . .
Advanced carcinoma						
Type 1	1	0	. . .	0	0	. . .
Type 2	1	8	<.05	7	7	. . .
Type 3	4	9	. . .	6	11	<.05
Type 4	2	2	. . .	7	7	. . .
Type 5	7	1	<.05	17	3	<.01

Table 4.—DNA Ploidy and Lymph Node Metastasis According to Depth of Invasion

Depth of Invasion	Lymph Node Metastasis*: Low Ploidy (n=152)	High Ploidy (n=102)
Differentiated type		
Mucosa	2/24 (8.3)	0/18
Submucosa	2/22 (9.1)	12/33 (36.4)†
Muscularis propria	1/9 (11.1)	2/7 (28.6)
Serosa	3/6 (50.0)	13/13 (100)†
Undifferentiated type		
Mucosa	8/33 (24.2)	0/0
Submucosa	6/21 (28.6)	1/3 (33.3)
Muscularis propria	4/13 (30.6)	4/7 (57.1)
Serosa	13/24 (54.2)	18/21 (85.7)†

*Number in parentheses indicates percentage.
†Significantly different from low ploidy (*P*<.05).

(Fig 1). There were no significant differences in the frequency of the aneuploid tumor population. Conversely, the UT was free of high-ploidy cases at the stage confined to the mucosa, while the frequency remarkably increased with progression of the tumor. The rate was 46.7% for serosal carcinoma. There were significant differences between events related to serosa and those related to the mucosa (*P*<.01) and between the serosa and the submucosa (*P*<.01).

DNA Ploidy and Tumor Size According to Depth of Invasion

Size of the tumors in each layer of the gastric wall is given in Table 2. The mean sizes were approximately equal in the layers of mucosa, submucosa, and muscularis propria, except in the case of UT classed as high ploidy. The size of the carcinoma invading the serosal layer was significantly larger than that of carcinoma limited to the muscularis propria (*P*<.05 in the low-ploidy group [DT] and *P*<.01 in the high-ploidy group [DT and UT]). Thus,

UT classed as high ploidy was dominant with regard to increases in tumor size, in proportion to invasion into the deeper layers.

DNA Ploidy and Gross Appearance

In the case of DT, the high-ploidy group frequently had elevated lesions at the early stage ($P<.01$), and type 2 lesions were the most common gross types of advanced carcinoma ($P<.05$) (Table 3). Conversely, depressed lesions of early carcinoma ($P<.01$) and type 5 lesions of advanced carcinoma ($P<.01$) were most commonly seen in the low-ploidy group. In cases of UT, gross appearance of an early carcinoma classed as high ploidy included one elevated lesion and two depressed lesions. On gross inspection of the advanced carcinoma, the high-ploidy cases were predominant in type 3 lesions ($P<.05$) and less frequent in type 5 lesions ($P<.01$). Advanced carcinoma classed as type 4 (the diffusely infiltrative type), most of which was histologically undifferentiated, belonged to the high-ploidy group as frequently as to the low-ploidy group. Characteristically, the carcinoma of type 4 involving the entire stomach was observed in four (44.4%) of nine cases of low ploidy and in seven (77.8%) of nine cases of high ploidy.

Metastatic Potential

The incidence of lymph node metastasis was higher in the high-ploidy group than in the low-ploidy group at the stage of invasion beyond the mucosa (Table 4). In case of DT, the difference in the incidence of nodal involvement was significant in cases of invasion confined to the submucosa and also in cases of invasion extending to the serosa in the high-ploidy group ($P<.05$). In cases of UT, a significant difference was evident only in carcinoma invading the serosa ($P<.05$). The DT classed as high ploidy had a lymph node metastasis even in cases of submucosal carcinoma, while in 18 of 21 with UT lesions and lymph node metastasis, the carcinoma had invaded the serosa.

Prognosis

There were four patients with an early carcinoma and a postoperative recurrence, including one with low ploidy and three with high ploidy. All four patients with a DT lesion had died five years after the operation. The ten-year survival rates of low- and high-ploidy groups with DT lesions were 94.4% and 88.4%, respectively (no statistically significant difference), while patients with UT lesions had a good clinical course regardless of the DNA ploidy. The postoperative survival curves for patients with advanced carcinoma are shown in Fig 2. The five-year survival rates of low- and high-ploidy groups were, respectively, 58.9% and 49.5% for patients with DT lesions and 77.5% and 37.5% for patients with UT lesions. In cases of UT, the difference was statistically significant ($P<.01$).

The relationship among mode of recurrence, postoperative survival time, and depth of invasion in the high-ploidy group is summarized in Fig 3. In 12 patients with DT lesions, the mucosa was invaded in two, the submucosa was invaded in one, the muscularis propria was invaded in two, and the serosa was invaded in seven. Of these patients, two with mucosal carcinoma died six years six months and nine years six months after operation with recurrences in the lung and liver, respectively. A patient with submucosal carcinoma died of multiple bone metastasis five years seven months after the operation. The mode of recurrence was confirmed in four of nine patients with advanced carcinoma. Liver metastasis occurred in three patients, including one with a lesion invading the muscularis propria and two with serosal carcinoma. Another patient with serosal invasion died of disseminating metastasis. Conversely, 16 of 17 with carcinoma classed as UT had a lesion extending to the serosa and died soon after operation. The mode of recurrence in 16 with serosal carcinoma included nine with disseminating metastasis, with or without liver metastasis, three with liver metastasis, one with a local recurrence in the remnant stomach, and three with an unknown pattern. Therefore, hematogenous metastasis usually occurred in patients with the DT carcinoma of aneuploidy, even when the invasion was confined to the mucosa or to the submucosa. Disseminating metastasis occurred more frequently in those with the UT carcinoma of aneuploidy extending to the serosa.

Multivariate Analysis of Prognostic Factors

A multivariate analysis was performed for 226 patients who underwent curative surgery. The variables analyzed included age, sex, tumor size, gross type, histologic types, depth of invasion, growth pattern, vessel invasion, lymphatic involvement, lymph node metastasis, extent of lymph node dissection, stage of disease, and DNA ploidy. Age of patients was classified into three types: under 49, 50 to 69, or over 70 years. Size of the tumor was also classified into three types: under 4.0, 4.1 to 8.0, or over 8.1 cm. Growth pattern was classified into the following three types: expansive, intermediate, or infiltrative. Vessel invasion and lymphatic involvement were classified into two categories: present or absent. Lymph node metastasis was classified into four categories: (1) no evidence of regional lymph node metastasis; (2) primary nodal involvement along the lesser or greater curvatures; (3) secondary nodal involvement, including that along the left gastric, splenic, celiac, and common hepatic arteries; or (4) tertiary nodal involvement, such as involvement of the hepatoduodenal, retropancreatic, and mesenteric nodes. The extent of lymph node dissection was classified into two categories: complete removal of the primary lymph node or complete removal of primary and secondary lymph nodes with or without dissection of tertiary nodes. Stage of the disease was classified into four types according to the histopathologic classification of the Japanese staging system.[18] Of these variables, DNA ploidy significantly influenced the prognosis ($P<.05$, $\chi^2=4.42$), as did the sex ($P<.01$, $\chi^2=7.27$), gross type ($P<.05$, $\chi^2=4.34$), vessel invasion, ($P<0.05$, $\chi^2=4.31$), extent of lymph node dissection ($P<.01$, $\chi^2=9.01$), and stage of disease ($P<0.01$, $\chi^2=6.90$).

COMMENT

There is general agreement that aneuploid tumors usually are related to an advanced disease. The involvement of surrounding tissues, metastasis, and a poor prognosis have been noted in cases of carcinoma of the colon,[1] esophagus,[2] and prostate.[3] In our study of gastric carcinoma, we noted an aneuploid carcinoma preponderance associated with lymph node metastasis, tumor invasion, and prognosis. The high-ploidy group had a greater population in the advanced stage than in the early stage and showed a stronger metastastic potential than the low-ploidy group,[15] resulting in a poorer prognosis.

We found a distinct difference in the mode of development between aneuploid tumors consisting of the DT and those of the UT. In the case of the DT with an abnormal DNA content, early carcinoma with an elevated form was frequent and often led to an advanced carcinoma of the ulcerating, circumscribed type (type 2). Conversely, in the case of the UT, the ulcerating infiltrative type (type 3) and diffusely infiltrative type (type 4) of advanced carcinoma may occur, although little is known of the aneuploid tumor origin. Characteristically, the UT with an abnormal DNA content gave rise to a remarkable increase in frequency of aneuploid tumors, tumor size, and the metastatic potential during the progression from the early to the advanced stage. These findings are attributed to (1) a difference in growth rate between DT and UT or (2) a change in cytogenetic profile during the progression of the UT.

According to the DNA analysis, aneuploid carcinoma was present even in a lesion confined to the mucosa and less than 5 mm in diameter.[16] In such cases, there was a preponderance of the DT, and UT with an aneuploid profile was not included. The DNA characteristics did not change in the case of tumor progression into the gastric wall, as determined in a comparative study between primary and recurrent gastric carcinomas.[21] Hence, it is reasonable to consider that the UT featured by aneuploidy is rapid in growth and less likely to be detected until the advanced stage, thereby supporting the first hypothesis.

With regard to the second hypothesis, Hattori et al[22] reported that the diffuse type of carcinoma would be kinetically more heterogeneous than the intestinal type of carcinoma, because the former type showed differences in distribution of the tritiated thymidine–incorporated cells in the gastric wall. The cancer cells were not located in the superficial layer but rather were in the deeper layer. Haraguchi et al[17] obtained evidence of heterogeneous DNA ploidy in a small number (30%) of the UT of serosal carcinoma. In such cases, low-ploidy patterns were evident in the mucosal layer, and high-ploidy patterns were seen in some parts of the deeper layer. In light of these findings, a more malignant transformation may occur in a small number of cases during the progression of UT carcinoma of diploid origin from early to advanced stages.

In the multivariate analysis, DNA ploidy proved to be a major independent factor. In this respect, DNA analysis is useful for predicting the prognosis of patients who undergo curative surgery. We observed that the behavioristic features of aneuploid carcinoma are governed by the individual histologic types. A differentiated carcinoma with aneuploid profile was associated with nodal involvement and hematogenous metastasis, even at the early stage of disease. Conversely, the metastatic potential in the case of undifferentiated carcinoma was usually inhibited when the lesion was confined to the proper muscle layer. However, the prognosis was extremely poor when the carcinoma had invaded the serosa. Death seemed to relate to the occurrence of peritoneal dissemination. Well-planned treatment, including radical surgery, anticancer chemotherapy, and careful follow-up, will lead to more satisfactory results in treating patients with aneuploid gastric carcinoma.

This investigation was supported in part by the Grant-in-Aid for General Scientific Research 62480284 and for Encouragement of Young Scientists 63770990 from the Japanese Ministry of Education, Science, and Culture.

References

1. Banner BF, Vega JETL, Roseman DL, et al: Should flow cytometric DNA analysis precede definitive surgery for colon carcinoma? *Ann Surg* 1985;202:740-744.

2. Matsuura H, Sugimachi K, Ueo H, et al: Malignant potentiality of squamous cell carcinoma of the esophagus predictable by DNA analysis. *Cancer* 1986;57:1810-1814.

3. Frankfult OS, Chin JL, Englander LS, et al: Relationship between DNA ploidy, glandular differentiation and tumor spread in human prostate cancer. *Cancer Res* 1985;45:1418-1423.

4. Frankfult OS, Slocum HK, Rustum YM, et al: Flow cytometric analysis of DNA aneuploidy in primary and metastatic human solid tumors. *Cytometry* 1984;5:71-80.

5. Dowle CS, Owainati A, Robins A, et al: Prognostic significance of the DNA content of human breast cancer. *Br J Surg* 1987;74:133-136.

6. Matsusaka T, Kodama Y, Soejima K, et al: Recurrence in early gastric cancer: A pathologic evaluation. *Cancer* 1980;46:168-172.

7. Kodama Y, Inokuchi K, Soejima K, et al: Growth patterns and prognosis in early gastric carcinoma: Superficially spreading and penetrating growth types. *Cancer* 1983;51:320-326.

8. Inokuchi K, Kodama Y, Sasaki O, et al: Differentiation of growth patterns of early gastric carcinoma determined by cytophotometric DNA analysis. *Cancer* 1983;51:1138-1141.

9. Czerniak B, Herz F, Koss LG: DNA distribution patterns in early gastric carcinomas: A Feulgen cytometric study of gastric brush smears. *Cancer* 1987;59:113-117.

10. Petrova AS, Subrichina GN, Tschistjakova OV, et al: Flow cytofluorometry, cytomorphology and histology in gastric carcinoma. *Oncology* 1980;37:318-324.

11. Ribeiro MM, Simoes MAS, Bastos J: Analysis of 242 cases of gastric carcinoma. *World J Surg* 1981;5:97-102.

12. Sugano H, Nakamura K, Kato Y: Pathological studies of human gastric cancer. *Acta Pathol Jpn* 1982;32(suppl):329-347.

13. Naora H: Microspectrophotometry of cell nucleus stained by Feulgen reaction: I. Microspectrophotometric apparatus without Schwarzchild-Villiger effect. *Exp Cell Res* 1955;8:259-278.

14. Mendersohn ML: The two-wavelength method of microspectrophotometry: II. A set of tables to facilitate the calculations. *J Cell Biol* 1958;4:415-424.

15. Korenaga D, Okamura T, Saito A, et al: DNA ploidy is closely linked to lymph node metastasis, tumor invasion and prognosis in clinical gastric cancer. *Cancer* 1988;62:309-313.

16. Korenaga D, Mori M, Okamura T, et al: DNA ploidy in clinical malignant gastric lesions less than 5 mm in diameter. *Cancer* 1986;58:2542-2545.

17. Haraguchi M, Okamura T, Korenaga D, et al: Heterogeneity of DNA ploidy in patients with undifferentiated carcinomas of the stomach. *Cancer* 1987;59:922-924.

18. Japanese Research Society for Gastric Cancer: The general rules for the gastric cancer study in surgery and pathology. *Jpn J Surg* 1981;11:127-139.

19. Kaplan EL, Meier P: Nonparametric estimation from incomplete observation. *J Am Stat Assoc* 1958;53:457-481.

20. Cox DR: Regression models and life tables. *J R Stat Soc* 1972;343:187-220.

21. Korenaga D, Haraguchi M, Okamura T, et al: Consistency of DNA ploidy between primary and recurrent gastric carcinomas. *Cancer Res* 1986;46:1544-1546.

22. Hattori T, Hosokawa Y, Fukuda M, et al: Analysis of DNA ploidy patterns of gastric carcinomas of Japanese. *Cancer* 1984;54:1591-1597.

Prophylactic Antibiotherapy in Abdominal Surgery

First- vs Third-Generation Cephalosporins

Nelly Rotman, MD; Jean-Marie Hay, MD; François Lacaine, MD;
Pierre-Louis Fagniez, MD; the Association de Recherche en Chirurgie Cooperative Group

• To compare the efficiency of antibioprophylaxis by cefazolin sodium or cefotaxime sodium, 3137 consecutive patients undergoing abdominal surgery were included in a prospective, randomized, controlled, multicenter study. The patients were divided into four strata, according to the degree of contamination during the operation and the risk factors. Within each stratum, the patients were randomized into three groups of treatment: (1) cefazolin, (2) cefotaxime, and (3) nontreatment (control). Antibiotics were administered perioperatively in three intravenous doses of 1 g at eight-hour intervals. Patients undergoing colon surgery or with peritonitis at the time of the operation were excluded from the study. The wound abscess rate was significantly lower in the treated groups than in the control group, except in stratum 3 (contaminated surgery). The percentage of postoperative peritonitis was twice as low in the treated groups as in the control group. There was no difference between the groups receiving cefazolin or cefotaxime. The patients in the treated groups received significantly less postoperative antibiotics than the patients in the control group. In terms of cost, antibioprophylaxis by cefazolin seems to be warranted in all operations with a low anaerobic contamination.

(*Arch Surg* 1989;124:323-327)

In the last two decades, several studies have demonstrated the benefits offered by prophylactic antibiotherapy in some surgical settings, and these studies have helped to clarify the type, timing, and duration of antimicrobial prophylaxis.[1-4] The efficiency of prophylactic antibiotherapy is well established for gynecologic and high-risk biliary and gastric surgery, as well as for colorectal surgery.[3] However, controversy remains concerning the usefulness of antibioprophylaxis in surgical procedures with spontaneous, minimal postoperative infection.[5] Another question concerns the choice of the more appropriate prophylactic antibiotic, which has been complicated since third-generation cephalosporins have become available. Because of their broad-spectrum effectiveness against the digestive tract pathogens and their minimal adverse effects, cephalosporins are commonly administered for prophylaxis in patients undergoing surgery. In a prospective evaluation of antimicrobial prophylaxis, Crossley et al[6] showed that more than half of the patients received a cephalosporin. Although second- and third-generation cephalosporins have an expanded spectrum, their superiority over first-generation cephalosporins for surgical prophylaxis has not been demonstrated.[7-10] The aim of this study on 3137 consecutive patients undergoing abdominal surgery was to evaluate the benefits of prophylactic antibiotherapy by comparing treated and untreated patients and to compare the efficiency of a first-generation (cefazolin) and a third-generation (cefotaxime sodium) cephalosporin in preventing postoperative infection.

Accepted for publication May 16, 1988.

From the Service de Chirurgie Digestive, Hôpital Henri-Mondor, Creteil, France (Drs Rotman and Fagniez), the Service de Chirurgie Digestive, Hôpital Louis-Mourier, Colombes, France (Dr Hay), and the Service de Chirurgie Digestive, Hôpital Tenon, Paris (Dr Lacaine).

A complete listing of participants in the Association de Recherche en Chirurgie Cooperative Group appears at the end of this article.

Reprint requests to Association de Recherche en Chirurgie, 8 Avenue des Peupliers, 92270 Bois-Colombes, France (Dr Rotman).

PATIENTS AND METHODS

During a four-year period (June 1982 through June 1986), 3137 consecutive patients were included in a prospective, randomized, controlled, multicenter study.

Patient Selection

All patients undergoing intra-abdominal or parietoabdominal surgery were included in the study. The patients were divided into three strata, according to the degree of contamination of the operation. This distribution was made according to the classification of the National Research Council.[11] Stratum 1 included operative procedures in which neither the digestive nor the genitourinary tracts were entered (clean). Stratum 2 included the operations with a low contamination (clean-contaminated), and stratum 3 included operative procedures in which more endogenous organisms were likely to be encountered (contaminated). A fourth stratum was designed to include patients with a high risk of infection whatever the operation. The classification of patients according to surgical procedure was as follows:

Stratum 1
- Abdominal and groin hernia (elective procedures)
- Hiatal hernia
- Hyperselective vagotomy
- Staging, exploratory laparotomy
- Vascular surgery
- Ovarian cyst

Stratum 2
- Cholecystectomy
- Elective gastrectomy (cancer and/or stenosis excluded)
- Hepatectomy
- Pancreatectomy (acute pancreatitis excluded)
- Hysterectomy

Stratum 3
- Small-bowel obstruction
- Small-bowel resection
- Common bile duct surgery
- Appendectomy
- Gastrectomy (cancer and/or stenosis)

Stratum 4
- Diabetes mellitus
- Ascites
- Obesity (>20%)
- Weight loss (>15%)
- Abdominal radiotherapy
- Steroids } within 6 mo before surgery
- Chemotherapy }

Excluded preoperatively from the study were (1) patients who had received antimicrobial therapy within 15 days before surgery, (2) patients with a known allergy to cephalosporins or renal failure, and (3) patients undergoing colon surgery. These latter patients were excluded because their allocation in a nontreatment group is unethical.[12]

Only patients undergoing vascular procedures without prosthetic material were included in the study. The patients with peritonitis or intra-abdominal abscesses, discovered at the time of operation, were given curative antibiotherapy and thus were withdrawn from the study. The patients who received postoperative curative antibiotherapy for a postoperative intra-abdominal or extra-abdominal infection were not excluded from the study.

The age, sex, type of surgical procedure, length of operation, and duration of hospital stay were recorded for each patient.

Methods

Patients were given either cefazolin, cefotaxime (treated groups), or no antibiotherapy (control group). The allocation to one of the three groups was performed by a computer-generated randomization. The random assignment was balanced within each center. A form was filled out for each patient. The type of treatment to be performed was concealed in the upper-right-hand corner of the form that was unsealed by the anesthetist in the operating room. This method was preferred to that of sealed envelopes, to avoid nonsequential allocation when the order of the envelopes became mixed.[13] Each drug was administered intravenously in three doses for a total dose of 3 g. The first dose was given 20 minutes before the anesthetic induction. The subsequent doses were administered at eight-hour intervals.

Skin preparation was done in the operating room, using either povidone-iodine (Betadine) or tincture of chlorhexidine gluconate (Hibitane). Local irrigation of the wound and/or the peritoneal cavity was performed in all the cases with the antiseptic used for skin preparation.

The study was approved by the Comité d'Ethique of the Paris XII University.

Criteria for Evaluation of Efficiency of Prophylactic Antibiotherapy

Failure of prophylactic antibiotherapy was defined as the occurrence of an infection at the operative site. Patients were examined daily during their hospital stay by a physician unaware of the prophylactic antimicrobial regimen. All the patients underwent a physical examination 30 to 40 days after they were discharged from the hospital, in order not to overlook a late wound abscess. The main criterion for the evaluation of prophylactic antibiotherapy was the presence of a wound abscess at the site of operation. A wound abscess was defined on clinical grounds as a purulent exudate. The occurrences of intra-abdominal or extra-abdominal infectious complications (pulmonary infection, urinary tract infection, or septicemia), as well as noninfectious complications (myocardial infarction, phlebitis, pulmonary embolism, liver failure, or neurologic disorders), were also recorded.

Statistical Analysis

The number of patients necessary for the study was defined so as to obtain a reduction in the wound abscess rate from 7% (with no antibiotherapy) to 3.5% (with antibiotherapy), with a type I error of 0.05 and a type II error of 0.05. The estimation of the wound abscess rate was made according to the study of the Ad Hoc Committee on Trauma.[14] The calculated number of patients necessary for the study was 1015 in each group (two-sided test). The χ^2 and Student's t tests were used to compare the characteristics of the three groups.[15]

	Stratum 1		
	Control	Cefazolin	Cefotaxime Sodium
No. of patients	276	230	239
Mean ± SD age, y	48.2 ± 17.8	49.5 ± 17.0	47.7 ± 18.0
Sex, M/F	201/75	164/66	187/52
Type of operation, No.			
Digestive	126	113	112
Vascular	9	8	5
Gynecologic	14	15	8
Urologic	1	2	3
Other	129	96	114
Mean ± SD length of operation, min	68.8 ± 49.1	73.6 ± 53.1	69.2 ± 51.7
Mean ± SD hospital stay, d	16.1 ± 39.6	15.5 ± 40.6	18.5 ± 53.9

RESULTS

After randomization, the following were withdrawn from the study: 187 patients with an intra-abdominal abscess or peritonitis at the time of operation, 17 patients who had received preoperative antibiotherapy, and 19 patients with an inadequate prophylactic regimen.

Clinical data and follow-up were available in 3137 patients. The clinical data of the patients are listed in Table 1. The number of operations on the digestive tract, the length of operation, and the duration of the hospital stay were not different among the three groups within each stratum. In stratum 4, there were significantly more men, and the patients were significantly younger in the control than in the treated groups. In stratum 3, there were significantly more women in the control than in the cefotaxime-treated group.

The number of patients undergoing skin preparation with povidone-iodine or chlorhexidine was not different in each group of treatment, except in stratum 3 of the cefotaxime-treated group, in which significantly more patients had skin preparation with chlorhexidine (Table 2).

Postoperative Complications

In stratum 4, independent of the treatment group, the rate of infectious and noninfectious complications, as well as the mortality, were significantly higher ($P<.001$) than in strata 1, 2, and 3 (Table 3).

Parietal Infection

The incidence of wound abscesses was significantly lower in the groups receiving prophylactic antibiotherapy than in the control group ($P<.001$) (Table 4). When analysis was carried out separately in each stratum, antibioprophylaxis was effective in clean operations, with a decrease in the

Table 1.—Clinical Data per Treatment Group and Strata*

Stratum 2			Stratum 3			Stratum 4		
Control	Cefazolin	Cefotaxime	Control	Cefazolin	Cefotaxime	Control	Cefazolin	Cefotaxime
205	198	204	251	264	268	328	336	338
						$P<.001$ (Control vs Cefazolin)		
48.6±15.7	48.8±15.2	49.0±15.8	36.6±21.7	37.7±23.0	38.8±23.6	51.1±15.3	54.6±11.3	56.0±15.7
							$P<.001$ (Control vs Cefotaxime)	
						$P<.05$ (Control vs Cefazolin)		
64/141	62/136	60/144	98/153	116/148	130/138	176/152	152/184	155/183
				$P<.05$ (Control vs Cefotaxime)			$P<.05$ (Control vs Cefotaxime)	
165	144	153	221	237	246	229	245	249
1	1	0	4	4	6	12	17	11
37	45	49	9	14	10	25	30	37
6	9	7	4	4	5	11	11	7
0	2	3	15	12	8	60	41	48
101.8±52.5	99.8±48.0	105.1±50.3	80.2±81.0	79.0±78.7	78.6±70.4	123.4±90.9	123.9±86.2	114.4±68.3
15.2±10.6	21.5±44.5	23.2±64.9	17.4±35.4	20.5±48.5	17.9±35.0	26.6±55.5	24.0±40.2	24.5±50.6

*Some patients had more than one procedure during the same operation. No statistical difference has been found, unless specified.

Table 2.—Skin Preparation per Strata and Treatment Groups*

	Treatment Group, No. of Patients					
	Control		Cefazolin		Cefotaxime Sodium	
Stratum	Tincture of Chlorhexidine Gluconate	Povidone-Iodine	Tincture of Chlorhexidine Gluconate	Povidone-Iodine	Tincture of Chlorhexidine Gluconate	Povidone-Iodine
1	129	147	113	117	117	122
2	105	100	98	100	102	102
3	123	128	130	134	147	121
					$P<.05$	
4	167	161	177	159	169	169

*No statistical difference has been found, unless specified.

wound abscess rate from 4% in the untreated group to 0.4% in the treated groups. Similar results were found in strata 2 and 4. In stratum 3, there was no statistically significant difference between the treated and untreated groups, although the percentage of wound abscesses was lower in the treated groups. There was no statistically significant difference for wound abscess between the groups receiving cefazolin or cefotaxime.

Intra-abdominal Infectious Complications

The percentage of postoperative intra-abdominal infection (generalized or localized peritonitis) was twice as low in the groups receiving prophylactic antibiotics as in the control group. However, this result was statistically significant only in the cefotaxime-treated group. There was no statistical difference between the groups receiving cefazolin or cefotaxime (Table 5).

Extra-abdominal Infectious Complications

The rate of urinary tract infection was significantly lower in the cefotaxime-treated groups ($P<.02$) as compared with the cefazolin-treated group (Table 5). There was no significant difference between the control group and the treated groups.

The postoperative pulmonary infection rate was significantly lower in the group receiving cefazolin than in the control and cefotaxime-treated groups ($P<.05$). The number of septicemias was not different in the three groups.

Three hundred sixty-six patients (11.6%) were given postoperative curative antibiotherapy for an extra-abdominal or intra-abdominal infection. The patients treated by prophylactic antibiotics required significantly less postoperative antibiotherapy than the patients in the control group. There was no statistically significant difference between the groups receiving cefazolin or cefotaxime. There was no statistically significant difference between the three groups of treatment concerning the mortality. *Noninfectious complications* were not different in the three groups (Table 5).

COMMENT

Numerous studies have been carried out on antibioprophylaxis in patients undergoing surgery, but in most of them, the number of patients is too low for the study to be

Table 3.—Postoperative Complications per Stratum (Independent of Treatment Groups)*

	No. (%)			
	Stratum 1 (n=745)	Stratum 2 (n=607)	Stratum 3 (n=783)	Stratum 4 (n=1002)
Intra-abdominal and extra-abdominal infectious complications	35 (4.7)	86 (14.2)	99 (12.6)	284 (28.3)*
Noninfectious complications	22 (3)	31 (5.1)	35 (4.5)	108 (10.8)*
Mortality	1 (0.1)	3 (0.5)	13 (1.6)	53 (5.3)*

*$P<.001$, when stratum 4 is compared with each of the other strata.

Table 4.—Number of Wound Abscesses per Stratum and per Treatment Group*

	Treatment Group, No. (%)		
Stratum	Control (n=1060)	Cefazolin (n=1028)	Cefotaxime Sodium (n=1049)
		$P<.01$	
1	11 (4)	1 (0.4)	1 (0.4)
	$P<.01$		
		$P<.05$	
2	9 (4)	2 (1)	2 (1)
	$P<.05$		
3	8 (3.2)	5 (1.8)	8 (2.9)
		$P<.01$	
4	29 (8.9)	13 (3.9)	12 (3.6)
	$P<.02$		
		$P<.001$	
Total	**57** (5.4)	**21** (2)	**23** (2.2)
	$P<.001$		

*No statistically significant difference has been found, unless specified.

conclusive.[16] This prospective, randomized, controlled, multicenter study on prophylactic antibiotherapy in abdominal surgery was undertaken to evaluate the actual efficiency of cephalosporins in preventing postoperative infectious complications and to compare first- and third-generation cephalosporins on a sufficient number of patients.

Cephalosporins were selected as the antimicrobial agent because this class of antibiotics is effective against potentially pathogenic microorganisms encountered in abdominal surgery, ie, gram-positive cocci and gram-negative aerobes. The mode of administration of prophylactic antibiotherapy used in the present study relied on well-established principles: there is no need to give antibiotics before the induction of anesthesia,[17,18] and a prolonged course of treatment offers no advantages compared with a 24-hour course.[3,4]

The surgical procedures were graded in clean, clean-contaminated, and contaminated operations. We thought it was necessary to create another stratum for "at-risk" patients, whatever the type of operation. Age, diabetes, obesity, and malnutrition increase the wound abscess rate.[18,19] This stratum was individualized to obtain an even distribution of at-risk patients in each of the treatment

Table 5.—Postoperative Complications in Three Treatment Groups (Independent of Strata)*

	Treatment Group, No. (%)		
	Control (n=1060)	Cefazolin (n=1028)	Cefotaxime Sodium (n=1049)
		$P<.05$	
Generalized or localized peritonitis	21 (2)	11 (1.1)	10 (0.95)
Urinary tract infection	69 (6.5)	74 (7.2)	50 (4.7)
			$P<.02$
		$P<.05$	
Pulmonary infection	41 (3.9)	22 (2.1)	39 (3.7)
			$P<.05$
Septicemia	34 (3.2)	29 (2.8)	26 (2.5)
		$P<.001$	
Postoperative antibiotherapy	153 (14.4)	112 (10.9)	101 (9.6)
		$P<.02$	
Noninfectious complications	59 (5.6)	66 (6.4)	71 (6.8)
Mortality	23 (2.2)	29 (2.8)	18 (1.7)

*No statistically significant difference has been found, unless specified.

groups, as recommended by Solomkin et al.[20] The rate of postoperative complications (infectious and noninfectious) was significantly higher in stratum 4 compared with the other strata. This result highlights the importance of the host condition in the occurrence of postoperative complications. Within each stratum, the three groups of treatment were not significantly different with regard to the type and length of the operation and the hospital stay. The extended hospital stay in stratum 1 may result from the duration of preoperative hospitalization, with most of the preoperative investigations being performed in the hospital.

A wound abscess was chosen as the main criterion for the evaluation of antibioprophylaxis, because the occurrence of a wound abscess is usually said to be responsible for an extended hospital stay and an increase in the overall costs. The patients were followed up for at least 30 days after their discharge from the hospital to avoid overlooking a late wound abscess that could have been delayed by the use of prophylactic antibiotherapy and could have resulted in a bias in the study. The results of the study demonstrate that a first-generation cephalosporin (cefazolin) is as effective as a third-generation cephalosporin (cefotaxime) in decreasing the overall wound abscess rate, when compared with the untreated group of patients. This is in accordance with the results of the randomized trial by Jones et al,[10] who compared antibioprophylaxis with cefazolin and cefotaxime in various elective surgical procedures.

When analysis is carried out separately in each stratum, antibioprophylaxis is effective in decreasing the wound abscess rate in clean operations. Similar results are found in clean-contaminated (stratum 2) and at-risk (stratum 4) groups. In the contaminated group (stratum 3), there was no statistically significant difference between the treated and untreated groups, although the wound abscess rate was lower in the treated groups. This can be explained by the fact that stratum 3 included bowel resection and appendectomy, with both operations being contaminated by a more important proportion of anaerobes against which the cephalosporins used in the study have a modest activity.[7] If prophylactic antibiotherapy is considered for these types of operations, another antibiotic regimen should be used.[21] Antibioprophylaxis in clean surgery is strongly questioned, because the postoperative infection rate is spontaneously low and can be lowered by simple skin preparation.[18,22] In clean surgical cases, prophylactic antibiotherapy can be of benefit if the cost of antibiotics is lower than the cost of treatment of a wound abscess. In our study, there was no difference in the hospital stay of the patients, whether they received prophylactic antibiotics or not, with all the wound abscesses being treated at the outpatient department. The cost of an eight-day treatment of a wound abscess, with two dressings per day by a specialized nurse, amounts to $217. The overall cost of wound abscess treatment in the control group (57 wound abscesses for 1060 patients) amounts to approximately $12 400. The cost of prophylaxis with cefotaxime sodium in 1049 patients, with a 3-g regimen, amounts to $21 075. When the cost of treatment of the wound abscesses that occurred in this group is added up, the total cost reaches $26 000. When the same calculation is made for prophylaxis by cefazolin, the total cost is $9200. Furthermore, the patients in the control groups received significantly more postoperative antibiotherapy compared with the patients given cefazolin or cefotaxime perioperatively. The cost of postoperative antibiotherapy cannot be evaluated from the data collected in this study, but it is not unlikely that some benefit in cost can be obtained by a 24-hour course of cefazolin, even in the clean-surgery group.

The number of cases of localized or generalized postoperative peritonitis was lower in the groups receiving prophylaxis than in the control group. This is in accordance with previous reports that have shown a beneficial effect of antibioprophylaxis on postoperative intra-abdominal sepsis.[2,12] Nevertheless, although the postoperative peritonitis rate in the cefazolin- and cefotaxime-treated groups was half that of the control group, this result is statistically significant only for cefotaxime. This result must be interpreted cautiously, as statistical significance would be reached for the cefazolin-treated group with only one more patient. For this reason, the superiority of cefotaxime over cefazolin in preventing postoperative intra-abdominal sepsis is not likely.

Antibioprophylaxis has a less clear-cut effect on extra-abdominal infectious complications. The type of organisms responsible for the pulmonary and urinary tract infections are not available for all the patients, and their susceptibility to the antibiotics used for prophylaxis cannot be assessed. In our series, the mortality is similar in the three groups. This result may be related to the exclusion of patients undergoing colon surgery, for which it is well established that antibioprophylaxis decreases the mortality.[12] Up to now, there has been no evidence of the superiority of third-generation over first-generation cephalosporins.[7-10] The results of our study confirm this finding: cefazolin is as effective as cefotaxime in decreasing the postoperative wound abscess rate, and both prophylactic regimens decrease the rate of postoperative peritonitis. The present study was started in 1982 at a time when the duration of antibioprophylaxis exceeded 48 hours,[6] and its results have confirmed that a 24-hour course of antibiotics is sufficient to decrease the postoperative wound infection rate. Since our study, recent investigations have shown that a single-dose prophylactic regimen, using newer antimicrobial agents, could be all that is necessary for the prevention of wound abscesses.[10] Nevertheless, more studies on large groups of patients are required to establish the best single-dose prophylactic regimen. For this reason, in 1987, we started a study comparing a one-dose prophylaxis with ceftriaxone vs a three-dose regimen with cefazolin.

The Association de Recherche en Chirurgie includes the following coworkers in France: Bernard Fethi, MD (Sens), Jean-Louis Bernard, MD (Orléans), Jacques Chipponi, MD (Clermont-Ferrand), Bernard Descottes, MD (Limoges), Gérard Desvignes, MD (Montargis), André Elhaddad, MD (Aulnay), Jacques Emer, MD (Flers), Pierre Louis Fagniez, MD (Créteil), Abe Fingerhut, MD (Poissy), Yves Flament, MD (Colombes), Jacques Françin, MD (Quimperlé), Serge Hannoun, MD (Saint-Brieuc), Jean-Marie Hay, MD (Colombes), Henri Hennet, MD (Romorantin), Daniel Keller, MD (Strasbourg), Gérard Kohlman, MD (Corbeil), Matthias Kracht, MD (Créteil), François Lacaine, MD (Paris), Jean Noel Maillard, MD (Colombes), Christian Mathon, MD (Lyons), Philippe Oberlin, MD (Poissy), Xavier Pouget, MD (Limoges), Xavier Pouliquen, MD (Argenteuil), François Poulton, MD (Saint-Brieuc), Jean Pourcher, MD (Poissy), Michel Rodary, MD (Orsay), Nelly Rotman, MD (Créteil), François Rouffet, MD (Juvisy), Michel Sage, MD (Auxerre), Jean Louis Sicard, MD (Nice), and Christian Thomsen, MD (Créteil).

References

1. Hirschman JV, Inui TS: Antimicrobial prophylaxis: A critique of recent trials. *Rev Infect Dis* 1980;2:1-22.
2. Guglielmo BJ, Hohn DC, Koo PJ, et al: Antibiotic prophylaxis in surgical procedures: A critical analysis of the literature. *Arch Surg* 1983; 118:943-955.
3. Kaiser AB: Antimicrobial prophylaxis in surgery. *N Engl J Med* 1986;315:1129-1138.
4. Stone HH, Haney BB, Kolb LD, et al: Prophylactic and preventive antibiotic therapy: Timing, duration and economics. *Ann Surg* 1979;189: 691-699.
5. Nichols RL: Use of prophylactic antibiotics in surgical practice. *Am J Med* 1981;70:686-692.
6. Crossley K, Couch-Gardner L, and the Task Force on Prophylactic Antibiotics in Surgery: Antimicrobial prophylaxis in surgical patients. *JAMA* 1981;245:722-726.
7. Fry DE: Third-generation cephalosporin antibiotics in surgical practice. *Am J Surg* 1986;151:306-313.
8. DiPiro JT, Bowden TA, Hooks VH: Prophylactic parenteral cephalosporins in surgery: Are the newer agents better? *JAMA* 1984;252:3277-3279.
9. Scher KS, Jones CW: Which cephalosporin for wound prophylaxis? An experimental comparison of three drugs. *Surgery* 1985;98:30-33.
10. Jones RN, Wojeski W, Bakke J, et al: Antibiotic prophylaxis of 1036 patients undergoing elective surgical procedures: A prospective, randomized comparative trial of cefazolin, cefoxitin, and cefotaxime in a prepaid medical practice. *Am J Surg* 1987;153:341-346.
11. Ad Hoc Committee on Trauma, National Research Council, Division of Medical Sciences: Organization, methods, and physical factors. *Ann Surg* 1964;160(suppl):19-31.
12. Baum ML, Anish DS, Chalmers TC, et al: A survey of clinical trials of antibiotic prophylaxis in colon surgery: Evidence against further use of no-treatment controls. *N Engl J Med* 1981;305:795-799.
13. Cancer Research Campaign Working Party: Trials and tribulations: Thoughts on the organisation of multicentre clinical studies. *Br Med J Clin Res* 1980;281:918-920.
14. Ad Hoc Committee on Trauma, National Research Council, Division of Medical Sciences: Factors influencing the incidence of wound infection. *Ann Surg* 1964;160(suppl):32-81.
15. Schwartz D, Flamant R, Lellouch J: *Clinical Trials.* Orlando, Fla, Academic Press Inc, 1980, pp 96-98.
16. Evans M, Pollock AV: Trials on trial: A review of trials of antibiotic prophylaxis. *Arch Surg* 1984;119:109-113.
17. Burke JF: The effective period of preventive antibiotic action in experimental incisions and dermal lesions. *Surgery* 1961;50:161-168.
18. Cruse PJE, Foord R: A five-year prospective study of 23 649 surgical wounds. *Arch Surg* 1973;107:206-210.
19. Pruitt BA: Host-opportunist interactions in surgical infection. *Arch Surg* 1986;121:13-22.
20. Solomkin JS, Dellinger EP, Christou NV, et al: Design and conduct of antibiotic trials: A report of the Scientific Studies Committee of the Surgical Infection Society. *Arch Surg* 1987;122:158-163.
21. Greenall MJ, Bakran I, Pickford IR, et al: A double-blind trial of a single intravenous dose of metronidazole as prophylaxis against wound infection following appendicectomy. *Br J Surg* 1979;66:428-429.
22. Olson M, O'Connor M, Schwartz ML: Surgical wound infections: A five-year prospective study of 20 193 wounds at the Minneapolis VA administration medical center. *Ann Surg* 1983;199:253-259.

When patients with active peptic ulcers are also critically ill…

CONTROL THE ACID RISK

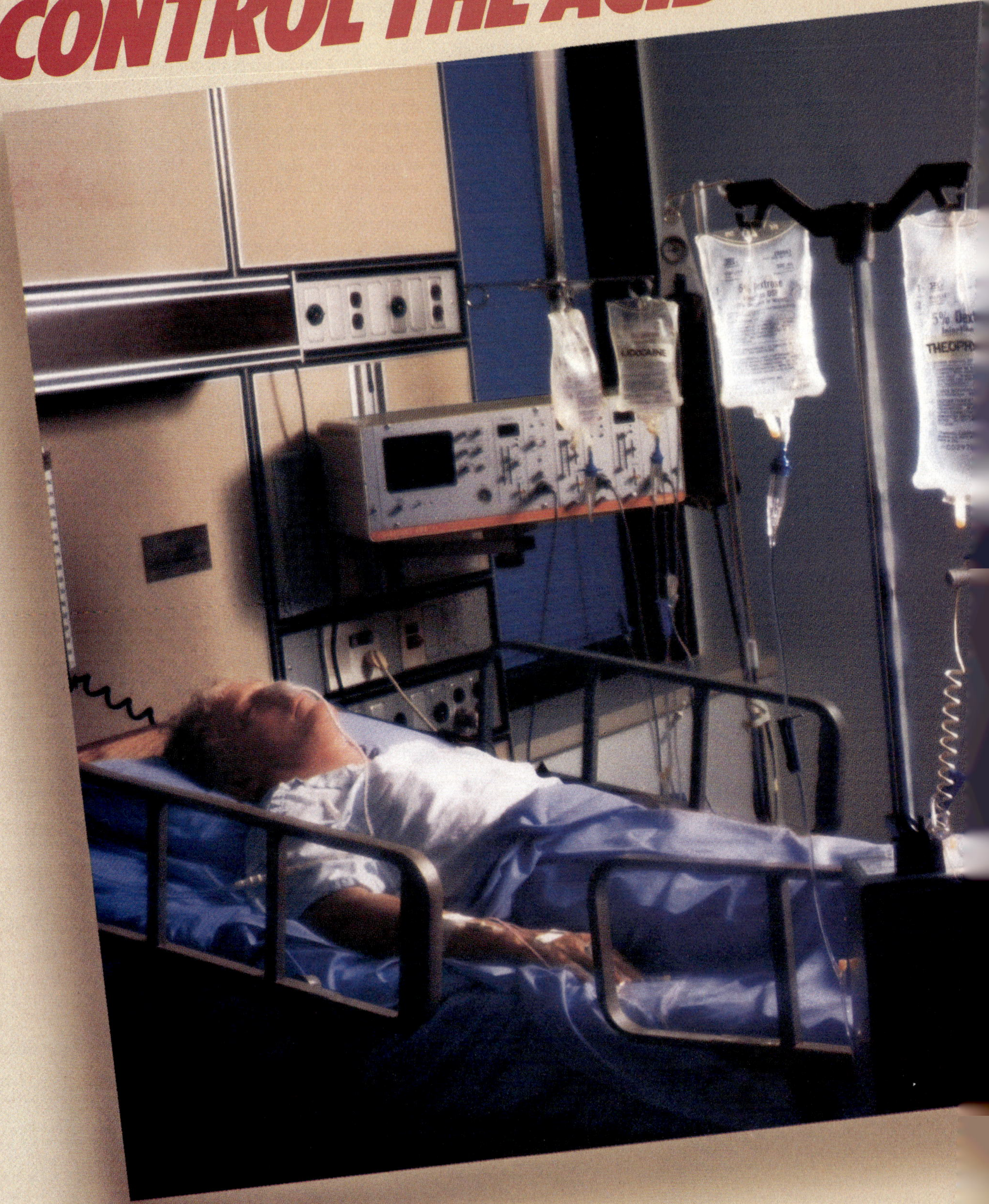

Guidelines for Practical Utilization of Intraoperative Frozen Sections

Marianne U. Prey, MD; Thomas Vitale, MD; Scott A. Martin, MD

• We reviewed 4057 intraoperative frozen sections from 1980 through 1984 to assess the accuracy, strengths, and weaknesses of this technique. Breast, lymph node, and skin comprised half of the sites evaluated. Frozen-section and final diagnoses agreed in 91.5% and disagreed in 6.8% of the cases; 1.7% of the cases were deferred. False-negative frozen-section diagnoses were due to pathologist sampling or judgment errors and surgeon sampling errors. There were eight (0.15%) false-positive diagnoses, none of which altered patient treatment. We recommend that lymph nodes for lymphoproliferative disorders and breast tissue for which a malignant diagnosis will not result in an immediate mastectomy not be submitted for frozen-section diagnosis. Appropriate studies of these tissues can be carried out without an intraoperative diagnosis; such a policy will increase the cost-effectiveness of frozen sections without compromising patient care.

(*Arch Surg* 1989;124:331-335)

The technique of freezing tissue to cut slices thin enough to be interpreted by light microscopy has been used for over 100 years.[1] Technological advances have simplified the process, making the frozen section rapid interpretation a readily available procedure. This ease, however, should not justify the performance of the procedure. From numerous reports of frozen-section data in the literature, it is widely asserted that the only reasonable request for an intraoperative frozen section is to obtain a diagnosis that will direct the course of surgery or affect immediate (within 24 hours) postoperative patient care.[2-5] Notwithstanding these reports, it is our opinion that some frozen sections continue to be requested even when the results will not influence the immediate management of the patient.

The purpose of this study was twofold. First, we assessed the accuracy of frozen-section diagnoses and identified strengths and weaknesses with this technique. Second, we analyzed the patterns of frozen-section utilization by tissue site to establish practical guidelines for the use of the intraoperative frozen section.

Accepted for publication Dec 18, 1987.

From the Departments of Pathology, St Louis University (Dr Prey) and St John's Mercy Medical Center (Drs Prey and Martin), St Louis; and the Department of Surgery, Holmes Regional Medical Center, Melbourne, Fla (Dr Vitale). Dr Prey is now with SmithKlein Bio-Science Laboratories, St Louis.

Reprints not available.

As additional ancillary techniques for tissue study become more numerous and complex, the allocation and handling of specimens by the pathologist for diagnostic procedures is critical. It is necessary, therefore, that the pathologist and the surgeon be fully aware of the limitations of intraoperative frozen sections so that the procedure is used only judiciously and that specimens are not wasted, particularly when they are of limited size or volume.

MATERIALS AND METHODS

Surgical pathology accessions at St John's Mercy Medical Center, St Louis, that included intraoperative frozen-section consultations during a five-year period from 1980 through 1984 were reviewed. The final pathology reports from 4057 cases provided the database for this report. Frozen-section diagnoses that were stated in the reports were classified as benign, malignant, or deferred and were then compared with the final diagnoses in the reports. Actual histologic sections were not reviewed, since one of the objectives of the study was to assess the accuracy of our reported intraoperative frozen-section diagnoses. An audit of the accuracy of our final diagnoses was not an objective. In the absence of a deferral, the intraoperative diagnosis either agreed or disagreed with the final diagnosis. When there was disagreement, the reviewers (M.U.P. and S.A.M.) classified the frozen-section diagnosis as false positive, false negative, or other diagnostic discrepancy.

Designation of a false-positive result required an erroneous malignant frozen-section diagnosis and a benign final interpretation of the same specimen. Designation of a false-negative result required an erroneous benign frozen-section diagnosis and a malignant final diagnosis. The "other" category was employed when the frozen-section diagnosis differed from the final diagnosis but the discrepancy was neither a false-positive nor a false-negative result. For example, an ovarian carcinoma diagnosed as papillary serous cystadenocarcinoma by frozen section and as endometrioid carcinoma in the final diagnosis would be classified under other diagnostic discrepancy.

Additional information was recorded about the frozen-section diagnosis. Benign diagnoses were further categorized as follows: (1) no pathologic diagnosis or diagnostic tissue received, (2) inflammatory or reactive process, (3) hyperplastic or proliferative process, (4) hamartoma or malformation, (5) benign neoplasm, or (6) nondiagnostic specimen. Similarly, malignant diagnoses were further designated as carcinoma, sarcoma, melanoma, lymphoma or lymphoproliferative, glial neoplasm, or malignant neoplasm, final diagnosis deferred.

Factors contributing to a discrepancy between frozen-section interpretation and final diagnosis were classified as follows: (1)

Table 1.—Distribution of Total, Benign, Malignant, and Deferred Frozen-Section Diagnosis by Tissue Site

Site	Total, No. (%)	Benign, No. (%)	Malignant, No. (%)	Deferred, No. (%)
Breast	**1262** (23.0)	844 (66.9)	404 (32.0)	14 (1.1)
Lymph node	**724** (13.2)	515 (71.1)	185 (25.6)	24 (3.3)
Skin	**689** (12.5)	495 (71.8)	187 (27.1)	7 (1.0)
Soft tissues	**369** (6.7)	205 (55.6)	149 (40.4)	15 (4.1)
Endometrium	**322** (5.9)	314 (97.5)	6 (1.9)	2 (0.6)
Thyroid gland	**300** (5.5)	273 (91.0)	20 (6.7)	7 (2.3)
Ovary	**282** (5.9)	234 (83.0)	48 (17.0)	0 (0)
Lung	**260** (4.7)	148 (56.9)	105 (40.4)	7 (2.7)
Nervous system	**213** (3.9)	136 (63.8)	73 (34.3)	4 (1.9)
Colon, rectum, and anus	**136** (2.5)	88 (64.7)	46 (33.8)	2 (1.5)
Parathyroid gland	**120** (2.2)	120 (100.0)	0 (0)	0 (0)
Pancreas, gallbladder, and biliary tract	**101** (1.8)	57 (56.4)	42 (41.6)	2 (2.0)
Lip, tongue, mouth, and pharynx	**87** (1.8)	56 (64.4)	28 (32.2)	3 (3.4)
Liver	**80** (1.5)	26 (32.5)	54 (67.5)	0 (0)
Stomach and esophagus	**74** (1.3)	51 (68.9)	22 (29.7)	1 (1.4)
Uterine cervix	**545** (1.0)	40 (74.1)	14 (25.9)	0 (0)
Salivary gland	**51** (0.9)	45 (88.2)	6 (11.8)	0 (0)
Small intestine	**47** (0.9)	34 (72.3)	13 (27.7)	0 (0)
Bone and joint	**45** (0.8)	29 (64.4)	13 (28.9)	3 (6.7)
Prostate	**44** (0.8)	19 (43.2)	24 (54.4)	1 (2.3)
Kidney	**24** (0.4)	11 (45.8)	13 (54.2)	0 (0)
Pleura	**21** (0.4)	14 (66.7)	7 (33.3)	0 (0)
Larynx	**21** (0.4)	12 (57.1)	8 (38.1)	1 (4.8)
Nose, nasopharynx, and paranasal sinus	**12** (0.2)	9 (75.0)	2 (16.7)	1 (8.3)
Spleen	**6** (0.1)	4 (66.7)	2 (33.3)	0 (0)
Eye and orbit	3 (0.1)	3 (100.0)	0 (0)	0 (0)
Vagina	**2** (<0.1)	2 (100.0)	0 (0)	0 (0)
All other sites	**144** (2.6)	106 (73.6)	35 (24.3)	2 (1.4)
Total	**5493 (100)**	**3890** (70.8)	**1506** (27.4)	**96** (1.7)

sampling error by the pathologist, (2) sampling error by the surgeon, (3) judgment error by the pathologist, and (4) other.

A sampling error by the pathologist occurred when the lesion was present in the tissue received intraoperatively but was either not specifically selected by the pathologist for frozen section or not observed in the actual frozen-section slides. In the latter case, diagnostic tissue was subsequently detected in deeper sections from the same frozen-section tissue block. A sampling error by the surgeon resulted when the tissue submitted intraoperatively for consultation was not diagnostic, but subsequently submitted tissue from the same site for permanent section evaluation did contain the lesion of interest. A judgment error by the pathologist occurred when the surgical pathology report stated that the diagnostic pathologic process was present in the frozen-section slides examined but was not interpreted correctly during the intraoperative consultation.

Information derived from a review of the pathology reports was encoded for computer-assisted sorting and retrieval. The two-digit Systematized Nomenclature of Medicine system was used for tissue site classification. Some closely related tissue sites were grouped together for convenience.

RESULTS

A total of 70 834 cases were accessioned in the surgical pathology files from 1980 through 1984 at St John's Mercy Medical Center. Of these cases, 4057 (5.7%) had intraoperative frozen sections performed. Many cases required evaluation of more than one tissue block, resulting in a total of 5493 frozen sections that were actually performed.

Table 1 summarizes the distribution of frozen sections by tissue site. Breast, lymph node, and skin account for almost half (48.7%) of the cases. Some individual sites were grouped for convenience; for example, the nervous system included the brain, meninges, pituitary gland, and pineal, spinal, and cranial nerves. In other instances, the grouping was chosen on the basis of the anatomic proximity or histologic similarity of sites in which pathologic processes often obscured certainty of specific site identification. All other sites included those that individually had few frozen sections and neither false-positive nor false-negative diagnoses.

The numbers of benign, malignant, and deferred diagnoses are also given in Table 1. The number of benign frozen-section diagnoses were more often greater than the number of malignant diagnoses except for the liver, in which two thirds of the frozen-section diagnoses were malignant.

The results of the comparison of the frozen-section interpretations with the final pathologic diagnoses are given in Table 2. There was absolute agreement in 5024 (91.5%) of all the sections examined. Frozen-section and final diagnoses disagreed in 373 (6.8%) of the cases. The 96 (1.7%) frozen-section diagnoses that were deferred for permanent sections were excluded from this analysis.

The distribution of the diagnostic discrepancies into false-positive and false-negative categories is given in Table

Table 2.—Comparison of Frozen-Section Interpretations With Final Diagnoses

Site	Agree, No. (%)	Disagree, No. (%)
Breast	1197 (94.8)	51 (4.0)
Lymph node	651 (89.9)	49 (6.8)
Skin	640 (92.9)	42 (6.1)
Soft tissues	331 (89.7)	23 (6.2)
Endometrium	296 (91.9)	24 (7.5)
Thyroid gland	265 (88.3)	28 (9.3)
Ovary	257 (91.1)	25 (8.9)
Lung	237 (91.2)	16 (6.2)
Nervous system	190 (89.2)	19 (8.9)
Colon, rectum, and anus	122 (89.7)	12 (8.8)
Parathyroid gland	108 (90.0)	12 (10.0)
Pancreas, gallbladder, and biliary tract	80 (79.2)	19 (18.8)
Mouth, lip, tongue, and pharynx	78 (89.7)	6 (6.9)
Liver	79 (98.8)	1 (1.3)
Stomach and esophagus	69 (93.2)	4 (5.4)
Uterine cervix	51 (94.4)	3 (5.6)
Salivary gland	48 (94.1)	3 (5.9)
Small intestine	44 (93.6)	3 (6.4)
Bone and joint	35 (77.8)	7 (15.6)
Prostate	36 (81.8)	7 (15.9)
Kidney	23 (95.8)	1 (4.2)
Pleura	17 (81.0)	4 (19.0)
Larynx	18 (85.7)	2 (9.5)
Nose, nasopharynx, and paranasal sinus	9 (75.0)	2 (16.7)
Spleen	4 (66.7)	2 (33.3)
Eye and orbit	2 (66.7)	1 (33.3)
Vagina	0 (0)	2 (100.0)
All other sites	137 (95.1)	5 (3.5)
Total	**5024** (91.5)	**373** (6.8)

Table 3.—Categorization of Diagnostic Discrepancies

Site	False-positive Diagnoses, No. (%)	False-negative Diagnoses, No. (%)
Breast	0 (0)	15 (1.2)
Lymph node	2 (0.3)	29 (4.0)
Skin	1 (0.1)	31 (4.5)
Soft tissues	0 (0)	4 (1.1)
Endometrium	0 (0)	0 (0)
Thyroid gland	0 (0)	8 (2.7)
Ovary	1 (0.4)	6 (2.1)
Lung	1 (0.4)	3 (1.2)
Nervous system	0 (0)	7 (3.3)
Colon, rectum, and anus	0 (0)	7 (5.1)
Parathyroid gland	0 (0)	0 (0)
Pancreas, gallbladder, and biliary tract	0 (0)	18 (17.8)
Mouth, lip, tongue, and pharynx	0 (0)	2 (2.3)
Liver	0 (0)	1 (1.3)
Stomach and esophagus	2 (2.7)	2 (2.7)
Uterine cervix	0 (0)	1 (1.9)
Salivary gland	0 (0)	2 (3.9)
Small intestine	0 (0)	0 (0)
Bone and joint	0 (0)	5 (11.1)
Prostate	0 (0)	4 (9.1)
Kidney	0 (0)	1 (4.2)
Pleura	0 (0)	3 (14.3)
Larynx	0 (0)	2 (9.5)
Nose, nasopharynx, and paranasal sinus	1 (8.3)	0 (0)
Spleen	0 (0)	1 (16.7)
Eye and orbit	0 (0)	1 (33.3)
Vagina	0 (0)	1 (50.0)
All other sites	0 (0)	0 (0)
Total	**8** (0.1)	**154** (2.8)

3. Most discrepancies represented minor, insignificant differences in interpretation. Less than half of the cases in which the frozen-section and final diagnoses disagreed were classified as false negative or false positive. False-negative diagnoses were more common for lesions of the lymph node, skin, colorectum, pancreas, and sites that were infrequently evaluated.

The types of error resulting in false-negative frozen-section diagnoses are enumerated in Table 4. Overall, most of the errors (42%) were due to the pathologist's sampling of the specimen. The pathologist's judgment accounted for 40% of the false-negative interpretations. Finally, the surgeon's sampling of tissue was responsible for 18% of the false-negative errors. The sites most prone to sampling problems for the surgeon were the pancreas, bone, joint, and prostate. The pathologist had greatest difficulty in selecting the diagnostic tissue for the frozen-section examination when dealing with sites such as the breast, ovary (especially when large and cystic), lung, and colon. Skin lesions were prone to sampling errors mainly due to the focal positivity of surgical margins.

Of 5493 total frozen sections, there were only eight false-positive diagnoses (0.15%). Table 5 lists the sites of false-positive frozen sections. All but one of these diagnoses were due to judgment errors by pathologists. The single exception resulted from contamination of a lymph node specimen by tissue adherent to the cold probe in the cryostat from a prior case. The other false-positive lymph node diagnosis was due to misinterpretation of a hilar lymph node with anthracotic carbon deposition as metastatic carcinoma. This lymph node accompanied a pneumonectomy specimen that contained squamous cell carcinoma. The one false-positive frozen section of skin was the result of interpretation of actinic keratosis as squamous cell carcinoma in situ. This lesion was at the surgical margin of a specimen that contained a basal cell carcinoma. Further marginal excision was not carried out in this case. An ovarian tumor diagnosed as a borderline mucinous tumor on frozen section was judged to be a mucinous cystadenoma after examining permanent sections. No additional surgery was performed on the basis of the frozen-section diagnosis. A case of organizing pneumonia was misdiagnosed as alveolar carcinoma. The tissue initially submitted for this intraoperative consultation was a specimen obtained by lobectomy. Additional surgery included only a pleural biopsy. There was one case of gastric lymphoid hyperplasia ("pseudolymphoma") associated with ulcer, which was thought to be malignant lymphoma at the time of frozen section. The operative procedure in this case was a subtotal gastrectomy for antral ulcers. A

Table 4.—Summary of Errors Resulting in False-negative Frozen-Section Interpretations

Site	Sampling Error by Pathologist, No. (%)	Sampling Error by Surgeon, No. (%)	Judgment Error, No. (%)
Breast	9 (60.0)	3 (20.0)	3 (20.0)
Lymph node	9 (31.0)	0 (0)	20 (69.0)
Skin	24 (77.4)	4 (12.9)	3 (9.7)
Soft tissues	2 (50.0)	0 (0)	2 (50.0)
Thyroid gland	3 (37.5)	1 (12.5)	3 (37.5)
Ovary	4 (66.7)	0 (0)	2 (33.3)
Lung	2 (66.7)	1 (33.3)	0 (0)
Nervous system	0 (0)	2 (28.6)	5 (71.4)
Colon, rectum, and anus	5 (71.4)	0 (0)	2 (28.6)
Pancreas, gallbladder, and biliary tract	2 (11.1)	8 (44.4)	8 (44.4)
Mouth, lip, tongue, and pharynx	1 (50.0)	0 (0)	1 (50.0)
Liver	0 (0)	0 (0)	1 (100.0)
Stomach and esophagus	1 (50.0)	0 (0)	1 (50.0)
Uterine cervix	0 (0)	0 (0)	1 (100.0)
Salivary gland	1 (50.0)	0 (0)	1 (50.0)
Bone and joint	0 (0)	5 (100.0)	0 (0)
Prostate	1 (25.0)	2 (50.0)	1 (25.0)
Kidney	0 (0)	0 (0)	1 (100.0)
Pleura	1 (33.3)	0 (0)	2 (66.7)
Larynx	0 (0)	0 (0)	2 (100.0)
Spleen	0 (0)	1 (100.0)	0 (0)
Eye and orbit	0 (0)	0 (0)	1 (100.0)
Vagina	0 (0)	0 (0)	1 (100.0)
Total	**65** (42.2)	**27** (17.5)	**61** (39.6)

case of pseudoepitheliomatous hyperplasia of the esophagus was diagnosed with frozen section as squamous cell carcinoma. This diagnosis was rendered on the proximal margin of a partial esophagectomy specimen that was removed for squamous cell carcinoma. An additional 1.5-cm portion of esophagus was resected based on this intraoperative diagnosis. Last, a nasal specimen diagnosed as papilloma with focal squamous cell carcinoma in situ intraoperatively was actually an inverted papilloma. Tissue was resected from the nasal cavity, ethmoid sinus, and maxillary sinus in this procedure, and all sites contained inverted papilloma.

COMMENT

The false-positive and false-negative rates, 0.15% and 2.8%, respectively, of our five-year frozen-section audit were below most of the rates previously published.[2,6-8] The overall utilization rate of 5.7% was also in keeping with the recommended rate of 10% or less.[3] The distribution of cases according to tissue site was comparable with other reports in that most of our frozen sections were performed on breast, lymph node, and skin.[4,5,8] The large number of breast and skin frozen sections can be expected, since these two tissue sites together account for 30% of the cases of cancer per year.[9]

Examination of the surgical margins of cutaneous lesions is a necessary intraoperative procedure when surgical cure is to be accomplished with a single visit to the operating room. Similarly, the presence of metastatic tumor in lymph nodes is vital information for most surgical procedures for cancer. Detection of metastases may determine the placement of clips for marking irradiation portals and may influence the extent of surgical procedures.

Table 5.—False-positive Frozen-Section Diagnoses

Site	Total, No. (%)	Judgment Error, No. (%)
Lymph node	2 (0.3)	1 (50.0)
Skin	1 (0.1)	1 (100.0)
Ovary	1 (0.4)	1 (100.0)
Lung	1 (0.4)	1 (100.0)
Stomach and esophagus	2 (2.7)	2 (100.0)
Nose, nasopharynx, and paranasal sinus	1 (8.3)	1 (100.0)
Total	**8** (0.1)	**7** (87.5)

We believe that the distinction between a benign and malignant lymphoproliferative process is not appropriate at the time of frozen section. Diagnostic difficulties encountered with lymph nodes not altered by metastatic carcinoma or easily recognized infectious processes have been emphasized by other authors.[5,10] In such instances, the pathologist's role should be to determine whether adequate material has been sampled to permit accurate diagnosis on evaluation of properly fixed sections with optimal cytologic presentation.

We anticipated a decrease in the proportion of intraoperative frozen sections performed on breast tissue in comparison with previously published reports,[2,4,5,7,10] since the approach to the patient with breast disease has changed. It is now uncommon, at least in our institution, for patients to undergo a mastectomy following a frozen-section diagnosis of carcinoma from an incisional biopsy during the same anesthesia. Rather, most of our patients with breast lesions initially have an excisional biopsy on an outpatient basis. Further surgery, if required, is done at a later date following discussion of the results of the final pathology report with the patient. Before definitive surgery, alternative methods of management are also considered by the patient and surgeon. The final pathology report of the excisional biopsy specimen is usually available within 24 hours; when surgery is performed on Saturday, the report is available on Monday. Despite these practices, frozen sections are still routinely and unnecessarily requested on breast tissue. The opportunity to obtain fresh tissue for estrogen and progesterone receptors is not missed if a frozen section is not requested. In actual practice, all breast tissue received in our laboratory is examined in the fresh state. Our specimens are transported by way of a mechanical transport system, with a transit time of three minutes from the operating room to the gross pathology laboratory. The pathologist is notified when a breast biopsy specimen is received, and the pathologist then decides whether it is necessary to reserve tissue for hormone receptor analysis. Many breast cancers are grossly obvious and do not require microscopic confirmation. In instances of uncertainty, sufficient tissue for hormone receptor analysis is reserved at −70°C until permanent sections of grossly similar tissue adjacent to the reserved tissue are evaluated. This protocol has eliminated freezing artifact of lesions that are difficult to interpret. The tissue reserved for receptor analysis can be thawed and examined histologically when a diagnosis remains equivocal.

Frozen-section evaluation of breast lesions, therefore, can be an unnecessary expense that may actually hinder the pathologist from rendering an accurate diagnosis. This is especially true when the quantity of tissue is limited. In addition, every frozen section has a small chance of giving a false-negative diagnosis. With this in mind, frozen-section diagnoses rendered for breast lesions that are clinically or mammographically suspicious are accompanied by a word of caution. No breast lesion can be considered completely benign until the entire specimen has been examined by permanent sections. It seems unnecessary, therefore, to jeopardize an accurate diagnosis and subject the patient to a potential false-negative diagnosis when immediate care will not be affected.

In situations where the lesion is small and cannot be divided for histologic examination and special studies, cytologic preparations are helpful and often diagnostic.[11,12] Either touch preparations or smears of cells exfoliated from the cut surface of the specimen can be used for intraoperative diagnosis, thus sparing the solid tissue for hormone receptor analysis in the case of specimens of breast cancer. In other instances, this same approach is useful to triage tissue for microbiologic culture, special fixatives, procurement for immunocytochemistry, electron microscopy, or whatever is deemed necessary to arrive at a correct final diagnosis.

Another consideration, as addressed by Kindschi,[3] is one of simple economics. Current procedural terminology[13] identifies the activity of intraoperative consultation, intraoperative consultation with frozen section, and performance of each additional frozen section as codes 88329, 88331, and 88332, respectively. The pathologist's professional fees and institutional technical charges associated with these codes will vary. They may add appreciably to patient costs, particularly when multiple frozen sections are required.

The information derived from review of our frozen-section cases agreed with previous similar studies. When confronted with difficult diagnostic decisions, pathologists tend to be appropriately conservative. Our review showed that false-positive diagnoses did not result in excessive additional surgery.

We propose that the most practical and effective use of frozen section will occur in the circumstances in which the surgeon views the pathologist as a consultant and the pathologist is sensitive to the needs of the surgeon. When the pathologist is appropriately informed of pertinent historical information, the therapeutic considerations, and intraoperative findings, an optimal utilization of tissue for accurate diagnosis can be achieved. When a request for an intraoperative frozen section diagnosis is appropriate, the surgeon can be assured that the diagnosis rendered is accurate.

Susie Oberlander prepared the manuscript, Scott W. Prey, MS, provided computer expertise, and B. Balfour Kraemer, MD, and Frederick T. Kraus, MD, provided editorial advice.

References

1. Wright JR: The development of the frozen section technique, the evolution of surgical biopsy, and the origins of surgical pathology. *Bull Hist Med* 1985;59:295-326.
2. Dehner LP, Rosai J: Frozen section examination in surgical pathology. *Minn Med* 1977;60:83-94.
3. Kindschi FW: Frozen sections their use and abuse. *JAMA* 1984;251:2559-2560.
4. Ackerman LV, Ramirez GA: The indications for and limitations of frozen section diagnosis. *Br J Surg* 1959;46:336-350.
5. Saltzstein SL, Nahum AM: Frozen section diagnosis: Accuracy and errors; uses and abuses. *Laryngoscope* 1973;83:1128-1143.
6. Dahlin DC: Seventy-five year experience with frozen sections at the Mayo Clinic. *Mayo Clin Proc* 1980;55:721-723.
7. Holaday WJ, Assor D: Ten thousand consecutive frozen sections. *Am J Clin Pathol* 1974;61:769-777.
8. Kaufman Z, Lew S, Griffel B, et al: Frozen-section diagnosis in surgical pathology. *Cancer* 1986;57:377-379.
9. Silverberg E, Lubera J: Cancer statistics, 1987. *CA* 1987;37:2-19.
10. Nakazawa H, Rosen P, Lane N, et al: Frozen section experience in 3000 cases. *Am J Clin Pathol* 1968;49:4151.
11. Silva EG, Kraemer BB: Preparing and evaluating frozen tissue sections, in *Techniques and Cytology in Intraoperative Pathologic Diagnosis: Frozen Section and Other Techniques.* Baltimore, Williams & Wilkins, 1987.
12. Godwin JT: Rapid cytologic diagnosis of surgical specimens. *Acta Cytol* 1976;20:111-115.
13. Fanta CM, Finkel AJ, Kirschner CG, et al: *Physicians' Current Procedural Terminology,* ed 4. Chicago, American Medical Association, 1987.

Editorial Comment

The study by Prey et al in the accompanying article reconfirms the accuracy of frozen-section diagnosis done in a qualified institution. Of the 0.15% false-positive diagnoses, none involved breast samples, which made up 23% of the sample, and none affected the surgical care of the patients. Frozen section in 1988 is an accurate diagnostic technique on which sound surgical judgment can be made intraoperatively.

The popularity of the two-stage mastectomy, as described by the authors, may be less now than in the recent past. In my practice, more and more women are requesting a breast biopsy and definitive treatment as a single procedure. The patient enters the hospital as an outpatient for the breast biopsy and, if the frozen section gives abnormal results, at that time undergoes the indicated oncologic procedure. Certainly efficient use of medical resources is better served by this process.

Frozen section should be used when the knowledge gained is necessary to direct intraoperative management, such as adequate margins of resection, adequate sampling of lesions that require an operative approach to gain access, and appropriate pathologic study of the fresh tissue. Otherwise, frozen section is not often necessary and should not jeopardize the ability to determine permanent section diagnosis, unless the knowledge gained is critical to immediate surgical care.

Edward M. Copeland III, MD
Gainesville, Fla

DEFINING A NEW STANDA

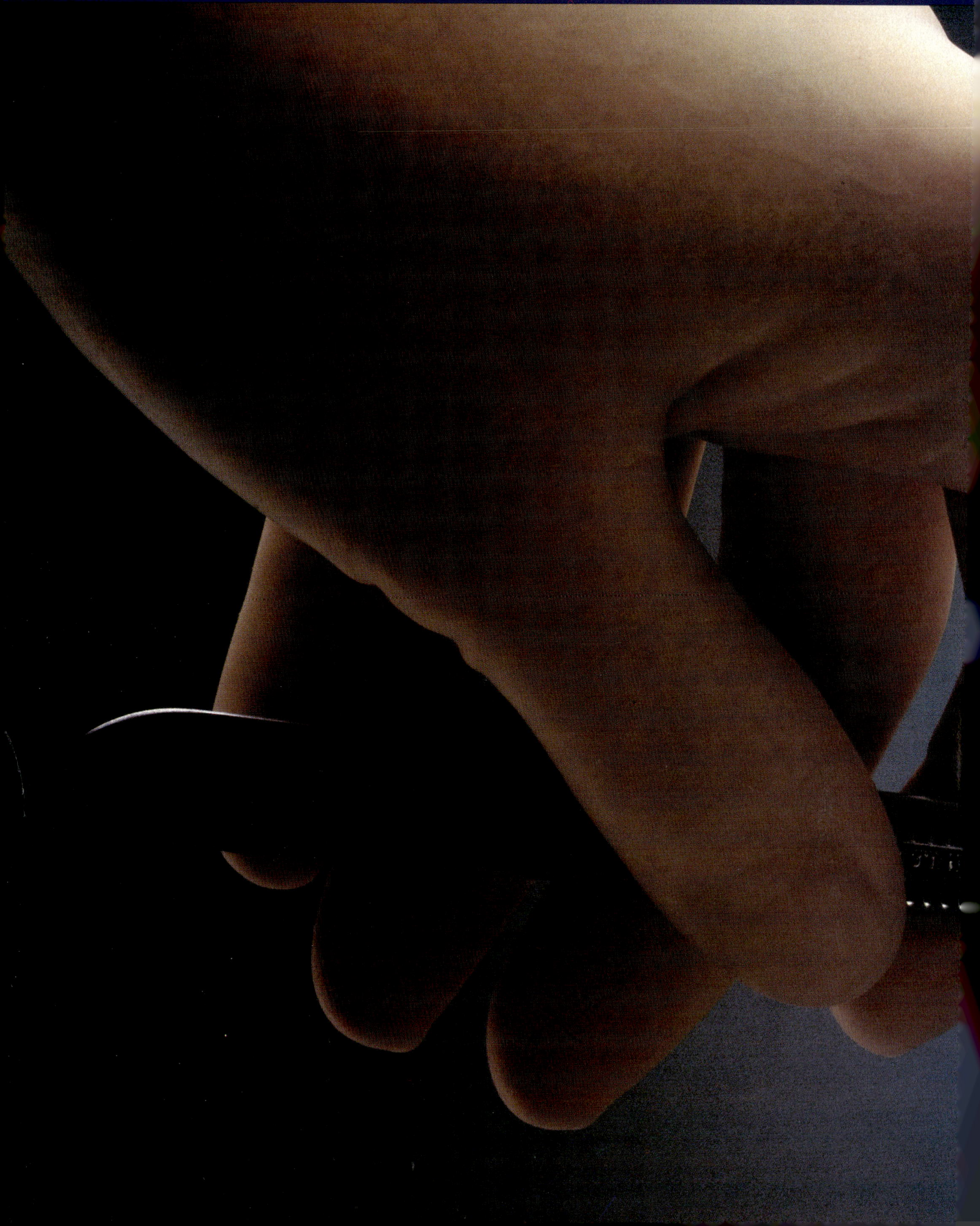

Comparison of Antibody Response With Delayed Hypersensitivity in Severely Injured Patients

Michael J. Hershman, FRCS; William G. Cheadle, MD; Sarah H. Appel; Christopher D. George, FRCS; Pattie F. Davidson, RN; Karen M. Cost, PhD; Hiram C. Polk, Jr, MD

• Twenty-seven severely injured patients had antibody response to gram-negative organisms measured of whom 25 also had skin testing. Twenty-three patients (92%) were anergic at admission. Injury Severity Scores were greater in patients who remained anergic for three weeks compared with patients whose skin tests became positive. Patients with major infection had longer anergy duration than uninfected patients. Twenty-two (81%) of 27 anergic patients mounted antibody responses. Initial bacterial contamination determined the clinical outcome and antibody response. Six of eight patients with moderate contamination mounted IgM responses to all organisms and/or an IgG response to *Escherichia coli*, and they remained uninfected. Of the other two patients, one died, and the other developed chronic infection. Seven of eight patients with heavy contamination developed major sepsis despite mounting several antibody responses. Six patients without contamination mounted no antibody responses and remained uninfected.

(*Arch Surg* 1989;124:339-341)

Trauma is the most common cause of death in patients under 35 years of age and the fourth leading cause among all age groups.[1] Despite advances in surgical techniques and antimicrobial therapy, infection remains the major cause of late death following trauma.[2] Inability to eradicate sepsis has turned the surgeon's attention to host-defense mechanisms, and these studies have shown that components of both cell-mediated and humoral immunity systems are affected by trauma.[3]

Cell-mediated immunity may be assessed clinically by using delayed-type hypersensitivity of skin to recall test antigens, and anergy has been associated with both trauma and sepsis.[4,5] Cost et al[6] have previously described a modification of the enzyme-linked immunosorbent assay (ELISA) technique that can be used clinically to detect antibody against whole bacterial organisms. We have previously shown that antibody responses to *Staphylococcus aureus* have correlated well with clinical infection due to this organism and subsequent recovery.[7] The ELISA technique has now been applied to two additional organisms that are representative of those recovered in clinical gram-negative infection, *Escherichia coli* and *Pseudomonas aeruginosa*. These bacteria are common pathogens that affect patients with trauma, and the strains used were isolated from our surgical intensive care unit. This study aimed to define further the role of anergy following trauma and to determine whether trauma and anergy are associated with an inability to mount specific antibody responses to these particular gram-negative organisms. We also aimed to assess serially the gram-negative antibody responses in patients with severe trauma in an attempt to define healthy responses better.

Accepted for publication March 15, 1988.

From the Price Institute of Surgical Research, Department of Surgery, University of Louisville School of Medicine.

Reprint requests to Department of Surgery, University of Louisville, Louisville, KY 40292 (Dr Polk).

PATIENTS AND METHODS

Twenty-seven consecutive patients who were admitted to Humana Hospital University, Louisville, and who sustained major trauma that resulted in an Injury Severity Score (ISS) of at least 20, were studied. Patients with a medical history of myocardial infarction, organ failure, neoplastic disease, or current immunosuppressive therapy (steroids or cytotoxic drugs) were excluded. Patients who were transferred from other centers after initial stabilization were accepted; however, those patients who were transferred after prolonged care were excluded. Informed consent was obtained from the patient or relatives in all cases. There were 13 patients who sustained blunt trauma, 12 who sustained penetrating trauma, and two who had major burns.

To allow more meaningful comparisons between equivalent injuries in patients of different ages, the concept of expressing the ISS as a percentage of the 50% lethal dose of injury for age was used.[8,9] Using a probit fit of burn mortality, Bull[8] developed LD_{50} values for three separate age ranges. Individual percentage of these LD_{50} values were calculated by dividing the ISS for each patient by the appropriate LD_{50} for age and expressed as a percentage ($\%LD_{50}$). Contamination that was present at the time of admission or surgery was graded: massive soft-tissue contamination or large-bowel spillage (2+); minor soft-tissue, intrathoracic, or abdominal contamination (1+); or no contamination (0).

Infectious events in these patients were classified into major and minor groups by usual clinical criteria. Major events included every example of bacteremia, all of which were associated with definable clinical problems, major wound infection, intra-abdominal or other serous cavity abscess, and any situation in which reoperation for suspected infection was undertaken. Minor events included urinary tract infections and minor wound sepsis. Some positive cultures of pathogenic bacteria from orifices or sites that were unassociated with any sign of clinical sepsis were reported but not classified as an infectious event. Infections were categorized as "early," that is, occurring within the first week following trauma, or "late," occurring after the first week.

Venous blood samples were obtained for immunological studies from each patient within 24 hours of admission and at weekly intervals during their hospital course or until a positive skin test was elicited. The three recall antigens used were *Candida albicans* (Center Laboratories, New York), tuberculin purified protein derivative (Aplisol, Parke-Davis, Morris Plains, NJ), and *Trichophyton* (Berkeley Biological, Berkeley, Calif). Intradermal injections of 0.1 mL of each antigen were administered and read by the same person 24, 48, and 72 hours later. A skin test was considered positive if the diameter of induration was greater than 5 mm for *Candida* and *Trichophyton*, and greater than 10 mm for tuberculin purified protein derivative. Patients were classified as normal if they demonstrated a positive response to any one of the recall antigens. Patients with no positive responses were classified as anergic.

The IgG and IgM antibodies to one strain of *E coli* and three strains of *P aeruginosa* (0 serotypes: M, E, and EG) were detected with the use of an ELISA technique. In the development of the ELISA technique, we had shown that both IgG and IgM responses to several strains of *E coli* were quantitatively very similar; therefore, strain O*;K*:NM was considered to be representative of the entire *E coli* species. Antibody response to various *Pseudomonas* strains were more variable; thus, three strains of this organism were used.[6] These organisms were clinical isolates from our surgical intensive care unit. The ELISA procedure that was

Patient	ISS	$\%LD_{50}$	Major Infection†	Early ELISA Response‡: IgG to *Escherichia coli*	Early ELISA Response‡: PAN IgM	Anergy Duration, d§
Patients With No Contamination						
1	33	83	None	−	−	+13
2	25	63	None	−	−	+0
3	41	103	None	−	−	>22
4‖	41	141	Early and late	−	−	+28
5	50	125	None	−	−	+42
6	29	73	None	−	−	>9
7	41	103	None	−	−	+35
8	34	85	None	+	−	+14
9	50	125	Late	+	−	+0
10	47	103	Early	−	+	>48
11	24	60	Early	+	+	>11
Patients With Moderate Contamination (1+)¶						
12‖	43	108	Early	−	−	>20
13	34	85	Early and late	−	−	+15
14	34	85	Late	+	−	+25
15	42	105	None	+	−	>10
16	41	141	None	+	−	>39
17	50	125	None	−	+	>11
18	25	86	None	−	+	>11
19	34	85	None	+	+	>15
Patients With Severe Contamination (2+)¶						
20‖	50	125	Early and late	−	−	>16
21‖	50	125	None	−	−	...
22	29	73	Early and late	−	−	+12
23	35	88	Early and late	−	−	+86
24	38	95	Early and late	+	−	+14
25	29	100	Early	+	+	+24
26	38	95	Early	−	+	+36
27‖	50	125	Early and late	−	+	...

Tabular Analysis of Patient Observations*

*ISS indicates Injury Severity Score; $\%LD_{50}$, percent lethal dose of injury for age; ELISA, enzyme-linked immunosorbent assay; and PAN, response of *all* four IgM antibodies.

†Early indicates occurring within the first week of trauma; late, occurring after one week of trauma.

‡Minus sign indicates negative response; plus sign, positive response.

§Plus sign indicates injury day that skin test became positive; greater than sign, duration of recorded anergy.

‖Patient died.

¶1+ indicates minor soft-tissue, intrathoracic, or abdominal contamination; 2+, massive soft-tissue contamination or large-bowel spillage.

used was modified from a method that was developed and validated in our laboratory.[6] The assay was performed in flat-bottomed, 96-well polystyrene microtest plates (Flow Laboratories, Inc, Hamden, Conn). Formaldehyde solution–killed bacterial suspensions of the test organisms in carbonate buffer (0.05 mol/L, pH 9.6) were added to the wells in 200-μL aliquots and incubated for three hours at 37°C. After washing the plate with phosphate-buffered saline solution with 0.02% sodium azide added, this solution with 0.5% bovine serum albumin (BSA) was added to each well and incubated for 90 minutes at 27°C. After a second wash with phosphate-buffered saline solution with 0.05% polysorbate 20 (Tween 20) and 0.02% sodium azide (PTA), 200 μL of test serum, diluted 1:200 in PTA:BSA, was added to each well and incubated for two hours at 27°C. After a third wash with PTA, alkaline phosphatase–labeled goat anti–human IgG and IgM (Sigma Chemical Co, St Louis) were added in a 1:1000 dilution in PTA-BSA and incubated for 15 to 18 hours at 27°C. After a final wash with PTA, 200 μL of nitrophenol substrate (Sigma), 1 mg/mL in carbonate buffer with 0.001-mol/L magnesium chloride was added to each well. The plates were incubated for 60 minutes at 27°C, and the reaction then was stopped by the addition of 50 μL of 1N sodium hydroxide to each well. The optical density (OD) of each well was measured photometrically at 410 nm with a rapid microplate reader (Mini-Reader, Dynatech Laboratories, Inc, Alexandria, Va) as originally reported by Cost et al.[6] Controls for each plate included wells with antigen but no serum and wells with reference serum and antigen. The control serum was obtained from a healthy laboratory worker whose immunoglobulin levels were documented within the normal range as tested by radial immunodiffusion (Kallestead Laboratories, Chaska, Minn). This laboratory worker was also shown to have antibodies present to all test organisms that were used. Patients' sera were tested in quadruplicate for each of the three antibody classes against each of the four organisms, and the mean OD was recorded.

To minimize intrinsic variation with the ELISA, the following standardization procedure was used. The OD that was recorded for the reference serum in the first assay that was performed was designated as a standard and used to correct data from all subsequent assays. In cases in which the OD reading was off scale, the assay was repeated by using patient's serum and control serum, diluted to 1:400 in PTA-BSA.

A twofold increase in OD units, with the second value reaching a minimum of 0.5 OD units, was defined as a positive response. This had to occur within two weeks for IgM and within three weeks for IgG measurements. A threefold increase of IgG in three weeks was considered a positive response. Responses were divided into early, which commenced within the first week after injury, or late, which commenced subsequent to the first week after injury. The late responses were classified as appropriate or inappropriate to the documented infection. Wilcoxon rank-sum tests were used to compare median anergy duration, and Student's t tests were used to compare mean ELISA scores.

RESULTS

Twenty-seven patients were studied. The mean ISS was 38 (range, 24 to 50), and the $\%LD_{50}$ was 108 (range, 60 to 141). Fourteen patients developed a major infection, ten developed a minor infection, and three had no infection.

Skin-testing data were available for 25 patients, as two patients sustained severe burns, which precluded application of the tests. Trauma was associated with anergy, as 23 patients (92%) were anergic at admission to the hospital. Increasingly severe injury was associated with a longer duration of anergy. Of the 23 patients who were anergic at admission, seven had skin tests that became positive within three weeks of injury, ten patients remained anergic for longer than three weeks, and six patients were not tested for as long as three weeks. The $\%LD_{50}$ of patients whose skin tests became positive within three weeks (median = 80) was significantly less than the $\%LD_{50}$ of the patients who remained anergic for greater than three weeks (median = 103) ($P<.04$). Twelve patients who were anergic at admission developed major sepsis, two had minor septic episodes, and nine had no infection. Although absence of response to the recall antigens at admission did not predict septic episodes, major sepsis was associated with prolonged anergy. When the last recorded day of anergy was considered, the group of patients who had a major infection had a duration of anergy (median = 22) that was significantly greater than the no-infection group (median = 13) ($P<.05$). Both groups had similar median $\%LD_{50}$ values, which were 87 for the septic group and 86 for the no-infection group.

Comparison with the ELISA data (Table) showed that patients were able to mount antibody responses in the face of continuing skin test anergy. One patient mounted multiple antibody responses despite remaining anergic for 86 days. Twenty-two (82%) of the 27 patients had early antibody responses. Of those 22 patients, 19 had IgM responses, ten had IgG responses, and seven had both. The 22 patients had a total of 61 separate early antibody responses, of which 14 (23%) were IgG, and 47 (77%) were IgM. The early IgG responses were usually to *E coli* (nine of 14 responses), while the early IgM responses were usually to one of the *Pseudomonas* organisms (34 of 47 responses). All patients who developed a major infection had either *E coli* or *Pseudomonas* isolated by culture.

We observed the importance of degree of contamination and identified specific antibody responses that occurred in patients who coped with their infection well. These included an IgG response to *E coli* alone and IgM responses to all four organisms. Six patients in the no-contamination group had no antibody response and did not develop infection. Six of eight patients in the moderate-contamination group mounted antibody responses either to *E coli* or IgM to all four organisms and did not develop early infection. Of the other two patients in this group, one died and the other developed chronic infection of six months' duration. All patients with severe contamination became infected, except one who died three days after injury.

There were 20 late ELISA responses that were defined as commencing at least one week after injury. Fourteen of these responses occurred synchronously with infection.

COMMENT

Trauma[10] and operation[11,12] have both been shown to depress cell-mediated immunity as demonstrated by absence of response to recall skin test antigens (anergy). The results of our study confirmed that severe trauma was associated with anergy, as 23 (92%) of these patients were anergic as compared with 12% of a routine elective surgical population.[5] We found that the duration of the anergic response correlated closely to the $\%LD_{50}$ for our patient population. The degree of anergy has been associated with both age[13] and severity of trauma.[10,13]

These results indicate that the presence of anergy at admission was not predictive of subsequent major septic episodes following severe trauma, as almost all patients were anergic but only half of them developed a major infection. In fact, one of the two patients who were reactive at admission developed major sepsis. Conflicting reports are available in the literature that both support an association of anergy with septic episodes[4,5,13] and others that have shown no predictive value of anergic skin tests.[14,15] Our data would suggest, though, that major sepsis does prolong the anergic state. Also, the duration of anergy correlates with injury severity and the age of the patient as shown by the $\%LD_{50}$. The recall antigens that were used in this study reliably assessed anergy in repetitive testing. Our decision not to use two other commonly used antigens, streptokinase-streptodornase (Varidase) and mumps, was based on previously voiced reservations regarding their value and reliability in repetitive skin testing.[12]

The presence of anergy did not impair the ability of most patients to mount an antibody response, as early antibody production against *E coli* and the three *Pseudomonas* organisms was seen in 22 of the 27 patients. Most patients had IgM responses (19/22), and about half of them demonstrated IgG responses to *E coli* (10/22). Only two patients developed IgG responses to *Pseudomonas*. The degree of bacterial contamination at initial injury was a major determinant of antibody response and clinical outcome. In the group with no contamination, six patients did not mount an antibody response against the organisms tested, nor developed infection. Antibody response may have been unnecessary in these patients as they would not have become infected. All patients with severe contamination, however, developed infection irrespective of antibody response, except the one patient who died early after admission. In the presence of moderate contamination, IgG response to *E coli* and/or IgM responses to all four organisms may have been beneficial, as six patients had such responses and did not develop early infection. Of the other two patients in this particular group who did not mount such antibody responses, one died and the other developed chronic infection of six months' duration. Confirmation of the apparent protective nature of these responses in the face of moderate contamination will require further study.

The ELISA reported in this article appeared to characterize reliably antibody response to *Pseudomonas* and *E coli*. Indeed, ELISA techniques have recently gained acceptance in the clinical setting as sensitive methods for the determination of antibodies to a wide variety of bacterial antigens. The advantages over conventional techniques, such as agglutination and complement fixation, include relative simplicity, high sensitivity, and the ability to detect antibodies of specific immunoglobulin classes.[6,16] Future developments in ELISA techniques may be extended to immunoglobulin subclasses, specific defects of which have been associated with recurrent infections.[17]

The ability of patients with depressed cellular immunity, as measured by skin testing, to mount an antibody response demonstrates a potentially beneficial aspect of humoral immunity in the prevention of infection following major trauma. The level of contamination present at admission is of paramount importance, although age and severity of injury as shown by $\%LD_{50}$ are also critical. The IgM response to moderate contamination appears to be beneficial in the prevention of early infection. This may be of greater predictive value in larger groups of patients than delayed hypersensitivity skin testing, which appears to be depressed in severely injured patients.

The authors wish to acknowledge Lloyd MacLean, MD, professor of surgery, McGill University and surgeon in chief, Royal Victoria Hospital, Montreal, for his help in review of this manuscript.

References

1. *Injury in America: A Continuing Public Health Problem.* Washington, DC, National Academy Press, 1985.
2. Goris RJA, Draaisma J: Causes of death after blunt trauma. *J Trauma* 1982;22:141-146.
3. MacLean LD: Significance of immunoreactivity in trauma. *Acta Chir Scand Suppl* 1985;522:151-170.
4. Wolfe JHN, Wu AVO, O'Connor NE, et al: Anergy, immunosuppressive serum and impaired lymphocyte blastogenesis in burn patients. *Arch Surg* 1982;117:1266-1271.
5. Pietsch JB, Meakins JL, MacLean LD: The delayed hypersensitivity response: Applications in clinical surgery. *Surgery* 1977;82:349-355.
6. Cost KM, West CS, Brinson D, et al: Measurement of human antibody activity against *Escherichia coli* and *Pseudomonas aeruginosa* using formalin treated whole organisms in an ELISA technique. *J Immunoassay* 1985;6:23-43.
7. Hershman MJ, Appel SH, George CD, et al: The use of a new assay for detecting antibody to *Staphylococcus aureus* in severely injured patients. *J Trauma*, in press.
8. Bull JP: Measures of severity of injury. *Injury* 1976;9:184-187.
9. Polk HC Jr, George CD, Wellhausen SR, et al: A systematic study of host defense processes in badly injured patients. *Ann Surg* 1986;204:282-299.
10. Christou NV, McLean ADH, Meakins JL: Host defense in blunt trauma: Interrelationships of kinetics of anergy and depressed neutrophil function, nutritional status and sepsis. *J Trauma* 1978;20:240-247.
11. Christou NV, Rode H, Larsen D, et al: The walk in anergic patient: How best to assess the risk of sepsis following elective surgery. *Ann Surg* 1984;199:438-444.
12. Slade MS, Simmons RL, Yunin E, et al: Immunodepression after major surgery in normal patients. *Surgery* 1975;78:363-372.
13. Meakins JL, McLean APH, Kelly R, et al: Delayed hypersensitivity and neutrophil chemotaxis: Effect of trauma. *J Trauma* 1978;18:240-247.
14. Johnson WC, Ulrich R, Mequid MM, et al: Role of delayed hypersensitivity in predicting postoperative morbidity and mortality. *Am J Surg* 1970;137:536-542.
15. Brown R, Bancewicz J, Hamid J, et al: Failure of delayed hypersensitivity skin testing to predict postoperative sepsis and mortality. *Br Med J Clin Res* 1982;284:851-853.
16. Ritzmann SE: Relative sensitivity of assays for antigens and antibodies, in *Behring Diagnostics Manual on Proteinology and Immunoassays*, ed 2. La Jolla, Calif, Behring Diagnostics, 1977, pp 5-59.
17. Heiner DC: Recognition and management of IgG subclass deficiencies. *Pediatr Infect Dis* 1987;6:235-238.

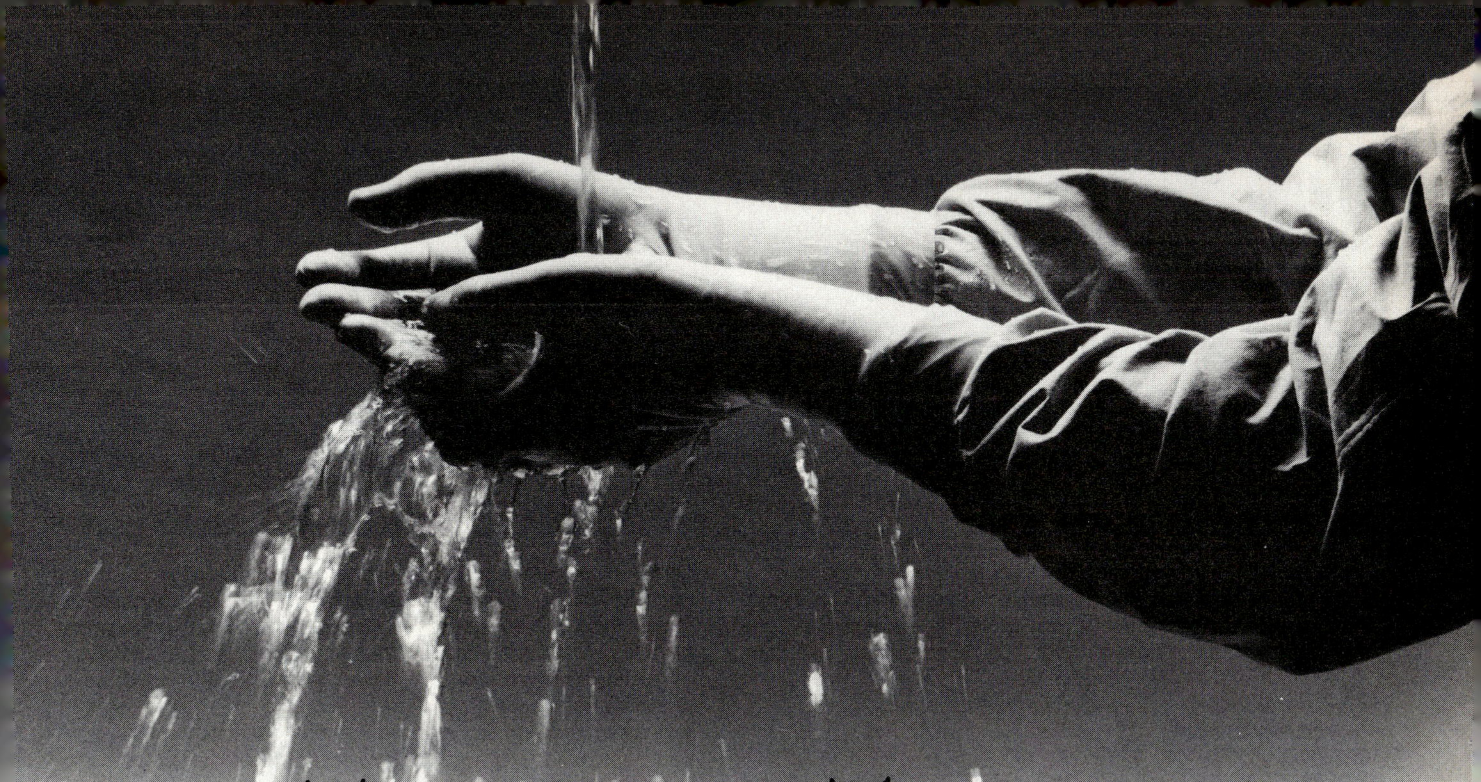

THE DIRTY TRUTH ABOUT SURGICAL GLOVES

All surgical gloves are sterile. That's a fact. But, the truth is that most gloves must be "scrubbed" or wiped thoroughly before surgery. The reasons? Actually, there is only one reason. Powder.

Whether used on the inside or outside surface, talc, starch, silica or other powders are linked to a variety of complications: granulomatous reactions, peritonitis, adhesions and increased incidence of infection in the patient and dermatitis for the physician and nurse. Powders also contaminate OR equipment, sutures, microscope lenses and test procedures.

The only way to eliminate powder-related problems is to eliminate powder. While some powders are the residue of the manufacturing process, most gloves require powder as a donning lubricant. And, powders can leak from the interior through perforations and tears, can spill from the cuff or escape during a glove change. Regardless of how powder gets on the glove, before surgery it must be removed.

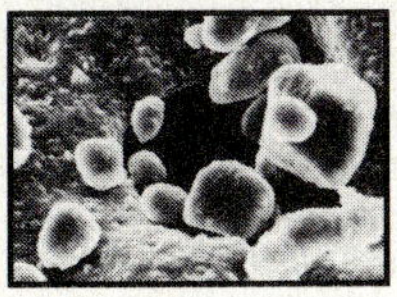

SEM (1000X) of surface of commercially available glove showing cornstarch particles and a surface perforation.

Methods used to remove powder can actually introduce new particulates or may compromise sterility. And, routine glove scrub methods can leave residual powder clinging to the glove surface.

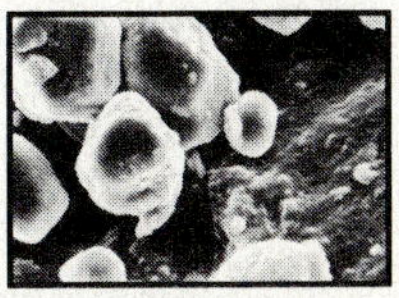

Before scrub: SEM (1000X) of surface of commercially available glove employing cornstarch.

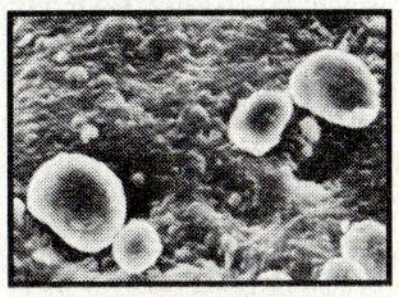

After scrub: SEM (1000X) of same brand glove following 30–40 second warm water scrub followed by wipe with a lint-free towel. SEM shows residual cornstarch particles on the surface.

So, considering the potential risks, why use powder at all?

Now there is PRISTINE,™ the powder-free surgical glove. With a patented, friction-resistant inner surface, donning is smooth and simple. And, with no powders, talcs, starches, silicas or donning lubricants of any kind, using PRISTINE means no glove scrub, powder dermatitis or powder-related post-op complications.

PRISTINE's pure latex construction is durable yet thin enough to give you the tactile sensitivity you need for handling the most delicate instruments. And, the texturized exterior ensures maximum control.

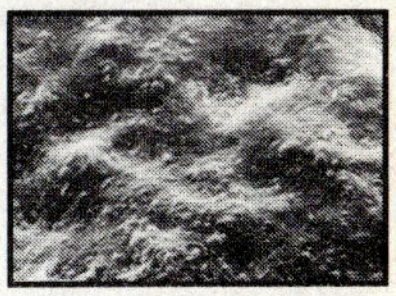

Surface of a PRISTINE powder-free surgical glove. SEM (1000X) shows no foreign body or particulate contamination.

So, for a free sample of PRISTINE gloves, mail the coupon below. To order and for more information, contact World Medical Supply, (800) 545-5475, in CA (800) 547-3366.

Try PRISTINE and discover the glove that is missing only one thing—powder.

PRISTINE.™ The Surgeon's Glove.

Yes. I would like to try PRISTINE gloves.

Please send me a free sample pair in size ______________.

Name ______________

Address ______________

City ______ State ______ Zip ______

Phone ______________

World Medical Supply (USA), Inc.
4340 Stevens Creek Boulevard, Suite 110
San Jose, California 95129 (408) 985-8822
(800) 545-5475, in CA (800) 547-3366

Computed Tomography and Diagnostic Peritoneal Lavage in Blunt Abdominal Trauma

Their Combined Role

Paul A. Kearney, Jr, MD; Thomas Vahey, MD; Richard E. Burney, MD; Gary Glazer, MD

• We reviewed medical records and films of all 196 trauma patients who underwent computed tomography (CT) between June 1982 and October 1986 to see whether CT achieved the level of accuracy attributed to it, whether diagnostic peritoneal lavage (DPL) performed in conjunction with CT was a useful diagnostic test for blunt abdominal trauma, and whether laparotomy was mandatory when pelvic fluid collections were seen by CT after blunt trauma. A total of 36 patients underwent DPL, 29 before and seven after CT. There were seven false-negative CTs that were clinically significant. Diagnostic peritoneal lavage was positive in three patients who had false-negative CTs. Although overall accuracy was excellent, CT was not reliable in detecting bowel injury. Diagnostic peritoneal lavage was helpful in detecting injuries missed by CT. Most stable patients with moderate or large intraperitoneal fluid collections on CT accompanying solid viscus injury were treated successfully without laparotomy.

(*Arch Surg* 1989;124:344-347)

Since it became widely available after 1980, abdominopelvic computed tomographic (CT) scanning has rapidly gained in popularity as a method of examining the multiply injured patient[1] and has been reported to be replacing all other tests commonly used for the diagnosis of blunt abdominal trauma, including diagnostic peritoneal lavage (DPL).[2] Proposed advantages of CT scanning over DPL include organ specificity, improved diagnosis of extra-abdominal injuries, and a reduction in unnecessary laparotomies for blunt trauma.[3-5] At the same time, delay, cost, lack of sensitivity for hollow viscus injuries, and unavailability of high-resolution equipment or personnel experienced in interpretation have all been cited as potential weaknesses of CT scanning.[6-8] A high rate of false-negative CT findings has been reported by other investigators,[6,7,9] who have advocated the continued use of peritoneal lavage. There is, as a result, lack of agreement regarding the appropriate roles of CT and DPL in the diagnostic evaluation of the abdomen in the multiply injured patient.

We have used CT with *increasing* frequency and DPL with *decreasing* frequency in the evaluation of blunt abdominal trauma since 1982. The chief purpose of this study was to evaluate whether CT achieved the high sensitivity, specificity, and reduction in the nontherapeutic laparotomy rates that have been attributed to it. In addition, we wished to find out whether DPL performed in conjunction with CT was a useful diagnostic test in patients with blunt abdominal trauma, and whether moderate to large pelvic fluid collections detected by CT in injured patients were a mandatory indication for laparotomy.

PATIENTS AND METHODS

The records of all 199 patients undergoing CT scanning for blunt abdominal trauma between June 1, 1982, and Oct 31, 1986, were searched. Both the medical records and the CT films were available for review in 196 (98%) of the patients. Data collection included mechanism of injury, indication for CT scan and/or DPL, presence of a pelvic fluid collection on CT scan, quality of scan, and outcome. The sensitivity, specificity, and diagnostic accuracy of both peritoneal lavage and CT scan were determined by laparotomy, clinical outcome, and/or repeated CT.

All CT scans were performed according to a standard protocol, which calls for oral contrast medium to be administered 30 to 40 minutes prior to scanning, followed by a bolus of intravenous (IV) and oral contrast media at the time of the CT scan. Scans were taken at 1-cm intervals through the lower part of the chest, the abdominal cavity, and the pelvis. Scan quality was recorded at the time of the scan, as were all scans in which oral and/or IV contrast agents were omitted. All scans were reviewed by experienced staff radiologists, if not at the time the scan was done, then within 12 hours. A small number (5%) of the CT scans early in the period of study were performed on an early-model scanner (GE 8800), which has a scan time of 5.6 s. The majority of scans were done on the more rapid late-model scanner (GE 9800), which has a scan time of 2 s.

Accepted for publication April 29, 1988.

From the Departments of Surgery (Drs Kearney and Burney) and Radiology (Drs Vahey and Glazer), University of Michigan, Ann Arbor. Dr Kearney is now with the Department of Surgery, University of Kentucky, Louisville.

Reprint requests to the University of Michigan Hospitals, BIC255 University Hospital, Box 0014, 1500 E Medical Center Dr, Ann Arbor, MI 48109-0014 (Dr Burney).

Diagnostic peritoneal lavage was performed using an open lavage technique. Both the bladder and stomach were decompressed prior to insertion of the lavage catheter. If initial aspiration for blood was negative, 1 L of Ringer's lactate was infused through a peritoneal dialysis catheter directed into the pelvis under direct vision. Criteria for a positive lavage were those generally considered significant for intra-abdominal injury.[10]

RESULTS

Of the 196 scans available for review, 119 (61%) were of adults and 77 (39%) were of children. All patients were stable (86%) or rapidly stabilized (14%) in the emergency department prior to abdominopelvic CT scan. Motor vehicle collisions accounted for two thirds of the injuries in patients who underwent CT evaluation. Other causes of injury included pedestrian accidents, falls, motorcycle and bicycle accidents, assaults, and other accidents. The most common indications for CT were altered mental status (39%), equivocal abdominal examination results (37%), and age less than 16 years (19%). The remaining examinations were done in patients with acute spinal cord injury (3%) and patients with hematuria (2%).

The distribution of injuries and accuracy of detection by CT scan are shown in Table 1. There was one false-positive diagnosis, an apparent ruptured diaphragm that was not present at operation (the patient also had splenic rupture correctly identified by CT). There were seven false-negative scans. Sensitivity of CT was 96.5%, specificity 99.5%, and accuracy 96%.

Thirty-six patients underwent DPL as well as CT. For 29 patients, DPL was done *prior to* CT, usually because of a high index of suspicion of intraperitoneal hemorrhage on admission or initially unstable vital signs. The remaining seven patients underwent DPL *after* CT, usually because of a change in clinical signs or symptoms. There were three false-negative results and no false-positives.

Table 2 summarizes all of the instances in which significant intra-abdominal injuries were missed by CT, DPL, or both. Diagnostic peritoneal lavage was performed in five patients with false-negative CT scans: before CT in three and after CT in two. In three of these patients DPL was positive, but in the other two, DPL was falsely negative. One of the patients with false-negative results by both CT and DPL had a ruptured spleen, the other had a diaphragmatic tear and an inferior vena cava laceration. In the latter patient, however, CT scan correctly identified a splenic injury for which the patient underwent exploratory surgery, which led to the other diagnoses.

The one remaining instance in which DPL results were false-negative occurred in a 54-year-old motor vehicle accident victim. A CT scan done following DPL demonstrated an injury to the distal ileum, which was repaired in the operating room.

The two other false-negative CT scans occurred in patients who did not have DPL. One patient had a sigmoid hematoma discovered incidentally during a laparotomy for a ruptured spleen. This sigmoid lesion was identifiable on CT but had been overlooked on the initial interpretation. Another patient, although never requiring operation, had a clinical course consistent with traumatic pancreatitis. Initially his scan was interpreted as normal, but retrospective review identified a pancreatic contusion.

Bowel injuries occurred in five patients in this series (2.5%): three had perforations of the small bowel and two had mesenteric injuries. However, CT scan detected only one of the five; DPL was carried out on four of these patients and detected three of these injuries.

Table 1.—Intra- and Extra-abdominal Injuries Identified by Abdominopelvic Computed Tomographic (CT) Scan and Operation

	CT				
	True-Positive	True-Negative	False-Positive	False-Negative	Operation False-Negative
Spleen	22	172	0	1	1*
Liver	21	173	0	1†	1*
Bowel	1	191	0	4	0
Diaphragm	1	193	1	1‡	0
Kidney	28§	168	0	0	...
Pancreas	2	193	0	1	...
Lung	42	154	0	0	...
Bone	46	150	0	0	...

*Clearly identified by CT but not identifiable at operation.
†Also had ruptured mesenteric hematoma.
‡Also had a missed inferior vena cava laceration.
§Includes four incidental renal lesions: one hypernephroma, one angiolipoma, and two renal cysts.

Two patients were considered to have false-negative surgical results. One patient had a large intrahepatic hematoma with contusion by CT scan that could not be identified at laparotomy (for ruptured spleen). The second patient had intrasplenic hematoma and diaphragm rupture identified by CT. At laparotomy, no superficial splenic injury could be identified. Follow-up CT scans, however, clearly showed a resolving intrasplenic hematoma.

A moderate fluid collection on CT was defined as fluid present in more than one paracolic gutter or perihepatic or subdiaphragmatic space. A large fluid collection was defined as filling the pelvis and at least one other gutter or space. There were 23 patients who had the CT findings of liver and/or splenic injury accompanied by moderate to large amounts of pelvic fluid. Only one (12%) of eight children in this group and six (40%) of 15 adults required surgical exploration for their injuries. The blood transfusion requirement of those who did not require surgery was significantly less (2.6 ± 1.5 U) than that of those who were operated on (6.5 ± 3 U; $P = .005$).

The overall outcome in this group of patients was good. One hundred sixty-two patients (83%) were discharged alive and well. Twenty-six patients (13%) had poor outcomes, in most instances secondary to significant head or spinal cord injuries. Significant morbidity because of a delay in diagnosis or treatment occurred in only two patients (patients 1 and 5, Table 2). There were eight deaths (4%), none the direct result of an incorrect CT scan or DPL interpretation.

Scan quality was judged to be good or excellent in 190 (96%) of the studies. The majority of scans were performed on the faster scanner (95%). All of the false-negative CT scans except one (patient 3, Table 2) occurred while using the faster scanner. Ninety percent of the patients received oral contrast medium and 95% received IV contrast medium. Both contrast agents were omitted in only two patients (1%). This contributed to a false-negative study in one patient (patient 3, Table 2). No nontherapeutic laparotomies were performed.

The charge for abdominopelvic CT scanning is $946. The average time from ordering of scan to completion averaged 2.5 to three hours, with actual scan times ranging from 30 to 60 minutes. The charge for DPL is $146; the average time to completion was 30 minutes.

COMMENT

The unreliability of physical examination in detecting the intra-abdominal injury in the multiply injured patient is well recognized.[10,11] Liberal use of DPL substantially reduced the morbidity and mortality of unrecognized abdominal hemorrhage, while maintaining an acceptable rate for nontherapeutic laparotomy.[10,12-14] Nevertheless, DPL remains an invasive procedure and does not provide the kind of specific information about the location or extent of organ injury that became available with CT scanning.[1,3-5] It has been a matter of debate whether CT can or should completely replace DPL for the diagnosis of abdominal trauma in stable, multiply injured patients.

A protocol was developed by us in 1982, calling for DPL to be carried out after CT in stable patients, to address the question of whether CT could replace DPL in the diagnosis of blunt abdominal trauma. We soon discovered that DPL and CT were being carried out for different reasons, and that it was hard to convince participants that DPL was necessary in patients with a normal CT scan, making completion of the protocol impossible. We also discovered that, depending on the setting and clinical course, both DPL and CT might be called for.

This study was undertaken first to assess the accuracy of CT in the diagnosis of stable trauma patients and, second, to find out what the contribution of DPL had been in the evaluation of these patients. The findings suggest that, despite the excellent results of CT in detecting most intra-abdominal injuries, a small but clinically important number of critical injuries were missed by CT. In our hands, despite the increasing enthusiasm for CT, DPL remained an important adjunctive procedure, particularly in the detection of bowel injury. This was true regardless of whether DPL was carried out before or after CT.

Federle[4,5,15] has reported a high sensitivity and specificity for CT scanning in detecting hollow viscus injury. We were unable to confirm this finding. Four of five bowel injuries were missed by CT, despite good-quality images and interpretation by experienced radiologists. Even retrospective review of these scans failed to change the original interpretation. We concur with Marx et al[7] that CT scanning is unreliable for hollow viscus injury. When there has been a focal concentration of force against the abdomen, as with a high-riding seat belt or the direct blow of a handlebar or a nightstick, we would recommend performing DPL in addition to CT because of the higher incidence of bowel injury in these situations.

Another important finding of this study is that pelvic fluid collections seen on CT scan in association with hepatic or splenic injury are not necessarily a mandatory indication for laparotomy, as has been suggested by a study in which need for operation was analyzed on the basis of quantification of hemoperitoneum by CT scan.[16] In that report, only 11 of 273 patients with small amounts of intraperitoneal blood required operation, whereas 28 of 30 with moderate or large intraperitoneal hemorrhage did. This was particularly true in the presence of hepatic injury.[4,5,17,18] Fluid collections confined to the perisplenic, perihepatic, or subhepatic space (Morison's pouch) or to the left or right paracolic gutter were all considered to be small intraperitoneal collections. Moderate hemoperitoneum consisted of blood in two or more of these locations. Intraperitoneal fluid collections were considered large (500 mL or more) when pelvic fluid was accompanied by blood in one or more of the above locations.

We did not find quantification of intraperitoneal hemorrhage to be as useful in determining the need for surgical intervention. Hemodynamic stability, transfusion requirement (significantly less in those patients treated nonoperatively), and clinical course were better indicators. Only 13 (7%) of 197 patients in this study required laparotomy for their injuries. Seven of these had moderate to large intraperitoneal fluid collections as indicated by CT. Had the rule of mandatory laparotomy for moderate or large intraperitoneal fluid collections been followed, 16 additional laparotomies would have been done, most likely without benefit. Only six (40%) of 15 adults and one of eight children with liver and/or spleen injuries and with moderate to large abdominal fluid collections required laparotomy.

Table 2.—Patients With False-negative Computed Tomography (CT) or Diagnostic Peritoneal Lavage (DPL) Results

Patient/ Age, y	CT Scan Result	DPL Result	Findings at Surgery
1/73	False-negative	Positive after CT	Lacerated jejunum
2/48	False-negative*	Positive before CT	Ruptured duodenum
3/3 mo	False-negative†	Positive after CT	Ruptured mesenteric hematoma, contusion caudate lobe, liver
4/54	Positive	False-negative before CT	Lacerated distal ileum
5/73	False-negative	False-negative before CT	Ruptured spleen
6/41	False-negative*	False-negative before CT	Ruptured diaphragm, lacerated inferior vena cava
7/57	False-negative*	Not done	Sigmoid mesenteric hematoma
8/36	False-negative	Not done	Pancreatic contusion

*Other positive intra-abdominal findings.
†No oral or intravenous contrast medium used.

Computed tomographic scanning for blunt abdominal trauma was not a rapid study in our hands, because of the requirement for oral contrast medium and because of the delays inherent in scheduling and moving multiply injured patients to the radiology suite and back. Intravenous and oral contrast enhancement is important, however, to get the most information from a CT scan, particularly when injury to the pancreas, duodenum, or small bowel is in question.[1-5] One of the seven false-negative evaluations in this study probably resulted from the omission of administration of oral and intravenous contrast media.

It has been recommended that CT scanning precede DPL, because the presence of lavage fluid in the peritoneal cavity may interfere with scan interpretation.[2,5] This has discouraged the use of DPL in situations in which it might be helpful but CT was also likely to be done, as in a patient with blunt trauma, abdominal pain, and hematuria. In this series, when DPL preceded CT it did not interfere with interpretation of the CT scan. There were no false-negative or false-positive results that could be attributed to prior DPL, even after retrospective review. The radiologist was informed that DPL had been carried out, and liberal use of density readings helped to differentiate lavage fluid from blood or intestinal contents. Computed tomographic scan correctly diagnosed a distal ileal laceration in a patient with a prior false-negative lavage by using density readings to identify intestinal contents in the pelvis.

There have been a number of attempts to compare abdominal CT and DPL.[6,7,9,19] The issue remains controversial because direct comparison of CT and DPL is probably not possible, except for a very small number of narrowly defined diagnostic questions. The two tests are called for in similar but not identical situations and provide different kinds of information. The results of this study suggest that there are frequent situations in which additional information can be gained from one study even though the other has been done. Neither appears to be completely reliable in the detection of occult bowel injury, but the combination detects more injuries than either study alone. This suggests that CT scanning and DPL are more complementary than they are competing procedures, and they should be thought of and used in this way.

In summary, the results of this study of 196 patients with blunt abdominal trauma or multiple injuries confirm the overall accuracy of CT to be excellent for both intra- and extra-abdominal injuries, but because not all patients can wait for CT, and because a small number of critical injuries may still be missed, DPL should continue to play an important adjunctive role, particularly when bowel injury is suspected. While CT should generally be performed first, the combination can be used effectively in either order. We have not found the presence of moderate to large peritoneal fluid collections associated with solid organ injury to be a reliable indication for laparotomy in the stable trauma patient, and we believe that other clinical indications and clinical course remain the best determinants.

References

1. Federle MP, Goldberg HI, Kaiser JA, et al: Evaluation of abdominal trauma by computed tomography. *Radiology* 1981;138:637-644.
2. Wing VW, Federle MP, Morris JA, et al: The clinical impact of CT for blunt abdominal trauma. *AJR* 1985;145:1191-1194.
3. Federle MP, Crass RA, Jeffrey RB, et al: Computed tomography in blunt abdominal trauma. *Arch Surg* 1982;117:645-650.
4. Federle MP: CT of upper abdominal trauma. *Semin Roentgenol* 1984;19:269-280.
5. Federle MP: Computed tomography of blunt abdominal trauma. *Radiol Clin North Am* 1983;21:461-474.
6. Davis RA, Shayne JP, Max HM, et al: The use of computerized axial tomography versus peritoneal lavage in the evaluation of blunt abdominal trauma: A prospective study. *Surgery* 1985;98:845-849.
7. Marx JA, Moore EE, Jorden RC, et al: Limitations of computed tomography in the evaluation of acute abdominal trauma: A prospective comparison with DPL. *J Trauma* 1985;25:933-946.
8. Peitzman AB, Makaroun MS, Slasky BS, et al: Prospective study of computed tomography in initial management of blunt abdominal trauma. *J Trauma* 1986;26:585-592.
9. Fabian TC, Mangiante EC, White TJ, et al: A prospective study of 91 patients undergoing both computed tomography and peritoneal lavage following blunt abdominal trauma. *J Trauma* 1986;26:602-608.
10. Fischer RP, Beverlin BC, Engrav LH, et al: Diagnostic peritoneal lavage 14 years and 2586 patients later. *Am J Surg* 1978;136:701-704.
11. Wilson CB, Vidrine A, Rives JD: Unrecognized abdominal trauma in patients with head injuries. *Ann Surg* 1965;161:608-613.
12. Alyono D, Perry JF: Significance of repeating diagnostic peritoneal lavage. *Surgery* 1982;91:656-658.
13. Perry JF, DeMeules JE, Root HD: Diagnostic peritoneal lavage in blunt abdominal trauma. *Surg Gynecol Obstet* 1970;146:795-796.
14. Thal ER, Shires GT: Peritoneal lavage in blunt abdominal trauma. *Am J Surg* 1973;125:64-69.
15. Donohue JH, Federle MP, Griffiths BG, et al: Computed tomography in the diagnosis of blunt intestinal and mesenteric injuries. *J Trauma* 1987;27:11-17.
16. Federle MP, Jeffrey RB: Body computed tomography: Hemoperitoneum studied by computed tomography. *Radiology* 1983;148:187-192.
17. Meyer AA, Crass RA, Lim RC, et al: Selective nonoperative management of blunt liver injury using computed tomography. *Arch Surg* 1985;120:550-554.
18. Moon KL, Federle MP: Computed tomography in hepatic trauma. *AJR* 1983;141:309-314.
19. Goldstein AS, Sclafani SJA, Kupferstein MH, et al: The diagnostic superiority of computerized tomography. *J Trauma* 1985;25:938-944.

Invited Editorial Comment

The issue of CT scanning vs DPL in the evaluation of abdominal trauma remains highly controversial. From 1982 to 1986, largely as a result of impressive data emerging from the San Francisco General Hospital, the pendulum swung from an aggressive DPL policy to one of exclusive CT scanning in many regions of the United States. During this learning curve, there was greater patient morbidity resulting from delayed laparotomy due to lack of CT sensitivity than to unnecessary laparotomy due to lack of DPL specificity. The above clinical review joins other recent studies emphasizing that these diagnostic tests are not mutually exclusive but rather complementary. There is no question that DPL is extremely reliable in confirming free intraperitoneal bleeding but that it does not quantitate or qualify the source of hemorrhage. Moreover, DPL will not signal those injuries confined to the retroperitoneum. On the other hand, CT scanning has consistently failed with acute pancreatic trauma as well as hollow visceral disruption. Thus, the germane issue is not CT scanning vs DPL, but rather when to employ these tests and how to use the information provided by them. The authors propose that free intraperitoneal blood identified in the pelvic cul-de-sac by CT (>500 mL) does not preclude nonoperative management of liver and splenic injuries. Clearly the long-term risks of blood transfusion must be factored into the cost-benefit equation. But the same logic should apply to the hemodynamically stable patient from whom free blood is aspirated in the emergency department. Further chemical analysis of this blood may identify otherwise occult gut injury. Considering the added expense and obligatory time for CT scanning, the corollary is why not employ DPL as the screening test and reserve CT to further characterize suspected visceral injury? In either case, the above review underscores the prevailing consensus that ultimate patient care will improve with recognition of the complementary rather than competitive roles of CT scanning and DPL.

Ernest E. Moore, MD
Denver

The Training and Utilization of Surgical Physician Assistants

A Retrospective Study

Linda Ballard Brandt; Malcolm S. Beinfield, MD; Horace A. Laffaye, MD; Arthur E. Baue, MD

• A community hospital's search for qualified surgical house staff in 1975 led to the development of a postgraduate residency program in surgery for physician assistants. Eleven years after its inception, the program's purpose and structure were reviewed, and its alumni, goals, and contributions were evaluated. A 1987 alumni survey provided data to assess the value of residency training to current employment and job satisfaction.

(*Arch Surg* 1989;124:348-351)

When approval of its physician surgical residency program was disallowed in 1975, Norwalk (Conn) Hospital was faced with the dilemma of providing surgical house staff for inhouse patient care.[1] Its solution was the exclusive use and training of physician assistants (PAs) in surgery.

The decision to develop a postgraduate program to recruit and train PAs as surgical house staff was not made lightly by this 427-bed community hospital in southwestern Connecticut. Members of Norwalk Hospital's Department of Surgery, the chief executive officer, and the chairman of the Department of Nursing joined forces with the chairman of the surgical department and Section of Plastic Surgery at Yale University School of Medicine, New Haven, Conn, to identify the hospital's needs and goals and to assess the role of the PA in other settings. A training program specific to PAs that would expand on their undergraduate PA education was considered essential. This involved identifying inherent differences between the training and utilization of physician residents and that of PA residents. Whereas the physician surgical resident trains to develop the skills necessary to become an independent operating surgeon, the surgical PA is trained to develop skills and judgment as a surgeon's assistant, a qualified team member.[2]

When Norwalk Hospital developed its PA Surgical Residency Program, the PA profession was little more than ten years old. In 1974, about 75% of all PAs worked in primary care settings. Of those employed in specialty areas, approximately 19% were in surgery.[3] A primary care medical background was considered essential in preparing these individuals for the decision-making process involved in the management of surgical patients.[3] Norwalk Hospital's first class of PA surgical residents in 1976 was handpicked for interpersonal skills, academic excellence, and leadership abilities.

The general feeling was that PAs could be trained to perform most surgical house staff functions, ie, admit patients, take histories, perform physical examinations, write preoperative and postoperative orders at the direction of the attending surgeon, provide first or second assistance in the operating room, and assist in the management of the patient on the floors, in the recovery room, in the intensive care unit (ICU), and in the emergency room. This is how surgical PAs currently function at Norwalk Hospital.[4] The residency program was designed to provide the entering PA with the knowledge, skills, and experience to perform these functions. Emphasis is placed on understanding the pathophysiology of disease necessary for patient management.

ORDER WRITING

It was apparent early on that a key factor in the utilization of PAs as surgical house staff was closely linked to their abilities to write orders. Criteria were set up so that all orders were written at the direction of the attending surgeon and were countersigned within 24 hours. Orders written at the direction of the attending surgeon represent either the transmittal of direct orders or, as is often the case, orders that are in keeping with the pattern of care for each individual surgeon. Although permitting nonphysicians to write orders was difficult for many attending physicians in other disciplines to accept, the experience at Norwalk Hospital has indicated that it enables the surgical service to function in a manner consistent with proper patient care.

The director of the pharmacy at Norwalk Hospital reported in 1985 that "the overall quality of drug therapy orders written by PAs has proven to be generally quite good" and that "the number of orders requiring confirmation, clarification, or modification at the request of our pharmacists is comparable to those written by house staff or attending physicians." He additionally noted that "the spirit of cooperation and accessibility of the PAs has resulted in an excellent working relationship with the pharmacy staff."

OBJECTIVES

The objectives of Norwalk's PA Surgical Residency Program are simply stated: (1) to maintain excellence of surgical patient care through the use of well-trained surgical PAs who perform the functions of surgical house

Accepted for publication June 20, 1988.

From the Department of Surgery, Norwalk (Conn) Hospital (Ms Brandt and Drs Beinfield and Laffaye); Department of Surgery, Yale University School of Medicine, New Haven, Conn (Drs Beinfield and Laffaye); and Office of the Vice President, St Louis University Medical Center (Dr Baue).

Reprint requests to Norwalk/Yale PA Surgical Residency Program, Norwalk Hospital, Norwalk, CT 06856 (Ms Brandt).

officers and (2) to involve the surgical attending staff in an ongoing educational program.

STRUCTURE

The program was developed during the summer of 1976 and was initiated that September with a class of 12 PAs. The current structure encompasses a full calendar year divided into trimesters: one on rotation at Yale University School of Medicine and two on the surgical service at Norwalk Hospital. The didactic curriculum at each institution is ongoing with the clinical experience.

During the eight months at Norwalk Hospital, the curriculum consists of over 90 hours of general surgical and specialty lectures, teaching rounds, patient management problem sessions, a review of selected surgical readings, medical writing, medical ethics, and journal club. A paper suitable for publication is required. Clinically, PA residents are trained as assistants to the surgeons in the preoperative and postoperative management of patients on the floors and as first assistants in the operating room. They function as surgical house staff, taking inhouse call on nights and weekends.

The four-month Yale rotation, developed to complement the Norwalk experience, stresses the pathophysiology of surgery in three major courses: anatomy with cadaver dissection; animal surgery; and physiology. An oral research presentation is required. Clinical rotations are required in anesthesiology and emergency medicine. A choice of two electives is offered in any discipline, including burns/plastic and reconstructive surgery, orthopedics, cardiothoracic and vascular surgery, cardiology, pediatric surgery, or radiology. The strengths of both institutions, Norwalk Hospital and Yale University School of Medicine, are used to maximum advantage.

The career objectives of the PAs who enter the surgical residency also help determine the program's structure. A diverse surgical subspecialty clinical curriculum makes available all disciplines at Norwalk Hospital, Yale–New Haven Hospital, and the West Haven (Conn) Veterans Hospital. An elective rotation in cardiothoracic surgery was established at the University of Massachusetts Medical Center, Worcester. Thus, Norwalk's PA surgical residents train for specific employment opportunities while meeting the service needs of the hospital.

ADMISSIONS

A formal admissions process was developed in 1978. A committee composed of the program's directors, three general surgeons, including the department chairman, and a representative of the surgical PA staff reviews each completed application and interviews selected candidates. Applicants invited for interviews spend a full day touring both Norwalk Hospital and Yale University School of Medicine, meeting with the admissions committee and talking with members of the current class. This approach enables applicants to make a more informed choice and reinforces a "match" between candidates selected and the residency program. To date, only two of the PAs entering the residency have failed to complete the program.

As of August 1987, the PA Surgical Residency has graduated 110 surgical PAs. On average, 90% of the PAs entering the residency have at least baccalaureate degrees. Most graduated in the top 10% of their respective PA schools. Although applicant numbers fluctuated widely during the first years of the program, they currently remain fairly constant, averaging 7.5 applicants per residency position. An increase in employment of PAs in surgery, specifically as surgical house staff in hospital settings and in cardiothoracic private practice groups, has been noted nationally.[5] If the market trend toward specialty employment of PAs continues, the demand for postgraduate specialty training should remain stable or experience a growth. Predicted increases in the numbers of practicing physicians has failed to impact negatively on the employment of PAs in the specialty areas.

Table 1.—Division of Total Work Time of Respondents by Surgical Work Setting*

	Mean % of Total Time (No. Reporting in Each Category)		
Category	Hospital (n=25)	Private Practice (n=19)	University Medical Center (n=6)
Clinical	79.2 (25)	83.4 (19)	84.2 (6)
Administrative	9.6 (11)	9.2 (11)	10.0 (1)
Patient education	12.6 (19)	11.6 (12)	15.0 (2)
Teaching PAs	12.3 (12)	5.5 (2)	. . .
Research	5.4 (5)	6.4 (5)	11.7 (3)

*PA indicates physician assistant. N=50.

EVALUATION

The program's 11-year experience was evaluated on the basis of the following questions: (1) Have the initially stated objectives been met? (Are the PAs performing most functions of surgical house staff in a satisfactory manner and is the attending staff actively involved in a teaching program?); (2) Do the program's alumni feel that their training was worthwhile?; (3) Are the alumni satisfied with their employment and career choice?

Since 1977, the surgical service at Norwalk Hospital has continued exclusively to use surgical PAs in house staff positions. The number of permanent staff PA positions has increased from six in 1977 to 14 in 1987 due to an increase in the service needs of the institution. Of the 110 PAs who have completed the program through 1987, 35% (39) have served in the Department of Surgery at Norwalk as staff surgical PAs. Replacements for staff PA positions are always recruited from the current residency class. The average length of employment beyond the residency year as a staff PA at Norwalk is four years, but several surgical PAs remain on staff after more than ten years, providing continuity for the surgical team.

Of the 62 surgeons currently on active staff at Norwalk Hospital (excluding oral surgeons), 42 are actively involved in the didactic curriculum of the program, presenting lectures, chairing teaching conferences, and making daily bedside rounds. Additionally, 25 attending physicians from other disciplines, including medicine, cardiology, radiology, pathology, respiratory therapy, obstetrics/gynecology, and pediatrics, present lecture material in their various specialties. Five surgeons help plan the didactic curriculum, clinical evaluation methods, and tests. Staff PAs are responsible for a series of 20 lectures for student PAs who rotate on the surgical service. The team approach to patient care and education is reinforced by assigning a staff PA, a PA resident, and a student PA to each group of surgeons.

ALUMNI SURVEY

To determine the alumni's assessment of their training and to follow up their employment, a decriptive questionnaire was mailed in July 1987 to 99 physician assistants who completed the PA Surgical Residency Program. Job networking and various alumni functions enable the PA surgical residency office to maintain an up-to-date address file on most graduates. The survey was designed to obtain demographic information, as well as to determine relationships between current employment, PA surgical residency training, and job satisfaction. Seventy-seven questionnaires (77.8%) were returned. Three of these were excluded because the subjects were no longer working as PAs (one physician, one

Table 2.—Division of Clinical Work Time of Respondents by Surgical Work Setting*

Type of Work	Hospital (n=25)	Private Practice (n=19)	University Medical Center (n=6)
	Mean % of Clinical Time (No. Reporting in Each Category)		
Preoperative care	19.9 (21)	25.9 (17)	24.2 (6)
OR assistance	42.8 (23)	26.7 (18)	41.7 (6)
Postoperative care	30.0 (23)	24.3 (18)	20.8 (6)
ICU care	15.0 (13)	13.3 (8)	16.3 (4)
Emergency care	8.1 (9)	5.2 (6)	7.5 (2)

*OR indicates operating room; ICU, intensive care unit. N=50.

student, and one retired PA). Therefore, 74 responses (74.75%) were considered for this report.

RESULTS

Surgical Specialty and Setting

The survey revealed that 52 (71%) of the respondents were employed in surgical settings: 22 (30%) in general surgery; 19 (26%) in cardiothoracic and vascular surgery; eight (11%) in orthopedics; and three (4%) in other surgical subspecialties. Although 22 (29%) were employed in nonsurgical areas, nine (12%) worked in emergency medicine or trauma, where their surgical skills were used.

Hospitals (35 [47%]) and university medical centers (nine [12%]) employed 44 (59%) of these graduates, while private practice groups employed 22 (30%). The remaining eight (11%) worked in corporations, health maintenance organizations, clinics, and PA programs. Cardiothoracic and orthopedic groups employed 18 (90%) of the privately employed surgical PAs, while only seven (28%) of the hospital-based surgical PAs worked in these two specialties. Thirty-three percent (two) of the university medical center–employed respondents worked in cardiothoracic surgery; none worked in orthopedic surgery. The majority of hospital-based surgical PA respondents (17 [68%]) worked in general surgery. Ten (28.5%) hospital-employed respondents worked in nonsurgical specialties, seven of these in emergency departments.

Work Categories

Since Norwalk's training program emphasizes operative, intraoperative, and postoperative aspects of surgical patient care, division of work time by type of work was specifically asked on the questionnaire. All respondents identified as working in a surgical specialty regardless of setting spent the majority of their time performing clinical duties (Table 1). Two surgically employed respondents were excluded from these tables: one employed by a health maintenance organization and one privately employed cardiothoracic surgical PA who did not respond completely to the breakdown of work time. The tables therefore represent the responses of 50 surgical PA respondents. When broken down by specific type of work, clinical time was predominantly divided between preoperative, intraoperative, and postoperative care (Table 2). More than half of the respondents employed in surgical hospital or university medical center settings also spent time managing patients in an ICU. Slightly less than half of the privately employed surgical PAs worked in an ICU.

Whereas almost half of the hospital-employed surgical PAs teach PAs, none of the university medical center surgical PA respondents spent time in this category. Patient education occupied about 12% of the time for 76% of the hospital-based surgical PAs and 63% of the privately employed surgical PAs. One third of the surgical PAs working in university medical centers were active in patient education.

Working Hours

The questionnaire asked the average number of hours worked per week and the number of "on-call" hours. Considering only full-time respondents and including on-call hours, the survey revealed that 51 (75%) worked between 40 and 60 hours per week, six (9%) worked less than 40 hours per week and were still considered full-time employees, and 11 (16%) worked in excess of 60 hours per week. Six respondents considered part-time workers were excluded from these figures. Forty-nine (66%) took call: 34 (69%) of these from home by beeper, 15 (31%) inhospital. Of those required to take call, 30 (62%) were compensated for their on-call time: 19 (63%) of these received additional salary and 11 (37%) were given compensatory time off.

Acceptance of Orders by Nursing Staff

Writing patient orders is an important aspect of the PA Surgical Residency Program. Acceptance of these orders by the nursing staff is essential to the surgical PA's job performance. Eighty-nine percent of the survey's respondents reported that they were permitted to write orders: 79% of these stated that they never encountered difficulties with acceptance by nursing staff, 18% rarely had problems, and only 3% said that nursing staff refused to accept their orders.

Salaries

Fifty-two (77%) of the 68 responding full-time employed alumni reported annual salaries between $30 000 and $49 000; nine (13%) earned more than $50 000. These figures include all respondents working full-time regardless of length of employment. The survey indicated that most full-time and part-time respondents (70 [94.6%]) received time off and reimbursement for continuing medical education in addition to their salary and vacation time.

Value of Training

Particularly encouraging were responses to questions regarding the value of the PA surgical residency training. All respondents indicated the positive value of their surgical residency training; 98.6% indicated value to current employment (82.4% very much and 16.2% moderately so), and 1.4% reported that the training was not relevant to their current employment but was important for employment in the surgical specialties. Ninety-five percent would recommend the Norwalk/Yale PA Surgical Residency Program to PAs interested in surgery, and 95% stated that postgraduate training was important to the PA profession, particularly in the specialties.

Job Satisfaction

When asked to rate current level of job satisfaction from high to unsatisfactory, 84% of the responding alumni indicated a good to high degree of satisfaction. Ninety-one percent were always, with few exceptions, regarded by their employing physicians as professional members of the health care team.

COMMENT

Comparison with a 1981 survey by the Association of Physician Assistant Programs shows that Norwalk Hospital/Yale alumni closely follow the national trend in surgical subspecialty employment. The survey lists general surgery (37.3%), orthopedics (23.6%), and cardiothoracic surgery (19.2%) as the top three surgical subspecialties.[6] Our survey indicated the same three leading employment specialties, although more respondents work in cardiothoracic surgery than orthopedics.

The survey finding that the majority of responding alumni not only valued their postgraduate surgical training but also would recommend the program to PAs interested in surgery combined with the high degree of job satisfaction and professional respect spoke well for the future of postgraduate training in the specialties. The high percentage of respondents reporting the importance of postgraduate education to the PA profession further supports the continuation of postgraduate specialty training for PAs. Survey respondents commented that formal postgraduate specialty training provided them with the "fastest way to get the broadest exposure" in surgery and the subspecialties, allowing them to build confidence and competence. Additional comments indicated the need for postgraduate training in the specialties as an option for primary care PAs to provide growth in their level of responsibility. Many respondents indicated that being well trained in surgery opened doors and expanded employment opportunities.

Division of clinical work time corresponded with the structure and emphasis of the program in the total management of the surgical patient. Most responding alumni working in surgical settings are using their skills and knowledge in the preoperative, intraoperative, and postoperative areas of care.

Salary ranges among survey respondents confirm studies that identify surgery as one of the highest paid areas of employment for PAs. Ninety percent of the responding alumni earned more than $30 000 annually, whereas a 1984 American Academy of Physician Assistants survey showed approximately 60% of PAs nationally to be earning $20 000 to $30 000 per year.[7] Reasonable working hours, including on-call time, were also reported by 74% of the respondents, dispelling fears of long "residency" hours. No doubt these factors—salary, working hours, and full use of skills—influenced the reported high degree of job satisfaction.

SUMMARY

The Norwalk Hospital/Yale University School of Medicine PA Surgical Residency Program is one solution to the increasing problem of providing adequate coverage of surgical patients in hospitals without physician surgical residents. Employment of surgeons as permanent house staff is professionally unattractive and financially prohibitive. Appropriately trained PAs are able to fulfill most house staff service requirements whether they are employed exclusively or in conjunction with physician residents. It is, however, a mistake to employ PAs as alternate house staff unless the educational and professional differences between physician residents and PAs are recognized. Unlike physician residents, surgical PAs have a limited upward mobility. Adjustments must be made to provide appropriate scheduling, compensation, and training to accommodate the surgical PA's permanent employment situation. A commitment must be made to provide surgical PAs with support, supervision, and continuing education appropriate to their profession and their function as members of the surgical team. Review of Norwalk's experience indicates that the postgraduate surgical residency for PAs has benefited both the hospital, in meeting its service and educational requirements, and the surgical PA, who enjoys an advantage in an increasingly specialized PA job market.

References

1. Heinrich JJ, et al: The physician's assistant as resident on surgical service. *Arch Surg* 1980;115:310-314.
2. Beinfield MS: The surgical PA: A community hospital resource. *Conn Med* 1980;44:823-824.
3. Perry HB, Detmer DE, Redmond EL: The current and future role of surgical physician assistants. *Ann Surg* 1981;193:132-137.
4. Carson C, Beinfield MS: The surgical physician assistant functioning in the role of the junior surgical house officer in a community hospital, in Carter RD, Perry HB (eds): *Alternatives in Health Care Delivery: Emerging Roles for Physician Assistants.* St Louis, WH Green, 1984, chap 34.
5. Schafft GE, Cawley JF: Specialization and career mobility, in Schafft GE, Cawley JF (eds): *The Physician Assistant in a Changing Health Care Environment.* Rockville, Md, Aspen Systems Corp, 1987, chap 9.
6. Perry HB, Carter RD: Physician assistants working in surgery: An overview, in Carter RD, Perry HB (eds): *Alternatives in Health Care Delivery: Emerging Roles for Physician Assistants.* St Louis, WH Green, 1984, pp 95-96.
7. Schafft GE, Cawley JF: The development of a profession, in Schafft GE, Cawley JF (eds): *The Physician Assistant in a Changing Health Care Environment.* Rockville, Md, Aspen Systems Corp, 1987, p 10.

Invited Editorial Comment

Progressive changes in various aspects of health care provision for inpatients and outpatients are continuing to develop, and as informed health care providers we must all keep abreast of these changes and their impact on our daily activities. The article by Brandt et al describes a one-year surgical training program for PAs. While the authors emphasize the educational value of the experience, we are provided with limited objective information about the quality of the educational experience. We are told of the characteristics of subsequent employment and remuneration of individuals finishing the educational program; however, we are not informed of any educational objectives that have been accomplished. For example, how do the graduates fare on certifying and recertification examinations?

The issue of order writing by PAs remains controversial. The Joint Review Committee for Physician's Assistants approved by the American College of Surgeons indicates that PA tasks to be performed "include transmission and execution of the surgeon's orders." In the program described by Brandt et al, this is interpreted as orders written "that are in keeping with the pattern of care for each individual surgeon."

Considerable difficulty exists with defining roles, and even more difficulty exists in defining needs in the provision of health care. The PA appeared as a physician surrogate in a period of perceived physician shortages. Currently, we have no evident physician shortage but have resident physician shortages for which surgical PA programs are being advocated. Current nursing manpower needs have been highlighted by a recent decision by the American Medical Association to begin a program to train "registered care technologists" to function somewhere between nurses' aides, licensed practical nurses, registered nurses, and nurse clinicians. The tasks performed by PAs in the article by Brandt et al are in other circumstances performed by nurses. The exact role of all of these health care workers is obscure.

Physicians' assistants are not likely to remain *dependent* health care providers and neither are surgical PAs. As recently stated in *Alternatives in Health Care Delivery* (Carter RD, Perry HB [eds], St Louis, WH Green, p 312), PAs are capable of providing *interdependent* rather than physician *dependent* health care and should be accepted as being "fiscally autonomous providers." Fiscally autonomous, *interdependent* surgical physician assistants could eventually seek hospital staff and operating privileges and create another class of surgeons to replace the disappearing general practitioners that operate.

Donald L. Kaminiski, MD
St Louis

Physiologic Effects of Steep Positioning in the Surgical Intensive Care Unit

Loren D. Nelson, MD, Hans B. Anderson, RRT

• **Ten hemodynamically stable patients requiring mechanical ventilation for radiographically symmetric acute lung disease were studied during steep lateral positioning and continuous rotation in a Roto Rest kinetic treatment bed. There were no significant hemodynamic or ventilatory differences among the four positions (supine, right side down, left side down, and rotating). In four patients, arterial oxygen pressure (Pa_{O_2}) decreased 16% to 49% in the lateral position when compared with the supine position. Continuous rotation restored the Pa_{O_2} toward the supine value in each patient. In six patients, Pa_{O_2} increased 11% to 35% during lateral positioning. In five of the six patients, the increase in Pa_{O_2} differed between sides, suggesting asymmetric lung disease. Continuous rotation did not significantly alter the Pa_{O_2} from the supine values in these patients. Adverse effects on oxygenation caused by positional changes may be reversed by continuous rotation using the Roto Rest kinetic bed.**
(*Arch Surg* 1989;124:352-355)

Steep positional changes are commonly used in postoperative patients to help prevent pulmonary complications. These changes in position may affect pulmonary gas exchange by altering both ventilation and perfusion.[1] The alterations produced by position changes may have therapeutic implications in patients with mismatching of ventilation and perfusion. Though positional variation in pulmonary gas exchange may be more pronounced in patients with unilateral disease,[2] it may also occur in patients with radiographically symmetric disease.[3]

The Roto Rest kinetic bed has been used since before 1974 with only anecdotal reports regarding its physiologic effects. The purpose of this study is to evaluate the effects of steep positional therapy using the Roto Rest kinetic bed on pulmonary gas exchange and hemodynamics in patients with radiographically symmetric acute lung disease.

Accepted for publication Dec 3, 1987.
From the Department of Surgery, University of Miami, and the Surgical Intensive Care Unit, Jackson Memorial Medical Center, Miami. Dr Nelson is now with the Section of Surgical Sciences, Vanderbilt University School of Medicine, Nashville, Tenn.
Reprint requests to St Thomas Hospital, PO Box 380, 4220 Harding Rd, Nashville, TN 37202 (Dr Nelson).

PATIENTS AND METHODS

Ten patients admitted to the surgical intensive care unit (SICU) at Jackson Memorial Medical Center, Miami, were studied. All were hemodynamically stable, had a functioning pulmonary arterial catheter, and were receiving mechanical ventilatory support for radiographically symmetric acute lung disease. The patients were awake and alert so as to be able to give informed consent. No patients were receiving inotropic support at the time of study, but three were receiving low-dose dopamine hydrochloride (<3 μg/kg/min), two were receiving intravenous aminophylline, and one was receiving sodium nitroprusside (<1 μg/kg/min; Table 1). The administration rate of these medications was unchanged during the study. The primary diagnosis at the time of admission to the SICU and initial chest roentgenographic findings are summarized in Table 1.

Measurements of intravascular pressures, cardiac output, arterial and mixed venous blood gases, oxygen consumption ($\dot{V}O_2$), and carbon dioxide production ($\dot{V}CO_2$) were made after 30-minute periods of stabilization in each of four positions: supine, right side down, left side down, and rotating. The order of position changes was determined by a random numbers table. Each position was achieved using the Roto Rest kinetic bed. During the rotating mode, the patient was turned from side to side through an arc of 124° approximately every 3½ minutes. The mean time required to complete the measurements was 3.7 ± 0.9 hours.

Pressure transducers were calibrated to the level of the left atrium before each measurement. During continuous rotation, pressures were measured and cardiac output injections were performed as the rotating bed crossed the horizontal position. No attempt was made to estimate intrathoracic pressure, and therefore transmural pressures were not recorded. Cardiac output was measured in triplicate by the thermodilution technique using 10 mL of room-temperature 5% dextrose in water. The $\dot{V}O_2$ and $\dot{V}CO_2$ values were measured by inspired and expired gas analysis using a metabolic gas monitor (MGM/TWO).

All patients were receiving mechanical ventilatory support via an artificial airway. Inspired oxygen concentration was maintained at 0.45, and positive end-expiratory pressure was titrated to achieve an arterial oxygen pressure (Pa_{O_2}) of greater than 65 mm Hg in the supine position. Mechanical tidal volume was set at 12 to 15 mL/kg. Intermittent mandatory ventilation was adjusted to keep the arterial carbon dioxide pressure (Pa_{CO_2}) between 35 and 45 mm Hg and pH greater than 7.35. Ventilator settings were not altered during the study period. Arterial and venous blood gas analysis was performed using an automated blood gas analyzer (Corning 178). Venous oxygen saturation was measured using an Oximetrix (Oximetrix-3) continuous in vivo analyzer, an American-Optical Unisat cooximeter, or an Instru-

Table 1.—Demographics, Medications, Roentgenographic Results, and Ventilator Settings*

Patient No./Age, y/Sex	Diagnosis	BSA, m^2	Vasoactive Medications	Chest Roentgenography	IMV	PEEP
1/58/F	Small-bowel obstruction	1.4	Dopamine hydrochloride, <3; sodium nitroprusside, <1	Bilateral effusions; diffuse interstitial infiltrate	. . .	5
2/62/M	Abdominal aneurysmectomy	1.8	Dopamine, <3; sodium nitroprusside, <1; aminophylline, 20	Bilateral effusions	2	8
3/75/F	Biliary sepsis	2.0	Dopamine, <3	Clear	4	5
4/58/F	Perforated duodenal ulcer	1.5	None	Bilateral effusions	2	5
5/41/F	Perforated colon	1.4	None	Diffuse interstitial infiltrate and effusions	2	5
6/27/F	ARDS	1.6	Aminophylline, 25	Diffuse interstitial infiltrates	2	35
7/77/M	Carcinoma of mouth	1.6	None	Bilateral subsegmental collapse	2	5
8/65/F	Mesenteric embolism	1.6	None	Bilateral effusions	2	5
9/80/M	Multiple trauma	1.9	None	Diffuse reticular infiltrates	6	5
10/48/F	Biliary pancreatitis	2.0	None	Diffuse interstitial infiltrate	2	5

*BSA indicates body surface area; IMV, intermittent mandatory ventilation rate (breaths per minute); PEEP, positive end-expiratory pressure (centimeters of water); ARDS, adult respiratory distress syndrome. Dopamine and sodium nitroprusside are given in micrograms per kilogram per minute, aminophylline in milligrams per hour. For all patients, fraction of inspired oxygen was 0.45.

mentation Laboratories 282 cooximeter. Derived hemodynamic and pulmonary variables were calculated using standard formulas.[4]

Serial portable chest roentgenograms were done daily while the patients remained intubated. The films were reviewed by radiologists who were unaware of the study results.

Measured and calculated variables were compared using a χ^2 analysis or paired t test. P values of less than .05 were considered to be statistically significant. This study was approved by the University of Miami Subcommittee for the Protection of Human Subjects.

RESULTS

There were no statistically significant differences in mean arterial pressure, cardiac index, central venous pressure, pulmonary artery occlusion (wedge) pressure, systemic vascular resistance, pulmonary vascular resistance, or left ventricular stroke work index during any of the four positionings (Table 2).

There were no statistically significant differences in spontaneous ventilatory rate, spontaneous tidal volume, total minute ventilation, $Paco_2$, $\dot{V}co_2$, dead space–tidal volume ratio (Vd/Vt), or effective dynamic compliance among the various positions (Table 2). The $Paco_2$ increased more than 10% above the supine value in the lateral positions in two patients and during continuous rotation in two patients, but in no case was the increase more than 8 mm Hg. The increase in $Paco_2$ was due to an increase in $\dot{V}co_2$ in three instances and an increase in Vd/Vt in the fourth instance.

The Pao_2 varied more than any other value studied during the positionings (Table 2 and Fig 1). In four of ten patients, Pao_2 decreased by more than 10% (range, 16% to 49% [24 to 65 mm Hg]; mean decrease, 28% [46 mm Hg]) in both of the lateral positions when compared with the supine position (Fig 2). The mean supine Pao_2 in these patients was 143 mm Hg and the mean lateral Pao_2 was 97 mm Hg ($P<.025$). In one patient the decrease in Pao_2 was associated with an increase in right-to-left physiologic shunt (Qsp/Qt), in two with an increase in $\dot{V}o_2$, and in one an increase in both $\dot{V}o_2$ and Qsp/Qt. Continuous rotation restored the Pao_2 toward the supine value (mean, 136 mm Hg) in each of these four patients. No patient who had a significant decrease in Pao_2 in the lateral positions developed asymmetric progression of infiltrates on serial chest roentgenograms.

In six of ten patients, Pao_2 increased by more than 10% (range, 11% to 35% [15 to 27 mm Hg]; mean increase, 22% [21 mm Hg]; $P<.001$) in one lateral position compared with supine (Fig 3). In five of these six patients, the increase in Pao_2 differed between the two lateral positions by more than 10% (range, 11% to 33% [17 to 27 mm Hg]; mean difference, 24% [22 mm Hg]), suggesting asymmetric lung disease. Three of these five patients later developed asymmetric progression of their pulmonary infiltrates on serial chest roentgenograms. The increase in Pao_2 was associated with a decrease in Qsp/Qt in four patients. In the other two patients the increase in Pao_2 was not associated with a decrease in Qsp/Qt or $\dot{V}o_2$, or an increase in mixed venous oxygen saturation. Continuous rotation through the entire 124° arc did not significantly alter the Pao_2 from the supine values in patients whose Pao_2 increased in the steep lateral positions ($P>.05$).

COMMENT

A major cause of arterial hypoxemia is mismatching of ventilation and perfusion.[1] Both ventilation and perfusion, to some degree, depend on patient position. Since the normal perfusion pressure of the pulmonary circulation is low and the relative hydrostatic pressure differences due to gravity are high (especially in the upright position), changes in the distribution of blood flow occur with position changes. There is also a redistribution of ventilation with position changes. However, the changes in the distribution

Table 2.—Hemodynamic, Ventilatory, and Oxygenation Results in Ten Patients*

Value	Supine	RSD	LSD	Rotating
Hemodynamic Results				
MAP, mm Hg	95±14	99±16	94±18	93±13
CI, L/min/m²	3.7±1.0	3.8±0.8	3.7±0.8	3.5±0.6
CVP, mm Hg	15±5	11±4	15±7	12±3
PAOP, mm Hg	17±5	15±5	18±6	16±4
SVR, dyne•s•cm⁻⁵	1109±372	1200±392	1098±351	1156±321
PVR, dyne•s•cm⁻⁵	144±77	161±57	167±68	148±59
LVSWI, g•m/m²	36±8	38±9	36±10	34±8
Ventilatory Results				
VR (spon), breaths/min	16±9	19±8	21±10	18±8
Vt (spon), mL	231±60	238±62	223±88	224±77
Ve (spon), L/min	3.9±2.5	4.7±2.0	4.9±2.2	4.1±1.9
Pa_{CO_2}, mm Hg	42±6	44±8	43±7	44±7
$\mathring{V}_{CO_2}$, mL/min	183±44	196±33	196±41	193±27
Vd/Vt	0.43±0.10	0.42±0.09	0.44±0.09	0.44±0.10
EDC, mL/cm H_2O	26±9	25±9	25±8	27±10
Oxygenation Results				
Pa_{O_2}, mm Hg	112±39	105±39	103±28	108±34
Qsp/Qt	0.21±0.13	0.23±0.12	0.20±0.07	0.20±0.11
$\mathring{V}_{O_2}$, mL/min	191±55	213±50	206±50	200±40
D_{O_2}, mL/min	981±282	995±253	974±257	928±222

*RSD indicates right side down; LSD, left side down; MAP, mean arterial pressure; CI, cardiac index; CVP, central venous pressure; PAOP, pulmonary artery occlusion (wedge) pressure; SVR, systemic vascular resistance; PVR, pulmonary vascular resistance; LVSWI, left ventricular stroke work index; VR (spon), spontaneous ventilatory rate; Vt (spon), spontaneous tidal volume; Ve (spon), spontaneous minute ventilation; Pa_{CO_2}, arterial carbon dioxide pressure; $\mathring{V}_{CO_2}$, carbon dioxide production; Vd/Vt, dead space–tidal volume ratio; EDC, effective dynamic compliance; Pa_{O_2}, arterial oxygen pressure; Qsp/Qt, physiologic intrapulmonary shunt fraction; $\mathring{V}_{O_2}$, oxygen consumption; D_{O_2}, oxygen delivery. Values are mean±SD. There were no statistically significant differences between mean values obtained in the different positions.

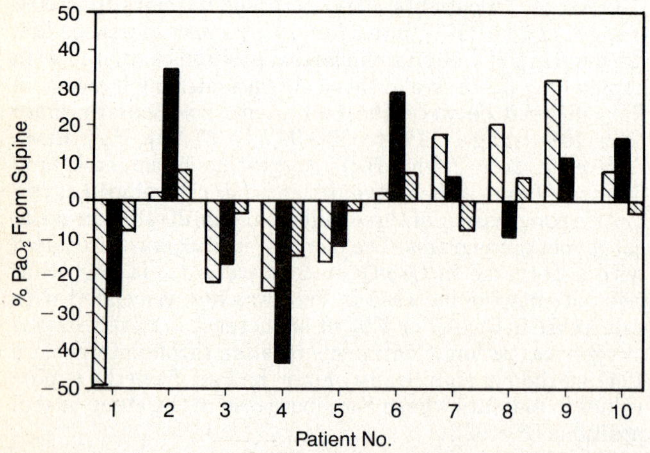

Fig 1.—Percent changes from supine arterial oxygen pressure (Pa_{O_2}) values in ten patients during steep lateral positioning and continuous rotation using Roto Rest kinetic bed. Broadly hatched bars indicate right side down; black bars, left side down; closely hatched bars, rotating.

of perfusion are greater than the changes in regional ventilation. Since relative matching of ventilation and perfusion is required for optimal gas exchange (especially oxygenation), position changes may have a major effect on

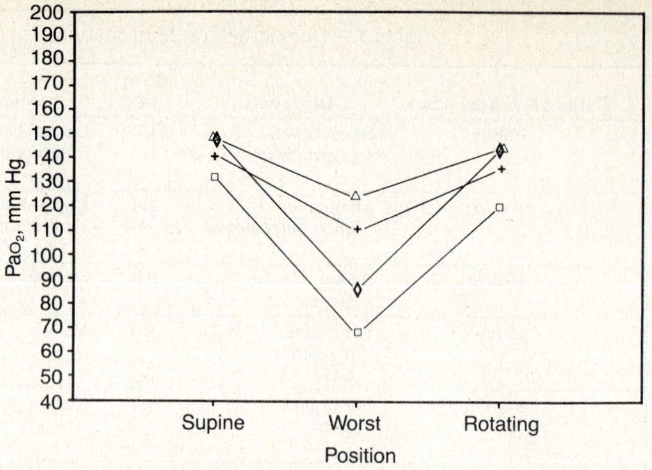

Fig 2.—Decreases in arterial oxygen pressure (Pa_{O_2}) during steep lateral positioning (seen in four patients) were corrected during continuous rotation therapy.

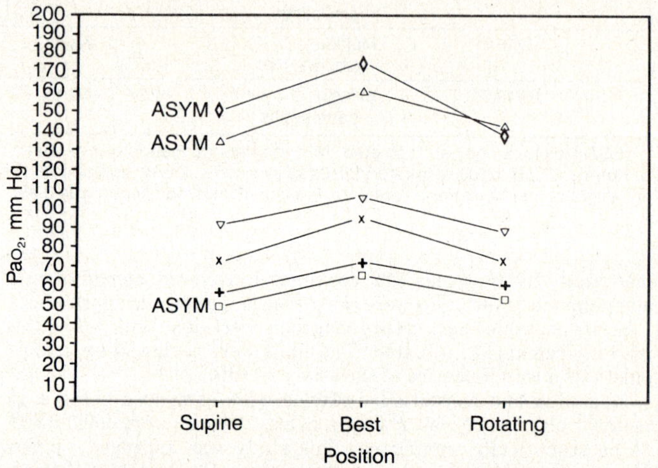

Fig 3.—Increases in arterial oxygen pressure (Pa_{O_2}) during steep lateral positioning (seen in six patients) were less than decreases noted in Fig 2. Continuous rotation in these patients did not alter Pa_{O_2} from supine values. ASYM indicates three patients who later developed asymmetric infiltrates on chest roentgenograms.

arterial oxygenation. This is especially true in situations where normal compensatory mechanisms are impaired.

Unilateral pulmonary disease is a situation where lateral positioning has been shown to have major effects on oxygenation.[2,3,5-7] However, differences in oxygenation produced by position changes also occur in patients with radiographically symmetric pulmonary disease.[3] In patients with no evidence of acute pulmonary disease, the effect of positional changes on oxygenation is minimal.[3]

Frequent position changes and early ambulation of postoperative patients have long been the standard of care to prevent pulmonary complications. Patients who are confined to bed because of injuries or critical illness have been difficult to manage and have a high incidence of pulmonary complications. Use of the Roto Rest kinetic treatment bed has been advocated as a means to minimize problems related to immobility.

The Roto Rest bed has been shown to be effective in improving oxygenation in patients with acute unilateral pulmonary injury.[8] This study was performed to evaluate the effect of steep lateral positioning and continuous rotation between lateral positions on hemodynamics and gas exchange in critically ill patients with radiographically symmetric acute pulmonary disease.

We found no significant effect of steep lateral positioning or continuous rotation on cardiac index, arterial blood pressure, pulmonary arterial pressure, central venous pressure, pulmonary arterial occlusion (wedge) pressure, or the derived parameters of systemic and pulmonary vascular resistance and ventricular work. Though these patients were preselected to be hemodynamically stable and were not receiving significant inotropic or vasopressor support, their status, at some point in their SICU admission, was in sufficient question to warrant placement of a pulmonary artery catheter. These findings are significant in that kinetic therapy has in the past been withheld for fear of precipitating adverse hemodynamic effects. Adverse hemodynamic effects were not seen in any patient in this study.

We also found no significant effects on total ventilation; ie, there were no statistically significant changes in $Paco_2$ or the direct determinants of $Paco_2$ ($\dot{V}co_2$, alveolar ventilation, ventilatory rate, minute ventilation, tidal volume, or Vd/Vt). We cannot say from this study whether there were effects on regional ventilation of the lung or atelectasis.

The major effect of short-term steep positional and kinetic therapy was on oxygenation. In four patients, Pao_2 decreased 16% to 49% in one of the lateral positions. The decreases in Pao_2 were not predictable from radiographic data. Continuous rotation restored the Pao_2 toward the supine value in all four patients. This suggests that in patients who require position changes but develop hypoxemia in the lateral position, kinetic therapy has a good chance of improving the hypoxemia.

On the other hand, six of ten patients demonstrated an increase in Pao_2 in the lateral position, and five of these six patients had a difference in Pao_2 between the lateral positions, suggesting asymmetric lung disease. Three of these five patients later demonstrated asymmetric lung disease on serial chest radiographs. In these patients there was no significant difference in oxygenation between rotating and supine positions. However, if these findings are substantiated in a larger series, the Roto Rest may prove to be useful in predicting which patients may develop asymmetric lung disease and in treating hypoxemia resulting from asymmetric lung disease.

The differences in Pao_2 between supine and lateral positions were associated with a change in Qsp/Qt in six of the ten patients. In two patients whose Pao_2 decreased in the lateral position, the decrease was at least partially explained by an increase in $\dot{V}o_2$ rather than changes in the distribution of pulmonary blood flow. In two patients whose Pao_2 increased in the lateral positions, the increase could not be explained by changes in the common determinants of Pao_2: cardiac output, Qsp/Qt, mixed venous oxygen saturation, or $\dot{V}o_2$.

This study has addressed only the immediate, short-term effects of positional therapy on hemodynamics and pulmonary function. Whether or not the effects noted in this study will be substantiated by larger studies and whether the effects on oxygenation will be of lasting clinical or therapeutic significance remains to be seen. It is conceivable that the effects on oxygenation may become more pronounced over time, but it is also possible that these effects may be negated by adaptive physiologic changes or additional pathologic insults.

We express our thanks to the nurses and staff of the SICU for their support in completing this study.

References

1. West JB: *Pulmonary Pathophysiology: The Essential.* Baltimore, Waverly Press, 1977.
2. Ibanez J, Raurich JM, Abizanda R, et al: The effect of lateral positions on gas exchange in patients with unilateral lung disease during mechanical ventilation. *Intensive Care Med* 1981;7:231-234.
3. Zack MB, Pontoppidan H, Kazemi H: The effect of lateral positions on gas exchange in pulmonary disease: A prospective evaluation. *Am Rev Respir Dis* 1974;110:49-55.
4. Nelson LD, Snyder JV: Technical problems with data acquisition, in Snyder JV (ed): *Oxygen Transport in the Critically Ill Patient.* Chicago, Year Book Medical Publishers Inc, 1987, pp 205-234.
5. Katz JD, Barash PG: Positional hypoxemia following post-traumatic pulmonary insufficiency. *Can Anaesth Soc J* 1977;24:346-352.
6. Rivera D, Artucio H, Arcos J, et al: Positional hypoxemia during artificial ventilation. *Crit Care Med* 1984;12:436-438.
7. Hasan FM, Beller TA, Sobonya RE, et al: Effect of positive end-expiratory pressure and body position in unilateral lung injury. *J Appl Physiol* 1982;52:147-154.
8. Schimmel L, Civeta JM, Kirby RR: A new mechanical method to influence pulmonary perfusion in critically ill patients. *Crit Care Med* 1977;5:277-279.

In Other AMA Journals

ARCHIVES OF PATHOLOGY & LABORATORY MEDICINE

The Effect of Digital Rectal Examination on Serum Levels of Prostatic-Specific Antigen

Michael K. Brawer, MD; Ron B. Schifman, MD;
Frederick R. Ahmann, MD; Marie E. Ahmann; Karen M. Coulis

Serum prostate-specific antigen (PSA) and acid phosphatase (AP) levels were measured before and after digital rectal examination in 26 patients with varying genitourinary complaints. Prostate examination had no effect on the level of these markers. However, AP levels demonstrated greater within-day, intraindividual variance than PSA levels. Digital rectal examination does not appear to be a source of preanalytical error for serum PSA or AP determinations (*Arch Pathol Lab Med* 1988;112:1110-1112).

Reprint requests to the Department of Surgery, University of Arizona Health Sciences Center, Tucson, AZ 85724 (Dr Brawer).

Nosocomial Abscess

Results of an Eight-Year Prospective Study of 32 284 Operations

Mary M. Olson, RN, BSN, Melody O'Connor Allen, MD

• This article details the results of 114 abscesses found after 32 284 operations during a 30-day prospective infection surveillance. Abscesses occurred more often after gastric/esophageal (3.6%), colonic/appendiceal (2.8%), and pancreatic/biliary (1.5%) operations. Abscesses were intra-abdominal (58%), pelvic/perineal (31%), and retroperitoneal (3%). The most common pathogens were *Escherichia coli*, enterococci, and *Bacteroides* organisms. Abscess symptoms appeared 10 ± 6 days (mean ± SEM) after surgery and were drained 8 ± 8 days after onset of symptoms. Hospital stay from onset of symptoms to discharge was four times greater than that for wound infection. Twenty-seven patients (28%) died. Mortality was increased in patients older than 50 years and in those with renal failure or multiple abscesses. Nosocomial abscesses had a greater morbidity than wound infection. Excessive expense and high mortality warrant infection surveillance for both wound infection and ongoing nosocomial abscesses.
(*Arch Surg* 1989;124:356-361)

Prospective infection surveillance is an established means of ensuring early identification and treatment of postoperative wound infections.[1-6] Surveillance at our institution resulted in a steady decline in overall wound infection rates with significant reduction in the number of infection-related hospital days and costs.[1] Knowing that the rates of morbidity and mortality of postoperative abscess far exceed those of simple wound infection,[5,7] we undertook to assess the value of infection surveillance as a means of reducing hospital costs related to nosocomial abscess. We describe herein our eight-year experience with prospective surveillance of over 30 000 operations for postoperative abscesses. Clinical factors associated with high risk of death from abscess were sought. The impact of infection surveillance on time to diagnosis and incidence of wound infection and nosocomial abscess were determined by comparing results during each year of surveillance with the year in which surveillance was initiated (1977).

PATIENTS AND METHODS

Data Collection

Postoperative infection surveillance was carried out by one of us (M.M.O.), a nurse epidemiologist, after 32 284 operations performed at the Minneapolis Veterans Administration Medical Center from 1977 to 1985. Patients with wound infections and abscesses were identified during daily visits to surgical wards and by monitoring all culture results. A wound was considered clearly infected if pus discharged from it. Wounds with serous or nonpurulent drainage and negative cultures were considered infected only if significant physical signs of sepsis were present concurrently (warmth, erythema, induration, and pain) and if infection was diagnosed medically. Wounds with cellulitis and no drainage and suture abscesses were not considered as being infected. *Postoperative abscesses* were defined as any circumscribed assemblance of pus defined at operation, during percutaneous drainage, or at autopsy, or when the abscess cavity was clearly demonstrated on contrast roentgenography. Only those abscesses noted within 30 days of initial operation that were *not* present at that operation were included in the study.

Operations were classified as clean, clean-contaminated, or contaminated according to criteria established by the American College of Surgeons.[8] Clinical data were collected regarding the initial and all subsequent operations. Specific data were collected regarding methods of detection, type, and results of treatment of abscesses. *Mortality* was defined as death occurring during this hospital admission. One patient was discharged and readmitted, and death occurred within 30 days of the initial surgery.

Data Analysis

Clinical variables prior to initial operation, operative data, and postoperative course were compared between survivors and nonsurvivors. Comparisons were performed using Student's t test and Fischer's exact test, χ^2 analysis, or comparison of two percentages based on large samples when groups were appropriately large.[9] Results for all years during infection surveillance (1978 through 1984) were compared with those from the first year of surveillance (1977).

Cost Analysis

Costs related to the complication of nosocomial abscess occurring after operation were estimated for each year of the study. Estimates of cost per wound infection were calculated using an average increase of ten hospital days per patient with infection.[2] Estimates of cost per abscess were calculated using an average increase of 44 hospital days per patient based on abscess data obtained from the present study. Minnesota Hospital Association estimates of cost per day were used (estimates published yearly in *Minneapolis Star Tribune*).

RESULTS

Demographic Data

Ninety-seven patients (92 men and two women) developed 114 abscesses during the eight-year study period.

Accepted for publication Nov 4, 1987.
From the Department of Surgery (112), Veterans Administration Medical Center, Minneapolis.
Reprint requests to Department of Surgery (112), Veterans Administration Medical Center, 54th Street and 48th Avenue S, Minneapolis, MN 55417 (Ms Olson).

The majority of abscesses occurred in patients older than 50 years, with a mean (±SEM) age of 60±15 years (Fig 1). Fifty-seven percent of patients had a history of cancer, 24% were alcoholic, 17% were diabetic, and 8% had undergone either radiotherapy or chemotherapy. At the time of initial operation, four patients had respiratory failure, 12 had renal failure, and three had shock.

Initial Operation

The median duration of hospitalization prior to initial operation was ten days, with a range from zero to 71 days. Ninety percent (87/97) of patients received preoperative antibiotics. Of these patients, 68% received a cephalosporin within four hours of operation, while the remaining patients received oral neomycin sulfate plus erythromycin stearate (36%), an aminoglycoside (29%), ampicillin sodium (13%), or clindamycin phosphate (13%). The largest number of abscesses occurred on the general surgery services (71 of 97). Nearly one third of all abscesses occurred after colonic or rectal surgery, followed next in frequency by gastric, pancreatic/biliary, and urologic surgery (Fig 2).

Ten percent of operations in 97 patients who developed nosocomial abscess were classified as clean, 57% as clean-contaminated, and 33% as contaminated. The majority of operations were elective (78%). Wound closure following operation was primary in 88% of patients. Drains were inserted in 26 of 97 patients at the initial operation.

The number of wound infections and abscesses in different wound classes were compared (Table 1). The highest incidence of abscess formation (1.0%) comprised 32 of 3251 operations in the contaminated classification.

Infectious Complications Other Than Abscess After Initial Operation

Infectious complications other than abscess occurred in 56 of 97 patients. In 38 patients, this "other site" infection had the same pathogen as the abscess. The most common type of infection was bacteremia (24%). Eleven patients (11%) had wound infections compared with an overall wound infection rate of 2.5% in 32284 patients who underwent operations during the study period. Wound dehiscence occurred in 10% of patients with abscess, the median day of dehiscence being postoperative day 6 (range, three to 12 days). Pneumonia and urinary tract infection occurred in 11% of patients.

Abscess Data

The majority of abscesses were located in the abdominal cavity (58%), with 31% in the perineum or pelvis and 3% in the retroperitoneum (Table 2). The median time from initial operation to clinical presentation of all 114 abscesses was eight days (range, three to 29 days). The incidence of wound infection and nosocomial abscess by type of operation was calculated for the eight-year study period (Table 3). Signs and symptoms of abscess formation included a white blood cell count greater than 10×10^9/L (81%), a temperature greater than 37.8°C (78%), localized pain and tenderness (61%), ileus (38%), diarrhea (33%), abdominal distention (27%), nausea and vomiting (23%), bacteremia (24%), confusion (13%), palpable mass (8%), and shock (7%). *Bacteroides* bacteremia occurred in 13 patients. Renal failure following surgery was present in 13% and respiratory failure in 10% of patients. Radiographic data obtained in patients with abscess were presented as the number of abnormal findings (ie, diagnostic of abscess) out of the total number of studies performed on the 97 patients (Table 4).

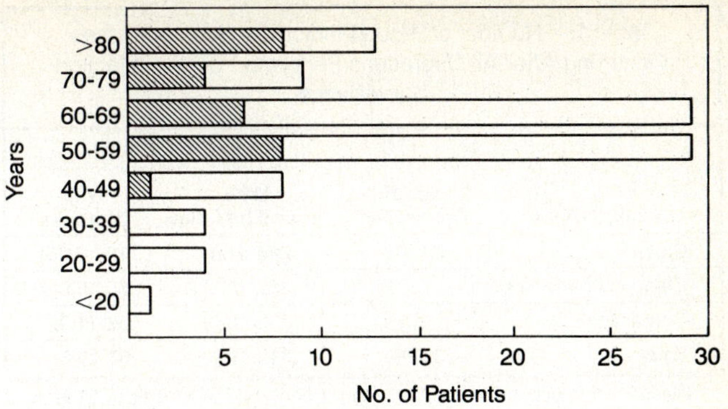

Fig 1.—Number of nosocomial abscesses by decade of life in 97 patients. Shaded bars indicate deaths.

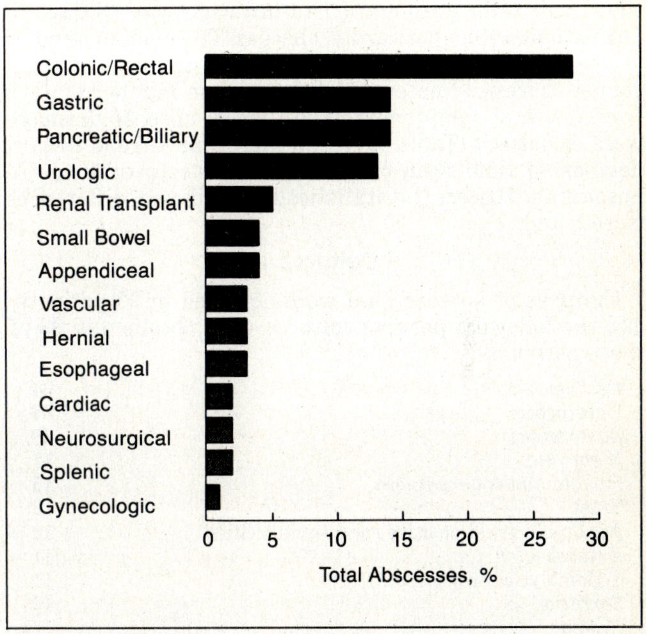

Fig 2.—Distribution of abscesses by type of operation in 97 patients.

Ninety patients underwent drainage of abscess. Twenty-nine of the patients whose abscesses required drainage had anastomotic leaks. Three patients had small abscesses adjacent to an anastomotic leak; these abscesses were not drained. Four patients died before drainage could be performed. Seventy-three patients had one operation for drainage, 11 patients had two operations, five patients had three operations, and one patient had four operations. Percutaneous computed tomographic (CT)–guided abscess drainage was the primary procedure performed in three patients. One patient first underwent operative drainage and then repeated drainage via the percutaneous method. All patients were treated with antibiotics, which were given from two to 110 days (median, 16 days) after clinical presentation of abscess. Eighty-eight percent of patients received an aminoglycoside, while 55% received ampicillin and clindamycin, and 49% received cephalosporin. "Triple antibiotics" (ampicillin, clindamycin, and aminoglycoside) were used in 34 of the 97 patients.

The median time from presentation of abscess symptoms to drainage was four days (range, zero to 43 days). Drainage was performed from four to 50 days (median, 14 days) after the initial operation. Of the 90 patients in whom abscesses were drained, nine patients underwent the drainage pro-

Table 1.—Number of Wound Infections and Abscesses Occurring After All Operations Performed During Infection Surveillance

		No. (%) of Patients	
Wound Class*	No. of Operations	With Wound Infection	With Abscess
Clean	20162	280 (1.4)	10 (0.05)
Clean-contaminated	8871	252 (2.8)	55 (0.6)
Contaminated	3251	278 (8.6)	32 (1.0)
Total	**32284**	**810** (2.5)	**97** (0.3)

*Classification according to criteria established by the American College of Surgeons.[8]

cedure on the same day as clinical presentation. The longest time span from presentation to drainage was 43 days in one patient with a pericardial abscess. The median number of hospital days from original operation to onset of nosocomial abscess symptoms and the median number of days from onset of symptoms to the time of abscess drainage were calculated (Table 5). While there was a trend toward decreasing time from onset of symptoms to drainage of nosocomial abscess, no statistically significant differences were noted.

Cultures

Cultures of abscess fluid were obtained in 90 patients, and the following positive cultures were obtained in 88 of these patients:

Escherichia coli	34
Enterococci	34
Bacteroides	28
Klebsiella	17
Pseudomonas aeruginosa	15
Yeast	13
Anaerobic gram-positive cocci (unidentified)	12
Enterobacter	11
α-Hemolytic streptococci	11
Serratia	10
Proteus	7
Clostridium perfringens	5
Staphylococcus epidermidis	4
Clostridium species	4
Citrobacter	4
β-Hemolytic streptococci	3
Fusobacterium	2
Anaerobic gram-positive bacilli (unidentified)	1
Anaerobic gram-negative bacilli (unidentified)	1
Eubacterium	1
Acinetobacter anitratum	1
Neisseria	1
S aureus	1

The most common pathogens were *E coli*, enterococci, and *Bacteroides* organisms. In the 24 patients who had a single pathogen in pure culture, *E coli* and *P aeruginosa* were found most often. *Staphylococcus epidermidis*, α-hemolytic streptococci, and diptheroids were not considered pathogens unless they were found in pure culture.[10] Fifty-eight percent of abscesses contained only aerobes, while 9% contained only anaerobes and 33% contained a mixture of both types (Fig 3). Pathogens were sensitive to preoperative antibiotics in 50% of cases. Pathogens resistant to all aminoglycosides except amikacin sulfate were present in 9% of cultures.

Mortality

Twenty-seven (28%) of 97 patients died. The vast majority of deaths occurred in patients older than 50 years (Fig 1). Total hospital stay until death ranged from 11 to 212 days (median, 34 days). Time from drainage to death ranged from one to 160 days (median, ten days). The most common cause of death was sepsis (21 of 27 patients). Each of the remaining six deaths was due to cardiac arrest, pulmonary embolus, cancer, thrombosis of the superior mesenteric artery, massive gastrointestinal tract bleeding, or an unknown cause. Persistent abscesses were present in 11 (41%) of 13 patients at autopsy. New abscesses were found in two patients who died.

Evaluation of *preoperative clinical data* showed that prolonged prothrombin time (>13 s), renal failure, and age greater than 50 years were more common in patients who died ($P<.01$). Alcoholism, diabetes, cancer, radiation treatment, shock, respiratory failure, and abnormal values of white blood cell count ($>10\times10^9$/L), bilirubin (>21 μmol/L), albumin (<30 g/L), and hemoglobin (<75 g/L) were not common variables in patients who died. Evaluation of *operative data* failed to reveal any variable that was more common among patients who died. The variables studied included blood loss of greater than 2000/cm^3, emergent operation, gross fecal soilage, unprepared bowel, and duration of operation of greater than four hours.

Table 2.—Anatomic Location of 114 Nosocomial Abscesses

Location	No. of Abscesses
Abdomen	
Abdominal	30*
Subphrenic	24
Subhepatic	11
Hepatic	1
Total (%)	**66** (58)
Pelvis/perineum	
Pelvic	27
Pouch of Douglas	1
Rectal	2
Perineal	5
Total (%)	**35** (31)
Retroperitoneum	
Retroperitoneal	1
Perinephric	1
Peripancreatic	1
Total (%)	**3** (3)
Other	
Cranial	1
Pericardial	2
Neck	1
Prostate	1
Groin	1
Abdominal wall	1
Corpus cavernosum	1
Retropharyngeal	1
Subcutaneous	1
Total (%)	**10** (9)

*Exact location of abscess was not specified by the surgeon.

Table 3.—Comparison of Overall Wound Infection Rate With Abscess Rate

	Rate, (%)	
Type of Operation	Wound Infection	Abscess
Pancreatic	5.5	6.0
Esophageal	12.5	5.0
Colonic	5.0	3.0
Gastric	6.0	3.0
Appendiceal	6.5	2.0
Biliary tract	2.5	0.8
Hernial	1.0	0.1

Table 4.—Accuracy of Radiographic Tests in Diagnosis of Nosocomial Abscesses*

Location of Abscess	No. of Cases in Which Abscess Was Diagnosed/Total Studies Performed: Plain Abdominal X-ray Film	CT Scan	Echogram	Barium Contrast Enema	Gallium Scan	UGI Series	IVP	Sinogram	T-Tube Cholangiogram	Lateral Neck X-ray Film
Abdomen										
Abdominal	19/35	5/7	3/5	3/11	7/10	4/7	...	2/2	0/1	...
Subphrenic	17/29	3/3	3/6	2/2	5/6	4/8	...	...	1/1	...
Subhepatic	6/15	3/4	1/1	2/2	1/2	0/1	...	...	...	...
Hepatic	0/2	...	0/1	...	1/1	...	...	...	...	...
Pelvis/perineum										
Pelvic	16/29	15/16	2/5	5/6	4/7	1/1	7/7	1/1	...	...
Rectal	0/2	2/2	0/1	...	...	...	...	1/1	...	...
Perineal	0/2	1/1	0/1	2/2	...	...	...	...	...	...
Retroperitoneum										
Retroperitoneal	0/1	...	...	...	...	...	...	...	...	...
Perinephric	0/1	...	1/1	...	...	...	1/1	...	...	...
Peripancreatic	...	1/1	1/1	...	...	...	...	...	...	...
Other										
Cranial	...	1/1	...	...	...	...	...	...	...	...
Pericardial	...	1/1	...	...	...	...	...	...	...	...
Neck	...	...	...	...	...	2/2	...	...	...	...
Corpus cavernosum	0/1	...	...	...	...	...	...	...	...	...
Retropharyngeal	...	...	...	...	...	...	...	...	...	2/2
Subcutaneous	...	0/1	...	...	...	...	...	...	...	...
Total (%)	**58/117** (50)	**32/37** (87)	**11/22** (50)	**14/23** (61)	**18/26** (69)	**11/19** (58)	**8/8** (100)	**4/4** (100)	**1/2** (50)	**2/2** (100)

*Thirteen patients had findings counted more than once, eg, one computed tomographic scan positive for two abscesses (subphrenic and subhepatic). CT indicates computed tomographic; UGI, upper gastrointestinal tract; and IVP, intravenous pyelogram.

Table 5.—Time to Diagnosis and Treatment of Abscess*

	Median Hospital Days: 1977 (n=18)†	1978 (n=20)	1979 (n=13)	1980 (n=14)	1981 (n=7)	1982 (n=3)	1983 (n=12)	1984 (n=10)
Original operation to onset of symptoms	7	7	9	5	11	7	7	10
Onset of symptoms to abscess drainage	6	3	4	4	4	3	6	1

*Values in parentheses indicate number of patients with abscesses.
†First year of institution of prospective infection surveillance.

In the *postoperative data*, multiple abscess, renal and respiratory failure, urinary tract and respiratory tract infection, and peritonitis were more common in patients who died ($P<.05$). Factors not significantly different between survivors and nonsurvivors were bacteremia, wound infection or dehiscence, number of drainage procedures, number of days from onset of symptoms to drainage, and recurrent abscess.

Cost Analysis

A significant decline in incidence of wound infection during the seven-year period of infection surveillance was noted when compared with the 1977 incidence (Table 6). While the incidence of nosocomial abscess formation was less than or equal to the 1977 incidence in six of seven years of infection surveillance, the incidence of nosocomial abscess was significantly lower ($P<.01$) compared with that of the first year of surveillance in only one of the years studied (1982). The mean (±SEM) time from onset of abscess symptoms to discharge was 44±32 days.

The cost related to abscess was also evaluated (Table 7). Data were calculated on the assumption that all hospital days subsequent to onset of symptoms of abscess were complication related. Cost per abscess was $13 354, while the minimal cost per patient for wound infection was $3085.[1] The number of abscesses (97) was one eighth that of wound infections (810), but the cost was at least one half less ($1 295 316 vs $2 498 750).

COMMENT

Classic articles dealing with the subject of abscess combine results of patients having primary abscess with those of patients who develop abscesses after surgical procedures, ie, nosocomial abscesses.[5,11,12] Authors quote overall mortalities from 20% to 40%, noting that patients with postoperative abscess frequently require multiple operations, have prolonged hospital stays, and have the highest risk of death. In a five-year prospective study, Krukowski et al[13] described a 0.8% incidence of intra-abdominal sepsis after abdominal operation but made no comment as to mortality or morbidity specific to that complication. The purpose of the present study was to

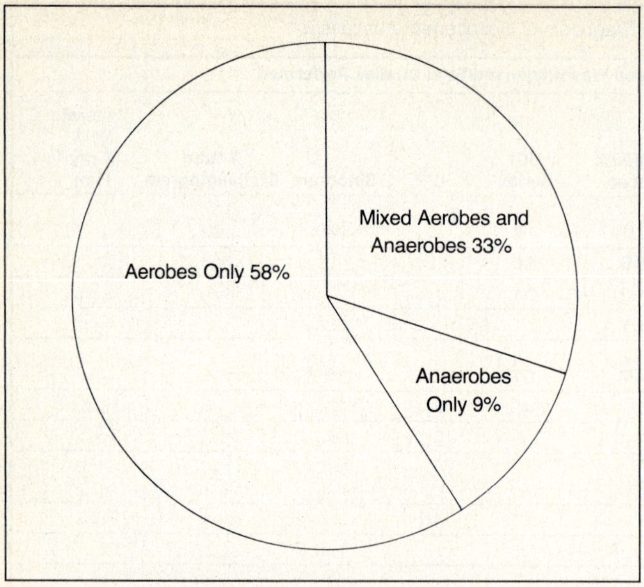

Fig 3.—Types of organisms in abscess culture.

describe morbidity and mortality of nosocomial abscesses and to assess the value of prospective infection surveillance as a means of minimizing the incidence of this complication.

One hundred fourteen nosocomial abscesses were detected in 97 patients during an eight-year period of prospective infection surveillance after 32 284 operations. Abscesses occurred most frequently in elderly patients with multiple medical problems. The highest incidence of nosocomial abscess was in patients with contaminated operations (1%). It is pertinent to note that our method of classification includes "dirty" class IV operations[8] in the contaminated classification. Our results compare favorably with those of Krukowski et al,[13] who reported a rate of 3.8% for patients with either contaminated or dirty operations.

The majority of nosocomial abscesses were located in the abdominal cavity or pelvis (89%), while only 3% were located in the retroperitoneum. Our data are consistent with those of Hinsdale and Jaffe,[14] who described 87 patients who underwent reoperations for abdominal sepsis; the authors found that 45 of 47 nosocomial abscesses were intraperitoneal. Our results differ from studies that include primary abscesses, in which nearly one third of abscesses were located in the retroperitoneum.[12] The majority of nosocomial abscesses occur after operations on the gastrointestinal tract.[13,15,16] In our study the highest rate of abscess occurred after pancreatic operations (6%), followed by esophageal (5%), colonic (3%), and gastric (3%) operations.

The diagnosis of nosocomial abscess was made using a combination of clinical (leukocytosis, fever, and pain) and radiologic findings. The most accurate radiologic tests for diagnosing abdominal abscesses were CT (79%) and gallium (74%) scanning. When a draining sinus tract was present, the sinogram was uniformly successful in diagnosing abscess. As in other studies, CT scanning was the most useful diagnostic test for pelvic and perineal abscesses.[16-18] These data are consistent with those of Saini et al,[16] who described a 92% diagnostic accuracy with CT scanning, 77% with ultrasonography, and 75% with gallium scanning in a series of 100 consecutive abscesses.

Ninety of 97 patients in our study underwent operative drainage of abscess; of these patients 17 required more than one drainage procedure. Percutaneous CT–guided drainage was used as the primary procedure in only three patients. Several recent articles have demonstrated excellent results with percutaneous drainage of single, uncomplicated abscesses.[19-21] We anticipate more frequent use of this technique in carefully selected cases.

Death occurred in 28% of our patients, most often due to continued sepsis. Mortality was significantly associated with age greater than 50 years, preoperative renal failure or prolonged prothrombin time, multiple abscesses, postoperative renal or respiratory failure, postoperative peritonitis, and urinary or respiratory tract infection ($P<.05$). These findings are consistent with those of other authors who have found increasing age, delay in diagnosis, organ failure, generalized peritonitis, and multiple or recurrent abscess to be highly associated with mortality.[5,14-16]

The high cost of surgical complications has been well documented.[22-24] In a one-year prospective survey to identify adverse outcomes of surgery, Couch et al[22] determined a cost of nearly $50 000 per patient in whom significant mishap occurred. They concluded that continuous monitoring of surgical results would help to identify the prevalence of avoidable complications and to potentially minimize their incidence. In our institution, prospective infection surveillance clearly correlated with early detection and a steady decline in yearly incidence of wound infection during the eight-year study period. During the same period, however,

Table 6.—Overall Incidence of Wound Infection and Abscess

Year	No. of Operations	Incidence, % (% of Change)*: Wound Infection	Abscess
1977	4476	4.2 . . .	0.4 . . .
1978	4335	2.8 (↓33)	0.5 (↑25)
1979	3969	2.4 (↓43)	0.4 . . .
1980	3808	2.7 (↓36)	0.3 (↓25)
1981	3624	1.9 (↓56)	0.2 (↓50)
1982	3898	1.8 (↓57)	0.08 (↓80)
1983	3914	1.8 (↓57)	0.3 (↓25)
1984	4260	2.2 (↓48)	0.3 (↓25)

*Descending arrows indicate percent decrease in incidence of either wound infection or abscess compared with incidence in 1977 (year surveillance was initiated); ascending arrow, percent increase in incidence.

Table 7.—Dollar Cost Over Eight Years

Year	No. of Patients With Abscesses	Additional Hospital Days*	Cost/d, $†	Total Cost, $
1977	18	792	171	135 432
1978	20	880	185	162 800
1979	13	572	257	147 004
1980	14	616	292	179 872
1981	7	308	365	112 420
1982	3	132	403	53 196
1983	12	528	489	258 192
1984	10	440	560	246 400
. . .	. . .	. . .	. . .	**1 295 316**

*Average hospitalization from onset of abscess symptoms to discharge was 44 days.

†Cost per day in a Minneapolis–St Paul hospital, as estimated by the Minnesota Hospital Association Estimators.

there was no significant decrease in occurrence or time to diagnosis of nosocomial abscess. We feel that the decline in wound infection rates was related not only to institution of infection surveillance, but also to several improvements in operative procedures made during the period.[1] Notably, better bowel preparation technique for colonic surgery and modification in choice of perioperative antibiotics, suggested by the work of Condon et al,[25] contributed to diminished wound infection rates. Our failure to note a concomitant decline in incidence of nosocomial abscess in these patients suggests that technical factors related to anastomotic healing are critical determinants in the development of this postoperative complication.

Nosocomial abscess significantly lengthened hospital stay, resulting in the need for operative drainage in the majority of patients, and led to abscess-related hospital costs of over $1 million. While infection surveillance by a nurse epidemiologist failed to significantly shorten time to diagnosis or time from onset of symptoms to abscess drainage, we feel that such surveillance helps to identify adverse institutional trends and lapses in technique that might otherwise go unnoticed. Most important, the surgeon must recognize that the signs and symptoms of nosocomial abscess are often subtle. A high level of suspicion must be maintained in high-risk patients to identify and to treat nosocomial abscess as rapidly as possible.

References

1. Olson M, O'Connor MJ, Schwartz ML: A five-year prospective study of 20193 wounds at the Minneapolis VA Medical Center. *Ann Surg* 1984;199:253-259.
2. Cruse PJE, Foord R: The epidemiology of wound infection: A ten-year prospective study of 62939 wounds. *Surg Clin North Am* 1980;60:27-40.
3. Garner JS: *Guideline for Prevention of Surgical Wound Infections,* publication 99-2381. Atlanta, Centers for Disease Control, 1985.
4. Centers for Disease Control: Nosocomial infection surveillance, 1983. *CDC Surveillance Summaries* 1984;33(No. 2SS):9SS-21SS.
5. Fry DE, Garrison RN, Heithsch RC, et al: Determinants of death in patients with intra-abdominal abscess. *Surgery* 1980:88:517-523.
6. Condon RE, Schulte WT, Malangoni MD, et al: Effectiveness of a surgical wound surveillance program. *Arch Surg* 1983;118:303-307.
7. Pitcher WD, Musher DM: Critical importance of early diagnosis and treatment of intra-abdominal infection. *Arch Surg* 1982;117:328-333.
8. American College of Surgeons Committee on Control of Surgical Infections: *Manual on Control of Infection in Surgical Patients,* ed 2. Philadelphia, JB Lippincott, 1982, pp 27-30.
9. Peavy JV, Dyal WW: *Analytical Statistics,* publication 00-1839. Atlanta, Centers for Disease Control, 1972.
10. *NNIS Site Definitions Manual* (protocol). Atlanta, Centers for Disease Control, 1975, p 71.
11. Ochsner A, Debakey M: Subphrenic abscess: Collective review and analysis of 3608 collected and personal cases. *Surg Gynecol Obstet* 1938;66:426-438.
12. Altemeier WA, Culbertson WR, Fullen WD, et al: Intra-abdominal abscess. *Am J Surg* 1973;125:70-79.
13. Krukowski ZH, Stewart MPM, Alsayer HM: Infection after abdominal surgery: Five-year prospective study. *Br Med J* 1984;288:278-280.
14. Hinsdale JG, Jaffe BM: Reoperation for intra-abdominal sepsis. *Ann Surg* 1984;199:31-36.
15. Doberneck RC, Mittleman J: Reappraisal of the problems of intra-abdominal abscess. *Surg Gynecol Obstet* 1982;154:875-879.
16. Saini S, Kellum JM, O'Leary M, et al: Improved localization and survival in patients with intra-abdominal abscesses. *Am J Surg* 1983;145:136-142.
17. Norwood SH, Civetta JM: Abdominal CT scanning in critically ill surgical patients. *Ann Surg* 1985;202:166-174.
18. Dobrin PB, Gully PH, Greenlee HB, et al: Radiologic diagnosis of intra-abdominal abscess. *Arch Surg* 1986;121:41-46.
19. Gerzof SG, Robbins SG, Johnson AH: Percutaneous catheter drainage of abdominal abscesses: A five-year experience. *N Engl J Med* 1981;305:653-657.
20. Aeder MI, Wellman JL, Haaga JR, et al: Role of surgical and percutaneous drainage in the treatment of abdominal abscesses. *Arch Surg* 1983;118:273-280.
21. Martin EC, Karlson KB, Fankucken EI, et al: Percutaneous drainage of postoperative intra-abdominal abscesses. *AJR* 1982;138:13-15.
22. Couch NP, Tilney NL, Rayner AA, et al: The high cost of low-frequency events. *N Engl J Med* 1981;304:634-637.
23. Mason LB, García AG: Hospital costs of surgical complications. *Arch Surg* 1984;119:1065-1066.
24. Drucker WR, Gavett JW, Kirshner R, et al: Toward strategies for cost containment in surgical patients. *Ann Surg* 1983;198:284-300.
25. Condon RE, Bartlett JG, Greenlee H, et al: Efficacy of oral and systemic antibiotic prophylaxis in colorectal operation. *Arch Surg* 1983;118:496-502.

In Other AMA Journals

ARCHIVES OF INTERNAL MEDICINE

Prevention of Amphotericin B–Induced Renal Impairment: A Review on the Use of Sodium Supplementation

Robert A. Branch, MD

Amphotericin B is the treatment of choice for most deep-seated mycoses; however, doses may have to be limited because of concern over adverse effects such as nephrotoxicity. Evolving evidence suggests that the extent of amphotericin B–induced renal impairment may be modified via alteration of a normal physiologic feedback response that further contributes to changes due to direct nephrotoxicity. As such, renal impairment has a substantial theoretically preventable and reversible element. In animals exposed to amphotericin B, sodium loading interferes with this response. Mounting clinical evidence also supports the usefulness of sodium supplementation to prevent as well as to reverse amphotericin B–induced nephrotoxicity. At this time, the use of sodium supplementation (eg, intravenous saline and/or ticarcillin disodium, which contains 5.2 mEq of sodium per gram of drug) along with avoiding dehydration appears to be a safe and effective means of reducing the risk of nephrotoxicity associated with amphotericin B administration; however, it is not known whether renal changes can be entirely prevented. These preliminary observations merit confirmation in a prospective, randomized clinical trial (*Arch Intern Med* 1988;148:2389-2394).

Reprint requests to Department of Pharmacology, Vanderbilt University School of Medicine, Nashville, TN 37232 (Dr Branch).

Determinants of Urea Nitrogen Production in Sepsis

Muscle Catabolism, Total Parenteral Nutrition, and Hepatic Clearance of Amino Acids

Mauro Pittiruti, MD; John H. Siegel, MD; Gabriele Sganga, MD; Bill Coleman; Charles E. Wiles III, MD; Robert Placko

• The major determinants of urea production were investigated in 26 patients with multiple trauma (300 studies). The body clearances (CLRs) of ten amino acids (AAs) were estimated as a ratio of muscle-released AAs plus total parenteral nutrition–infused AAs to their extracellular pool. While clinically septic trauma (ST) patients without multiple-organ failure syndrome (MOFS) had a higher level of urea nitrogen production (25.6±13.4 g of N per day) compared with nonseptic trauma (NST) patients (14±7.5 g of N per day) and with ST patients with MOFS (4.28±1.5 g of N per day), in all groups urea N production was found to be a function of muscle protein degradation (catabolism), total parenteral nutrition–administered AAs, and the ratio between leucine CLR and tyrosine CLR (L/T) (r^2=.82, *P*<.0001). Since tyrosine is cleared almost exclusively by the liver, the L/T ratio may be regarded as an index of hepatic function. The significant differences between urea N production in ST and NST patients lay in an increased positive dependence on muscle catabolism and increased negative correlation with L/T in the ST group. At any L/T ratio, urea N production was increased in ST patients over NST patients, but in ST patients with MOFS, it fell to or below levels of NST patients. These data show that the ST process is associated with enhancement of ureagenesis, due to increased hepatic CLR of both exogenous and endogenous AAs. In sepsis with MOFS, a marked inhibition of urea synthesis occurs, partially explained by a decreased hepatic CLR of non-branched-chain AAs.
(*Arch Surg* 1989;124:362-372)

The physiologic response to injury is characterized by a net loss of body nitrogen, as evidenced by the increased urinary excretion of N primarily in the form of urea. It has been shown that the main source of this N loss is from the skeletal muscle[1] due to the effect of mediators released in response to injury,[2] to the altered hormonal milieu,[3,4] and to the direct effect of injury on muscle metabolism.[5,6] This muscle proteolysis is associated with an increased release of amino acids (AAs) into the plasma; these AAs appear to be then utilized by liver and other tissues,[7] either for protein synthesis,[8,9] or for oxidative catabolism. However, regardless of the catabolic pathway, the ammonia N is detoxified through synthesis of urea; thus, ureagenesis is increased. When sepsis occurs after major trauma, proteolysis is enhanced in skeletal muscle[7,8] and lipogenesis and gluconeogenesis from the deaminated AAs released are increased in the liver,[10,11] leading to a generalized protein depletion, with a state of acute protein malnutrition.[5] While muscle proteolysis cannot be totally inhibited by the administration of intravenous AA solutions, there is evidence that partial or complete N balance can be achieved.[12] However, a significant portion of the AAs infused will be catabolized in the liver, along with those AAs already available from proteolysis. As a result, there is increased N to be disposed of as urea.

Previous studies of sepsis suggest that as septic severity progresses, there is a relative impairment of hepatic function,[13] which may lead to overt liver failure in the multiple-organ failure syndrome (MOFS). This liver failure is associated with a decrease in clearance (CLR) of those AAs utilized by the liver.[14] When this happens, many of the synthetic processes that occur in the hepatocytes may be compromised, including urea synthesis. The present study is an investigation of the relative influence of muscle protein degradation and the AA CLRs as major determinants of urea production (as estimated by urea N excretion) after multiple trauma, and its modulation by posttraumatic sepsis and septic MOFS with a hepatic component.

PATIENTS AND METHODS

Patients

Urea production, muscle protein degradation (catabolism), and the body CLR of ten AAs were estimated in 26 patients with

Accepted for publication April 12, 1988.
From the Maryland Institute for Emergency Medical Services Systems (MIEMSS) and the Department of Surgery, University of Maryland, Baltimore. Drs Pittiruti and Sganga were MIEMSS Consiglio Nationale de Researche fellows of the Centro di Studio per la Fisiopatologia dello Shock, Università Cattolica, Rome.
Reprint requests to Maryland Institute for Emergency Medical Services Systems, University of Maryland, 22 S Greene St, Baltimore, MD 21201 (Dr Siegel).

Table 1.—Age, Weight, BSA, and ISS[42] in Nonseptic and Septic Posttrauma Patients*

	Mean ± SD	
	Nonseptic Trauma Patients (n = 16)	Septic Trauma Patients (n = 10)
Age, y	30.8 ± 13.5	29 ± 15
Weight, kg	70.5 ± 8.5	73.7 ± 16.6
BSA, m²	1.77 ± .17	1.85 ± .25
ISS	20 ± 10.4	23.3 ± 8.9

*BSA indicates body surface area; ISS, Injury Severity Score.

multiple trauma (300 studies) who were receiving intravenous support without oral intake before and during total parenteral nutrition (TPN). The detailed clinical characteristics of this patient population have been presented previously.[15] All but three of the nonseptic trauma (NST) group and all but two of the septic trauma (ST) group were patients with multiple trauma secondary to motor vehicle accidents. The rest had major single-system injuries. The mean values for the two groups with regard to age, body weight, body surface area, and Injury Severity Score are shown in Table 1. No statistically significant differences could be found between the ST group and the NST group.

Sixteen of the 26 posttrauma patients had clinical courses uncomplicated by any septic episode or by renal failure; two patients in the NST group died (one of brain death and one following a cardiorespiratory arrest). Ten of the 26 posttrauma patients developed clinical sepsis according to the following criteria: (1) intra-abdominal purulent collection, which required drainage; or (2) severe extra-abdominal infection with positive blood cultures and systemic physiologic involvement, as demonstrated by persistent hyperpyrexia and a hyperdynamic cardiovascular response associated with low vascular resistance and increased oxygen consumption typical of the septic A state.[16]

In this group, sepsis developed between days 3 and 8 following injury. In 94% of the cases, it was evident by day 6. Seven of these patients survived the ST process. Three patients died: all of them developed progressive, overwhelming sepsis with MOFS, as defined by evidence of two or more organ failures (lung, liver, kidney, cardiac, or coagulation system), according to the criteria of Faist et al.[17] Using conventional clinical and biochemical criteria, all of these ST patients with MOFS showed some evidence of hepatocellular dysfunction during their clinical course. Renal failure (serum creatinine level, >2 μmol/L) developed late in three ST patients, in two ST nonsurvivors, and in one ST survivor. Studies during renal failure have not been included in the present analysis. All patients were in a state of good health before their injury, with the exception of one patient (a 16-year-old male), who had chronic cystic fibrosis, including cirrhotic changes. This patient underwent a splenectomy for a traumatic splenic rupture in the postinjury period: he became septic and later died of MOFS.

Serial studies of the biochemical and physiologic variables described below were begun on each patient on the day of trauma, or on the first day after trauma, and were continued on an eight-hour basis. All patients were given TPN (10% to 25% glucose solution containing 4.3% AAs). Studies were continued until TPN support was discontinued and oral feeding was started, or until death. During each eight-hour study period, several data were collected simultaneously (plasma and urine levels of AAs, urea, and 3-methylhistidine [3MH]; cardiac output and oxygen consumption by thermodilution and/or indocyanine green dilution; blood gas levels; renal CLR of urea and creatinine; hematologic and coagulation measurements; plasma levels of acute-phase-response proteins; and standard biochemical measurements). The results of the analysis of other aspects of these data are presented in detail in other communications.[14,15]

In the data analysis, the clinical course of each patient, either ST or NST, was divided into two periods: (1) early (less than or equal to five days after injury) and (2) late (more than five days after injury). Since in most patients of the ST group, sepsis became clinically evident between the fourth and sixth days after trauma, "early sepsis" roughly corresponds to the latent, preclinical, or

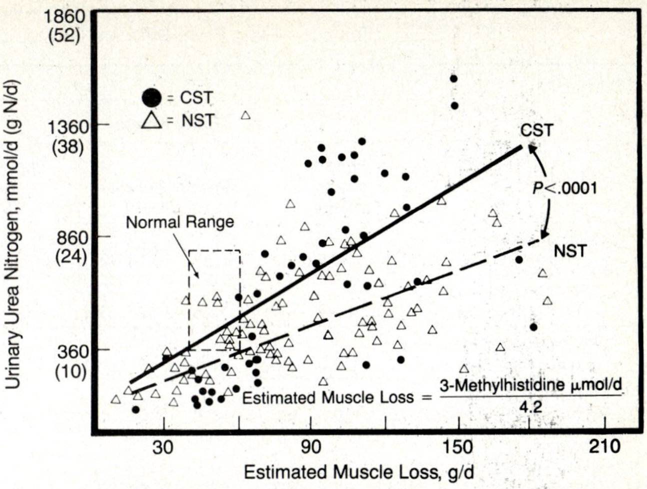

Fig 1.—Dependence of urinary urea nitrogen (N) production on estimated muscle loss in clinically septic trauma (CST) vs nonseptic trauma (NST) patients. **Urinary Urea (g N/d) = 0.111 (Muscle Loss) + 0.073 (Muscle Loss × Sepsis) + 3.48.** n = 166; r^2 = .47; $F(2,163)$ = 72.3; and P<.0001. Range of normal from literature (dotted box). Difference between CST and NST slopes significant by Scheffé S method (P<.0001). Muscle catabolism (grams per day) equals urinary 3-methylhistidine (micromoles per day) divided by 4.2.

very early phase of the ST process, while "late sepsis" identifies the clinically overt ST state. The rationale for this time-related subdivision has also been confirmed by the previous analyses of data collected from this patient population.[15]

Biochemical Methods

The separation and estimation of free AAs in plasma and 3MH in urine was carried out after deproteinization, using an AA analyzer (Beckman 6300). The estimation of urea N, creatinine, and glucose in blood and urine was performed on an analyzer (Beckman Astra-4, Beckman Instruments, Anaheim, Calif).

Urea Production

In our patient population, renal function was normal in all studies considered; urea production was estimated by the measurement of urea N excretion in the urine during each eight-hour study period. The rate of urea excretion may differ from the rate of urea synthesis for several reasons[18]: (1) renal excretion may be impaired due to prerenal causes or to renal disease; (2) a minor proportion of urea may diffuse through the body water compartments, and its excretion may be delayed, especially when sudden changes in the urea synthesis rate take place, but the studies of Long et al[19] with labeled urea indicate that in ST patients, the breakdown and recycling of urea is negligible.

Muscle Protein Degradation (Catabolism)

The amount of skeletal muscle protein degradation during each study period was estimated by the measurement of the urinary excretion of 3MH, according to the method developed by Bilmazes and coworkers.[20] The validity of this assumption has been recently questioned, since experiments performed in the rat show that a significant amount of urinary 3MH may originate from tissues other than the skeletal muscle, such as smooth muscle of the gastrointestinal tract.[21,22] However, the gut origin of a major fraction of 3MH in the rat has been challenged,[23] and the applicability of these rat data to human studies has been recently criticized.[24,25]

The use of the 3MH method to estimate human muscle protein degradation (ie, muscle catabolism) has been shown in other studies on critically ill patients to give results physiologically compatible with data obtained with more invasive techniques.[26] Also, in the human, no more than 60 μmol/d of the urinary 3MH appear to be of nonskeletal muscle origin[27] (or <15% of our mean

Table 2.—Data From Different Groups of Patients, Early and Late in Clinical Course*

	Mean ± SD					
	Early Phase			Late Phase		
	Nonseptic Trauma Patients	Septic Trauma Survivors	Septic Trauma Deaths (MOFS)	Nonseptic Trauma Patients	Septic Trauma Survivors	Septic Trauma Deaths (MOFS)
Muscle protein degradation, g/d	79.56 ± 36.52 (67)	98.26 ± 39.75 (27)	67.77 ± 10.66 (4)	62.01 ± 33.4 (23)	98.05† ± 40 (40)	39.86‡ ± 16 (8)
Urea nitrogen production, g/d	11.8 ± 5.44 (97)	14.6 ± 8.92 (54)	8.99 ± 2.36 (7)	14 ± 7.5 (41)	25.65§ ± 13.45 (71)	4.28‖¶ ± 1.5 (16)
Intravenous amino acid intake, g/d	43.2 ± 16.3 (26)	49.5 ± 26.5 (32)	30.3 ± 20.2 (10)	65.8 ± 26.7 (31)	102§ ± 34 (36)	42.8‖¶ ± 13.4 (32)
Plasma glucose, mg/dL	133.8 ± 30 (80)	142.9 ± 44.5 (52)	166.9† ± 66.5 (15)	121.5 ± 17 (35)	182.4† ± 62.4 (77)	192.8† ± 71.1 (27)
Oxygen consumption, mL/min/m²	183.5 ± 42.5 (27)	199.4 ± 44.6 (30)	179.4 ± 23.8 (8)	176.5 ± 38.1 (12)	230.8† ± 49.3 (47)	205.7 ± 29.5 (15)
Cardiac index, L/min/m²	5.20 ± 1.38 (30)	5.53 ± 1.11 (35)	4.15‡ ± .65 (9)	4.08 ± .73 (13)	5.44¶ ± 1.20 (55)	4.90 ± 1.72 (16)
Total peripheral resistance, dyne × s × cm^{-5}	916 ± 370 (30)	723.8 ± 197.5 (35)	839 ± 141.8 (9)	976.5 ± 211.4 (13)	818.5 ± 350.8 (55)	721.3 ± 193.5 (16)
Body temperature, °C	37.84 ± 0.66 (67)	38.03 ± 0.91 (50)	38.56¶ ± 0.41 (15)	37.66 ± 0.69 (40)	38.14¶ ± 0.80 (68)	38.20 ± 0.49 (14)
White blood cell count (× 10⁹/L)	9.33 ± 3.84 (83)	7.34 ± 2.91 (49)	5.78†‡ ± 1.28 (13)	12.87 ± 2.53 (32)	16.43† ± 5.21 (80)	18.69† ± 6.68 (25)

*Number of observations in parentheses throughout. Statistical significances simultaneously tested by Scheffé S method for early phase (less than five days) and late phase (more than five days) after trauma.
†Differences vs nonseptic trauma patients ($P<.005$).
‡Differences between septic trauma survivors vs septic trauma deaths ($P<.05$).
§Differences vs nonseptic trauma patients ($P<.0001$).
‖Differences between septic trauma survivors vs septic trauma deaths ($P<.005$).
¶Differences vs nonseptic trauma patients ($P<.05$).

total of 413 μmol/d in ST patients). Even if the proportion of 3MH coming from nonskeletal muscle was quantitatively of importance, this would not interfere with the main objective of our study, which is to correlate the amount of AA released from muscle protein degradation to the rate of urea synthesis. Since actin and myosin in skeletal muscle and smooth muscle have comparable AA compositions,[28] we can expect the same qualitative uptake of plasma AAs by the liver, independently of the type of muscle from which they were released.

AA CLR

The body CLR of ten AAs (leucine, isoleucine, valine, alanine [ALA], methionine, proline, phenylalanine, tyrosine, asparagine plus aspartate, and glutamine plus glutamate [GLUT]) was estimated as a ratio of muscle-released AAs plus TPN-infused AA to the size of their extracellular pool, estimated from the plasma AA levels, according to the method that has been previously presented.[14] This computation of AA CLR is an estimate of the total-body CLR, which differs from the estimate proposed by Clowes et al,[7,12] which relies on the leg arteriovenous difference of AA multiplied by the estimated ratio of leg blood flow to total cardiac output. Nevertheless, the striking finding of these data is that there is virtually no difference in the estimated magnitude of effect, or in the nature of the responses, where they can be compared, between our data[14] and those of Loda et al[29] and Clowes and his associates.[30]

Statistical Methods

Statistical analyses were by means of linear regression analysis, and interpretation was as previously outlined.[31] The Scheffé S method[32] was used to test simultaneously the significance of any differences between regression coefficients and the differences between the pairs of regression coefficients characterizing the ST and NST groups.

The bar diagrams shown in the two figures illustrate the working out of such equations for a "typical" patient who just happened to have all of the average values for his group of each of the independent variables. The quantity of the dependent variable predicted by the regression would be the sum, as indicated by the bars, of the regression coefficients for each significant independent variable relationship times the corresponding mean values for that variable. This effectively converts the mean value of each independent variable into proportionate units of the dependent variable and thus allows a direct visual comparison of the magnitude and direction of each effect. All formulas and procedures were as described by Seber.[32]

RESULTS

Considering data obtained from the entire course in the critical care unit (Fig 1), both NST and clinically ST patients showed increased muscle protein degradation (estimated from urinary 3MH excretion) and increased urinary urea production compared with the normal range. However, as also shown in Fig 1, the rate of urea production per gram of estimated muscle protein loss was significantly higher ($P<.0001$) by the Scheffé S method in the patients who became clinically septic.

The interpretation of this increased muscle protein degradation and increased urea production in the ST survivors is not immediately clear, since compared with the NST patients, the surviving ST patients (but not the ST MOFS deaths) received significantly higher levels of TPN-administered AAs due to their increased hyperdynamic, hypermetabolic state with increased cardiac output, oxygen consumption, and temperature (Table 2). However, in the ST patients with MOFS, excessive hyperglycemia and circulatory intolerance to large fluid volumes forced a reduction in the magnitude of TPN support (Table 2). The

Table 3.—Plasma Levels of Ten Amino Acids in Different Groups of Patients, Early and Late in Clinical Course*

	Mean ± SD						
	Early Phase				Late Phase		
	Nonseptic Trauma Patients No AA (83)	Nonseptic Trauma Patients (22)	Septic Trauma Survivors (15)	Septic Trauma Deaths (MOFS) (8)	Nonseptic Trauma Patients (32)	Septic Trauma Survivors (95)	Septic Trauma Deaths (MOFS) (45)
Alanine, μmol/L	90.72 ± 35.28	86.86 ± 20.97	115.9† ± 31.93	117.8 ± 25.56	115.8 ± 31.24	180.2† ± 58.02	231.7‡ ± 197.4
Asparagine, μmol/L	25.65 ± 11.19	31.40 ± 18.82	28.05 ± 9.525	42.13 ± 10.76	20.84 ± 7.278	32.58 ± 13.09	67.31§‖ ± 85.30
Glutamine, μmol/L	174.1 ± 46.19	170.8 ± 40.07	190.5 ± 66.34	169.0 ± 39.39	201.7 ± 27.13	253.1 ± 53.43	322.0§¶ ± 257.0
Proline, μmol/L	46.44 ± 20.59	42.43 ± 17.15	54.87† ± 25.77	62.63 ± 16.68	69.50 ± 18.30	119.3 ± 64.43	147.6§ ± 154.0
Isoleucine, μmol/L	22.86 ± 10.53	23.99 ± 9.42	26.03 ± 8.32	14.50¶ ± 4.50	24.40 ± 9.94	33.70† ± 11.24	30.98 ± 17.88
Leucine, μmol/L	63.29 ± 19.27	58.98 ± 24.69	75.88 ± 19.29	56.75 ± 7.166	65.12 ± 16.96	75.49 ± 16.60	68.35 ± 30.86
Valine, μmol/L	102.7 ± 29.55	101.3 ± 47.14	155.2† ± 44.63	107.6 ± 14.15	117.6 ± 30.22	150.4‡ ± 30.53	114.0# ± 39.62
Methionine, μmol/L	9.2 ± 2.9	12.14 ± 4.38	14.49 ± 6.25	9.250 ± 4.20	18.72 ± 5.81	27.68 ± 10.83	55.64‡# ± 53.19
Phenylalanine, μmol/L	35.72 ± 8.0	37.75 ± 6.889	54.29§ ± 15.08	54.00† ± 10.58	55.89 ± 14.62	82.03§ ± 24.34	93.80‡ ± 42.69
Tyrosine, μmol/L	28.21 ± 6.05	22.22 ± 6.54	34.93§ ± 14.62	32.88 ± 5.94	34.76 ± 5.12	39.36 ± 11.85	56.57‡# ± 26.26

*Mean ± SD. Number of observations in parentheses. All studies during amino acid (AA) total parenteral nutrition (TPN) infusion, except for those labeled No AA, which received glucose only. Patient values for No AA obtained within three days of initial traumatic injury and before initiation of AA TPN. Statistical significances simultaneously tested by Scheffé S method for early phase (less than five days) and late phase (more than five days) after trauma.
†Differences vs receiving AA TPN in nonseptic trauma patients ($P<.05$).
‡Differences vs receiving AA TPN in nonseptic trauma patients ($P<.0001$).
§Differences vs receiving AA TPN in nonseptic trauma patients ($P<.005$).
‖Differences of septic trauma survivors vs septic trauma deaths ($P<.005$).
¶Differences of septic trauma survivors vs septic trauma deaths ($P<.05$).
#Differences of septic trauma survivors vs septic trauma deaths ($P<.0001$).

present multivariable analysis was undertaken to sort out the relative influence of all these factors (muscle proteolytic catabolism with endogenous AA release, TPN-administered AAs, and hepatic dysfunction related to development of overt or occult organ failure).

AA Uptake as a Determinant of Urea Production

Table 3 shows the mean and SDs of the plasma levels of each AA studied in the three different groups of patients (NST, ST survivors, and ST deaths) in the early and late phase of the posttrauma response. This table shows that as sepsis progresses, both in time as well as in severity (MOFS), the plasma levels of the neutral, sulfur-containing, and aromatic AAs rise significantly, while the branched-chain AA plasma levels either rise slightly or actually fall in the patients with late MOFS compared with other ST patients.

To investigate the importance of AA metabolism as a source of urea N production in trauma and sepsis, the uptake of each of the ten AAs noted in the "Patients and Methods" section was studied. Figure 2 shows the multiple regression of urea N production from the total uptake of the two AAs that are quantitatively most important for liver gluconeogenesis: ALA and glutamine plus glutamate (GLUT). Urea N production is expressed in this figure in millimoles per hour, to allow a quantitative evaluation of the relationship between ureagenesis and uptake of AAs. (It must be remembered that each millimole of urea represents the N from two amino groups.) It is interesting that while the uptakes of GLUT and ALA do not equal the urea N, they can explain almost 66% of the urea N production variability ($r^2=.655$; $P<.0001$), if the effect of sepsis is considered (Fig 2). This suggests that ureagenesis from other AAs bears a fairly constant relationship to that derived from these two AAs. However, the critical aspect of this analysis is that, for any level of ALA uptake and any level of GLUT uptake greater than 0.5 mmol/h, the presence of sepsis is associated with a significant increase in expected production of urea N ($P<.05$ by the Scheffé S method). This is consistent with the increased urea N production rate per gram of estimated proteolysis shown in Fig 1 and suggests a resetting of the oxidative catabolic machinery in sepsis. Alanine and glutamine (via transamination in the gut to ALA)[33,34] are major gluconeogenic precursors, and as a result, the plasma glucose levels are seen to rise in this group of ST patients. This is shown in Fig 3, where the levels of plasma glucose and the estimated extracellular water (ECW) pool of glucose in ST and NST patients are seen to increase as an inverse function of the glucose input rate (ratio of glucose infusion rate to the plasma glucose level, corrected to estimated ECW pool size) and as a direct function of the ALA uptake. At the lower ranges of glucose uptake and at the higher ranges of alanine uptake, the regression predicts that the ST patients have a larger glucose pool than the NST patients. In a patient with an average ECW (17.2 L), 1 mmol/L of glucose represents a bit more than 1 mg/dl of plasma glucose: thus, the ST patients with very large glucose pools are also very hyperglycemic. These data are consistent with observations that demonstrate a higher rate of ALA gluconeogenesis[35] and a reduced level of glucose oxidation in sepsis[36] so that turnover and pool size increase.[11]

These data (Figs 2 and 3) suggest that the diversion of ALA to gluconeogenesis may be a major source of AA N

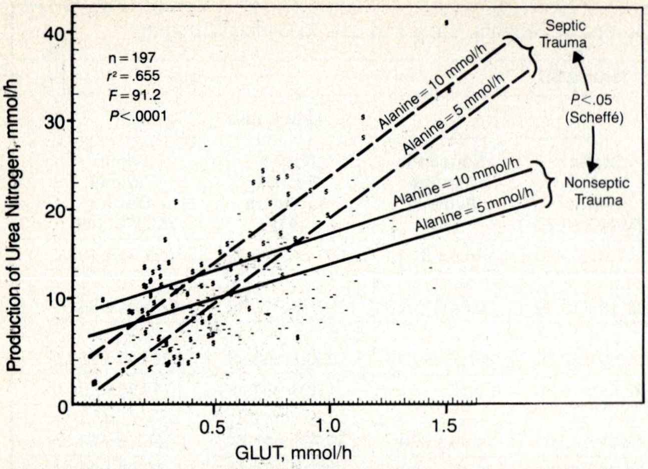

Fig 2.—Dependence of urea nitrogen production on central uptakes of alanine (ALA) and glutamate plus glutamine (GLUT). **Urea N (millimoles per hour) = 0.61 (ALA millimoles per hour) + 7.76 (GLUT millimoles per hour) + 9.26 (GLUT millimoles per hour) × (Sepsis) − 4.39 (Sepsis) + 2.45.** Statistical significance of covariance effect of sepsis was tested by Scheffé S method and showed significant effect ($P<.0001$) both on intercept and on slope. Septic trauma patient points shown by S. Nonseptic trauma patient points by minus sign.

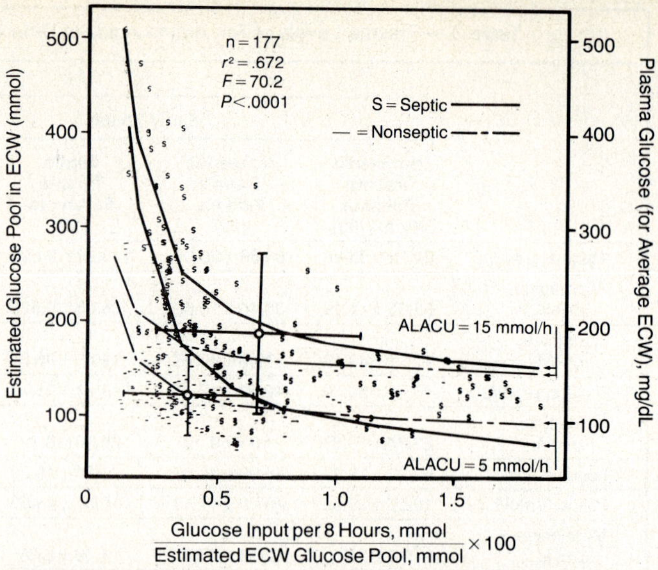

Fig 3.—Prediction in septic trauma (ST) and nonseptic trauma (NST) patients of variability of estimated glucose pool size (total millimoles of glucose in extracellular water [ECW] volume) by the eight-hour glucose input (GLI [in millimoles]) as percent of total estimated ECW pool of glucose (GLECW = mean eight-hour plasma glucose [in millimoles per liter] × estimated ECW [in liters]) and by central uptake of alanine (ALACU [in millimoles per hour]). **Glucose Pool (mmol) = 57.5 (Sepsis) + 4.686 (ALACU) + 3.217 (ALACU) × (Sepsis) + 9.54 / (GLI/GLECW) + 32.72 / (GLI/GLECW) × (Sepsis) + 75.59.** Scale at right shows estimated level of plasma glucose (milligrams per deciliter) corresponding to each value of estimated glucose pool size (millimoles), using mean estimated ECW volume of all patients (17.2 L). Since inputs were quantified on an eight-hour basis, eight-hour glucose input (GLI) is quantity of glucose infusion during each eight-hour period (millimoles) to maintain observed mean level of plasma glucose. Central uptake of alanine (ALACU) is mean quantity per hour of total parenteral nutrition alanine infusion (millimoles per hour) plus estimated quantity of alanine release (millimoles per hour) per gram of muscle protein degradation to maintain observed plasma level of alanine.[14] Estimated glucose pool size was derived from mean plasma glucose level during GLI period times estimated ECW as previously described.[14] Increase in the magnitude of estimated ECW glucose pool in ST over NST for given GLI and ALACU reflects increase in GLECW due to endogenous gluconeogenesis with additional glucose release into pool above that infused and to sepsis mediated reductions in glucose utilization from pool during GLI period. In sepsis GLI/GLECW ratio falls to greater extent than NST because GLECW is increased.

for potential ureagenesis, and that the effect of the increased glucose synthesis is greatest in the sicker ST patients, since proportionately less glucose is being oxidized, so that plasma glucose levels increase. In the ST patients with MOFS studied, this generally resulted in a clinical reduction in the rate of TPN-infused glucose, to reduce the excessive hyperglycemia shown in Fig 3 and in Table 2.

Muscle Catabolism and AA Infusion as Determinants of Urea Production

Figure 4 shows the multiple regression-covariance analysis of the dependence of urea N production on muscle protein degradation, with its presumed release of AAs, and on AA infusion from TPN. In the total patient population (ST and NST), AA infusion and muscle proteolytic catabolism (estimated from 3MH), which are the sources of exogenous and endogenous AAs, respectively, explain 79% of the variability of urea N production ($r^2=.791$, $P<.0001$). However, by the use of the bar diagram technique, in which the mean value of each variable is multiplied by its regression coefficient, the relative effect of each independent variable (catabolism and AA infusion) can be assessed with regard to its effect on urea N production in NST patients and in ST patients. The Scheffé S method,[32] for the simultaneous contrast of all differences, was used to determine the significant differences between these two groups of patients.

Septic trauma patients (including both early and late courses, survivors, and nonsurvivors) have a higher estimated mean value of urea N production (743 mmol/d) than NST patients (439 mmol/d) due to the effect both of the increased AA infusion rate and of the increased muscle protein degradation (ie, increased total supply of AAs). However, despite the increased TPN-AA infusion rate in sepsis, a significant ($P<.05$ by the Scheffé S method) *difference* between ST and NST patients was found in the increased *relative* effect of muscle catabolism on ureagenesis. Counterbalancing this, there is a significant ($P<.01$) *negative* effect of sepsis on the urea N production intercept value, which accounts for the remaining unexplained variability in urea production. This seems to be associated with the septic insult itself, and will be partially explained when Fig 7 is discussed below.

In summary, in sepsis, the actual value of urea N production is the result of the interaction of the positive effect of TPN-AA infusion and of the increased muscle catabolism, but the significant increment due to sepsis appears to be correlated with the sepsis-enhanced proteolysis. However, there is also a negative *additional* effect due to sepsis. There appears to be no difference in the regressions testing this effect of sepsis if only ST survivors or ST deaths are considered, with the difference in urea N production being explainable by differences in the above independent variables.

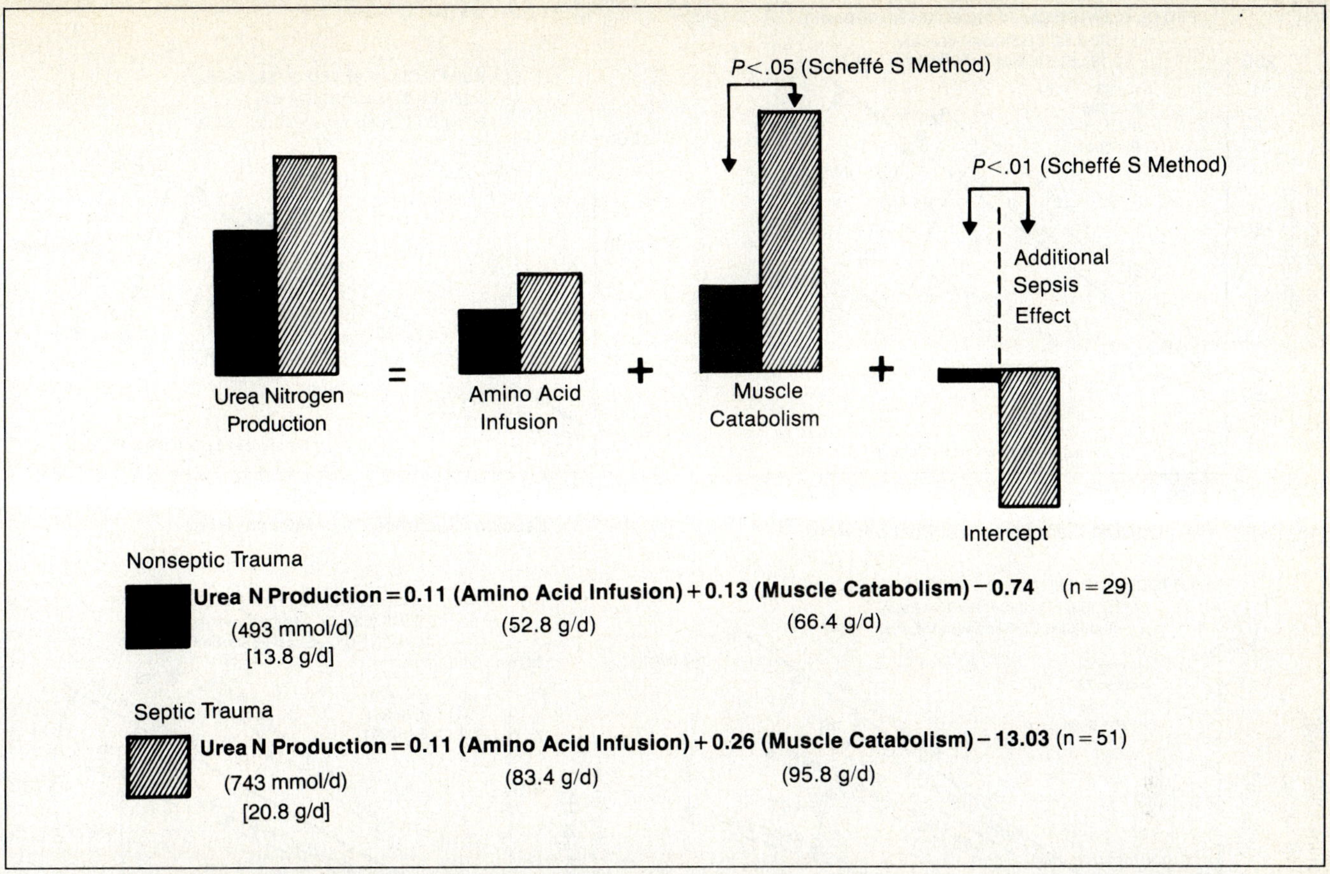

Fig 4.—Relative dependence of urea nitrogen (N) production (mean value estimated from regression) on amino acid infusion and muscle catabolism, in septic trauma and nonseptic trauma patients. See "Statistical Methods" section for explanation of bar graph. All regression coefficients were obtained from multiple regression covariance analysis: n = 80; $r^2 = .791$; $F(4,75) = 70.8$; and $P < .0001$. Covariance differences between septic trauma and nonseptic trauma tested by Scheffé S method.

Effect of Differential AA CLRs on Urea Production

To analyze further the additional negative effect of sepsis on urea N production demonstrated in Fig 4, the relative CLRs of each of the AAs studied were compared with the CLR of leucine. This was done because earlier studies[14] suggested that the leucine/tyrosine CLR ratio (L/T ratio) obtained at a constant leucine to tyrosine TPN infusion ratio was a functional index of hepatic impairment in sepsis and ST MOFS. Representative leucine to other AA CLR ratios are shown in Fig 5, with regard to the simultaneous statistical comparisons among NST patients, early ST survivors (less than five days after trauma), late ST survivors (more than five days after trauma), and ST MOFS deaths. A decrease in the slope of the clearance relationship means a rise in the leucine-AA CLR ratio. Except for the aromatic AA, progression of sepsis from early to late caused an increase in the leucine-AA CLR ratio compared with NST patients for all nonbranched AAs studied (of which proline and methionine are shown). However, there was no further leucine-AA CLR ratio increase between late ST survivors and ST MOFS deaths. Only when the aromatic AAs, phenylalanine and especially tyrosine, were considered was there a further increase in the leucine-AA CLR ratio as the MOFS developed. Since in these comparisons, the percent pool appears in both ordinate and abscissa, any error due to pool size estimation cancels out. This is an important observation with relevance to hepatic function in sepsis, since while leucine is cleared by both peripheral tissues and liver, tyrosine is almost entirely metabolized in the liver.[14,37] Thus, the L/T ratio provides a sensitive index that can be used to investigate the role of sepsis-induced hepatic dysfunction in modulating the posttraumatic ureagenic response to muscle proteolysis and TPN-AA infusion.

Figure 6 shows the relationship between urea N production and the L/T CLR ratio. This regression covariance analysis demonstrates a negative correlation between the two measurements, both in ST and NST survivors following trauma, with urea N production falling as the L/T ratio increases. Since the coefficient for sepsis is significantly positive (17.44), this indicates that for the same value of the L/T ratio, ST survivors have a consistantly higher rate of urea N production. The secondary lines show the 95% confidence limits of the regression lines for ST and NST survivors.

Thus, the effect of progressive or sustained sepsis, in the absence of the MOFS with hepatic dysfunction, is to produce an increased efficiency of ureagenesis for each level of hepatic CLR of AAs. This difference between ST and NST is highly significant ($P < .0001$ by the Scheffé S method). However, these data also suggest that at any given level of control (sepsis vs nonsepsis), increasing hepatic dysfunction, as measured by using the L/T ratio,[14] reduces the liver's ability to synthesize urea.

The ST nonsurvivors with clinical MOFS were not included in the regression for ST survivors, but their data are plotted on the graph. At any level of the L/T CLR

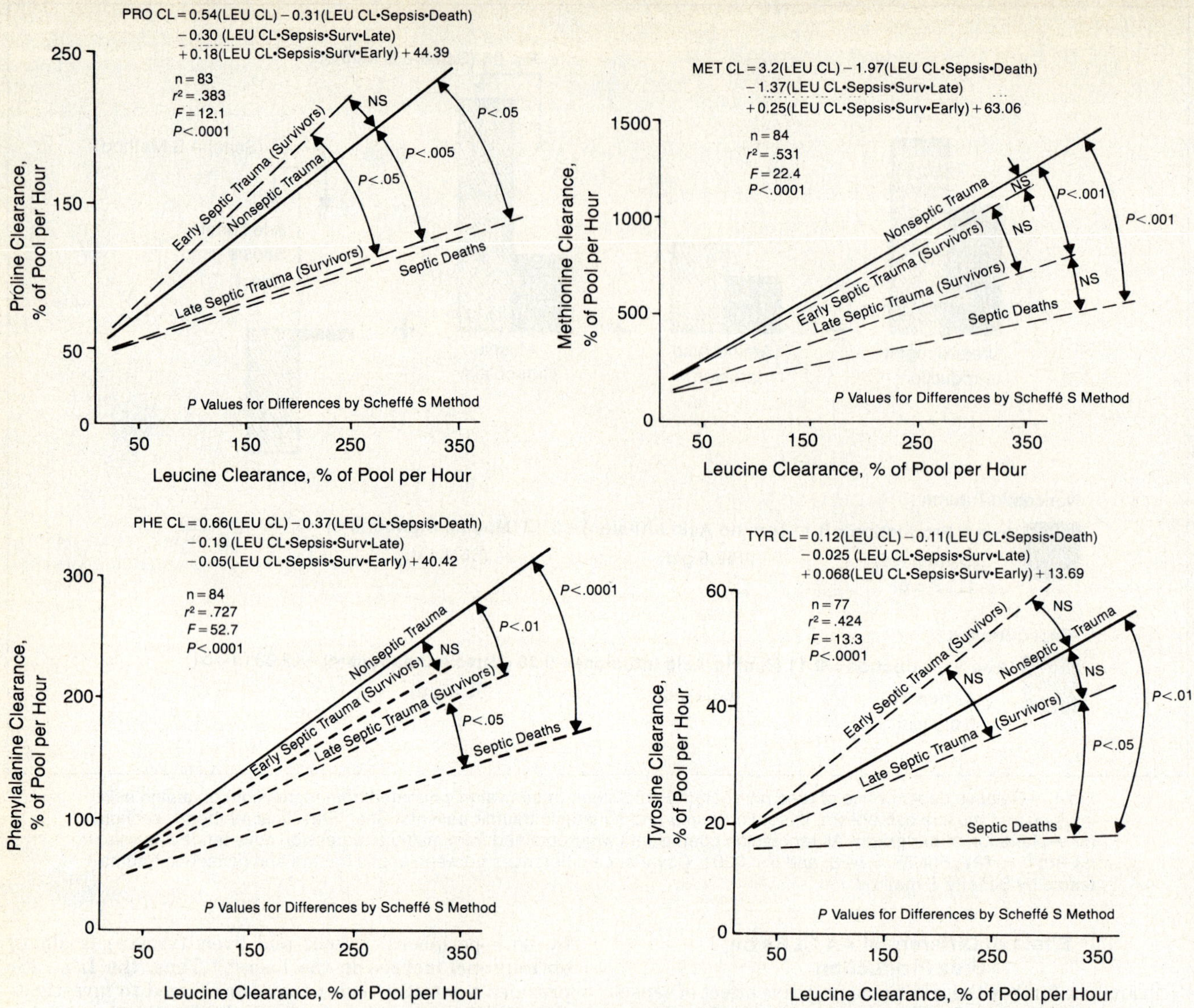

Fig 5.—Representative amino acid (AA) clearances (CLRs) as compared with leucine CLR **early** and **late** in nonseptic patients after trauma, in septic trauma (ST) survivors, and in ST multiple-organ failure syndrome (MOFS) deaths. Although total amount of AA varied somewhat during clinical course, all patients were given total parenteral nutrition with **constant** leucine to tyrosine concentration ratio as standard total parenteral nutrition. All slope differences tested by Scheffé S method of simultaneous contrasts. Note that only in leucine CLR to aromatic AA CLR relationships is there significant difference between **late** ST survivors and ST MOFS deaths. All regressions shown in figure are highly significant ($P<.0001$). Covariance differences tested for significance by Scheffé S method, P values as shown. NS indicates not significant.

ratio, their production of urea was abnormally low, both early and late in their clinical course. A second effect in the ST MOFS deaths is that, with time, they also trend to higher L/T CLR ratios and, consequently, lower levels of urea N production (Fig 7). This suggests that in the ST MOFS, the decrease in ureagenesis is due not only to a lower hepatic CLR of AAs from the plasma but also to a direct inhibition of ureagenesis, appearing quite early in the course of ST patients with MOFS, even when the level of hepatic dysfunction appears to be quite minimal on clinical grounds.

The interaction of all these factors (muscle protein degradation with release of AAs, TPN-AA infusion, and the impaired CLR of tyrosine relative to the total-body CLR of leucine [L/T ratio] at a constant TPN infusion ratio) is shown in Fig 7 for ST and NST patients, with regard to whether they were studied *early* or *late* in their clinical course. This diagram is generated from a single significant ($P<.0001$) multiple regression, with a covariance analysis that takes into account both the effect of sepsis and the effect of time (early vs late) on each regression coefficient and on the intercept value for that group. The mean values for each variable are shown in parentheses below each effect. The significance of the differences in the coefficients of the regression (double asterisks) and the significance of the coefficients themselves (single asterisk) were all simultaneously tested by the Scheffé S method.

For each type of study (early or late; ST or NST), the bar diagram, in which the mean values are multiplied by their respective regression coefficients, displays the *relative* effect of each of the components of urea production, as estimated by the global multiple regression. In all patients, ST or NST, early or late in their course, both AA infusion

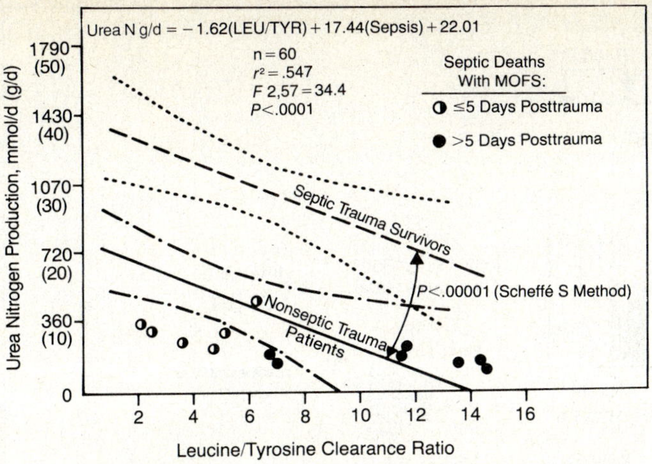

Fig 6.—Regression between urea nitrogen (N) production and leucine clearance/tyrosine clearance ratio in septic trauma survivors and in nonseptic trauma patients; covariance effect of sepsis significant by Scheffé S method. Secondary lines indicate 95% confidence limits of regression lines. Septic trauma patients with multiple-organ failure syndrome (MOFS) are also plotted, but were excluded in regression analysis. **Urea N g/d = −1.62 (Leucine/Tyrosine) + 17.44 (Sepsis) + 22.01.**

and muscle protein degradation are significant determinants of urea N production.

As already noted in the regression of Fig 4, there is an increased relative effect of muscle catabolism in enhancing urea N production in sepsis. This analysis shows it to be significantly different from that seen in NST patients *only* during the late ST period, even though the mean value of muscle catabolism is increased in early sepsis (111 g/d) to a greater extent than in late sepsis (89.5 g/d).

On the other hand, the introduction of an additional variable, which accounts for the relative efficiency of the peripheral AA CLR to the hepatic AA CLR (the L/T CLR ratio) yields important information concerning possible mechanisms of urea synthetic control in sepsis. This ratio, as might be expected from Fig 6, is *negatively* related to urea N production, suggesting that it reflects an inhibitory effect on urea synthesis.

In addition, Fig 7 makes it clear that the unexplained negative effect of sepsis, shown by the intercept value in the bar diagram of Fig 4, is now largely explained by this new independent variable, the index of hepatic AA CLR (L/T CLR ratio). This strongly suggests that in the ST state, the enhancement of ureagenesis due to the increased hepatic gluconeogenesis and oxidative catabolism of AA, is partly counterbalanced by a relatively impaired efficiency of the liver in clearing plasma AAs for metabolism.

COMMENT

Both trauma and sepsis independently can induce muscle protein degradation, with an increased loss of urinary N associated with an accelerated gluconeogenesis and ureagenesis. The mechanism of this accelerated proteolysis in the skeletal muscle has been extensively studied.[1] While some authors have stressed the role of increased circulating levels of catabolic hormones (catecholamines, corticosteroids, and glucagon)[4] or catabolic mediators,[2] others[5,16,36] have explained proteolysis by a peripheral impairment of glucose oxidation (postreceptor insulin resistance), which would compel the skeletal muscle to use alternative fuels, including the keto acids derived from the branched-chain AAs of its own structural proteins.

The possibility that this may be mediated by a host-defense–related response has been explored by Clowes et al[2] and Loda et al,[29] who have isolated a humoral factor that appears to be the stable circulating cleavage product of interleukin I. This substance can induce both proteolysis in the skeletal muscle and acute (TNF)-phase protein synthesis in the liver. Tumor necrosis factor has also been implicated as a possible causative agent.

The humorally mediated muscle protein degradation (proteolysis) releases AAs in proportion to their molar ratio in actin and myosin. However, in the presence of an impairment of skeletal muscle glucose oxidation, which occurs in sepsis,[6,36] the branched-chain AAs are preferentially oxidized by muscle itself.[33,35] This oxidation, whose first step involves deamination to α-keto acids, is coupled with the synthesis of ALA from muscle pyruvate, which accepts the transaminated amino N.[6,33,34] At the same time, a net synthesis of glutamine also occurs by a similar mechanism of acceptance of amino N by transamination from muscle glutamate. Since skeletal muscle cannot synthesize urea, the synthesis of ALA and glutamine represents the means of disposal of muscle protein–derived AA N. As a result, the final mixture of AAs released from the muscle into the plasma is qualitatively different from the composition of the muscle protein,[33-35] since it is enriched in ALA and glutamine, but it contains less branched-chain AAs. While the plasma ALA is mostly taken up by the liver, a large amount of glutamine is extracted not only by the liver but also by the gut,[33,34] which transaminates it to ALA.

In the normal postabsorptive state, ALA is responsible for only about 10% of glucose production by the liver, but it becomes a more important gluconeogenic precursor in starvation (25%),[33] and other data suggest that it may be even more important after trauma, or during sepsis.[7,9,10,14,16,35] After lactate, ALA appears to be the most important source of carbon for gluconeogenesis; a quantitatively lesser role is played by the other gluconeogenic AAs.[33,34] In particular, the increase in gluconeogenesis during sepsis seems to be accounted for by the utilization of ALA, derived from skeletal muscle protein and lactate.[35] Also, studies with labeled ALA have confirmed the major contribution of ALA to the accelerated gluconeogenesis in ST patients.[35] Furthermore, in sepsis, it appears that gluconeogenesis from ALA cannot be suppressed by exogenous glucose infusion.[11] In experimental sepsis,[10,35] the rate of increase of glucose synthesis appears to correlate only with the availability of sufficient substrate, indicating that the gluconeogenic capacity of the liver is not a limiting factor in ALA uptake. These data are compatible with our observations shown in Fig 3 that the increase in the plasma glucose level at any glucose uptake rate can be correlated with the ALA uptake so as to explain more than 67% of the variability in plasma glucose.

During accelerated gluconeogenesis, the amino group of ALA contributes importantly to the synthesis of urea. Quantitatively, the increased utilization of gluconeogenic AAs as substrate for gluconeogenesis in the liver is sufficiently large that the amino N generated can account for most of the increase in urea formation during trauma and/or sepsis.[35] However, while most of the ALA uptake is accounted for by the liver, the "central" uptake of glutamine is due to an overall *splanchnic* uptake (gut, kidney, and liver). Nevertheless, the weight of glutamine uptake in predicting urea production (Fig 2) is not surprising, since part of the amino N carried by glutamine may finally reach the liver as ALA (synthesized by the gut and kidney) or as serine (synthesized by kidney).

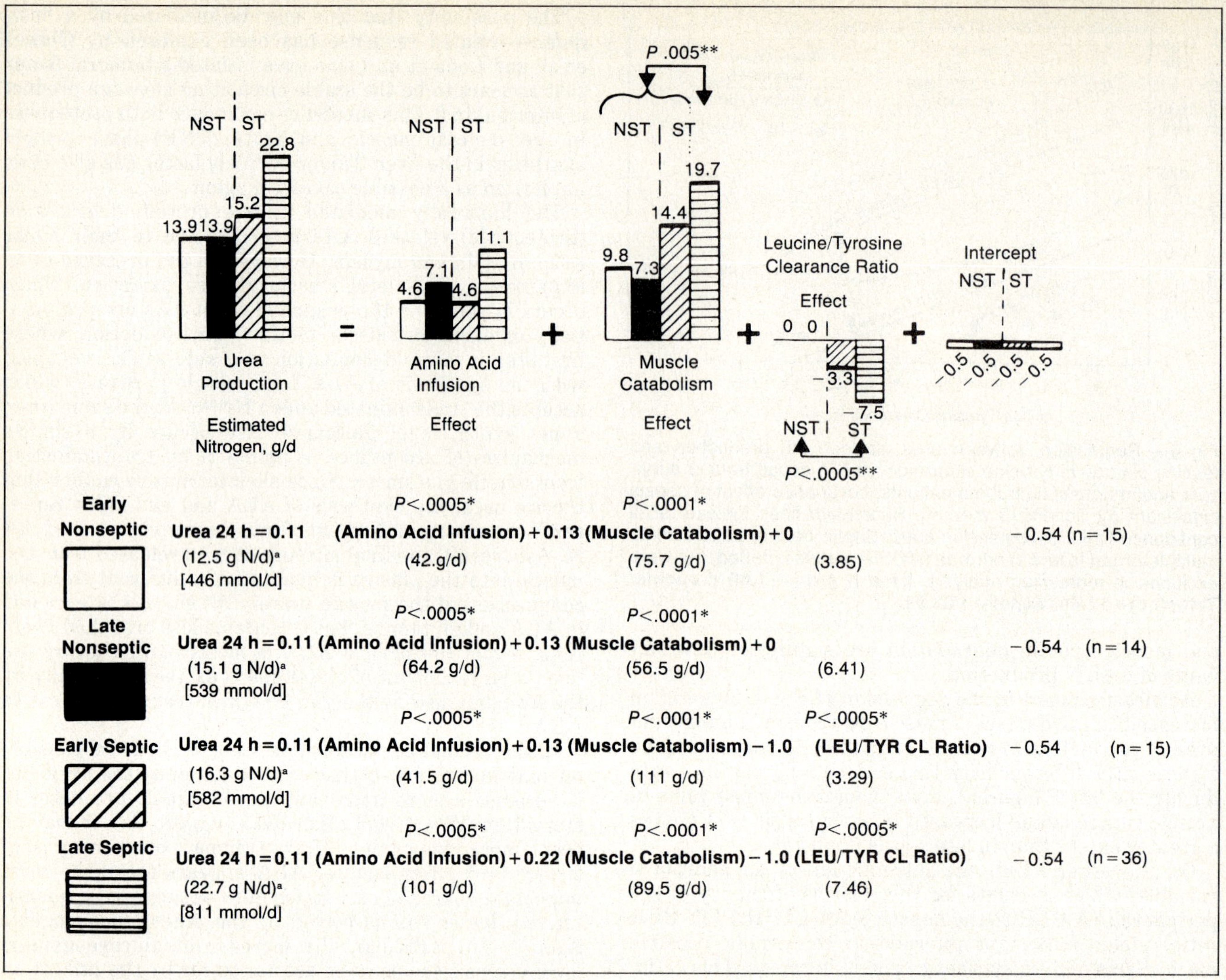

Fig 7.—Relative dependence of urea nitrogen production on amino acid infusion, muscle catabolism, and leucine/tyrosine clearance ratio in septic trauma (ST) and nonseptic trauma (NST) patients, **early** (less than five days) and **late** (more than five days) after injury. See "Statistical Method" section for explanation of bar graph. All regression coefficients obtained from multiple regression covariance analysis on combined groups: n = 80; $r^2 = .821$; $F(4,75) = 86$; and $P<.0001$. Coefficients of regression (single asterisk) and differences in coefficients (double asterisks) are simultaneously significant by Scheffé S method. Regression derived estimated nitrogen (grams per day) **above** compared to actual mean values in parentheses **below** designated by [a]. Mean values for AA infusion and muscle catabolism given in parentheses in grams per day.

Quantitatively, in sepsis, ALA appears to be much more important than glutamine. Indeed, some of our late ST patients had a mean hourly uptake of ALA of over 12 mmol/h, which could theoretically yield 12 mmol/h of urea N or nearly 30% of the mean urea N production. This is, in part, due to the fact that all our patients were supported by TPN, so that they were utilizing both the muscle-released and the TPN-infused ALA, while glutamine was not administered in the TPN. In our data, the combined ALA and GLUT uptake plus the effect of sepsis explain 66% of the variability of urea N production. More important, these data (Fig 2) show that sepsis per se may significantly increase the mean rate of urea N production from ALA.

It must be emphasized that the AAs that are cleared by the liver may also be utilized for protein synthesis. In patients who have undergone trauma, and especially if sepsis occurs, the proportion of AAs utilized for synthesis of enzymes, liver structural proteins, plasma proteins, and acute-phase reactants may be higher than the proportion of AAs whose carbon is used for glucose production or for oxidation to energy. Clowes et al[7] found that in ST patients who were fasting, the release rate of AAs from the muscle was increased three times over normal, while the total-body loss of N was increased by only 30%, suggesting that a large part of these AAs were utilized for protein synthesis. However, our data suggest that competition for AAs between oxidative catabolism and protein synthesis may be responsible for the acute-phase protein reprioritization seen in sepsis.[15] Furthermore, in the prediction of the variability of urea formation, there were two other important factors to be considered, the *sepsis effect* and the *death effect* due to the development of a fatal ST MOFS with hepatic dysfunction.

Effect of Sepsis

As noted above, if compared with NST patients, ureagenesis was enhanced in ST survivors: this increase in ureagenesis appears to be related to the increase in AA-derived gluconeogenesis, through the increased supply of AAs from the peripheral tissue and from TPN. However, our data show that despite the high rate of TPN given to the ST patients, increased catabolic muscle protein degradation played the major role in causing a higher urea N production (Fig 4).

This dependence of urea production on increased proteolysis seems to be a phenomenon typical of the overt, clinical phase of sepsis, even though the highest mean values for muscle catabolism were reached earlier in the clinical course, during the first few days after the injury. This is clearly shown by the bar diagram in Fig 7. If one compares the relative effect of muscle catabolism on ureagenesis, between the pre-ST period and the overt ST period, it can be seen that the largest significant effect is during the *late* phase of sepsis, despite the fact that muscle catabolism is generally higher during the *early* phase. One explanation may be the increased production of interleukin I, which occurs in sepsis.[2] Its degradation product, proteolysis-inducing factor, has been shown to increase both muscle catabolism and hepatic protein synthesis.[29] This may imply that urea synthesis may be directly or indirectly coupled to the monokine–mediated proteolysis and thus statistically more dependent on muscle catabolism–released AA than on AA administered by TPN, which may not be in phase with interleukin I (or TNF) production.

In addition, there may also be an increased "efficiency" of ureagenesis by direct hormonal stimulation of gluconeogenesis and/or ureagenesis. It is known that high plasma levels of ALA can stimulate glucagon secretion, which is a gluconeogenic hormone.[34] It is also known that usually the coupling of gluconeogenesis and ureagenesis is optimal, despite the fact that these two processes have been shown in vitro to depend on, and compete for, adenosine triphosphate.[38] However, in vivo studies in nonseptic animals show that ureagenesis is generally not decreased, even when the rate of gluconeogenesis is relatively high.[35,38] On the contrary, overstimulation of ureagenesis (in the nonseptic liver) can reduce the gluconeogenic activity, because of competition for adenosine triphosphate or aspartate.[38]

As long as there are adequate oxygen consumption and energy availability and adequate stimulation by an increased supply of gluconeogenic substrates and by a high glucagon-insulin ratio, experimental studies suggest that the normal liver can go on producing glucose and synthesize urea at maximal rates,[10] while, at the same time, synthesizing proteins required for immunologic defense and maintenance of organ function.[8,9] This is what appears to happen in the compensated response to human trauma, in the absence of sepsis and ST MOFS, where acute-phase protein reprioritization occurs.[15]

However, as a limiting factor to sepsis-induced increased ureagenesis, the hepatotoxic effect of sepsis (as measured by the L/T ratio[14]) selectively alters the liver's ability to catabolize AAs, causing a relative negative effect on urea synthesis. The latter factor appears to become more prominent in late sepsis as the MOFS develops fully, but it is significant in all late ST patients, regardless of whether fatal MOFS occurs or not.

Effect of MOFS (Septic Death Effect)

In our study, ST patients with MOFS were strikingly different from ST survivors, since their clinical course showed a progressive decrease of urea excretion and a decrease in muscle catabolism. In the late course of ST patients with MOFS, muscle protein degradation (catabolism) was significantly lower, if compared with ST survivors. However, it was not significantly different from the muscle catabolism value in NST patients. Nevertheless, the ST patients with MOFS had a mean production of urea N that was less than one third of the urea N production in the NST patients.

The reduced muscle catabolism might be explained as an adaptive mechanism due to liver failure and the MOFS, in that the increased circulating plasma levels of AAs, due to the reduced AA CLR by the liver in MOFS, may inhibit further muscle proteolysis. It is also possible that some aspect of ST MOFS may directly inhibit production of the proteolysis-initiating factors, as suggested by G.H.A. Clowes, MD (oral communication, June 1987).

On the liver side of urea metabolism, the decrease in urea synthesis may be due to the reduced muscle protein degradation, reflecting a lower muscle catabolism; to the failure of hepatic uptake of AAs; and to the iatrogenic reduction in the TPN infusion rate, because of the observed insulin-resistant hyperglycemia. However, the main significant effect that is evident in the multiple correlation shown in Fig 7 is that *all* ST patients (including both survivors and patients with MOFS) share an inhibiting effect on urea production due to a relative impairment of all hepatic AA CLRs, except for the branched-chain AAs,[14] as expressed by the L/T CLR ratio. This effect becomes even more important in the setting of MOFS, when the source of circulating AAs due to muscle catabolism (and TPN) is decreased. A similar finding was reported by Loda et al[29] and Pearl et al,[30] who found in both ST patients and cirrhotic patients[39] undergoing surgical procedures that nonsurvivors were characterized by significantly lower central CLRs of AAs if compared with survivors.

The reduced ureagenesis may be also due to a failure of gluconeogenesis. In recent experimental studies,[40] hepatic gluconeogenic capability was found to be depressed in severe, late sepsis. However, since this was evident *before* the final onset of depressed, oxidative capability, the mechanism of this selective failure of gluconeogenesis remains obscure. However, hypoglycemia did not occur in any of our clinical patients with MOFS, but rather hyperglycemia, which suggests a different mechanism than the terminal failure of glucose synthesis seen with endotoxemia.

There may be a relative energy failure, since ureagenesis is a synthetic pathway that requires energy (approximately 147 to 168 kJ are required for the synthesis of 1 mol of urea),[35,38] and gluconeogenesis from AAs (more important quantitatively in ST patients) consumes more energy than gluconeogenesis from lactate or pyruvate.[34] At the same time, the ST liver also appears to be maximally stimulated to the synthesis of a variety of proteins, especially acute-phase reactants, at a rate that might be expected to require large amounts of energy.[15,29] However, oxygen consumption, while reduced in some patients with late MOFS,[16,41] was not significantly lower than that in surviving ST patients in this group.

All studies were carried out in accordance with the guidelines of the Human Investigations Committee of the University of Maryland School of Medicine, Baltimore.

References

1. Ryan TN: Metabolic adaptations for energy production during trauma and sepsis. *Surg Clin North Am* 1976;56:1073-1090.
2. Clowes GHA, George BC, Villee CA, et al: Muscle proteolysis induced by a circulating peptide in patients with sepsis or trauma. *N Engl J Med* 1983;308:545-552.

3. Alberti KGMM, Batstone GF, Path MRC, et al: Relative role of various hormones in mediating the metabolic response to injury. *JPEN* 1980;4:141-146.
4. Bessey PQ, Watters JR, Aoki TT, et al: Combined hormonal infusion simulates the metabolic response to injury. *Ann Surg* 1984;200:264-281.
5. Border JR, Chenier R, McMenamy RH, et al: Multiple systems organ failure–muscle fuel deficit with visceral protein malnutrition. *Surg Clin North Am* 1976;56:1147-1169.
6. O'Donnell TF, Clowes GHA, Blackburn GL, et al: Proteolysis associated with a deficit of peripheral energy fuel substrates in septic man. *Surgery* 1976;80:192-200.
7. Clowes GHA, Randall HT, Cha CJ: Amino acid and energy metabolism in septic and traumatized patients. *JPEN* 1980;4:195-205.
8. Beisel WR: Magnitude of the host nutritional responses to infection. *Am J Clin Nutr* 1977;30:1236-1247.
9. Wannemacher RW: Key role of various individual amino acids in host response to infection. *Am J Clin Nutr* 1977;30:1269-1280.
10. Imamura M, Clowes GHA, Blackburn GL, et al: Liver metabolism and gluconeogenesis in trauma and sepsis. *Surgery* 1975;77:868-880.
11. Long CL, Kinney JM, Geiger JW: Nonsuppressibility of gluconeogenesis by glucose in septic patients. *Metabolism* 1976;25:193-201.
12. Clowes GHA, Heideman M, Lindberg B, et al: Effects of parenteral alimentation on amino acid metabolism in septic patients. *Surgery* 1980;88:531-543.
13. Cerra FB, Siegel JH, Border JR, et al: The hepatic failure of sepsis: Cellular versus substrate. *Surgery* 1979;86:409-422.
14. Pittiruti M, Siegel JH, Sganga G, et al: Increased dependence on leucine in post-traumatic sepsis: Leucine/tyrosine clearance ratio as indicator of hepatic impairment in septic multiple organ failure syndrome. *Surgery* 1985;98:378-387.
15. Sganga G, Siegel JH, Brown G, et al: Reprioritization of hepatic plasma protein release in trauma and sepsis. *Arch Surg* 1985;120:187-199.
16. Siegel JH, Cerra FB, Coleman B, et al: Physiological and metabolic correlations in human sepsis. *Surgery* 1979;86:163-193.
17. Faist E, Baue AE, Dittmer H, et al: Multiple organ failure in polytrauma patients. *J Trauma* 1983;23:775-787.
18. Walser M, Bodenlos LJ: Urea metabolism in man. *J Clin Invest* 1959;38:1617-1626.
19. Long CL, Jeevanandam M, Kim BM, et al: Whole body protein synthesis and catabolism in septic man. *Am J Clin Nutr* 1977;30:1340-1344.
20. Bilmazes C, Uavy R, Haverberg LN, et al: Muscle protein breakdown rates in humans based on N-methylhistidine (3-methylhistidine) content of mixed proteins in skeletal muscle and urinary output of N-methylhistidine. *Metabolism* 1978;27:525-530.
21. Wassner SJ, Li JB: N-Methylhistidine release: Contributions of rat skeletal muscle, GI tract, and skin. *Am J Physiol* 1982;243:E293-E297.
22. Rennie MJ, Millward DJ: 3-Methylhistidine excretion and the urinary 3-methylhistidine/creatinine ratio are poor indicators of skeletal muscle protein breakdown. *Clin Sci* 1983;65:217-225.
23. Brenner H, Herbertz L, Thul P, et al: The contribution of small gut to the 3-methylhistidine metabolism in the adult rat. *Metabolism* 1987;36:416-418.
24. Ballard FJ, Tomas FM: 3-Methylhistidine as a measure of skeletal muscle protein breakdown in human subjects: The case for its continued use. *Clin Sci* 1983;65:209-215.
25. Harris CI: Reappraisal of the quantitative importance of non-skeletal muscle source of N-methylhistidine in urine. *Biochem J* 1981;194:1011-1014.
26. Young VR, Munro HN: N-Methylhistidine (3-methylhistidine) and muscle protein turnover: An overview. *FASEB J* 1978;37:2291-2300.
27. Afting EG, Bernhardt W, Janzen RWC, et al: Quantitative importance of non-skeletal muscle N-methylhistidine and creatine in human urine. *Biochem J* 1981;200:449-452.
28. Haverberg LN, Omstedt PT, Munro HN, et al: N-Methylhistidine content of mixed proteins in various rat tissues. *Biochim Biophys Acta* 1975;405:67-71.
29. Loda M, Clowes GHA, Dinarello CA, et al: Induction of hepatic protein synthesis by a peptide in blood plasma of patients with sepsis and trauma. *Surgery* 1984;96:204-213.
30. Pearl R, Clowes GHA, Hirsh EF: Prognosis and survival as determined by visceral amino acid clearance in severe trauma. *J Trauma* 1985;25:777-783.
31. Coleman B, Siegel JH: Statistical interpretation, in Peters RM, Pencock EE, Benfield JR (eds): *The Scientific Management of Surgical Patients.* Boston, Little Brown & Co Inc, 1983, pp 445-480.
32. Seber GAF: *Linear Regression Analysis.* New York, John Wiley & Sons Inc, 1977.
33. Felig P: The glucose-alanine cycle. *Metabolism* 1973;22:179-207.
34. Ruderman NB: Muscle amino acid metabolism and gluconeogenesis. *Annu Rev Med* 1975;26:245-258.
35. Beisel WR, Wannemacher RW: Gluconeogenesis, ureagenesis, and ketogenesis during sepsis. *JPEN* 1980;4:277-285.
36. Vary T, Siegel JH, Nakatani T, et al: Effect of sepsis on activity of pyruvate dehydrogenase complex in skeletal muscle and liver. *Am J Physiol* 1986;250:E634-E640.
37. Williams IH, Sugden PH, Morgan HE: Does metabolism of the aromatic amino acids interfere with their use as monitors of protein turnover? *Am J Physiol* 1981;240:E677-E681.
38. Krebs HA, Lund P, Stubbs M: Interrelations between gluconeogenesis and urea synthesis, in Hanson RW, Mehlman MA (eds): *Gluconeogenesis: Its Regulation in Mammalian Species.* New York, John Wiley & Sons Inc, 1976, pp 269-291.
39. Clowes GHA, McDermott W, Williams LF, et al: Amino acid clearance and prognosis in surgical patients with cirrhosis. *Surgery* 1984;96:675-685.
40. Guillem JG, Clemens MG, Chaudry IH, et al: Hepatic gluconeogenic capability in sepsis is depressed before changes in oxidative capability. *J Trauma* 1982;22:723-729.
41. Siegel JH, Vary TC: Sepsis, abnormal metabolic control, and the multiple organ failure syndrome, in Siegel JH (ed): *Trauma: Emergency Surgery and Critical Care.* New York, Churchill Livingstone Inc, 1987, pp 441-501.
42. Joint Committee on Injury Scaling: *The Abbreviated Injury Scale (1980 Revision).* Des Plaines, Ill, American Association for Automotive Medicine, 1980.

In Other AMA Journals

ARCHIVES OF INTERNAL MEDICINE

An Ecogenetic Hypothesis for Lung Cancer in Women

Ralph I. Horwitz, MD; Laurie F. Smaldone, MD; Catherine M. Viscoli, MPhil

Epidemiologic studies have established a strong association between cigarette smoking and lung cancer, but the risk estimates for women are less impressive than for men. We assessed the possible role of family history and its interrelationship with cigarette smoking as risk factors for lung cancer in women by conducting a case-control study. Among 112 cases, 7% had a primary family member with lung cancer compared with only 3% of 224 controls for an odds ratio of 2.8. Cigarette smoking was present for 87% of the cases and 41% of the controls for an odds ratio of 11.3. The ecogenetic interrelationship of cigarette smoking and family history was supported by the gradient in the odds ratio for lung cancer created by the two variables: patients who never smoked but had a positive family history had an odds ratio of 5.7; patients who smoked but had a negative family history had an odds ratio of 15.1; and patients who smoked and had a positive family history had an odds ratio of almost 30. We conclude that family history may be an important risk factor for lung cancer in women, and that the ecogenetic interrelationship of family history with cigarette smoking may help explain the occurrence of this disease in women (*Arch Intern Med* 1988;148:2609-2612).

Reprint requests to Yale University School of Medicine, Room IE-61 SHM, PO Box 3333, New Haven, CT 06510 (Dr Horwitz).

Isolated Regional Perfusion in the Treatment of Subungual Melanoma

Peter C. Baas, MD; Harald J. Hoekstra, MD, PhD; Heimen Schraffordt Koops, MD, PhD; J. Wolter Oosterhuis, MD, PhD; Jan Oldhoff, MD, PhD

• Subungual melanoma is rare and represents only 1% to 3% of all diagnosed melanomas in Western countries. The tumor is frequently mistaken for a benign lesion and the delay in diagnosis and final treatment may be responsible for the high local recurrence rate and the low disease-free survival rate. From 1965 to 1982 the combined-modality therapy of amputation and adjuvant isolated regional perfusion with melphalan with or without dactinomycin was used in the treatment of 22 patients with subungual melanoma. Disease was staged according to the M. D. Anderson classification, as follows: stage I (primary melanoma), 11 patients; stage IIIA (in-transit metastases and/or satellitosis), three patients; stage IIIB (regional lymph nodes), seven patients; and stage IIIAB (in-transit metastases and/or satellitosis and regional lymph nodes), one patient. There were no cardiovascular complications and no treatment mortality. During a follow-up of at least 4.5 years, 12 patients (55%) developed distant metastases, including four patients with stage I disease (36%) and eight patients with stage III disease (73%). There were no locoregional recurrences. The median survival was three years (range, 0.5 to 12.5 years) and the overall five-year survival was 40%, with 56% of patients having stage I disease and 27% having stage III disease. The prognosis of subungual melanoma is determined by the stage of the disease. Isolated regional perfusion may prolong disease-free survival in patients with subungual melanoma compared with previously published data.

(*Arch Surg* 1989;124:373-376)

In 1834, Boyer[1] described a 57-year-old man with a subungual melanotic neoplasm located at the tip of the left little finger and an enlarged lymph node in the axilla. A subungual "black line" under the nail remained stationary for 28 years but started to grow slowly and caused pain. In the course of the next two years the pigmented area widened, became inflamed and painful, and bled on the slightest touch. Finally, an amputation through the middle phalanx was performed for a tumor the size of a chicken egg located at the fingertip. The axillary lymph node remained untouched and subsequently disappeared; during follow-up there was no recurrence. In 1855 Demargnay and Monod[2] described a 69-year-old woman with an easily bleeding black tumor on the left thumb that originated from the nail bed and lifted the nail. Shortly after cauterization of the tumor a local recurrence developed with enlarged axillary lymph nodes and an amputation of the thumb was performed.[2] It was Hutchinson[3] who published the first important clinical description of a subungual melanoma in 1857 in an article entitled "Melanotic Disease of the Great Toe, Following a Whitlow of the Nail." In a classic report called "Melanosis Often Not Black: Melanotic Whitlow,"[4] Hutchinson stated that melanoma may occur subungually, that it is a malignant neoplasm, and therefore the primary treatment should be amputation of the involved finger or toe.[4]

Since these early reports, more than a century has passed and only a few case reports and clinical series have been published. Although the incidence of melanoma is increasing and is approximately four per 100 000, subungual melanoma is very rare and represents only approximately 1% to 3% of all diagnosed melanoma in Western countries. A higher proportion of subungual melanoma is diagnosed in dark-skinned patients.[5,6] Subungual melanoma is still frequently mistaken for benign conditions such as subungual hematoma, chronic paronychia, onchymycosis, glomus tumor, and pyogenic granuloma.[7] Amelanotic subungual melanoma exists, but is rarely diagnosed.[8] The delay in diagnosis is believed to be responsible for the low five-year survival rate associated with subungual melanoma in comparison with the survival rate from melanoma at other locations. Improvement in survival can be achieved by early recognition and proper surgical treatment.

Subungual melanomas are close to the underlying periosteum and therefore exarticulation of at least the involved phalanx is the treatment of choice. Axillary or inguinal lymph node dissection is mandatory when the lymph nodes are involved, while some surgeons perform elective node dissections.

From 1965 to 1982 we treated 22 patients with a combination of amputation and adjuvant isolated regional perfusion for subungual melanoma. In all patients with a subungual melanoma of the upper extremity an elective or therapeutic axillary dissection was performed to enable better perfusion. In the lower extremity only therapeutic lymph node dissections were performed. To gain some insight into the results of our treatment, the patients with subungual melanoma treated in this way were evaluated and the existing literature was reviewed.

PATIENTS AND METHODS

Thirty-one patients with a primary subungual melanoma of the finger or toe in the period 1965 through 1982 were evaluated for this combined-modality therapy of surgery and adjuvant isolated regional perfusion at the Division of Surgical Oncology, Groningen (the Netherlands) University Hospital. Of these 31 patients, eight were excluded from perfusion treatment because of distant metastases or unstable heart disease. One patient refused perfusion treatment. Twenty-two patients were treated by isolated regional perfusion with melphalan, with or without dactinomycin, and amputation of the involved finger or toe at the metacarpophalangeal joint or metatarsophalangeal joint. There were 13 female and nine male patients with a mean age of 57 years (median age, 62 years; range, 21 to 81 years). As Table 1 illustrates, the fingers were involved more often than the toes. Five melanomas appeared at the fingers, ten appeared at the thumb, six appeared at the great toe, and one appeared at the second toe.

All patients with a subungual melanoma of the upper extremity

Accepted for publication Dec 3, 1987.

From the Division of Surgical Oncology (Drs Baas, Hoekstra, Schraffordt Koops, and Oldhoff) and the Department of Pathology (Dr Oosterhuis), University Hospital, Groningen, the Netherlands.

Presented during the 1987 Joint Annual Meeting of the Association of Head and Neck Oncologists of Great Britain, British Association of Surgical Oncology, Society of Head and Neck Surgeons, and Society of Surgical Oncology, London, April 25, 1987.

Reprint requests to Division of Surgical Oncology, Groningen University Hospital, PO Box 30.001, 9700 RB Groningen, the Netherlands (Dr Hoekstra).

Table 1.—Clinical Details, Staging, Treatment, and Follow-up

Patient No./ Age, y/Sex	Year Treated	Site	Clark/Breslow Microstaging (Thickness, mm)	M. D. Anderson Staging System*	Treatment†	Follow-up, mo (Outcome)‡	Metastases, mo
1/69/M	1965	R thumb	V (15)	IIIB	1+2	9 (DOD)	8
2/55/M	1971	R thumb	IV (6)	IIIB	1+2	5 (DOD)	3
3/66/F	1972	L thumb	IV (4)	IA	1+2	15 (DOD)	14
4/65/M	1974	R-hand finger	IV (9)	IIIB	1+2	11 (DOD)	11
5/42/F	1974	R-hand finger	IV (6)	IA	1+2	161 (NED)	...
6/66/M	1974	R thumb	IV (4)	IA	1+2	81 (DHI)	...
7/59/M	1975	L great toe	IV (15)	IA	1+3	80 (DCC)	...
8/48/F	1976	R great toe	V (10)	IA	1+3+5	32 (DOD)	30
9/55/F	1976	L thumb	IV (8)	IA	1+2	41 (DOD)	30
10/35/F	1977	R great toe	IV (5)	IA	1+3+5	115 (NED)	...
11/66/F	1977	R great toe	IV (4-5)	IA	1+3+5	25 (DOD)	15
12/65/F	1978	R great toe	V (9)	IIIB	1+3+4	21 (DOD)	19
13/60/F	1978	R-hand finger	V (5)	IIIB	1+2	12 (DOD)	8
14/49/F	1978	L-hand finger	V (5)	IIIB	1+2	24 (DOD)	12
15/66/M	1979	L thumb	IV (4)	IIIB	1+2	99 (NED)	...
16/44/F	1979	R great toe	IV (6)	IIIA	1+3+4	33 (DOD)	33
17/81/M	1980	R thumb	IV (7)	IIIAB	1+2	8 (DOD)	8
18/43/M	1980	R thumb	IV (1.5)	IA	1+2	89 (NED)	...
19/64/F	1982	R-hand finger	IV (1.4)	IIIA	1+2	63 (NED)	...
20/76/M	1982	L-foot toe	... (2.9)	IIIA	1+3	56 (NED)	...
21/21/F	1982	L thumb	IV (4.5)	IA	1+2	55 (NED)	...
22/65/F	1982	L thumb	IV (5)	IA	1+2	64 (NED)	...

*M. D. Anderson staging system: stage IA, primary melanoma; stage IIIA, satellitosis and/or in-transit metastases; stage IIIB, regional node metastases; and stage IIIAB, satellitosis and/or in-transit metastases and regional node metastases.

†1 indicates amputation; 2, axillary perfusion; 3, iliac perfusion; 4, femoral perfusion; and 5, popliteal perfusion.

‡DOD indicates dead of disease; NED, no evidence of disease; DHI, dead of heart infarct; and DCC, dead of colon carcinoma.

were treated with axillary lymph node dissection for technical reasons, followed by an isolated regional axillary perfusion and amputation of the thumb or finger. Patients with lower extremity subungual melanoma were treated with isolated regional iliac perfusion and amputation of the toe, followed six weeks later by a second popliteal perfusion. In two patients with suspect inguinal lymph nodes, an inguinal lymph node dissection with femoral perfusion was performed instead of popliteal perfusion.

The histologic specimens were reexamined by one of us (J.W.O.) and microstaged according to Clark et al[9] and Breslow.[10] Sixteen patients' lesions were staged as Clark IV and five as Clark V; one patient's lesion could not be staged according to Clark's classification. The median Breslow thickness was 5 mm (range, 1.4 to 15 mm). The disease was classified according to the M. D. Anderson classification, as follows: stage IA (primary tumor), 11 patients; stage IIIA (satellitosis and/or in-transit metastasis), three patients; stage IIIB (regional node metastases), seven patients; and stage IIIAB (satellitosis and/or in-transit metastasis with regional lymph node metastasis), one patient. The follow-up was at least 4.5 years for the living patients. Clinical data, microstaging, tumor stage according to the M. D. Anderson classification, treatment, and follow-up are summarized in Table 1. When a median number is mentioned, this number is determined from real data. For the statistical analysis we used the Kaplan-Meier method.

Hypothermic or normothermic isolated regional perfusions were performed from 1965 to 1969, while all perfusions performed since then have been under hyperthermic conditions.

For perfusions of the lower extremity a lower abdominal incision paralleling the inguinal ligament or through a paramedian incision was used. The vessels were approached through the retroperitoneal space. An iliac lymph node dissection was always performed for technical reasons. The inferior epigastric and obturator vessels were ligated. After general heparinization (heparin sodium, 3.3 mg/kg of body weight) the internal iliac artery was temporarily occluded. The external iliac artery and vein were cannulated. The collateral circulation was blocked by means of a tourniquet placed around the thigh as high as possible to prevent leakage of cytostatics to the systemic circulation. For perfusion of the upper extremity an axillary lymph node dissection was performed for technical reasons, the axillary artery and vein were exposed and cannulated, and the collateral circulation was blocked using a tourniquet around the arm.[11] The extremity was perfused with the aid of a pump oxygenator; the perfusate (350 mL of dextran, 500 mL of blood, and 30 mL of 8.4% sodium bicarbonate and heparin sodium) was heated for the hyperthermic perfusions with a heat exchanger in the oxygenator. Adequate tissue oxygenation could be obtained and maintained only when the perfusion pressure was no lower than 15 mm Hg below the systemic mean arterial pressure.[12] The extremity temperature was monitored by four thermistor probes inserted through the skin into the subcutaneous tissue and the muscles of the upper and lower ends of the upper and lower extremities. Administration of the drug(s) was started when the subcutaneous tissue temperature of the lower part of the extremity reached 38°C. Leakage from or to the systemic circulation was checked with the aid of a scanner placed over the heart using radioactive iodine (^{131}I) bound to human albumin as an isotope. The duration of the perfusion was 60 minutes. After its completion the extremity was washed out with an inert fluid, whereupon the catheters were removed, the vessels were closed, and the heparin was antagonized with protamine chloride. After completion of the perfusion the thumb, finger, or toe was amputated at the metacarpophalangeal or metatarsophalangeal joint. A fasciotomy was performed to prevent a compartment syndrome.[13] For femoral perfusions, first a superficial inguinal lymph node dissection was performed, followed by cannulation of the femoral vessels immediately below Poupart's ligament. When popliteal perfusion was performed, the cannulae were introduced at the level of the adductor canal. The technique for femoral and popliteal perfusion was the same as described above.

Melphalan (L-phenylalanine mustard) was used in dosages of 1 to 1.5 mg/kg of body weight for the lower extremity and 0.5 to 0.7 mg/kg of body weight for the upper extremity. Since 1982, the melphalan dosage has been calculated on the basis of the extremity volume.[14] Melphalan was given at a dosage of 10 mg/L of perfused tissue. For patients with stage I lesions, melphalan alone was used as the cytostatic drug for perfusion. For satellitosis or in-transit metastases at stage IIIA or IIIAB, 0.5 to 1 mg of dactinomycin was added to the perfusion fluid (maximum, 0.006 and 0.014 mg/kg of body weight for the upper and lower extremity, respectively). Anticoagulation was started the day after perfusion and continued until full mobilization was achieved. Antimicrobial agents were not routinely given either preoperatively or postoperatively.

RESULTS

There were no complications during the perfusion treatment or during the 30-day postoperative period. No patient died as a result of this therapy. The median survival was three years (range, 0.5 to 12.5 years); the overall five-year survival according to the Kaplan-Meier test was 40%; for stage I disease it was 56% and for stage III disease it was 27% ($P<.05$) (Fig 1). During a follow-up of at least 4.5 years, 12 patients (55%) developed distant metastases, including four patients (36%) with stage I disease and eight patients (73%) with stage III disease, after a median time of 13 months (range, three to 33 months). There were no locoregional recurrences in the extremities (Fig 2).

Tissue reaction by the extremity was seen approximately two days after hyperthermic perfusion. The perfused extremity was red, warm, and slightly edematous. Cardiovascular complications during the surgical perfusion procedure or in the postoperative period were not observed, and no patient died as a result of this therapy. Two patients (9%) developed complications. During follow-up one patient

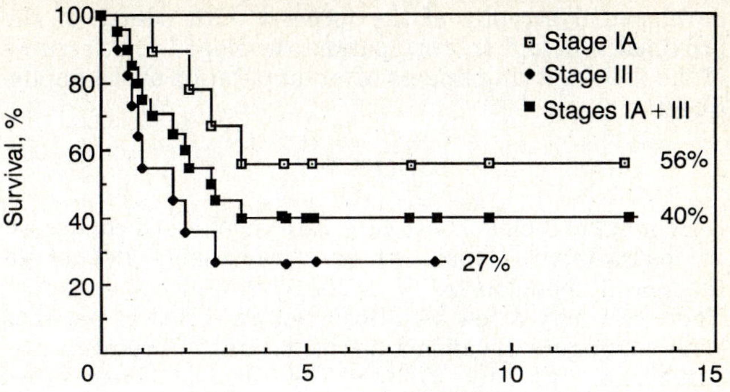

Fig 1.—Survival.

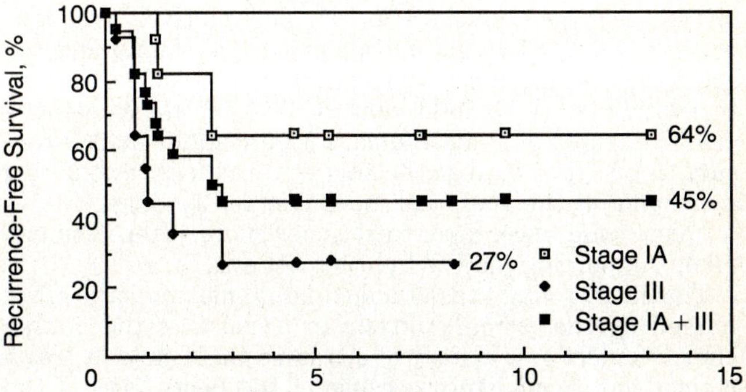

Fig 2.—Recurrence-free survival.

Table 2.—Overview of Clinical Details of Patients With Subungual Melanoma

Study, y	No. of Patients	Mean (Median) Age, y	Sex, F/M	Site, No. of Patients: Fingers	Toes	Thumb	Great Toe	Trauma, No. of Patients
Das Gupta and Brasfield,[5] 1965	34	... (...)	20/14	20	14	10	8	...
Pack and Oropeza,[6] 1967	72	57 (...)	32/40	40	32	18	29	...
Welvaart and Schraffordt Koops,[16] 1978	25	64 (...)	12/13	...	...	...	...	...
Patterson and Helwing,[17] 1980	66	61 (64)	22/44	31	35	17	33	19
Panizzon and Krebs,[18] 1980	12	57 (...)	5/7	4	8	1	7	6
Papachristou and Fortner,[19] 1982	52	... (65)	27/25	18	34	8	24	...
Takematsu et al,[15] 1985	16	56 (58)	4/12	11	5	8	3	7
Japanese series,[15] 1985	63	... (...)	.../...	46	17	32	16	...
Present study, 1987	22	57 (62)	13/9	15	7	10	6	...
Overall	362	± 59	45%/55%	55%	45%	56%	83%	34%

Table 3.—Overview of Therapy and Survival of Patients With Subungual Melanoma

Study, y	No. of Patients	M. D. Anderson Staging	Treatment	Local Recurrence, %	5-y Survival, %
Das Gupta and Brasfield,[5] 1965	34	I, II, III	Amputation ± lymph node dissection	...	38
Pack and Oropeza,[6] 1967	72	I-IV	Amputation ± lymph node dissection	...	48
Welvaart et al,[16] 1978	25	I-IV	Amputation ± lymph node dissection ± regional perfusion	...	...
Patterson and Helwing,[17] 1980	66	I + III	Amputation ± lymph node dissection	...	16
Panizzon and Krebs,[18] 1980	12	I + III	Amputation ± radiotherapy ± chemotherapy ± lymph node dissection	...	25
Papachristou and Fortner,[19] 1982	52	I + III	Amputation ± lymph node dissection	29	53
Takematsu et al,[15] 1985	16	I + III	Amputation + lymph node dissection + chemotherapy	0	40
Present study, 1987	22	I + III	Amputation ± lymph node dissection + regional perfusion	0	40

developed dystrophy of the forearm with edema of the proximal arm and another patient developed contractures of the little and ring fingers after amputation of the middle finger.

COMMENT

Subungual melanoma is very rare in Western countries, in contrast with Japan, where it represents 19% of all diagnosed melanomas.[5,6,15] It is a slow-growing tumor. There are only a few well-documented series of patients with subungual melanoma published in the literature, as summarized in Table 2.[5,6,15-19] The tumor is most often diagnosed in the sixth decade.

The fingers are more often involved than the toes. In nearly three fourths of all patients it was either the thumb or the great toe that was affected. The relatively frequent occurrence of subungual melanoma in the thumb and the great toe is unexplained and intriguing. Extreme exposure to ultraviolet (UV) light may be one of the exogenous causes of subungual melanoma. Fingers suffer more exposure to UV light than do the shoe-covered toes. Subungual melanoma of the toes was more frequently diagnosed in women,[5] who wear open-toed shoes more often, than in men,[1] supporting the UV light hypothesis.

The clinical diagnosis of a subungual melanoma is often missed by the primary physician because of the benign clinical aspect or a history of a trauma that causes a treatment delay. Most likely because of the delay, 50% of the patients already had local or regional metastases. There is no causal relationship between trauma or chronic infection and subungual melanoma, although trauma has been mentioned in 34% of cases of subungual melanoma.[15,17,18]

The prognosis of a melanoma depends on the histopathologic features of the primary, based on the depth of invasion and thickness of the tumor, and the presence of local, regional, or distant metastasis at the time of diagnosis. It is very difficult for a pathologist to describe the depth of invasion and the tumor thickness of a subungual melanoma based on a small biopsy specimen. Adequate histologic staging requires a partial amputation to provide an adequate biopsy specimen. Nail destruction and invasion of bone are specific prognostic factors for a subungual melanoma.[19] All subungual melanomas in this series were high-risk tumors at Clark stages IV and V and with a Breslow thickness greater than 1.5 mm.

When a subungual melanoma finally is diagnosed, how should this unusual tumor be treated? How wide should local excision of the tumor be? In their first article Pack and Adair[7] advocated amputation in the metacarpophalangeal or metatarsophalangeal joint. Later Pack and Oropeza,[6] as well as Papachristou and Fortner,[19] asserted that any amputation below the carpometacarpal or tarsometatarsal level was inadequate as far as local recurrence is concerned. We administered isolated regional perfusion followed by amputation at the metacarpophalangeal joint or metatarsophalangeal joint and no local recurrences were diagnosed. Patients with clinically palpable nodes should undergo lymph node dissection. The question of whether an elective or prophylactic regional lymph node dissection is of any value is still controversial.[19]

In the majority of the published series only the five-year survival rate, but not the rate of locoregional control, is mentioned (Table 3). It seems that in our series hyperthermic isolated regional perfusion did not improve the survival of the patients with a subungual melanoma, but 100% locoregional control was achieved without severe morbidity and no mortality.

Isolated hyperthermic regional perfusion in the treatment of melanomas of the extremities is still controversial. At this writing, a prospective randomized trial to investigate the value of hyperthermic isolated regional perfusion in the treatment of a primary extremity melanoma with a thickness of 1.5 mm or more was under way in Europe. As has been suggested by Franklin et al,[20] those patients with a subungual melanoma without distant metastases might benefit from perfusion therapy, just like those patients with local recurrence, satellitosis, or in-transit metastases from a nonsubungual extremity melanoma without distant metastases.

We thank Leo T. van der Weele for the statistical analysis of the data.

References

1. Hertzler ZE: Fungus hematodes du petit doight. *Gazette Med Paris,* 1834, p 212.
2. Demargnay, Monod: Cancer mélanique du ponce et de baissell. *Gaz Hop,* 1855, p 415.
3. Hutchinson J: Melanotic disease of the great toe, following a whitlow of the nail. *Trans Pathol Soc Lond* 1857;8:404.
4. Hutchinson J: Melanosis often not black: Melanotic whitlow. *Br Med J* 1886;1:491.
5. Das Gupta TK, Brasfield R: Subungual melanoma: Twenty-five-year review of cases. *Ann Surg* 1965;161:545-552.
6. Pack GT, Oropeza R: Subungual melanoma. *Surg Gynecol Obstet* 1967;124:571-582.
7. Pack GT, Adair EE: Subungual melanoma: The differential diagnosis of tumors of the nail bed. *Surgery* 1939;5:47-72.
8. Braitman M: Subungual malignant melanoma. *Cutis* 1979;23:617-623.
9. Clark WH, From L, Bernardino EA, et al: The histogenesis and biologic behavior of human malignant melanoma of the skin. *Cancer Res* 1969;29:705-727.
10. Breslow A: Tumor thickness, level of invasion and node dissection in stage I cutaneous melanoma. *Ann Surg* 1975;182:572-575.
11. Schraffordt Koops H, Oldhoff J, Oosterhuis JW, et al: The role of isolated limb perfusion for regional metastases of the extremities, in Balch CM (ed): *Pigment Cell.* New York, S Karger AG, 1985, pp 146-169.
12. Fontijne W, de Vries J, Mook P, et al: Improved tissue perfusion during pressure-regulated hyperthermic regional isolated perfusion in dogs. *J Surg Oncol* 1984;26:69-76.
13. Schraffordt Koops H: Prevention of neural and muscular lesions during hyperthermic regional perfusion. *Surg Gynecol Obstet* 1972;135:401-403.
14. Van Os J, Schraffordt Koops H, Oldhoff J: Dosimetry of cytostatics in hyperthermic regional isolated perfusion. *Cancer* 1985;3:698-701.
15. Takematsu H, Tomita Y, Kato T, et al: Subungual melanoma: A clinico-pathologic study of 16 Japanese cases. *Cancer* 1985;55:2725-2731.
16. Welvaart K, Schraffordt Koops H: Subungual malignant melanoma: A nail in the coffin. *Clin Oncol* 1978;4:309-315.
17. Patterson RH, Helwing EL: Subungual melanoma: A clinical pathological study. *Cancer* 1980;46:2074-2087.
18. Panizzon R, Krebs A: Das subunguale maligne Melanom. *Hautarzt* 1980;31:132-140.
19. Papachristou DN, Fortner JG: Melanoma arising under the nail. *J Surg Oncol* 1982;21:219-222.
20. Franklin HR, Schraffordt Koops H, Oldhoff J, et al: To perfuse or not to perfuse? A retrospective comparison study to evaluate the effect of adjuvant isolated regional perfusion in patients with stage I extremity melanoma with a thickness of 1.5 mm or more. *J Clin Oncol* 1988;6:701-708.

Editorial Comment

Although this is a rare melanoma, the authors emphasize that the diagnosis is made late because this tumor is confused with benign conditions. Since the survival rate is determined by the stage of the disease, a high index of suspicion is essential to detect lesions in early stages. Treatment with amputation and adjuvant isolated regional perfusion did not improve survival, but substantial palliation was achieved with no instances of local or regional recurrence. Since this is a rare tumor, a randomized control trial would take too long to conduct. With the authors' report of excellent locoregional control, further studies with this treatment regimen are indicated.

LaSalle D. Leffall, Jr, MD
Washington, DC

Influence of Estrogen Receptors on Survival and Recurrence in Patients With Breast Cancer Without Lymph Node Metastases

Hope S. Maki, MD, James L. Hoehn, MD

• A retrospective chart review was conducted to determine the prognostic effect of estrogen receptor (ER) protein in patients with node-negative operable breast cancer. One hundred nine patients with breast cancer whose tumors underwent ER analysis and whose lymph node negativity was established histologically were studied. Based on life-table analysis, the overall survival at six years was 92.7% for ER-positive patients, 95.3% for ER-negative patients, and 94.4% for ER-borderline patients. The disease-free survival was 83.3%, 92.8%, and 71.4%, respectively. Survival and disease-free survival were also correlated to menopausal status. The difference in survival was not statistically significant at six years. We conclude that in node-negative primary operable breast cancer, ER status should not be used as a discriminant for adjuvant treatment.

(*Arch Surg* 1989;124:377-380)

Since the early 1970s, estrogen receptor (ER) determinations on breast cancer specimens have become standard practice. Initially, ER positivity was equated with a more favorable prognosis.[1-11] Recently, other reports have indicated that ER status may have prognostic significance only in a select patient population.[12-15]

The present study was undertaken to review our experience with patients with node-negative breast cancer during a five-year period. In particular, overall survival and disease-free survival (DFS) were examined and correlated with ER status.

PATIENTS AND METHODS

From January 1975 through December 1979, 424 patients were treated surgically for primary breast cancer. From this group, 109 tumors were identified that had no axillary node involvement confirmed on histologic examination and that had undergone ER determinations. Inoperability, metastatic disease, and bilaterality were grounds for elimination from the study. All patients underwent either a radical (11 patients) or modified radical (98 patients) mastectomy.

Estrogen receptor protein analysis was done using a modification of the dextran-coated charcoal procedure described by Liskowski and Rose[16] and previously reported from our institution.[17] The samples were immediately taken to the pathology laboratory, where a portion was sectioned for histologic examination and a portion was quick frozen in liquid nitrogen and stored at −70°C until it was assayed. All ER assays were performed within one week of specimen collection. Specific ER sites are expressed as femtomoles of receptor per milligram of protein. Results were expressed as positive (>10 fmol/mg of protein), negative (<3 fmol/mg of protein), or borderline (3 to 10 fmol/mg of protein). Overall survival and DFS were measured from the date of the pathologically confirmed diagnosis.

Statistical analysis was done according to Kaplan-Meier life-table methods. For comparisons of survival rates where survival was 100% in one of the groups, the confidence limits for the group with less than 100% survival were compared with exact confidence limits from the binomial with zero failures in n trials, where n is the number of patients who were followed up for at least six years. In addition, Cox proportional-hazards regression analysis was used to study the effects of other variables on survival.

RESULTS

Of the 109 patients included in the study, only one was male. The median age was 62 years (range, 28 to 88 years). Twenty-one patients were premenopausal and 87 patients were postmenopausal. The average size of the 104 tumors that were measured was 2.3 cm (range, 0.5 to 7.0 cm). Fifty-two tumors were 2.0 cm in diameter or less, 51 were more than 2 cm and less than or equal to 5.0 cm in diameter, and one tumor was more than 5.0 cm in diameter. Estrogen receptor protein analysis showed 46 patients to be positive, 43 to be negative, and 20 to be borderline. Thirty-three patients had received adjuvant therapy (29 of them with adjuvant postoperative radiation therapy) primarily for medial or central lesions and four patients had received chemotherapy based on a protocol study being conducted at the time. Seventy-six patients were treated with surgery alone.

The mean follow-up time for the entire group was 77.0

Accepted for publication Feb 18, 1988.

From the Department of Surgery, Marshfield (Wisc) Clinic and Marshfield Medical Research Foundation.

Reprint requests to Department of Surgery, Marshfield Clinic, 1000 N Oak Ave, Marshfield, WI 54449 (Dr Hoehn).

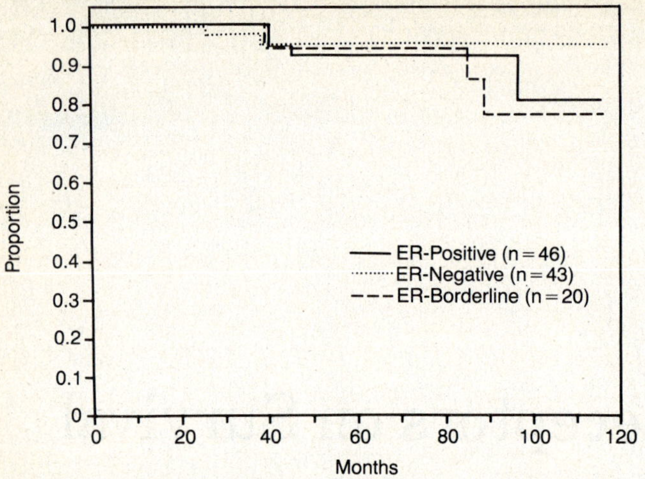

Fig 1.—Life-table analysis of overall survival for entire group. Differences are not statistically significant.

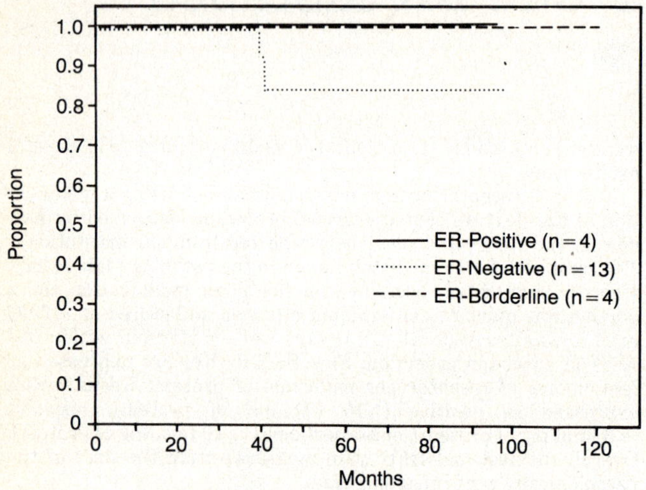

Fig 2.—Life-table analysis of overall survival for premenopausal patients. Differences are not statistically significant.

Fig 3.—Life-table analysis of overall survival for postmenopausal patients. Differences are not statistically significant.

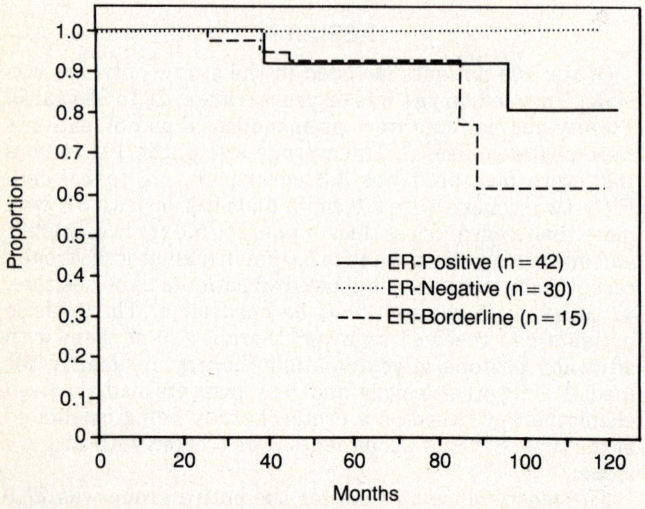

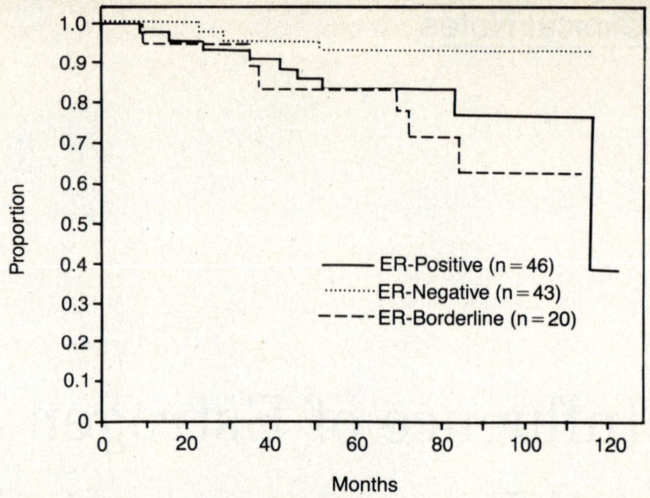

Fig 4.—Life-table analysis of disease-free survival for entire group. Differences are not statistically significant.

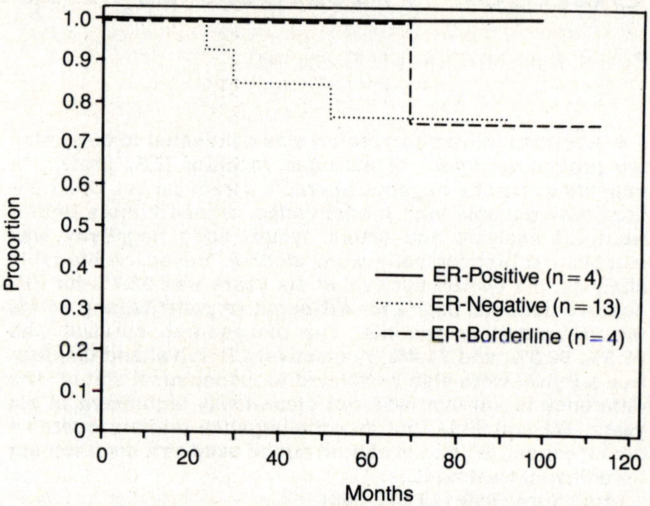

Fig 5.—Life-table analysis of disease-free survival for premenopausal patients. Differences are not statistically significant.

Fig 6.—Life-table analysis of disease-free survival for postmenopausal patients. Differences are not statistically significant.

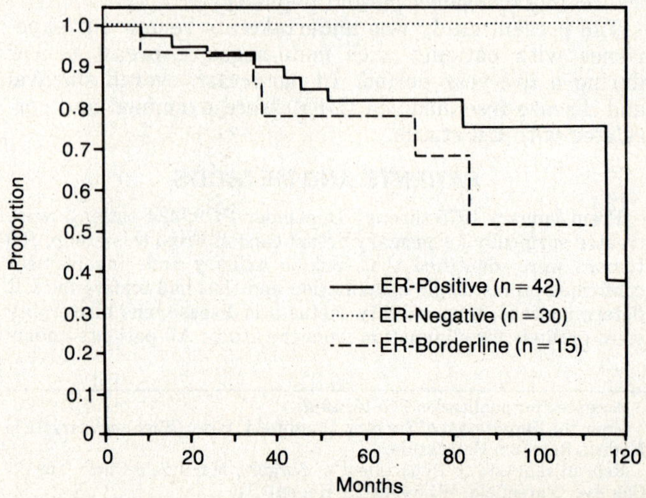

Table 1.—Recurrence and Survival

Menopausal Status	Estrogen Receptor Status, No. (%) of Patients*: Positive	Negative	Borderline
Recurrence			
Premenopausal	0/4 (0)	3/13 (23)	1/4 (25)
Postmenopausal	9/42 (21)	0/30 (0)	5/15 (33)
Total	9/46 (20)	3/43 (7)	6/20 (30)
Survival			
Premenopausal	4/4 (100)	10/13 (77)	4/4 (100)
Postmenopausal	31/42 (74)	27/30 (90)	12/15 (80)
Total	39/46 (85)	40/43 (93)	14/20 (70)†

*Included are patients dying of other cancer.
†Including the one male patient.

Table 2.—Cox Proportional-Hazards Analysis of Estrogen Receptor Levels

Independent Variable	Overall Survival: Coefficient Estimate	Overall Survival: Z*	Disease-Free Survival: Coefficient Estimate	Disease-Free Survival: Z*
Age, y	.02560	0.63	−.00571	−0.21
Tumor size, cm	−.27544	−0.78	−.14240	−0.59
Menopausal status (0 = premenopausal; 1 = postmenopausal)	−.66081	−0.53	−.16029	−0.19
Estrogen receptor level	−.00107	−0.09	.00303	0.49

*No coefficient was statistically significant.

months. All patients were available for follow-up. The mean DFS was 72.3 months. At the time of chart review, nine patients were alive with disease, nine had died of disease, and 15 had died of other causes. The remaining 76 patients had no evidence of disease.

The mean DFS was 67.2 months for the ER-positive patients, 77.4 months for the ER-negative patients, and 73.1 months for the ER-borderline patients. For patients receiving no adjuvant therapy, the mean DFS was 72.3 months, for those undergoing radiation therapy it was 69.7 months, and for the four patients receiving chemotherapy it was 91.8 months. Table 1 lists the overall survival and recurrence for all patients according to menopausal status at the time of chart review.

Survival and DFS were correlated to ER status using life-table analysis. Figure 1 depicts the overall survival according to ER status. At six years, survival was 92.7% for the ER-positive patients, 95.3% for the ER-negative patients, and 94.4% for the ER-borderline group. Figures 2 and 3 show the overall survival according to menopausal status. The number of premenopausal patients is small (four ER-positive, 13 ER-negative, and four ER-borderline). Respective overall survivals were 100%, 84%, and 100% at six years. Respective survivals among the postmenopausal patients were 92% for the ER-positive, 100% for the ER-negative, and 92.3% for the ER-borderline groups at six years. The differences in survival are not statistically significant.

The DFS for the entire group is shown in Fig 4. At six years 83.3% of the ER-positive, 92.8% of ER-negative, and 71.4% of ER-borderline patients were free of disease. The DFS probability for the ER-negative group was greater than for the ER-positive and ER-borderline groups at six years. The difference between the ER-negative and ER-borderline group was of borderline significance ($Z = 1.84$). The DFS according to menopausal status was examined. Among the premenopausal patients, DFS was 100%, 76.2%, and 75%, respectively, at six years for the ER-positive, ER-negative, and borderline groups. The differences were not significant because of the small numbers in the subgroups (Fig 5). Among the postmenopausal patients, the DFS was 81.6%, 100%, and 68.1% for ER-positive, ER-negative, and borderline groups, respectively, during the same time period (Fig 6). The DFS probability for ER-negative postmenopausal patients was greater than for ER-positive or ER-borderline patients at six years, but the difference was not statistically significant.

Because the patients with breast cancer were of a variety of ages and had differences in tumor size and menopausal status, Cox proportional-hazards regression analyses were performed to see whether adjustment for these factors would influence the survival patterns with regard to the ER level. The best-fitting models as determined by the likelihood ratio test were those using the continuous measurement of the ER level, rather than classification as positive, negative, or borderline. Table 2 shows the estimated regression coefficients for overall survival and disease recurrence. In both cases the coefficient for the ER level is very close to zero and is not statistically significant. When patients were classified as ER-positive, ER-negative, or ER-borderline, the coefficient for the ER-negative group was negative and approached statistical significance in all analyses, suggesting that these patients as a group had a more favorable prognosis compared with the ER-borderline and ER-positive patients. These analyses support the life-table results.

Additional regression analyses were done using only postmenopausal patients, with no change in the results. In an attempt to control for the effect of differences in treatment, an additional set of analyses was done using only those patients who had undergone a modified radical mastectomy and who did not receive initial adjuvant treatment. Again, the results were unaffected.

It is important to recognize that the analyses in the present report are based on a relatively small sample of patients. Nevertheless, there was no evidence from any of the analyses that positive ER status was associated with improved survival. In fact, there was evidence that ER-negative patients enjoyed a more favorable prognosis.

COMMENT

When the ER protein assay gained widespread use in the early 1970s, it was noted that ER-positive patients with metastatic breast cancer as a group had a more favorable response to endocrine therapy than those patients with ER-negative determinations.[1] Shortly thereafter, Walt and coworkers[2] reported that ER positivity was also associated with an improved survival. Knight et al[3] noted a statistically significant increase in early recurrence in ER-negative patients that was independent of age, tumor size, location, or axillary lymph node status. Allegra and coworkers[4] in 1979 reported similar results that also were independent of age, menopausal status, tumor size, and nodal status. Furmanski et al[5] confirmed their earlier finding that patients with ER-positive tumors survived longer and had a longer DFS.[6] Numerous other reports of similar findings have been published.[7-11]

Several studies have recently proposed that this association between ER status and prognosis does not pertain to all subgroups of patients. In 1980, Hilf et al[12] studied

ER status as a prognostic factor for recurrence as well as response to chemotherapy. The likelihood of recurrence was based on nodal and menopausal status, not ER level. A Norwegian study conducted by Aamdal et al[13] showed that ER status influenced survival and DFS only in patients with positive lymph nodes. Furthermore, during the study period this influence only persisted in the premenopausal women with axillary metastases. A point should be made, however, that in 58 patients (25%) lymph node status was based only on findings from the clinical examination. Axillary dissections were not performed because these patients were older. In 1982 Shapiro et al[14] found that the presence or absence of axillary lymph node metastases, and not ER status, was the most important prognostic variable for patients with breast cancer. Finally, in 1985 Butler et al[15] looked specifically at the same question that the present report examines: Does ER status have prognostic significance in overall survival or DFS in node-negative disease? Five hundred fifty-six patients were followed up for a median period of 75 months. The overall survival and DFS in the entire group and in premenopausal and postmenopausal patients did not change significantly according to ER status. Butler and colleagues[15] concluded that adjuvant chemotherapy should not be considered for patients with ER-negative tumors and histologically negative lymph nodes.

Major advances in the study of the prognosis of breast cancer based on ER protein determinations have been made in the past decade. The hope has been that subgroups of patients will be identified who would benefit from adjuvant treatment following initial surgical intervention. In patients with histologically negative lymph nodes, we failed to demonstrate an effect of ER status on outcome, including either DFS or overall survival. Our results are based on a lengthy follow-up in a stable patient population. However, the study did include a small number of premenopausal patients who may benefit from further study.

Pat Pierce, Steven Broste, MS, and Brian Weiler provided assistance with statistical analysis and Shirley Thompson provided assistance with the figures.

References

1. McGuire WL: Current status of estrogen receptors in human breast cancer. *Cancer* 1975;36:638-644.
2. Walt AJ, Singhakowinta A, Brooks SC, et al: The surgical implications of estrophile protein estimations in carcinoma of the breast. *Surgery* 1976;80:506-512.
3. Knight WA, Livingston RB, Gregory EJ, et al: Estrogen receptor as an independent prognostic factor for early recurrence in breast cancer. *Cancer Res* 1977;37:4669-4671.
4. Allegra JC, Lippman ME, Simon R, et al: Association between steroid hormone receptor status and disease-free interval in breast cancer. *Cancer Treat Rep* 1979;63:1271-1277.
5. Furmanski P, Saunders DE, Brooks SC, et al: The prognostic value of estrogen receptor determinations in patients with primary breast cancer: An update. *Cancer* 1980;46:2794-2796.
6. Rich MA, Furmanski P, Brooks SC, et al: Prognostic value of estrogen receptor determinations in patients with breast cancer. *Cancer Res* 1978;38:4296-4298.
7. Cooke T, Shields R, George D, et al: Estrogen receptors and prognosis in early breast cancer. *Lancet* 1979;1:995-997.
8. Gapinski PV, Donegan WL: Estrogen receptors and breast cancer: Prognostic and therapeutic implications. *Surgery* 1980;88:386-392.
9. Osborne CK, Yochomowitz MG, Knight WA, et al: The value of estrogen and progesterone receptors in the treatment of breast cancer. *Cancer* 1980;46:2884-2888.
10. Singhakowinta A, Saunders DE, Brooks SC, et al: Clinical applications of estrogen receptor in breast cancer. *Cancer* 1980;46:2932-2938.
11. Neifeld JP, Lawrence W, Brown PW, et al: Estrogen receptors in primary breast cancer. *Arch Surg* 1982;117:753-757.
12. Hilf R, Feldstein ML, Gibson SL, et al: The relative importance of estrogen receptor analysis as a prognostic factor for recurrence or response to chemotherapy in women with breast cancer. *Cancer* 1980;45:1993-2000.
13. Aamdal S, Bormer O, Jorgensen O, et al: Estrogen receptors and long-term prognosis in breast cancer. *Cancer* 1984;53:2525-2529.
14. Shapiro CM, Schifeling D, Bitran JD, et al: Prognostic value of the estrogen receptor level in pathologic stage I and II adenocarcinoma of the breast. *J Surg Oncol* 1982;19:119-121.
15. Butler JA, Bretsky S, Menendex-Botet C, et al: Estrogen receptor protein of breast cancer as a predictor of recurrence. *Cancer* 1985;55:1178-1181.
16. Liskowski L, Rose DP: Experience with a simple method for estrogen receptor assay in breast cancer. *Clin Chim Acta* 1976;67:175-182.
17. Hoehn JL, Plotka ED, Dickson KB: Comparison of estrogen receptor levels in primary and regional metastatic carcinoma of the breast. *Ann Surg* 1979;190:69-71.

Editorial Comment

Patients with breast cancer who have negative lymph nodes have a relatively favorable prognosis, but some will not be cured by local therapy. A growing number of oncologists consider tumor ER negativity sufficient reason for recommending systemic adjuvant chemotherapy for these patients and this is supported by a recent clinical trial. Maki and Hoehn have found that ERs have no prognostic value and highlight the controversy that continues to exist on this issue. One cannot help but speculate that differing case selection, laboratory methods, numbers of cases, and duration of follow-up, as well as the influence of potent covariables, are contributing to this controversy. To complicate the matter further, the prognosis of node-negative patients varies considerably between institutions and is remarkably good at some, possibly because of earlier diagnosis and more complete staging. The five-year DFSs in excess of 90% regardless of ER status reported by Maki and Hoehn make it plain that the population at high risk for failure may be very small and a challenge to identify. Estrogen receptor status is only one of several prognostic factors in node-negative patients and is likely not the most reliable; it may be a better marker of how to treat than of whom to treat. Nuclear grade, histologic differentiation, intramammary lymphatic permeation, and skin involvement are others. The most promising factors, however, are objective measures of aggressive tumor growth, ie, thymidine labeling index and flow cytometric measurements of S-phase fraction and DNA ploidy. Future decisions for adjuvant therapy will likely be made on these bases.

William L. Donegan, MD
Milwaukee

A Foregut Carcinoid Tumor Causing Zollinger-Ellison Syndrome

Gordon B. Werbel, MD; Suzanne P. Nelson, MD; Philip G. Robinson, MD; John Anastasi, MD; Raymond J. Joehl, MD; Robert V. Rege, MD

• A patient had severe peptic ulcer disease complicated by gastric outlet obstruction and choledochoduodenal fistula. Serum gastrin levels were elevated preoperatively to 340 ng/L. A 1.5-cm histologically benign carcinoid tumor of the antrum of the stomach was found at surgery, and surgical resection of the tumor resulted in normalization of serum gastrin levels and amelioration of the peptic acid diathesis. The patient remains asymptomatic at one year. Immunohistochemical staining demonstrated that the carcinoid indeed contained gastrin along with chromogranin, cholecystokinin, and neuron-specific enolase. This is a case of Zollinger-Ellison syndrome caused by a benign foregut carcinoid (gastric carcinoid-gastrinoma).

(*Arch Surg* 1989;124:381-384)

Carcinoid tumors are most commonly found in the appendix, small intestine, and colon, but they may arise in the stomach, pancreaticoduodenal region, gallbladder and bile ducts, ovary, and pulmonary bronchial tree.[1] These neoplasms arise from enterochromaffin or enterochromaffinlike cells and have the potential to secrete vasoactive substances and hormones. The clinical, histochemical, and biochemical behavior of these tumors varies widely, and their behavior frequently depends on their site of origin.

Kulchitsky's cell tumor or carcinoid tumor of the stomach is a rare gastric tumor. It was originally described by Askanazy[2] in 1923 and accounts for less than 3% of gastrointestinal carcinoids and only 0.3% of all gastric tumors.[1,3,4] Although these tumors histologically resemble other gastrointestinal carcinoids, they are microscopically and clinically most similar to carcinoids of the lung, another foregut derivative. In general, they do not produce the carcinoid syndrome but, if they do, it is an atypical syndrome caused by the secretion of 5-hydroxytryptophan and histamine.[5] Most often, gastric carcinoids are clinically silent or are associated with atrophic gastritis and pernicious anemia,[6-8] while others have been reported to produce acid hypersecretion[8-10] and a syndrome indistinguishable from that described by Zollinger and Ellison.[11]

The following case report illustrates the effects of a gastrin-secreting carcinoid tumor of the gastric antrum. This tumor was associated with severe peptic ulcer disease complicated by gastric outlet obstruction and choledochoduodenal fistula.

REPORT OF A CASE

A 72-year-old man presented to the Veterans Administration Lakeside Medical Center, Chicago, with a three-week history of postprandial nausea and vomiting, anorexia, and weight loss. Peptic ulcer disease had been documented on several occasions over the previous eight-year period by upper gastrointestinal endoscopy and contrast roentgenograms. Fifteen months prior to hospital admission, the patient was hospitalized for gastric outlet obstruction and responded rapidly to administration of an H_2 receptor antagonist, which he took thereafter intermittently for symptoms of dyspepsia and abdominal pain. Other medications included aspirin and sulindac, which were administered for symptomatic rheumatoid arthritis. He also had a 45-pack-year history of cigarette smoking, but he had quit smoking 15 years ago. He denied alcohol ingestion, abdominal pain, flushing, or diarrhea. A fasting serum gastrin level, performed six years prior to hospital admission when he was asymptomatic, was elevated at 200 ng/L (limits of normal [fasting], 50 to 155 ng/L).

On physical examination, the patient was cachectic and profoundly dehydrated. In the supine position, blood pressure was 100/60 mm Hg and heart rate was 100 beats per minute, and, in the sitting position, 70 mm Hg systolic (palpable) and 120 beats per minute; temperature was 36.3°C. Findings from head, neck, chest, and cardiac examinations were unremarkable; the sclera were nonicteric. The abdomen was scaphoid, nontender, and without masses or hepatosplenomegaly. Bowel sounds were active. Rectal examination demonstrated occult blood in the stool.

Several diagnostic tests were performed. Results of a complete blood cell count were normal. Serum electrolytes demonstrated a severe hypokalemic, hypochloremic metabolic alkalosis (potassium, 2.7 mmol/L; chloride, 65 mmol/L; bicarbonate ion, 56 mmol/L); arterial blood gas determinations showed a metabolic alkalosis with partial respiratory compensation (pH, 7.55; carbon dioxide pressure, 54 mm Hg; oxygen pressure, 51 mm Hg; base excess, 29 mmol/L). Ketones were in the urine. Chest and abdominal roentgenograms were remarkable for a markedly distended

Accepted for publication Sept 6, 1988.

From the Departments of Surgery (Drs Werbel, Nelson, Joehl, and Rege) and Pathology (Drs Robinson and Anastasi), Veterans Administration Lakeside Medical Center and Northwestern University Medical School, Chicago.

Reprint requests to Department of Surgery, Northwestern Memorial Hospital, 250 E Superior St, Chicago, IL 60611 (Dr Rege).

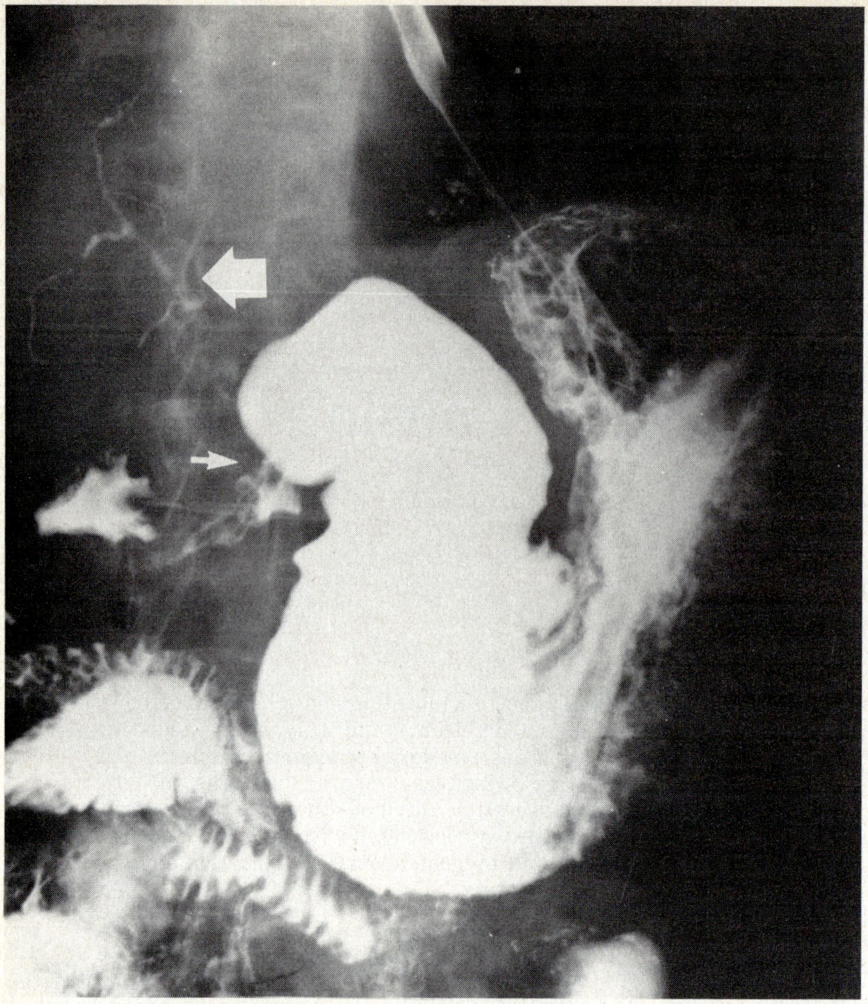

Fig 1.—Upper gastrointestinal series in our patient demonstrates two abnormalities: markedly deformed duodenal bulb with partial gastric outlet obstruction (small arrow) and presence of barium sulfate in biliary tree (large arrow).

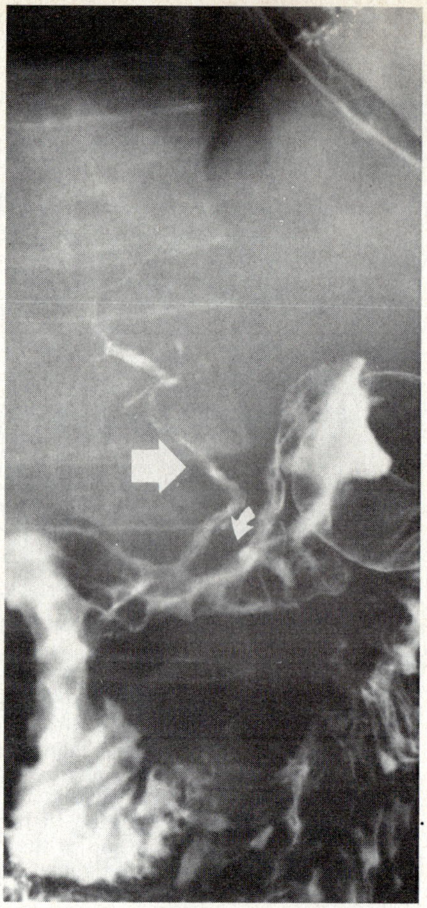

Fig 2.—Magnification view of duodenum demonstrates duodenal ulcer (small arrow) and choledochoduodenal fistula (large arrow). Barium sulfate flowed freely from duodenum into common duct. Upper endoscopy confirmed presence of active peptic ulcer disease.

stomach, and air was in the biliary tract. An upper gastrointestinal tract series demonstrated a pyloric channel ulcer with gastric outlet obstruction and narrowing of the first portion of the duodenum; a choledochoduodenal fistula was confirmed by free flow of barium sulfate from the duodenum into the common bile duct (Figs 1 and 2). Upper endoscopy showed a benign prepyloric ulcer with surrounding edema; the endoscope could not be advanced into the duodenum.

Fluid and electrolyte abnormalities were corrected by intravenous administration of 2.6 L of balanced salt solutions containing supplemental potassium chloride. A nasogastric tube was inserted to decompress the stomach, and intravenous hyperalimentation was administered. The peptic ulcer was treated with 1600 mg/d of cimetidine hydrochloride by continuous intravenous infusion. The nasogastric tube drained 3 to 4 L/d from the stomach during ten days of treatment. A fasting serum gastrin level, which was drawn after stabilization of the patient's condition with decompression of the stomach by nasogastric suction, was elevated to 340 ng/L. Although Zollinger-Ellison syndrome was considered, performance of a secretin stimulation test was contraindicated by the patient's condition. Furthermore, he was not a candidate for a total gastrectomy. The patient was taken to surgery for exploratory laparotomy and treatment of his gastric outlet obstruction and biliary fistula.

At operation, a benign stricture of the pyloric channel was found. No duodenal, pancreatic, or omental masses were found. A 1.5-cm submucosal mass was palpated in the gastric antrum along the lesser curvature, 1 cm proximal to the pylorus. No hepatic or intra-abdominal metastases were found. A vagotomy and antrectomy, which included the antral mass and adequate margins of resection, were performed. Gastrointestinal continuity was restored with a gastrojejunostomy (Billroth II anastomosis), and the choledochoduodenal fistula was not disturbed. The patient's postoperative course was uncomplicated, and he ate a general diet on his sixth postoperative day. Repeated serum gastrin level was 40 ng/L four weeks after the operation.

On gross examination the antral mucosa demonstrated a 1.5-cm intramural, submucosal, yellow-brown lesion; the lesion had a well-defined border but was not encapsulated. Microscopically, the tumor cells were small and regular; also, the tumor cells had a moderate amount of acidophilic cytoplasm and round regular nuclei with a stippled chromatin pattern (Fig 3). No evidence of tissue infiltration existed. The lymph nodes had no evidence of metastases. There was no evidence of G-cell hyperplasia in the remainder of the gastric antrum. A Grimelius stain showed argyrophilic granules while a Fontana-Masson stain was negative for argentaffinity, indicating that this was a tumor of foregut origin (Table). Thus, the histologic appearance was consistent with a benign carcinoid tumor of the stomach.

Immunohistochemical stains were performed on the formaldehyde-fixed, paraffin-embedded tumor using the peroxidase method of Sternberger[12] as modified by Taylor.[13] Special stains for gastrin as well as chromogranin, cholecystokinin, and neuron-specific enolase were positive. Stains for glucagon, insulin, S100 protein, keratin, somatostatin, serotonin, human pancreatic polypeptide, and corticotropin (ACTH) were negative. The case was

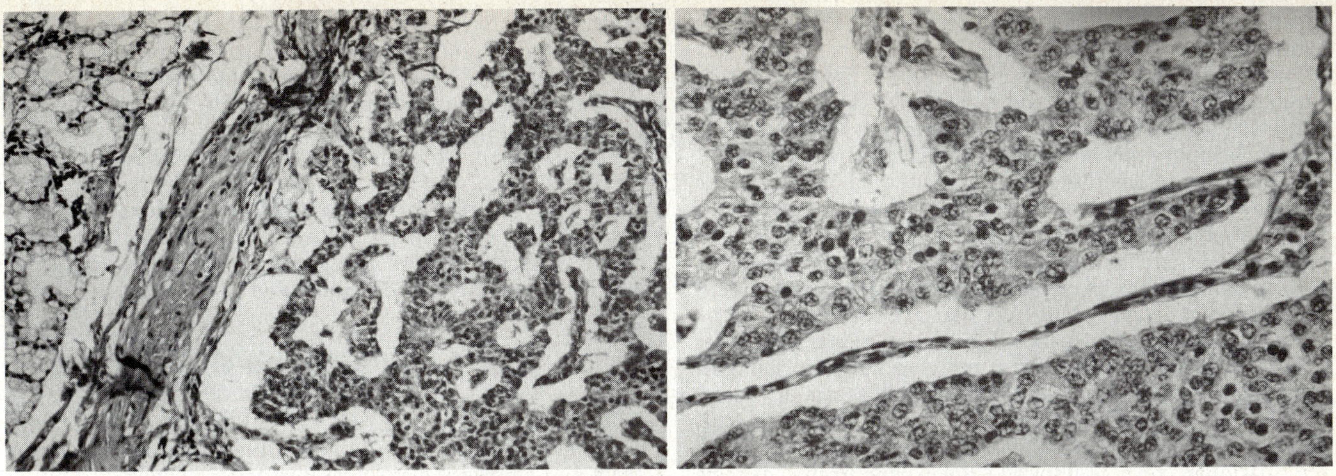

Fig 3.—Left, Pale-staining duodenal Brunner's glands in upper left corner. Note small, regular cells with acidophilic cytoplasm and round, regular nuclei and stippled chromatin (hematoxylin-eosin, original magnification ×40). Right, Higher magnification shows thick cords of neoplastic cells with thin intertwining blood vessels, consistent with benign carcinoid tumor (hematoxylin-eosin, original magnification ×250).

Types of Intracellular Granules in Carcinoid Tumors of the Gastrointestinal Tract*

Derivation of Carcinoid	Argyrophilic Granules	Argentaffinic Granules
Foregut	Present	Absent
Midgut	Present	Present
Hindgut	Absent	Absent

*The types of intracellular granules found in carcinoid tumors are derived embryologically from the foregut, midgut, or hindgut. Note that the carcinoid tumor reported herein stained for argyrophilic but not argentaffinic granules. Thus, it is a typical gastric carcinoid of foregut origin.

reviewed by the Armed Forces Institute of Pathology (Washington, DC), Gastrointestinal Branch, and they agreed with the diagnosis and the immunochemistry findings.

COMMENT

A variety of names have been used to describe carcinoid tumors that secrete gastrin, including carcinoid-islet cell tumor,[14] gastrinoma,[15] and apudoma.[16] The term *apudoma* originated shortly after Pearse[17,18] recognized that endocrine cells were dispersed throughout the body and that these cells shared certain cytochemical and ultrastructural characteristics, including a high *a*mine content, a capability for amine *p*recursor *u*ptake, and the presence of *d*ecarboxylase enzyme (APUD). The name APUD was given to these cells, and the term *apudoma* was used to describe neoplasias or hyperplasias of these cells. All apudomas contain polypeptide hormones, and some are capable of secreting them. The cells of the APUD system and their neoplastic counterparts are found in the pituitary, pineal gland, hypothalamus, pancreas, stomach, intestine, thyroid, parathyroid, carotid body, skin, adrenal glands, lung, and urogenital tract; hence the term *apudoma* is not a morphologic diagnosis but rather a conceptual diagnosis. It does not apply to a specific histologic type of tumor.

Gastrinoma is the clinical term for neuroendocrine (APUD) tumors that secrete gastrin. This diagnosis is based on clinical grounds, including a history of severe peptic ulcer disease, often with complications, and elevated serum gastrin levels. The term *gastrinoma* describes the clinical state of the patient, but it does not define the morphologic and pathologic characteristics of the tumor. It does not indicate whether the tumor is benign or malignant, or whether the tumor arises from pancreatic islet cells (most common site) or from extrapancreatic organs. If the tumor is removed surgically and stained immunochemically, it may show the presence of multiple hormones, including gastrin.[19] The term *carcinoid-islet cell tumor* was therefore proposed in 1967 by Weichert et al[14] because carcinoid tumors and islet cell tumors have similar structures. However, the term *carcinoid-islet cell tumor* has not become popular among either pathologists or surgeons because it adds little to either the pathologic or clinical diagnosis.

Therefore, the term *carcinoid tumor* persists because it is well understood by physicians and it represents a specific histologic diagnosis. Contrary to popular belief, the presence of serotonin in the tumor is not required for the diagnosis of carcinoid tumor; as previously stated, it is rare in carcinoids derived from the foregut. If the clinical presentation suggests the overproduction of a specific vasoactive substance or polypeptide hormone, the tumor can be stained immunochemically for a variety of neuroendocrine markers, including insulin, glucagon, vasoactive intestinal polypeptide, somatostatin, pancreatic polypeptide, and gastrin. The pathologist then reports these neuroendocrine lesions of the gastrointestinal tract as carcinoids with a note indicating the location of the tumor and the immunochemical stains that were performed and whether they were positive or negative. With this in mind, the lesion in our patient can be best described as a gastric (or antral) carcinoid-gastrinoma, which describes both its histologic and clinical features.

In contrast to the benign behavior of carcinoids of the appendix,[20-23] carcinoid tumors in the stomach have a high propensity to metastasize and should be considered potentially malignant. In a review of 2837 carcinoid tumors, Godwin[1] found that 55% of patients with gastric carcinoids had metastases and, subsequently, only 50% survived five years. He also found a 2% incidence of multicentric gastric carcinoids. Several more recent reports have shown a higher incidence of multicentricity (14% to 50%), less frequent metastases (18% to 36%), and longer survival.[6-8,24] Nevertheless, the size of the primary tumor is closely correlated with the incidence of metastases and may have more significance than site of origin. Carcinoids less than 1 cm in diameter have a 2% incidence of metastasis, whereas those greater than 2 cm are associated with an 80% to 100% incidence of metastases.[22,25]

Since the clinical presentation of patients with a gastric carcinoid can be variable and most patients are asymptomatic or have minimal symptoms, many are found incidentally on barium swallow roentgenograms, upper endoscopy, and laparotomy. In others, an atypical carcinoid syndrome may develop and is characterized by a severe and prolonged vasodilatory facial flush, hypotension, periorbital edema, and lacrimation.[26] Other symptoms, including Zollinger-Ellison syndrome,[9,10] have been reported depending on the biochemically active compounds that are secreted.

Recommended treatment of gastric carcinoid includes wide local excision for small tumors or subtotal gastrectomy for larger lesions; resection of metastasis is recommended in selected patients who are suitable candidates. Metastatic disease is poorly controlled with chemotherapy, but patients with Zollinger-Ellison syndrome can be treated with high-dose histamine receptor blockers or by total gastrectomy, and flushing episodes have been successfully ameliorated by the serotonin antagonists, methysergide and cyproheptadine. In addition, a report[27] on the treatment of Zollinger-Ellison syndrome with somatostatin analogue indicates that this may be a safe, effective method of controlling peptic ulcer diathesis.

The operation we performed in this patient resected the carcinoid, bypassed the gastric outlet obstruction, and permitted spontaneous closure of the choledochoduodenal fistula (the latter most certainly a complication of his duodenal ulcer). His prognosis is good because the tumor was less than 2 cm in diameter and postoperative plasma gastrin level is normal.

CONCLUSION

Gastric carcinoid is a rare clinical entity, and the diagnosis is often difficult and sometimes obscure. However, early and aggressive surgical intervention should improve prognosis and survival of these patients since smaller tumors are less likely to recur or act in a malignant manner.

References

1. Godwin JD: Carcinoid tumors: An analysis of 2837 cases. *Cancer* 1975;36:560-569.
2. Askanazy M: Zur Pathogenese der Magenkrehse und über ihren gelegentlichen Ursprung aus ange horenen epithelialen keimen in der Magen wand. *Dtsch Med Wochenschr* 1923;49:49-51.
3. Sanders RJ, Axtell HK: Carcinoids of the gastrointestinal tract. *Surg Gynecol Obstet* 1964;119:369-381.
4. MacDonald RA: A study of 356 carcinoids of the gastrointestinal tract. *Am J Med* 1956;21:867-878.
5. Friesen SR: Tumors of the endocrine pancreas. *N Engl J Med* 1982;306:580-590.
6. Solcia E: Gastric carcinoids and related endocrine growths. *Digestion* 1986;35:3-22.
7. Carney JA: The syndrome of gastric argyrophil carcinoid tumors and nonantral gastric atrophy. *Ann Intern Med* 1983;99:761-766.
8. Wilander E: Histopathology of gastric carcinoids: A survey of 42 cases. *Histopathology* 1984;8:183-193.
9. Bhagavan BS: Zollinger-Ellison syndrome: Ultrastructural and histochemical observations in a child with endocrine tumorlets of gastric antrum. *Arch Pathol Lab Med* 1974;98:217-222.
10. Goodrick WJM: Zollinger-Ellison syndrome: Associated gastric tumor showing islet cell features. *Minn Med* 1963;46:634-639.
11. Zollinger RM, Ellison EH: Primary peptic ulceration of the jejunum associated with islet cell tumors of the pancreas. *Ann Surg* 1955;142:719-728.
12. Sternberger LA: The unlabeled antibody-enzyme method of immunohistochemistry. *J Histochem Cytochem* 1970;18:315-333.
13. Taylor CR: Immunoperoxidase techniques: Practical and theoretical aspects. *Arch Pathol Lab Med* 1978;102:113-121.
14. Weichert R, Reed R, Creech O Jr: Carcinoid-islet cell tumors of the duodenum. *Ann Surg* 1967;165:660-669.
15. Carlei F, Bloom SR, Polak JM: Regulatory peptides of the gastrointestinal tract and their derivative tumors, in Cohens S, Soloway RD (eds): *Hormone-Producing Tumors of the Gastrointestinal Tract.* New York, Churchill Livingstone Inc, 1985, pp 1-24.
16. Welbourn RB: Apudomas of the gut. *Am J Surg* 1977;55:115-125.
17. Pearse AGE: Common cytochemical and ultrastructural characteristics of cell-producing polypeptide hormones (the APUD series) and their relevance to thyroid and ultimobranchial C cells and calcitonin. *Proc R Soc Lond* 1968;170:71-80.
18. Pearse AGE: The diffuse neuroendocrine system and the APUD concept: Related endocrine peptides in brain, intestine, pituitary, placenta and anuran cutaneous glands. *Med Biol* 1977;55:115-125.
19. Mukai K, Greider MH, Grotting JC, et al: Retrospective study of 77 pancreatic endocrine tumors using the immunoperoxidase method. *Am J Surg Pathol* 1982;6:387-399.
20. Oberndorfer S: Karzinoide Tumoren des Dunnderma. *Z Pathol* 1907;1:426-432.
21. Ritchie MB: Carcinoid tumors. *Am J Med Sci* 1956;232:311-328.
22. Moertel CG: Carcinoid tumors of the vermiform appendix. *Cancer* 1968;21:270-278.
23. Ryden S: Carcinoid tumors of the appendix in children. *Cancer* 1975;36:1538-1542.
24. Borch K: Gastric endocrine cell hyperplasia and carcinoid tumors in pernicious anemia. *Gastroenterology* 1985;88:638-648.
25. Glasser CM, Bhagavan BS: Carcinoid tumors of the appendix. *Arch Pathol Lab Med* 1980;104:272-275.
26. Kaplan EL: The carcinoid syndromes, in Friesen SR (ed): *Surgical Endocrinology: Clinical Syndromes.* Philadelphia, JB Lippincott, 1978, pp 120-147.
27. Ellison EC, O'Dorisio TM, Sparks J, et al: Observations on the effect of a somatostatin analogue in the Zollinger-Ellison syndrome: Implications for the treatment of apudomas. *Surgery* 1986;100:437-444.

In Other AMA Journals

ARCHIVES OF INTERNAL MEDICINE

Calf Deep Venous Thrombosis: A Wolf in Sheep's Clothing?

John T. Philbrick, MD, Daniel M. Becker, MD, MPH

To determine the natural history of calf deep venous thrombosis (C-DVT), an analytic review of the 20 relevant English-language papers published since 1942 was performed. Remarkably little methodologically sound research on this subject was found. However, available evidence suggests that C-DVT propagates to the thigh in up to 20% of cases and that propagation invariably occurs before embolization. No fatal emboli were reported in patients presenting with isolated C-DVT. Traditional anticoagulation treatment with heparin sodium and warfarin sodium of symptomatic patients with C-DVT appears to prevent extension, embolization, and early recurrence. There is no convincing evidence that C-DVT leads to chronic venous insufficiency or whether the risks of anticoagulation exceed the risks of no treatment. As an option to anticoagulation, physicians may choose to follow patients with C-DVT with serial impedance plethysmography, treating only if there is evidence of proximal extension (*Arch Intern Med* 1988;148:2131-2138).

Reprint requests to University of Virginia School of Medicine, Box 494, Charlottesville, VA 22908 (Dr Philbrick).

Technique

Fibrin Glue Achieves Hemostasis in Patients With Coagulation Disorders

Harry B. Kram, MD; Ragu C. Nathan, MD; Frederick J. Stafford, MD; Arthur W. Fleming, MD; William C. Shoemaker, MD

• Fibrin glue (FG), made with highly concentrated human fibrinogen and clotting factors, was used to achieve parenchymal organ hemostasis in patients with disordered coagulation secondary to massive transfusion, chronic disease, and disseminated intravascular coagulation; it was effective in controlling liver hemorrhage in seven patients and in the performance of a splenorrhaphy in one other patient. The coagulation profile was grossly abnormal in all patients, and the mean ± SD intraoperative blood loss was 5.1 ± 4.2 L; patients received 14 ± 10 U of blood perioperatively. The amount of FG required to achieve hemostasis varied directly with the extent of injury and intraoperative blood loss ($r = .84$), and all patients with a blood loss greater than 4 L required at least 25 mL of FG to stop bleeding. Two patients died postoperatively secondary to cardiac arrest and adult respiratory distress syndrome. Because FG does not depend on adequate platelet or clotting factor levels to be effective, it is especially useful in patients with parenchymal organ hemorrhage and disordered coagulation.

(*Arch Surg* 1989;124:385-387)

The development of disordered coagulation in the acutely injured patient who requires emergency surgery is associated with increased mortality.[1,2] In addition, the failure to effect intraoperative hemostasis rapidly may result in iatrogenic injury, resulting from attempts to control hemorrhage in an operative field obscured by rapidly pooling blood. Conventional topical hemostatic agents, which enhance normal clotting by providing a matrix around which blood clots can form or entrap platelets, are usually ineffective in the bleeding patient with deficient clotting factors and thrombocytopenia.

The use of highly concentrated human fibrinogen, in combination with thrombin, factor XIII, and calcium chloride, has been shown to result in the formation of a fibrin glue (FG) that is effective in establishing hemostasis of parenchymal organs, sealing anastomoses, and promoting normal wound healing after surgery.[3-7] Moreover, experimental studies revealed that FG was effective in hemostatically sealing vascular graft anastomoses in an anticoagulated canine model.[8] In the present study, FG was used to achieve hemostasis of liver and splenic injuries in patients with disordered coagulation secondary to massive transfusion, chronic disease, and disseminated intravascular coagulation.

MATERIALS AND METHODS

FG

Fibrin glue is made from four components: (1) highly concentrated fibrinogen (total protein approximately 120 mg/mL); (2) aprotinin (3000 KIU/mL) (1 KIU is equivalent to 1.111×10^{-3} trypsin inhibitor U); (3) dried thrombin (500 US [NIH] U/mL) (1 US [NIH] U is comparable with 1 IU of the first national standard); and (4) calcium chloride (400 μmol/mL). The fibrinogen is obtained from human donor plasma. After preheating to 37°C, the fibrinogen is dissolved in aprotinin, and the dried thrombin is reconstituted in calcium chloride. The two solutions are then drawn up into separate syringes that are loaded onto a double-barreled syringe holder designed to mix and apply the components simultaneously. The reconstitution procedure takes ten to 15 minutes, and the components should be used within four hours. The reconstituted adhesive contains 70 to 100 mg/mL of fibrinogen, 2 to 7 mg/mL of fibronectin (cold-insoluble globulin), 10 U/mL of factor XIII (1 U is that amount of factor XIII that is contained in 1 mL of citrated, pooled human plasma), and 35 mg/L of plasminogen.

On application, the components mix to form a clear, viscous solution that firmly adheres to wound surfaces and sets into a white, rubberlike mass within seconds. The adhesive continues to gain in tensile strength over the course of time; 70% of the maximum tensile strength is achieved in ten minutes.[9] During the subsequent course of wound healing, the adhesive slowly dissolves by fibrinolysis and is eventually completely removed from the body; aprotinin is added to slow the fibrinolytic process. The essential reactions after mixing of the components are proteolysis, fibrin cross-linking, and, finally, lysis and absorption of the clot material during the wound-healing process.

Clinical Data

The use of FG to control parenchymal organ hemorrhage was successfully performed in eight patients with coagulation disorders (Figs 1 through 4); the causes of injury are listed in Table 1. The coagulation profile was grossly abnormal in all patients, and the mean ± SD intraoperative blood loss was 5.1 ± 4.2 L; patients received 14 ± 10 U of blood perioperatively. Fibrin glue was used to achieve liver hemostasis in seven patients and in the performance of a splenorrhaphy in one other patient (Table 2). Of the eight patients in the series, seven experienced varying periods of intraoperative hypotension.

RESULTS

Fibrin glue was immediately effective in achieving hemostasis in all patients, including one patient with a 9-L blood loss secondary to a gunshot wound of the liver that failed to be controlled using mattress sutures, microcrystalline collagen, and clamping of the portal vessels (Pringle maneuver). The amount of FG required to achieve hemostasis varied directly with the extent of injury and intraoperative blood loss ($r = .84$), and all patients with a blood loss greater than 4 L required at least 25 mL of FG to stop bleeding (Fig 5).

One patient with continued disseminated intravascular coagulation underwent reexploration because of hemoperitoneum 24 hours after successful resection of a ruptured hepatic tumor and sealing of the resected liver margin with FG; at reexploration, the FG patch was found to be completely intact, and no bleeding source was identified. The patient recovered without rebleeding. One other patient with multiple injuries of the colon, small intestine, stomach, lung, and diaphragm developed multiple intra-

Accepted for publication May 11, 1988.

From the Department of Surgery, Martin Luther King, Jr-Charles R. Drew Medical Center, Los Angeles, and the UCLA School of Medicine.

Reprint requests to Department of Surgery, Martin Luther King Jr-Charles R. Drew Medical Center, 12021 S Wilmington Ave, Los Angeles, CA 90059 (Dr Kram).

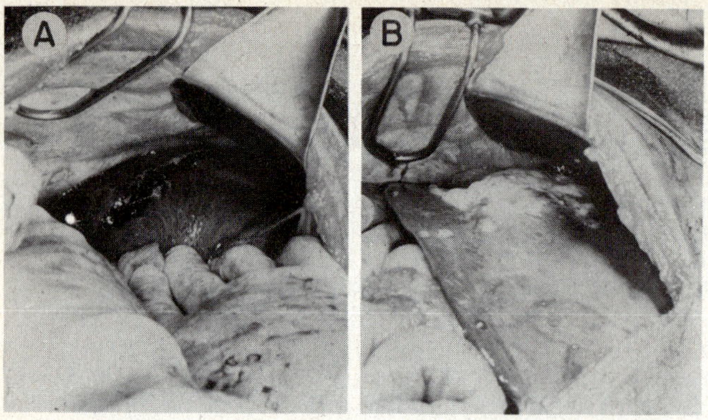

Fig 1.—Gunshot wound of liver in patient with coagulopathy sealed using fibrin glue. A indicates before fibrin glue application; B, after fibrin glue application.

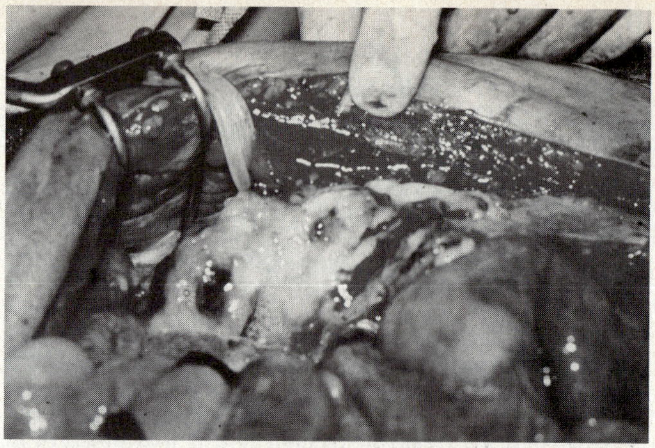

Fig 2.—Resection of ruptured hepatic tumor in patient with disseminated intravascular coagulation sealed using fibrin glue.

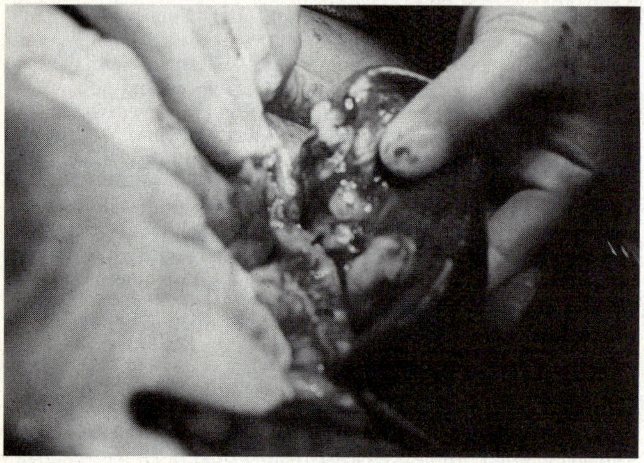

Fig 3.—Multiple splenic hilar injuries secondary to blunt trauma in patient with thrombocytopenia sealed using fibrin glue.

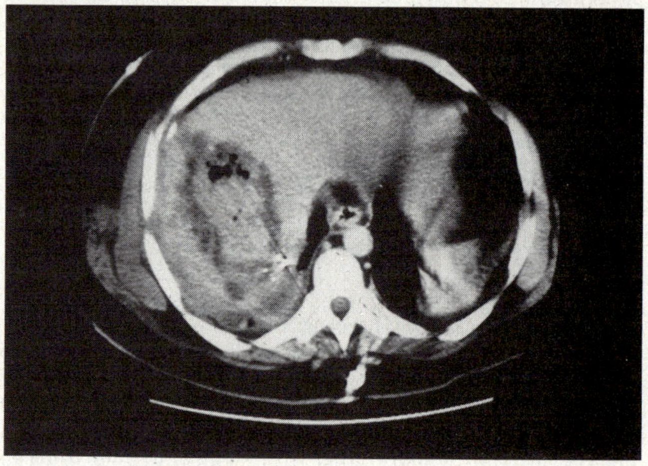

Fig 4.—Computed tomographic scan five days following fibrin sealing of high-velocity gunshot wound through the liver in patient with severe dilutional coagulopathy.

Table 1.—Clinical Data of Eight Patients With Coagulation Disorders

Patient/Age, y/Sex	Cause	Additional Diagnoses*	Prothrombin Time (Actual/Control), s	Partial Thromboplastin Time (Actual/Control), s	Platelet Count $\times 10^9$/L
1/31/M	Gunshot wound	None	16/10	66/34	60
2/34/M	Gunshot wound	Alcoholic hepatitis, chronic pancreatitis	20/10	180/30	37
3/20/M	Gunshot wound	DIC	24/10	180/30	77
4/40/M	Gunshot wound	None	17/9	68/31	220
5/26/M	Gunshot wound	None	15/10	53/30	121
6/20/M	Motor vehicle accident	None	15/10	41/20	59
7/72/M	Ruptured hepatic tumor	Metastatic cancer, COPD, DIC	70/10	180/30	37
8/31/F	Assault	Chronic anemia, thrombocytopenia	14/10	32/31	65

*DIC indicates disseminated intravascular coagulation; COPD, chronic obstructive pulmonary disease.

Table 2.—Perioperative Data of Eight Patients With Coagulation Disorders

Patient	Organ Treated With Fibrin Glue	Additional Injuries	Intraoperative Blood Loss, mL	Blood Transfused, U	Complications	Outcome
1	Liver	Diaphragm, lung	9000	16	None	Survived
2	Liver	Spleen, stomach, diaphragm, lung	3500	13	Delirium tremens	Survived
3	Liver	Colon, small intestine, gallbladder, iliac vein, lung, ribs	13 000	22	Cardiac arrest	Died on postoperative day 1
4	Liver	Colon, stomach, gall-bladder, lung	5800	24	Adult respiratory distress syndrome, necrosis of colostomy	Died on postoperative day 5
5	Liver	Colon, small intestine, stomach, diaphragm, lung	1250	4	Cardiac arrest, multiple intra-abdominal abscesses	Survived
6	Liver	Liver, lung, ribs	2000	4	None	Survived
7	Liver	None	5150	28	Hemoperitoneum	Survived
8	Spleen	Ribs	1100	3	None	Survived

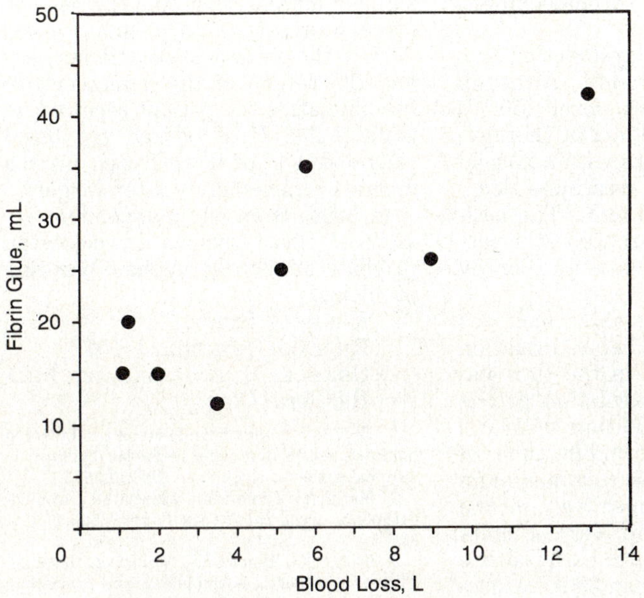

Fig 5.—Relationship between intraoperative blood loss and amount of fibrin glue (FG) required to achieve hemostasis in patients with coagulation disorders. Note that amount of FG used varied directly with extent of hemorrhage ($r=.84$) and that all patients with blood loss greater than 4 L required at least 25 mL of FG to achieve hemostasis.

abdominal abscesses following extensive fecal contamination, cardiac arrest, and multiple operations.

COMMENT

These studies evaluated the efficacy and safety of FG in achieving parenchymal organ hemostasis in patients with coagulation disorders. No complication attributable to FG was seen, and its use was deemed lifesaving in several patients. The amount of FG required to achieve hemostasis was directly related to the extent of injury and blood loss.

Fibrin glue was found to control bleeding of deep, as well as superficial, parenchymal organ injuries. This allows for a wider spectrum of indications for use when compared with conventional topical hemostatic agents made of collagen, gelatin, or cellulose; use of the latter agents is usually limited to superficial capsular tears in easily accessible areas. Packing of hemostatic material into a deep injury may increase the size of the defect or lead to subcapsular hematoma formation.[10] Completely filling in the defect with a fibrin plug, on the other hand, may help to avoid these complications. No cases of intravascular embolization of FG occurred despite its injection into deep wounds; the use of a high thrombin concentration (500 U/mL) in preparing FG results in the adhesive solidifying within seconds of application, avoiding this complication.

Because FG does not depend on adequate platelet or clotting factor levels, it is effective in patients with dilutional or disease-related coagulation disorders. Previous animal studies revealed that FG was superior to oxidized regenerated cellulose in controlling hemorrhage in a heparinized model.[8] Similarly, FG was successful in achieving hemostasis in all patients with coagulation disorders in the present series. In conclusion, FG provides hemostasis of superficial and deep parenchymal organ injuries, reduces the need for parenchymal sutures, is effective in the presence of deficient platelets and clotting factors, has good local and systemic compatibility, and promotes normal wound healing. Its use may be lifesaving in the critically ill surgical patient with exsanguinating parenchymal organ hemorrhage.

The fibrin glue used in this study was supplied as Fibrin Sealant by Immuno AG, Vienna.

References

1. String T, Robinson AJ, Blaisdell FW: Massive trauma: Effect of intravascular coagulation on prognosis. *Arch Surg* 1971;102:406-411.
2. Phillips TF, Soulier G, Wilson RF: Outcome of massive transfusion exceeding two blood volumes in trauma and emergency surgery. *J Trauma* 1987;27:903-910.
3. Redl H, Schlag G, Dinges H, et al: Background and methods of 'fibrin sealing,' in Winter GD, Gibbons DF, Plenk H (eds): *Biomaterials.* New York, John Wiley & Sons Inc, 1982, pp 669-696.
4. Kram HB, Shoemaker WC, Hino ST, et al: Splenic salvage using biologic glue. *Arch Surg* 1984;119:1309-1311.
5. Kram HB, Reuben BI, Fleming AW, et al: Use of fibrin glue in hepatic trauma. *J Trauma* 1987;27:825.
6. Kram HB, Shoemaker WC, Hino ST, et al: Tracheal repair with fibrin glue. *J Thorac Cardiovasc Surg* 1985;90:771-775.
7. Kram HB, Garces MA, Klein SR, et al: Common bile duct anastomosis using fibrin glue. *Arch Surg* 1985;120:1250-1256.
8. Kram HB, Nugent P, Reuben BI, et al: Fibrin glue sealing of polytetrafluoroethylene (PTFE) vascular graft anastomoses: Comparison with oxidized cellulose. *J Vasc Surg*, in press.
9. Guttmen T: *Untersuchungen eines Fibrinklebers fur die Anwendung in der shirugie periper Nerven: Diplomarkiet Inst F Botanik, technische mikroscopie Organ: Rohstofflehre.* Vienna, Technische Universität Wien, 1978.
10. Morgenstern L: Microcrystalline collagen used in experimental splenic injury: A new surface hemostatic agent. *Arch Surg* 1974;109:44-47.

Cefotetan-Associated Coagulopathies

To the Editor.—Two patients from our hospital (Hartford [Conn] Hospital) who developed coagulopathies supposedly from cefotetan were recently described in the ARCHIVES.[1] Having had the opportunity to evaluate these cases in detail, and having a view different from that of the author (Dr Holt), we felt obliged to write this letter. While there was a temporal relationship between cefotetan therapy and the development of hypoprothrombinemias in these patients, there were a number of other reasons for the development of coagulopathies (ie, malignant neoplasm, poor nutritional status, concurrent use of agents that effect hemostasis, and renal or hepatic dysfunction).

During cefotetan therapy the nutritional status of both patients deteriorated. The first patient was without oral intake for the initial six days of her eight-day course of treatment with cefotetan and received no enteral feedings or hyperalimentation during this period. The second patient was without oral intake for the majority of his treatment with cefotetan (17 of 27 days) and for the remainder of the period his oral intake was poor. He received hyperalimentation beginning on the 23rd day of therapy. Not surprisingly, both patients had significant weight loss during the initial three weeks of hospitalization (8.2% and 7.7% loss from initial weight, respectively). Moreover, the initial total serum albumin concentrations were low (21 and 23 g/L, respectively) in both patients. The first patient did not have repeated serum albumin concentrations measured until after discontinuation of cefotetan therapy. In the second patient both the serum albumin and total protein concentrations remained abnormally low throughout his hospitalization. This indicates that the nutritional status of both patients was less than optimal immediately before and during cefotetan therapy. Adding to the overall debilitation of the first patient was the presence of metastatic carcinoma.

Each patient received medications that have been proven to effect hemostasis. Parenteral ranitidine (50 mg every eight hours), which can cause thrombocytopenia,[2-5] was administered to both patients concurrent with cefotetan therapy. In fact, in the second case, the platelet count dropped to 93×10^9/L on the fourth day of cefotetan therapy. This patient also received concurrent therapy with dipyridamole, an antiplatelet agent used in the prevention of thromboembolic events.[6]

Evidence of renal dysfunction was present in both patients. Although the serum creatinine level (50 to 60 μmol/L during cefotetan therapy) of the first patient was within normal limits, her estimated creatinine clearance was only 52 mL/min. The estimated creatinine clearance of the second patient during cefotetan therapy was only 36 mL/min.

The initial prothrombin time was slightly elevated just before initiation of cefotetan therapy in the first patient. Her initial coagulation profile showed a prothrombin time of 13.8 s and a partial prothrombin time of 26 s; these values rose to a maximum of 26.2 s and 48 s, respectively, on the seventh day of therapy. Normal limits in patients at Hartford Hospital are 11 to 13 s and less than 38 s, respectively. Values returned to baseline after three daily administrations of 10 mg of phytonadione intramuscularly.

The second patient was transferred to our hospital via helicopter with the preliminary diagnosis of active gastrointestinal tract bleeding secondary to the formation of an aortoduodenal fistula. He received 7 U of packed red blood cells during and immediately after emergency surgery to correct the situation. His hematocrit and hemoglobin level at this time were 0.35 and 120 g/L, respectively (normal values for men range from 0.45 to 0.52 and 130 g/L to 180 g/L, respectively). This patient had high initial coagulation values (ie, prothrombin time of 14.1 s and a partial thromboplastin time of 52 s). Coagulation values maximized on the 12th day of cefotetan therapy at 28 s and 88 s, respectively. During the next two weeks transfusions were given every few days, for a total of 6 U of packed red blood cells. The hematocrit and hemoglobin level continued to decline during this period to minimum values just before the second surgery of 0.21 and 73 g/L, respectively.

This led us to conclude that the patient had a small, active bleeding process occurring throughout this two-week interval. Providing further support for this view was the need to oversew a suture on a small vessel during the patient's second surgery and the return of the hematocrit to baseline after the patient received an additional 8 U of packed red blood cells and 4 U of fresh-frozen plasma during or immediately after surgery.

In brief, from our independent review of these two cases, cefotetan played a minor role in their bleeding problems.

KAREN S. SMITH
RICHARD QUINTILIANI, MD
CHARLES H. NIGHTINGALE, PHD
Hartford, Conn

1. Holt J: Hypoprothrombinemia and bleeding diathesis associated with cefotetan therapy in surgical patients. *Arch Surg* 1988;123:523.
2. Mann AJ: Cimetidine associated thrombocytopenia. *Drug Intell Clin Pharm* 1983;17:126-128.
3. Gafter U, Komlos L, Weinstein T, et al: Thrombocytopenia, eosinophilia, and ranitidine. *Ann Intern Med* 1987;106:477.
4. Gibson PR, Pidcock ME: Immune-mediated thrombocytopenia associated with ranitidine therapy. *Med J Aust* 1986;145:661-662.
5. Spychal RT, Wickham NW: Thrombocytopenia associated with ranitidine. *Br Med J* 1985;291:1687.
6. Dipyridamole package insert. Ridgefield, Conn, Boehringer Ingelheim Pharmaceuticals Inc, 1985.

Effect of β-Adrenergic Blockade on the Growth Rate of Abdominal Aortic Aneurysms

To the Editor.—I read the recent article in the ARCHIVES by Leach et al[1] with great interest. The effect of propranolol hydrochloride on other types of aneurysmal disease could also be explored. For example, the incidence of coronary artery aneurysms in a coronary artery surgery study of 20 087 patients was 5%.[2] The cause was primarily atherosclerotic or congenital, with over half secondary to atherosclerosis. The main complications reported were rupture with sudden death, thrombosis, and myocardial infarction secondary to embolization. Medical treatment generally consists of the use of antithrombotic drugs. Often a patient has associated coronary artery stenosis and poststenotic dilation and aneurysm formation. Often these patients are receiving propranolol for treatment of associated disease, such as hypertension, angina pectoris, and the control of certain types of cardiac arrhythmias. Therefore, in a large medical center such as Yale (New Haven, Conn), where many coronary angiographic studies are done, patients with coronary artery aneurysms could participate in a prospective clinical study with propranolol and be followed up angiographically. Recent coronary aneurysm studies[3] in Japan on patients with a history of Kawasaki disease have examined the distensibility of coronary aneurysms with the vasodilator dipyridamole and found a decrease in the distensibility when compared with normal coronary arteries. Distensibility studies could be combined with propranolol treatment studies. Another potential area of interest is treatment of intracranial aneurysms with propranolol, because connective-tissue disorders and hypertension may contribute to the causation of intracranial aneurysms.

KATHIE M. DALESSANDRI, MD
Martinez, Calif

1. Leach SD, Toole AL, Stern H, et al: Effect of β-adrenergic blockade on the growth rate of abdominal aortic aneurysms. *Arch Surg* 1988;123:606-609.
2. Swaye PS, Fisher LD, Litwin P, et al: Aneurysmal coronary artery disease. *Circulation* 1983;67:134-138.
3. Matsumara K, Yasuyaki O, Tsunao I, et al: Coronary angiography of Kawasaki disease with the coronary vasodilator dipryridamole: Assessment of distensibility of affected coronary arterial wall. *Angiography* 1988;39:141-147.

Spontaneous Renal Rupture in Pregnancy

To the Editor.—Spontaneous renal rupture is a rare complication of pregnancy, but is hazardous to both the mother and the infant. It seems hardly possible to initially diagnose spontaneous renal rupture in a pregnant woman, mainly because it presents the symptoms of acute abdomen, and because the incidence of the disease is rare. We report a case of a pregnant women with spontaneous renal rupture in whom renal arteriography confirmed the diagnosis.

Report of a Case.—A 31-year-old pregnant woman, in the third trimester, was admitted to the hospital on June 15, 1986, because of severe left flank pain of sudden onset that was accompanied by shock.

When she recovered from the shock by means of multiple infusions, her blood pressure was 134/80 mm Hg, and her heart rate was 90 beats per minute. Fetal heart sounds were not audible. Marked tenderness was found in the lower left abdominal quadrant and left flank. There was no vaginal bleeding or discharge. The chest roentgenogram showed a mild left pleural effusion.

She denied having any recent blunt trauma to her back or abdomen. She reported no blood in her stool or urine, and showed no urinary symptoms. This was her first pregnancy.

A complete blood cell count yielded the following: red blood cell count, 2.2×10^{12}/L; white blood cell count, 19.0×10^{9}/L; hemoglobin level, 61 g/L; and hematocrit, 0.192. Urinalysis showed occasional red blood cells and no white blood cells per high-power field.

The provisional diagnosis of premature separation of the normally implanted placenta causing intrauterine fetal death was made. On June 16, she delivered vaginally a dead male infant weighing 1940 g. Four days after admission, she again complained of abdominal pain, accompanied by the progression of anemia. Computed tomography of the abdomen disclosed an extensive retroperitoneal hematoma around the left kidney (Fig 1). The left kidney was not seen on the intravenous pyelogram. Blood transfusions maintained her circulatory stability, but on June 25, she once again became hemodynamically unstable with further progression of anemia and an increase of abdominal circumference. For the detection of the bleeding origin, aortography and left renal arteriography were performed (Fig 2). The renal arteriography elucidated a large subcapsular hematoma of the left kidney. A left-sided nephrectomy and drainage of the retroperitoneal giant hematoma were urgently performed.

The left kidney measured 25 cm from the upper pole to the lower pole, 15 cm in frontal diameter, and 10 cm in sagittal diameter. The capsule ruptured at the lower pole. Pathologically, arterial malformation of the kidney was suspected.

Postoperatively, the course of recovery was uneventful.

Comment.—Retroperitoneal hemorrhage originating from spontaneous rupture of the kidney should be considered as a differential diagnosis of acute abdomen in pregnancy.[1] However, as the incidence of the disease in pregnant women seems extremely small, the correct diagnosis can hardly be obtained preoperatively, according to reported cases in the English literature.[1,2] In our case, the diagnosis was confirmed by renal arteriography, which had been performed during the hemodynamically unstable period. We feel that renal arteriography can be safely performed to establish the diagnosis of spontaneous renal rupture in pregnancy.

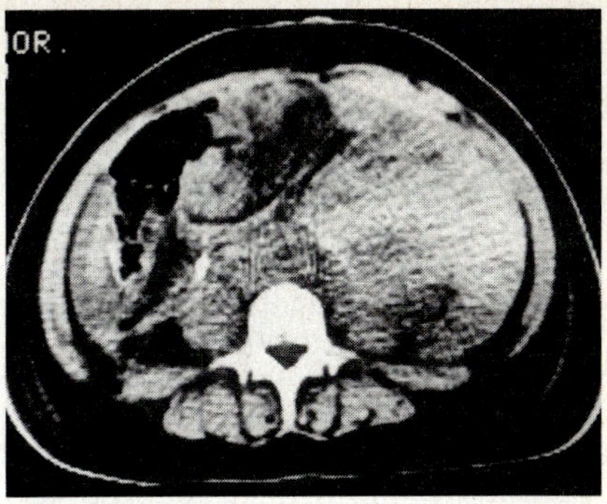

Fig 1.—Computed tomogram of abdomen. Large retroperitoneal hematoma is present around left kidney.

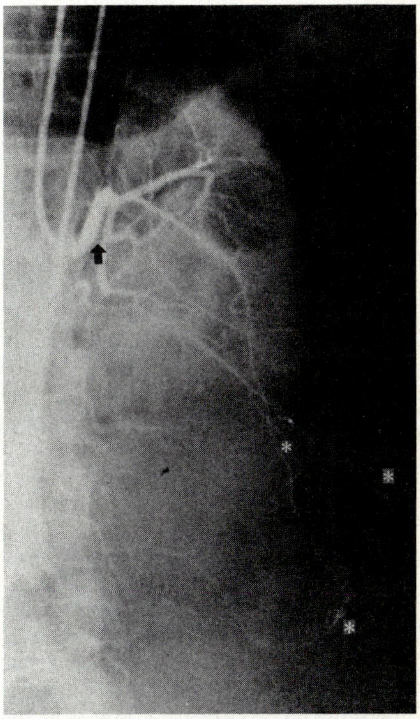

Fig 2.—Renal arteriogram showing left renal trunk shifted cephalad (arrow). Capsular arterial branches (asterisks) run away from renal parenchyma, suggesting large subcapsular hematoma.

Renal arteriography is an informative diagnostic tool useful in treating a pregnant woman who has retroperitoneal hematoma.

HIROSHI IZUMOTO, MD
HISAHIRO MATSUI, MD
HIROSHI HAYASHI, MD
RYOICHI KONDO, MD
SHIGERU TERAMOTO, MD
Okayama, Japan

1. Kiser DM, McGannon PT, Sinclair AB: Massive retroperitoneal hemorrhage from spontaneous rupture of hamartoma of the kidney in pregnancy. *Am J Obstet Gynecol* 1964;88:545-546.
2. Joachim GR, Becker EL: Spontaneous rupture of the kidney. *Arch Intern Med* 1965;115:176-183.

Essentials of Surgery, edited by Peter F. Lawrence, Merril Dayton, Richard Bell, and Marcia Bilbao, 410 pp, $27, Baltimore, Williams & Wilkins, 1988.

Any attempt by experienced surgeons to improve methods of teaching medical students deserves serious examination. This book, edited by surgeons from the University of Utah and a radiologist from the University of South Carolina, so qualifies. The softcover book is the core of a multimedia effort by members of the Association of Surgical Education to combine modern teaching techniques with new technology for better medical education. The 88 authors of this book are primarily young academic surgeons who are concerned about this frequently neglected responsibility of academic surgery. The book brings back memories of three decades ago when some of us introduced educational subjects for the first time into the program of the Society of University Surgeons and created a Committee on Surgical Education.

The authors are, for a change, not the old guard whose names are usually associated with textbook chapters. In their place is the younger generation of experts. The result is refreshing and innovative.

The textbook is the core of the multimedia program around which the editors have created a variety of peripherals that can be purchased separately. The book itself is relatively inexpensive ($27), but the entire package costs $1900. For this considerable sum one gets all the technical props needed for teaching medical students, including videotapes for teaching essential surgical skills, a computer software package of patient management problems, a bank of 1100 written questions, a group of multiple-choice questions intended for use in an oral examination, and a set of 198 35-mm slides to be used in lecture presentations.

Only about 10% of all medical students will end up practicing surgery or a surgical specialty. The challenge in writing a text for students is to identify the concepts and data important for all students. This involves identifying principles and omitting nonessentials. In general, *Essentials of Surgery* is remarkably successful due to Lawrence's preliminary survey of a wide variety of surgeons asking them what they considered essential for students to learn. The authors were well briefed, I am certain, before they signed on. A few seemed to ignore their fathometer and either plunged too deeply or remained too near the surface of their assigned subject.

A case in point is the question of what data a student should know concerning surgical disease and management. It seems to me that three sets of data so qualify. First, what are the numbers defining normalcy? These, like multiplication tables, simply must be memorized or be kept at hand. The second aspect pertains to frequency, which is difficult to understand until one can establish by experience a personal database. What diseases occur frequently and what are the signs and symptoms associated with them? Not yet within the curriculum but, in my opinion, soon to be included are the performance characteristics of diagnostic tests. The third type of data is a numerical characteristic of prognosis. Undoubtedly, some harsh editorial supervision was needed to achieve the proper subject depth for students. Perhaps that is why the editors selected young colleagues as authors. One problem with the book is that there are too many authors (88) for this 410-page volume. Some of the chapters have detectable crevices where one author left off and another took over.

An appealing feature of the book is its limited length. This is in contrast to the current trend in textbooks, which increasingly have come to resemble hardcover dinosaurs, understandably frightening away many students. This book can be read and understood within the limited time now available in most medical school curricula devoted to surgery.

As the title of the book indicates, this volume covers general surgery, which quite properly is the core of medical student teaching. I understand that a subsequent volume is being prepared for surgical specialties.

Each chapter, be it devoted to a general subject or to a specific disease or anatomic area, is similarly organized. This makes it easier to read and check references. The first part of each chapter contains a short paragraph entitled "Assumptions." These are what the student is expected to know before proceeding. Next comes a highlighted half page entitled "Objectives." This skeleton is fleshed out in the bulk of the chapter that follows. At the end of each chapter are the feathers and appendages: a list of essential operative skills and often descriptions of how to perform them, a list of no more than 20 references for in-depth reading, and, finally, some study questions. The book has a nonthreatening "user-friendly" tone.

The text is liberally sprinkled with good algorithms, which, like most of the tables, are well chosen and clean. Line drawings are good, except for some glaring exceptions (eg, the chapter on the small bowel). The quality of x-ray reproductions and their descriptive legends varies.

The book starts with a chapter on health care issues, a trend that reflects the interests of modern students. I was disappointed that there was only passing reference to surgical decision making. Perhaps the editors assumed that students were familiar with this important aspect of clinical medicine. If they made such an assumption, they were mistaken!

This is an important and imaginative book for medical students and those responsible for their surgical education. Taken alone it will be a valuable textbook for junior and senior students. Purchased with its peripherals of slides, tapes, and computer software, it will be expensive but valuable.

Teaching is an art as well as a science, but as with other art forms, the best master the scientific fundamentals. *Essentials of Surgery* demonstrates modern trends in surgical education for medical students.

B. Eiseman, MD
Denver

Liver Transplantation: Clio Chirurgica, by T. E. Starzl, C. G. Groth, and L. McKowka, 363 pp, $45, Austin, Texas, Silvergill Inc, 1988.

Carlyle believed that unique individuals are of prime importance in shaping the course of human history. It was a theory of history much in vogue during the Victorian era but was superseded by an emphasis on economic and political power as determinants. Carlyle's thesis is debatable for history in general, but few can doubt the importance of unique individuals in changing the course of surgical history. Carlyle calls the historic leaders "heroes." Starzl, the senior author of this volume, and Roy Calne are, of course, the two heroes who have taken liver transplantation from theory to clinical reality.

Clio was the Greek goddess of history and this book is one of a series of monographs each devoted to the history of some aspect of surgery. It is unique in that the entire history of liver transplantation is concentrated within 25 years.

Starzl and his colleagues provide 41 seminal articles that trace the development of liver transplantation. Each is put in its historic perspective by a few pages of commentary, which indicates the question the reported laboratory or clinical data answers and how the article provided a step forward. The connecting commentaries provide a balance of scholarly reporting and personal interests of those who contributed.

It is difficult for those of us who lived through and, in various ways, participated in this exciting era of surgical advancement to be dispassionate by either the way that progress was made or the exciting personalities involved. Scientific progress made at this breakneck speed is usually controversial and surrounded by great excitement. Reading this or any other history of science, one finds that each new step seems to be a logical progression of that which went before. Those who participated, however, know this is far from fact. Many blind alleys, such as plasmapheresis, lymph duct drainage, or splenectomy, were probed at a great expenditure of time, energy, and money before being abandoned. A good scientist knows when to quit as well as when to press on in the dogged fashion that characterizes those who advanced liver transplantation. Not recorded in this history of liver transplantation are the harsh comments of deans, hospital administrators, the press, and even lesser faculty members "bumped" from the operating schedule when a patient receiving a transplant needed care. Many eggs and egos were broken in making the transplantation omelette.

The authors demonstrated good judgment in the selection of papers to be reprinted and photographs of the contributing pioneers. Several unsung contributors were mentioned. One example is Jack Cannon whose paragraph in the 1956 *Transplantation Bulletin* suggested that liver transplantation might someday be possible. Another appropriate homage went to Stewart Welch, who, though unsuccessful, pioneered liver transplants in animals.

An obvious question is how the Pittsburgh group of editors handled the almost equally important contributions of Calne and his colleagues in Cambridge and London. The two groups have been neck and neck in an exciting scientific race for 25 years. Only four of the 41 articles chosen for reprint were written by Sir Roy Calne. However, Starzl, Groth, and McKowka give effusive praise and recognition to Calne and simply admit that it would not be possible to include all of his contributions. It is a reflection of the friendly rivalry that has existed between Starzl and Calne over two decades. Invariably, they shared their experiences with each other so that the most efficient rate of progress could be made. It is a relationship of which surgery can be proud.

At best, history has two benefits: it records events and by accurately tracing the pattern by which events occur helps us understand how progress can be made. This book has worth on both counts. It illustrates how talented, well-trained, disciplined, and dedicated people can develop ideas and turn them into reality. To those of us who knew both groups of players in this exciting field, it also illustrates how dogged dedication to an idea can prove successful.

One can only pity students of surgery who cannot be a part of a scientific environment on the cutting edge of surgical progress. Sharing, even vicariously, the excitement of progress broadens the young surgeon's entire education. Providing such excitement is one of the many contributions made by the authors of this book. It is the highest form of education.

Accepted wisdom in the press emphasizes "breakthroughs" in science as though everything is at a standstill until one day a brilliant new idea strikes an investigator, who, in one form or another, shouts "Eureka!" and proclaims his idea to the world. Such nonsense is dispelled by this carefully documented scholarly history of liver transplantation. Progress is slow, hesitating, and frustrating even by such heroes as those who wrote this book.

B. Eiseman, MD
Denver

Calendar of Events

March

Central Surgical Association, March 8-11, Calgary, Alberta, Canada.

April

Association College of Surgeons, (Spring), April 2-6, Boston, Mass.
Association for Surgical Education, April 5-8, Tampa, Fla. Local Coordinator: Dr Charles Cox, University of South Florida.
Society for Clinical Vascular Surgery, April 5-9, Innisbrook, Tarpon Springs, Fla.
Association for Surgical Education, April 6-8, Harbour Island Hotel, Tampa, Fla.
American Surgical Association, April 10-12, Broadmoor, Colorado Springs, Colo.
Surgical Infection Society, April 13-14, The Broadmoor, Denver, Colo.
Southwestern Surgical Congress 41st Annual Meeting, April 23-26, Hyatt Regency, Monterey, Calif.

May

American Association for Thoracic Surgery, May 8-10, Sheraton/Hynes, Boston, Mass.
The Society of Surgical Oncology Inc, May 21-24, Westin St Francis, San Francisco, Calif.

June

Society for Vascular Surgery/International Cardiovascular Society, June 18-21, Hilton, New York, NY.
Western Thoracic Surgical Association, June 21-25, Hyatt Regency, Monterey, Calif.

September

Society of Thoracic Surgeons, September 10-13, Convention Center, Baltimore, Md.
33rd World Congress of Surgery, September 10-16, Toronto, Canada. Contact: Congress Canada, 73 Richmond St W, Suite 300, Toronto, Ontario, Canada M5H 1Z4.

October

American Association for the Surgery of Trauma, October 5-7, Chicago, Ill.
American Society of Anesthesiologists, October 14-16, New Orleans, La.
American College of Surgeons (Congress), October 15-20, World Congress Center, Atlanta, Ga.
American College of Chest Physicians, October 30-November 3, Boston, Mass.

November

Western Surgical Association, November 11-14, St Louis, Mo.
American Heart Association, November 13-16, New Orleans, La.

The Veterans Administration and Surgical Education in the United States

This issue of the *Archives of Surgery* contains reports presented at the 12th Annual Meeting of the Association of Veterans Administration (VA) Surgeons. Since its founding in 1930, the VA has played an increasingly important role in the American medical care system. The VA system of care developed slowly until the conclusion of World War II. There were 97 VA hospitals, mainly located in rural America, caring for patients with chronic medical problems. Following World War II, the rapid downsizing of a huge military medical system created a need for the VA to care for a large number of patients transferred from the military. The simultaneous reestablishment of full activity of the medical schools created a need for training sites and teachers. Over the next 45 years this affiliation was to become an excellent marriage.

President Harry S Truman appointed GEN Omar N. Bradley to head the VA. Paul R. Howley, MD, was named VA chief medical director, and Paul B. Magnusen, MD, chairman of the department of orthopedic surgery at the Northwestern University School of Medicine in Chicago, was selected as his aide. Dr Magnusen's concept of affiliations between the VA and medical schools was implemented promptly at the Hines VA Hospital in Chicago, where 56 residents (many medical veterans returning from the service) from Northwestern University and University of Illinois schools of medicine completed their training.[1] These affiliations were followed by similar agreements with medical schools in Minneapolis, Minn, Boston, Mass, New York, NY, and San Francisco, Calif. The number of medical centers in the VA system increased to 172 by the 1980s, of which 134 are affiliated with 102 medical schools.

The development and monitoring of these affiliations is the function of the dean's committee, chaired by the dean of the school of medicine and composed of top management of the VA medical center and the chairs of the departments utilizing the facility for medical student and resident physician training. The hospital provides the plant, equipment, personnel, patients, salary support, research space, and monies; the school helps to recruit faculty, staff, and residents. The VA is responsible for quality assurance and utilization review of patient care, and the school is responsible for the quality of the educational and research programs.

This metamorphosis of the VA and its marriage with the medical schools has not been without controversies. However, without this interdependent relationship, both would be very different organizations in terms of mission, quality of patient care, teaching, and research productivity.

Over 50% of all physicians practicing in the United States have received part of their education in VA medical centers. During fiscal year 1989-1990, the VA is supporting 8328.9 full-time resident positions (12.7% of the total resident positions in the United States). This includes 884 general surgery staff positions (11% of the US total) and 1072 residents in the surgical specialties (13.6% of the US total). Extensive VA-supported training also exists for medical students, nurses, dentists, pharmacists, psychologists, social workers, and a full complement of other medical providers and support personnel. During the 1987 academic year, there were 105 000 people from 1000 professional schools in training at VA medical centers.

Medical school affiliations caused the rapid growth of the research program in the VA system. This critical program affects the ability to successfully recruit and retain academic personnel. The total dollar allocation for research by the VA system exceeds $500 million per year, thus constituting a major component of American medical research.[2] The VA is also a major source of faculty salary support. Its patients present a spectrum of diseases essential to increasing the depth and scope of clinical experience needed to maintain a well-balanced training program.

American surgical education and research would change significantly if VA resources were not present. Furthermore, the flexibility offered medical schools by this relationship allows the schools a greater ability to change in this time of major funding challenges (ie, training programs and less financial support for research). The need for support of these two partners has never been more critical to their continued success.

James M. Guernsey, MD, FACS
Martinez, Calif

1. Worthen DM. The affiliation partnership between US medical schools and the Veterans Administration. *Ala J Med Sci.* 1982;24:83-88.
2. Gronvall JA. The VA's affiliation with academic medicine: an emergency post-war strategy becomes a permanent partnership. *Academic Med.* 1989;64:61-66.

Papers Read Before the 12th Annual Surgical Symposium of the Association of Veterans Administration Surgeons, Minneapolis, Minn, May 12 to May 16, 1988

Common Bile Duct Healing

Do Different Absorbable Sutures Affect Stricture Formation and Tensile Strength?

Kenneth W. Sharp, MD; Charles B. Ross, MD; Vicki N. Tillman; John F. Dunn, MD

• Few basic investigations have addressed the problem of common bile duct strictures. We systematically investigated the healing canine end-to-end choledochal anastomosis and tested the hypothesis that common bile duct anastomoses sutured with monofilament polyglyconate absorbable suture would heal with less stricture formation and greater tensile strength than those sutured with braided polyglactin 910 and chromic catgut sutures. Seventy-six canines, randomized to control vs sutured groups, underwent either mobilization (controls) or transection of the mid–common bile duct and were allowed to heal 5, 10, 15, or 50 days postoperatively before sacrifice. The type of absorbable suture used to construct a common bile duct anastomosis was found to have no major effect on anastomotic strictures nor on anastomotic breaking strength. Polyglyconate suture caused significantly less perianastomotic inflammation than did chromic suture, with polyglactin 910 sutures evoking an intermediate inflammatory response. Surgeons may safely choose sutures for biliary procedures based on the clinical circumstances and personal preference.

(*Arch Surg.* 1989;124:408-414)

Biliary strictures are a complex surgical problem with high recurrence rates, yet little basic research has focused on their pathogenesis.[1-4] A variety of methods for repair of common bile duct (CBD) injuries and strictures have been reported,[5-9] but many controversies still exist over anastomotic techniques, stenting, and the use of absorbable vs nonabsorbable sutures. Nonabsorbable sutures have fallen into disfavor because of erosion into the duct lumen where they have served as a nidus for the collection of biliary debris and stones.[10-12] A range of absorbable sutures are now available for use in biliary surgery, including the more recently introduced monofilament polyglyconate (PGN) suture (Maxon), which retains tensile strength longer while inciting less inflammation than chromic catgut and earlier synthetic absorbable sutures.[13] The monofilament configuration of this suture also offers the advantage of less drag and sawing when used in delicate, friable tissues. Although CBD stricture formation may depend on many factors, differences in suture composition, structure, degradation, and handling properties, as well as the tissue inflammatory response to the suture, may influence healing and stricture formation in the CBD.

We systematically investigated the biomechanical properties of the healing end-to-end canine CBD anastomosis in this study and tested the hypothesis that CBD anastomoses sutured with monofilament PGN would heal with less stricture formation and greater tensile strength than anastomoses sutured with chromic catgut (chromic) or braided polyglactin 910 (PGA-910) sutures.

Accepted for publication December 16, 1988.

Presented as a poster exhibit at the 12th Annual Surgical Symposium of the Association of Veterans Administration Surgeons, Minneapolis, Minn, May 13-14, 1988.

From the Departments of Surgery, Nashville Veterans Administration Medical Center (Drs Sharp, Ross, and Dunn), and Vanderbilt University Medical Center (Drs Sharp, Ross, and Dunn and Ms Tillman), Nashville, Tenn.

Reprint requests to Department of Surgery, Nashville Veterans Administration Medical Center, 1310 24th Ave S, Nashville, TN 37212 (Dr Sharp).

MATERIALS AND METHODS

Design

Seventy-six adult mongrel dogs of both sexes (average weight, 29 kg) were randomly assigned to a healing period (5, 10, 15, or 50 days) and suture vs control groups, as shown in Table 1. Two dogs served as control animals for each healing period, and five additional dogs were studied at healing period 0 as controls not operated on.

Operative Procedure

Preoperatively, dogs were fasted for 24 hours with water allowed ad libitum. Dogs were anesthetized intravenously with sodium pentobarbital, 30 mg/kg, and were endotracheally intubated. A blood sample was taken for the determination of the serum total bilirubin and alkaline phosphatase levels. Dogs randomized to suture groups underwent laparotomy, cholecystectomy, and transection of the mid–CBD using minimal periductal dissection. End-to-end CBD anastomosis was next accomplished using interrupted, simple 5-0 sutures with atraumatic needles of equivalent sizes. Dogs randomized to control groups underwent laparotomy, cholecystectomy, and mobilization of the mid–CBD with minimal periductal dissection and without CBD transection. Postoperatively, dogs were allowed access to fresh water ad libitum. Regular chow was resumed on the second postoperative day. The protocol for the operative procedure and care of these animals was approved and monitored by the Nashville (Tenn) Veterans Administration

Medical Center animal care committee under the guidelines of the American Association for the Accreditation of Laboratory Animal Care.

Sacrifice

A blood sample was taken for the determination of serum total bilirubin and alkaline phosphatase levels, following which the dogs were weighed and then sacrificed by intravenous barbiturate overdose. Laparotomy was performed and the peritoneal contents were inspected for gross or contained bile leaks, abscesses, and adhesions. The hepatic hilum, CBD, and duodenum were removed en bloc and submitted for study.

Cholangiography

A cannula was inserted into a proximal hepatic duct, and all other proximal ducts were ligated. The specimen was placed lying flat directly on the film cassette to minimize magnification. A cholangiogram was taken after the distal CBD was occluded, and contrast medium was injected into the CBD via the cannula to a pressure of 25 cm contrast, as measured manometrically.

The CBD width was measured at the anastomosis (Fig 1) and the area of mobilization in controls, as well as 1.5 cm proximal and 1.5 cm distal to the anastomosis. A dilatation ratio (proximal width to distal width) was derived as an indication of proximal duct dilatation or functional obstruction. A stricture ratio (anastomotic width to distal width) was derived as an indication of the true anastomotic stricture relative to a normal duct. In controls not operated on, ie, day 0, the smallest portion of the mid–CBD was considered the area of mobilization.

Tensiometry

Standard specimen strips 3 mm wide and 4 cm long were prepared and vertically mounted in a tensiometer (Model 1130, Instron Inc, Canton, Mass) with an electronic load-weighing system synchronously linked to a strip-chart recorder. The distance between the edges of the clamps was set at 1 cm. A distracting force was constantly applied at 5 cm/min and charted as load vs time. Breaking strength was determined as the maximal load required to pull the strip specimen apart and was reported as grams per millimeter of strip width. Strips were cut for tensiometric analysis so that sutures were excluded or the sutures were cut or removed.

Histologic Grading

Standard specimens were fixed in Bouin's solution and stained with hematoxylin-eosin. Perianastomotic inflammation was qualitatively assessed by an investigator who had no knowledge of sutures and healing periods. A grading scale from 1 to 4 was employed. Grade 1 represented no discernible inflammation, grade 2 represented minimal inflammatory cellular infiltration mainly confined to an area 500 μm to either side of the anastomosis, grade 3 inflammation represented a heavier infiltrate confined to an area 1000 μm to either side of the anastomosis, and grade 4 inflammation was most severe with a diffuse and heavy cellular infiltrate spreading greater than 1000 μm from either side of the anastomosis.

Statistical Analysis

Mean values and SEMs were calculated for all variables. Main effects due to healing periods and types of suture on the dilatation ratio, stricture ratio, breaking strength, and inflammatory grade were evaluated by a 4×4 ANOVA, with $P<.05$ considered significant. Multiple comparisons between groups at individual healing periods and within groups over time were made using the Student Neuman-Keuls Test (NK), with $P<.05$ considered significant.[14] The Student t test for independent samples was likewise used where appropriate, with P adjusted as necessary to correct for the multiple use of single data groups for comparison.[14] Pearson's correlations were used to evaluate the relationship between inflammation and anastomotic stricture ratio and breaking strength, with $P<.05$ considered significant.

RESULTS

Seventy-six dogs were required to complete the study. Three dogs developed free anastomotic leaks within the first 2 weeks postoperatively (two sutured with PGA-910 and one with chromic sutures) and were excluded from further analysis. These technical failures all occurred early in the course of the study. All other animals tolerated their operative procedures well with no statistically significant differences in postoperative weight changes between sutured vs control animals. Serum alkaline phosphatase levels were more frequently elevated (>80 U/L) in animals sacrificed within 15 days of operation and decreased with time. Total bilirubin levels followed the same trend, but none of the control animals had elevated total bilirubin levels (> 9 μmol/L). Laboratory results are summarized in Table 2.

Table 1.—Experimental Design*

Healing Period, d	Controls	Suture Type: Chromic	PGA-910	PGN
0 (not operated on)	5	0	0	0
5	2	5	5	5
10	2	5	5	5
15	2	5	5	5
50	2	5	5	5

*Values represent the total number of animals in each group. PGA-910 indicates polyglactin 910; PGN, polyglyconate.

Cholangiographic analysis revealed the presence of proximal ductal dilatation (proximal width to distal width ratio, >1.0) in all suture groups and control groups not operated on at all healing periods (Table 3). Proximal ducts of animals sacrificed earlier tended to be more dilated than those of animals allowed to heal for 50 days and sacrificed later, but overall, no statistically significant effects were attributable to treatment, ie, control and suture types ($P=.296$), or to the healing period ($P=.211$). Visual inspection of the data revealed minor differences within suture groups, with chromic-sutured bile ducts substantially more dilated at 10 days compared with those allowed to heal 50 days.

Cholangiographic analysis of the stricture ratio was done to assess true narrowing at the anastomosis compared with a normal duct. No statistically significant main effect was found due to treatment, ie, control vs suture type ($P=.701$), but these results were affected by the healing period ($P<.001$) (Table 4). Overall, strictures were significantly more severe at 5 days compared with those present at 15 days (NK, $P<.05$). Ten-day animals gave intermediate results with no significant differences between their stricture ratios and those of either the 5- or 15-day groups. Strictures at day 50 were significantly less severe than the strictures at all other healing periods (NK, $P<.05$ for all comparisons).

Visual inspection of the data for stricture ratios suggested the presence of minor differences within groups even though the 4×4 ANOVA showed no overall suture effects, so the NK was used to compare stricture ratios present at different healing periods within each suture group (Table 5). Fifty-day chromic CBD anastomoses were significantly less strictured than the 5-day chromic group (NK, $P<.05$) but no different compared with 10- or 15-day chromic groups. No major differences were present between the stricture ratios at any of the healing periods in the PGA-910–sutured animals. The PGN-sutured dogs, however, had significantly less CBD anastomotic stricture at 50 days compared with 5, 10, or 15 days (NK, $P<.05$ for all comparisons). The CBD anastomoses sutured with PGN

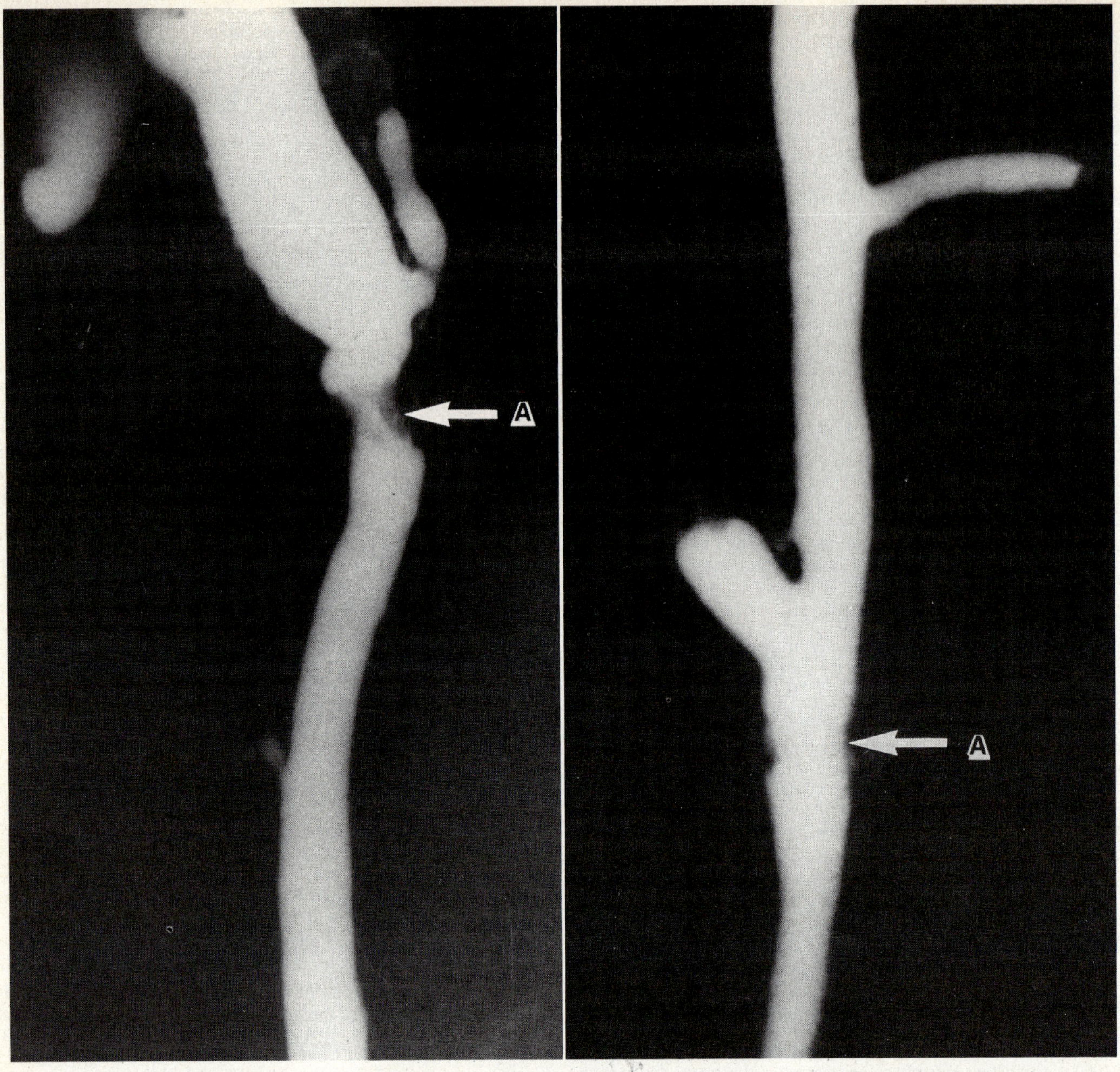

Fig 1.—Examples of specimen cholangiograms. A indicates the anastomosis. Left, A 15-day polyglactin 910–sutured anastomosis. Right, A 50-day polyglactin 910–sutured anastomosis.

also were significantly less strictured at 50 days compared with PGA-910–sutured 50-day anastomoses.

Analysis of CBD anastomotic breaking strength data revealed a significant effect due to treatment, ie, control vs sutured bile ducts ($P<.001$). This effect was observed because the breaking strength of intact CBD strips (controls) was significantly greater than the breaking strengths of sutured anastomoses (NK, $P<.05$ for all comparisons) at all of the healing periods tested. However, no significant differences emerged between the types of suture used to construct CBD anastomoses (Table 6).

Overall, CBD anastomotic breaking strength also was significantly affected by the healing period ($P<.001$), with breaking strength rising with longer healing times, as one would expect (Table 4). The CBD anastomotic breaking strength was significantly weaker in animals allowed to heal for 5 days compared with all other healing periods (NK, $P<.05$). The CBD anastomotic breaking strength was greatest in 50-day animals compared with all earlier healing period groups (NK, $P<.05$ for all comparisons).

A more detailed inspection of the breaking strength data revealed slightly different patterns of healing depending on the particular type of suture (Table 6). The CBD anastomoses sutured with chromic had no significant differences in breaking strength at 5, 10, or 15 days. For chromic-sutured animals, however, statistically significant increased breaking strength only was present when comparing the 50-day group with either the 5-, 10-, or 15-day groups (NK, $P<.05$ for all comparisons). The CBD anastomoses sutured with PGA-910 were significantly stronger at 15 days compared with 5 days (NK, $P<.05$), had intermediate strength at 10 days, and had significantly greater strength at 50 days compared with the 5- and 10-day but not the 15-day PGA-910–sutured groups (NK,

Table 2.—Laboratory Assessment at Sacrifice*

Healing period, d	Total Bilirubin, % <9 μmol/L	Total Bilirubin, % >9 μmol/L	Alkaline Phosphatase, % <80 U/L	Alkaline Phosphatase, % 80-250 U/L	Alkaline Phosphatase, % >250 U/L
0 (controls not operated on) (n=5)	100	0	100	0	0
5					
Controls (n=2)	100	0	0	100	0
Sutured (n=15)	80	20	33	20	47
10					
Controls (n=2)	100	0	50	0	50
Sutured (n=15)	80	20	53	14	33
15					
Controls (n=2)	100	0	50	50	0
Sutured (n=15)	100	0	60	0	40
50					
Controls (n=2)	100	0	50	50	0
Sutured (n=15)	93	7	80	20	0

*Values represent the percentage of animals whose laboratory values fell within the specified range.

Table 3.—Dilatation Ratios (Proximal Width to Distal Width) for Healing Periods and Suture Groups*

Healing Period, d	Control	Suture Type: Chromic	PGA-910	PGN
5	1.59±0.42	2.11±0.40	2.05±0.77	1.49±0.27
10	1.51±0.07	2.46±0.55†	1.66±0.21	1.55±0.19
15	1.16±0.02	1.63±0.23	1.83±0.18	1.35±0.10
50	1.02±0.02	1.17±0.20	1.32±0.11	1.98±0.19

*Values represent mean±SE for that group. Dilatation ratio greater than 1.0 represents proximal dilatation. PGA-910 indicates polyglactin 910; PGN, polyglyconate.

†Number is significantly different from the dilatation ratio of 50-day chromic animals ($P<.05$ by Neuman-Keuls Test).

$P<.05$ for 50-day vs 5- and 10-day comparisons). Anastomoses sutured with PGN were significantly stronger at 50 days compared with 5 days (NK, $P<.05$), but intermediate CBD anastomotic breaking strengths were present at 10 and 15 days, not significantly different from either the 5- or 50-day groups.

To develop a broader understanding of CBD healing in terms of anastomotic breaking strength as it relates to the breaking strength of undisrupted bile duct, sutured animals in each healing period were combined into single groups and compared with the day 0 control group not operated on. Student's t test was used, with $P<.0125$ considered significant to correct for multiple uses of the single set of control data from animals not operated on.[14] The CBD breaking strength in these controls was 515.4±38.4 g/mm compared with 221.6±18.8 g/mm in animals allowed to heal for 50 days. Hence, CBD anastomotic breaking strength in sutured animals never returned to control levels during the course of this study, only regaining 43% of the strength of intact tissue by 50 days.

Perianastomotic inflammation was qualitatively graded based on both the degree of inflammatory cellular infiltrate present and the area around the anastomosis where the infiltrate was a predominant finding. Inflammatory changes were most severe in the animals sacrificed earlier, but particularly at 5 days, the inflammatory response in chromic anastomoses seemed most severe (Fig 2). Mononuclear cells and macrophages were the dominant inflammatory cells present in all groups at all healing periods, but neutrophils were seen frequently in animals sacrificed earlier. Chromic sutures tended to evoke a greater inflammatory foreign-body reaction than either PGA-910 or PGN. The foreign-body response to both PGA-910 and PGN was minimal.

Table 4.—Effect of Healing Period on Common Bile Duct Anastomotic Strictures and Breaking Strength*

Healing Period, d	Stricture Ratio (Anastomotic Width to Distal Width)	Breaking Strength, g/mm
5	0.53±0.06	62.9±8.0†
10	0.64±0.05	116.8±11.4
15	0.79±0.06‡	145.3±18.2
50	1.09±0.11§	221.6±18.8‖

*Values represent the mean±SE for the combined groups of sutured dogs (n=15) at each healing period.

†Value is significantly different from the breaking strengths of the 10-, 15-, and 50-day groups.

‡Value is significantly different from the stricture ratio of the 5-day group.

§Value is significantly different from the stricture ratios of the 5-, 10-, and 15-day groups.

‖Value is significantly different from the breaking strengths of the 5-, 10-, and 15-day groups (comparisons by the Neuman-Keuls Test, $P<.05$ is significant).

Table 5.—Stricture Ratios (Anastomotic Width to Distal Width) for Healing Periods and Suture Groups*

Healing Period, d	Control	Suture Type: Chromic	PGA-910	PGN
5	0.81±0.03	0.46±0.08	0.74±0.13	0.40±0.05
10	0.97±0.02	0.66±0.06	0.62±0.13	0.63±0.08
15	0.89±0.10	0.77±0.15	0.89±0.07	0.72±0.07
50	0.75±0.08	1.00±0.19†	0.91±0.26	1.37±0.21‡

*Values represent mean±SE for that group. Stricture ratio less than 1.0 represents anastomotic narrowing compared with normal duct. PGA-910 indicates polyglactin 910; PGN, polyglyconate.

†Value is significantly different from the stricture ratio of the 5-day chromic group.

‡Value is significantly different from the stricture ratios of the 5-, 10-, and 15-day polyglyconate groups and the 50-day polyglactin 910 group (comparisons by the Neuman-Keuls Test, $P<.05$ is significant).

Table 6.—Common Bile Duct Anastomotic Breaking Strength for Healing Periods and Suture Groups*

Healing Period, d	Control, g/mm	Suture Type: Chromic, g/mm	PGA-910, g/mm	PGN, g/mm
5	484.2±35.1	69.8±14.9	59.9±18.2	58.8±9.7
10	443.3±50.0	104.4±22.0	121.9±16.6	124.2±23.4
15	406.7±126.6	118.5±9.3	162.1±31.4†	155.3±46.0
50	471.3±91.3	207.8±32.3‡	238.6±28.3§	218.3±41.1‖

*Values represent mean±SE for that group. PGA-910 indicates polyglactin 910; PGN, polyglyconate.

†Value is significantly different from the 5-day polyglactin 910 group.

‡Value is significantly different from the 5-, 10-, and 15-day chromic groups.

§Value is significantly different from the 5- and 10-day polyglactin 910 groups.

‖Value is significantly different from the 5-day polyglyconate group (comparisons by the Neuman-Keuls Test, $P<.05$ is significant).

The overall perianastomotic inflammatory response was evaluated by 4×4 ANOVA. In general, all groups, including the controls, showed more inflammation in the earlier healing periods, with inflammation decreasing as the healing time increased (Table 7). Significant effects were due to treatment, ie, control and suture type ($P<.001$), as well as to the healing period ($P=.005$). Animals sutured with chromic had significantly greater perianastomotic inflammation than either control animals or those sutured with PGN (NK, $P<.05$ for both comparisons). Animals sutured with PGA-910 had an intermediate result, tending to have less inflammation than chromic, yet more than PGN, but not statistically different from either the chromic or PGN group. Fifty-day anastomoses were significantly less inflamed overall than either the 5-, 10-, or 15-day groups (NK, $P<.05$ for all comparisons).

Table 7.—Perianastomotic Inflammation for Healing Periods and Suture Groups*

Healing Period, d	Control	Suture Type: Chromic	PGA-910	PGN
5	2.0±0	3.60±0.25	2.75±0.25	2.0±0
10	2.50±1.5	3.0±0.32	2.20±0.20	2.0±0.32
15	1.0±0	2.75±0.48	3.0±0.32	2.40±0.51
50	1.0±0	2.20±0.20	2.0±0.32	1.60±0.25

*Values represent mean±SE for that group. Grade 1 indicates no discernible inflammation, whereas grade 4 indicates maximal inflammatory response. Overall, the inflammatory response incited by chromic suture tends to be greater than that incited by polyglactin 910 (PGA-910) suture (Neuman-Keuls Test, $P<.10$) and is significantly greater than the inflammatory reaction to polyglyconate (PGN) suture (Neuman-Keuls Test, $P<.05$). Overall, inflammation at 50 days is significantly less than that present at either 5, 10, or 15 days (Neuman-Keuls Test, $P<.05$ for all comparisons).

There was a weak negative correlation between inflammation and anastomotic stricture ratio ($r=-.26$, $P=.02$; more inflamed anastomoses tended to have tighter strictures). The correlation between inflammation and anastomotic breaking strength was weakly positive ($r=.29$, $P=.007$; anastomoses with greater degrees of inflammation tended to have greater strength).

COMMENT

The pathogenesis of biliary strictures represents an important fundamental problem in general surgery. It is surprising that more basic investigation of bile duct healing has not been done since virtually hundreds of articles have

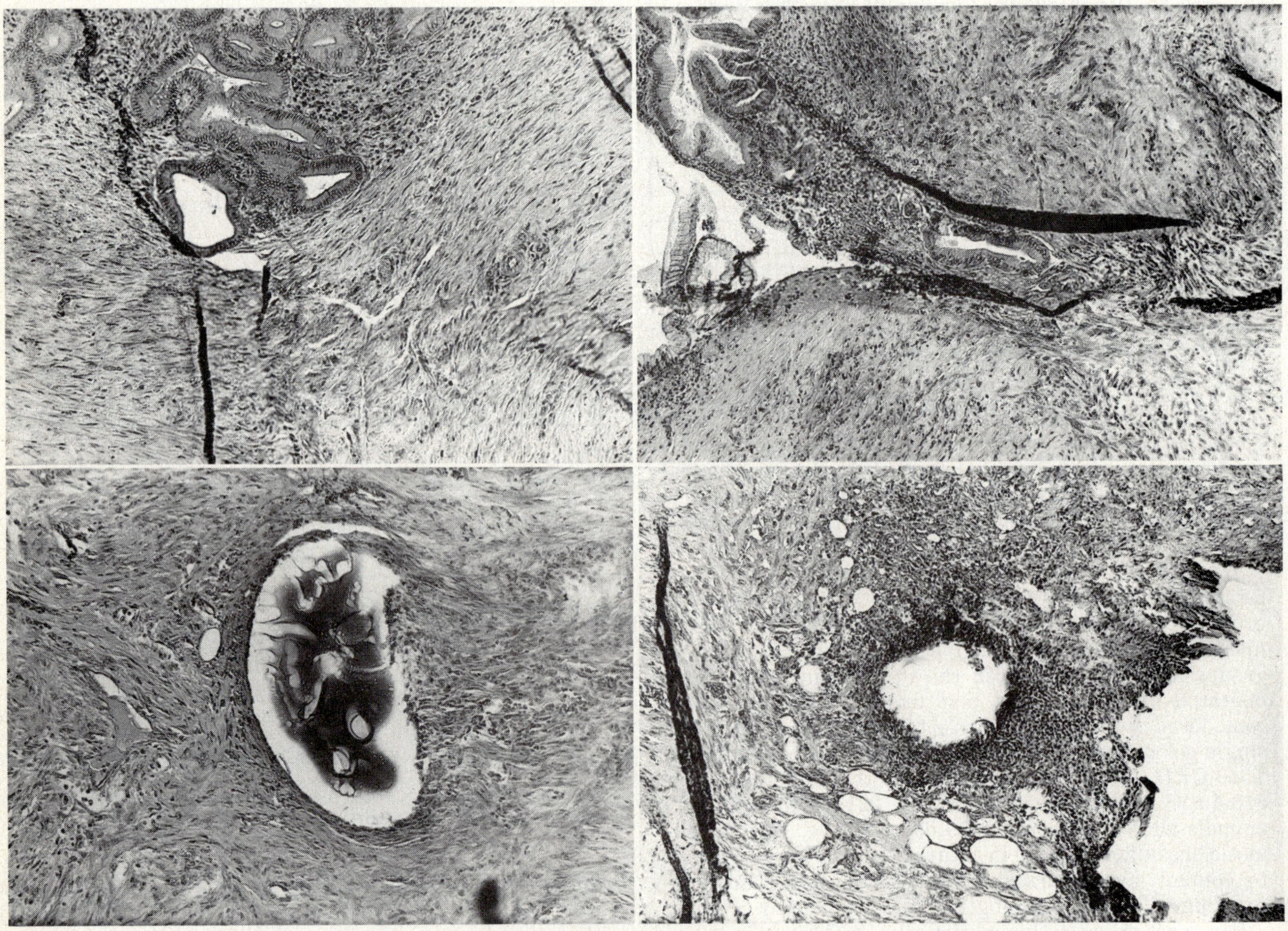

Fig 2.—Perianastomotic inflammation and tissue reaction to sutures in 5-day common bile duct anastomoses. Top left, A polyglactin 910–sutured anastomosis. A mild inflammatory reaction, grade 2, is present. Top right, A chromic-sutured anastomosis demonstrating a more intense, grade 4, inflammatory response. Bottom left, A polyglyconate suture eliciting a minimal foreign-body reaction. Bottom right, A vigorous inflammatory response to chromic suture at 5 days. (The suture was removed during processing of the specimen.) See the text for an explanation of inflammation grades (hematoxylin-eosin, original magnification ×35).

been published on intestinal anastomotic healing and anastomotic techniques. No standard method for the repair of CBD injuries and strictures exists. Individual surgeons and institutions favor techniques that yield good results in their practices, yet no technique has uniformly produced results so superior to others that it makes them obsolete. The issues of whether to stent and for how long, whether to do an end-to-end choledochal or some type of biliary-enteric diversion, and what type of sutures to use are controversial. Perhaps least controversial at this time is the general acceptance that absorbable sutures are preferable to nonabsorbable ones, because of the tendency of the latter to erode into the duct lumen, where they may cause recurrent episodes of obstructive jaundice and cholangitis.[10-12] Differences in the type of absorbable sutures available and their relative evaluation in biliary surgery have been minimally addressed.[15]

This study was done to address the main question of whether the type of absorbable suture used to construct an end-to-end choledochal anastomosis makes any difference in terms of CBD anastomotic stricture formation and tensile strength, as well as to add more basic information about wound healing in the bile duct. Absorbable sutures available for surgical use are continually changing, with newer sutures being used that are ideally designed to maintain tensile strength during the early phases of wound healing, while simultaneously eliciting minimal foreign-body inflammatory reaction. Catgut suture elicits a strong foreign-body inflammatory response in tissue. Degradation of chromic catgut is by enzymatic proteolysis, and, when exposed to bile, it loses 60% of its initial tensile strength after 7 days.[15] The PGA-910 suture is a braided synthetic one, consisting of a copolymer of glycolic and lactic acids present in a ratio of 90:10, which is slowly hydrolyzed by water and elicits less inflammation than catgut.[16] This suture loses 40% to 50% of its initial tensile strength by 7 days when immersed in bile.[15] The PGA-910 suture represents the first generation of synthetic absorbable sutures available for widespread clinical use. This suture handles much like silk because of its braided construction, and it is pliable and easy to tie with knots that go down smoothly and lie flat. However, also because of its braided construction, this type of suture has a high degree of drag when being pulled through tissues and tends to saw delicate, friable tissues, a particular disadvantage when suturing bile ducts.

The latest generation of absorbable suture is composed of a synthetic polymer of polyglyconate, which consists of glycolic acid and trimethylene carbonate combined in a 2:1 ratio.[13] This monofilament suture is more slowly degraded and absorbed and retains its tensile strengths in tissue longer than the first-generation absorbables.[13] It also evokes minimal foreign-body inflammatory reaction and is slowly absorbed by nonenzymatic hydrolysis. This suture offers the quality of less tissue drag and sawing than earlier synthetic absorbable sutures. Because tissue inflammation has been reported to be less around suture materials with low capillarity (monofilaments compared with braided sutures), available evidence suggests that the tissue inflammatory response to this newer synthetic absorbable suture would be less than that elicited by braided ones.[17]

The relationship of tensile strength and tissue inflammation to function, integrity, and subsequent stricture formation of an anastomosis is incompletely understood. It seems reasonable to assume that increased tissue inflammation due to an inflammatory suture, compared with a suture that elicits a minimal inflammatory response, would result in increased stricture formation. It also is tempting to speculate that increased inflammation would lead to greater scar formation with increased tensile strength, but this is also unknown. Hence, we included an evaluation of perianastomotic inflammation associated with different sutures in this study to see if inflammation would have a major effect on the clinically important variables of anastomotic stricture and tensile strength. Although the correlations were weak, there was a notable negative relationship between perianastomotic inflammation and the anastomotic stricture ratio, which indicated that more inflamed anastomoses also tended to have tighter strictures. Likewise, there was a substantial positive relationship between anastomotic breaking strength and perianastomotic inflammation, with more severely inflamed anastomoses having greater anastomotic breaking strength. These relationships provide evidence that favorably supports the use of a suture that inherently maintains tensile strength longer, yet elicits a minimal inflammatory response for procedures involving the CBD.

Our cholangiographic data showed generally expected results—that animals sacrificed earlier showed edematous anastomoses with dilated proximal ducts, and that this improved with time. The relationships between inflammation and stricture and inflammation and breaking strength were not as clear when the data for individual suture groups were evaluated by ANOVA. The more inflammatory suture did not greatly increase stricture formation, but there was a trend toward less-strictured anastomoses in 50-day PGN-sutured animals. Our data on tensile strength also failed to show differences in anastomotic breaking strength between the suture groups. Thus, the function and integrity of choledochal anastomoses appeared to be influenced by factors other than or in addition to those assessed in this study.

The CBD anastomotic breaking strength never returned to that of intact tissues, even after 50 days of healing. This finding conflicts with that of Northover and associates,[1] who reported that the breaking strength of pig end-to-end CBD anastomoses returned to normal values by 15 days and greatly exceeded the strength of intact CBD tissue at 50 days. This difference may be due to species variation, especially since it relates to the blood supply of the bile ducts in these animals. Our finding that the CBD anastomosis has not reached even half of the strength of intact CBD tissues by 50 days of healing also may reflect a basic difference between healing of the bile duct and that of other tissues, such as stomach or colon, which reach approximately 70% of strength of normal tissues by 21 days.[16,18,19] Earlier studies implicated bile as the cause of impaired healing in the CBD compared with the stomach or intestine.[20] In the study by Douglass and associates,[20] canine CBD anastomoses healed with less stricture formation when bile was completely diverted away from the healing CBD anastomosis. However, the biomechanical properties of these anastomoses were not assessed in their study, so the role of bile as a mediator of altered CBD healing and stricture formation remains speculative.

Perianastomotic inflammation was significantly affected by both the type of absorbable suture used to construct a CBD anastomosis and the duration of healing. We found that inflammation decreased with time, and that PGN suture evoked much less perianastomotic inflammation than chromic suture and tended to cause less than PGA-910 suture. We believe that the increased inflammation present in PGA-910–sutured anastomoses was likely due to the increased capillarity of the braided suture, which may have allowed more bile to seep into the tissue than may have occurred around a monofilament suture. It might have been useful to assay collagen synthesis to determine if there was a correlation between increased collagen synthesis and increased inflammation as a potential mediator of stricture formation, but previous work by Casey and Peacock[4] suggested that wound contraction, not collagen synthesis, is the fundamental biological process leading to stricture of a repaired CBD.

Experience gained from the present study has reemphasized the critical importance of the standard surgical principles of gentle tissue handling, maintenance of blood supply, precise hemostasis, and the creation of a tensionless anastomosis when operating on the CBD. Ultimately, suture choice depends on the surgeon's confidence in the suture as well as its appropriateness for a given clinical situation. The surgeon's confidence in a suture clearly is affected by its tendency to drag or saw through tissue, the security of knots tied, the number of knots needed for security, and overall ease of "handling." Our data support the use of any of the three sutures in this study based on no functional anastomotic differences in short-term analysis, but our preference remains for a monofilament suture that does not cut through inflamed tissues, yet ties easily and securely. A monofilament suture is generally preferable in situations demanding low tissue drag (eg, when suturing inflamed or edematous ducts) but is not as easily handled or tied as PGA-910.

In conclusion, our results demonstrate that the type of absorbable suture used to construct an end-to-end choledochal anastomosis does not affect the formation of CBD anastomotic strictures or tensile strength. A PGN suture causes substantially less perianastomotic inflammation than chromic suture and tends to cause less than PGA-910 suture, but a clinical advantage to this property in terms of CBD anastomotic stricture or tensile strength was not apparent in this short-term study. Further basic investigations clearly are needed to study the effects of biliary stents on CBD healing, to study the effects of alterations in blood supply on the healing CBD anastomosis, to clarify the effect of bile on CBD healing, and to characterize the healing biliary-enteric anastomosis.

This work was supported by the National Institutes of Health (Bethesda, Md) grant BRSG RR 05424 24-40, and a grant provided by the American Cyanamid Company, Wayne, NJ. The study was conducted at the Nashville (Tenn) Veterans Administration Medical Center research facility, and the support and assistance rendered to us by the research staff there is appreciated. We wish to thank Lillian Nanney, PhD, and Mary McKissock for technical support in the histologic preparation of our specimens. Cheri Premeau, MA, of Statistical Research Consultants Inc, Nashville, Tenn, provided statistical consultation and support.

References

1. Northover JMA, Hickman R, Watson RGK, Terblanche J. Healing of the bile duct anastomosis after transverse choledochotomy or transplantation in the pig. *Surg Gynecol Obstet.* 1985;160:33-36.
2. Kram HB, Garces MA, Klein SR, Shoemaker WC. Common bile duct anastomosis using fibrin glue. *Arch Surg.* 1985;120:1250-1256.
3. Lamesch AJ, Dociu N. Microsurgical reconstruction of the biliary duct: experimental study in rats and dogs. *Microsurgery.* 1986;7:46-52.
4. Casey WJ, Peacock EE Jr. Some factors affecting pathophysiology of bile duct stenosis. *Surg Forum.* 1977;28:414-416.
5. Blumgart LH, Thompson JN. The management of benign strictures of the bile ducts. *Curr Probl Surg.* 1987;24:1-66.
6. Wheeler ES, Longmire WP Jr. Repair of benign stricture of the common bile duct by jejunal interposition choledochoduodenostomy. *Surg Gynecol Obstet.* 1978;146:260-262.
7. Braasch JW, Bolton JS, Rossi RL. A technique of biliary tract reconstruction with complete follow-up in 44 consecutive cases. *Ann Surg.* 1981;194:635-638.
8. Way LW. Biliary stricture. In: Way LW, Pelligrini CA, eds. *Surgery of the Gallbladder and Bile Ducts.* Philadelphia, Pa: WB Saunders Co; 1987: 419-436.
9. Smith RS. The Rodney Smith method of biliary stricture repair. In: Way LW, Pelligrini CA, eds. *Surgery of the Gallbladder and Bile Ducts.* Philadelphia, Pa: WB Saunders Co; 1987:429-436.
10. Mackie DB, Haynes S, May RE. Unabsorbable suture material: a rare cause of recurrent stones in the common bile duct. *Br J Surg.* 1973; 60:23-24.
11. Lewis JW, Caleta LF. Stone formation on silk suture after choledochoduodenostomy. *South Med J.* 1981;74:1280-1281.
12. Galletti G, Ussia G, Bertoni R, Ruscelli P, Salerno A. Comparison of the effects of polyglycolic acid and monofilament nylon sutures in the common bile duct of pigs. *Ital J Surg Sci.* 1984;14:111-117.
13. *A New Synthetic Monofilament Absorbable Suture.* Surrey, England: Davis & Geck, American Cyanamid Co; 1986.
14. Godfrey K. Statistics in practice: comparing the means of several groups. *N Engl J Med.* 1985;313:1450-1456.
15. Sugimachi K, Sufian S, Weiss MJ, Pavlides CA, Matsumoto T. Evaluation of absorbable suture materials in biliary tract surgery. *Int Surg.* 1978;63:135-139.
16. Peacock EE Jr. Collagenolysis and the biochemistry of wound healing. In: Peacock EE Jr, ed. *Wound Repair.* 3rd ed. Philadelphia, Pa: WB Saunders Co; 1984:102-140.
17. Blomstedt B, Osterberg B. Suture materials and wound infection: an experimental study. *Acta Chir Scand.* 1978;144:269-274.
18. Hastings JC, Van Winkle W Jr, Barker E, Hines D, Nichols W. Effect of suture materials on healing wounds of the stomach and colon. *Surg Gynecol Obstet.* 1975;140:701-707.
19. Gottrup F. Healing of incisional wounds of the stomach and duodenum: a biomechanical study. *Am J Surg.* 1980;140:296-301.
20. Douglass TC, Dounsbury BF, Cutter WW, Wetzel N. An experimental study of healing in the common bile duct. *Surg Gynecol Obstet.* 1950;91:301-305.

In Other AMA Journals

ARCHIVES OF INTERNAL MEDICINE

Changing Concepts in Surgical Management of Renovascular Hypertension

John A. Libertino, MD; Thierry A. Flam, MD; Leonard N. Zinman, MD; Christopher Y. Ying, MD; Donald J. Breslin, MD; Neil W. Swinton, Jr, MD; M. D. Phelps, Jr, MD; Nicholas P. Tsapatsaris, MD; Bartholomew O'B. Woods, MD

As newer surgical techniques and concepts have emerged, including revascularization of the totally occluded renal artery and alternatives to aortorenal bypass (hepatic, splenic, or iliac artery to renal artery grafts), our patient population has changed. Patients with diffuse atherosclerotic disease, bilateral renal artery stenosis, totally occluded renal arteries, and azotemia are being referred for renal revascularization, thereby changing the indications for operation and the results that can be anticipated. Although our results in patients operated on solely for uncontrollable hypertension or renal failure have been successful, much work needs to be done to improve the results obtained when patients have a combination of uncontrollable hypertension and renal failure (*Arch Intern Med* 1988;148:357-359).

Reprint requests to Department of Urology, Lahey Clinic Medical Center, 41 Mall Rd, Burlington, MA 01805 (Dr Libertino).

Epidural Anesthesia in Patients Undergoing Thoracic Surgery

Barbara K. Temeck, MD; Paul W. Schafer, MD; Woo Y. Park, MD; John W. Harmon, MD

• Epidural anesthesia has been reported to exert beneficial effects in surgical procedures. Over the past 3 years at the Veterans Administration Medical Center in Washington, DC, thoracic surgical procedures have been done using a combined technique of epidural anesthesia with light general anesthesia. A retrospective review of this experience from January 1984 to November 1987 was done in 90 consecutive patients. Postoperative extubation of patients was accomplished immediately in 32%, within 1 hour in 34%, within 3 hours in 28%, within 18 hours in 4%, and was prolonged in only 1% of patients. Mortality was 2% and morbidity was 3%. This analysis indicates that the technique of epidural anesthesia with light general anesthesia provided satisfactory anesthesia with low mortality and morbidity in a high-risk group of patients undergoing surgery.

(*Arch Surg.* 1989;124:415-418)

Epidural anesthesia has been used successfully for lower abdominal, peripheral vascular, and major orthopedic procedures.[1-3] Potential advantages of the epidural anesthesia technique in these procedures include a reduction in cardiac preload and afterload,[4] higher postoperative pulmonary flow rates with improved oxygenation,[5,6] decreased incidence of venous thromboembolism[7] as well as blood loss,[8,9] better suppression of stress responses,[10] and a positive effect on postoperative nitrogen balance.[11] Potential disadvantages include the time required to establish the epidural anesthesia, volume needed to avoid decrease in blood pressure, and potential for technical complications such as epidural hematoma. Questions can be raised as to what the overall influence would be of the block on respiration, ie, inhibition or facilitation. Although postoperative pain relief could improve pulmonary function, the high level of epidural block could paralyze some of the ventilatory muscles; also, fluid requirements to maintain blood pressure might predispose to later congestive heart failure.

Epidural anesthesia alone was successfully used for thoracic surgical procedures on awake spontaneously breathing patients by Crawford et al.[12] However, the usual approach in the United States is to perform general thoracic surgery under general anesthesia with endotracheal ventilatory support. Advantages of general anesthesia are ease of administration, satisfactory relaxation, ability to control the depth of anesthesia, and good hemodynamic stability, which, however, can be affected by cardiorespiratory depressant effects of some agents. The disadvantage is a central depressant of respiration that can extend into the postoperative period in a patient who can awaken in pain and require longer postoperative intubation.

A combination of epidural anesthesia with light general anesthesia might offer a method of anesthesia that would maximize the benefits of each form of anesthesia. The purpose of this study was to examine the outcome of this technique for a group of patients operated on over the past 3 years at the Veterans Administration Medical Center in Washington, DC.

PATIENTS, MATERIALS, AND METHODS

Ninety consecutive patients underwent thoracic surgical procedures while receiving epidural anesthesia with light general anesthesia from January 1984 to November 1987. This retrospective study examines several categories of information concerning these patients.

For each patient the following factors were examined: age, sex, disease category (benign or malignant), stage and histologic features of malignant disease, and operative procedures with a risk assessment evaluation using the American Association of Anesthesiology (ASA) classification[13] and the analysis of Goldman et al.[14] The pulmonary status was examined by history and physical examination, chest roentgenogram, and data, when available, from pulmonary function tests.

Perioperative and Operative Data

No patient had a contraindication to the epidural anesthesia. In each patient, a No. 17 Tuohy needle was inserted into one of the lower thoracic intravertebral spaces. The epidural space was identified and with the bevel of the needle cephalad, a test dose of 3 mL of 0.5% bupivacaine hydrochloride with epinephrine (1:200 000) was injected followed after 2 minutes by the main dose of local anesthetic solution (10 to 12 mL) given at the rate of 0.7 mL/s. An epidural catheter was then inserted and fixed. The

Accepted for publication Dec 20, 1988.

From the Departments of Surgery (Drs Temeck, Schafer, and Harmon) and Anesthesiology (Dr Park), Veterans Administration Medical Center and Georgetown University School of Medicine, Washington, DC.

Read before the 12th Annual Surgical Symposium of the Association of Veterans Administration Surgeons, Minneapolis, Minn, May 13, 1988.

Reprint requests to Department of Surgery, Veterans Administration Medical Center, 50 Irving St NW, Washington, DC 20422 (Dr Temeck).

analgesia level achieved was usually from T2-4 to S1-3. After confirming adequacy of the epidural anesthesia for the surgery, anesthesia was induced with thiopental (Pentothal) sodium, succinylcholine, or pancuronium bromide and a Robert Shaw or Carlens endobronchial tube was inserted. Anesthesia was maintained using a low concentration (0.25% to 0.5%) of either enflurane or isoflurane, nitrous oxide (50%), fentanyl citrate, and pancuronium. All patients received 100% oxygen during one lung ventilation. At the end of the surgical procedure, all patients received 1 to 2.5 mg of neostigmine (Prostigmine) bromide and 0.4 to 1.2 mg of atropine sulfate for reversal of neuromuscular blockage. During the operative procedure, monitoring of hemodynamic status included mean arterial blood pressure, central venous pressure, and mean blood loss. Postoperative assessment included recording the time at which each patient was extubated and the mean time elapsing prior to the administration of the first postoperative analgesic.

Clinical Outcome

Major clinical outcome was analyzed with regard to several variables. The first was mortality and morbidity. Mortality was defined as a death within 30 days of the operative procedure; morbidity was defined as cardiovascular problems such as myocardial infarction, ischemia, congestive heart failure, or arrhythmias. Respiratory problems were defined by the need for mechanical ventilation for more than 24 hours postoperatively or by the decision to reintubate a patient. Also considered were infections, such as development of pneumonia or wound infection, and renal, gastrointestinal, and neurological problems developing in the 30-day postoperative period.

RESULTS

There were 89 men and 1 woman with an age range from 32 to 80 years (median, 61 years). Twelve patients (13.3%) had benign disease with 2 excisions of bullae, one lobectomy, and 9 wedge resections. Table 1 outlines the treatment, stage of disease, and type of surgical procedures for the 78 patients with malignant disease (83% were epidermoid and the remainder were adenocarcinoma) as evaluated by the TNM staging system.[15]

The overall risk assessment of the patients indicated a mean ASA classification of II with 7 class I, 61 class II, 18 class III, and 4 class IV patients. The cardiac risk assessment of the patients by the index of Goldman et al[14] was 9.77 (SD = 3.53), which is the Goldman class II. The pulmonary risk factors are presented below.

Pulmonary Risk Factors	% (Proportion)
History of cigarette smoking (average, 60 pack-years)	97 (87/90)
Preoperative history of chronic obstructive pulmonary disease	69 (62/90)
Preoperative purulent productive cough	6 (5/90)
Forced expiratory volume in 1 s (FEV_1) less than 2 L	68 (45/66)
Maximal ventilatory volume less than 50% predicted	55 (36/66)

Seventy-three percent of the patients had pulmonary function tests with mean spirometric values of FEV_1 of 1.83 L (SD = 0.33), a forced vital capacity (FVC) of 2.97 L (SD = 0.57), an FEV_1/FVC ratio of 62% predicted, and a mean maximal ventilatory volume of 48% predicted.

Perioperative Data

No patient required more than light general anesthesia as a supplement to the epidural anesthesia. Stable hemodynamics as followed by continuous intra-arterial and central venous monitoring were maintained without vasopressors or afterload reducers except for one patient who required administration of one dose of ephedrine (5 mg) intravenously. The mean arterial pressure was 87 mm Hg with a normal range being 80 to 90 mm Hg; the average amount of fluid administered was 2800 mL, including blood products of which 1200 mL was given during the first hour of fluid administration. The mean duration of the operation was 4 hours. The following outlines the time period to accomplish extubation.

Table 1.—Treatment and Stage of Disease

Treatment at Thoracotomy	Total	Stage of Disease I	II	III
Pneumonectomy	**4**	3	1	...
Lobectomy	**22**	11	6	5
Wedge resection				
Wedge only	**50**	42	5	3
Wedge and chest wall resection	**1**	...	...	1
Exploratory thoracotomy	**1**	...	...	1
No. (%) of patients	**78**	**56** (72)	**12** (15)	**10** (13)

Table 2.—Cardiac Risk Index

Class*	Point Total	Life-Threatening Complications, %	Cardiac Death, %
I	0-5	0.7	0.2
II	6-12	5	2
III	13-25	11	2
IV	26	22	56

*According to the point system of Goldman et al.[14]

Time to Extubation	No. (%) of Cases
Immediate	29 (32)
1 hour	31 (34)
3 hours	25 (28)
18 hours (morning after)	4 (4)
>24 hours	1 (1)

First postoperative analgesia was given at 6.7 hours; thus, the mean duration of epidural analgesia was 10.7 hours. None of the patients required diuresis for pulmonary edema. The epidural catheter was removed on the first postoperative day.

Clinical Outcome

The mortality for the group of patients was 2.2% (2/90) due to myocardial infarction occurring on postoperative days 3 and 4. Morbidity developed in 3 (3.3%) of the 90 patients, including the 48-hour requirement for mechanical ventilation in 1 patient and pneumonia in 2 other patients. No adverse effects relating to epidural anesthesia resulted other than the previously described use of one dose of ephedrine for 1 patient.

COMMENT

This review was carried out to assess the results of epidural anesthesia with light general anesthesia for thoracic surgical procedures. The study indicates that the technique described provided effective and safe intraoperative anesthesia and early postoperative analgesia in these patients. Cardiovascular stability was maintained without a requirement for excessive fluid administration. The time to extubation was not prolonged. Mortality and morbidity were better than predicted by the ASA classification[13] and criteria of Goldman et al.[14] We suggest that to maximize the potential surgical benefits of this technique for other patients, careful preoperative risk assessment be emphasized to anticipate potential complications with the goal of preoperative preparation, such as volume correction, to prevent the complications. With regard to the anesthetic technique, it is recommended that the epidural anesthetic be given at the dermatome level where the operation is performed as at T7-8 for a sixth intercostal space incision to avoid hypotension that can occur at high levels of thoracic epidural anesthesia. Titration of the amount of local anesthetic should be done to avoid total sympathetic blockade. There should be slow induction of general anesthesia and the anesthesia should be maintained lightly just to allow toleration of the endotracheal tube with the anesthesia for the intraoperative and postoperative period provided by the epidural anesthesia.

In the series of patients under investigation, the patients were demonstrated to be at high risk for postoperative complications as defined by their pulmonary and cardiac risk factors. Postoperative pulmonary complications have been identified with the following risk factors[16] (the percentages or data in parentheses relate each factor to the patients in the study group): thoracic, upper abdominal surgery (100% of operations); preoperative chronic obstructive pulmonary disease (69% of patients); preoperative purulent cough (6% of patients); anesthesia time exceeding 3 hours (mean operative time 4 hours); cigarette smoking (87% of patients, average 60 pack-years); and age greater than 60 years (median age, 61 years).

Hodgkin[17] proposed the spirometric values listed below as indicating risk of postoperative pulmonary complications. The patients in this series were at high risk according to these criteria: (1) FEV_1 less than 2.0 L or 50% of predicted; (2) FVC_1 less than 50% of predicted; (3) FEV_1/FVC_1 less than 50% of predicted; (4) FEV_1 less than 1.0 L; (5) FVC less than 1.5 L; (6) FEV_1/FVC less than 35% of predicted; and (7) maximal ventilatory volume less than 50% of predicted.

The fact that there was no mortality and only 3.3% morbidity related to pulmonary problems is remarkable considering the pulmonary risk factors in the series reported herein. The surgical risk of the patients was also high as a result of their cardiac status.[16,18] The following ASA classification of physical status is the best available predictor of overall mortality from cardiac and noncardiac causes and is a fair predictor of cardiac deaths: I, a normal healthy patient for elective operation; II, a patient with mild systemic disease; III, a patient with severe systemic disease that limits activity but is not incapacitating; IV, a patient with incapacitating systemic disease that is a constant threat to life; and V, a moribund patient not expected to survive 24 hours with or without operation.

The patients in ASA class II have a predicted mortality of 1.3% for elective risk procedures, 1.7% for elective medium-risk procedures, and 5.4% for elective high-risk procedures.[13] However, computation of the cardiac risk index as described by Goldman et al[14] is more accurate in assessing the risk of cardiac death in patients undergoing surgery. Goldman identified nine independent factors that correlate with significant life-threatening and fatal complications in noncardiac surgical procedures:

Criteria	Points
History of myocardial infarction within 6 months	10
Age over 60 years	5
Physical examination	
S_3 or jugular venous distention	11
Important aortic stenosis	3
Electrocardiogram	
Rhythm other than sinus or sinus plus atrial premature beats on last preoperative electrocardiogram	7
More than five premature ventricular contractions per minute at any time preoperatively	7
Poor general medical status	3
Intraperitoneal, intrathoracic, or aortic surgery	3
Emergency operation	4
Total	**53**

Each factor was assigned a specific number of points. Patients could be separated into four classes of significantly different risk according to the point system of Goldman et al[14] (Table 2).

For the group of patients in this series, the 2.2% mortality corresponded to the cardiac risk index (class II) of Goldman et al.[14] However, the predicted cardiac morbidity of 5% did not occur.

The satisfactory outcome for the patients in this series despite their severe risk factors was probably influenced by several different factors. The level of central depression under the combined technique is slight as compared with that of general anesthesia alone so that breathing can be considered tranquil, which means similar to that of normal physiological sleep. The ventilation achieved is the "controlled respiration" described by Guedel and Treweek[19] in which maintenance of a careful degree of hypocapnia suppresses spontaneous respiration that can return as soon as the carbon dioxide level is allowed to become normal. Another explanation for the satisfactory pulmonary outcome of these patients is the influence of this technique on postoperative pulmonary function. General anesthesia with muscle relaxants does not relieve the depressant effects of early postoperative pain. Vital capacity and lung compliance fall, leading to the accumulation of bronchial secretions.[20] Under epidural analgesia with light general anesthesia, static compliance has been shown to decrease less.[21] There is enhancement of postoperative pulmonary function.[22]

With regard to the reduced incidence of cardiovascular complications, studies have shown a decrease in the size of the myocardial infarctions due to improvement in regional endocardial perfusion to the ischemic site by epidural analgesia as compared with general anesthesia.[4] Mechanisms thought to be involved are afferent sensory blockage, decreased adrenergic tone, and coronary and systemic vasodilatation with a decrease in cardiac preload and afterload.[23] The metabolic stability afforded by epidural analgesia may also blunt the surgical stress response with the stoppage of nociceptive spinal excitability and the inhibition of release of catecholamines.[10]

An additional advantage of the epidural part of the combined technique is the low blood loss that has been demonstrated under regional techniques for surgical procedures possibly as a result of the low central venous pressure associated with epidural anesthesia.[8,9] For the operations reviewed, an average of 300 mL of blood loss occurred.

The potential for decreased blood pressure with epidural anesthesia must be considered and adequate volume support given. All patients in this series had preoperative assessment of their volume status by clinical and laboratory criteria and correction of deficits. This was done without using a Swan-Ganz central venous catheterization prior to operation, although a central venous line was placed intraoperatively in all patients. This retrospective analysis indicated that this approach was adequate. Stable intraoperative hemodynamics were achieved except for one episode of hypotension responding to ephedrine. There were no other complications associated with the epidural analgesic technique. Mention should be made of the potential complication of epidural hematoma; this complication is rare. In the series of Bonica and Anderson,[24] the risk was less than 0.01%. It did not occur in this series.

In conclusion, the combined technique of epidural analgesia with light general anesthesia provided satisfactory anesthesia for thoracic operations in a high-risk group of patients undergoing thoracic surgical procedures. This approach may be preferable to general anesthesia alone, but only a prospective randomized study could definitively demonstrate such superiority.

References

1. Hole A, Terjesen T, Brevik H. Epidural versus general anaesthesia for total hip arthroplasty in elderly patients. *Acta Anaesthesiol Scand.* 1980;24:279-287.
2. Raggi R, Dardik H, Mauro AL. Continuous epidural anesthesia and postoperative epidural narcotics in vascular surgery. *Am J Surg.* 1987;154: 192-197.
3. Cunningham FO, Egan JM, Inahara T. Continuous epidural anesthesia in abdominal vascular surgery. *Am J Surg.* 1980;139:624-627.
4. Vik-Mo H, Ottensen S, Renck H. Cardiac effects of thoracic epidural analgesia before and during acute coronary artery occlusion in open chest dogs. *Scand J Clin Lab Invest.* 1978;38:737-746.
5. Shulman M, Sandler N. Post thoracotomy pain and pulmonary function following epidural and systemic morphine. *Anesthesiology.* 1984;61:569-575.
6. Pflug AE, Murphy TM, Butler SH, Tucker GT. The effects of postoperative peridural analgesia on pulmonary therapy and pulmonary complications. *Anesthesiology.* 1974;41:8-17.
7. Modig J, Borg T, Karlstom G, Maripuu E, Sahlstedt B. Thromboembolism after total hip replacement: role of epidural and general anesthesia. *Anesth Analg.* 1983;62:174-180.
8. Parks WY, Poon KC, Macnamara YW. Epidural block for lumbar laminectomy. *Reg Anaesth.* 1987;12:48-49.
9. Moir DD. Blood loss during major vaginal surgery: a statistical study of the influence of general anaesthesia and epidural analgesia. *Br J Anaesth.* 1968;40:233-240.
10. Enquist A, Brandt MR, Fernandes A, Kehlet H. The blocking effect of epidural analgesia on the adrenocortical and hyperyglycaemic response to surgery. *Acta Anaesthesiol Scand.* 1977;21:330-335.
11. Kehlet H, Brandt MR, Prangehansen H, Albert GMM. Effect of epidural analgesia on metabolic profiles during and after surgery. *Br J Surg.* 1979;66:543-546.
12. Crawford OB, Ottosen P, Buckingham WW, Bradsher CA. Peridural anesthesia in thoracic surgery: a review of 677 cases. *Anesthesiology.* 1951;12:73-84.
13. Owens WD, Felts JA, Spitznagel EL Jr. ASA physical status classification: a study of consistency of rating. *Anesthesiology.* 1978;49:239-243.
14. Goldman L, Caldera DL, Nussbaum SR, et al. Multifactorial index of cardiac risk in noncardial surgical procedures. *N Engl J Med.* 1977; 297:845-850.
15. American Joint Committee on Cancer, Task Force on Lung. Staging of lung cancer 1979: American Joint Committee for Cancer staging and end results reporting task force on lung. Chicago, Ill: American Joint Committee on Cancer; 1979.
16. Houston MC, Ratcliff DG, Hays JT, Gluck FW. Preoperative medical consultation and evaluation of surgical risk: review article. *South Med J.* 1987;80:1385-1397.
17. Hodgkin JE. Preoperative assessment of respiratory function. *Respir Care.* 1984;29:496-505.
18. Rose SD, Corman LC, Mason DJ. Cardiac risk factors in patients undergoing non-cardiac surgery. *Med Clin North Am.* 1978;63:1271-1288.
19. Guedel AE, Treweek DN. Ether apneas. *Anesth Analg.* 1934;13:263-264.
20. Bromage PR. Physiology. In: Bromage PR, ed. *Epidural Analgesia.* Philadelphia, Pa: WB Saunders Co; 1978:415-420.
21. Bromage PR. Spirometry in assessment of analgesia after abdominal surgery. *Br Med J.* 1955;2:589-593.
22. Bromage PR. Surgical applications. In *Epidural Analgesia.* Philadelphia, Pa: WB Saunders Co; 1978:449-454.
23. Yeager MP, Glass DD, Neff RK, et al. Epidural anesthesia analgesia in high-risk surgical patients. *Anesthesiology.* 1987;66:729-736.
24. Bonica J, Anderson C. Peridural block: analysis of 3637 cases and a review. *Anesthesiology.* 1957;18:723-784.

Use of Sequential B-Mode Ultrasonography to Manage Abdominal Aortic Aneurysms

Fred N. Littooy, MD; George Steffan, PA; Howard P. Greisler, MD; Theresa L. White, RN; William H. Baker, MD

• The utility and safety of sequential B-mode ultrasonography to treat male patients with small (<6.0 cm in diameter) abdominal aortic aneurysms (AAAs) were studied retrospectively in 149 consecutive patients. Sixty-three of these patients have had operative repair of the AAA. Eighty-six remain unoperated on. Mean growth rate was 0.79 cm/y (1.06 cm/y in the operated-on group and 0.36 cm/y in the unoperated-on group). Seven patients sustained rupture of the AAA during follow-up and 4 patients died as a consequence of elective repair, for a combined mortality rate of 7.4% (11/149). Only one AAA that was less than 5.0 cm ruptured. This has proved to be an effective way to manage AAAs in this population.

(*Arch Surg* 1989;124:419-421)

The decision to repair an abdominal aortic aneurysm (AAA) electively depends on the risk of that operative repair vs the risk that an untreated aneurysm will rupture. Most patients with AAAs are in the sixth and seventh decades of life, and many have debilitating diseases that limit life expectancy and increase the operative risk. Separate studies by Szilagyi et al[1] and Darling[2] pointed out that the risk of rupture increases as the diameter of the aneurysm increases. B-mode ultrasonography gives us an accurate diagnostic tool to determine the size of the aneurysm and to follow its growth over time. Elective operative repair of aneurysms, introduced in 1952 by Dubost et al,[3] is now carried out with a 1% to 5% mortality rate in many centers.[4-6] Using the information on the natural history of aortic aneurysms based on size of the aneurysm and the ability to diagnose and size the aneurysm accurately, the surgeon is better able to decide on operative vs nonoperative therapy. This study was undertaken to assess the usefulness and safety of this approach in a male population.

PATIENTS AND METHODS

For the years 1977 through 1987, we studied 149 consecutive male patients retrospectively from the Hines (Ill) Veterans Administration Medical Center. Each patient had a diagnosis of AAA and had at least two sequential B-mode abdominal ultrasonograms to evaluate that AAA. The abdominal aorta had to measure at least 3.0 cm in greatest diameter for that patient to be included in the study. Ultrasonography was performed with a commercial real-time sector scanner from 1982 to 1987. Prior to that, a static scanner was used. Anteroposterior and transverse diameters were measured, and we used the larger of the two measurements to size the aneurysm. Mean growth rates were determined by the change in size over time of the AAA between the first and last ultrasonographic measurements (centimeters per year). Patients with AAAs of less than 5.0 cm in greatest diameter were followed up every 3 to 6 months with serial ultrasonography and advised to have an elective repair of the aneurysm if it reached 5.0 cm in greatest diameter or if symptoms developed in the patient. In some patients who were considered to be high risk, we would often delay operative repair until the aneurysm reached 6.0 cm in diameter.

Accepted for publication December 29, 1988.

From the Loyola University Medical Center, Maywood, Ill (Drs Littooy, Greisler, and Baker); and the Hines (Ill) Veterans Administration Hospital (Drs Littooy and Greisler, Mr Steffan, and Ms White).

Read before the 12th Annual Surgical Symposium of the Association of Veterans Administration Surgeons, Minneapolis, Minn, May 12, 1988.

Reprint requests to Department of Surgery, Loyola University Medical Center, 2160 S First Ave, Maywood, IL 60153 (Dr Littooy).

We then examined expansion rates based on grouping by the initial size of the aneurysm (ie, 3.0 to 3.9 cm; 4.0 to 4.9 cm). We further broke this down into patients who have had operative repair vs those not yet operated on. Further study included the rate of rupture with this approach and the results of operative therapy. All operations were performed by general surgical residents at the fourth- or fifth-year level or by peripheral vascular fellows assisted by a trained vascular surgeon.

During the 10-year period (1977 through 1987), 149 male patients met the criteria for inclusion in the study. The mean age was 68.1 years (range, 48 to 92 years). Of the 149 patients, 86 have had only serial ultrasonography. The remaining 63 patients have undergone operative repair of the AAA.

RISK FACTORS

Atherosclerotic risk factors for the group as a whole included cerebrovascular accident in 30 (20.1%), congestive heart failure in 43 (28.9%), heart disease as defined by myocardial infarction (MI), angina pectoris, congestive heart failure, abnormal electrocardiogram, or arrhythmias in 103 (69.1%), hypertension as defined by diagnosed and medically treated hypertension in 92 (61.7%), smoking in 137 (91.9%), and diabetes mellitus in 18 (12.1%).

Other risk factors included chronic obstructive pulmonary disease in 47 (31.5%) and chronic renal failure (creatine value >141 μmol/L) in 36 (24.2%). Risk factors, particularly the presence of heart disease (79% vs 55%), creatine values greater than 141 μmol/L (31% vs 19%), and cerebrovascular accident (26% vs 11%), were more pronounced in the nonoperated-on patients.

DIAGNOSIS

Abdominal aortic aneurysms were detected by several means in our population of 149 patients. Ninety-four (63%) were picked up on physical examination. The remainder were found during workup for other diagnoses. Diagnostic roentgenograms of the abdomen, back, or pelvic regions detected calcium in the walls of the AAA in 22 patients (14.8%). Ultrasonographic studies in 24 patients (16.1%) and computed tomographic scans in 4 patients (2.7%) delineated the AAA. Angiography for occlusive disease or other problems revealed AAAs in 3 patients (2.0%). One additional AAA (0.7%) was found on exploration of the abdomen during surgery for other problems.

EXPANSION RATES BY SERIAL ULTRASONOGRAPHY

To date, 149 patients have had at least two serial ultrasound examinations. Eighty-six are in the unoperated-on group, and 63 have gone on to have operative repair. The expansion rate for the group as a whole and for the nonoperated-on and operated-on patients as separate groups is depicted in Table 1. The mean growth rate overall is 0.79 cm/y (range, 0 to 6.0 cm). In patients not yet operated on, the growth rate has been 0.36 cm/y vs 1.06 cm/y in the operated-on group. This difference in growth rates between operated-on and unoperated-on patients is noted throughout the different groups based on initial size of the aneurysm. In addition, initial size of the aneurysm had no effect on expansion rate in the patient population as a whole or when broken down into operated-on and unoperated-on patients. The increased expansion rate seen in patients coming to operation is likely not related to initial size, as 41 (65.1%) of the 63 operated-on patients had aneurysms of less than 5.0 cm in greatest diameter at the time of initial diagnosis. In fact, 24 of those patients had AAAs of less than 4.0 cm in diameter initially.

OUTCOME

In the 86 unoperated-on patients, the mean length of follow-up was 41.5 months (range, 1 to 156 months). Fifty-three (61.6%) are still alive after a mean follow-up of 44.8 months (range, 10 to 156 months). Thirty-three nonoperated-on patients with a mean follow-up of 36.2 months (range, 1 to 82 months) have died. Causes of death in this group are rupture of AAA in 4 (12.1%), coronary artery disease in 14 (42.7%), cancer in 5 (15%), other causes in 8 (24.2%), and unknown in 2 (6%). No patient died of a cerebrovascular accident. Of the patients who died because of a ruptured AAA, 2 had severe medical problems but were offered operative repair. They refused and died at 26 and 33 months, respectively, after their initial diagnosis and both had AAAs with a diameter of greater than 6.5 cm. Of the other 2 patients, 1 had severe medical risks (congestive heart failure and renal failure), and his AAA was only 4.6 cm in diameter. He represents the only AAA with a diameter of less than 5.0 cm known to have ruptured. The last patient had multiple medical problems with an AAA that eventually reached 5.5 cm in diameter and was not offered operative repair. He died 78 months after diagnosis.

Of the 63 patients who had operative repair, the mean time from diagnosis to operation was 25.4 months (range, 1 to 78 months). Indication for operative repair included the following: size alone in 43 patients (68.2%), symptomatic abdominal or back pain without rupture in 11 (17.4%), claudication in 4 (6.4%), renal-vascular hypertension in 2 (3.2%), and a ruptured aneurysm in 3 (4.7%). Of these indications, 58 patients underwent surgery that was considered purely elective. The repair in 2 patients was done in less than 24 hours after hospital admission for acutely symptomatic but nonruptured AAAs, and three repairs were done for ruptured AAAs. We were able to use tube graft replacement in only 9 patients (14.3%), and we had to extend the bifurcation replacement grafts to the level of the groin on at least one side in 16 patients (25.4%). There were only two long-term graft complications: one pseudoaneurysm and one aortoenteric fistula.

Operative mortality rates are summarized in Table 2. In the 58 patients who underwent elective surgery, there were two postoperative deaths (3.4%). One was due to an MI 2 weeks postoperatively in a patient with no previous coronary artery disease, and the other was secondary to bleeding complications intraoperatively. Both patients who underwent surgery urgently for acutely symptomatic but nonruptured AAAs died of MIs. Combining these two groups as some do yielded an operative mortality rate of 6.67% for nonruptured AAAs.

All three patients operated on for a ruptured AAA died: one because of an intraoperative MI, one because of refractory hypotension, and the other 33 days postoperatively from other medical conditions. The patient with the intraoperative MI was a high-risk patient who had a large thoracoabdominal aneurysm with severe visceral, renal, and peripheral occlusive disease. Previously he had been considered to have an inoperable aneurysm. In the second patient who died, the aneurysm ruptured during angiography in preparation for an elective repair. The third patient was severely debilitated in the hospital for 8 months and the aneurysm ruptured while he was in the hospital. Mean long-term follow-up in the 57 survivors was 42.8 months (range, 1 to 126 months). Forty-three (75.4%) remain alive. The cause of 14 late deaths include coronary artery disease in 5 (35.7%), carcinoma in 3 (21.4%), other in 5 (35.7%), and unknown in 1 (7.14%).

In summary, seven ruptured AAAs (4.7%) have occurred in the total population of 149 patients (Table 3). Three of the seven patients reached the operating room. It is likely that one of these ruptures was caused by the catheter during an aortogram being done to evaluate the aneurysm in a patient who was to undergo elective surgery. Two ruptures occurred in patients who were high risk and refused the offered surgical therapy. The other four ruptures occurred in patients who were not considered to be surgical candidates based on severe coexisting disease or functional status of the patient.

Table 1.—Expansion Rate of AAA by Serial Ultrasonography*

	Average Expansion Rate, Mean cm/y		
Initial Size of AAA, cm	**All Patients (N=149)**	**Nonoperative Repair (n=86)**	**Operative Repair (n=63)**
2.0-2.9	0.64 (3)	0.36 (1)	0.79 (2)
3.0-3.9	0.50 (63)	0.26 (41)	0.86 (22)
4.0-4.9	1.01 (50)	0.40 (33)	1.1 (17)
5.0-5.9	0.96 (22)	0.32 (7)	1.2 (15)
6.0-6.9	0.86 (6)	1.1 (2)	0.80 (4)
7.0-7.9	0.0 (2)	0.0 (1)	0.0 (1)
8.0-8.9	0.0 (2)	0.0 (1)	0.0 (1)
>9.0	2.2 (1)	...	2.2 (1)
Overall	0.79 **(149)**	0.36 **(86)**	1.06 **(63)**

*AAA indicates abdominal aortic aneurysm. Number in parentheses indicates number of patients.

Table 2.—Operative Mortality

	No. of Patients	Deaths, No. (%)
Nonruptured	60	4 (6.6)
Elective	58	2 (3.4)
Urgent	2	2 (100)
Ruptured	3	3 (100)

Table 3.—Summary of Patients Whose AAAs Rupture*

Patient	Size at Last Examination, cm	Total FU From Dx to Rupture, mo	Comments†
A	4.6	6	1, 5, 6
B	5.5	78	1, 3, 5
C	6.6	26	1, 2, 5
D	7.4	33	1, 2, 5
E	6.5	18	1, 3, 4, 5
F	6.3	24	1, 4, 5, 8
G	10.0	22	1, 3, 4, 5, 7

*AAA indicates abdominal aortic aneurysm; FU, follow-up; and Dx, diagnosis.

†1 indicates high medical risk; 2, refused surgery; 3, surgery not offered electively; 4, emergency repair; 5, died as consequence of rupture; 6, only AAA of less than 5.0 cm in size to rupture; 7, thoracoabdominal aneurysm; and 8, ruptured during aortogram.

COMMENT

Size of an AAA correlates closely with the lethal potential of that aneurysm. Assuming a 5% operative mortality rate, the risk of rupture of an AAA becomes greater than the risk of elective repair when the aneurysm reaches 5 cm in greatest diameter.[2] This is certainly true in basically healthy patients in whom the risk may be closer to 1% to 2% with careful perioperative management, as so well described by Whittemore et al.[4] Using these same principles, Hollier et al[7] treated very high-risk operative candidates with an exceptional operative mortality rate of 6%. Of course patients who are expected to die of their coexisting medical problems within the same time frame are not surgical candidates. Two recent studies, one by Cronenwett et al[8] and one by Sterpetti et al,[9] analyzed several variables that are associated with rupture or the enlargement rate of small AAAs. In the study of Cronenwett et al of actuarial rupture rates, only three covariables, diastolic blood pressure, initial aneurysm anteroposterior diameter, and degree of chronic obstructive pulmonary disease, were independently predictive of rupture. They noted an increase in rupture rate from 2% to 100% when these three risk factors were either all absent or all present, respectively. Sterpetti et al demonstrated only two variables to be independent predictors of mean enlargement rate: (1) absence of distal arterial occlusive disease and (2) the ratio of the diameter of the aneurysm to the diameter of normal aorta above the aneurysm. Although both of these studies are retrospective, they do indicate that predicting the possibility of rupture perhaps hinges on more than size of the aneurysm alone. Therefore, even a high-risk operative candidate with a small (<6.0-cm-in-diameter) AAA may still be better served with an operation if we had a better understanding of the other factors that may increase the potential for rupture of a particular AAA.

At the present time, size of the AAA is our guide to decisions in operative repair; therefore, it is important to have a reproducible, accurate, noninvasive, relatively inexpensive means of sizing the AAA. Proper preparation of the patient and use of B-mode ultrasonography by experienced examiners gives us that tool to make measurements within 3 mm of actual size.[10] Some advocate using computed tomographic scanning in this evaluation, because it is more accurate, gives more information about the thickness of the wall, relationship of the aneurysm to the renal or visceral vessels, existence of iliac aneurysms, etc.[11] Nevertheless, it is more expensive and uses radiation. Angiography, whether standard or digital subtraction,[12] is invasive, expensive, and occasionally nondiagnostic. For long-term follow-up of small AAAs, serial B-mode ultrasonography is the tool of choice in our hands.

Much has been learned about growth rates of AAAs from the longitudinal ultrasonographic studies of patients with small AAAs (3 to 6 cm in diameter) by Bernstein and Chan.[6] Their data on 99 high-risk patients followed up by ultrasonography documented a mean expansion rate of 0.4 cm/y. This rate has been documented by others as well.[8,9] Measurement of the growth rate of small aneurysms in our institution showed some surprising findings. Although the growth rate in 86 yet unoperated-on patients was 0.36 cm/y and very similar to the results of Bernstein and Chan, the growth rate in 63 patients eventually operated on was 1.06 cm/y. This made the growth rate for the study group of 149 patients as a whole 0.79 cm/y. Since nearly two thirds of the patients who underwent surgery had small aneurysms (3 to 5 cm) when initially seen, and because the growth rate was basically the same despite the grouping by initial size, it would appear that some other factors were at work. Although we did not analyze the potential risk factors, it should be noted that the incidence of hypertension, chronic obstructive pulmonary disease, and renal failure was actually higher in the unoperated-on group. Perhaps as suggested in work by Busittil et al,[13] increased collagenase activity may play a role in the increased expansion rate. Perhaps this increased activity is related to other risk factors that may increase proteolytic activity such as collagenase.

Finally, is it safe to base our treatment of patients with small AAAs (<5.0 cm in greatest diameter) on serial ultrasonography? Bernstein and Chan[6] used serial ultrasonography in the previously mentioned 99 high-risk patients with small aneurysms up to 6 cm in size and operated when the aneurysms reached 6.0 cm in size or when symptoms developed. Using that approach 4 (4%) have died of elective aneurysm repair or rupture. Only 3 of their patients had ruptures during follow-up: 2 had AAAs of less than 6.0 cm in size, one of which was less than 5.0 cm in size. His 5-year cumulative survival rate was 63.7%. Although we did not calculate cumulative survival rates, 61.6% of our nonoperated-on patients are alive after a mean follow-up of 44.8 months, and 68.3% of the operated-on patients are alive at a mean follow-up of 42.8 months.

In comparison, seven patients in our series (4.7%) had ruptures during follow-up. These were summarized earlier in Table 3. Our mortality rate in elective aneurysm repair was 3.4% (2/58) or 6.6% (4/60) if the urgent, unruptured aneurysms are included. The overall mortality rate from rupture or elective aneurysm repair of 7.4% (11/149) compares favorably with that of the series of Bernstein and Chan[6] of 4%. Using a threshold of 5.0 cm greatest diameter in the low- or medium-risk patient and 6.0 cm greatest diameter in the high-risk patient appears to be a safe approach in the treatment of these patients. As we gain a better understanding of the effect of risk factors other than size of the aneurysm and improve perioperative management, we believe we can treat these patients even more safely.

References

1. Szilagyi DE, Elliot JP, Smith RF. Clinical fate of the patients with asymptomatic abdominal aortic aneurysm and unfit for surgical treatment. *Arch Surg.* 1972;104:600-606.
2. Darling RC. Ruptured arteriosclerotic aneurysms: a pathologic and clinical study. *Am J Surg.* 1970;119:397-401.
3. Dubost C, Allary M, Oeconomos N. Resection of aneurysm of the abdominal aorta: re-establishment of the continuity by a preserved human arterial graft with result after 5 months. *Arch Surg.* 1952;64:405-408.
4. Whittemore AD, Clowes AW, Hechtman HB, Mannick JA. Aortic aneurysm repair: reduced operative mortality associated with maintenance of optimal cardiac performance. *Ann Surg.* 1980;192:414-420.
5. Crawford ES, Saleh SA, Babb JW, et al. Infrarenal abdominal aortic aneurysm: factors influencing survival after operation performed over a 25-year period. *Am Surg.* 1981;193:699-709.
6. Bernstein EF, Chan EL. Abdominal aortic aneurysm in high-risk patients: outcome of selective management based on size and expansion rate. *Ann Surg.* 1984;200:255-263.
7. Hollier LH, Reigel MM, Kazmier FJ, Pairolero PC, Cherry FC, Hallet JW Jr. Conventional repair of abdominal aortic aneurysm in the high risk patient: a plea for abandonment of nonresective treatment. *J Vasc Surg.* 1986;3:712-717.
8. Cronenwett JL, Murphy TF, Zelenock GB, et al. Acturial analysis of variables associated with rupture of small abdominal aortic aneurysms. *Surgery.* 1985;98:472-482.
9. Sterpetti AV, Schultz RD, Feldhaus RJ, Cheng SE, Peetz DJ Jr. Factors influencing enlargement rate of small abdominal aortic aneurysms. *J Surg Res.* 1987;43:211-219.
10. Leopold GR, Goldberger LE, Bernstein EF. Ultrasonic detection and evaluation of abdominal aortic aneurysms. *Surgery.* 1972;72:939-945.
11. Gomes MN, Choyke PL. Improved identification of renal arteries in patients with aortic aneurysms by means of high-resolution computer tomography. *J Vasc Surg.* 1987;6:262-268.
12. TurnipseedWD, Acher CW, Detmer DE, et al. Digital subtraction angiography and B-mode ultrasonography for abdominal and peripheral aneurysms. *Surgery.* 1982;92:619-626.
13. Busittil RW, Abou-Zanzam AM, Machleder HI. Collagenase activity of the human aorta: comparison of patients with and without abdominal aortic aneurysms. *Arch Surg.* 1980;115:1373-1378.

Pelvic Fracture Hemorrhage

Priorities in Management

B. Mark Evers, MD; Henry M. Cryer, MD; Frank B. Miller, MD

• Hemorrhage remains the leading cause of mortality in patients with severe pelvic fractures. To evaluate diagnostic and treatment priorities for this problem, we retrospectively reviewed 245 consecutive patients admitted to our institution with pelvic fractures. Supraumbilical diagnostic peritoneal lavage (DPL) was grossly positive in 27 patients, and eight (30%) of these had life-threatening intra-abdominal hemorrhage identified at laparotomy. No patient with a positive DPL by count alone had life-threatening intra-abdominal hemorrhage. Pelvic fracture stabilization with early external pelvic fixation was associated with less requirement for blood transfusion (10±1 U) than with the pneumatic antishock garment (17±3 U). Nine patients with pelvic arterial injuries underwent angiographic embolization, and eight patients died (89%). We conclude that pelvic angiography should be performed before laparotomy in hemodynamically unstable patients with pelvic fracture, unless the DPL is grossly positive.

(*Arch Surg* 1989;124:422-424)

Massive extraperitoneal hemorrhage from pelvic fracture remains a significant problem. Despite the institution of various protocols, including the use of the pneumatic antishock garment (PASG), pelvic external fixation, and angiography with selective embolization, there remains a subgroup of patients with severe pelvic fractures in whom the mortality ranges from 25% to 39%, with the majority succumbing to exsanguination.[1-5]

This challenging subgroup of multiply injured patients requires rapid evaluation, identification, and control of the source of major blood loss. Several authors have recently suggested that to decrease the mortality in this subset of patients, a more aggressive approach is necessary. Panetta and associates[6] have advocated the use of early angiography in all patients with pelvic fracture requiring more than 4 U of blood within 24 hours or more than 6 U within 48 hours. The Gilliland group[5] has proposed that angiography and selective embolization should precede laparotomy even when diagnostic peritoneal lavage (DPL) is positive. And Moreno et al[2] have submitted that angiography should precede laparotomy when a DPL is positive by count but that laparotomy should be performed first when the lavage is grossly positive. Though a more aggressive protocol is clearly indicated, the proper sequence of diagnostic and therapeutic maneuvers to determine the major source of bleeding remains controversial. The current study was undertaken to help clarify this important problem.

PATIENTS AND METHODS

Between January 1983 and December 1986, our institution admitted 245 consecutive patients with pelvic fractures, excluding isolated acetabular fractures. Patient charts were retrospectively reviewed for mechanism of injury, age, length of hospital stay, admission blood pressure and heart rate, results of DPL, transfusion requirements, treatment modality, and Injury Severity Score.

When intra-abdominal injury was suspected, DPL was performed supraumbilically using the open technique. The lavage was considered grossly positive when greater than 10 mL of blood was aspirated from the abdominal cavity and count positive when the red blood cell count exceeded 0.0001×10^{12}/L, or when the white blood cell count was greater than 0.0005×10^{9}/L in the lavage fluid. Laparotomy was considered positive when an intraperitoneal cause of bleeding was found.

Patients treated with PASG had the extremity compartments inflated to 50 mm Hg and the abdominal compartment to 40 mm Hg. The PASGs were deflated after eight hours if the patient remained hemodynamically stable and without the need for continued blood replacement. Patients treated with immediate external pelvic fixation instead of PASG had the external fixator applied within 12 hours of admission. Pelvic angiography was performed percutaneously using the Seldinger technique. Selective arterial embolization was performed using absorbable gelatin sponge (Gelfoam) and/or stainless steel coils.

Statistical analysis comparing transfusion requirements in the PASG and fixator groups was by the Behrens-Fisher t test, with Welch degrees of freedom, for groups of unequal size. Data were reported as the mean±SEM. To determine the association between DPL results and intra-abdominal injury, the Yates χ^2 was used and the degree of correlation quantitated with the φ_2 correlation coefficient.[7]

RESULTS

There were 153 men and 92 women with a mean age of 36 years (range, 14 to 87 years) in our patient group. Mechanism of injury was motor vehicular in 143 (58%), auto-pedestrian in 39 (16%), fall in 27 (11%), crush in 19 (8%), motorcycle in 14 (6%), bicycle in two, and sledding in one. Overall mortality was 14% (35/245), with hemorrhage the leading cause (Table 1). When hemorrhage was the cause of death, the primary site of bleeding was the pelvis in 61% (11/18) and the pelvis and the abdomen combined in 22% (4/18). The Injury Severity Score is correlated with mortality in Table 2.

No blood transfusion was required in 113 patients (46%). Fifty-one patients (21%) required 1 to 3 U of blood, 37 patients (15%) required 4 to 9 U of blood, and 10 U or more of blood were required for hemodynamic stability in 44

Accepted for publication Nov 7, 1988.
From the Department of Surgery, University of Louisville School of Medicine.
Read before the 12th Annual Surgical Symposium of the Association of Veterans Administration Surgeons, Minneapolis, May 13, 1988.
Reprint requests to Department of Surgery, University of Louisville, Louisville, KY 40292 (Dr Cryer).

Table 1.—Cause of Death	
Cause	**No. (%)**
Hemorrhage	18 (52)
Head injury	11 (31)
Sepsis	5 (14)
Myocardial infarction	1 (3)
Total	**35 (100)**

Table 2.—Correlation of Injury Severity Score With Mortality

Injury Severity Score	No. (% of Total)	Deaths (% of Group)
0-10	67 (27)	1 (1)
11-20	60 (24)	0 (0)
21-30	56 (23)	12 (21)
31-40	33 (13)	7 (21)
41-50	21 (9)	8 (38)
≥51	8 (3)	7 (88)
Total	**245 (100)**	**35** (14)

Table 3.—Intra-abdominal Injuries at Laparotomy

Indication*	No.	Spleen	Bladder	Liver	Diaphragm	Other
DPL positive (gross)	27	13 (3)†	5	9 (4)†	2	11 (1)†
DPL positive (count)	19	3	3	4	...	8
Other	14	3	9	1	1	5
Total	**60**	**19 (3)†**	**17**	**14 (4)†**	**3**	**24 (1)†**

*DPL indicates diagnostic peritoneal lavage.
†Severe hemorrhage from injury in parentheses.

patients (18%). Patients requiring 4 U or more of blood were considered to have a major hemorrhage.

Supraumbilical DPL was performed in 83 patients. The lavage was negative in 37 of these patients, with no false-negative examinations. The DPL was positive in 46 patients; no intra-abdominal injury was found at laparotomy in four of these patients (false-positive rate, 9%). In this group of patients with pelvic fracture, DPL had a sensitivity of 100% and a specificity of 91%. The χ^2 for DPL accuracy was 59.25 ($P<.001$), and the φ_2 correlation coefficient was .92, demonstrating an excellent association.

Intra-abdominal injuries in relation to DPL findings are given in Table 3. Twenty-seven of the 46 positive lavages were grossly positive, and life-threatening intra-abdominal hemorrhage was found at laparotomy in eight (30%). None of the 19 patients with a positive DPL by count alone had significant ongoing intra-abdominal hemorrhage at laparotomy. An additional 14 patients underwent exploratory laparotomy for indications other than a positive DPL. Nine of them had a positive cystogram and had laparotomy for bladder repair. Four patients underwent laparotomy based on clinical criteria, and an additional patient had laparotomy based on radiographic findings of a ruptured hemidiaphragm. None of these 14 patients had life-threatening intraperitoneal bleeding at laparotomy. There were eight negative laparotomies, including four false-positive lavages and four patients operated on for physical findings. Five (63%) of these eight patients with negative laparotomies died.

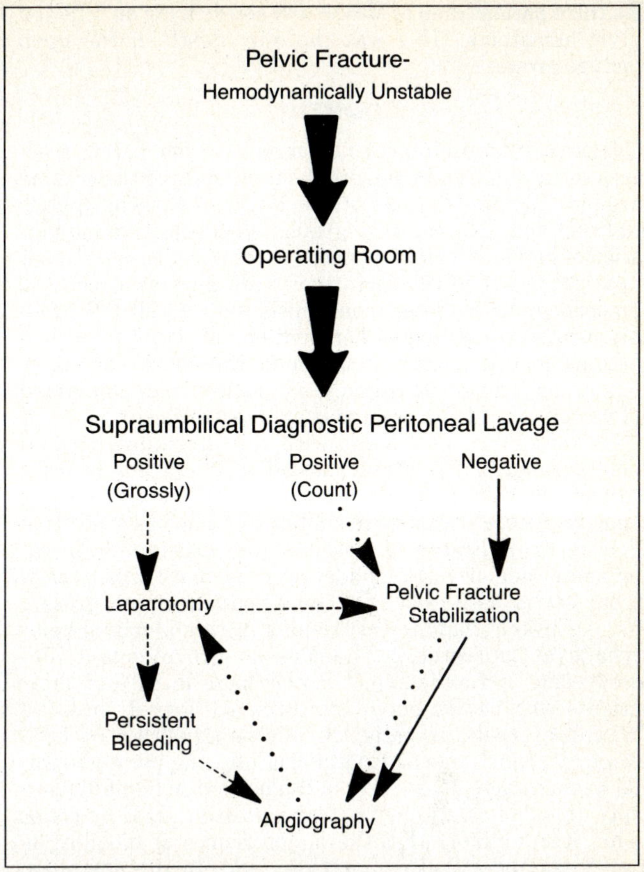

Management protocol for hemodynamically unstable patient with pelvic fracture.

After control of abdominal hemorrhage, we performed pelvic fracture stabilization to control bleeding from bony fragments by either PASG (24 patients) or immediate external pelvic fixation (23 patients). Mean blood transfusion requirements after fracture stabilization with PASG were 23 ± 3 U compared with 8 ± 1 U with the external fixator. However, these groups were not strictly comparable because the fixator was initially used on more patients in hemodynamically stable condition. In addition, all but one of the patients with pelvic arterial injuries were in the PASG group. When all patients who required less than 4 U of blood and all patients with major pelvic arterial injuries were excluded, 17 patients treated with PASG required 17 ± 3 U after fracture stabilization and six died of pelvic hemorrhage. On the other hand, the 14 patients treated with the external fixator required 10 ± 1 U ($P<.05$) and none died.

Sixteen patients had arteriography for continued hemodynamic instability after laparotomy and/or pelvic stabilization. Arterial injuries were identified in nine patients. Eight of these underwent successful embolization. Eight (89%) of the nine patients with pelvic arterial injury died. Four patients died early of exsanguination or persistent hemorrhagic shock and four died later of multiple system organ failure (MSOF) and sepsis.

Seven patients had open wounds communicating with the pelvic fracture. Three patients were bleeding massively from these wounds. Bleeding stopped with local wound packing alone in one patient; local wound packing plus pelvic fixation in a second patient; and local wound packing, PASG, and arteriographic embolization in the third patient.

The third patient died of MSOF and sepsis from an infected pelvic hematoma. This was the only death in the open fracture group.

COMMENT

Massive retroperitoneal hemorrhage from pelvic fractures remains a formidable problem confronting the trauma surgeon. Despite the use of the PASG,[1,8] external pelvic fixation,[9] and invasive angiography with selective embolization of pelvic arterial injuries,[6,10,11] there remains a subset of patients with pelvic fracture who die early as a result of hemorrhage or die later from sepsis-induced MSOF probably related to prolonged hemorrhagic shock. To improve outcome in this subset of patients, the source of major hemorrhage must be rapidly identified and controlled before massive blood loss and coagulopathy occur.

Our data were consistent with the literature[2,12-14] and demonstrated that peritoneal lavage is an extremely accurate test in ruling out intra-abdominal injury when it is negative. These data also indicated that a grossly positive DPL is an indicator of possible life-threatening intra-abdominal hemorrhage mandating immediate laparotomy. In our series, eight (30%) of the 27 patients with grossly positive lavages had life-threatening intra-abdominal hemorrhage at laparotomy. The Moreno group[2] found life-threatening intra-abdominal hemorrhage in 84% of their patients with severe pelvic fractures and grossly positive DPL. Conversely, no patient in our series with a positive lavage by count alone had significant ongoing intra-abdominal hemorrhage. Therefore, in the patient in hemodynamically unstable condition who has a positive DPL by count alone, it is unlikely that the major source of bleeding is from intra-abdominal hemorrhage, and, in this instance, we would advocate immediate fracture fixation followed by arteriography and then laparotomy.

The high mortality associated with negative laparotomy in patients in hemodynamically unstable condition with pelvic fracture has previously been emphasized.[5,13] Our 63% mortality with negative laparotomy confirms these reports. Four of these patients in hemodynamically unstable condition underwent exploratory laparotomy without a DPL for physical findings suggestive of intra-abdominal injury. Data suggested that physical examination of the abdomen in patients with pelvic fracture is unreliable. On the other hand, DPL has been extremely accurate in ruling out intra-abdominal injury in our patients and in all other series reported.[2,12-14] Therefore, we believe that a DPL should be performed before laparotomy in all patients in hemodynamically unstable condition with pelvic fractures.

Pelvic fracture stabilization has been shown to tamponade bleeding from multiple small- and medium-sized vessels within disrupted cancellous bone,[15] and we have previously reported a significant reduction in mortality with the use of PASG. There has been recent evidence that immediate external pelvic fixation is as good as or better than PASG for the control of pelvic hemorrhage.[2,9,16,17] In the present study the numbers were relatively small and the analysis was retrospective, but when attempts were made to make these two groups as comparable as possible, our data agreed with the growing concept that the external pelvic fixator may be more efficacious than PASG in stopping nonarterial pelvic fracture hemorrhage. The fixator has the added advantages of earlier patient mobilization and rehabilitation without interfering with any surgical procedures.[9,16,17]

Our results with arteriographic embolization of pelvic arterial injuries (89% mortality) are much worse than those reported by others. Matalon and associates[11] reported a 50% mortality in 20 patients who had angiographic embolization of pelvic arterial bleeding and noted that only one patient died of presumed continued pelvic hemorrhage. Panetta et al[6] reported 11 deaths (35%) in 31 patients who had pelvic arterial injuries treated by angiographic embolization. Four patients died of refractory hemorrhagic shock in spite of successful angiographic embolization in our series, which suggests that we were performing angiography too late. Additionally, we believe that a prolonged low-flow state secondary to persistent, uncontrolled hemorrhage contributed to the late development of MSOF and sepsis in four other patients. The mean elapsed time from admission to arrival in angiography in our series was 4 ± 0.5 hours. Therefore, our data suggest that earlier angiographic control of pelvic arterial hemorrhage is necessary to reduce mortality in this group of patients.

Based on our data, we have developed the following protocol to prioritize the management of patients in hemodynamically unstable condition with pelvic fractures (Figure). Supraumbilical DPL should be performed in the operating room and, if the lavage aspirate is grossly positive, then a rapid abdominal exploration with control of intra-abdominal bleeding should be performed. In our opinion, computer tomographic scanning is too time-consuming to be efficient in the evaluation of these complex patients. Pelvic fixation should be applied during or after laparotomy if a pelvic hematoma is present. Angiography with selective arterial embolization is then performed if hemodynamic instability persists or if a large and/or expanding retroperitoneal hematoma is found. If the lavage is positive by count alone, then pelvic fixation and immediate angiography should be performed first, followed by laparotomy. If the lavage is negative, patients should undergo immediate pelvic stabilization followed by angiography.

References

1. Flint IM, Brown A, Richardson JD, et al: Definitive control of bleeding from severe pelvic fractures. *Ann Surg* 1979;189:709-716.
2. Moreno C, Moore EE, Rosenberger A, et al: Hemorrhage associated with major pelvic fracture: A multispecialty challenge. *J Trauma* 1986;11:987-994.
3. Naam NH, Brown WH, Hurd R, et al: Major pelvic fractures. *Arch Surg* 1983;118:610-616.
4. Mucha P, Farnell MB: Analysis of pelvic fracture management. *J Trauma* 1984;24:379-386.
5. Gilliland MD, Ward RE, Flynn TC, et al: Peritoneal lavage and angiography in the management of patients with pelvic fractures. *Am J Surg* 1982;144:744-747.
6. Panetta T, Sclafani SJA, Goldstein AS, et al: Percutaneous transcatheter embolization for massive bleeding from pelvic fractures. *J Trauma* 1985;25:1021-1029.
7. Zar JH: *Biostatistical Analysis*, ed 2. Englewood Cliffs, NJ, Prentice-Hall International Inc, 1984.
8. Batalden DJ, Wickstrom PH, Ruiz E, et al: Value of the G suit in patients with severe pelvic fractures. *Arch Surg* 1974;109:326-328.
9. Gylling SF, Ward RE, Holcroft JW, et al: Immediate external fixation of unstable pelvic fractures. *Am J Surg* 1985;150:721-724.
10. Margolies MN, Ring EJ, Waltman AC, et al: Arteriography in the management of hemorrhage from pelvic fractures. *N Engl J Med* 1972;287:317-321.
11. Matalon TSA, Athanasoulis CA, Margolies MN, et al: Hemorrhage with pelvic fractures: Efficacy of transcatheter embolization. *AJR* 1979;133:859-864.
12. Murr PC, Moore EE, Lipscomb R, et al: Abdominal trauma associated with pelvic fracture. *J Trauma* 1980;20:919-923.
13. Hubbard SG, Bivins BA, Sachatello CR, et al: Diagnostic errors with peritoneal lavage in patients with pelvic fractures. *Arch Surg* 1979;114:844-846.
14. Maull KI, Sachatello CR: Management of pelvic fractures. *South Med J* 1976;69:1285-1289.
15. Huittinen VM, Slatis P: Postmortem angiography and dissection of the hypogastric artery in pelvic fractures. *Surgery* 1973;73:454-462.
16. Mears DC, Fu FH: Modern concepts of external skeletal fixation of the pelvis. *Clin Orthop* 1980;151:73-79.
17. Kellom JF, McMurtry RY, Paley D, et al: The unstable pelvic fracture. *Orthop Clin North Am* 1987;18:25-41.

Anastomotic Tensile Strength Following In Situ Replacement of an Infected Abdominal Aortic Graft

Raymond Vetsch, MD; Dennis F. Bandyk, MD; David D. Schmitt, MD; Thomas M. Bergamini, MD; James D. Storey, MD; Jonathan B. Towne, MD

• The tensile strength and histologic features of anastomotic bonding were studied prior to and following in situ replacement of aortic vascular prostheses infected by *Staphylococcus epidermidis*. Sterile (n=6) and infected (n=19) Dacron grafts were used to replace the abdominal aorta of 25 dogs. After five weeks, grafts were explanted, and peak tensile force (measured in kilograms) required for anastomotic disruption was measured using a linear gain tensiometer. Anastomotic tensile strength (mean±SEM) of infected grafts (5.4±0.5 kg) was decreased when compared with that of sterile, control grafts (9.0±0.9 kg). The decreased anastomotic tensile strength of infected grafts was the result of an inflammatory aortitis adjacent to the suture line. Only grafts infected with the study strain of bacteria demonstrated signs of infection. In 19 dogs, the graft infection was treated by graft excision, antibiotic administration, and in situ graft replacement (Dacron or polytetrafluoroethylene prostheses). After five weeks and 12 weeks, anastomotic tensile strength of polytetrafluoroethylene (10.6±0.6 kg) and Dacron (10.8±0.5 kg) replacement grafts was similar to that of uninfected control grafts. In situ replacement of vascular prostheses infected by *S epidermidis* can result in graft healing with normal anastomotic bonding.

(*Arch Surg* 1989;124:425-428)

Late-appearing graft infection and anastomotic pseudoaneurysm formation have not decreased as clinical problems of using vascular prostheses despite improvements in suture and graft fabrication and despite the routine use of perioperative antibiotic prophylaxis. Graft infection or anastomosis dehiscence develops in approximately 5% of patients after implantation of a vascular prosthesis.[1-3] The pathogenesis of late graft healing complications, especially those involving the common femoral artery, appear to be the result of infection caused by slime-producing strains of *Staphylococcus epidermidis*.[4,5] When vascular prostheses are colonized by low-virulence bacteria, such as *S epidermidis*, the microorganisms are harbored and survive within a biofilm adherent to the prosthetic surface. This bacterial biofilm incites a chronic inflammatory process adjacent to the prosthesis with autolysis of perigraft tissue and the adjacent artery wall, which, with time, results in the anastomotic and perigraft healing complications associated with late graft infection. The predilection of prosthetic implants for staphylococcal colonization, especially *S epidermidis*, is well documented. *Staphylococcus epidermidis* can be cultured from diseased artery walls and groin lymph nodes in one third of patients undergoing vascular prosthesis implantation,[6,7] from 75% of prostheses revised for anastomotic pseudoaneurysm,[8] and from 80% of aortofemoral prostheses removed because of infection.[4]

In a canine model of aortic graft infection due to *S epidermidis* that mimicked the anatomic and microbiologic characteristics of late graft infection in humans, we found that in situ replacement of infected grafts resulted in early (three weeks) graft healing, but positive cultures of replacement grafts were obtained in 30% of the animals.[9] The study did not address the late outcome of graft colonization or compare anastomotic bonding of infected grafts with that of in situ replacement grafts. Since life- and limb-threatening complications of *S epidermidis* graft infections are associated with suture-line dehiscence, measurements of anastomotic tensile strength are of critical importance in assessing the efficacy of in situ graft replacement as a treatment option for this prosthetic infection.

In this study, we utilized our canine model of *S epidermidis* prosthetic graft infection to evaluate the tensile strength of graft-to-artery anastomoses. Anastomotic tensile strength of sterile control, infected, and in situ replacement grafts was correlated with clinical signs of infection (eg, perigraft exudate, graft incorporation, anastomotic aneurysm), aortic wall histologic features, interval following graft replacement, and microbiologic evidence of infection. Confirmation of normal anastomotic binding following in situ graft replacement of an established *S epidermidis* graft infection would favor the use of this surgical approach, as compared with the increased morbidity associated with total graft excision, artery ligation, and extra-anatomic arterial bypass.

MATERIALS AND METHODS

Canine Model

Using sterile surgical technique, 25 female conditioned mongrel dogs (weighing 20 to 25 kg) underwent interposition grafting of the infrarenal aorta with a sterile (n=6) or infected (n=19) Dacron vascular prosthesis (6-mm diameter, 5-cm length). A commercially available double-velour, knitted Dacron graft (Meadox Medicals Inc, Oakland, NJ) was implanted. In situ replacement of the infected grafts was performed using an identical sterile Dacron graft or a 6-mm-diameter, expanded polytetrafluoroethylene (PTFE) (Gore-Tex, W. L. Gore & Associates Inc, Elkton, Md) vascular prosthesis. These graft types have been used in prior in vitro and in vivo studies of bacterial adherence to vascular prosthetic surfaces.[9] Of note, both graft types have been shown in a canine model to result in comparable graft-to-artery bonding strengths at three to nine months after implantation.[10] All animals received humane care and our methods complied with the *Principles of Laboratory Animal Care* and the *Guide for the Care and Use of Laboratory Animals* (National Institutes of Health [Bethesda, Md] publication No. 80-23, revised 1978).

The technique of graft colonization with a slime-producing strain

Accepted for publication Dec 2, 1988.

From the Surgical Service, Veterans Administration Medical Center, Milwaukee (Drs Vetsch, Bandyk, Storey, and Towne), and the Department of Surgery, The Medical College of Wisconsin, Milwaukee (Drs Bandyk, Schmitt, Bergamini, and Towne).

Read before the 12th Annual Surgical Symposium of the Association of Veterans Administration Surgeons, Minneapolis, May 13, 1988.

Reprint requests to Department of Surgery, MCMC, 8700 W Wisconsin Ave, Milwaukee, WI 53226 (Dr Bandyk).

Table 1.—Microbiologic, Anatomic, and Histologic Evidence of Infection Involving Primary Dacron Grafts and In Situ Replacement Grafts*

Graft Type	Recovery of *Staphylococcus epidermidis*	Anatomy: Graft Incorporation	Anatomy: Perigraft Cavity	Histologic Finding: Adjacent Aortitis
Primary Dacron				
Sterile, control	0/6	6/6	0/6	ND
Infected	16/16 (100)	0/19 (0)	17/19 (85)	9/19 (45)
In situ replacement				
5 wk				
Dacron	2/8	6/8	0/8	0/8
PTFE	0/4	4/4	0/4	0/4
12 wk				
PTFE	0/6	6/6	0/6	1/6
Total	**2/18** (11)	**16/18** (89)	**0/18** (0)	**1/18** (5)

*Data are expressed as number of positive findings/number of grafts tested. Numbers in parentheses are percents. ND indicates not determined; PTFE, polytetrafluoroethylene.

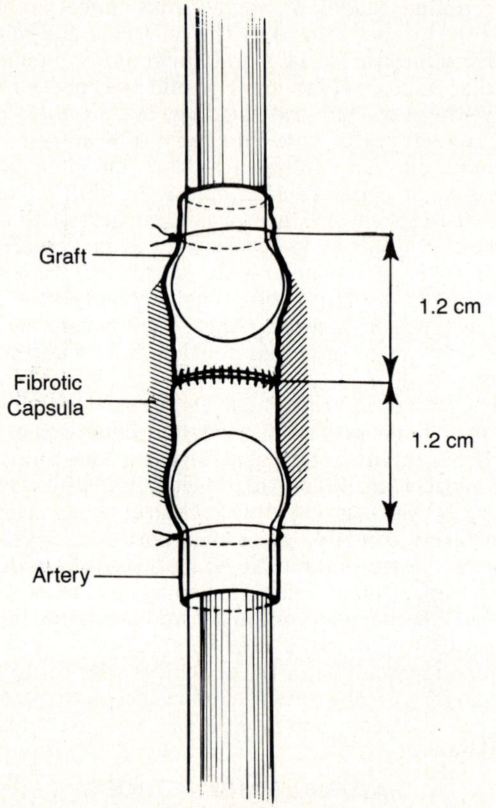

Diagram shows mounting of apparatus for tensiometer measurement of prosthetic graft-to-artery anastomotic bonding strength.

of *S epidermidis* (American Type Culture Collection 35983) has been previously described.[9] In brief, the Dacron grafts were immersed in the inoculating solution (7.0 $\log_{10}$ colony-forming units [CFUs] of *S epidermidis*) for 24 hours at room temperature prior to implantation. During the incubation period, a bacteria-laden biofilm formed on the prosthetic surface with a mean bacterial concentration of approximately 5×10^4 CFU/cm^2 of graft material.[9] The *S epidermidis* study strain was susceptible to cefazolin sodium (minimum inhibitory concentration, <0.25 mg/mL).

Graft Implantation

The dogs were anesthetized with intravenous pentobarbital sodium (20 mg/kg), intubated, and mechanically ventilated with a volume-cycled respirator. The abdominal wall was shaved, scrubbed with povidone-iodine detergent, painted with 1% povidone-iodine solution, and covered with povidine-iodine impregnated plastic drapes. No antibiotics were administered during the perioperative period. A midline incision was used for exposure of the infrarenal aorta. A 3-cm length of aorta was dissected from surrounding retroperitoneal structures, and lumbar arteries in the mobilized segment were ligated. Systemically administered heparin was not used during the period of aortic cross-clamping. Grafts were preclotted and anastomosed end-to-end to the transected aorta with continuous 6-0 polypropylene sutures, using ×2.5 optical magnification. The retroperitoneum was covered over the graft with a continuous suture (3-0 chromic catgut), and the midline wound was sutured closed.

Graft Explantation and Replacement

Five weeks after implantation, the control and infected aortic grafts were exposed through the previous midline incision using sterile surgical technique. Cefazolin sodium (25 mg/kg) was administered intravenously one hour before the operation to minimize colonization of replacement grafts. In addition, animals undergoing in situ replacement for five weeks were administered cefazolin sodium (25 mg/kg) intramuscularly at 12-hour intervals for ten days, while animals undergoing in situ PTFE replacement for 12 weeks were administered cefazolin sodium (25 mg/kg) intramuscularly at eight-hour intervals for one day (based on a prior study protocol[9]). No antibiotic was administered to dogs undergoing excision of sterile, control Dacron grafts.

After proximal and distal control of the grafted aorta was obtained, the Dacron graft was exposed and examined for signs of infection (eg, perigraft inflammation/fluid, perigraft cavity formation, and/or anastomotic dehiscence). Swabs of the perigraft fluid or the external graft surface were obtained and cultured aerobically on tryptic soy agar with 5% sheep's blood. The graft was then totally excised, including anastomotic sites and 1 cm of adjacent aorta, with care taken not to disrupt the fibrous capsule surrounding the anastomoses. A 1-cm length of graft without adherent thrombus, perigraft capsule, or adjacent aorta was placed in tryptic soy broth, ultrasonically oscillated at 20 kHz for ten minutes to mechanically disrupt the prosthetic surface biofilm, and incubated at 35°C, a technique previously shown to increase the recovery of bacteria from explanted vascular prostheses compared with broth culture alone.[11] One graft-to-artery anastomosis was used for measurement of anastomotic tensile strength, while the other anastomotic site was used for histologic and microbiologic studies. One-centimeter lengths of aorta (suture line included) were cultured in tryptic soy broth at 35°C and fixed in 2% glutaraldehyde for hematoxylin-eosin and Brown-Brenn tissue Gram's staining for histologic examination. Aorta wall histologic findings were interpreted by a pathologist in a blinded fashion.

Following total graft excision, the aorta was débrided to grossly normal artery wall, and aortic continuity was established by implantation (randomized) of double-velour Dacron or PTFE grafts in study animals to undergo reoperation after five weeks and only PTFE grafts in study animals reexamined 12 weeks after in situ replacement. All animals underwent graft replacement using similar graft-to-artery anastomotic technique with a 6-0 continuous polypropylene suture. The perigraft cavity surround-

Table 2.—Anastomotic Tensile Strength (Mean ± SEM) of Primary Dacron and In Situ Replacement Grafts

Graft Type	No. of Anastomoses Tested	Peak Tensile Force, kg
Primary Dacron		
Sterile, control	10	9.0±0.9
Infected	19	5.4±0.5*
Replacement		
5 wk		
Dacron	15	10.8±0.5
PTFE	8	10.7±0.5
12 wk		
PTFE	6	10.6±0.6

*P<.003 relative to other groups, Mann-Whitney U test.

ing primary infected Dacron grafts was débrided to adjacent retroperitoneal structures (duodenum and inferior vena cava). The replacement graft was covered with retroperitoneum and the midline incision closed.

Explantation of Replacement Grafts

Five and 12 weeks after in situ replacement of the established *S epidermidis* graft infection, the aortic grafts were exposed through the prior midline incision. No antibiotic was administered prior to or during the operation. The extent of replacement graft healing was noted, including the presence or absence of graft incorporation, perigraft cavity, and fluid. The grafts were totally excised, including the adjacent aorta, without disruption of anastomotic sites and surrounding fibrous tissue. The replacement graft and adjacent aorta were analyzed, using tensiometer, microbiologic, and histologic methods previously described, to assess anastomotic tensile strength and determine whether recurrent *S epidermidis* colonization had occurred.

Measurement of Anastomotic Tensile Strength

Tensile strength of intact graft-to-artery anastomoses was measured with a linear gain tensiometer calibrated to 22.5 kg full scale using an elongation speed of 0.25 cm/s. Anastomotic sites were mounted with the perigraft capsule intact and held within the testing apparatus over a specially designed mounting device with 21-gauge wire to avoid slippage of tissue (Figure). Tensiometer reading was recorded continuously until disruption of the anastomosis occurred, at which time peak tensile strength (measured in kilograms) was determined. Peak tensile strength was recorded for each anastomosis and analyzed according to graft type, presence of clinical signs of graft infection, results of graft cultures, and time of implantation.

Data Analysis

All cultures without growth after 14 days were considered sterile. Bacterial isolates were identified and staphylococcal species isolated with the API STAPH-IDENT system. *Staphylococcus epidermidis* isolates were evaluated for slime production to verify recovery of the study strain. Anastomotic tensile strength difference between groups was expressed as the mean ± SEM. To avoid assumptions about the distribution of the tensiometry data, statistical significance was assessed by the Mann-Whitney U test.

RESULTS

All animals survived the operative procedures and follow-up intervals. One PTFE replacement graft was thrombosed at the time of excision, 12 weeks after implantation. No pseudoaneurysms or anastomotic disruptions were observed in the sterile control and primary infected Dacron grafts.

Vascular Prosthesis Biofilm Infection

Five weeks after implantation of Dacron grafts colonized in vitro with the study strain of bacteria, all study animals had patent grafts with microbiologic and anatomic evidence of *S epidermidis* infection (Table 1). An inflammatory process was present in the retroperitoneum, surrounding the prosthetic graft, and involving adjacent structures (aorta, inferior vena cava, duodenum). A perigraft cavity containing fibrinopurulent exudate was present in 17 (89%) of 19 dogs. Histologic examination of the aorta adjacent to suture lines demonstrated acute inflammation (wall thickening and multiple foci of polymorphonuclear leukocytes) in nine (47%) of 19 animals. By 1 cm from the anastomosis, the artery wall was normal. Sterile, control Dacron grafts implanted five weeks prior had no anatomic signs of infection, graft cultures yielded no growth, and aortic histologic examination demonstrated only foreign-body reaction (infiltrates of giant cells and histocytes) adjacent to suture material.

The anastomotic tensile strength of infected Dacron grafts was significantly less (P<.003) than control Dacron grafts (Table 2). For all anastomoses tested, disruption occurred at the suture line in the aorta. The peak tensile force required to disrupt the graft-to-artery anastomosis in animals with infected grafts and aortitis at the opposite anastomotic site (4.5 ± 1.6 kg) was less but not statistically different from that of anastomotic sites without adjacent aortitis (6.4 ± 1.4 kg).

Results of Graft Replacement

In situ graft replacement resulted in perigraft healing without signs of infection in 16 (89%) of 18 study animals (Table 1). Two Dacron grafts explanted after five weeks were poorly incorporated with a perigraft cavity present, and one PTFE graft at 12 weeks demonstrated pseudoaneurysm formation at the distal anastomosis. Of note, culture of the artery wall adjacent to the disrupted anastomosis isolated the *S epidermidis* study strain, but culture of the PTFE graft yielded no bacterial growth, and the peak tensile force required to disrupt the opposite anastomosis was 12.2 kg. All replacement PTFE grafts at five weeks after implantation showed no anatomic signs of infection, were adherent to perigraft tissues, and required scalpel dissection for excision. *Staphylococcus epidermidis* was recovered from two (11%) of 18 replacement grafts. Positive cultures for the study strain were obtained from the two Dacron replacement grafts that demonstrated no graft incorporation. Tensile strengths of anastomoses from these grafts were 9.5 and 14.4 kg, respectively.

Anastomotic tensile strength of replacement grafts was similar to that of control Dacron grafts and significantly increased compared with Dacron grafts infected with *S epidermidis*. Anastomotic tensile strength of Dacron and PTFE replacement grafts was similar, and duration following in situ replacement did not influence PTFE anastomotic bonding.

COMMENT

Our study confirmed that *S epidermidis* colonization of a vascular prostheses as a bacterial biofilm can incite a perigraft inflammatory process that involves the adjacent artery wall and decreases anastomotic tensile strength. Although anastomotic dehiscence was not observed in the primary infected Dacron grafts, the absence of this complication was likely because of the short (five-week) duration of graft implantation. The cause of anastomotic aneurysms has largely been attributed to host vessel degeneration due to abnormal mechanical stress at the suture line, but the possibility that a low-grade infection contributes to these disruptive forces has not been fully explored. Using a sensitive microbiologic culture technique, we have previously documented that microorganisms can frequently be isolated from vascular prostheses that require revision for complications of thrombosis or anastomotic pseudoaneurysm.[8] *Staphylococcus epidermidis* was the prevalent organism recovered (69% of isolates), and slime production, a growth characteristic associated with prosthetic device infection in humans, was seen in 87% of strains isolated from grafts revised for anastomotic pseudoaneurysm. The canine model used in this study mimicked the anatomic and microbiologic characteristics of late graft infection in humans. Viable microorganisms were sequestered primarily within a biofilm on the prosthetic surface, and bacterial invasion of perigraft tissue and signs of graft sepsis were absent. Despite the localized nature of the infection and low virulence of the infecting *S epidermidis* organisms, graft colonization was recognized by host defenses, and a perigraft inflammatory process developed. If the artery wall adjacent to suture lines was involved either by inflammation and/or bacterial infection, anastomotic tensile strength was significantly less than the normal anastomotic bonding strength measured in grafts without clinical signs of infection. Of note, this canine model of *S epidermidis* graft infection demonstrated that the presence of arteritis adjacent to the suture line of grafts exhibiting clinical signs of infection was sporadic, occurring at one half (nine of 19) of anastomotic sites. When arteritis was documented, artery wall cultures yielded the *S epidermidis* study strain and anastomotic strength was significantly decreased. In only one animal was anastomotic dehiscence observed. These findings emphasize the importance of aortitis and artery wall infection as causes of aortic stump dehiscence following excision of an infected graft and as sources of infection of in situ replacement grafts.

The artery wall has been documented as a potential source for graft colonization and was in this study the likely origin of the PTFE replacement graft infection observed after 12 weeks of implantation.[7] Infection was manifest at an anastomotic site that previously demonstrated aortitis adjacent to an infected Dacron graft. Of importance, the PTFE graft exhibited no other signs of infection and the opposite anastomotic site had a normal tensile strength (12.2 kg). This observation suggests that infection of an in situ replacement graft may begin as an isolated process involving a single anastomotic site or segment of the prosthetic conduit. The decreased anastomotic tensile strength of grafts exhibiting perigraft inflammation is suggestive evidence that this process, if unabated, will eventually lead to anastomotic dehiscence. In contrast, the presence of normal anastomotic bonding (normal tensile strength and suture line histologic structure) following primary or in situ replacement is persuasive evidence that a suture line complication is unlikely to develop. Routine use of broth media for culture of vascular prostheses associated with anastomotic pseudoaneurysm and increased attention to the histologic structure of the artery wall adjacent to the prosthesis are required, if our understanding of this healing complication is to improve.

We have previously reported that in situ replacement of a graft with established *S epidermidis* infection resulted in graft healing without signs of infection.[9] The present study provides additional data that support the efficacy of in situ replacement for this infection. Graft healing was observed for three months after replacement and associated with normal anastomotic tensile strength. Persistent colonization was confirmed in only two (11%) of 18 replacement grafts, which was less than the one-third incidence observed after four weeks in a prior study.[9] The lower incidence of replacement graft colonization may have resulted from extended administration of antibiotics (ten days vs one day) following graft replacement, or the longer implantation time with resultant additional graft healing in animals with intact host defenses.

Anastomotic tensile strength was similar in PTFE and Dacron replacement grafts after five weeks and did not change in PTFE grafts implanted for 12 weeks. The tensile strength of graft-to-artery anastomoses measured in both control and replacement grafts was comparable with that measured by Quinones-Baldrich et al[10] in a similar canine model. The excellent perigraft healing and the low incidence of *S epidermidis* colonization of PTFE replacement grafts compared with Dacron grafts favor this prosthesis for in situ replacement of *S epidermidis* graft infections.

The diagnosis of graft infection caused by bacterial biofilms can frequently be made based on clinical presentation. Gram's stain of perigraft exudate typically demonstrates only polymorphonuclear leukocytes, and perigraft tissue culture is sterile. In contrast, infections caused by *Staphylococcus aureus* and gram-negative microorganisms are not confined to a surface biofilm but rather are associated with invasive infection of perigraft tissues and sepsis. In situ graft replacement should not be considered as a treatment option when Gram's stain shows microorganisms in the perigraft tissue/exudate, a manifestation of an invasive bacterial infection. When in situ graft replacement is utilized, the artery adjacent to the graft should be débrided to grossly normal wall. This procedure removes artery tissue weakened by arteritis and potentially colonized by *S epidermidis*, a source for graft reinfection. Antibiotics should be administered prior to and following in situ replacement to minimize bacterial adherence to and colonization of prosthetic surfaces, and to eradicate residual foci of bacterial arteritis.

Although our study demonstrates that normal anastomotic tensile strength is present three months following in situ replacement of aortic grafts infected with *S epidermidis*, late anastomotic complications may still develop. In situ replacement for *S epidermidis* graft infection mandates extended postoperative surveillance using anatomic diagnostic techniques, such as computed tomography, magnetic resonance imaging, or B-mode ultrasound capable of assessing perigraft healing and anastomotic integrity.

This research was supported by the Veterans Administration, Washington, DC.

We thank W. L. Gore & Associates and Meadox Medicals Inc for the generous donation of graft material. We acknowledge the excellent technical support of Holly Kelly, Candace Krepel, and James Budzinski.

References

1. Szilagyi DE, Smith RF, Elliott JP, et al: Anastomotic aneurysms after vascular reconstruction. *Surgery* 1975;78:800-816.

2. Nichols WK, Stanton M, Silver D, et al: Anastomotic aneurysms following lower extremity revascularization. *Surgery* 1980;88:366-374.

3. Berni GA, Thiele BL, Bodily KC, et al: Changing etiology of anastomotic aneurysms. *J Vasc Surg* 1982;16:76-85.

4. Bandyk DF, Berni GA, Thiele BL, et al: Aortofemoral graft infection due to *Staphylococcus epidermidis*. *Arch Surg* 1984;119:102-108.

5. Bandyk DF: Vascular graft infection: Epidemiology, bacteriology, and pathogenesis, in Bernhard VM, Towne JB (eds): *Complications in Vascular Surgery*, ed 2. New York, Grune & Stratton, 1985, pp 471-485.

6. Bunt TJ, Mohr JD: Incidence of positive inguinal lymph node cultures during peripheral revascularization. *Am Surg* 1984;10:522-523.

7. Macbeth GS, Rubin JR, McIntyre JE Jr, et al: The relevance of arterial wall microbiology to the treatment of prosthetic graft infections: Graft infection vs arterial infection. *J Vasc Surg* 1984;1:750-756.

8. Kaebnick HW, Bandyk DF, Bergamini TW, et al: The microbiology of explanted vascular prostheses. *Surgery* 1987;102:756-762.

9. Bergamini TW, Bandyk DF, Govostis D: Infection of vascular prostheses caused by bacterial biofilms. *J Vasc Surg* 1988;7:21-30.

10. Quinones-Baldrich WJ, Ziomek S, Henderson BA, et al: Primary anastomotic bonding in polytetrafluoroethylene grafts. *J Vasc Surg* 1987; 5:311-318.

11. Tollefson DF, Bandyk DF, Kaebnick HW, et al: Surface biofilm disruption: Enhanced recovery of microorganisms from vascular prostheses. *Arch Surg* 1986;122:38-43.

Hemodynamic Effects on Endothelial Cell Monolayer Detachment From Vascular Prostheses

Howard P. Greisler, MD; Eric D. Endean, MD; John J. Klosak, MD; Joan Ellinger; Scott C. Henderson; Si M. Pham, MD; Steven J. Durham, MD; David P. Showalter, MD; Jeffery Levine, PhD; Harvey S. Borovetz, PhD

• The establishment of an early blood-contacting endothelialized surface may improve the graft-host relationship. This study evaluated the adherence of indium 111–radiolabeled endothelial cells that were cultured to confluence on fibronectin-treated polyester elastomer (Hytrel) grafts that were perfused for two hours on a pulse duplicator apparatus under high- and low-shear conditions. Perfusate samples were serially assayed for radioactivity. After perfusion, grafts were sectioned into four segments and assayed for retained radioactivity. All graft segments were hematoxylin stained and examined under light microscopy for evaluation of cell density. Excellent endothelial cell adherence (90%) was observed under both hemodynamic conditions at 120 minutes, with most losses occurring within the first 15 minutes. No differences were seen between high- and low-shear conditions or proximal vs distal graft segments.

(*Arch Surg* 1989;124:429-433)

The need for improved small-diameter vascular prostheses has led to intense research on methods of optimizing the graft-host relationship. One suggested method of improving this relationship and optimizing the clinical efficacy of implanted grafts is the establishment of an early confluent endothelialized blood-contacting surface. The underlying assumption is that such an endothelialized surface would function to improve surface thrombogenicity and potentially inhibit subendothelial proliferative activity of fibroblasts and smooth-muscle cells and thereby decrease occlusions secondary to thrombosis and pseudointimal hyperplasia. Approaches to early endothelialization have included techniques for endothelial seeding,[1-5] the use of partially or totally bioresorbable grafts,[6-10] and the in vitro culturing of an endothelial cell monolayer on the prosthetic surface before implantation.[11] Investigations of endothelial cell attachment to treated and untreated prosthetic surfaces and resistance of this cell layer to detachment from the surface in circulation have yielded disparate results. A recent publication showed the loss of 30% of seeded cells after 30 minutes of perfusion and the loss of 83% of the cells after 24 hours,[12] while another recent study showed greater than 90% retention of endothelial cells cultured on either fibronectin-treated or collagen I/III–treated polymer surfaces after 30 minutes of 90-dynes/cm^2 shear stress.[13] Optimization of endothelial cell adherence to the surface and preservation of normal endothelial cell functional characteristics are critical to the development of clinically efficacious endothelialized prosthetic surfaces. The current study evaluates the adherence of endothelial cells that were cultured on fibronectin-treated prosthetic materials that were perfused in vitro under different pulsatile hemodynamic conditions.

MATERIALS AND METHODS

A single mongrel dog was anesthetized with intravenous thiamylal sodium and anesthesia was maintained with 0.8% methoxyflurane, 30% nitrous oxide, and 69.2% oxygen. Under sterile conditions, both external jugular veins were removed, carefully everted, and placed in Hanks' balanced salt solution (calcium and magnesium free). The veins were then placed in trypsin (0.05%)–edetic acid (EDTA) (0.02%) (pH, 8.0) and incubated at 37°C for ten minutes. The veins were removed and placed in 40 mL of collagenase (0.05%) (pH 7.0) and incubated for an additional ten minutes. The veins were then discarded, and the cell-containing enzyme solutions were centrifuged for ten minutes at 800 revolutions per minute. The cell pellets were reconstituted in complete media that contained M-199 culture media, 10% fetal bovine serum, beef lung heparin sodium (5 U/mL), and purified endothelial cell growth factor (5 ng/mL). Endothelial cell purity was documented by immunoperoxidase stains (Fig 1) with rabbit anti–human factor VIII antibody (DAKO Corp, Santa Barbara, Calif) and a goat anti–rabbit secondary antibody (Vector Laboratories, Burlingame, Calif). The cells were seeded in T-25 tissue culture flasks

Accepted for publication Dec 6, 1988.

From the Department of Surgery, Loyola University Medical Center, Maywood, Ill (Drs Greisler, Endean, and Klosak); the Department of Research, Hines (Ill) Veterans Administration Hospital (Dr Greisler, Ms Ellinger, and Mr Henderson); and the Departments of Surgery (Drs Pham, Durham, Showalter, and Borovetz) and Nuclear Medicine (Dr Levine), University of Pittsburgh School of Medicine.

Read before the 12th Annual Surgical Symposium of the Association of Veterans Administration Surgeons, Minneapolis, May 14, 1988.

Reprint requests to Loyola University Medical Center, 2160 S First Ave, Maywood, IL 60153 (Dr Greisler).

that were previously coated with fibronectin (10 μg/cm²). The cells were incubated at 37°C in a 5% carbon dioxide–humidified atmosphere. Culture media were changed every other day. When confluence was achieved, the cells were serially passaged three times, yielding 25 confluent T-75 flasks. The cells were then enzymatically removed and resuspended in phosphate-buffered saline, and cell counts were performed on both a Coulter counter and a hemacytometer. Oxine (100 μCi per million cells), labeled with indium 111, was added and incubated for 30 minutes at 22°C, followed by centrifugation at 1000 revolutions per minute for ten minutes. Phosphate-buffered saline washing was repeated three times to remove unattached ^{111}In. The final cell pellet was reconstituted in complete media in a volume four times that calculated to fill the grafts.

The grafts, 80×4 mm internal diameter, were composed of a polyester elastomer (Hytrel) that was translucent to light microscopy. The graft lumina were coated with fibronectin (0.01 mg/mL) before cell seeding. A stopper apparatus was fashioned on the ends of the grafts, and they were inoculated four times with the cell-containing media, with the total cell inoculum being 3.4×10^5 cells per square centimeter. The stoppers were then removed, and the endothelial cell–bearing grafts were placed in culture flasks that were submerged horizontally in complete media and incubated as previously described. They were rotated periodically to ensure circumferential coverage. The grafts were examined daily, and when confluence was visually achieved, the grafts were transported to a pulse-duplicating apparatus.

Endothelial cell-seeded grafts (Hytrel) were perfused in an in vitro perfusion circuit that was capable of simulating low-flow (30 to 300 mL/min) peripheral vascular hemodynamics. A computer-aided designed and machined disk cam and roller follower provided pulsatile pressure and flow waveforms at a frequency of 1 Hz.[14] In operation, the flow of perfusate (medium 199) passes through a prosthetic aortic valve and compliance chamber before entering the graft-housing chambers. Each housing chamber is filled with normothermic lactated Ringer's solution and contains one graft segment, along with various sensors (Fig 2). Hemodynamic parameters, measured at various locations within the housing chamber, include perfusion pressure, both proximal and distal to the graft segment (Mikro-Tip pressure transducers, model PC-360, Millar Instruments, Inc, Houston); fluid pressure (Millar Instruments Inc) within the housing chamber; and flow rate through the graft (model 501 flowmeter and model EP300A flow probe, Carolina Medical Electronics Inc, King, NC).[15] Fluid that exits the tissue chamber flows directly into a reservoir, thereby connecting the entire flow path in a closed loop.

The grafts were placed on the perfusion apparatus in pairs, and four runs were performed to perfuse all eight grafts. Before the runs, the distal 1-cm segments of each graft were excised to exclude the effect of the stoppers rubbing off cells, and 6 cm of each graft was exposed to the pulsatile-circulating media. Two hemodyamic conditions were established, and both grafts of each pair were subjected to one or the other condition. In one condition, each graft was subjected to pressures of 120/80 mm Hg and a mean flow of 90 mL/min with a shear rate of 240 inverse s. The alternate perfusion condition was 200/100 mm Hg and a mean flow of 195 mL/min with a shear rate of 520 inverse s. Shear rates were calculated according to Poiseuille's law. The grafts were maintained on the perfusion apparatus for 120 minutes. Periodic samples of the perfusate were obtained to ensure physiologic gases. Samples of perfusate were obtained at 5, 15, 60, and 120 minutes for radioactivity determination, representing ^{111}In shed during per-

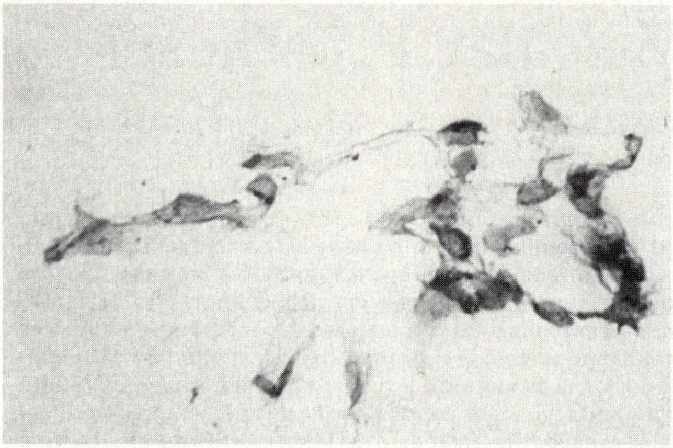

Fig 1.—Anti–factor VIII antibody immunoperoxidase stain of endothelial cells before graft inoculation (diaminobenzidine and Mayer's hematoxylin, ×40).

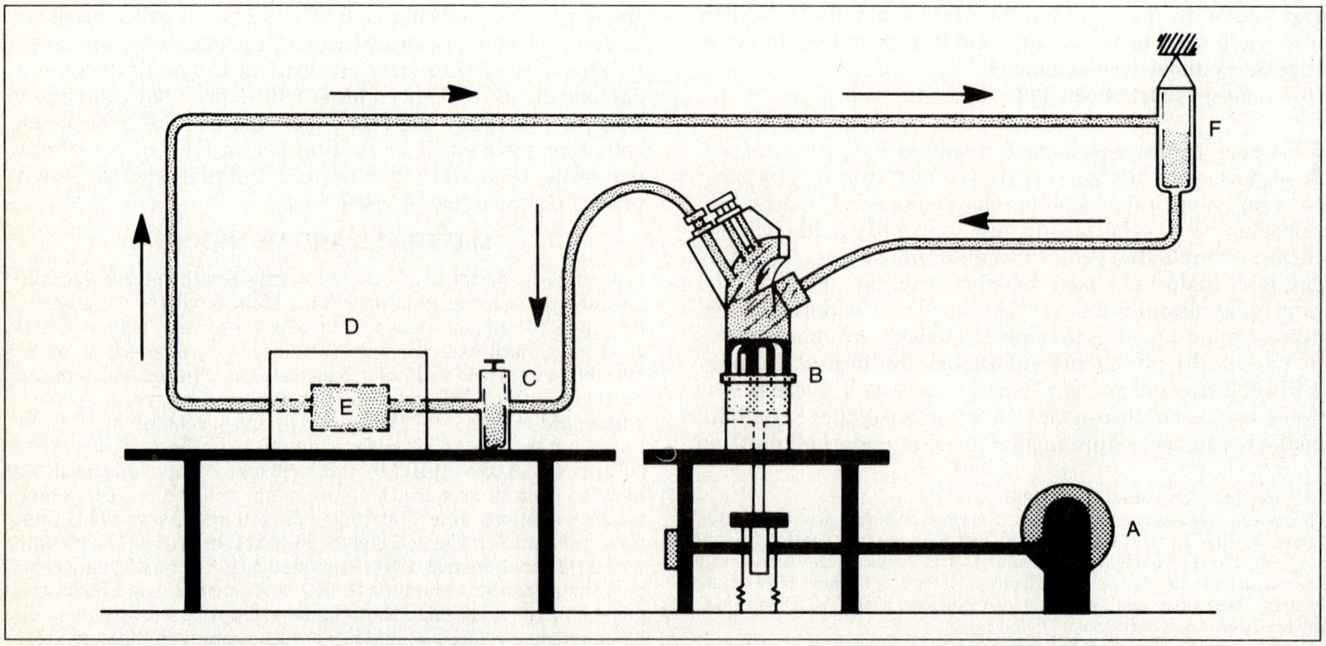

Fig 2.—Overview of perfusion circuit. A indicates variable speed motor; B, pulse duplicator and piston drive; C, compliance chamber; D, water bath; E, graft-housing tissue chamber and associated instrumentation; and F, perfusate reservoir (from Rogers et al[15]).

fusion. At the end of the 120 minutes, the grafts were removed from the perfusion apparatus and sectioned proximally to distally into the central four 1-cm segments, with the two end 1-cm segments being discarded to avoid artifact. Each segment was then placed into complete media and assayed for residual radioactivity. The specimens were then fixed in 40% formaldehyde solution and stained with Gill's hematoxylin for photography and evaluation of retained cell density. Three blinded experienced observers independently evaluated the grafts under light microscopy to determine the cell density on a qualitative scale, with 4+ as confluent, 3+ as nearly so, 2+ as nonconfluent, and 1+as scattered cells.

RESULTS

Figure 3 illustrates the activity of the perfusate vs time during the two low-flow/pressure runs. All four grafts (perfused in pairs) were utilized to generate these two curves. These bimodal curves demonstrate a relatively rapid initial rise in activity, indicating that most of the radioactivity cell loss occurred during the first 15 minutes. The slope of the curves then decreases substantially, becoming virtually asymptotic.

Figure 4 illustrates the activity of the perfusate vs time during the two high-flow/pressure runs. Again, four grafts (perfused in pairs) were utilized. Curves similar to those of Fig 3 were generated, revealing a relatively rapid initial loss of radioactivity with minimal loss thereafter.

Following perfusion, each 1-cm segment was assayed for residual radioactivity. The results are illustrated in Fig 5, which represents the four 1-cm segments of the grafts from proximal to distal. The residual radioactivity of each graft segment is shown under the schematic of its relative position along the length of the graft. There is no significant

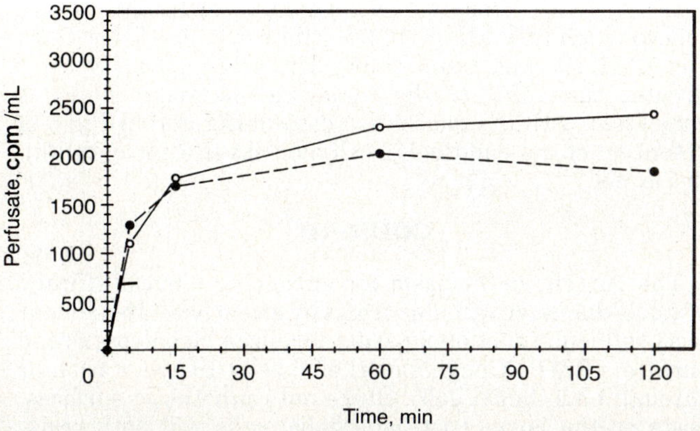

Fig 3.—Radioactivity of perfusate during low-flow–low-pressure runs. cpm indicates counts per minute.

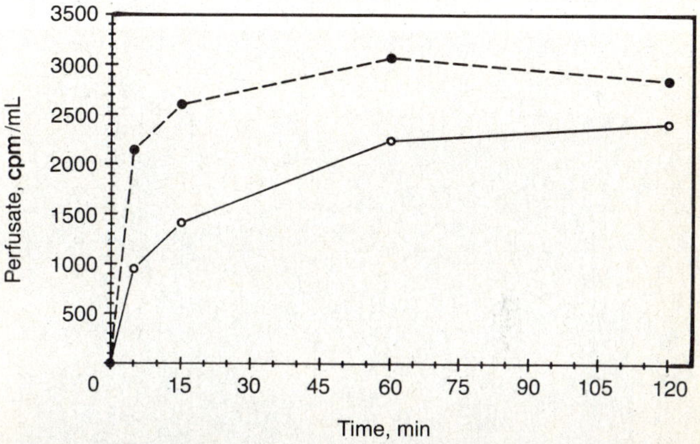

Fig 4.—Radioactivity of perfusate during high-flow–high-pressure runs. cpm indicates counts per minute.

Residual cpm on Graft Segments After Perfusion

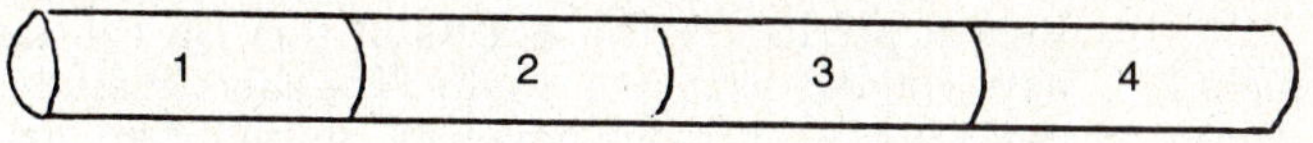

	1	2	3	4	Run	Flow
	1 370 165	1 227 434	1 126 199	1 189 888	Run 1	Low Flow
	1 787 373	1 669 282	1 608 490	1 542 754	Run 1	Low Flow
	1 327 209	1 384 312	1 297 732	1 356 559	Run 4	Low Flow
	1 187 425	1 339 516	1 286 041	1 257 502	Run 4	Low Flow
Mean ± SD	1 418 043 ± 223 680	1 405 136 ± 162 857	1 329 615 ± 174 688	1 336 675 ± 132 927		
	1 649 082	1 724 064	1 827 552	1 396 174	Run 2	High Flow
	1 246 101	1 327 308	1 175 698	1 294 040	Run 2	High Flow
	1 085 629	1 221 240	1 195 124	1 610 287	Run 3	High Flow
	1 302 095	1 397 275	1 290 597	1 190 647	Run 3	High Flow
Mean ± SD	1 320 726 ± 205 550	1 417 471 ± 187 778	1 372 242 ± 266 445	1 372 787 ± 155 184		

Fig 5.—Counts per minute (cpm) of postperfusion graft segments for each of eight grafts, arranged proximally to distally in respect to perfusate flow. Mean ± SD for each segment position is shown for both flow conditions.

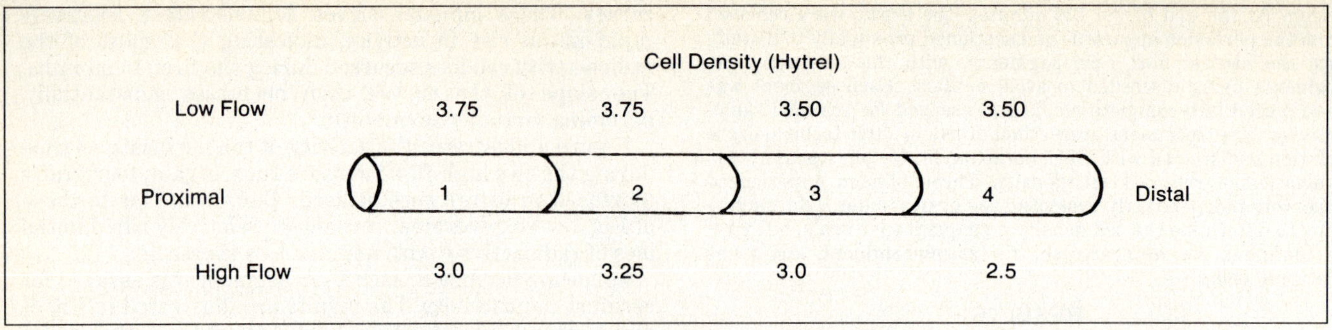

Fig 6.—Mean cell density scores of postperfusion Gill's hematoxylin–stained graft segments, determined by three blinded observers using light microscopy, with scores as follows: 4.0, confluent; 3.0, nearly so; 2.0, not confluent; and 1.0, scattered cells.

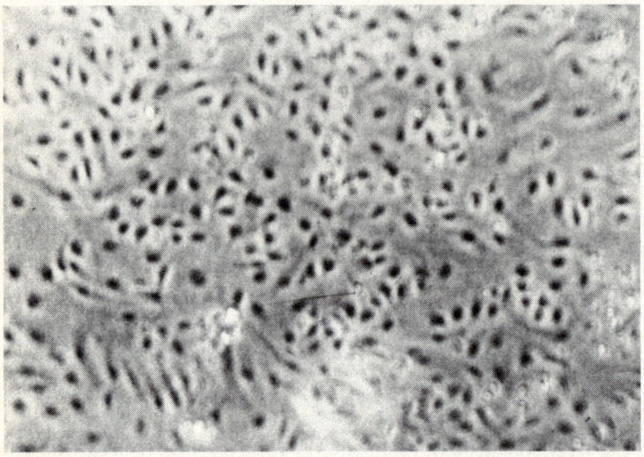

Fig 7.—Representative photomicrograph of Gill's hematoxylin–stained segment after high-flow/pressure graft. Hematoxylin stains only nucleus, with cytoplasm making up most of nonstained area (×10).

difference in retained radioactivity between the high- and the low-flow/pressure conditions.

Histologic evaluation of retained cell density is depicted in Fig 6, showing the mean scores given by the three blinded observers. A representative photomicrograph of a Gill's hematoxylin-stained segment following two hours of perfusion is shown in Fig 7. Gill's hematoxylin stains only the nucleus, with the cytoplasm occupying much of the remaining space. The blurred margins of the photomicrograph simply reflect focusing difficulty due to the convex nature of the specimen. The majority of the graft segments were considered to be near-confluent. Again, no significant differences are seen between the hemodynamic conditions or between graft segments.

The percentage of shed radioactivity during perfusion can be determined by calculating the radioactivity present on the grafts initially and comparing this with the residual activity on the grafts after each run. The initial activity could not be measured before perfusion directly because of the size of the graft, so the initial activity was calculated by summing the individual activity of the eight graft segments of each run and adding to this the total activity present in the perfusate at the end of each run. The activity present in the perfusate was calculated by multiplying the total volume in milliliters by the activity in counts per minute per milliliter of perfusate at 120 minutes. The calculated percent loss of endothelial cells (radioactivity) from the grafts during 120 minutes of perfusion of two grafts in both hemodynamic/pressure conditions was as follows: high flow: run 2, 10.2%, and run 3, 7.9%; low flow: run 1, 11.1%, and run 4, 9.5%. The percent loss is never greater than 12% of the initial radioactivity, which is consistent with the qualitative data illustrated in Fig 6 of retention of the endothelial cell monolayer at near-confluent levels.

COMMENT

The current enthusiasm for enhancing clinical efficacy of small-diameter vascular grafts by an early establishment of a confluent, functioning endothelialized blood-contacting surface, either through endothelial cell transplantation or through endothelial cell culture onto prosthetic surfaces, rests on the hopes that endothelial cells will both resist detachment under physiologic hemodynamic conditions and will function in a capacity, such that their procoagulant/anticoagulant and mesenchymal cell growth–regulating potentials are optimized. The adherence of an endothelial monolayer to a surface is dependent on the physical and biochemical characteristics of that surface. Studies attempting to optimize cell-surface attachment surface characteristics are currently under way in several laboratories. Recent studies of the effects of flow on cell detachment have yielded disparate results. The current study examines the effects of hemodynamics at the two extremes of physiologic conditions on cell adherence to fibronectin-coated polyester elastomer surfaces.

The results, whether measured quantitatively as retained radioactivity or semiquantitatively as retained cell numbers, show a remarkable retention of endothelial cells cultured on the material surface. No significant differences were found between high- and low-shear conditions. Essentially 90% of the initial confluent monolayer remained attached to the prosthetic surface following the two-hour perfusion. These results are consistent with the recent study by Schneider et al[16] in which 94% of endothelial cells remained adherent to a small-caliber prosthesis at one hour with flows of 100 mL/min. Our data further suggest that essentially no cell loss occurs following the initial 15 minutes of perfusion under these experimental conditions.

Previous work from our laboratory[17] in which endothelial cells were cultured on fibronectin-treated expanded polytef prostheses demonstrated a similar lack of effect of hemodynamics on percent cell loss but did demonstrate a shift of cell density from proximal to distal, interpreted as migration of cells in the direction of flow, intensified in the high-flow condition. This was not seen in the current study with polyester elastomer. An explanation for this discrepancy may be a difference in cell attachment forces to the two prosthetic materials. However, several methodologic differences were used in these two studies, and the former (expanded polytef) study requires confirmation to rule out methodologic reasons for the different results.

More important than documentation of cell retention by a prosthetic surface under physiologic hemodynamic conditions is the documentation of favorable endothelial cell functional characteristics. For example, Frangos and colleagues[18] reported augmentation of endothelial cell prostacyclin production in response to pulsatile flow conditions in culture. Sumpio et al[19] have reported augmented rates of endothelial cell proliferation in response to cyclic deformation, and quite likely, other mechanical stimuli and hemodynamic parameters can affect a wide variety of endothelial cell functional characteristics. Any alteration from normal cell-cycling behavior likely yields a modification of cellular synthetic activity of any of a large number of endothelial cell-derived effector substances. Much work is needed to evaluate endothelial cell function on different prosthetic surfaces in response to both hemodynamic conditions and cell-material interactions.

The results of this study confirm that canine jugular vein endothelial cells, grown to confluence on fibronectin-coated polyester elastomer small-diameter vascular prostheses, will be retained at 90% confluence by that surface following two hours of perfusion under the two extremes of physiologic hemodynamic parameters.

References

1. Herring MB, Gardner AL, Glover J: A single staged technique for seeding vascular grafts with autogenous endothelium. *Surgery* 1978;84:498.
2. Graham LM, Burkel WE, Ford JW, et al: Immediate seeding of enzymatically derived endothelium in Dacron vascular grafts: Early experimental studies with autologous canine cells. *Arch Surg* 1980;115:1289-1294.
3. Kempczinski RF, Roseman JE: Endothelial cell seeding of a new PTFE vascular prosthesis. *J Vasc Surg* 1985;2:424-429.
4. Jarrel BE, Williams SK, Stokes G, et al: Use of freshly isolated capillary endothelial cells for the immediate establishment of a monolayer on a vascular graft at surgery. *Surgery* 1986;100:392-399.
5. Douville EC, Kempczinski RF, Birinyi LK, et al: Impact of endothelial cell seeding on long term patency and subendothelial proliferation in a small-caliber highly porous PTFE graft. *J Vasc Surg* 1987;5:544-550.
6. Greisler HP: Arterial regeneration over absorbable prosthesis. *Arch Surg* 1982;117:1425-1431.
7. Greisler HP, Kim DU, Fenoglio C, et al: Arterial regenerative activity after prosthetic implantation. *Arch Surg* 1985;120:315-323.
8. Greisler HP, Ellinger J, Schwarcz TH, et al: Arterial regeneration over polydioxanone prosthesis in the rabbit. *Arch Surg* 1987;122:715-721.
9. Greisler HP, Endean ED, Klosak JJ, et al: Polyglactin 910/polydioxanone bicomponent totally resorbable vascular prostheses. *J Vasc Surg* 1988;7:607-705.
10. Greisler HP, Kim DU, Dennis JW, et al: Compound polyglactin 910/polypropylene small vessel prostheses. *J Vasc Surg* 1987;4:572-583.
11. Jarrell BE, Speicher L, Carabasi RA, et al: Use of an endothelial monolayer on a vascular graft prior to implantation. *Ann Surg* 1986;203:671-678.
12. Rosenman JE, Kempczinski RF, Pearce WH, et al: Kinetics of endothelial cell seeding. *J Vasc Surg* 1985;6:778-784.
13. Pratt KJ, Jarrell BE, Williams SK, et al: Kinetics of endothelial cell-surface attachment forces. *J Vasc Surg* 1988;7:591-599.
14. Brant AM, Chmielewski JF, Hung T-K, et al: Simulation in vitro of pulsatile vascular hemodynamics using a CAD/CAM designed cam disc and roller follower. *Artif Organs* 1986;10:419-421.
15. Rogers VJ, Teodori MF, Brant AM, et al: Characterization in vitro of the biomechanical properties of anastomosed host artery-graft combinations. *J Vasc Surg* 1986;4:396-402.
16. Schneider PA, Hanson SR, Price TM, et al: Durability of confluent endothelial cell monolayers on small-caliber vascular prostheses in vitro. *Surgery* 1988;103:456-462.
17. Greisler HP, in discussion, Pratt KJ, Jarrell BE, Williams SK, et al: Kinetics of endothelial cell-surface attachment forces. *J Vasc Surg* 1988;7:599.
18. Frangos JA, Eskin SG, McIntire LV, et al: Flow effects on prostacyclin production by cultured human endothelial cells. *Science* 1985;227:1477-1479.
19. Sumpio BE, Banes AJ, Levin LG, et al: Mechanical stress stimulates aortic endothelial cells to proliferate. *J Vasc Surg* 1987;6:252-256.

In Other AMA Journals

ARCHIVES OF INTERNAL MEDICINE

The Costs of Employee Smoking: A Computer Simulation of Hospital Nurses

Robert T. Swank, MA; Diane M. Becker, ScD, MPH; Catherine A. Jackson, MS

A computer simulation model of the economic impact of employee smoking on an employer was developed with a population of hospital nurses as the example. Net economic impact was calculated by estimating cumulative costs borne by the employer under various scenarios and comparing them with projected costs estimated from baseline data. The model included the following: baseline number of staff, baseline percentage of smokers, annual employee turnover rate, number of smokers interested in quitting, the cost of a smoking cessation program, expected success rate of a voluntary cessation program, smokers quitting spontaneously without a program, and employer-borne costs related to employee smoking. A variety of scenarios were constructed to generate a range of employer net economic impact figures and resulting percentages of smoking employees. Results showed that the benefits of a cessation program would be eliminated over several years, unless the prevalence of smoking in incoming employees was reduced. The most favorable scenario, combining a hospital cessation program and reduced smoking among new employees, generated cumulative savings, discounted at 5%, of $358 000 to $684 000 over an eight-year period (*Arch Intern Med* 1988;148:445-448).

Reprint requests to Department of Biostatistics, School of Hygiene and Public Health, Johns Hopkins University, 615 N Wolfe St, Baltimore, MD 21205 (Mr Swank).

Pentoxifylline Increases Extremity Blood Flow in Diabetic Atherosclerotic Patients

Richard W. Schwartz, MD; Nancy M. Logan; Paul J. Johnson, MD; William E. Strodel, MD; Joseph G. Fine, MD; Andris Kazmers, MD; Gordon L. Hyde, MD

• Pentoxifylline, a new trisubstituted methylxanthine derivative known for its hemorrheologic action, has been shown to improve exercise tolerance in atherosclerotic patients. We examined the response of diabetic atherosclerotic patients to pentoxifylline administration, measured by Doppler waveform analysis and exercise tolerance. Standard exercise tolerance and Doppler waveform analytic studies of the lower extremity, specifically the right dorsalis pedis artery, were performed before and after three months of pentoxifylline administration (400 mg three times a day). The study group comprised ten subjects (six men and four women) with a mean (±SD) age of 60±3.3 years. Data were analyzed using a paired Student *t* test. All ten subjects showed a significant increase in exercise tolerance after pentoxifylline treatment. Eight of ten subjects demonstrated a significant increase in right dorsalis pedis arterial flow.

(*Arch Surg* 1989;124:434-437)

A number of blood flow characteristics are reported to be altered in chronic arterial disorders such as atherosclerosis and diabetes mellitus, including increased blood plasma viscosity, decreased red blood cell deformability, increased fibrinogen level, decreased fibrinolytic activity, platelet hyperactivity, and plasma hypercoagulability.[1-9] Numerous investigators[10-16] have documented improvement in some or all of these pathophysiologic flow abnormalities in patients with both atherosclerosis and diabetes, following the administration of pentoxifylline (Trental). Pentoxifylline has also been shown to induce vasodilatation in the rabbit hindlimb[17] and to exert relaxing effects on vascular smooth muscle.[18] These reported improvements in hemorrheologic flow characteristics should decrease peripheral vascular resistance and theoretically result in an increased peripheral tissue blood flow. Because of these positive hemorrheologic effects, pentoxifylline has been commonly prescribed in Europe and North America for the treatment of chronic occlusive arterial disease (COAD).

Accepted for publication Dec 12, 1988.

From the Department of Surgery, University of Kentucky Chandler Medical Center, Lexington, Ky.

Read before the 12th Annual Surgical Symposium of the Association of Veterans Administration Surgeons, Minneapolis, May 16, 1988.

Reprint requests to Department of Surgery, University of Kentucky, 800 Rose St, Lexington, KY 40536-0084 (Dr Schwartz).

In the past decade, Porter et al[19] and others[20-24] have demonstrated the clinical efficacy of pentoxifylline in improving both initial claudication distance and absolute claudication distance in atherosclerotic patients with claudication. In the study conducted by Porter et al, these distances increased by as much as 100% in one third of the subjects taking pentoxifylline.

Not all investigators, however, have been able to show that pentoxifylline greatly improves either claudication distance or hemorrheologic characteristics in patients with intermittent claudication,[25] so it is clear that many questions about the usefulness of the drug remain unanswered. One weakness in the measurement of initial claudication distance is that it is somewhat subjective, because the investigator must rely on the subjects' signal at the onset of claudication. Total exercise time is less subjective, simply because the subjects walk until they cannot walk farther. It should be noted that Porter et al[19] attributed 50% of the improvement in claudication distances to placebo effect.

Given this lack of objective clinical evidence of improved blood flow following pentoxifylline therapy, the purpose of this study was to determine whether circulatory changes due to pentoxifylline administration could be assessed quantitatively via Doppler waveform analysis.

SUBJECTS AND METHODS

Subjects

Ten subjects (six men and four women) with a mean (±SD) age of 60±3.3 years were studied. The entry criteria included the following: (1) severe COAD as determined by physical assessment (eg, absence of or diminished peripheral pulses on palpation, minor trophic skin changes, elevation pallor of the lower limbs, and dependent rubor) and the results of noninvasive vascular testing (monophasic or biphasic Doppler waveforms and ankle/brachial [A/B] indexes <0.8); (2) intermittent claudication that had been stable for at least six months; (3) the ability to walk at least 20 m, but not farther than 200 m, on a treadmill before experiencing claudication; and (4) diabetes mellitus as defined by World Health Organization criteria, ie, fasting venous plasma glucose concentration greater than 7.8 mmol/L on at least two occasions, or a positive oral glucose tolerance test.

Criteria for initial exclusion included the following: (1) severe COAD as manifested by rest pain, lower-extremity ulcers, or

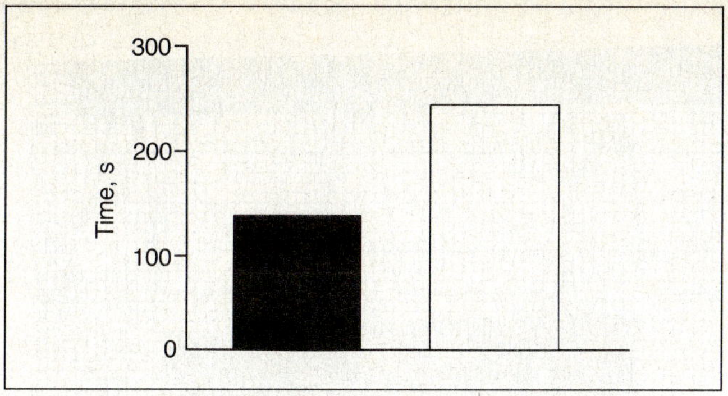

Fig 1.—Mean exercise tolerance before (solid bar) and after (open bar) pentoxifylline therapy.

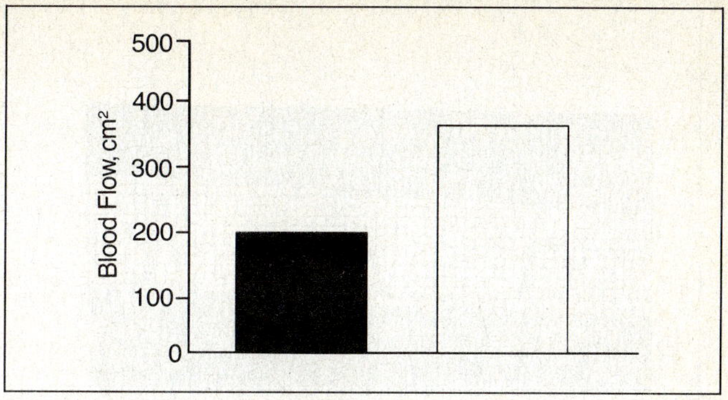

Fig 2.—Mean dorsalis pedis blood flow before (solid bar) and after (open bar) pentoxifylline therapy.

gangrene; (2) lumbar sympathectomy within the previous three months; (3) lower limb amputation; (4) serious concomitant cardiac, pulmonary, or malignant disease; (5) hypersensitivity to methylxanthine agents; and (6) previous use of pentoxifylline.

Study Design

Each subject participated in this study for a total of 16 weeks. The first four weeks constituted a "washout" phase, during which all medications (eg, vasodilators) being taken to treat intermittent claudication were discontinued. Pentoxifylline was not prescribed during this phase of the study. The purpose of the first phase was to verify the stability of the degree of intermittent claudication, which allowed each subject to serve as his/her own control, and to familiarize the patients with treadmill procedures.

At the start of the first phase (visit 1), each subject underwent a complete physical examination and electrocardiography. Lower-extremity vascular examination included Doppler waveform measurements at rest, and arterial pressures measured both at rest and after treadmill exercise. The Doppler equipment (Narcolab Arterial Diagnostic Unit, Narco Scientific Diagnostic Division, Huntington Valley, Pa) had an 8-mHz probe. To achieve the best Doppler measurement, the probe was tilted against the skin at an angle allowing the clearest audio signal (45°). Three experienced vascular technicians were trained for this study, although the data presented herein were collected, with few exceptions, by the same technician. The treadmill (Model 16-50, Quinton Instruments, Seattle, Wash) was set at a constant speed of 2.5 km/h and at a 12% grade.

During treadmill exercise, both the time interval to the onset of claudication and the total time that the subject was able to walk (total exercise time) were recorded. Symptoms accepted as representing claudication included lower-extremity pain, aches, cramps, and severe fatigue.

At the end of the washout phase (visit 2), the treadmill measurements were repeated. If the time interval to the onset of claudication measured at visits 1 and 2 differed by more than 20%, the subject was excluded from the study.

At this point, eligible subjects were then entered into the treatment phase of the study and were prescribed pentoxifylline (400 mg three times a day) for the remaining 12 weeks. To ensure that changes in exercise tolerance were due to pentoxifylline alone, subjects were instructed not to alter their smoking or exercise habits for the duration of the study. During the treatment phase, subjects were evaluated on four occasions (weeks 2, 4, 8, and 12). At each of these visits, they were monitored for concomitant medications, side effects, and health changes. The vascular examination at these visits included physical assessment, calculation of resting A/B indexes, measurements of the time interval to claudication, and the total exercise time. At the final visit (week 12), Doppler waveform measurements were also obtained.

Data Analysis

The response to treatment with pentoxifylline was assessed by changes in total exercise time (in seconds), A/B indexes, and Doppler waveforms. All lower-extremity arteries were analyzed qualitatively. Quantitative changes in Doppler waveforms of the dorsalis pedis artery were determined by calculating the area under each waveform curve using a computer (Systems III, Cromenco, Mountain View, Calif)/digitizer (Talos Systems Inc, Scottsdale, Ariz). The magnitude of the arterial flow pulse (technically referred to as the arterial blood bolus) from systole to systole was measured by calculating the integral area (in centimeters) under each waveform (the product of the y axis equals centimeters per second, and the x axis equals seconds). This is representative of the blood volume per heartbeat in the dorsalis pedis artery. The quantitative data were analyzed statistically using Student's t test. Significance was defined as $P<.05$.

RESULTS

Exercise Tolerance

Mean (±SE) exercise tolerance increased significantly from 140±20 s to 256±20 s following pentoxifylline administration ($P<.001$). This represented a mean increase of 101%±67% (Fig 1).

A/B Indexes

There was no significant change in dorsalis pedis pressure measurement following treatment. The mean initial dorsalis pedis arterial A/B index was 0.58±0.21; the mean posttreatment index was 0.60±0.15.

Doppler Waveforms

Nine of the ten subjects demonstrated improvement in waveforms after three months of treatment. Six of the subjects had a mean increase of 82%±57% in the magnitude of their dorsalis pedis waveform area measurements. Two subjects had no measurable dorsalis pedis signal before treatment but developed measurable signals following treatment. These eight subjects significantly ($P<.01$) increased their mean dorsalis pedis waveform from 206±74 cm to 372±85 cm (Fig 2). One subject increased his waveform tracing to such a point that it was consistently off the graph paper and subsequently could not be analyzed with the computer/digitizer. One subject demonstrated a decrease in waveform at the dorsalis pedis artery; she admitted being marginally compliant with the pentoxifylline regimen. Figure 3 demonstrates actual waveforms before and after three months of treatment in a subject who had demonstrated a measurable signal before treatment. Figure 4 shows the waveforms in a subject who had not had a measurable signal before treatment.

COMMENT

Pentoxifylline, a trisubstituted methylxanthine derivative, is the most well known of a new group of hemorrheo-

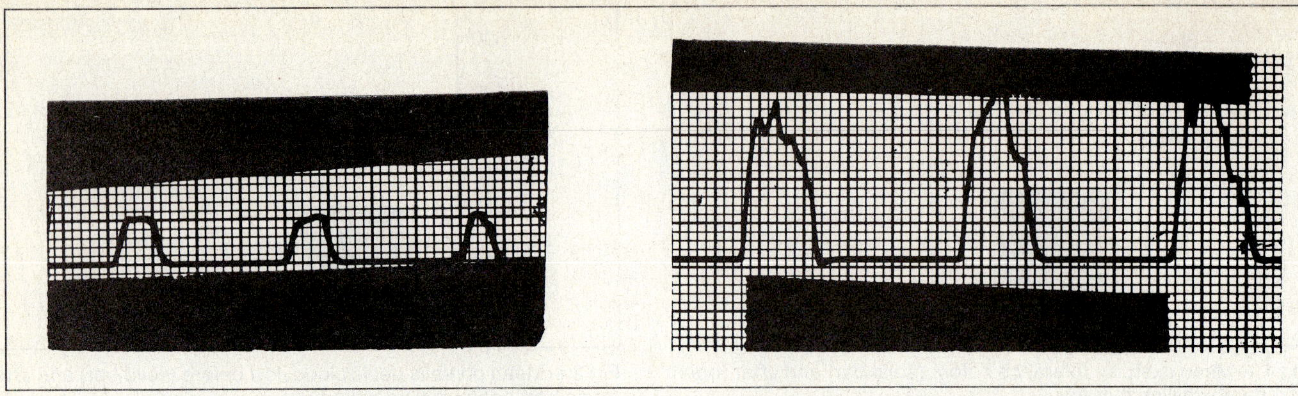

Fig 3.—Waveforms of one subject's left dorsalis pedis artery flow before (left) and after (right) three months of pentoxifylline therapy.

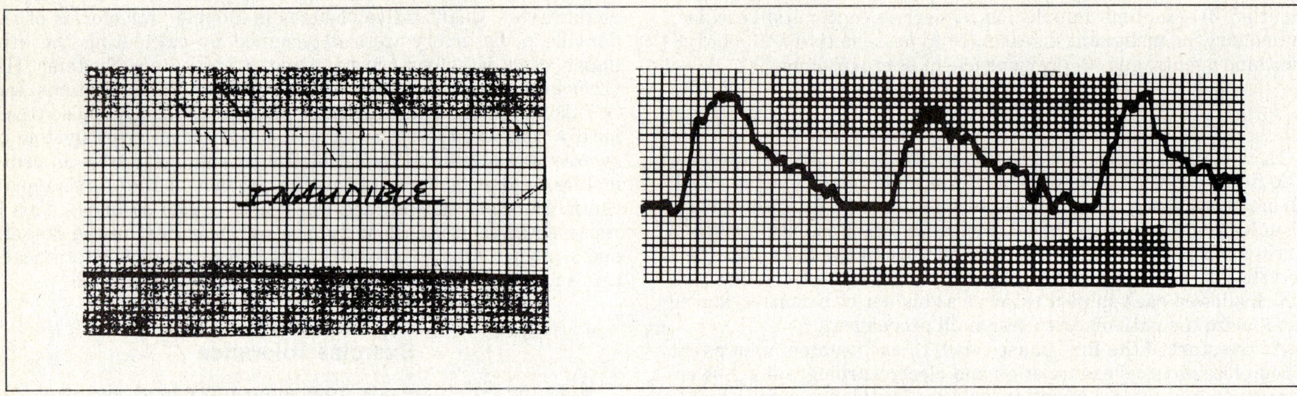

Fig 4.—Doppler waveforms from one subject's left dorsalis pedis artery before (left) and after (right) three months of pentoxifylline therapy. Doppler signal in this artery was inaudible before subject's participation in study.

logic agents. Several investigators[10-16] have shown that pentoxifylline therapy improves hemorrheologic abnormalities associated with diabetes and atherosclerosis. However, reports in the literature about the clinical improvement in patients taking pentoxifylline for the treatment of intermittent claudication have been contradictory.[19,21,23-25] To our knowledge, no studies have shown clear evidence that the use of this agent leads to improvement in distal extremity arterial flow as measured by noninvasive vascular tests.

The data presented in our pilot study demonstrate a mean 100% increase in claudication time. These findings are consistent with other reports in the literature.[19,21] The unique feature of this report is the significant ($P<.01$) change seen in the distal extremity arterial Doppler waveforms in seven subjects, and the reestablishment of dorsalis pedis flow in two subjects as measured by the digitizer method. This type of analysis calculates the area under the waveform curve (y axis equals centimeters per second, and x axis equals seconds). The actual measurement obtained is the length of blood bolus per heartbeat (measured in centimeters). Although only the dorsalis pedis artery waveforms were analyzed quantitatively by the digitizer method, each subject showed marked qualitative improvement in waveforms of other distal extremity arteries. The only subject who failed to demonstrate improvement on Doppler waveform testing was one who had poor compliance with the medication regimen. For the remaining subjects, although the waveform testing demonstrated marked improvement, A/B pressure indexes remained relatively unchanged. This latter finding was similar to the results found by other investigators.[26,27]

Our results may be explained by several independent mechanisms. First, clinical experience has shown that arterial waveforms may be a more sensitive indicator of changes in arterial flow than the A/B index.[26,27] Second, A/B indexes in diabetic patients are often unreliable, especially if COAD with significant arterial calcification exists. Third, since pressure is the product of flow and resistance (pressure equals flow times resistance), blood flow should increase if resistance decreases and arterial pressure remains stable. Pentoxifylline therapy may decrease resistance inherent to both COAD and diabetes by inducing vasodilatation and/or by improving the hemorrheologic disturbances. Diabetic patients with coexistent atherosclerosis might be particularly susceptible to the hemorrheologic effects of pentoxifylline, since this group may well have hemorrheologic abnormalities that are worse than those for either disease entity alone.

Our results demonstrate that the magnitude of the flow pulse (technically referred to as a blood bolus) in the dorsalis pedis artery from systole to systole is significantly increased. This measurement is representative of the increase in blood volume per heartbeat in the dorsalis pedis artery following pentoxifylline treatment.

In conclusion, pentoxifylline has been shown to produce variable amelioration of the hemorrheologic pathophysiologic problems associated with both atherosclerosis and diabetes mellitus. Both relaxation of smooth muscle and vasodilatation have been demonstrated in animal studies.

The exact mechanism by which pentoxifylline exerts its positive hemorrheologic effects in either the macrocirculation or the microcirculation has yet to be determined. However, the improvement in dorsalis pedis arterial flow demonstrated by this pilot study indicates that a randomized trial of pentoxifylline treatment may be appropriate in the diabetic atherosclerotic patient group.

This study was funded by Hoechst-Roussel Pharmaceuticals Inc, Somerville, NJ.

References

1. Angelkort B: Thrombozytenfunktion, plasmatische Blutgerinnung und Fibrinolyse bei chronisch arterieller Verschlusskrankheit. *Med Welt* 1979; 30:1239-1244.
2. Angelkort B, Maurin N, Boateng K: Influence of pentoxifylline on erythrocyte deformability in peripheral occlusive arterial disease. *Curr Med Res Opin* 1979;6:255-258.
3. Dormandy JA: Practical impact of hemorrheology on the treatment of chronic peripheral ischemia. *Angiology* 1981;32:710-712.
4. Ehrly AM: Verbesserung der Fliesseigenschaften des Blutes: Ein neues Prinzip zur medikamentösen Therapie chronischer peripherer arterieller Durchbluntungsstörungen. *Vasa* 1973;(suppl 1):1-18.
5. Reid HL, Dormandy JA, Barnes AJ, et al: Impaired red cell deformability in peripheral vascular disease. *Lancet* 1979;1:666-668.
6. Schmid-Schoenbein H: Blood rheology and physiology of microcirculation. *Ric Clin Lab* 1981;1(suppl 1):13-16.
7. Sternitzky R, Seige K: Hämorheologische Veränderungen und ihre klinische Bedeutung bei chronischarterieller Verschlusskrankheit. *Z Gesamte Inn Med* 1983;38:1-7.
8. Verstraete M: Drugs acting on the peripheral circulation, in Dukes MNG (ed): *Side Effects of Drugs Annual*, ed 4. Princeton, NJ, Excerpta Medica, 1980, pp 139-143.
9. Grigoleit HG, Lehrach F: Blutviskosität und Diabetes mellitus. *Med Monatsschr Pharm* 1973;27:353-356.
10. Ambrus JL, Ambrus CM, Gastpar M, et al: Studies on vaso-occlusive crisis of sickle-cell disease: I. Effect of pentoxifylline. *J Med* 1979;10:445-456.
11. Brevetti G, Abata S, Lavecchia G, et al: La pentossifillina nel trattamento delle arteriopatie obliteranti al secondo stadio. *Prog Med* 1979; 35:363-366.
12. Ehrly AM: The effect of pentoxifylline on the deformability of erythrocytes and on muscular oxygen pressure in patients with chronic arterial disease. *J Med* 1979;10:331-334.
13. Ehrly AM: Effects of orally administered pentoxifylline on muscular oxygen pressure in patients with intermittent claudication. *IRCS Med Sci* 1982;10:401-405.
14. Hess H, Franke I, Jauch M: Medicamentöse Verbesserung der Fliesseigenschaften des Blutes. *Fortschr Med* 1973;91:743-748.
15. Jarrett PEM, Moreland M, Browse NL: The effect of pentoxifylline on fibrinolytic activity and plasma fibrinogen levels. *Curr Med Res Opin* 1977;4:492-496.
16. Keller F, Leonhardt H: Amelioration of blood viscosity in sickle-cell anemia by pentoxifylline: A case report. *J Med* 1979;10:429-432.
17. Popendiker K, Boksay I, Bollman V: Zur Pharmakologie des neuen peripheren Gefässdilators 3,7-dimethyl-1-(5-oxohexyl)-Xanthin. *Arzneimittelforschung* 1971;21:1160-1171.
18. Stefanovich F: Effect of 3,7-dimethyl-1-(5-oxyhexyl)-xanthin and 1-hexyl-3,7-dimethyl xanthin on cyclic AMP phosphodiesterase of the human umbilical cord vessels. *Res Commun Chem Pathol Pharmacol* 1973;5:655-662.
19. Porter JM, Cutler BS, Lee BY, et al: Pentoxifylline efficacy in the treatment of intermittent claudication: Multicenter controlled double-blind trial with objective assessment of chronic occlusive arterial disease patients. *Am Heart J* 1982;104:66-72.
20. Roekharts F, Deleers L: Trental 400 in the treatment of intermittent claudication: Results of long-term, placebo-controlled administration. *Angiology* 1984;35:396-406.
21. Johnson WC, Sentissi JM, Baldwin D, et al: Treatment of claudication with pentoxifylline: Are benefits related to improvement in viscosity? *J Vasc Surg* 1987;6:211-216.
22. Reich T, Gillings D: Effects of pentoxifylline on severe intermittent claudication. *Angiology* 1987;38:651-656.
23. Lee BY, Berkowitz JP, Savitsky GS, et al: Pentoxifylline treatment of moderate to severe chronic occlusive arterial disease. *Clin Cardiol* 1985; 8:161-165.
24. Schubotz R: Double-blind trial of pentoxifylline in diabetics with peripheral vascular disorders. *Pharmatherapeutica* 1976;1:172-179.
25. Reilly D, Quinton DN, Barrie WW: A controlled trial of pentoxifylline (Trental 400) in intermittent claudication: Clinical, haemostatic and rheological effects. *NZ Med J* 1987;100:445-447.
26. Hurley JJ: Postoperative noninvasive evaluation of femorotibial bypass grafts, in Hershey FB, Barnes RW, Sumner DS (eds): *Noninvasive Diagnosis of Vascular Disease.* Pasadena, Calif, Appleton-Davies Inc, 1984, pp 43-55.
27. Sladen JG, Gilmour GL: Vein graft stenosis: Characteristics and effect of treatment. *Am J Surg* 1981;141:549-553.

In Other AMA Journals

ARCHIVES OF INTERNAL MEDICINE

Who Gets Screened for Cervical and Breast Cancer? Results From a New National Survey

Rodney A. Hayward, MD; Martin F. Shapiro, MD, PhD; Howard E. Freeman, PhD;
Christopher R. Corey, MA

To evaluate the adequacy of cervical and breast cancer screening in the United States, data were analyzed from a 1986 nationwide telephone survey (n = 4659). Papanicolaou smears within the recommended three- to five-year interval were reported by 79% of women aged 20 years or older. Within the preceding year, 55% of women aged 40 years or older had breast examinations performed by physicians, and 20% of women aged 50 years or older had mammograms. Women who were uninsured or lower in socioeconomic status were less likely to have each of these three preventive measures, independent of the age, health status, and frequency of physician visits of the respondent. In addition, women aged 50 years or older were less likely to have had Papanicolaou smears (63% vs 89%) and breast examinations (52% vs 68%) than those women aged 20 to 49 years. These findings suggest that women who are older, uninsured, or lower in socioeconomic status are at an increased risk for not receiving preventive care, and that screening mammography, although more common than a decade ago, is still markedly underused (*Arch Intern Med* 1988;148:1177-1181).

Reprint requests to B-973 Louis Factor Bldg, UCLA School of Medicine, Los Angeles, CA 90024-1685 (Dr Hayward).

Microvascular Free-Tissue Transfer

The Atlanta Veterans Administration Medical Center Experience

Grant W. Carlson, MD, John J. Coleman III, MD

• The entire microvascular tissue transfer experience from 1977 through 1987 at the Atlanta Veterans Administration Medical Center has been reviewed. Seventy-four free flaps were done in 68 patients. Assessable records were available in 52 patients who had 58 reconstructive procedures. The most frequently used flaps were jejunum in 15 patients (25.8%), latissimus dorsi in 11 patients (18.9%), rectus abdominis in eight patients (13.8%), and gracilis in seven patients (12.1%). Major complications occurred in 43.1% of the cases. Total flap loss occurred in eight patients (13.8%); from 1977 through 1982, four (28.6%) of 14 patients had total flap loss, and from 1983 through 1987, four (9.1%) had total flap loss. Partial flap loss occurred in four cases (6.9%). Of the 52 patients, 43 had their problems resolved expeditiously by free-tissue transfer. We conclude that in a university-affiliated Veterans Administration medical center, microvascular reconstruction is an important and necessary surgical tool. Failure rates have decreased markedly with time and increasing experience. Definition of new anatomic microvascular units for transfer has increased the number of reconstructive choices.

(*Arch Surg* 1989;124:438-440)

Microvascular tissue transplantation has undergone explosive growth and development since its reintroduction approximately 15 years ago.[1] Technical improvements in operating microscopes and an increased interest in cutaneous and muscular vascular anatomy led to a large number of new sources of tissue, some of which are easier to identify and more reliable than previous free flaps.

The advantages of free-tissue transfer are numerous. Many reconstructions can be done in one stage, eliminating costly multiple hospitalizations and operations. Consecutive procedures can be carried out with multiple flaps as required, without enlarging the local defect as is the danger with regional flaps. Free-tissue transfer minimizes the limitations of size and arc of rotation imposed by regional flaps. Distant donor sites allow greater flexibility in the design and transfer of composite tissue. The independent blood supply enables free flaps to be useful in compromised wounds over large avascular areas, such as bone or foreign body, and permits the vascular anastomosis to be performed outside the zone of injury or tumor involvement.[2]

In this study, the evolution of free-tissue transfer was examined from 1977 through 1987. Changing indications and results were reviewed with respect to the development of new types of free flaps.

PATIENTS AND METHODS

The entire microvascular tissue transfer experience from 1977 through 1987 at the Atlanta Veterans Administration Medical Center (VAMC) was reviewed. Seventy-four free flaps were done in 68 patients. Assessable records were available in 52 patients who had undergone 58 reconstructive procedures. Patient medical charts were reviewed to determine free-flap type, indications, results, complications, and long-term results. The review was divided into two time periods—1977 through 1982 and 1983 through 1987—to examine better the progression of free-tissue transfer.

The average age of patients was 51.3 years. There were 51 men and one woman. The majority of patients had underlying medical problems, including tobacco abuse in 28 patients, alcohol abuse in 16 patients, systemic arterial hypertension in nine patients, and atherosclerotic heart disease in seven patients.

RESULTS

As new techniques were developed and refined, the type of free flap and the indications varied in frequency. The most common flaps in 1977 through 1982 were latissimus dorsi in six patients (42.9%), jejunum in two patients (14.3%), and deep circumflex iliac artery (DCIA) osteomusculocutaneous flaps in two patients (14.3%). During 1982 through 1987, there was a change in distribution to the jejunum in 13 patients (29.5%), rectus abdominis in eight patients (18.2%), gracilis in seven patients (15.9%), radial forearm flap in five patients (11.4%), and latissimus dorsi in five patients (11.4%) (Fig 1). Over the entire decade, the most frequently used flaps were the jejunum in 15 patients (25.8%), latissimus dorsi in 11 patients (18.9%), rectus abdominis in eight patients (13.8%), and gracilis in seven patients (12.1%) (Fig 2). Complications occurred in 25 of 58 free-flap procedures (43.1%), including total free-flap loss in eight procedures (13.8%), partial flap loss in four procedures (6.9%), donor site problems in four patients (6.9%), and reexploration for hematoma or anastomotic problems in four procedures (6.9%). The total free-flap loss was 28.6% (4/14) during the first six years of the review but improved to 9.1% (4/44) during the second five-year period. One death (1.7%) occurred.

Donor site problems included three wound hematomas (5.2%) and one failed skin graft over the radial forearm donor site. Reexploration was performed in four cases, two of these for graft ischemia. Both grafts were salvaged with anastomotic revision. Wound hematomas were evacuated in two cases without jeopardy to the free flaps.

Orocutaneous fistulas occurred in three cases (5.2%) of jejunal free-flap reconstruction of the hypopharynx. Two fistulas closed spontaneously, and one required a sternocleidomastoid flap.

In the complex reconstructions that necessitate microvascular tissue transfer, an inadequate result can be secondary to some technical misadventure or to inappropriate use or expectations of the method. Three failures occurred in patients with large ventral hernias reconstructed with tensor fasciae latae free flaps. Recurrent herniation occurred in all three patients. Although it provides an ample amount of soft tissue, the tensor fasciae latae is probably not strong enough for definitive abdominal wall reconstruction above the umbilicus.

Numerous studies have demonstrated the ability of well-vascularized muscle to minimize the effects of bacterial colonization and improved wound healing in an otherwise unfavorable environment.[3,4] As our experience has increased, however, we have learned the limitations of the

Accepted for publication Oct 4, 1988.

From the Atlanta Veterans Administration Medical Center.

Read before the 12th Annual Surgical Symposium of the Association of Veterans Administration Surgeons, Minneapolis, May 12, 1988.

Reprint requests to 25 Prescott St, NE, Suite 3420, Atlanta, GA 30308 (Dr Coleman).

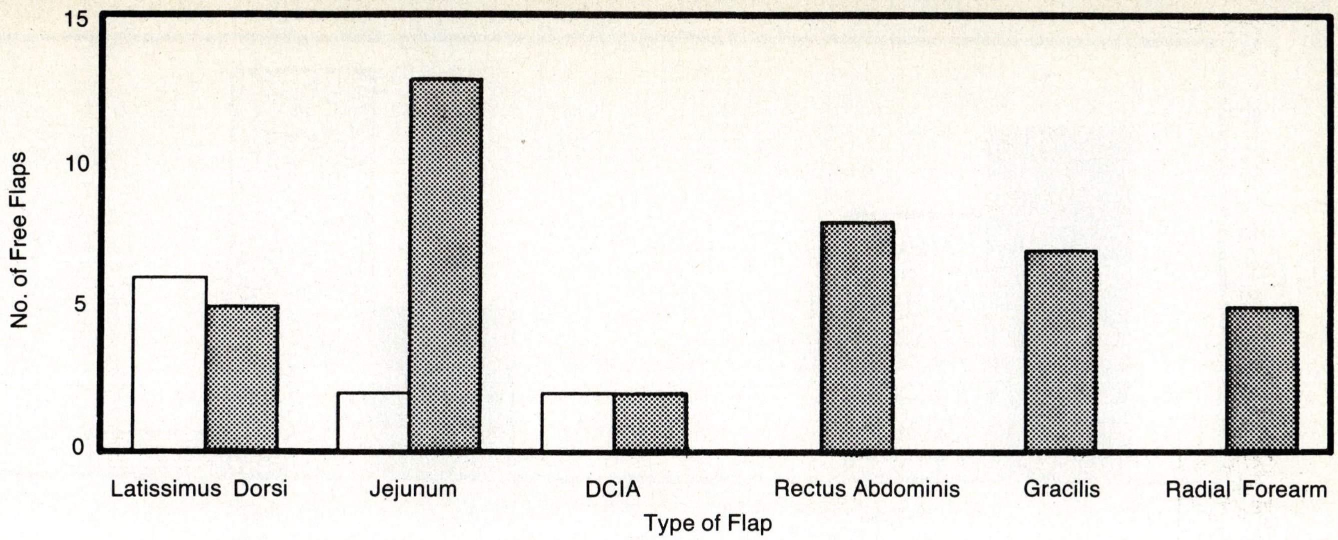

Fig 1.—Free flaps at the Atlanta Veterans Administration Medical Center, 1977 through 1982 (open bars) vs 1983 through 1987 (dotted bars). DCIA indicates deep circumflex iliac artery.

muscle in the infected and ischemic extremity. In three extremity reconstructions, the repair was inadequate. One patient with a massive injury to the hip required disarticulation after a latissimus muscle flap, and repeated débridements failed to control sepsis in the wound. In two patients, osteomyelitis persisted despite adequate coverage, probably secondary to residual foreign body, sequestrum, or hardware.

Free flaps to the head and neck accounted for three operative failures. One failure was the result of a patient avulsing a radial forearm flap reconstruction of a traumatic facial defect. Another failure occurred after two attempts at jejunal flap reconstruction of the hypopharynx. The initial failure was the result of kinking of the artery. The cause of the second failure was unknown but was assumed to be of technical origin. The pectoralis major tube flap was constructed as a salvage procedure, which failed to function, and the patient died of aspiration. The third operative failure occurred in a patient who had a resection of a craniofacial tumor. A latissimus dorsi free-flap reconstruction failed because of poor arterial inflow resulting from extracranial cerebrovascular disease.

Anatomic discoveries and the availability of a greater number of versatile flaps resulted in the addition of more complex head and neck reconstructions to extremity coverage as an indication for free-tissue transfer. During 1977 through 1982, lower-extremity reconstruction required eight (57.1%) of 14 and head and neck reconstruction required six (42.9%) of 14 of the microvascular tissue transfers. The period 1983 through 1987 saw head and neck reconstruction become the major reason for free-tissue transfer. Free-tissue transfer made up 65.9% (29/44) of the total reconstruction, with extremity reconstruction falling to 27.3% (12/44). During 1983 through 1987, the tensor fasciae latae free flap was introduced for abdominal wall reconstruction and was used in three (6.8%) of 44 patients (Fig 3).

Composite free flaps of skin, muscle, and bone were a major part of reconstruction in seven cases (12.1%), including DCIA in three cases, free fibula in two cases, serratus osteomusculocutaneous flap in one case, and radial osteofasciocutaneous flap in one case. Osseous nonunion in two complex tibial fractures complicated by osteomyelitis was successfully resolved by contralateral vascularized fibula

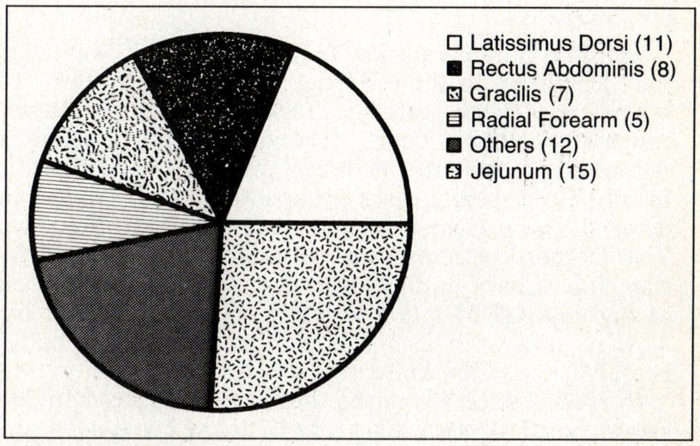

Fig 2.—Fifty-eight free flaps at the Atlanta Veterans Administration Medical Center, 1977 through 1987.

transfer. After composite resection of the oral cavity (three cases) and trauma secondary to gunshot wound (one case), the mandible was reconstructed with good bony union and with soft-tissue lining provided with the DCIA flap (two cases), serratus osteomusculocutaneous flap (one case), and radial forearm osteofasciocutaneous flap (one case). A complex three-dimensional defect resulting from radical hemimaxillectomy was repaired with a DCIA flap.

COMMENT

The last decade has seen the rapid development of microvascular free-tissue transfer. Refinement in technique, recapitulation of the axial blood supply to muscle, and the discovery of new cutaneous vascular territories have expanded the usefulness of this modality. Our experience at the Atlanta VAMC parallels this evolution. From 1977 through 1982, lower-extremity reconstruction was the major indication for free-tissue transfer. The resurgence of the jejunal free flap, first described in 1959,[5] and the description of the radial forearm fasciocutaneous flap have made microvascular tissue transfer an important and reliable method in head and neck reconstruction. From 1983 through 1987, head and neck reconstruction became the major indication for free-tissue transfer.

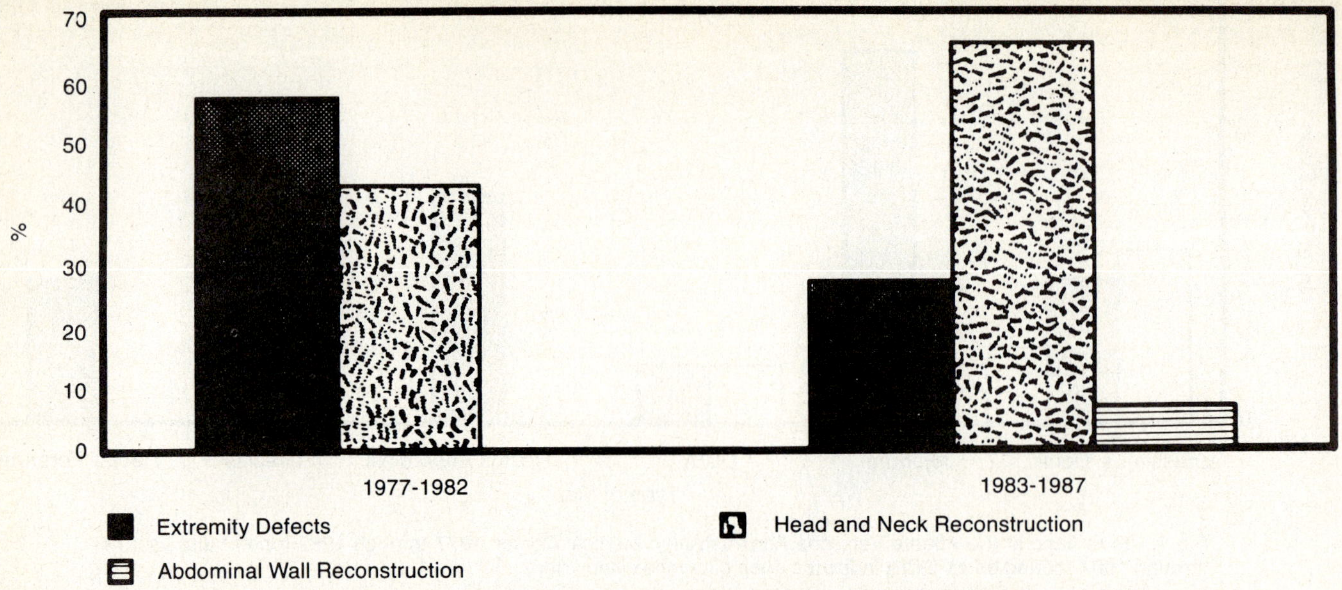

Fig 3.—Indications for microvascular free-tissue transfer, 1977 through 1982 vs 1983 through 1987.

The flap failure rate for 1977 through 1982 was 28.6% but decreased to 9.1% during 1983 through 1987. The overall flap failure rate of 13.8% is similar to previous reports.[2,6,7] In this series, the type of free flap did not determine failure rate. Technical problems were identified in four (50%) of eight cases of flap loss (causes: one patient, arterial; two patients, venous; and one patient, unknown). Two of these patients were salvaged with a second free flap. Inadequacy of donor vessels resulted in three cases of flap loss (37.5%), two of which were attempts at limb salvage in severely ischemic extremities. Lack of patient compliance was the cause in one case.

Operative success can no longer be measured in free-flap survival. Success must now be defined as resolution of the serious wound or restoration of function—be it restoration of gastrointestinal tract continuity or treatment of osteomyelitis. The operative success of microvascular free-tissue transfer at the Atlanta VAMC was 82.7%; 43 of 52 patients had satisfactory resolution of their problem. Our retrospective study has shown that as experience with microvascular tissue transfer increases, both the technical failures and inappropriate indications decrease. Reconstructive problems indigenous to our VAMC have been chronic osteomyelitis, ischemic limb problems, and head and neck cancer resections. Other problems amenable to microvascular repair include hand and extremity trauma, facial reanimation, or penile reconstruction. Continued investigation and evaluation of functional results will improve our abilities to select the proper reconstructive method and employ it to the patient's best benefit.

There has been a steady increase in anatomic information concerning the vascular supply to muscle, skin, and bone over the last 15 years that has translated directly into useful reconstructive methods. Early work by Ger[8] and others on muscle flaps in the lower extremities stimulated interest that resulted in a codification of useful muscle and musculocutaneous units by Mathes and Nahai[9] and McCraw et al.[10] Although the initial approach has emphasized local transposition of tissue, it soon became apparent that these units could be transferred by microvascular technique to satisfy complicated distant tissue demands with minimal donor site morbidity. The obvious utility and efficiency of these methods led to further experimental and clinical endeavors resulting in composite osseomusculocutaneous flaps, such as those of the DCIA described by Taylor et al,[11] and the fibula. Ponten[12] and others provided better understanding of the previously described axial cutaneous flaps, such as the groin flap, with the elucidation of the fasciocutaneous vascular system and its subsequent contributions, the radial forearm flap and scapula flap, both of which can carry vascularized bone as well as skin and fascia. Not only have these contributions provided a greater variety of tissues for microvascular transfer, but they also have defined vascular pedicles that have a larger diameter and are, therefore, more reliable for anastomosis. The increased success rate, both technical and functional, that has been seen in this review reflects these advances and, it is hoped, will continue in parallel with future discovery.

References

1. McLean D, Buncke H: Autotransplant of omentum to a large scalp defect, with microsurgical revascularization. *Plast Reconstr Surg* 1972;49:268-274.
2. Shaw WW: Microvascular free flaps: The first decade. *Clin Plast Surg* 1983;10:3-20.
3. Mathes SJ, Alpert BS, Chang N: Use of the muscle flap in chronic osteomyelitis: Experimental and clinical correlation. *Plast Reconstr Surg* 1982;69:815-828.
4. Weiland AJ, Moore JR, Daniel RK: The efficacy of free tissue transfer in the treatment of osteomyelitis. *J Bone Joint Surg Am* 1984;66:181-192.
5. Seidenberg B, Rosenak SS, Hurwitt ES, et al: Immediate reconstruction of the cervical esophagus by a vascularized isolated jejunal segment. *Ann Surg* 1959;149:162-171.
6. Coleman JJ, Searles JM, Hester TR, et al: Ten years experience with free jejunal autograft. *Am J Surg* 1987;154:394-398.
7. Swartz WM, Mears DC: The role of free-tissue transfers in lower extremity reconstruction. *Plast Reconstr Surg* 1985;76:364-373.
8. Ger R: The operative treatment of the advanced stasis ulcer: A preliminary communication. *Am J Surg* 1966;111:659-663.
9. Mathes S, Nahai F: *Clinical Atlas of Muscle and Musculocutaneous Flaps.* St Louis, CV Mosby Co, 1979.
10. McCraw JB, Dibbell DG, Carraway JH: Clinical definition of independent myocutaneous vascular territories. *Plast Reconstr Surg* 1977;60:341-352.
11. Taylor GI, Townsend P, Corlett RJ: The superiority of the deep circumflex iliac vessels as the supply for free groin flaps: Clinical work. *Plast Surg* 1979;64:745-759.
12. Ponten B: The fasciocutaneous flap: Its use in soft tissue defects of the lower leg. *Br J Plast Surg* 1981;34:215-220.

The Role of Isolated Profundaplasty for the Treatment of Rest Pain

David M. McCoy, MD; Alan P. Sawchuk, MD; James J. Schuler, MD; Joseph R. Durham, MD; Jens Eldrup-Jorgensen, MD; Thomas H. Schwarcz, MD; Joseph P. Meyer, MD; D. Preston Flanigan, MD

• This study was undertaken to determine the efficacy and durability of profundaplasty and define preoperative factors predictive of success. The hospital charts, vascular laboratory data, and arteriograms of 20 patients having 21 isolated profundaplasties for ischemic rest pain between 1979 and 1987 were reviewed. Follow-up extended to 72 months (mean, 26 months). Early success was achieved in 12 extremities (57%) and life-table analysis showed continued success to six years in 11 extremities (55%). Of the multiple preoperative factors assessed, only a low-thigh/ankle gradient pressure index (TAGI) of less than 0.55 was predictive of success. Life-table analysis for limbs with a TAGI of less than 0.55 showed an 89% success rate at six years compared with only a 32% success rate for limbs with a TAGI of more than 0.55. Isolated profundaplasty for the treatment of ischemic rest pain can be an efficacious and durable procedure when patients are selected based on objective hemodynamic measurements.

(*Arch Surg* 1989;124:441-444)

The profunda femoris artery is the primary source of collateral flow to the lower extremity in the presence of superficial femoral and/or popliteal occlusion. Arterial reconstruction of the profunda femoris to relieve limb-threatening ischemia was first reported by Morris et al[1] in 1961. Profundaplasty is now usually employed in conjunction with aortofemoral or femoral-femoral bypass in patients with combined aortoiliac and superficial femoropopliteal occlusive disease. Profundaplasty is infrequently employed as an isolated procedure to relieve limb-threatening ischemia, and the limb salvage rate following isolated profundaplasty has varied from 23%[2] to 83%.[3] This article reports our experience with profundaplasty as a sole procedure for the relief of limb-threatening ischemic rest pain and assesses the accuracy of various preoperative hemodynamic measurements used as predictors of limb salvage.

PATIENTS, MATERIALS, AND METHODS

Between 1979 and 1987, 20 patients underwent 21 isolated profundaplasties for relief of ischemic rest pain on the vascular surgery services at the University of Illinois, Westside Veterans Administration, and Cook County hospitals, Chicago. Demographic and atherosclerotic risk factors are included in Tables 1 and 2. Patients were admitted to the hospital with a chief complaint of rest pain, and no patient had tissue loss when profundaplasty was performed. The duration of rest pain extended from two weeks to five months with a mean duration of 36 days. Fourteen patients had previously undergone 15 vascular reconstructive procedures related to the involved limb (Table 3).

Preoperative evaluation consisted of Doppler-derived blood pressures at the high-thigh, low-thigh, calf, and ankle levels. Three segmental pressure gradient indexes were then calculated from the Doppler-derived segmental pressures for each patient: (1) the low-thigh/ankle gradient pressure index (TAGI) calculated as the (low-thigh pressure–ankle pressure)/low-thigh pressure; (2) the profundapopliteal collateral index (PPCI) calculated as the (low-thigh pressure–calf pressure)/low-thigh pressure; and (3) the tibial gradient index (TG) calculated as the (calf pressure–ankle pressure)/calf pressure (Fig 1).

Fourteen of the 21 preoperative angiograms were obtained and evaluated using the recommendations of the Ad Hoc Committee on Reporting Standards of the Society for Vascular Surgery, to assess the quality of runoff arteries.[4] This system grades both the degree of stenosis and the relative contribution to outflow of each vessel, with the scale of disease ranging from 1 to 10 (with 1 signifying the least amount of disease and 10 signifying the greatest amount of disease). Oblique and lateral angiograms of the profunda femoris artery were not routinely performed preoperatively and, therefore, a calculation of the percent of stenosis of the profunda femoris artery could only be roughly estimated by evaluation of the anteroposterior roentgenograms.

A successful outcome was defined as the relief of rest pain and continued limb salvage for at least three months postoperatively. Patients who achieved a successful outcome (group A) were then compared with patients who did not achieve a successful outcome (group B).

The short- and long-term effects of isolated profundaplasty on rest pain and limb salvage were statistically analyzed by life-table and log-rank analyses (SAS).[5] Preoperative factors possibly predicting a successful outcome were analyzed using the Cox proportional hazards model of logistic regression (SAS). Results were interpreted as being statistically significant when $P<.05$.

RESULTS

There was no operative mortality, and the only complication consisted of one superficial wound infection. In the immediate postoperative period, 14 (67%) of 21 patients reported an improvement in rest pain, six patients (28%) reported no improvement in rest pain, and one patient (5%) reported a worsening of rest pain. There were 11 patients in group A (successful) and nine patients in group B (failure). One patient who reported immediate improvement in rest pain was subsequently unavailable for follow-up. Ten (91%) of 11 patients in group A reported immediate and continued improvement in rest pain, whereas three (33%) of nine patients in group B reported immediate improvement in rest pain that was not sustained at three months.

All nine patients in group B required at least one subsequent operative procedure. The procedures required consisted of one above-knee and five below-knee amputations, two femorotibial bypasses, and one femoropopliteal bypass. These procedures were performed between the first and 90th postoperative day with a mean of 26 days between the initial profundaplasty and the subsequent

Accepted for publication Oct 6, 1988.

From the Department of Surgery, Division of Vascular Surgery, University of Illinois College of Medicine at Chicago; and Westside Veterans Administration Medical Center and Cook County Hospital, Chicago. Dr Flanigan is now in private practice in Orange, Calif.

Read before the 12th Annual Surgical Symposium of the Association of Veterans Administration Surgeons, Minneapolis, May 12, 1988.

Reprint requests to Division of Vascular Surgery (m/c 957), University of Illinois at Chicago, 1740 W Taylor St, Suite 2200, Chicago, IL 60612 (Dr Schuler).

Table 1.—Demographic Factors

Factors	Patients, No. (%)
Age, y	
>60	16 (80)
<60	4 (20)
M	16 (80)
F	4 (20)

Table 2.—Risk Factors

Factors	Patients, No. (%)
Smoking	18 (90)
Diabetes	8 (40)
Hypertension	9 (45)

Table 3.—Previous Vascular Procedures

Procedure	No. of Patients
Aortobifemoral bypass	4
Femoropopliteal bypass	6
Superficial femoral artery angioplasty	1
Superficial femoral artery endarterectomy	1
Femoroinfrapopliteal bypass	3

procedure. The indications for additional procedures were continued or worsening rest pain in all nine patients, with four of the nine patients also exhibiting signs of early forefoot gangrene.

Follow-up extended to 72 months (mean, 26 months) and was 95% complete. The overall limb salvage rate for the 21 profundaplasties performed was 71%. Early success, as defined by relief of rest pain and continued limb salvage to at least three months postoperatively, was achieved in 12 extremities (57%). Life-table analysis showed continued success to six years in 11 extremities (55%) (Fig 2).

Possible preoperative predictors of success were evaluated and statistically analyzed using Cox proportional hazards multivariate logistic regression. The mean duration of rest pain (46 days, group A; 26 days, group B) and the presence or absence of diabetes or hypertension had no significant effect on the outcome ($P=.19$, .62, and .35, respectively). For all patients in the study, the mean preoperative low-thigh brachial index was 0.54, the mean calf brachial index was 0.26, the mean ankle brachial index was 0.21, and the mean foot brachial index was 0. Table 4 includes the mean preoperative pressure indexes at the low-thigh, calf, and ankle levels for groups A and B as well as the calculated P values for each anatomic level. None of the preoperative pressure indexes had a statistically significant effect on outcome of the procedure.

Evaluation of the preoperative angiograms revealed that eight patients had a runoff score of less than 5 at the popliteal level whereas six patients had a score of more than 5 at this level. Evaluation of the trifurcation and distal tibial vessels showed that all 14 patients had a score of more than 5 with a mean value of 8.5 signifying significant distal runoff disease. The mean runoff scores for preoperative angiograms at the popliteal and trifurcation and distal levels were 5.5 and 8.0 for group A and 6.8 and 9.2 for group B, respectively. Neither of these angiographic scores at these two levels had any effect on outcome ($P=.97$ and .26, respectively). The mean percent of stenosis at the origin of the profunda femoris artery was 53% for group A vs 50% for group B with no effect on outcome ($P=.72$).

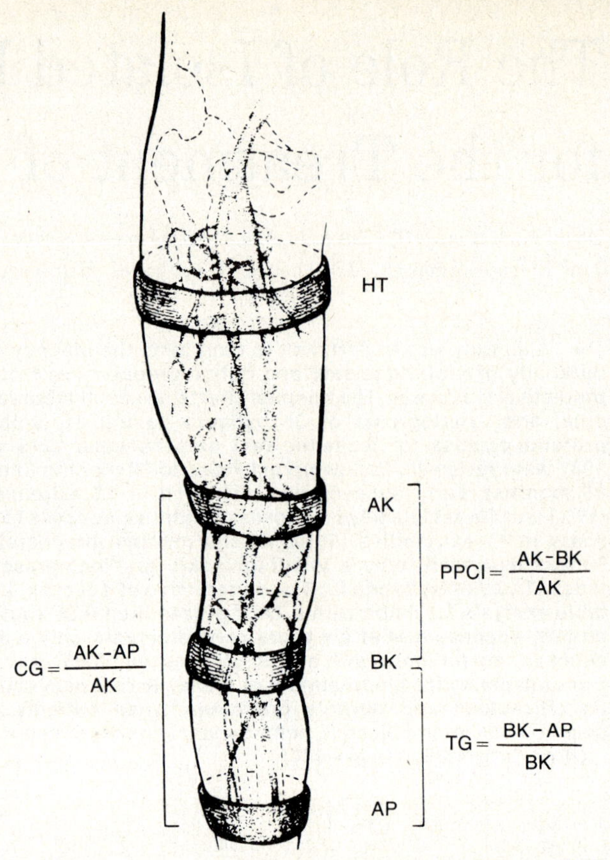

Fig 1.—Determination of segmental pressure gradient indexes from preoperative segmental pressure measurements. CG indicates combined gradient index; PPCI, profundapopliteal collateral index; TG, tibial gradient index; AK, above-knee pressure; BK, below-knee pressure; HT, high thigh; and AP, ankle pressure. CG = thigh/ankle gradient pressure index (from Boren et al[7]).

Intraoperative records showed that the mean length of the profundaplasty performed was 5.6 cm, with 50% of the profunda arteries being endarterectomized. Saphenous vein, polytef (PTFE), endarterectomized superficial femoral artery, or Dacron was used to patch the profunda artery. Neither the length of the profundaplasty nor whether an endarterectomy was performed nor the type of patch material used had any bearing on outcome ($P=.49$, .43, and .45, respectively).

The mean PPCI for all patients was 0.43, and the mean TG for all patients was 0.17. The mean PPCI for group A was 0.28 compared with 0.64 for group B. This index had a P value tending toward significance when evaluated for its effect on outcome ($P=.10$). The mean TG was 0.14 for group A and 0.27 for group B. Multivariate logistic regression showed this index also tended toward predicting a significant effect on outcome ($P=.13$).

The mean TAGI for all patients was 0.53 (SD, 0.37). However, the mean TAGI in group A was 0.39 compared with 0.79 in group B. Multivariate logistic regression showed that the difference between those patients who had a successful outcome (group A) and those who failed (group B) had a calculated P value that was statistically significant ($P=.043$, likelihood ratio test for significance), implying that the lower the TAGI, the better the chances of achieving a successful outcome. Eight of 11 patients in group A had a TAGI of less than 0.55, whereas six of seven patients in

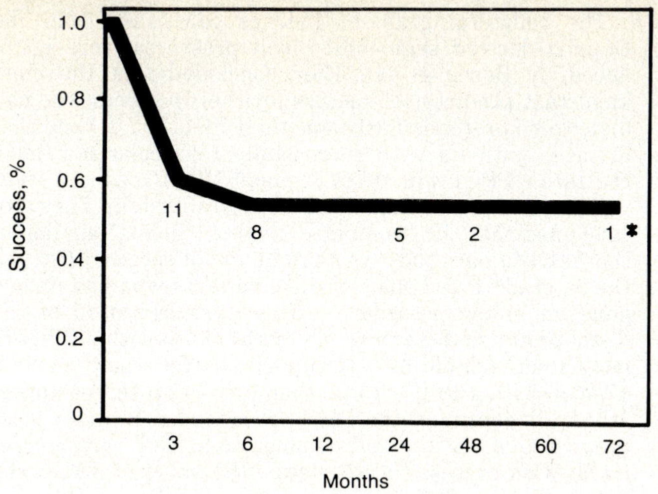

Fig 2.—Life-table analysis for all patients who underwent profundaplasty. Asterisk indicates effective size of patient population.

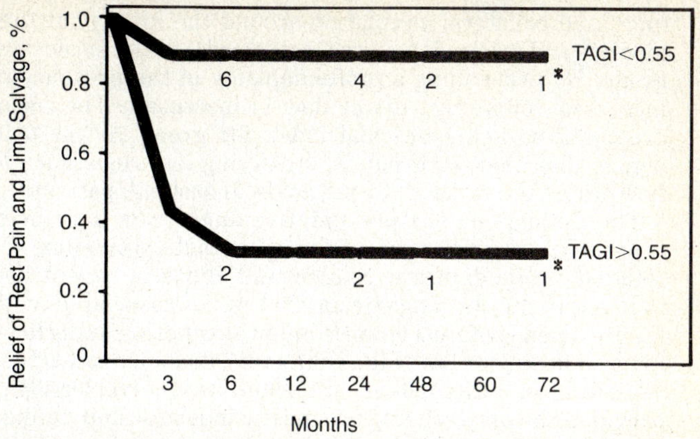

Fig 3.—Life-table comparison of thigh/ankle gradient index (TAGI). Asterisk indicates effective size of patient population. $P = .01$ (log-rank test).

Table 4.—Preoperative Factors*

Factors	Group A	Group B	*P*
Rest pain duration, d	46	26	.19
Diabetes, No. of patients	5	3	.62
Hypertension, No. of patients	5	4	.35
Low-thigh brachial index	0.48	0.60	.13
Calf brachial index	0.33	0.22	.17
Ankle brachial index	0.29	0.13	.11

*Cox proportional hazards model of logistic regression (SAS[5]).

Table 5.—Success Rates of Isolated Profundaplasty

Source	Year	%
Martin and Jamieson[15]	1974	67
Thompson et al[17]	1976	54
Modgill et al[3]	1977	83
Ward and Morris-Jones[13]	1977	40
Hull et al[6]	1978	33
Mitchell et al[11]	1979	50
Sladen and Burgess[10]	1980	67
Boren et al[7]	1980	48
Taylor et al[12]	1981	71
Towne et al[8]	1981	23

group B had a TAGI of more than 0.55. Life-table analysis for limbs with a TAGI of less than 0.55 showed an 89% success rate at six years compared with only a 32% success rate for limbs with a TAGI of more than 0.55 ($P = .01$ log-rank test) (Fig 3). Decision matrix analysis showed that a TAGI of less than 0.55 had a sensitivity of 89%, a specificity of 67%, an accuracy of 78%, a positive predictive value of 73%, and a negative predictive value of 86%.

COMMENT

Isolated profundaplasty is considered a relatively easy operation with minimal morbidity and mortality even when performed in high-risk patients who have undergone previous vascular procedures. This fact is borne out in our study in which 21 profundaplasties resulted in no mortality and a morbidity of 5%.

Hull et al,[6] Boren et al,[7] and Towne et al[8] stated that the possible benefit of profundaplasty may very well be to lower the amputation level from the above-knee to the below-knee level by increasing collateral flow through the profunda sytstem in patients in whom profundaplasty fails to achieve limb salvage. The overall mean increase in the calf brachial index in our study following profundaplasty was 0.23. Those patients in group B who subsequently required a below-knee amputation had a mean increase in the calf brachial index of 0.21, thus lending support to the concept that even if the limb cannot be salvaged, profundaplasty does substantially increase below-knee pressures probably enough to retain the knee and heal a below-knee amputation.

In our study, isolated profundaplasty for the relief of rest pain resulted in a success rate of 55% and a limb salvage rate of 71%. These rates agree with those in other reported series in the literature that indicate that the success rate of profundaplasty varies from 23% to 83% (Table 5).

Therefore, as can be seen from various series, isolated profundaplasty for rest pain/limb salvage has approximately a 50% chance of being successful. Because of this relatively low success rate, a variety of preoperative clinical, hemodynamic, and angiographic criteria have been evaluated in an attempt to predict which patients would achieve long-term limb salvage following isolated profundaplasty.[7,9-11]

The mean duration of rest pain was 20 days longer in group A than in group B. Although this preoperative variable did not have a statistically significant effect on outcome ($P = .18$), one may speculate that the longer the duration of symptoms preoperatively, the better the development of a collateral bed around the knee joint. Contrary to this, the small series of Rutledge and Burnham[9] (eight patients with rest pain) showed that the only patients who achieved a successful outcome from the procedure (two patients) were those who presented with the acute onset of rest pain.

Although the preoperative Doppler-derived segmental blood pressures had no statistically significant predictive value on the outcome of the procedure, it is interesting to compare the mean preoperative calf and ankle brachial indexes in groups A and B. The mean preoperative calf brachial index for group A was 0.13 higher than that for group B. This higher pressure at the calf level signifies increased collateral circulation around the knee joint (geniculate and profundapopliteal collaterals) in the successful group. By performing a profundaplasty in the presence of increased collaterals, distal flow is increased. The mean preoperative ankle brachial index for group A was 0.16 higher than that for group B, signifying less resistance to flow from the low thigh to the ankle in group A patients.

The findings on the preoperative angiogram have been reported to be important as far as predicting outcome for isolated profundaplasty. Sladen and Burgess[10] identified four signs on the angiogram that were associated with failure: open profunda femoris inflow, competing superficial femoral flow, poor low-thigh collaterals, and poor calf artery visualization. Mitchell et al[11] found that arteriography provided the only reliable prognostic indicator and defined the following favorable signs: profunda orifice stenosis, minimal distal profunda occlusive disease, disease-free profunda collaterals, reconstitution of collaterals into a patent superficial femoral or popliteal artery, and good popliteal outflow. Taylor et al[12] noted that the complete absence of collateral vessels around the knee was associated with an unsuccessful result. Contrary to this, Ward and Morris-Jones[13] stated that the degree of preoperative profunda stenosis and distal runoff had no influence on the clinical outcome. Berguer et al,[14] analyzing the geometry of the profunda femoris artery, stated that in the presence of an occluded superficial femoral artery, even an apparently undiseased deep femoral artery represents an inflow stenosis of 50% and that even minimal disease in the deep femoral artery (0.5- to 1.0-mm thickening) considerably increases the percent of stenosis. Therefore, they concluded that the apparent absence of disease at the deep femoral artery on the preoperative angiogram is not a contraindication to performing a profundaplasty.

Unfortunately, we were unable to accurately measure percent of profunda stenosis on the preoperative angiogram. We do believe, however, that profundaplasty performed on a deep femoral artery with a higher percent of stenosis should result in a better outcome. Also, although this was not performed routinely in our patients intraoperatively, measurement of the pressure gradient between the area immediately proximal to the deep femoral artery stenosis and the area distal to this stenosis should reveal valuable information as to the applicability of performing a profundaplasty. The higher the pressure gradient, the better the results of the procedure should be. We believe a high pressure gradient along with adequate collateral outflow around the knee distally are prerequisites for the relief of rest pain and limb salvage following profundaplasty. The runoff status of the popliteal and trifurcation system of group B was worse than that of group A on the preoperative angiogram (6.8 and 9.2 vs 5.5 and 8.0, respectively) and although this difference was not statistically significant, one would expect that a less diseased popliteal and distal runoff system improves the chances that the procedure will work.

This study shows that those patients who reported an immediate improvement in rest pain postoperatively attained long-term success from the procedure (ten of 11 patients, 91% in group A), whereas in those patients who reported no improvement or worsening of their rest pain postoperatively (six of nine patients, 67%) in group B, the procedure was ultimately a failure. We have found no mention of this specific postoperative subjective indicator in the literature except by Martin and Jamieson,[15] who stated that it becomes necessary to rely on the patients' symptoms to ascertain the success of the operation and that this index is not very reliable.

The collateral gradient indexes calculated from the Doppler-derived segmental blood pressures were introduced by Boren et al.[7] They concluded that the most important predictor of success for their patients who had undergone profundaplasty was the PPCI ($P<.01$) and that in those patients with successfully revascularized limbs the mean PPCI was 0.18. A small PPCI means a well-vascularized profundapopliteal collateral system. They also concluded that the "combined gradient index," similar to the TAGI in our study, was predictive of success ($P<.01$). Ouriel et al[16] found that, of their patients who had undergone an inflow procedure with revascularization of the distal profunda femoris artery, eight of ten with a PPCI of more than 0.25 did not attain a successful result whereas 17 of 20 with a PPCI of less than 0.25 improved postoperatively. In our study, the TAGI proved to be the index most predictive of success and demonstrated an inverse correlation with success, ie, the lower the value of TAGI, the better the chance of relief of rest pain following isolated profundaplasty ($P=.04$). By calculating the TAGI, one is able to estimate the resistance of the tibial vessels. If the resistance between the vessels of the low thigh and the ankle is low, more nutrient blood will be carried to the foot and, therefore, increase the probability of alleviating rest pain. Those patients whose TAGI was less than 0.55 and who also experienced relief of their rest pain benefited from the procedure for up to six years.

Our results tend to agree with those of other series, ie, approximately 50% of patients who undergo an isolated profundaplasty for rest pain will be benefited by the procedure. Because of this less than acceptable success rate, the task facing vascular surgeons is to define those subsets of patients who will benefit most from isolated profundaplasty by careful evaluation of preoperative hemodynamic factors.

References

1. Morris G, Edwards W, Cooley DA, et al: Surgical importance of the profunda femoris artery. *Arch Surg* 1961;82:32-37.
2. Morris-Jones W, Jones CDP: Profundaplasty in the treatment of femoropopliteal occlusion. *Am J Surg* 1974;127:680-686.
3. Modgill VK, Humphrey CS, Shoesmith JH, et al: The value of profundaplasty in the management of severe femoropopliteal occlusion. *Br J Surg* 1977;64:362-364.
4. Rutherford RB, Flanigan DP, Gupta SK, et al: Suggested standards for reports dealing with lower extremity ischemia. *J Vasc Surg* 1986;4:80-94.
5. *SAS User's Guide*. Cary, NC, SAS Institute, 1985.
6. Hull DA, Babcock GK, Hyde GL, et al: Femoral artery profundaplasty. *Am J Surg* 1978;136:356-358.
7. Boren CH, Towne JB, Bernhard VM, et al: Profundapopliteal collateral index: A guide to successful profundaplasty. *Arch Surg* 1980;115:1366-1372.
8. Towne JB, Bernhard VM, Rollins DL, et al: Profundaplasty in perspective: Limitations in the long-term management of limb ischemia. *Surgery* 1981;6:1037-1045.
9. Rutledge R, Burnham SJ: Profundaplasty in the ischemic extremity. *J Cardiovasc Surg* 1983;24:107-110.
10. Sladen JG, Burgess JJ: Profundaplasty: Expectations and ominous signs. *Am J Surg* 1980;140:242-245.
11. Mitchell RA, Bone GE, Bridges R, et al: Patient selection for isolated profundaplasty. *Am J Surg* 1979;138:912-918.
12. Taylor LM, Bauer GM, Eidemiller LR, et al: Extended profundaplasty. *Am J Surg* 1981;141:539-542.
13. Ward S, Morris-Jones W: The long-term results of profundaplasty in femoropopliteal arterial occlusion. *Br J Surg* 1977;64:365-367.
14. Berguer R, Higgins RF, Cotton LT: Geometry, blood flow, and reconstruction of the deep femoral artery. *Am J Surg* 1975;130:68-73.
15. Martin P, Jamieson C: The rationale for measurement after profundaplasty. *Surg Clin North Am* 1974;54:95-109.
16. Ouriel K, DeWeese JA, Ricotta JJ, et al: Revascularization of the distal profunda femoris artery in the reconstructive treatment of aortoiliac disease. *J Vasc Surg* 1987;6:217-220.
17. Thompson BW, Read RC, Campbell GS, et al: The role of profundaplasty in revascularization of the lower extremity. *Am J Surg* 1976;132:710-715.

Recombinant Human Tumor Necrosis Factor Produces Hemodynamic Changes Characteristic of Sepsis and Endotoxemia

William J. Schirmer, MD; James M. Schirmer; Donald E. Fry, MD

• Tumor necrosis factor (TNF) is a macrophage-derived peptide mediator released during endotoxemia and sepsis. We examined the systemic and visceral hemodynamic response to low doses of human recombinant TNF in rats. Each animal received a 30-minute intravenous infusion of either saline solution (n=8) or TNF (n=8) in a dose of 0.25 mg/kg or 1.0 mg/kg. Thermodilution cardiac output, blood pressure, pulse, vascular resistance, effective hepatic blood flow (galactose clearance), and effective renal plasma flow (*p*-aminohippurate clearance) were determined at time=2 hours. The 0.25-mg/kg dose had no apparent effect on systemic hemodynamics. The 1.0-mg/kg dose produced a hyperdynamic systemic circulatory response with an elevated cardiac output, tachycardia, and a diminished systemic vascular resistance. Effective hepatic blood flow was exquisitely sensitive to even the lowest dose of TNF, with a 29% reduction despite the normal cardiac output. Renal flow was unaffected by either dose. Tumor necrosis factor–induced systemic and visceral hemodynamic changes are remarkably similar to those seen in gram-negative sepsis, suggesting that TNF may occupy a proximal position in the pathogenesis of overwhelming infection.

(*Arch Surg* 1989;124:445-448)

Bacterial endotoxin administration produces a characteristic sequence of metabolic and hemodynamic alterations, culminating in widespread organ dysfunction, shock, and death. It is becoming increasingly evident that endotoxin itself does not directly damage host tissue; organ injury is the consequence of the ensuing activation of multiple humoral and cellular inflammatory mediators. Macrophages appear to occupy a pivotal position in this pathologic process. It has been shown that agents that stimulate reticuloendothelial hyperplasia render animals more susceptible to the lethal effects of endotoxin.[1] Furthermore, when harvested macrophages from endotoxin-sensitive mice are exposed to endotoxin, they produce a soluble factor that kills endotoxin-resistant mice.[2]

Tumor necrosis factor (TNF) is a macrophage-derived peptide mediator, the release of which is stimulated by endotoxin.[3] Animals given large doses of TNF develop hemodynamic collapse, hemoconcentration, metabolic acidosis, and widespread tissue damage.[4,5] Rats passively immunized against TNF are protected against endotoxin's lethal effects.[6] These observations suggest that TNF may be a primary mediator of shock and tissue injury during endotoxemia.

Whether TNF is a significant pathologic mediator during sepsis is not clear. In gram-negative sepsis, cardiac output is elevated and systemic vascular resistance is reduced, the reverse of what happens during endotoxemia. Lactic acidemia emerges prior to, rather than after, circulatory collapse.[7] Sepsis is further characterized by a redistribution of blood flow with reductions in hepatic and renal perfusion, which precede and appear to precipitate organ failure.[8,9] This study was undertaken to determine whether sublethal doses of TNF produce the earlier and more subtle perfusion abnormalities characteristic of hyperdynamic sepsis.

MATERIALS AND METHODS

Female Sprague-Dawley rats weighing 250 to 350 g were anesthetized with ketamine hydrochloride (5 mg/kg) and xylazine hydrochloride (37.5 mg/kg) by intraperitoneal injection. The right external jugular vein was cannulated with a 15-cm length of saline solution–filled polyethylene tubing passed centrally to the level of the right atrium. Each rat received a 1-mL/kg intravenous infusion of either saline (n=8) or human recombinant TNF (H-rTNF) in doses of 0.25 μg/g (n=8) or 1.0 μg/g (n=8) over a 30-minute period. Hemodynamics were determined by methods outlined below at time=2 hours after infusion.

Systemic Hemodynamics

A thermistor (YSI-511, Yellow Springs Instruments, Yellow Springs, Ohio) was inserted into each rat's aortic arch via the left

Accepted for publication Oct 6, 1988.

From the Departments of Surgery, Veterans Administration Medical Center and Case Western Reserve University Hospitals, Cleveland. Dr W. J. Schirmer is a Dudley P. Allen Fellow in surgical research of Case Western Reserve University Hospitals. Dr Fry is now with the Department of Surgery, University of New Mexico, Albuquerque.

Read before the 12th Annual Surgical Symposium of the Association of Veterans Administration Surgeons, Minneapolis, May 12, 1988.

Reprint requests to Department of Surgery 112W, Veterans Administration Medical Center, 10701 East Blvd, Cleveland, OH 44106 (Dr W. J. Schirmer).

Systemic Hemodynamics*

TNF Dose, mg/kg	Cardiac Output,† mL/min/100 g	Mean Arterial Pressure, mm Hg	Heart Rate, Beats per Minute	Systemic Vascular Resistance, mm Hg/mL/min/100 g	Hematocrit
Sham control	38.0±1.1	96.5±8.2	291.0±6.3	2.55±0.23	0.409±0.006
0.25	39.5±1.4	97.5±5.7	292.3±6.0	2.51±0.23	0.417±0.005
1.0	44.9±1.5†	88.9±3.6	325.5±9.2†	2.00±0.12‡	0.405±0.012

*Summary of changes in systemic hemodynamic variables at t = 2 hours induced by graded, sublethal doses of human recombinant tumor necrosis factor (TNF). While the lower TNF dose had no appreciable effect on systemic hemodynamics, the higher dose produced a hyperdynamic response characterized by an elevated cardiac output, tachycardia, and a diminished systemic vascular resistance. Values are given as mean ± SEM.

†$P<.01$ vs both other groups.

‡$P<.05$ vs both other groups.

common carotid artery shortly after the beginning of the intravenous infusion. Core body temperature was maintained within a range of 37°C ± 0.5°C by means of an infrared lamp. Thermodilution cardiac output (CO) was determined by the method of Isoyama et al[10] at time = 2 hours. A 0.15-mL bolus of room-temperature saline solution was rapidly injected via the central venous line, and the thermodilution curve was recorded from the thermistor tip to a dynagraph (Beckman R612, Beckman Instruments, Anaheim, Calif). Cardiac output was calculated as previously described by averaging duplicate curves and was expressed as milliliters per minute per 100 g of body weight.[10]

The aortic thermistor was removed and replaced with saline solution–filled polyethylene tubing. Mean arterial pressure (MAP) and heart rate (HR) were recorded via strain gauge to the dynagraph. Mean arterial pressure is expressed in millimeters of mercury and HR in beats per minute. Systemic vascular resistance was calculated by dividing MAP by CO, expressed in millimeters of mercury per milliliter per minute per 100 g of body weight. Hematocrit value was determined by centrifugation of a microcapillary tube of arterial blood. External body temperature was maintained within a range of 36°C ± 0.5°C.

Effective Hepatic and Renal Blood Flows

Effective hepatic blood flow (EHBF) was determined by the recently validated technique of galactose clearance at low concentrations.[8,11] Effective renal blood flow (ERBF) was determined by clearance of *p*-aminohippurate (PAH). Each rat received a priming intravenous dose of galactose (2.6 mg) and PAH (3.2 mg) combined in a 1.0-mL solution of saline at time = 90 minutes, followed immediately by a continuous intravenous infusion of galactose (13 mg/mL) and PAH (3.2 mg/mL) in saline solution via a Harvard pump at 0.04 mL/min.

Immediately following determination of systemic hemodynamics, five 100-μL arterial blood samples were collected into 1.1 mL of 62 mmol/L of sodium fluoride at five-minute intervals. The samples were centrifuged and the supernatant was frozen at −70°C until assay for galactose, which was performed by a manual adaptation of the automated fluorometric method of Henderson and Fales as described elsewhere.[8,12] Effective hepatic blood flow was calculated utilizing the Fick principle by the following equation: EHBF = I/css, where I indicates the infusion rate of galactose and css indicates the steady-state galactose concentration. Values are expressed in milliliters per minute per 100 g of body weight.

Four arterial blood samples were similarly collected at ten-minute intervals following a minimum of 60 minutes of equilibration for PAH assay. The 100-μL samples were immediately deproteinized in 200 μL of 5.1% perchloric acid. After centrifugation, the supernatants were frozen at −70°C until assay. The concentration of PAH was determined by spectrophotometric techniques described elsewhere.[13] Renal plasma flow was determined in a fashion analogous to that for EHBF, with the PAH infusion rate and concentration substituted for those of galactose in the preceding equation.

Statistics

Data are reported as the mean ± SEM. Between-group differences were determined by an analysis of variance followed by a Newman-Kuels multiple range test. Differences are reported as significant at either $P<.05$ or $P<.01$ confidence levels.

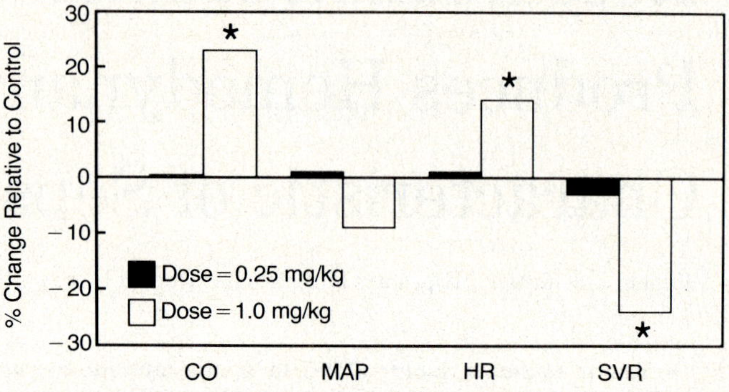

Fig 1.—Summary of percent change in systemic hemodynamic variables induced by graded, sublethal doses of tumor necrosis factor relative to sham control. Elevated cardiac output (CO) and pulse and diminished systemic vascular resistance (SVR) following higher tumor necrosis factor dose mimic hemodynamic pattern in gram-negative septicemia. Asterisks indicate $P<.01$ or $P<.05$ vs sham control (see Table for numerical data); MAP, mean arterial pressure; and HR, heart rate.

RESULTS

The systemic hemodynamic responses to the two doses of H-rTNF are compared with sham control values in the Table. The 0.25-mg/kg dose of H-rTNF had no appreciable effect on systemic hemodynamics. The 1.0-mg/kg dose caused a significant elevation in CO ($P<.01$) and HR ($P<.01$), and a reduction in systemic vascular resistance ($P<.05$). Mean arterial pressure remained relatively stable and the hematocrit value was unaffected, suggesting that fluid shifts were minor and, therefore, an unlikely influence on hemodynamics. Figure 1 graphically demonstrates how similarly the hemodynamic pattern induced by the higher H-rTNF dose mimics the hyperdynamic response typical of gram-negative sepsis, ie, tachycardia, elevated CO, and reduced peripheral vascular resistance.

The effects of the two H-rTNF doses on EHBF are graphically compared with a sham control value in Fig 2. Unlike systemic hemodynamics, EHBF appears to be exquisitely sensitive to even small doses of H-rTNF. The lowest dose of H-rTNF resulted in hepatic blood flow reduction ($P<.01$), despite the normal CO. In absolute terms, the higher dose affected EHBF to roughly the same degree as the lower dose, although relative to CO, EHBF seemed to be even further reduced. In contradistinction to liver flow, ERBF is unaffected by either dose of H-rTNF (Fig 3). Indeed, the trend suggested that H-rTNF may increase ERBF, although the differences did not achieve statistical significance.

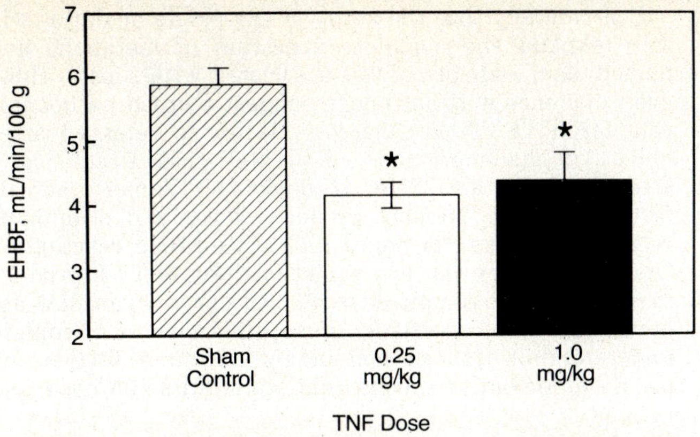

Fig 2.—Effective hepatic blood flow (EHBF) plotted as function of tumor necrosis factor (TNF) dose. Effective hepatic blood flow appears to be exquisitely sensitive to TNF, as indicated by fall in EHBF following lower TNF dose despite fact that systemic hemodynamics were unaffected. Fall in EHBF following higher TNF dose is more dramatic given fact that cardiac output actually increased. Asterisks indicate $P<.01$ vs sham control.

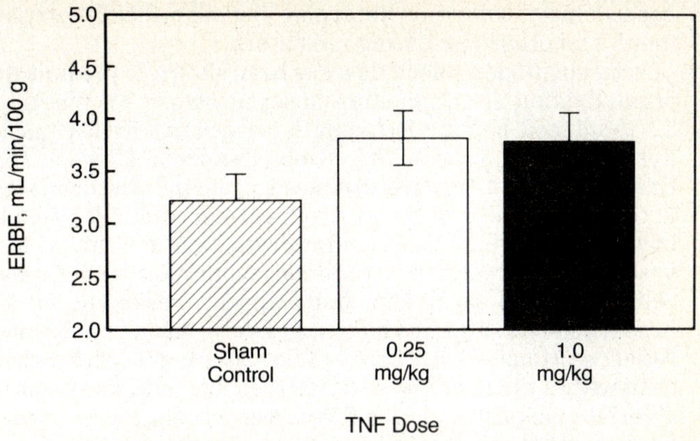

Fig 3.—Effective renal blood flow (ERBF) plotted as function of tumor necrosis factor (TNF) dose. Unlike liver flow, ERPF remained unaffected by either dose of TNF.

COMMENT

Sepsis can be divided into various phases, beginning with the introduction of the offending organism into the circulatory system, followed by the initial activation of circulating inflammatory systems, and, finally, the full-blown activation of the host-defense response. Multiple organ injury does not become apparent until well after the full-blown response has been activated.[14] Macrophage-derived products may be particularly important mediators of the preorgan failure state. It is well documented that fever during gram-negative sepsis is mediated by interleukin 1, another macrophage-derived biologic response modifier.[15] Evidence is mounting that suggests that TNF is also a critical mediator of the septic response.

Tracey et al[4,5] reported that high TNF doses produce hemodynamic collapse, hemoconcentration, metabolic acidosis, and multiple organ injury in both rats and dogs. Typical histopathologic changes reported after TNF administration include extensive acute inflammation, capillary thrombosis, and focal necrosis in multiple vital organ beds.[4,5,16] It was suggested that the syndrome of lethal shock and multiple organ injury, which occurs during endotoxemia, could be elicited by TNF.[5] However, both the biochemical and histologic abnormalities were seen only with large TNF doses and only after profound alterations in systemic perfusion. It is quite plausible that the peripheral disturbances were simply the result of systemic circulatory collapse. Such a pattern is much different from that observed during true gram-negative sepsis, in which organ dysfunction and organ injury emerge in the face of an elevated, rather than a depressed, CO.

In our study, TNF given in sublethal doses produced the more-subtle hemodynamic alterations characteristic of sepsis. The 1.0-mg/kg TNF dose produced an elevated CO and a depressed systemic vascular resistance, and at the same time, reduced EHBF—a blood flow pattern remarkably similar to early sepsis.[8,9] Such a hyperdynamic state can also be produced by giving carefully titrated doses of endogenously administered endotoxin. Tumor necrosis factor is released during endotoxemia and bacteremia.[17,18] Our study suggests that TNF may occupy a proximal position in the pathogenesis of both sepsis and endotoxemia.

Hepatic blood flow appears to be exquisitely sensitive to TNF. In studies of septic rats, we found that EHBF fell despite a normal to elevated CO.[8,9,19] The role of impaired nutrient flow in the cause of organ dysfunction in sepsis has been previously established.[8,9,19-21] Mediators, including arachidonic acid metabolites, complement components, oxygen radicals, the coagulation system, neutrophils, and platelets, seem to be involved to one degree or another in these hepatic flow changes. The question naturally arises whether TNF contributes significantly to the pathologic changes during sepsis. Studies concerning the interruption of TNF synthesis or the inhibition of its action are required to clarify this issue.

The effects of TNF appear to be organ specific, ie, EHBF is reduced while ERBF remains unaffected. Other studies have shown that the lung appears to be another target organ for TNF-induced injury.[4,5] The liver and lung differ from the kidney in that they are reticuloendothelial organs that harbor large resident macrophage populations. Tumor necrosis factor may either act directly on or perhaps regulate the macrophage release of other pathogenic mediators, the effects of which are felt most keenly within the microenvironment in which they are released. It is of some interest that the acute hemodynamic effects of large doses of TNF are remarkably similar to those of another biological response modifier, interleukin 2. Interleukin 2 causes a vascular leak syndrome that primarily targets the lung, liver, spleen, and thymus.[22] Clarification of the causes of these organ-specific effects may help define the role of TNF in multiple organ systems failure.

In previous studies, we found that infusion of zymosan produced a hemodynamic profile similar to sepsis, ie, elevated CO and reduced hepatic flow, which correlated with the degree of complement activation.[23] However, in subsequent studies in which cobra venom factor was used to activate complement, hepatic blood flow was reduced but systemic hemodynamics remained unaffected.[24] In addition to activating complement, zymosan may stimulate TNF release by both complement-dependent and complement-independent activation of macrophages. Tumor necrosis factor stimulates neutrophil adherence to endothelial cells and enhances leukocyte-mediated killing of infectious organisms, well-organized properties of complement.[25,26] The true explanation for the hemodynamic changes following zymosan infusion (and perhaps for the changes during sepsis) may involve an interplay between TNF, complement, and other circulating mediators.

Altered nutrient blood flow has been shown to precipitate organ dysfunction and failure in septic rats.[8,9,19-21] Whether TNF-induced hepatic ischemia is associated with hepatic dysfunction requires further study. Remick et al[16] reported that TNF given to mice produced profound disturbances in the endothelium of the gastrointestinal tract. The small-bowel villi were flattened and necrotic, and a study of the vasculature revealed neutrophil accumulation, endothelial cell blebs, gap formation, and exposed basement membrane. The measured reduction in EHBF in our study may reflect a primary disturbance of flow at the gut level rather than within the liver per se (EHBF equals nutrient hepatic arterial plus portal venous flow). A great deal of attention has recently been focused on bacterial translocation across the gut as a potential source of ongoing sepsis during multiple organ systems failure.[27,28] The results of our observations of possible gut flow disturbance and endothelial disruption suggest that TNF deserves to be considered a mediator of organ failure.

It is unlikely that the study of any single mediator will fully explain the complete spectrum of metabolic and hemodynamic abnormalities associated with sepsis. However, evidence is mounting to suggest a broad pathogenic role for TNF. Tumor necrosis factor is released after endotoxin challenge, and endotoxin's lethal effects can be attenuated by anti-TNF antibodies.[6,18] Tumor necrosis factor given to humans produces fever and stimulates release of stress hormones and acute-phase reactants.[29] Our study shows that low, sublethal doses of TNF produce systemic hemodynamic changes and early organ flow abnormalities characteristic of sepsis. A more complete understanding of the pathogenic significance of TNF awaits the development of specific inhibitors of its synthesis and actions.

This investigation was supported in part by US Veterans Administration.
Human recombinant tumor necrosis factor was a gift of Genetech Inc, South San Francisco, Calif.

References

1. Vogel SN, Moore RN, Sipe JD, et al: BCG-induced enhancement of endotoxin sensitivity in C3H/HeJ mice. *J Immunol* 1980;124:2004-2009.
2. Cerami A, Ikeda Y, Le Trang N, et al: Weight loss associated with an endotoxin-induced mediator from peritoneal macrophages: The role of cachectin (tumor necrosis factor). *Immunol Lett* 1985;11:173-179.
3. Torti FM, Dievkmann B, Beutler B, et al: A macrophage factor inhibits adipocyte gene expression: An in vitro model of cachexia. *Science* 1985;229:867-869.
4. Tracey KJ, Beutler B, Lowry SF, et al: Shock and tissue injury induced by recombinant human cachectin. *Science* 1986;234:470-474.
5. Tracey KJ, Lowry SF, Fahey TJ, et al: Cachectin/tumor necrosis factor induces lethal shock and stress hormone responses in the dog. *Surg Gynecol Obstet* 1987;164:415-422.
6. Beutler B, Milsark IW, Cerami AC: Passive immunization against cachectin/tumor necrosis factor protects mice from lethal effect of endotoxin. *Science* 1985;229:869-871.
7. Seigel JH, Cerra FB, Coleman B, et al: Physiologic and metabolic correlations in human sepsis. *Surgery* 1979;86:163-193.
8. Schirmer WJ, Townsend MC, Schirmer JM, et al: Galactose elimination kinetics in sepsis: Correlations of hepatic blood flow with function. *Arch Surg* 1987;122:349-354.
9. Townsend MC, Hampton WW, Haybron DM, et al: Effective organ blood flow and bioenergy status in murine peritonitis. *Surgery* 1986;100:205-213.
10. Isoyama T, Soto T, Tanaka J, et al: Measurement of cardiac output in small animals by a thermodilution method. *J Surg Res* 1982;33:153-164.
11. Schirmer WJ, Townsend MC, Schirmer JM, et al: Galactose clearance as an estimate of effective hepatic blood flow: Validation and limitations. *J Surg Res* 1987;41:543-556.
12. Henderson JM, Fales FW: Continuous flow fluorometry of low galactose concentrations in blood or plasma. *Clin Chem* 1983;26:129-132.
13. Smith HW: Measurement of renal clearances, in Smith HW (ed): *Principles of Renal Physiology.* New York, Oxford University Press Inc, 1956, appendix S.
14. Carrico CJ, Meakins JL, Marshall JC, et al: Multiple-organ-failure syndrome. *Arch Surg* 1986;121:196-208.
15. Dinarello CA: Interleukin-1. *Rev Infect Dis* 1984;6:951-984.
16. Remick DG, Kunkel RG, Larrick JW, et al: Acute in vivo effects of human recombinant tumor necrosis factor. *Lab Invest* 1987;56:583-590.
17. Beutler B, Mahoney J, Le Trang N, et al: Purification of cachectin, a lipoprotein lipase suppressing hormone secreted by endotoxin-induced raw 264.7 cells. *J Exp Med* 1985;161:984-995.
18. Beutler B, Milsark IW, Cerami A: Cachectin/tumor necrosis factor. *J Immunol* 1985;135:3972-3979.
19. Hampton WW, Townsend MC, Haybron MC, et al: Effective hepatic blood flow and bioenergy status in murine peritonitis. *J Surg Res* 1987;42:33-38.
20. Asher EF, Rowe RL, Garrison RN, et al: Experimental bacteremia and nutrient hepatic blood flow. *Circ Shock* 1986;20:43-49.
21. Machiedo GW, Hurd T, Rush BF, et al: Temporal relationship of hepatocellular dysfunction and ischemia in sepsis. *Arch Surg* 1988;123:424-427.
22. Rosenstein M, Ettinghausen SE, Rosenberg SA: Extravasation of intravascular fluid mediated by the systemic administration of recombinant interleukin-2. *J Immunol* 1986;137:1735-1742.
23. Schirmer WJ, Schirmer JM, Naff GB, et al: Systemic complement activation produces hemodynamic changes characteristic of sepsis. *Arch Surg* 1988;123:316-321.
24. Schirmer WJ, Schirmer JM, Naff GB, et al: Visceral perfusion abnormalities following complement activation: Clues to the mediators of organ ischemia in trauma and sepsis. *Am Surg* 1988;54:687-692.
25. Pohlman TH, Stanness KA, Beatty PG, et al: An endothelial cell surface factor(s) induced in vitro by lipopolysaccharide, interleukin-1, and tumor necrosis factor increases neutrophil adherence by a CDw18-dependent mechanism. *J Immunol* 1986;136:4548-4553.
26. Djeu JY, Blanchard DK, Halkias D, et al: Growth inhibition of *Candida albicans* by human polymorphonuclear neutrophils: Activation by interferon-gamma and tumor necrosis factor. *J Immunol* 1986;137:2980-2984.
27. Marshall JC, Christou NV, Horn R, et al: The microbiology of multiple organ failure: The proximal gastrointestinal tract as an occult reservoir for pathogens. *Arch Surg* 1988;123:309-315.
28. Deitch EA, Bridges W, Baker J, et al: Hemorrhagic shock-induced bacterial translocation is reduced by blocking xanthine-oxidase mediated activity. *Surgery* 1988;104:191-198.
29. Michie H. Spriggs D, Revhaug A, et al: Does tumor necrosis factor mediate the metabolic responses to septicemia/endotoxemia in humans? *Surgery* 1988;104:280-286.

The Association of *Escherichia coli* Virulence and Pulmonary Microvascular Damage

Roderick A. Barke, MD; David L. Dunn, MD, PhD; Agustin P. Dalmasso, MD; Melody O'Connor-Allen, MD; Richard L. Simmons, MD; Edward W. Humphrey, MD, PhD

• **Bacterial virulence indicates the degree of pathogenicity of a given strain of microbe for a given host. The effect of *Escherichia coli* virulence on lung microvascular permeability was studied in sheep with chronic pulmonary lymph fistulas following peritoneal contamination. The study was divided into four groups: (1) wild-type *E coli* (WT group, 2.5×10^9 colony-forming units [CFUs]/kg); (2) virulent *E coli* (PV group, 2.3×10^9 CFUs/kg); (3) nonvirulent *E coli* (PNV group, 2.6×10^9 CFUs/kg); (4) high-inoculum wild-type *E coli* (HIWT group, 6.1×10^9 CFUs/kg). In the late period (two to six hours), the increase in lung lymph flow in the PV group was significantly greater than the WT, PNV, and HIWT groups, with no difference noted among groups with respect to the pulmonary artery pressure, pulmonary wedge pressure, or albumin lymph/plasma ratio. It was concluded that (1) increased *E coli* virulence results in increased lung microvascular damage and (2) increased lung microvascular damage as a function of *E coli* virulence may not be solely due to increased bacterial numbers as a function of time.**

(*Arch Surg* 1989;124:449-452)

Adult respiratory distress syndrome (ARDS) represents a final common pathway with multiple possible disease states as possible causal factors. One important causal factor is gram-negative bacterial sepsis. It is well known, however, that not all patients with gram-negative bacterial sepsis develop ARDS. Bacterial virulence is defined as the degree of pathogenicity of a given strain of microbe for a given host. Bacteria with various degrees of virulence may coexist in equilibrium with the host in a truce that is occasionally broken when factors that upset the delicate equilibrium come into play (immunosuppression, trauma, malnutrition, etc). We hypothesized that bacterial virulence factors may contribute to the incidence and severity of ARDS in gram-negative bacterial sepsis. To examine this question, we isolated three strains of *Escherichia coli* with different virulence as determined by 72-hour mortality in a rat peritonitis model. We then studied these three *E coli* strains in a sheep model and compared (1) damage to the pulmonary microvasculature, (2) hemodynamic failure, (3) neutropenia, and (4) classic and alternative pathway complement consumption.

MATERIALS AND METHODS

We prepared 23 yearling sheep (weight range, 35 to 55 kg) with chronic pulmonary lymph fistulas as described by Staub et al.[1] The experimental animal was allowed to recover from the operative procedures for at least two days. On the experimental day, the sheep was obtunded with pentobarbital sodium and placed on a volume-cycled ventilator with oxygen supplementation. The experimental animal was maintained in a paralyzed, obtunded state during the experimental period using pancuronium hydrochloride (0.1 mg/kg every four hours) and morphine sulfate (0.1 mg/kg every four hours). A Swan-Ganz catheter was passed into the pulmonary arterial circulation, and a polyethylene catheter was passed into the central aortic circulation. A central venous catheter was placed for intravenous fluid administration. Arterial blood gas and pH values were obtained with the ventilator, and oxygen supplementation was adjusted to obtain a baseline pH of 7.35 to 7.45, arterial oxygen pressure of 90 to 150 mm Hg, and arterial carbon dioxide pressure of 35 to 45 mm Hg. A 10 F pediatric feeding tube was placed in the right upper quadrant for injecting *E coli* into the peritoneal cavity. A right-upper-quadrant catheter placement was chosen based on previous experiments that indicated that this position yielded the most consistent response to *E coli* peritoneal contamination.[2]

Throughout every experiment, data were recorded with the sheep in the right lateral decubitus position. Pulmonary lymph volume was measured by accumulating lymph in heparinized, tared plastic vials during five- to ten-minute periods. The experimental groups were divided as follows: the passaged virulent *E coli* group (six sheep, PV group); the wild-type *E coli* group (six sheep, WT group); the passaged nonvirulent *E coli* group (six sheep, PNV group); and the high-inoculum wild-type *E coli* group (five sheep, HIWT group). The time during which data were collected was divided into a baseline period and an experimental period. The baseline period began after the experimental animal entered a steady state, as determined by constant pulmonary lymph flow and constant hemodynamic parameters. During this period, the following data were recorded: mean pulmonary artery pressure, mean pulmonary wedge pressure, mean aortic pressure, cardiac output, arterial blood gas and pH determinations, white blood cell count with the differential cell count, classic (CH_{50}) and alternative pathway (AH_{50}) hemolytic complement, lung lymph flow, and lung lymph and plasma for albumin concentration. These data were sampled at least four times throughout the one- to two-hour baseline interval.

After the baseline period, the experimental period was initiated by the injection of approximately 2.0×10^9 *E coli* per kilogram of body weight (PV, PNV, and WT groups) or 6.0×10^9 *E coli* per kilogram of body weight (HIWT group) into the peritoneal cavity through the previously placed right-upper-quadrant catheter. In addition to the continuous hemodynamic measurements, the data collected during the experimental period were as follows: cardiac output every 60 minutes; arterial blood gas and pH values every 30 minutes; pulmonary lymph flow every 30 minutes for two hours and then every hour; white blood cell count with the differential cell count; and CH_{50} and AH_{50} blood samples at 1, 3, 5, and 6 hours after peritoneal contamination. The duration of the experimental period was seven hours. Each animal in the PV, PNV, and WT groups was given 1 L of 0.9% normal saline solution during the six-hour experimental period. In the pilot studies, marked third-space losses in the HIWT group, in comparison with the other groups, resulted in a lower pulmonary wedge pressure and pulmonary artery pressure, resulting in the groups being noncomparable with respect to the hydrostatic component of pulmonary lymph flow. Accordingly, each animal in the HIWT group was given 0.9% normal saline solution at a rate such that the pulmonary wedge pressure as a function of time would match historical controls for the WT group.

Albumin concentrations were determined using the bromocresol green dye–binding method of Doumas and Biggs[3] and expressed in grams per deciliter. The arterial pH and arterial oxygen and carbon dioxide pressures were measured using a blood gas analyzer (Corning). The white blood cell count was performed using a hemacytometer (Neubauer). The blood cell differential count

Accepted for publication Nov 14, 1988.

From the Departments of Surgery (Drs Barke, Dunn, O'Connor-Allen, Simmons, and Humphrey), Pathology (Dr Dalmasso), and Laboratory Medicine (Dr Dalmasso), The University of Minnesota, Minneapolis, and the Veterans Administration Medical Center, Minneapolis (Drs Barke, Dalmasso, O'Connor-Allen, and Humphrey).

Read before the 12th Annual Surgical Symposium of the Association of Veterans Administration Surgeons, Minneapolis, May 12, 1988.

Reprint requests to Department of Surgery (112), Minneapolis Veterans Administration Medical Center, Minneapolis, MN 55417 (Dr Barke).

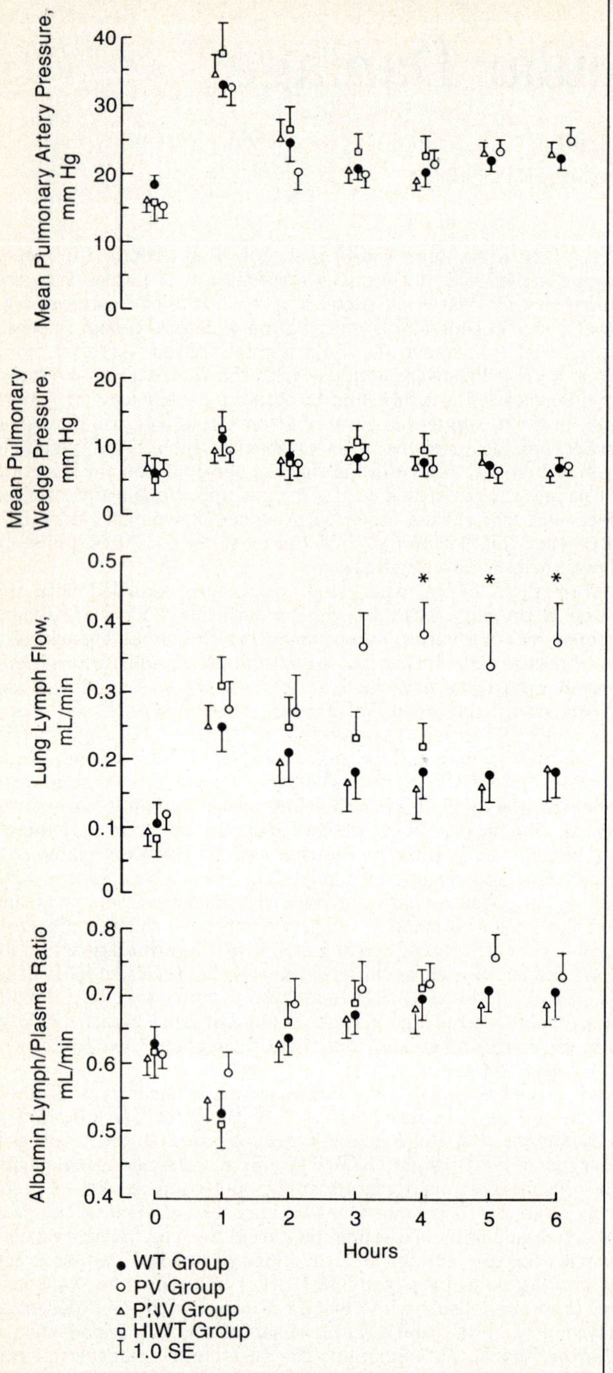

Fig 1.—Effect of *Escherichia coli* virulence (passaged virulent, [PV], wild-type [WT], and passaged nonvirulent [PNV] groups) or increased inoculum (high-inoculum wild-type [HIWT] group) on pulmonary artery pressure, pulmonary wedge pressure, lung lymph flow, and albumin lymph/plasma ratio. Lung lymph flow (asterisks) in PV group greater than in either HIWT, WT or PNV groups ($P<.05$).

was performed on a blood smear using Wright's stain. The classic hemolytic complement pathway was measured by the method of Barta et al,[4] and the alternative complement pathway was measured according to the method of Platt-Mills and Ishizaka.[5]

A clinical isolate of *E coli*, obtained initially from a human peritoneal infection at the University of Minnesota Hospitals,

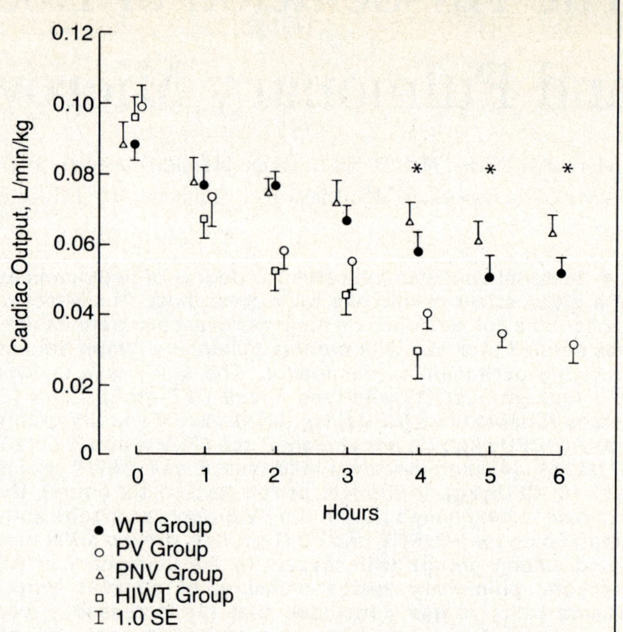

Fig 2.—Effect of *Escherichia coli* virulence (passaged virulent [PV], wild-type [WT], and passaged nonvirulent [PNV] groups) or increased inoculum (high-inoculum wild-type [HIWT] group) on cardiac output. Cardiac output (asterisks) in WT or PNV group greater than either PV or HIWT group ($P<.05$).

Minneapolis, was used for the WT group. A more virulent form of this strain was obtained by injection of 2×10^8 colony-forming units (CFUs) intraperitoneally into rats with reisolation of the organisms after streak plating of swabs obtained from the peritoneal cavity of moribund animals after eight hours. This sequence was repeated eight times to obtain the isolate used in the PV group. A less virulent form of the WT group strain was obtained by streaking the initial isolate onto agar plates, followed by isolation of individual colonies. This sequence was repeated eight times. Each strain, thus prepared, was kept as frozen isolates and thawed out before each experiment. Each of the three isolates was grown overnight in brain-heart infusion broth and inoculated intraperitoneally into rats. The dose that produced 50% lethality was determined after 72 hours by the method of Reed and Muench[6] and was found to be as follows: PV group, 5.8×10^7 CFUs; WT group, 1.5×10^8 CFUs; and PNV group, 1.2×10^9 CFUs.

For each experimental animal, a loop sample from a stock plate culture from the appropriate experimental group was inoculated into brain-heart infusion broth and incubated in a shaker bath for 18 hours at 37°C. The *E coli* broth was then subjected to three cycles of centrifugation (1600 for ten minutes), with each cycle followed by resuspension in 0.9% normal saline solution. Initial approximation of bacterial numbers on the day of experimentation was made using a Klett-Summerson densitometer. Serial dilutions were then performed, agar pour plates were made, and exact enumeration was established by viable colony counting. Blood samples were obtained from each experimental group at 1, 3, 5, and 6 hours after inoculation and tested for the presence of *E coli*.

The initial number of *E coli* used in each experimental group was as follows: WT group, $2.5\pm0.4\times(10^9)$ CFUs/kg; PV group, $2.3\pm0.5\times(10^9)$ CFUs/kg; PNV group, $2.6\pm0.4\times(10^9)$ CFUs/kg; and HIWT group, $6.1\pm0.6\times(10^9)$ CFUs/kg. No significant difference among the initial number of bacteria among the WT, PV, or PNV groups was observed. The HIWT group inoculum was significantly greater ($P<.05$) than the other groups.

The mean and SE of the mean pulmonary artery pressure, mean pulmonary wedge pressure, albumin lymph/plasma ratio, lymph flow, and absolute neutrophil count were calculated as a function of time for each experimental group. The cardiac output was normalized per kilogram of body weight in each experiment, and

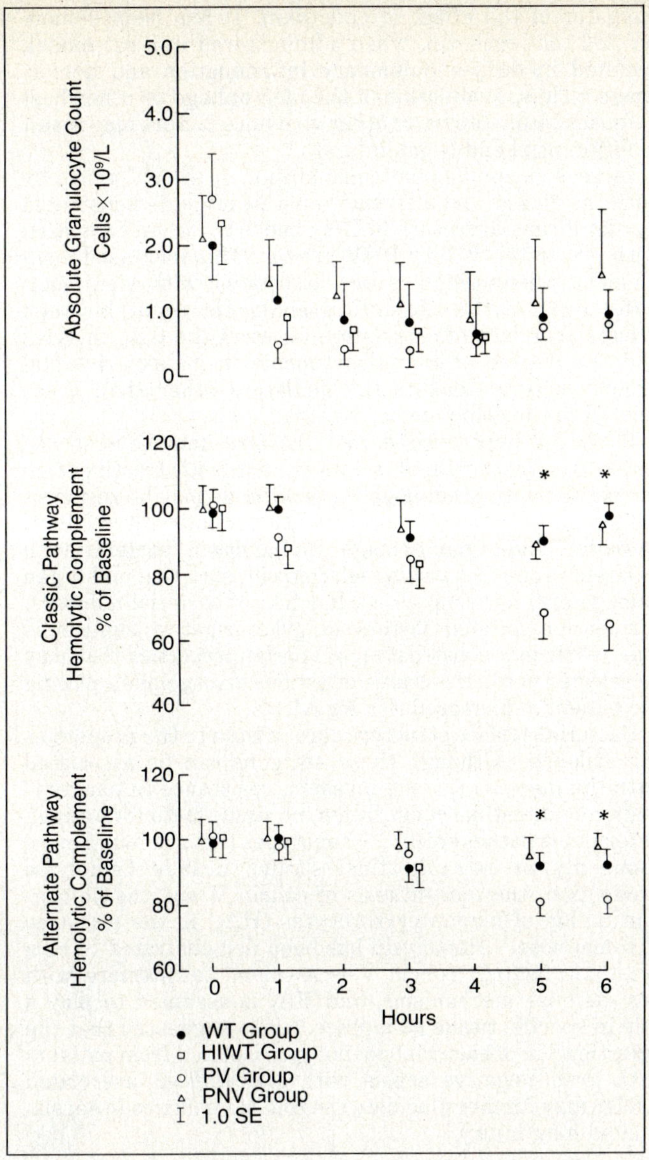

Fig 3.—Effect of *Escherichia coli* virulence (passaged virulent [PV], wild-type [WT], and passaged nonvirulent [PNV] groups) or increased inoculum (high-inoculum wild-type [HIWT] group) on absolute granulocyte count, CH_{50}, and AH_{50}. CH_{50} or AH_{50} (asterisks) in PV group less than either WT or PNV group ($P<.05$).

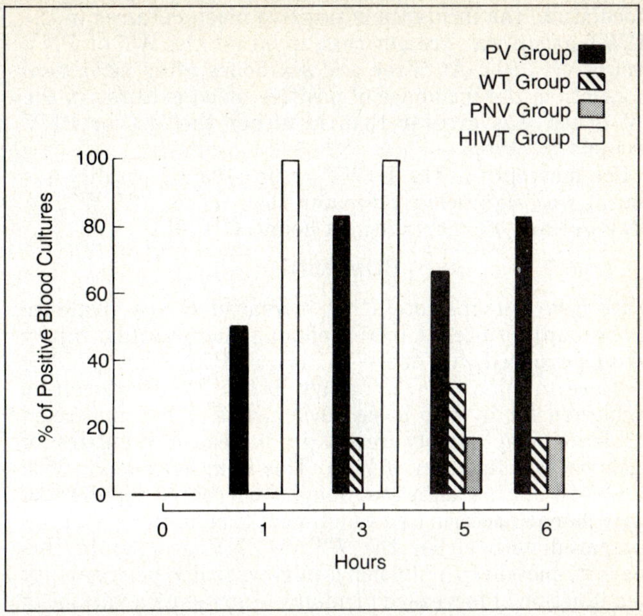

Fig 4.—Effect of *Escherichia coli* virulence (passaged virulent [PV], wild-type [WT], and passaged nonvirulent [PNV] groups) or increased inoculum (high-inoculum wild-type [HIWT] group) on incidence of positive blood cultures as function of time: one hour, HIWT greater than WT and PNV groups ($P<.01$); three hours, PV greater than WT and PNV groups ($P<.05$); three hours, HIWT greater than WT and PNV groups ($P<.01$); and six hours, PV greater than WT and PNV groups ($P<.05$).

the mean and SE were calculated as a function of time for each experimental group. Since the baseline measurements of classic and alternative hemolytic complement varied significantly among the experimental groups, CH_{50} and AH_{50} were normalized in each experiment to the average baseline values and expressed as a percent of baseline. The PV group was then tested as a function of time against either the WT group, the PNV group, or the HIWT group using a *t* statistic for two means with significance accepted at the *P* less than .05 level. In addition, the PNV and HIWT groups were tested against the WT group as a function of time using a *t* statistic for two means. No animal in the HIWT group survived six hours, and since some animals in this group became moribund after four hours, no data were tested as a function of time beyond four hours in this group. The HIWT group survival distribution was compared with the PV group survival distribution using Gehan's generalized Wilcoxon test[7] with significance accepted at the *P* less than .05 level. Blood culture data were tested as a function of time using a Fisher's exact test with significance accepted at the *P* less than .05 level.

RESULTS

During the following discussion, the time following the *E coli* peritoneal contamination has been divided into an early period (zero to two hours) and a late period (two to six hours).

During the early period (Fig 1), no significant difference in pulmonary hypertension, pulmonary wedge pressure, increased lung lymph flow, or the albumin lymph/plasma ratio was noted among the experimental groups. During the early period, no difference was noted among the groups with respect to cardiac output (Fig 2), granulocytopenia, and CH_{50} or AH_{50} (Fig 3). At one hour, the percent of positive blood cultures in the HIWT group was significantly greater than either the WT group or the PNV group.

During the late period (Fig 1), it is observed that no difference is noted among the WT, PNV, and HIWT groups with respect to pulmonary artery pressure, pulmonary wedge pressure and the albumin lymph/plasma ratio, noting that no data points are available after four hours in the HIWT group due to the animals' conditions. However, the lung lymph flow in the PV group was significantly greater ($P<.05$) than that of either the PNV, WT, or HIWT group. The cardiac output (Fig 2) in the WT and PNV groups was significantly greater ($P<.05$) than in either the PV or HIWT groups at four hours. In addition, the cardiac output in the WT and PNV groups was significantly greater ($P<.05$) than the PV group at five and six hours. During the late period (Fig 3), no significant difference is noted among the groups with respect to the absolute granulocyte count; however, the CH_{50} and AH_{50} in the PV group at five and six hours were significantly less ($P<.05$) than the CH_{50} and the AH_{50} in the PNV or WT groups.

The incidence of positive *E coli* blood cultures as a function of time in each experimental group is compared in Fig 4. At one hour and three hours after peritoneal inoculation, the incidence of positive blood cultures in the HIWT group was greater than in either the WT or PNV groups ($P<.01$). At three and six hours after peritoneal inoculation, the incidence of positive blood cultures in the PV group was greater than in either the WT or PNV groups ($P<.05$).

The mortality in the HIWT group (100% mortality, six hours) was significantly greater than in the PV, WT, or PNV groups (0% mortality, six hours) ($P<.05$).

COMMENT

We have demonstrated that increased *E coli* virulence (PV group) resulted in increased lung microvascular injury when compared with the WT, PNV, or HIWT groups. The increase in microvascular injury in the PV group can be accounted for by two basic mechanisms. First, increased virulence may simply result in increased numbers of bacteria as a function of time. This is in agreement with the blood culture data that suggest increased numbers of blood-borne bacteria as a function of time in the PV group compared with either the WT or PNV groups. In this respect, increased pulmonary microvascular permeability as a function of increased virulence represents a variant of a dose-response curve.

A second possible mechanism for the observed increase in lung injury in the PV group is an intrinsic property of the PV group *E coli*, independent of increased bacterial numbers, that results in increased lung damage. This is suggested by the comparison of the PV group with the HIWT group. In the HIWT group, an initial inoculum was chosen that would result in an increased mortality compared with the PV group. Indeed, the mortality in the HIWT group was 100% six hours after inoculation. This increase in inoculum (HIWT group) and associated increased mortality did not result in comparable lung injury when compared with the PV group. Increased animal mortality as a function of increased inoculum is a well-described phenomenon and is usually attributed to increased bacterial numbers as a function of time following inoculation. This suggests that the increased lung microvascular injury observed in the PV group may have resulted not only secondary to increased bacterial numbers as a function of time but to an additional property intrinsic to the PV group *E coli*.

A possible explanation for the decreased lung injury in the HIWT group when compared with the PV group would be vascular derecruitment in the HIWT group secondary to cardiac failure, resulting in a decreased perfused membrane surface area. Although this may be contributory, the fact that the cardiac output in the HIWT group is not significantly different from the PV group at four hours after inoculation suggests that the perfused membrane areas are comparable.

Thus, while the increased lung injury observed in the PV group is certainly related to the increased bacterial numbers as a function of virulence, an intrinsic bacterial factor independent of bacterial numbers may be present. Such an intrinsic bacterial factor would have to modulate the mechanism(s) of lung injury in such a manner as to create a disproportional degree of lung injury compared with its effect on other organ systems, resulting in a mortality differential. If one assumes the macrophage to have a central role in the mechanism of injury following *E coli* sepsis and endotoxemia, then modulation of the response of the macrophage to endotoxin by a factor in the PV group *E coli* could explain such differences in injury as observed in this study. One recently implicated possible factor is cachetin. Produced by endotoxin-activated macrophages, cachetin has been thought to be an important mediator of the effect of endotoxin. It has been demonstrated that cachetin, when administered in a rat model, resulted in diffuse pulmonary inflammation and hemorrhage.[8] Thus, modulation of the macrophage or other host defenses by endotoxin or other virulence factors may result in differential end-organ injury.

Increased complement consumption in the PV group by both the classic and alternative pathways is demonstrated by significant decreases in CH_{50} and AH_{50} when compared with either the WT or PNV groups. This increased complement consumption is not associated with significant differences in the absolute granulocyte count between groups. The lack of correlation between the CH_{50} or AH_{50} and the degree of granulocytopenia in all experimental groups suggest leukotactic mediators other than those related to the complement cascade.

It can be hypothesized that the host-immune response and/or treatment-related factors (ie, antibiotic treatment) in the patient with gram-negative septicemia may be responsible for the selection of more virulent strains with resultant increased end-organ damage. In addition, bacteria with different properties may be selected out, such that end-organ damage may not simply be a function of bacterial numbers. Virulence-associated factors in gram-negative septicemia may result in a constellation of special properties that may be selected out in the course of patient management, placing the patient at increased risk for ARDS.

Bacterial surface structures are related to the properties of virulence. Although these antigens can be associated with the degree of tissue invasion, resistance to phagocytosis, and intestinal colonization, no single factor or antigen determines pathogenicity.[9] Phenotypes that are found more commonly in extraintestinal strains include hemolysin production, the biosynthesis of colicin V, and the hemagglutination of human erythrocytes (HA_h) in the presence of D-mannose.[10] Hemolysin has been demonstrated to be a cytotoxic factor,[11] colicin V is assumed to interfere with host-defense mechanisms, and HA_h is assumed to play a role in specific tissue adherence.[10] It is suggested that the investigation of bacterial phenotypes isolated from patients with gram-negative sepsis with and without associated ARDS may further elucidate the role of virulence in sepsis-related lung injury.

This study was supported by Postdoctoral Fellowship Grant 5f32HL06278-02 from the National Institutes of Health, Bethesda, Md, and by Veterans Administration Medical Research Funds, Minneapolis.

References

1. Staub NC, Bland R, Brigham KL, et al: Preparation of chronic lung lymph fistulas in sheep. *J Surg Res* 1975;19:315-319.
2. Barke RA, Dunn DL, Dalmasso AP, et al: Comparative pulmonary effects of intraperitoneal inoculation of live vs dead *Escherichia coli*. *Arch Surg* 1984;119:173-179.
3. Doumas BT, Biggs HG: Determination of serum albumin, in Cooper GA (ed): *Standard Methods of Clinical Chemistry.* Orlando, Fla, Academic Press Inc, 1972, vol 7, p 175.
4. Barta O, Barta V, Shiley RA, et al: Haemolytic assay of sheep serum complement. *Zentralbl Veterinarmed B* 1975;22:254-262.
5. Platt-Mills TAE, Ishizaka K: Activation of the alternative pathway of human complement by rabbit cells. *J Immunol* 1974;113:348-353.
6. Reed LJ, Muench H: A simple method of estimating 50% end points. *Am J Hyg* 1938;27:493-497.
7. Lee ET: *Statistical Methods for Survival Data Analysis.* Monterey, Calif, Wadsworth Inc, 1980, p 123.
8. Tracey KJ, Beutler B, Lowry SF, et al: Shock and tissue injury induced by recombinant human cachectin. *Science* 1986;2:470-474.
9. Smith H: Microbial surfaces in relation to pathogenicity. *Bacteriol Rev* 1977;41:475-500.
10. Minshew BH, Jorgensen J, Swanstrum M, et al: Some characteristics of *Escherichia coli* strains isolated from extraintestinal infections of humans. *J Infect Dis* 1978;137:648-654.
11. Pruett TL, Chenoweth DE, Feigel VD, et al: *Escherichia coli* and human neutrophils. *Arch Surg* 1985;120:212-216.

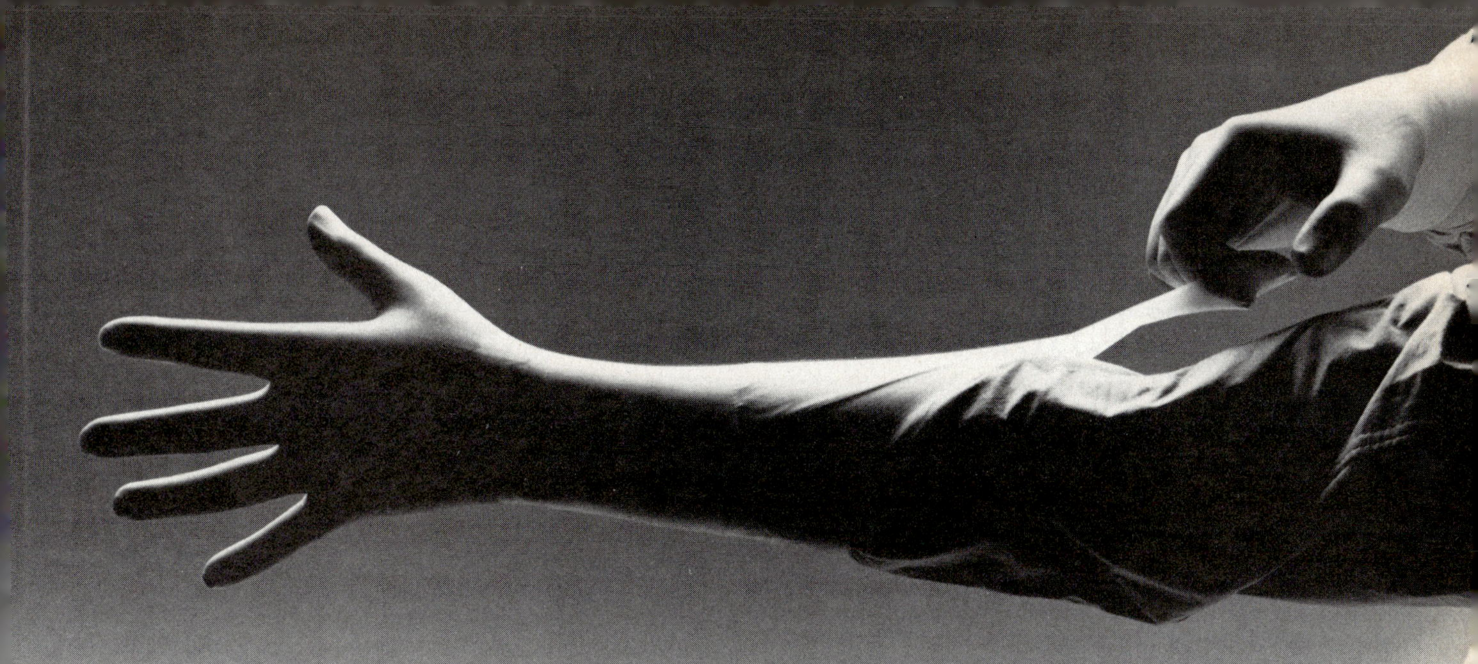

POWDER-FREE SURGICAL GLOVES CAN SAVE YOU MORE THAN TIME AND MONEY.

It's a fact. Using PRISTINE™ powder-free surgical gloves can save you time and money. No powders mean no valuable time spent performing a glove scrub, no basins, no wiping and no costly OR delays. And, because the highest quality, pure latex construction means maximum durability with fewer glove changes, you save money while gaining unequalled tactile sensitivity and excellent fit.

But, more than that, using PRISTINE powder-free gloves means the elimination of risks associated with all glove powders, and more protection for you and your patient.

HYPOALLERGENIC to protect your hands, PRISTINE gloves are 100% free of the powders, starches, talcs and silicas found on most other surgical gloves. And, by eliminating these powdered substances, PRISTINE gloves protect your hands from the chapping and cracking associated with powder-related dermatitis and hypersensitivity reactions.

Eliminate powder-related dermatitis and granulomatous reactions.

Even more important, no powder can mean no irritation or broken skin that could increase the potential for infection or the risk of other complications.

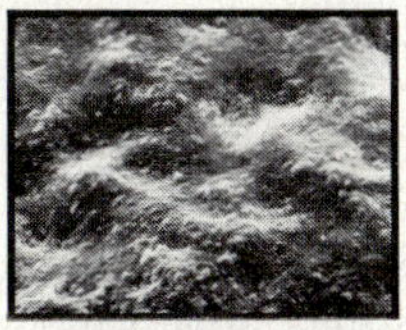

Surface of a PRISTINE powder-free surgical glove SEM (1000X) shows no foreign body or particulate contamination.

NO POWDER means fewer problems in the OR, too. No interior or exterior powders and no donning lubricants to leak from cuffs or escape during glove changes to contaminate equipment, test procedures or instruments.

For the patient, no powders in the OR mean none of the post-op complications such as granulomatous reactions, adhesions or peritonitis commonly linked to glove powders.

PRISTINE is the only glove with a patented friction-resistant interior surface for easy donning. Requires no donning lubricants and uses absolutely no powder.

To order, call (800) 545-5475, in CA (800) 547-3366. Complimentary samples may be requested by phone or by using the coupon below.

PRISTINE.™ The Surgeon's Glove.

Yes. I would like to try PRISTINE gloves.

Please send me a free sample pair in size ______

Name ______

Address ______

City ______ State ______ Zip ______

Phone ______

World Medical Supply (USA), Inc.
4340 Stevens Creek Boulevard, Suite 110
San Jose, California 95129 (408) 985-8822
(800) 545-5475, in CA (800) 547-3366

Effect of Eflorithine on Intestinal Regeneration

Jon S. Thompson, MD; Shailendra K. Saxena, MD, MS; John G. Sharp, PhD

• Patching intestinal defects with adjacent serosal surfaces results in the growth of new intestinal mucosa. Since polyamine biosynthesis is associated with cellular growth and differentiation, it may be important in this regenerative process. Our aim was to determine the effect of eflorithine (difluoromethylornithine), a specific inhibitor of polyamine synthesis, on intestinal regeneration. Forty-eight New Zealand white rabbits had 2 × 5-cm ileal defects patched with adjacent cecal serosal surface. One half of the animals took 2% eflorithine in drinking water postoperatively. Six animals in each group were killed 7, 14, 21, and 28 days after patching. There was no significant difference in neomucosal growth at any time. Villous height, disaccharidase activity, and crypt cell production were significantly lower in the eflorithine-treated animals. Eflorithine-treated animals had significantly lower ornithine decarboxylase activity and polyamine levels. Despite the inhibitory effect of eflorithine on polyamine synthesis and proliferative activity, epithelialization and contraction of the patched defect were not affected. These findings suggest that polyamine synthesis is important in proliferation and differentiation of cells in the neomucosa but does not influence cell migration in intestinal regeneration.

(*Arch Surg* 1989;124:454-457)

Patching intestinal defects with adjacent serosal surfaces results in the growth of new intestinal mucosa, termed *neomucosa*.[1] Growing neomucosa has been evaluated as a possible surgical therapy for patients with the short-bowel syndrome.[1-6] Neomucosal growth occurs by cell proliferation in the crypts in the surrounding normal mucosa and by migration of cells across the defect. The patched defect contracts to less than one half its initial size during the first week after patching. Presumably, intestinal transection is the initial stimulus for regeneration, but several factors affect the rate of this process, including size of the defect, luminal nutrition, intestinal location, and growth factors.[2-6]

The polyamines are intracellular cations that are important in cellular growth and differentiation.[7,8] Ornithine decarboxylase (ODC) is the rate-limiting enzyme of polyamine biosynthesis and therefore highly regulates the polyamine concentration. While increased polyamine synthesis occurs during mucosal cell proliferation, it is unclear whether it is essential to this process.[9] If ODC-mediated polyamine biosynthesis is important in intestinal regeneration, then stimuli that increase polyamine production might enhance this regenerative process.[5,10] The purpose of this study was to determine the effect of eflorithine (difluoromethylornithine), a specific inhibitor of ODC, on the growth of new intestinal mucosa after intestinal patching.

MATERIALS AND METHODS

Forty-eight male New Zealand white rabbits weighing 1.9 to 4.0 kg were included in the study. Two 2 × 5-cm ileal defects were patched with the adjacent colon serosal surface in each animal (Fig 1). One half of the animals took water and rabbit chow ad libitum. The other half took 2% eflorithine in drinking water and rabbit chow ad libitum. These animals drank an average of 190 mL of water per day, with an average dose of eflorithine of 1426 mg/kg/d. Six animals in each group were killed 7, 14, 21, and 28 days after operation. Neomucosal growth was determined by gross and microscopic measurements, including determinations of villous height. Tissue ODC activity, polyamine levels, and crypt cell production rate were measured to assess proliferative activity. Neomucosal function was evaluated by measuring in vitro glucose uptake and disaccharidase activity.

Operations were performed after an overnight fast using a sterile technique. Anesthesia was achieved with intramuscular ketamine hydrochloride and xylazine hydrochloride. Intestinal patching was performed by identifying the distal ileum and making two 5-cm incisions on the antimesenteric border, the first beginning 20 cm proximal to the ileocecal junction and the second beginning 10 cm proximal to the ileocecal junction. The defects were closed with a 2 × 5-cm patch of adjacent colon serosal surface with a continuous inverting 4-0 silk suture. The abdomen was irrigated with 10 mL of sterile water containing 100 mg of ampicillin sodium, and the incision was closed. The animals received 100 mg of ampicillin sodium intramuscularly preoperatively and twice daily for three days after operation. One hundred milliliters of 5% dextrose water was administered subcutaneously following the operation. The animals took nothing by mouth the first postoperative day, received fluids the second day, and took full alimentation after the third postoperative day.

After the animals were killed, the size of the patched defect and percentage of the defect covered with neomucosa were determined by measuring the transverse and longitudinal diameters and calculating the area of the ellipse ($\pi r_1 r_2$). Contraction was calculated by determining the patched area at death and expressing it as the percentage of the initial defect size (2 × 5 cm). Samples of

Accepted for publication Oct 6, 1988.

From the Omaha Veterans Administration Medical Center (Dr Thompson); the Departments of Surgery (Dr Thompson) and Anatomy (Drs Saxena and Sharp), University of Nebraska Medical Center, Omaha; and the Department of Surgery (Dr Thompson), Creighton University School of Medicine, Omaha.

Read before the 12th Annual Surgical Symposium of the Association of Veterans Administration Surgeons, Minneapolis, May 12, 1988.

Reprint requests to Department of Surgery, University of Nebraska Medical Center, 42nd and Dewey Avenue, Omaha, NE 68105 (Dr Thompson).

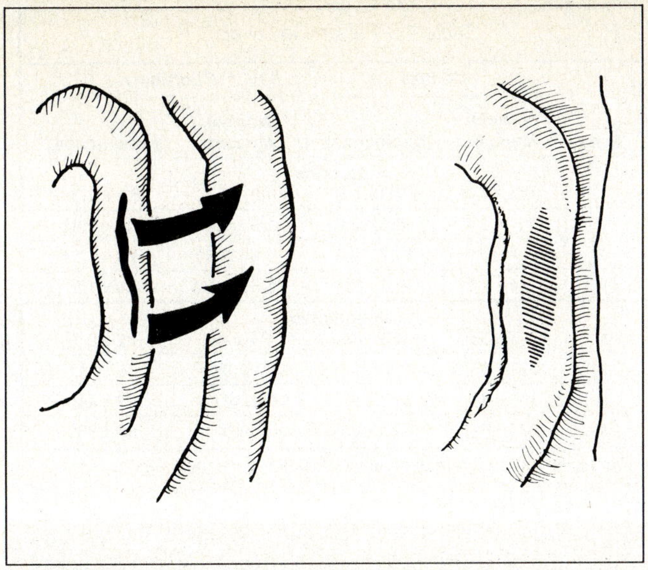

Fig 1.—Intestinal patching is performed by incising intestine on its antimesenteric border and patching this defect with adjacent serosal surface to create a 2 × 5-cm mucosal defect within intestinal lumen (from Thompson et al[19]).

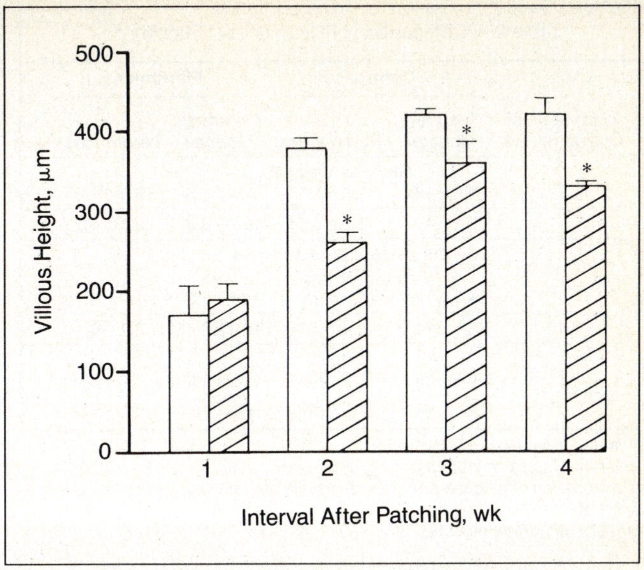

Fig 2.—Comparison of villous height in neomucosa of control animals (open bars) and animals treated with eflorithine (shaded bars). Asterisk indicates statistical significance of $P<.05$.

Table 1.—Comparison of Neomucosal Growth

Interval After Operation, wk	% Coverage Defect		% Initial Defect Size		Neomucosal Area, mm²	
	Control	Eflorithine	Control	Eflorithine	Control	Eflorithine
1	36 ± 11	39 ± 9	51 ± 5	46 ± 8	152 ± 53	136 ± 43
2	95 ± 1	96 ± 1	37 ± 2	36 ± 2	270 ± 17	271 ± 13
3	98 ± 1	98 ± 1	42 ± 2	45 ± 2	326 ± 14	346 ± 14
4	99 ± 1	99 ± 1	44 ± 3	49 ± 2	341 ± 25	381 ± 17

neomucosa were processed histologically and stained with hematoxylin-eosin. The measurement of villous height was made using an eyepiece micrometer.

Crypt cell production rate was determined by using a metaphase arrest technique.[5] Vincristine sulfate (1 mg) was administered by intraperitoneal injection two hours prior to killing. The mucosal sample was fixed in Carnoy's fixative and then hydrolyzed at 60°C for five minutes with Schiff's reagent. Crypts and villi were separated from the underlying connective tissue, and the crypts were dissected free using a dissecting microscope. Samples of crypts were transferred to a glass slide in 15% glacial acetic acid and were squashed for determination of the number of metaphases per crypt in a minimum of ten crypts. The mean of the metaphase counts of the crypts was taken as the reading for each sample. Crypt cell production rate was calculated assuming a linear accumulation for two hours.

Determination of net glucose uptake rates for both neomucosa and normal ileal mucosa was made using a double-isotope counting system with glucose labeled with carbon 14 and tritiated polyethylene glycol, where tritiated polyethylene glycol is the adherent fluid marker as described previously.[2] Three 5 × 5-mm disks of tissue were analyzed. The incubation medium included 10 mmol/L of glucose to which 15 μL of glucose labeled with carbon 14 (specific activity, 250 mCi/mmol/L) was added. Net uptake was expressed as nanomoles of glucose per minute per milligram of dry tissue weight. Disaccharidase activity in the neomucosa and normal mucosa was determined according to the method of Dahlquist.[11] Disaccharidase activity was expressed as micromoles of glucose per gram of protein per minute.

Polyamine levels were assayed in a mucosal homogenate containing 100 mg of mucosa in 50 mmol/L of potassium phosphate. The polyamines were separated by reverse-phase, ion-pair, high-performance liquid chromatography using a C18 column and quantitated by fluorescent detection after postcolumn derivatization with *o*-phthalaldehyde.[5] The mobile phases used in this separation consisted of two buffers: buffer A contained 85% 0.1 mol/L of acetic acid, 15% methyl alcohol, and 10 mmol/L of heptanesulfonic acid; buffer B contained 75% 0.25 mol/L of acetic acid and 25% methyl alcohol. The program was two minutes of 100% buffer B, which pumped for an additional 20 minutes. The height of the peak at the appropriate retention time was determined and concentrations were calculated based on a standard curve. Polyamine levels were expressed as picomoles per milligram of mucosa. Ornithine decarboxylase activity was determined by a radiometric technique in which the amount of ornithine labeled with carbon 14 was estimated.[6] Ornithine decarboxylase activity was expressed as picomoles of carbon dioxide per milligram of protein per 30 minutes.

Data are expressed as the means ± SEMs. The data were analyzed using one- and two-tailed Student's t tests, with $P<.05$ for significance levels.

RESULTS

Animals in both groups exhibited normal behavior. Control animals maintained body weight during the study. Animals receiving eflorithine lost 10% to 15% of body weight ($P<.05$) during the 14 days following operation, and body weight remained consistently below preoperative levels. Ten additional animals receiving eflorithine died during the first two weeks after operation and were noted to have markedly decreased oral intake. Bowel movements were of normal consistency in all animals. There were no complications related to the surgical procedure itself.

Table 2.—Comparison of Neomucosal Function*

Interval After Operation, wk	Control Normal Mucosa	Control Neomucosa	Eflorithine Normal Mucosa	Eflorithine Neomucosa
	Glucose Uptake†			
3	3.6±1.0	2.6±.02	4.9±1.6	5.1±1.0
4	6.2±4.1	3.3±1.0	5.7±2.8	6.1±1.2
	Disaccharidase Activity‡ Sucrase			
3	54.0±11.9	26.4±9.6	31.6±5.2	1.9±0.4§‖
4	83.1±16.0	40.4±4.7§	37.2±6.4§	2.7±0.7§‖
	Maltase			
3	346±60	272±48	200±14‖	17±3§‖
4	351±58	339±106	262±78	26±5§‖

*Values are means±SEMs.
†Nanomoles per minute per milligram.
‡Micromoles of glucose per gram of protein per minute.
§$P<.05$ vs control.
‖$P<.05$ vs normal mucosa.

Table 3.—Comparison of Proliferative Parameters*

Week	Control Normal Mucosa	Control Neomucosa	Eflorithine Normal Mucosa	Eflorithine Neomucosa
	Crypt Cell Production Rate, No./h			
1	7.5±0.9	8.9±1.1	7.9±0.6	8.9±1.8
2	14.9±1.7	17.7±2.1	12.6±0.7	9.3±1.7†‡
3	9.4±0.6	10.2±1.2	9.0±0.8	4.8±0.5†‡
4	9.7±1.3	13.5±1.7	8.6±0.6	5.5±0.4†‡
	Ornithine Decarboxylase Activity§			
1	235±95	488±89	154±52	173±31†
2	256±73	202±22	170±26	188±22
3	379±122	394±152	39±9†	107±21‡
4	101±4	264±80	31±7†	110±39

*Values are means±SEMs.
†$P<.05$ vs control.
‡$P<.05$ vs normal mucosa.
§Picomoles of carbon dioxide per milligram of protein per 30 minutes.

Table 4.—Polyamine Levels*

Week	Control Normal Mucosa	Control Neomucosa	Eflorithine Normal Mucosa	Eflorithine Neomucosa
	Putrescine			
1	10.5±7.6	7.3±5.9	4.8±2.0	3.8±1.3
2	7.1±1.4	8.6±2.6	1.6±0.7†	1.1±0.8†
3	8.7±0.9	10.4±2.8	4.8±1.0†	4.3±1.0†
4	5.4±1.5	9.8±2.1	5.4±0.9	6.0±1.5
	Spermidine			
1	45±33	83±49	34±16	12±2
2	317±35	249±32	11±3†	5±1†‡
3	366±96	182±40	155±47	109±44
4	294±27	227±25	166±51	95±38†

*Picomoles per milligram of mucosa. Values are means±SEMs.
†$P<.05$ vs control.
‡$P<.05$ vs normal mucosa.

There was no significant difference in neomucosal growth between the two groups at any time (Table 1). The defects were almost completely covered by neomucosa three weeks after operation and had contracted to less than half their initial size. Grossly, there was no difference in neomucosal area. Microscopically, however, villous height was significantly less in the eflorithine-treated animals (Fig 2).

There were significant differences in neomucosal function three and four weeks after operation (Table 2). Sucrase and maltase activities were significantly less in the neomucosa of eflorithine-treated animals compared with the adjacent normal mucosa and the neomucosa in the control group. Disaccharidase activity in the normal mucosa of the eflorithine-treated group was significanly lower than that of the control group. However, glucose uptake, measured in vitro, was similar in both the neomucosa and normal mucosa of the two groups of animals.

Proliferative activity in the crypts of both neomucosa and normal mucosa decreased with eflorithine administration. Crypt cell production rate was significantly lower in the neomucosa of eflorithine-treated animals compared with control animals 2, 3, and 4 weeks after operation. Crypt cell production rate was suppressed to a greater extent in the neomucosa than in adjacent normal mucosa in these animals.

Eflorithine-treated animals had lower ODC activity in both neomucosa and normal mucosa with significantly lower levels in neomucosa one week after operation and in adjacent normal mucosa three and four weeks postoperatively (Table 3). Putrescine and spermidine levels were also significantly lower in the eflorithine-treated animals, with the lowest levels attained in the second week after operation (Table 4).

COMMENT

Ornithine decarboxylase, the rate-limiting enzyme of polyamine biosynthesis that converts ornithine to putrescine, is irreversibly inhibited by the substrate analogue eflorithine.[7,8] Eflorithine, given enterally or parenterally, has been reported to cause a dose-dependent reduction in DNA and polyamine content of the intestinal mucosa. Villi become blunter and shorter and are lined by cuboidal to squamoid epithelium that frequently lacks a well-developed brush border.[12,13] The mucosal atrophy induced by eflorithine is transitory, indicating that intestinal cells are capable of compensating for the reduction in ODC-mediated polyamine synthesis.[12] Putrescine can be synthesized from spermidine, and this interconversion increases when the ODC pathway is inhibited.[14] Eflorithine abolishes the normal rise in ODC activity and mucosal polyamine content that accompanies intestinal adaptation resulting from intestinal resection and pancreaticobiliary diversion.[13,15,16] Eflorithine has also been shown to impair healing of gastric mucosal lesions caused by hypertonic saline, preventing the increased ODC activity that normally occurs during healing.[17] Thus, eflorithine might impair intestinal regeneration on patched intestinal defects.

In the present study, eflorithine suppressed polyamine synthesis and proliferative activity in neomucosa and normal adjacent intestinal mucosa beginning the second week after the patching procedure. Ornithine decarboxylase activity, mucosal polyamine content, and crypt cell production rate were all diminished in the eflorithine-treated animals. The 60% decrease in ODC activity was somewhat less than the 85% to 95% decrease reported by others with a similar dose of eflorithine.[13,18] The intestinal polyamine content in the eflorithine-treated animals was normal seven days after patching but decreased thereafter. This may be secondary to impaired absorption of eflorithine during the early postoperative period or the presence of stored polyamines that have not been depleted. Crypt cell production rate was highest 14 days after operation in the control animals, and eflorithine had a more pronounced inhibitory effect on the stimulated rather than basal proliferative activity.

The rate of epithelialization and extent of contraction of the patched defect were not affected by eflorithine administration. However, villi were shorter and brush border enzyme activity was less in the eflorithine-treated animals at each time point. These findings suggest that polyamine synthesis is important in proliferation and differentiation of cells in the neomucosa but is less important in cell migration and contraction during intestinal regeneration. Furthermore, proliferative activity in the intestinal crypts combined with cells made available by reducing villous size and cell populations is sufficient, even in the presence of eflorithine, to supply the epithelial cells necessary for continued cell migration onto the patched defect.

The findings of this study have implications for the mechanism of intestinal regeneration. This process involves migration of cells onto the patched defect, increased cellular proliferation in the crypts of the adjacent mucosa and then in the neomucosa, and contraction of the patched defect. The migrating cells proliferate and differentiate to form well-developed crypts and villi. Since epithelialization occurred at the normal rate in the eflorithine-treated animals, cell migration appears to be the rate-limiting factor rather than increased proliferative activity when sufficient cells are available for migration. This in turn implies that the ultimate determinant of intestinal epithelial regeneration is the perimeter of the normal epithelium surrounding any defect. However, we found previously that eflorithine partially inhibits urogastrone-stimulated epithelialization.[19] That observation suggests that increased cell proliferation is also an important factor in the rate of epithelialization. Contraction of the patched defect involves primarily subepithelial tissue responses, which is consistent with the failure of eflorithine to inhibit this process.[20]

This study was supported by grant DK36612 from the National Institutes of Health, Bethesda, Md.

The eflorithine was supplied by the Merrell Dow Research Institute, Cincinnati.

References

1. Thompson JS, Vanderhoof JA, Antonson DL, et al: Comparison of techniques of growing small bowel neomucosa. *J Surg Res* 1984;36:401-406.
2. Thompson JS, Vanderhoof JA, Davis SJ, et al: Effect of intestinal location on growth and function of neomucosa. *J Surg Res* 1985;39:68-75.
3. Thompson JS, Tempero MA, Haun JL, et al: The importance of luminal factors in neomucosal growth. *J Surg Res* 1986;40:126-132.
4. Bragg LE, Thompson JS: The influence of serosal patch size on the growth of small intestinal neomucosa. *J Surg Res* 1986;40:426-431.
5. Thompson JS, Sharp JG, Saxena SK, et al: Stimulation of neomucosal growth by systemic urogastrone. *J Surg Res* 1987;42:402-410.
6. Thompson JS: Growth of neomucosa after intestinal resection. *Arch Surg* 1987;122:316-319.
7. Pegg AE, McCann PP: Polyamine metabolism and function. *Am J Physiol* 1982;243:C212-C221.
8. Heby O: Role of polyamines in the control of cell proliferation and differentiation. *Differentiation* 1981;19:1-20.
9. Luk GB, Baylin SB: Polyamines and intestine growth: Increased polyamine biosynthesis after jejunectomy. *Am J Physiol* 1983;245:G656-G660.
10. Kingsworth AN, King WWK, McCann PP, et al: Putrescine dependence of epidermal growth factor–stimulated DNA synthesis in the mouse gastrointestinal tract. *Surg Forum* 1982;33:190-191.
11. Dahlquist A: Method of assay of intestinal disaccharidases. *Anal Biochem* 1961;7:18-25.
12. Yarrington JT, Sprinkle DJ, Loudy DE, et al: Intestinal changes caused by α-difluoromethylornithine (DFMO), an inhibitor of ornithine decarboxylase. *Exp Mol Pathol* 1983;39:300-316.
13. Kingsworth AN, Abu-khalaf M, LaMuraglia GM, et al: Inhibition of ileal and colonic ornithine decarboxylase activity by α-difluoromethylornithine in rats: Transient atrophic changes and loss of post resectional adaptive growth. *Surgery* 1986;99:721-727.
14. Seiler N, Bolkenius FN, Rennert OM: Interconversion, catabolism and elimination of the polyamines. *Med Biol* 1981;59:334-346.
15. Luk GB, Baylin SB: Inhibitors of intestinal epithelial DNA synthesis and adaptive hyperplasia after jejunectomy in the rat by suppression of polyamine biosynthesis. *J Clin Invest* 1984;74:698-704.
16. Hosomi M, Lirussi F, Stace NH, et al: Mucosal polyamine profile in normal and adapting (hypo and hyperplastic) intestine: Effects of DFMO treatment. *Gut* 1987;28:103-107.
17. Tabata K, Fitzpatrick LR, Johnson LR: Role of ornithine decarboxylase (ODC) in regeneration of damaged gastric mucosa in rats. *Gastroenterology* 1985;88:1604.
18. Alarcon P, Lebenthal E, Lee PC: Effect of difluoromethylornithine (DFMO) on small intestine of adult and weanling rats. *Dig Dis Sci* 1987;32:883-888.
19. Thompson JS, Saxena SK, Sharp JG: Difluoromethylornithine inhibits urogastrone stimulation of neomucosal growth. *J Surg Res* 1988;44:589-595.
20. Thompson JS, Hollingsed TC, Saxena SK: Prevention of contraction of patched intestinal defects. *Arch Surg* 1988;123:428-430.

Editor's Note

In this issue the first article(s) edited in accordance with our new style appears. For our current style, consult *American Medical Association Manual of Style*, eighth edition, available from the publisher, Williams & Wilkins, 428 E Preston St, Baltimore, MD 21202; 1-800-638-0672.

Effective Hepatic Blood Flow During Cardiopulmonary Bypass

William W. Hampton, MD; Michael C. Townsend, MD;
William J. Schirmer, MD; David M. Haybron, MD; Donald E. Fry, MD

• Hepatic dysfunction following cardiopulmonary bypass (CPB) is a relatively frequent finding, and jaundice occurring after CPB is associated with an increased mortality rate. Post-CPB jaundice may be a consequence of inadequate liver perfusion during CPB. To evaluate the potential impact of CPB on effective hepatic blood flow, 10 patients undergoing CPB for cardiac procedures were studied. Effective hepatic blood flow was measured in each patient during the operative procedure but before institution of CPB and during CPB as well. Effective hepatic blood flow was measured by the galactose clearance technique. Blood lactate and pyruvate levels were also measured before and during CPB. During CPB, effective hepatic blood flow was consistently reduced by an average of 19%. Although for most patients this reduction seems well tolerated, in a minority of patients it may contribute to postoperative hepatic dysfunction.

(*Arch Surg.* 1989;124:458-459)

Cardiac surgery necessitating cardiopulmonary bypass (CPB) has increased in scope and volume over the last 20 years. Although it has become an indispensable technique for most kinds of cardiac surgery, its use is not completely benign. Gastrointestinal complications of CPB contribute significant morbidity and mortality rates to the procedure,[1-3] and the incidence of post-CPB hyperbilirubinemia has been as high as 20% in large series.[1] Multiple studies have measured visceral blood flow during CPB in animals. Because of the different models used, there is really no consensus on the effects of CPB on visceral perfusion. Retrospective studies of patients undergoing CPB have implicated decreased organ perfusion during CPB or in the postoperative period, but difficulties in the measurement of hepatic blood flow have left this issue largely unexplored. In this study, we examined the effect of CPB on hepatic blood flow using the galactose clearance technique in patients undergoing cardiac procedures.

PATIENTS AND METHODS

Ten patients undergoing CPB were studied. Cardiopulmonary bypass was employed in each case using a roller pump (Pemco) with a disposable bubble oxygenator. Perfusion rates used in these 10 patients varied between 2.1 and 2.8 L/min per square meter. Hemodilution prime was used in all patients. In all but one patient, hypothermia of from 27°C to 29°C was employed. In one patient, normothermic CPB was used for the repair of an atrial septal defect. All patients in this study voluntarily signed an informed consent and the study was previously approved by the institutional review board at the Cleveland (Ohio) Veterans Administration Medical Center.

Twenty measurements of effective hepatic blood flow (EHBF) were made in 10 patients undergoing CPB for cardiac surgery. The first measurement was made after the patient was fully anesthetized and preparations were being made to begin CPB. The second measurement of EHBF was made for the patient after at least 30 minutes into the CPB procedure.

Measurement of EHBF was made by the method described by Henderson et al.[4] As soon as vascular access was obtained in each patient, blood samples were obtained for the analysis of baseline galactose levels. Patients were given an initial bolus of 12 mL of 5% D-galactose solution. This was followed by an infusion of D-galactose at 48 mL/h via a continuous infusion pump. While the patient was being draped, and more than 30 minutes after the bolus was administered, the first blood sample was obtained; thereafter, blood samples were obtained at 5- to 10-minute intervals for a total of five to nine blood samples for each patient. This group of blood samples was analyzed as described below to determine the pre-CPB EHBF. After each patient had been undergoing the CPB procedure for at least 30 minutes, a second set of six to nine blood samples was obtained at 5- to 10-minute intervals. This group of samples was analyzed for galactose concentration to determine the EHBF during CPB.

For each set of blood samples, the hematocrit was determined to allow for correction for hemodilution. Galactose concentration of each sample was determined by a manual modification of the automated fluorometric assay for galactose described by Henderson and Fales.[5] Plasma galactose concentration was then corrected to whole blood concentration by a factor of $1-(0.5\times\text{hematocrit})/100$. The steady-state concentraton of blood galactose was then determined from the average of each group of samples. The EHBF was calculated as follows: $\text{EHBF}=I/(C_{ss}-C_o)$, where I is the infusion rate of galactose; C_{ss}, mean steady-state blood galactose concentration; and C_o, baseline blood galactose concentration.

In addition, 8 of the 10 patients also had blood samples drawn near the middle of each EHBF measurement period for the determination of lactate and pyruvate levels. These blood samples were deproteinized immediately in perchloric acid and refrigerated until they could be assayed spectrophotometrically for blood lactate and pyruvate levels using specific kits (Sigma Chemical Co, St Louis, Mo).

RESULTS

In this group of patients, a consistent decrease in EHBF was demonstrated amounting to a 19% decrease during CPB. The data are summarized in Fig 1. All but one patient showed a decrease. On starting the CPB procedure, EHBF dropped from an average of 1468 ± 174 mL/min to 1190 ± 119 mL/min and the difference was statistically significant ($P<.05$; paired t test). During the period of CPB, the mean arterial pressure, hematocrit, and temperature were all reduced significantly, as seen below.

	Prior to CPB	During CPB
Mean arterial pressure, mm Hg	89.9 ± 2.9	72.7 ± 2.1
Hematocrit	0.334 ± 0.009	0.242 ± 0.011
Temperature, °C	35.6 ± 0.1	28.8 ± 0.9

During the period of operation before the CPB procedure began, the patients had a mean blood lactate level of 0.78 ± 0.13 mmol/L and mean pyruvate level of 0.112 ± 0.03 mmol/L. During CPB, mean blood lactate and pyruvate levels rose to 1.19 ± 0.18 and 0.142 ± 0.03 mmol/L as shown in Fig 2. While the increases in both lactate and pyruvate levels were statistically significant ($P<.05$), the lactate-pyruvate ratio remained constant.

COMMENT

The classic study of post-CPB jaundice by Sanderson et al[6] identified conditions related to development of this syndrome. They found that severity of cardiac disease,

Accepted for publication November 14, 1988.

From the Department of Surgery, Case Western Reserve University and the Cleveland (Ohio) Veterans Administration Medical Center. Dr Fry is now with the University of New Mexico School of Medicine, Albuquerque.

Read before the 12th Annual Surgical Symposium of the Association of Veterans Administration Surgeons, Minneapolis, Minn, May 13, 1988.

Reprint requests to Department of Surgery, University of New Mexico School of Medicine, 2211 Lomas Blvd NE, Albuquerque, NM 87131 (Dr Fry).

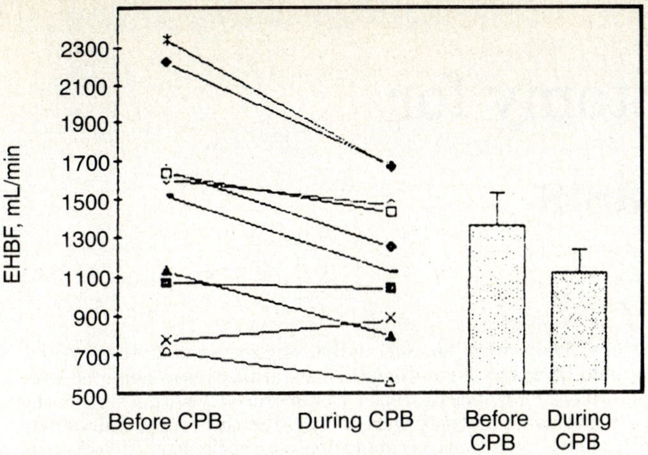

Fig 1.—The effective hepatic blood flow (EHBF) of 10 patients before and during cardiopulmonary bypass (CPB).

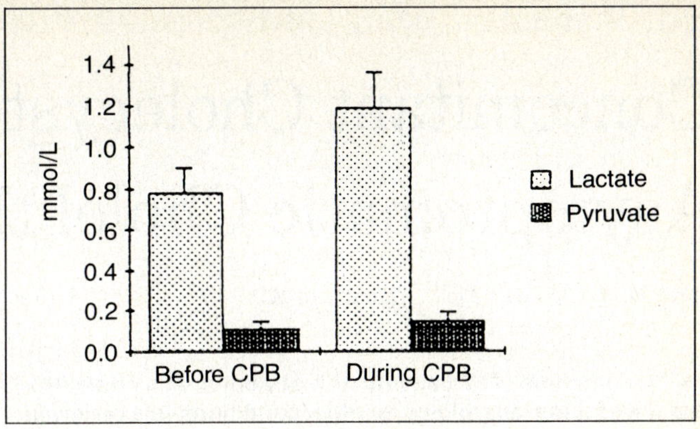

Fig 2.—Blood lactate and pyruvate concentrations before and during cardiopulmonary bypass (CPB) in 10 patients.

erythrocyte breakdown, plasma hemoglobin, duration of CPB, and halothane anesthesia did not correlate with the development of post-CPB jaundice. In their analysis, patients undergoing multiple-valve replacements were most likely to have this syndrome develop. They proposed that hepatic congestion or some other condition may have predisposed some patients to the ill effects of inadequate perfusion, postoperative low-flow states, anoxia, or vasopressor drugs. Other retrospective studies have imputed a variety of possible risk factors for this syndrome[1,3] and the cause is still unknown. The study of Collins et al,[1] carried out more recently, demonstrated that post-CPB jaundice is as frequent or more frequent than in the early days of CPB. They reported an incidence of this syndrome of 20% and a mortality rate of 25% in those patients who had post-CPB jaundice.

Several studies of visceral perfusion have been performed in animals. However, the applicability of the various animal models used to the human situation makes interpretation difficult. Lees et al[7] studied visceral perfusion extensively during CPB in rhesus monkeys and concluded that hepatic blood flow was adequate. Unfortunately, CPB in their study was performed at flow rates adjusted to approximate the normal cardiac output of the awake animals, and hypothermia and hemodilution were not employed. Waldhausen et al[8] determined hepatic blood flow in dogs during CPB and found that at normal perfusion rates, total hepatic blood flow was normal but hepatic blood flow fell markedly as total body perfusion was reduced.

We are not aware of any previous efforts to measure hepatic perfusion in humans during CPB. Schenk et al[9] measured hepatic blood flow in patients under anesthesia during the course of end-to-side portacaval shunts using an electromagnetic flow meter. In that study, mean hepatic blood flow was 1004 ± 322 mL/min, which is lower than the measurements in this study, but it was in a group of patients with severe liver disease. The galactose clearance technique used in our experiments has been very useful in measuring hepatic perfusion in a variety of settings.[10,11] The technique is particularly applicable to the conditions of this study because it is a noninvasive technique that could be easily carried out without impinging on the patient's care during the operation. The disadvantage of the technique is that it is not capable of making instantaneous measurements of hepatic blood flow, as EHBF is calculated from the steady-state levels of blood galactose obtained after a period of equilibration.

The data indicate that EHBF was significantly decreased during CPB. Steadily increasing blood lactate levels indicate that decreased perfusion to other areas of the body may be of metabolic significance. Increased blood lactate levels during CPB have been previously documented.[12] However, our data indicate that the lactate-pyruvate ratio remained constant. Since the lactate-pyruvate ratio represents a systemic expression of the cytoplasmic redox state, the constancy of this molar relationship may reflect that all tissues are not adversely affected by CPB and that lactate may actually be serving as an energy substrate for other tissues. Additional studies will need to address whether the flow abnormalities of CPB are tissue specific or are a generalized phenomenon.

None of the patients examined in this study developed post-CPB jaundice. Further studies either of groups at high risk for developing post-CPB jaundice or of larger numbers of patients undergoing routine bypass are needed to determine whether alteration in EHBF is a significant variable in the development of post-CPB jaundice. If so, the methodology of galactose clearance may be a valuable technique in monitoring the effects of newer regimens to correct visceral perfusion abnormalities.

References

1. Collins JD, Ferner R, Murray A, et al. Incidence and prognostic importance of jaundice after cardiopulmonary bypass surgery. *Lancet.* 1983;1:1119-1123.
2. Kingsley DPE. Hepatic damage following profound hypothermia and extracorporeal circulation in man. *Thorax.* 1966;21:91-98.
3. Lockey E, McIntyre N, Ross DN, et al. Early jaundice after open heart surgery. *Thorax.* 1967;22:165-169.
4. Henderson JM, Kutner MH, Bain RP. First order clearance of plasma galactose: the effect of liver disease. *Gastroenterology.* 1982;83:1090-1096.
5. Henderson JM, Fales FW. Continuous flow fluorometry of low galactose concentrations in blood or plasma. *Clin Chem.* 1983;26:129-132.
6. Sanderson RG, Ellison JH, Benson JA, et al. Jaundice following open heart surgery. *Ann Surg.* 1967;165:217-224.
7. Lees MH, Herr RH, Hill JD, et al. Distribution of systemic blood flow of the rhesus monkey during cardiopulmonary bypass. *J Thorac Cadiovasc Surg.* 1971;61:570-586.
8. Waldhausen JA, Lombardo CR, McFarland JA, et al. Studies of hepatic blood flow and oxygen consumption during total cardiopulmonary bypass. *Surgery.* 1959;46:1118-1127.
9. Schenk WG, McDonald JC, McDonald K, et al. Direct measurement of hepatic blood flow in surgical patients. *Ann Surg.* 1962;156:463-471.
10. Schirmer WJ, Townsend MC, Schirmer JM, et al. Galactose clearance as an estimate of effective hepatic blood flow: validations and limitations. *J Surg Res.* 1986;41:543-556.
11. Townsend MC, Hampton WW, Haybron DM, et al. Effective organ blood flow and bioenergy status in murine peritonitis. *Surgery.* 1986;100:205-213.
12.. Anderson MN, Norberg B, Senning A. Studies of liver function during extracorporeal circulation with low flow rate. *Surgery.* 1958;43:397-407.

Concomitant Cholecystectomy for Asymptomatic Cholelithiasis

Larry E. Bragg, MD, Jon S. Thompson, MD

• The outcome of 68 patients with asymptomatic cholelithiasis undergoing laparotomy for other conditions was reviewed to determine those most likely to become symptomatic postoperatively. Thirty-seven patients (54%) became symptomatic postoperatively. Eight patients (22%) required cholecystectomy within 30 days of operation or within the same hospitalization. These patients fasted for a longer period of time postoperatively (15±21 vs 4±3 days) than those undergoing later cholecystectomy. Significantly more of these patients required transfusion (38% vs 7%), mechanical ventilation (50% vs 11%), and total parenteral nutrition (50% vs 18%). Cholelithiasis frequently becomes symptomatic after laparotomy for other intra-abdominal conditions. Patients who require mechanical ventilation, transfusions, and parenteral nutrition and who are slow to resume enteral nutrition are more likely to require early cholecystectomy. Concomitant cholecystectomy adds minimal morbidity to other procedures and should be undertaken unless specific contraindications exist, particularly in this high-risk group.

(*Arch Surg* 1989;124:460-462)

Asymptomatic cholelithiasis is detected in 20% to 30% of individuals at the time of operation for an unrelated intra-abdominal problem.[1,2] If left untreated, symptoms will develop in a large percentage of these patients in the postoperative period that necessitate subsequent cholecystectomy.[1,3] For this reason, concomitant cholecystectomy is frequently performed for asymptomatic biliary calculi at the time of laparotomy.

Although the safety of concomitant cholecystectomy has been demonstrated,[4-6] concerns about adding a second procedure frequently remain in patients who are often elderly and undergoing extensive procedures, have a limited life expectancy, or are in hemodynamically unstable condition. It would be beneficial to identify which patients are most likely to require subsequent cholecystectomy. To address this question, we reviewed the outcome of a group of patients with asymptomatic cholelithiasis who were undergoing laparotomy. The group was analyzed to evaluate the safety of concomitant cholecystectomy and the natural history of untreated cholelithiasis following operation, and to detect variables predicting the need for subsequent cholecystectomy.

PATIENTS AND METHODS

From January 1979 to December 1987, 156 patients with asymptomatic cholelithiasis underwent laparotomy for non–biliary tract disease. There were 90 men and 66 women, aged 20 to 87 years. Patients in whom asymptomatic cholelithiasis was detected preoperatively, intraoperatively, or postoperatively within six months of a previous laparotomy were included in this study. Individuals with biliary symptoms preoperatively or acalculous cholecystitis postoperatively were excluded. Charts were reviewed to determine the primary diagnosis and operation, the management of cholelithiasis, and postoperative morbidity and mortality. Patients not undergoing concomitant cholecystectomy were further evaluated to determine subsequent development of biliary symptoms and to identify factors contributing to the eventual need for cholecystectomy. Variables evaluated included the presence of cancer, diabetes mellitus, obesity, or multiple stones and prolonged fasting, total parenteral nutrition, transfusion, or mechanical ventilation following the original operative procedure. Statistical comparisons were made using the χ^2 test with $P<.05$ for significance levels.

RESULTS

The primary operations are shown in Table 1. The most frequently performed procedures in patients undergoing concomitant cholecystectomy were colectomy, gastric resection, and fundoplication. Procedures were similar in those patients not undergoing cholecystectomy. The diagnosis of cholelithiasis was established preoperatively in 75 patients (48%), intraoperatively in 57 patients (37%), and postoperatively in 24 patients (15%). Cholecystectomy was significantly more likely to be performed when cholelithiasis was diagnosed preoperatively ($P<.005$) (Table 2). Thirty-four patients underwent primary procedures that were performed emergently, and only ten (29%) of these patients had concomitant cholecystectomy. In contrast, concomitant cholecystectomy was performed in 79 (65%) of 122 patients undergoing elective procedures ($P<.005$).

Eighty-eight of the patients (65%) with cholelithiasis discovered preoperatively or intraoperatively underwent cholecystectomy at the time of the original operation. Twenty patients (23%) had intraoperative cholangiography and one (1%) required common bile duct exploration. There were 27 postoperative complications (31%), one of which was directly related to the cholecystectomy (subhepatic abscess), and there were six deaths (7%) in this group. The number of complications and deaths was not significantly different in the patients who did not have concomitant cholecystectomy (18% and 9%, respectively).

Sixty-eight patients did not undergo concomitant cholecystectomy. The most common reason for not performing cholecystectomy at the original operation when the presence of cholelithiasis was determined preoperatively or intraoperatively was unstable condition (n = 16 [36%]), followed by a short life expectancy (n = 10 [23%]), inadequate incision (n = 9 [20%]), too much additional dissection (n = 6 [14%]), and concern for increasing risk of infection (n = 3 [7%]). Thirty-seven (54%) of these patients subsequently developed biliary symptoms and all but one required cholecystectomy. Twenty-six of the symptomatic patients (70%) required cholecystectomy within six months

Accepted for publication Nov 29, 1988.

From the Surgical Service, Omaha Veterans Administration Medical Center, and the Department of Surgery, University of Nebraska Medical Center and Creighton University School of Medicine, Omaha.

Read before the 12th Annual Surgical Symposium of the Association of Veterans Administration Surgeons, Minneapolis, May 12, 1988.

Reprint requests to Department of Surgery, University of Nebraska Medical Center, 42nd and Dewey avenues, Omaha, NE 68105 (Dr Bragg).

Table 1.—Primary Operations Performed in Patients With Asymptomatic Cholelithiasis			
Primary Operation	**Concomitant Cholecystectomy**	**No Cholecystectomy**	**Total**
Colectomy	32	19	**51**
Gastric resection	9	1	**10**
Fundoplication	9	0	**9**
Small intestine	8	11	**19**
Gynecologic	7	10	**17**
Vascular	6	8	**14**
Gastroplasty	4	2	**6**
Splenectomy	4	4	**8**
Other	10	12	**22**
Total	**89**	**67**	**156**

Table 2.—Outcome of Patients With Asymptomatic Cholelithiasis				
Time of Diagnosis	**n**	**Concomitant Cholecys-tectomy, No. (%)**	**No Cholecys-tectomy, No. (%)**	**Subsequent Biliary Symptoms**
Preoperative	75	59 (79)	16 (21)	3
Intraoperative	57	29 (51)	28 (49)	12
Postoperative	24	. . .	24	22
Total	**156**	**88**	**68**	**37**

of their original operation. Nine patients (28%) required common bile duct exploration. All patients 50 years of age or less (n = 15) eventually required cholecystectomy. There were no other significant differences between patients who remained asymptomatic and those who required cholecystectomy (Table 3).

Eight (22%) of the 68 patients required a second operation for cholecystectomy within 30 days of the original operation or within the same hospitalization. Sixty-two percent of patients requiring early reoperation for cholecystectomy had undergone emergent primary procedures, whereas only 17% of individuals later requiring cholecystectomy had emergent primary operations ($P<.05$). Additionally, these patients who required early cholecystectomy fasted for a longer period of time following the original operation and were more likely to require transfusion, mechanical ventilation, and total parenteral nutrition than those undergoing cholecystectomy at a later date (Table 4). Four patients (50%) developed acute cholecystitis, six patients (75%) experienced complications during the hospitalization, and there were four deaths (50%) in this group of patients who developed early symptoms postoperatively. The two groups were similar with respect to age and the presence of cancer, diabetes mellitus, obesity, postoperative shock, multiple stones, and peritonitis.

COMMENT

The decision to combine cholecystectomy with other intra-abdominal procedures in individuals with biliary symptoms is clearly justified. The advantages of combining procedures include avoiding a second anesthetic and in many cases a second incision. The safety of concomitant cholecystectomy has been well documented. Schreiber et al[4] performed cholecystectomy on 39 patients during

Table 3.—Outcome of Patients Not Undergoing Concomitant Cholecystectomy			
	Symptomatic, No. (%) (n=37)	**Asymptomatic, No. (%) (n=31)**	***P* Value***
Age <50 y	16 (100)	0	<.005
Multiple stones	19 (51)	18 (58)	NS
Cancer	10 (27)	12 (39)	NS
Diabetes	4 (11)	3 (10)	NS
Shock	6 (16)	9 (29)	NS
Emergency operation	10 (27)	10 (32)	NS
Transfusion	5 (13)	12 (39)	NS
Nothing by mouth postoperatively, d (mean ± SD)	5±2	6±3	NS
Total parenteral nutrition	10 (27)	5 (16)	NS
Mechanical ventilation	8 (22)	7 (23)	NS

*NS indicates not significant.

Table 4.—Comparison of Patients Undergoing Delayed Cholecystectomy			
	Early Cholecystectomy,* No. (%) (n=8)	**Late Cholecystectomy, No. (%) (n=29)**	***P* Value†**
Age <50 y	3 (38)	14 (48)	NS
Multiple stones	3 (38)	16 (55)	NS
Cancer	1 (12)	9 (31)	NS
Diabetes	1 (12)	3 (10)	NS
Shock	2 (25)	4 (14)	NS
Emergency operation	5 (62)	5 (17)	<.05
Transfusion	3 (38)	2 (7)	<.05
Nothing by mouth postoperatively, d (mean ± SD)	15±5	4±2	<.05
Total parenteral nutrition	4 (50)	6 (21)	<.05
Mechanical ventilation	4 (50)	4 (14)	<.05

*These patients required cholecystectomy within 30 days of the original operation or during same hospitalization.
†NS indicates not significant.

major abdominal operations with only one related complication. McSherry and Glenn[5] found little increase in the morbidity and mortality rates of patients undergoing cholecystectomy concomitant with another major intra-abdominal procedure. Kovalcik et al[6] likewise found that the rate of complications was only slightly increased when concomitant cholecystectomy was performed (14.3% vs 19.8%). Shennib et al[7] found no difference in outcome among patients undergoing elective colon resection and concomitant cholecystectomy, but they advised against combining cholecystectomy with emergent colon resections. In the present study, 88 patients underwent concomitant cholecystectomy with only one complication related to the biliary procedure.

The frequent utilization of abdominal ultrasonography

and computed tomography for the evaluation of intra-abdominal problems has resulted in the increasing identification of asymptomatic cholelithiasis. Studies of the natural history of asymptomatic gallstone disease have shown that biliary symptoms will develop in approximately 10% to 20% of these individuals.[8,9] We found previously that 70% of patients with asymptomatic gallstones developed symptoms within six months following laparotomy.[3] String[1] found that 65% of patients with asymptomatic gallstones developed symptoms following aortic reconstruction. In the present study, 37 (54%) of 68 patients with asymptomatic gallstones developed biliary symptoms following major abdominal operations.

Although many patients become symptomatic, it would be beneficial to avoid cholecystectomy in high-risk patients. Determination of factors predicting the development of symptomatic cholelithiasis would aid in the decision of whether to perform concomitant cholecystectomy. Identification of individuals most likely to become symptomatic would eliminate the need for cholecystectomy at a later date but would also avoid the potential complications of unnecessary cholecystectomy in individuals not at risk.

It is not known why the performance of a laparotomy alters the natural history of "silent" gallstones. Inflammation of the calculous gallbladder occurring postoperatively may be analogous to acute acalculous cholecystitis. The incidence of acalculous disease in patients in whom acute cholecystitis developed postoperatively has ranged from 35% to 62%.[10-12] The cause of inflammation remains unknown, but it is thought to be due to ischemia of the gallbladder wall or biliary stasis with distention of the gallbladder. Factors often present in the postoperative patient, and possibly predisposing to the development of acute cholecystitis, are hypotension, hypoxemia, fasting, dehydration, and blood transfusion.[10-15] The eight patients in this study who developed biliary symptoms during the original hospitalization displayed several of these characteristics that possibly placed them at risk for developing inflammation of the gallbladder. In comparison with the group in whom symptoms developed at a later date, significantly more patients with early symptoms fasted for a longer period of time and required total parenteral nutrition, mechanical ventilation, and transfusion.

Glenn[13] reported an association between prolonged fasting and acute cholecystitis. He proposed that in the absence of oral intake there is no stimulus for gallbladder contraction, and stagnation and inspissation of bile occur. This concept has been further supported by the demonstration of an increased frequency of cholelithiasis in patients receiving total parenteral nutrition and undergoing long periods of fasting.[16,17] Gafa et al[18] found that biliary tract sludge developed within nine days in five of 12 patients following gastrectomy and postoperative total parenteral nutrition. Positive pressure ventilation has been shown to result in bile stasis[19] and may also promote acute acalculous cholecystitis.[20] The increased bile pigment load resulting from blood transfusion was suggested as a mode of gallbladder injury by Lindberg et al.[21] The presence of calculi in the patients in whom early biliary symptoms developed in this study may also have contributed to the development of cholecystitis.

Operative procedures for symptomatic cholelithiasis occurring after laparotomy were frequently more extensive and associated with greater morbidity. Common bile duct exploration was required in nine patients (25%) undergoing cholecystectomy at a later date, whereas only one patient (1%) undergoing concomitant cholecystectomy required common duct exploration. Patients who required cholecystectomy during or within 30 days of the original hospitalization had significantly higher morbidity and mortality rates than patients undergoing concomitant cholecystectomy. Six (75%) of the eight patients requiring early reoperation experienced complications and four patients (50%) died. The increased morbidity and mortality rates in this group may have been related to the high incidence (50%) of acute cholecystitis in this group. The high complication rate associated with acute postoperative cholecystitis has been previously documented.[10-12]

Patients with asymptomatic cholelithiasis frequently develop biliary symptoms following an operation for unrelated intra-abdominal problems. Patients requiring mechanical ventilation, blood transfusions, and parenteral nutrition postoperatively and who are slow to resume enteral nutrition are more likely to require early cholecystectomy. Individuals who subsequently require cholecystectomy frequently undergo a more extensive biliary procedure. Since similar characteristics have been identified in patients in whom acalculous cholecystitis develops, the pathophysiologic mechanisms responsible for the development of cholecystitis in these patient populations may be similar. Concomitant cholecystectomy adds minimal morbidity to other procedures and should be undertaken unless specific contraindications exist, particularly in this high-risk group.

References

1. String ST: Cholelithiasis and aortic reconstruction. *J Vasc Surg* 1984; 5:664-669.
2. Herbst CA, Mittelstaedt CA, Staab EV, et al: Intraoperative ultrasonography evaluation of the gallbladder in morbidly obese patients. *Ann Surg* 1984;200:691-692.
3. Thompson JS, Philben VJ, Hodgson PE: Operative management of incidental cholelithiasis. *Am J Surg* 1984;148:821-824.
4. Schreiber H, Macon WL, Proies WJ: Incidental cholecystectomy during major abdominal surgery in the elderly. *Am J Surg* 1978;135:196-198.
5. McSherry CK, Glenn F: Biliary tract surgery concomitant with other intra-abdominal operations. *Ann Surg* 1981;193:169-175.
6. Kovalcik PJ, Burrell MJ, Old WJ: Cholecystectomy concomitant with other intra-abdominal operations. *Arch Surg* 1983;118:1059-1062.
7. Shennib H, Fried GM, Hampson LG: Does simultaneous cholecystectomy increase the risk of colonic surgery. *Am J Surg* 1986;151:266-268.
8. Gracie WA, Ransohoff DF: The natural history of silent gallstones: The innocent gallstone is not a myth. *N Engl J Med* 1982;307:798-800.
9. McSherry CK, Ferstenberg H, Calhoun WF, et al: The natural history of diagnosed gallstone disease in symptomatic and asymptomatic patients. *Ann Surg* 1985;202:59-63.
10. Ottinger LW: Acute cholecystitis as a postoperative complication. *Ann Surg* 1976;184:162-165.
11. Ziv Y, Feigenberg Z, Zer M, et al: Acute cholecystitis complicating unrelated disease: Etiologic considerations. *Am J Gastroenterol* 1987;82: 1165-1168.
12. Gately JF, Thomas EJ: Acute cholecystitis occurring as a complication of other diseases. *Arch Surg* 1983;118:1137-1141.
13. Glenn F: Acute acalculous cholecystitis. *Ann Surg* 1979;189:458-465.
14. Glenn F: Acute cholecystitis following the surgical treatment of unrelated disease. *Ann Surg* 1947;126:411-420.
15. Nobusawa S, Endo M: Prophylaxis of postoperative biliary stasis: A retrospective and prospective study. *Am J Gastroenterol* 1988;83:46-54.
16. Pitt HA, King W, Mann LL, et al: Increased risk of cholelithiasis with prolonged total parenteral nutrition. *Am J Surg* 1983;145:106-112.
17. Messing B, Bories C, Kunstlinger F, et al: Does total parenteral nutrition induce gallbladder sludge formation and lithiasis? *Gastroenterology* 1983;84:1012-1019.
18. Gafa M, Sarli L, Miselli A, et al: Sludge and microlithiasis of the biliary tract after total gastrectomy and postoperative total parenteral nutrition. *Surg Gynecol Obstet* 1987;165:413-418.
19. Johnson EE, Hedley-White J: Continuous positive pressure ventilation and choledochoduodenal flow resistance. *J Appl Physiol* 1975;39:937.
20. Long TN, Heimbach DN, Carrico CJ: Acalculous cholecystitis in critically ill patients. *Am J Surg* 1978;136:31-36.
21. Lindberg EF, Grinnan GLB, Smith L: Acalculous cholecystitis in Vietnam casualties. *Ann Surg* 1970;171:152-157.

Reversal of Pigment Gallstone Disease in a Canine Model

Lillian G. Dawes, MD; David L. Nahrwold, MD; Sanford I. Roth, MD; Robert V. Rege, MD

• Unlike dietary-induced cholesterol gallstones, which may disappear spontaneously when the lithogenic diet is withdrawn, little is known about the natural history of pigment gallstones. We examined whether pigment gallstone disease, which can be uniformly induced in the dog by six weeks of a methionine-deficient diet, can be reversed by return to normal diet. As previously reported, all dogs develop pigment gallstones as well as significant increases in biliary total calcium, free ionized calcium, and cholesterol concentrations after six weeks of a lithogenic diet. These changes are accompanied by a significant increase in the concentration of unconjugated bile salts in bile. In addition, histologic changes in the gallbladder wall occur that are consistent with a moderate degree of chronic cholecystitis. This study clearly demonstrates that return to a normal diet for six weeks allows bile composition to normalize, gallstones to disappear in 50% of dogs, and gallbladder histologic changes to return toward normal. Thus, it would appear that pigment gallstone disease in this model may be reversible, at least early during its course. Although the relevance of these findings to pigment gallstones in humans must be established, the potential for nonoperative treatment of pigment gallstones should not be discounted.

(*Arch Surg* 1989;124:463-466)

Gallstone disease is a common medical problem: 500 000 cholecystectomies are performed annually in the United States alone. It thus accounts for significant morbidity and mortality and has a major impact on health care costs, exceeding $5 billion in medical expenses each year. Although once considered a surgical disease, simple, safe, and inexpensive alternatives to surgery are being investigated. Some success has been achieved with cholesterol gallstone dissolution,[1] but the number of actual candidates for dissolution therapy has been limited by the frequent presence of gallstones with high calcium contents or with "calcium shells" that cannot be consistently dissolved with present techniques and agents.[2]

Pigment gallstones, found in 10% to 30% of patients with gallstones,[3] are largely composed of calcium salts of bilirubin, carbonate, phosphate, and free fatty acids[4] and are therefore usually not amenable to dissolution therapy. Unfortunately, this type of stone is also often seen in those patients who would benefit most from a nonoperative alternative, that is, in high-surgical-risk patients such as the elderly and patients with liver disease. If pigment gallstone disease were potentially reversible, the development of dissolution agents for pigment and for other calcium-containing gallstones would greatly increase the applicability of dissolution therapy.

Accepted for publication Nov 7, 1988.

From the Departments of Surgery (Drs Dawes, Nahrwold, and Rege) and Pathology (Dr Roth), Northwestern University Medical School, and Veterans Administration Lakeside Medical Center (Drs Dawes, Nahrwold, Roth, and Rege), Chicago.

Read before the 12th Annual Surgical Symposium of the Association of Veterans Administration Surgeons, Minneapolis, May 14, 1988.

Reprint requests to Department of Surgery, Suite 201, Wesley Pavilion, 250 E Superior St, Chicago, IL 60611 (Dr Dawes).

We herein examine whether pigment gallstone disease can be reversed in a dietary model. Dogs placed on a methionine-deficient, high-cholesterol diet (MDD) uniformly formed pigment stones that closely resembled human black pigment gallstones.[5,6] We have previously reported that 100% of dogs on this diet for six weeks develop alterations in bile composition and pigment gallstones.[7] In this study, we extend our previous work and examine the histologic changes that occur with stone formation. In addition, return to a regular diet reverses all alterations in bile composition, returns gallbladder histologic changes toward normal, and results in the disappearance of gallstones in 50% of dogs. Thus, pigment gallstone disease may be reversible, at least early during its course.

MATERIALS AND METHODS

Experimental Design

Bile samples from 12 mongrel dogs were collected at laparotomies performed before and during an MDD, which consistently produces gallstones.[5,6] The protocol for bile collection and the changes in bile composition that occurred after six weeks of MDD have previously been reported.[7] At the end of six weeks of MDD, each dog underwent laparotomy, aspiration of gallbladder bile, and palpation of the gallbladder for the presence of stones after it was emptied. Six dogs from our previous study were killed and their gallbladders were harvested for histologic examination. The remaining six dogs were allowed to recover from surgery, placed on a normal diet for an additional six-week period, and then killed. Bile was again collected for analysis, and the gallbladders were removed for microscopic evaluation. Comparisons were made for the presence and absence of stones, for gross and histologic evidence of cholecystitis, and for changes in bile composition among these dogs (MDD + N), dogs on a six-week lithogenic diet (MDD), and three dogs before MDD (normal).

Bile Analyses

Bile was immediately cultured for the presence of aerobic and anaerobic bacteria. The pH and carbon dioxide pressure (PCO_2) were anaerobically determined in a blood gas analyzer (Instruments Laboratory model 1301). Total calcium concentration was measured by fluorometric titration (Calcette calcium analyzer model 4008) and free ionized calcium with a Ca^{++}-sensitive electrode (ICA calcium analyzer). The proportions of conjugated and unconjugated bile salts were determined by thin-layer chromatography separation.[8] Each fraction was eluted from the gel with methanol for quantitative analysis. Total, conjugated, and unconjugated bile salt concentrations were then determined by the 3 α-hydroxysteroid dehydrogenase method.[9] The biliary electrolytes sodium and potassium were measured by flame photometry. Biliary phospholipid and cholesterol concentrations were determined by end-point enzymatic analysis (Wako phospholipid assay kit and Boehring Mannheim Biochemical cholesterol assay kit).

Gallbladder Histology

Gallbladders were opened longitudinally, examined grossly for the presence of stones, and immediately fixed in 10% formaldehyde solution. Paraffin-embedded sections were stained with hematoxylin-eosin, and coded slides were evaluated by a pathologist, without knowledge of the treatment of the individual dogs. Six histologic values of cholecystitis were scored: (1) cellular inflammation, (2) dilatation of mucosal crypts, (3) villous atrophy, (4) thickness of mucosal surface mucin, (5) fibrosis of the gallbladder

Table 1.— Histologic Changes in Gallbladder During Stone Formation*

	No. of Dogs With Stones	Mean Histologic Score
Normal	0/12	1±1
MDD	12/12	12±1†
MDD+N	3/6	5±2

*MDD indicates methionine-deficient diet; and MDD+N, MDD followed by a return to a normal diet.
†Significant difference from normal, $P<.05$.

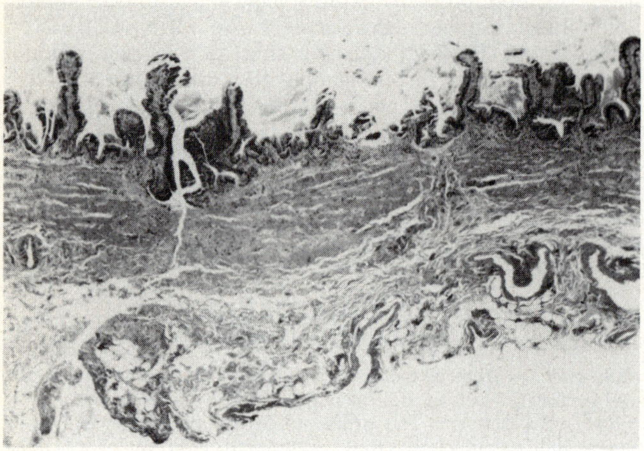

Fig 1.—Normal canine gallbladder. There are prominent villi with narrow crypts. Subepithelial tissues are relatively free of inflammatory cells. Muscularis is unremarkable. Serosa contains fibrous and adipose tissue without inflammation (hematoxylin-eosin, original magnification ×49).

wall, and (6) deposition of submucosal pigment. Each value was scored on a scale of 0 (normal) to 4 (severe changes), with a maximum possible score of 24.

Statistical Analysis

Differences between groups were analyzed by analysis of variance. Differences in bile composition and gallbladder histology between normal and MDD dogs and normal and MDD+N dogs were also analyzed by Student's *t* test. The statistical data reported for the comparisons were calculated by unpaired analysis. Paired analysis was also done to compare the six MDD+N dogs with themselves before and after MDD. Statistical significances were similar by all methods used. Results are reported as the mean±SEM.

RESULTS

All 12 dogs developed gallstones following six weeks of MDD (Table 1). Each dog had sludge and small stones in the aspirated bile, and, at laparotomy, larger stones were palpated in the gallbladder lumen. There was no perceivable difference between the six dogs that were killed immediately and the six dogs returned to a normal diet. Examination of the gallbladders harvested at six weeks of MDD contained multiple dark-brown to black, amorphous pigment gallstones ranging in size from 1 to 4 mm. The gallstones were accompanied in some cases by thick mucinous material and were embedded in biliary sludge. Bile cultures were sterile in all cases.

As would be expected, normal dogs showed no evidence of cholecystitis (Fig 1, Table 1), and the mean histologic score was correspondingly 1±1. With stone formation, the gallbladder walls were thickened, and each gallbladder wall showed varying degrees of submucosal lymphocyte and plasma cell infiltration, atrophy of villi, dilatation of the mucosal crypts, fibrosis of the gallbladder wall, and deposition of pigment in macrophages below the mucosa. An abundant amount of mucin was adherent to the mucosa of many of the gallbladders (Figs 2 and 3). These changes represent a moderate degree of chronic cholecystitis as reflected in the mean histologic score of 12±1.

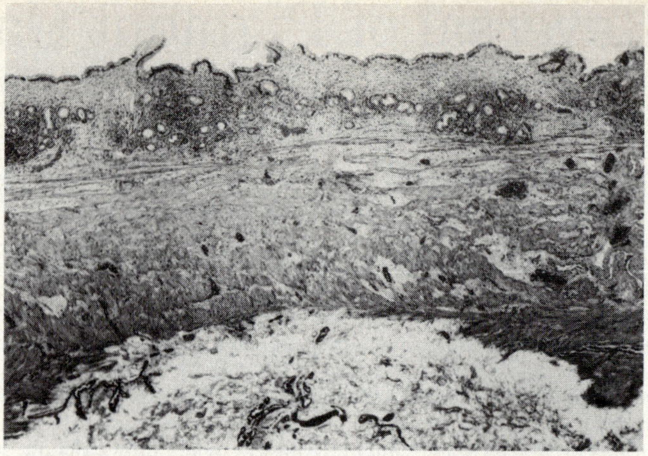

Fig 2.—Full-thickness section of canine gallbladder after six weeks of lithogenic (methionine-deficient) diet. Villi are absent. Crypts are increased in thickness. There is marked increase in mucosal thickness with accompanying increase in lamina propria. Severe chronic inflammatory infiltrate is seen in lamina propria, and mild infiltrate is present in muscularis mucosa and submucosa. Muscularis is thickened. There is mild increase in fibrosis of serosa (hematoxylin-eosin, original magnification ×49).

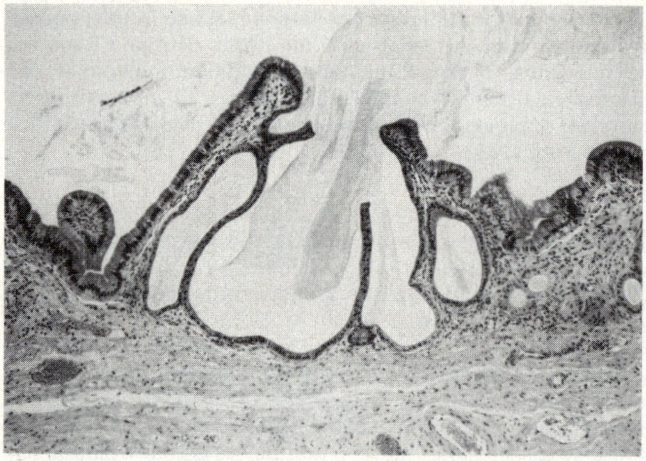

Fig 3.—Higher-power section of gallbladder from dog on lithogenic diet demonstrating mucus retention and dilatation of crypts. There is moderate chronic inflammation of widened lamina propria (hematoxylin-eosin, original magnification ×196).

Pigment gallstones were found in only three of six dogs that were returned to a normal diet for six weeks (Table 1), and their gallbladders appeared normal whether or not they contained gallstones. The stones that were present appeared more organized and were larger than those noted at six weeks of MDD, ranging from 2 to 8 mm. Moreover, there was marked improvement of the chronic cholecystitis (Fig 4, Table 1), reflected by a significant ($P<.05$) decrease in the mean histologic score to 5±2. This score was not significantly different from the score for normal gallbladders. Dogs without stones had the most impressive recov-

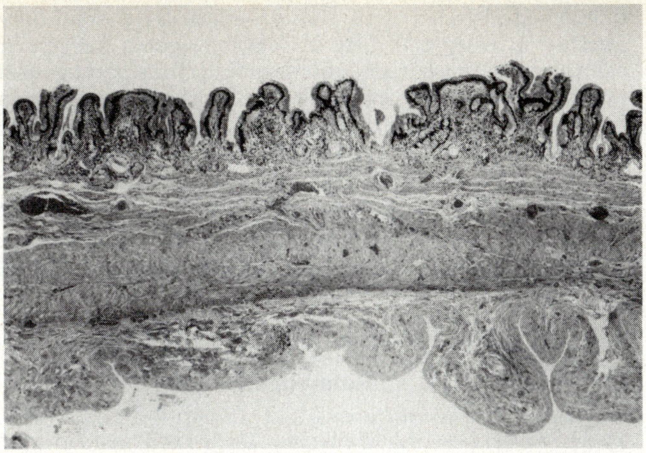

Fig 4.—Full-thickness section of gallbladder in dogs with gallstones returned to regular diet for six weeks. Villi are present, though there is still some dilatation of crypt areas. Lamina propria is widened, and there is mild chronic inflammation of lamina propria. Submucosa, muscularis, and serosa are near normal (hematoxylin-eosin, original magnification ×49).

Table 2.—Acidification and Concentration of Gallbladder Biles*

Biliary Value	Normal	MDD	MDD+N
pH	6.14±0.05	6.29±0.10	6.25±0.07
P_{CO_2}, mm Hg	56.9±2.5	79.7±7.0	60.4±4.4
Sodium, mmol/L	252±3	237±5	249±3
Potassium, mmol/L	11.3±0.3	11.3±0.3	10.8±0.2
Bile salts, mmol/L	257±7	241±9	243±12
Phospholipids, mmol/L	34.7±1.3	37.8±2.2	37.3±1.8

*MDD indicates methionine-deficient diet; MDD+N, MDD followed by a return to a normal diet; and P_{CO_2}, carbon dioxide pressure. All values for the normal and MDD groups were previously reported. All values are mean±SEM.

ery, with the mean histologic score decreasing to 3±1, whereas dogs with stones improved yet had some evidence of chronic cholecystitis, with a mean score of 8±3. Therefore, a return to a normal diet for six weeks resulted in resolving cholecystitis in all and the disappearance of stones in 50% of the dogs.

The results of bile analysis in MDD+N dogs were compared with previously published[7] data in these dogs before and after six weeks of MDD. Note that pH, P_{CO_2}, Na^+, K^+, bile salts, and phospholipid concentration remained normal after the restoration of a regular diet (Table 2). This was also true for dogs that continued to have gallstones in their gallbladders. There was no significant change in the ability of any dogs to concentrate or acidify bile at any time during the study. In contrast, the previously noted 29% and 23% increases in biliary Ca and Ca^{++}, and a twofold increase in cholesterol concentration after six weeks of MDD, were completely reversed when dogs were put back on a diet of regular dog chow for six weeks (Table 3). The Ca, Ca^{++}, and cholesterol concentrations of 9.88±0.25, 3.14±0.14, and 0.7±0.06 mmol/L, respectively, in MDD+N dogs were thus essentially the same as the values of 10.16±0.19, 3.02±0.07, and 0.7±0.03 mmol/L, respectively, in normal dogs. Also, there was a significant increase in the concentration of unconjugated bile salts in bile after six weeks of MDD, increasing from 0.5±0.5 to 13±4 mmol/L ($P<.05$). This was completely reversed by return to a normal diet; no unconjugated bile salts were detected in any MDD+N dog (Table 3).

Table 3.—Reversal of Bile Composition*

	Calcium Ion	Calcium	Cholesterol	Unconjugated Bile Salts
Normal	3.02±.07	10.16±0.19	0.7±0.03	0.5±0.5
MDD	3.71±0.17†	13.11±0.57†	1.4±0.10†	12.6±4.1†
MDD+N	3.14±0.15	9.88±0.27	0.7±0.06	Undetectable

*MDD indicates methionine-deficient diet; and MDD+N, MDD followed by a return to a normal diet. All values are millimoles per liter, mean±SEM.
†Significant difference from normal, $P<.05$.

COMMENT

Until recently, the presence of gallstones alone was an indication for cholecystectomy, and operations were frequently performed in asymptomatic or mildly symptomatic patients. However, clearer understanding of the pathogenesis and natural history of gallstones has led to radical changes in our attitude and approach toward gallstone disease. Expectant therapy for silent gallstones is common and believed to be as safe as, or safer than, operative therapy,[10] and alternatives such as oral dissolution therapy,[1] percutaneous cholecystostomy with contact dissolution,[11] and gallstone lithotripsy[12] are now being performed in selected patients. Gallstone disease is now increasingly viewed as a potentially reversible process.

The possibility of cholesterol gallstone dissolution arose in part from observations in animal studies documenting that diet-induced gallstones disappear when animals are returned to a normal diet.[13-16] As early as 1956, Christensen et al[13] showed that cholesterol gallstones in hamsters would disappear when they were placed on a nonlithogenic diet. Chang et al[14] later showed that disappearance of cholesterol crystals and gallstones in prairie dogs is associated with a decrease in biliary cholesterol levels, suggesting that the decrease in biliary cholesterol saturation was directly related to resolubilization of cholesterol crystals and gallstones. To our knowledge, similar observations have not been previously made for pigment gallstones in either humans or animals.

The canine dietary model of pigment gallstones was chosen because pigment gallstones of substantial size are uniformly produced in six weeks along with abnormalities in bile composition. Yet, at this time, gallbladder function is still relatively normal.[7] Although we approached this study with the idea that pigment gallstone disease is irreversible, we found that bile composition normalized, chronic cholecystitis improved, and gallstones disappeared in half of the dogs six weeks after return to a normal diet. The findings of these studies are thus analogous to the animal studies of cholesterol gallstone disease discussed above.

The fate of the pigment gallstones that disappeared during this study is not known. Since pigment gallstones are highly insoluble, containing a high proportion of calcium salts and an insoluble residue thought to be a tightly cross-linked network polymer,[17,18] spontaneous dissolution is unlikely. However, either partial or total dissolution of stones should not be discounted. It is possible that pigment gallstones are initially not so insoluble, but that later changes such as cross-linking of the polymer might render them resistant to dissolution. If this is the case, they could have been dissolved or decreased in size.

If stones did not dissolve, they must have passed from the gallbladder through the cystic duct, entering the duodenum via the common bile duct. Delius et al[19] recently implanted kidney stone fragments (insoluble in bile) ranging in size from 2 to 6 mm into normal canine gallbladders. At five weeks, the mean weight of stone fragments remaining in the gallbladders was one third of that implanted, and one third of dogs had gallbladders completely free of stone fragments. Thus, stones of size comparable with those seen in this study can spontaneously pass from the gallbladder into the duodenum in a relatively short time.

The fact that stones remained in some dogs after six weeks of normal diet may be a finding as important as stone disappearance. Despite normal bile composition and resolution of cholecystitis, gallstones were present in three of the dogs and these stones were more organized and slightly larger. Thus, although factors that resulted in pigment gallstones were present only transiently, gallstones persisted in several relatively normal gallbladders. One might speculate that pigment gallstones might form during transitory "lithogenic states" and perhaps, like cholesterol gallstones, could remain silent for long periods. In fact, at this early stage, these diet-induced gallstones may be analogous to biliary sludge. Similar to results seen herein, sludge in the gallbladder has been known to resolve or disappear when followed up by serial ultrasound examinations.[20,21] Although these speculations are intriguing, this short-term animal study was not designed to examine these issues.

Chronic cholecystitis has been noted histologically in this model at five and 12 months of the lithogenic diet,[6] yet this is the first report of cholecystitis as early as six weeks. The presence of these changes at this early stage suggests that they occur simultaneously with stone formation and are not secondary to the physical presence of gallstones. This is further supported by the partial resolution of cholecystitis in dogs that continued to harbor gallstones after six weeks of regular diet.

Histologic evidence of inflammation, cell proliferation, and mucin production has been previously reported before or early during stone formation in dietary models of gallstones.[22-25] Administration of the antibiotic lincomycin to guinea pigs causes early gallbladder inflammation and gallstone formation. In this model and in dihydrocholesterol-induced gallstones in rabbits, enhanced fluid transport across the gallbladder has been demonstrated even before the appearance of gallstones.[16] In addition, microscopic gallbladder changes have been found early during stone formation in rabbits fed dihydrocholesterol[16] and in mice fed a cholesterol–cholic acid diet.[25] As was seen in this model, cholecystitis improved in all these models when the lithogenic agent or diet was withdrawn.

Although the relevance of this animal study to humans must be established, these studies raise the possibility that pigment gallstone disease can be reversed at some point during its course. Thus, it is similar to early studies with cholesterol gallstones that, when combined with a thorough understanding of cholesterol solubility, led to successful cholesterol gallstone dissolution. However, it should be understood that it is not clear from this study whether the stones dissolved or passed from the gallbladder via the cystic duct. In either case, the potential for nonoperative treatment of pigment gallstones should not be discounted.

Although an acceptable agent for pigment gallstone dissolution has not yet been found, there are a few reports of successful dissolution of stones containing calcium salts. Calcium carbonate pancreatic stones in the dog have been experimentally dissolved with trimethadione,[26] and there has been some success with in vitro dissolution of calcium bilirubinate stones with sodium–edetic acid solutions.[27] Further investigation into dissolution agents for calcium salts along with a better understanding of the pathogenesis of pigment gallstones may lead to nonoperative alternatives for pigment gallstone disease. Moreover, if the gallstones disappeared after reversal of abnormalities in gallbladder bile composition by passage into the duodenum, rather than by dissolution, it might be possible to treat this type of gallstone by fragmentation (gallstone lithotripsy).

This work was supported by Merit Review grant from the Veterans Administration.

We thank Diane April for her careful assistance in preparation of the manuscript.

References

1. National Cooperative Gallstone Study Group: Chenodiol (chenodeoxycholic acid) for dissolution of gallstones: The National Cooperative Gallstone Study. *Ann Intern Med* 1981;95:257-282.

2. Bruchier IAD: The medical treatment of gallstones. *Annu Rev Med* 1980;31:59-77.

3. Trotman BW, Soloway RD: Pigment vs. cholesterol cholelithiasis: Clinical and epidemiological aspects. *Am J Dig Dis* 1975;20:735-740.

4. Moore EW: The role of calcium in the pathogenesis of gallstones: Ca^{++} electrode studies of model bile solutions and other biologic systems. *Hepatology* 1984;4:228s-243s.

5. Englert E, Harmon CG, Wales E: Gallstones induced by normal foodstuffs in dogs. *Nature* 1969;224:280-281.

6. Englert E, Harmon CG, Freston JW, et al: Studies on the pathogenesis of diet-induced dog gallstones. *Dig Dis* 1977;22:305-314.

7. Dawes LG, Nahrwold DL, Rege RV: Increased total and free ionized calcium in a canine model of pigment gallstones. *Surgery* 1988;104:86-90.

8. Chavez M, Krone C: Silicic acid thin-layer chromatography of conjugated and free bile acids. *J Lipid Res* 1976;17:545-547.

9. Talalay P: Enzymatic analysis of steroid hormones, in Glick D (ed): *Methods of Biochemical Analysis.* New York, Interscience, 1960, pp 119-143.

10. Gracie WA, Ransohoff DF: The natural history of silent gallstones: The innocent gallstone is not a myth. *N Engl J Med* 1982;307:798-800.

11. Allen MJ, Borody TJ, Bugliosi TF, et al: Cholelitholysis using methyl tertiary butyl ether. *Gastroenterology* 1985;1:122-125.

12. Sackmann M, Delius M, Sauerbruch T, et al: Shock-wave lithotripsy of gallbladder stones: The first 175 patients. *N Engl J Med* 1988;318:393-397.

13. Christensen F, Dam H, Kristensen G: Alimentary production of gallstones in hamsters: VI. Disappearance of cholesterol stones by treatment with a non-lithogenic diet. *Acta Physiol Scand* 1956;36:329-335.

14. Chang SH, Ho KJ, Taylor B: Cholesterol gallstone formation and its regression in prairie dogs. *Arch Pathol Lab Med* 1973;96:417-426.

15. Caldwell FT, Levitsky KI, Rosenberg B: Dietary production and dissolution of cholesterol gallstones in the mouse. *Am J Physiol* 1965;209:473-478.

16. Lee SP: Enhanced fluid transport across gallbladder mucosa in experimental cholelithiasis. *Am J Physiol* 1978;234:E575-E578.

17. Black BE, Carr SH, Ostrow JD, et al: Equilibrium swelling of pigment gallstones: Evidence for network polymer structure. *Biopolymers* 1982;21:601-610.

18. Ohkubo H, Ostrow JD, Carr SH, et al: Polymer networks in pigment and cholesterol gallstones assessed by equilibrium swelling and infrared spectroscopy. *Gastroenterology* 1984;87:805-814.

19. Delius M, Enders G, Brendel W: Passage of stone fragments from the gallbladder of dogs. *Surg Gynecol Obstet* 1988;166:241-244.

20. Lee SP, Maher K, Nicholls JF: Origin and fate of biliary sludge. *Gastroenterology* 1988;94:170-176.

21. Allen B, Bernhoft R, Blanchaert N, et al: Sludge is calcium bilirubinate associated with bile stasis. *Am J Surg* 1981;14:51-56.

22. Putz P, Willens G: Effect of a lithogenic diet on cell proliferation in the murine gallbladder epithelium. *Digestion* 1981;22:16-23.

23. Hayward AF, Freston JW, Bouchier IAD: Changes in the ultrastructure of gallbladder epithelium in rabbits with experimental gallstones. *Gut* 1968;9:550-556.

24. Lee SP, Thompsen LL: Toxin induced cell membrane injury in guinea pigs given lincomycin. *Pathology* 1982;14:317-322.

25. Lee SP, Scott AJ: The evolution of morphologic changes in the gallbladder before stone formation in mice fed a cholesterol–cholic acid diet. *Am J Pathol* 1982;108:1-8.

26. Noda AJ, Shibata T, Ogawa Y, et al: Dissolution of pancreatic stones by oral trimethadione in a dog experimental model. *Gastroenterology* 1987;93:1002-1008.

27. Nakamua Y, Suzuki N, Watanu T, et al: Study on dissolution and disintegration of calcium bilirubinate stone. *Tohoku J Exp Med* 1978;125:121-134.

Terminal Loop Cutaneous Ureterostomy in Cadaveric Kidney Transplantation

R. Neal Garrison, MD; Frederick R. Bentley, MD; Mohammad Amin, MD

• The presence of a nonfunctional bladder is a common finding in some patients with end-stage renal disease in whom transplantation is a proposed option. Over the last 20 years, we have performed six terminal loop cutaneous ureterostomies for urinary drainage during kidney transplantation. Neurogenic bladder in five patients and exstrophy in one patient prohibited use of the bladder. Four long-term graft survivors (19 months and 4, 10, and 20 years) experienced no short-term problems with the procedure, but two episodes of pyelonephritis have occurred. In our patients no graft dysfunction or loss could be attributed to infection, and no stomal stenosis or revision has occurred. We conclude that terminal loop cutaneous ureterostomy is feasible using normal-caliber ureters, and is a safe, effective means of urinary drainage during kidney transplantation when the bladder is not available. It also eliminates the necessity of preparatory bowel surgery that has its attendant risk of contamination in an immunocompromised patient.

(*Arch Surg* 1989;124:467-469)

A greater number of patients with nonfunctional lower urinary tracts are currently being considered as candidates for renal transplantation as immunosuppression has improved. Various methods of urinary drainage have been recommended as alternatives to the standard ureterovesical anastomosis when rehabilitation of the bladder is not possible. Using either long-term intermittent self-catheterization following a ureterovesical anastomosis or a cutaneous ileal conduit with a ureterointestinal connection are the techniques used most frequently.[1,2] Infection involving the upper urinary tract that leads to graft loss, and occasionally death, is a problem when utilizing these techniques, because differentiation between urosepsis and rejection can be difficult in a patient with chronic bacteriuria. In addition, preparatory intestinal surgery is needed several weeks prior to the transplantation when the ileal conduit technique is chosen, placing the patient at further risk for septic complications to occur.

Cutaneous ureterostomy was frequently used in the thigh or other sites when kidneys were initially transplanted.[3] Transplantation into the iliac fossa with end-ureterocutaneostomy was described by Kuss and associates[4] in 1951, although the results were disappointing due to the necrosis of the ureter in most of the cases. Martin and associates[5] utilized this technique in four patients, but the long-term function was apparently not good, since they saw no future for the technique. Amin and associates[6] reported on three patients in whom a new technique of terminal loop cutaneous ureterostomy was employed with good initial and long-term results. This report is a follow-up of these initial patients and three other patients. The first and second of these initial patients continue to have normal kidney function 20 and ten years, respectively, after kidney transplantation.

Accepted for publication Nov 7, 1988.

From the Department of Surgery, University of Louisville School of Medicine, Jewish Hospital, and the Surgical Service, Veterans Administration Medical Center, Louisville.

Read before the 12th Annual Surgical Symposium of the Association of Veterans Administration Surgeons, Minneapolis, May 12, 1988.

Reprint requests to Department of Surgery, University of Louisville School of Medicine, 529 S Jackson St, Louisville, KY 40202 (Dr Garrison).

PATIENTS AND METHODS

Patients

A review of the records of all patients who had received a kidney transplant from the University of Louisville Transplant Program at Jewish Hospital yielded six patients in whom a terminal loop cutaneous ureterostomy was the method used for urinary drainage. The individual patient records were reviewed and the patient group demographics listed. The indicating symptom that resulted in kidney transplantation was noted, along with the reason cutaneous drainage was utilized. The anatomic specifics of the donor organ and the type of immunosuppression used were noted, along with the morbidity and mortality for the transplantation. The long-term complications and the current status of the patient and graft were listed. Specific attention was given to the occurrence of upper urinary tract infection and complications directly related to the cutaneous drainage.

Technique

A standard oblique curvilinear kidney transplant incision in the lower quadrant of the abdomen is utilized, and the vascular anastomosis is completed with the available recipient vessels, as dictated by the donor vessel anatomy. An adequate length of donor ureter is necessary to reach the prechosen stomal site in a gentle sweep, and to fashion the terminal loop once the kidney is placed in the retroperitoneal iliac fossa. A length of ureter that reaches comfortably to the bladder is ample to avoid tension on the ureter at the stomal site. The site of the stoma is determined by previous scars and the topography of the abdominal wall, but is usually selected below the level of the umbilicus, and medial to the rectus sheath border. The distal end of the ureter is ligated securely with an absorbable ligature, and a small oval disk of skin, fascia, and muscle is excised at the stomal site so that the ureter can be brought out in a tension-free fashion. The ureter exits the skin in the form of a loop, leaving the terminal ligated segment buried in the abdominal wall, as pictured in the Figure. The fascia beneath the loop is closed for a short distance with absorbable suture so that retraction of the exposed ureter is prevented. The exterior loop of ureter is then incised in a longitudinal fashion, and the edges are sutured to the skin with 4-0 absorbable suture material.

A small 5-F pediatric feeding tube is used as a ureteral stent for several postoperative days to monitor function and bypass any obstruction that may result from early stomal edema. A temporary adhesive ostomy bag is fitted to the skin edges around the stomal site and stent, to be replaced with a permanent fitted ureterostomy appliance when healing has occurred. Prior to removal of the stent, a retrograde contrast study is performed to assure patency. The resultant stoma appears as a double-barrel ureterostomy with only the proximal end functional.

RESULTS

Over a 20-year period, six patients have undergone a terminal loop cutaneous ureterostomy at the time of kidney transplantation. The individual case outlines are listed in the Table. There were four male and two female patients, with an age range of 8 to 50 years. Five patients had a neurogenic bladder secondary to a variety of causes as the indication for utilizing cutaneous drainage, while one patient had exstrophy of the bladder as an indicator. All six patients had end-stage renal disease, which was secondary to chronic suppurative pyelonephritis, and had

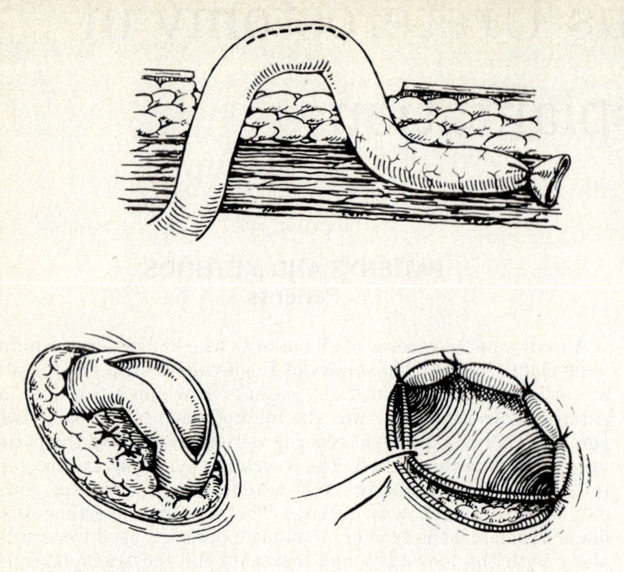

Technique of terminal loop cutaneous ureterostomy.

Case Outlines of Six Renal Transplant Recipients Who Underwent Cutaneous Ureterostomy			
Patient Age, y/Sex	Primary Urologic Abnormality	Graft Outcome	Patient Outcome
8/F	Neurogenic bladder	Functioning at 20 y	Alive
25/F	Meningomyelocele with neurogenic bladder	Functioning at 10 y	Alive
20/M	Paraplegia with neurogenic bladder	Functioning at death	Death at 52 d
29/M	Neurogenic bladder	Chronic rejection at 19 mo	Alive
50/F	Paraplegia with neurogenic bladder	Acute tubular necrosis at death	Death at 38 d
33/M	Exstrophy of bladder	Functioning at 4 y	Alive

undergone bilateral nephrectomy for infection control. Immunosuppression therapy consisted of azathioprine and prednisone, with cyclosporine added to form a triple-drug regimen in the patient with exstrophy.

Terminal loop cutaneous drainage was used as the planned primary procedure in all six cases. All grafts were from adult cadaver donors (five locally procured and one imported), had a single artery and vein as vascular conduits, and had more than an adequate length of single ureter to reach the skin surface. Three grafts had immediate function, while three experienced acute tubular necrosis and delayed function. No short-term complications could be attributed to the use of a cutaneous ureterostomy.

All short-term complications occurred in two patients and resulted in both patients dying. In one patient, a short-term rejection episode occurred in a zero-antigen matched graft ten days following transplantation. Treatment of this rejection allowed the return of renal function, but a subsequent gastrointestinal bleed required operative intervention for control. An invasive *Candida albicans* infection developed and led to the patient's death 52 days after the transplantation. The second death occurred in a similar manner, with treatment of a rejection episode leading to duodenal ulceration and perforation. A polymicrobial invasive peritonitis led to multiple organ system failure and death 38 days after the transplant procedure.

One patient experienced long-term rejection, and the patient resumed dialysis 19 months after the transplantation. Three functioning grafts were present 20, 10, and 4 years following the procedure. Two episodes of acute polynephritis have occurred in these functional grafts. One was associated with encrustations at the stomal site, which required simple débridement without revision of the stoma. The second incidence of invasive upper tract infection occurred in association with lymphocele obstruction of the ureter and was relieved with operative drainage of the lymphocele. No graft dysfunction or death has occurred secondary to pyelonephritis.

COMMENT

Most lower urinary tract problems that are encountered in potential renal transplant patients can be corrected, and the bladder can be made suitable for urinary drainage. However, a small group of transplant recipients may have an irreversibly damaged and nonfunctional bladder, and require an alternative method of drainage other than a ureterovesical connection. The patients in this latter group almost always have a congenital or acquired abnormality that abolishes adequate lower urinary tract function. The eligibility of these patients for renal transplantation is currently limited only by the enthusiasm of the transplant team. Once native kidney infection is controlled, there is usually no medical contraindication to kidney transplantation in this group of generally young and healthy patients.

Since the intestinal conduit was utilized by Kelley and associates[7] in 1966 for urinary drainage in renal transplantation, this procedure has been recommended by most authors. However, there is an apparent high complication rate and a significant mortality associated with this procedure. Stenzel and associates[1] reported that three of eight patients had ureteral stenosis requiring another operation. Glass and associates,[8] in a report of five patients and a review of the literature on renal transplantation using intestinal conduits, found that 22 (32%) of 68 patients suffered a total of 29 complications attributed to the conduit. Eighteen septic complications directly resulted in nine deaths in these 68 patients, and the sepsis was usually associated with strictures or ileal calculi. Patients with ileal conduits tend to form stones, and the resultant foreign-body obstruction affords bacterial loop colonization the opportunity for invasive infection of the upper urinary tract. In these patients, the differentiation between pyelonephritis and rejection can lead to critical delays and, at times, an inappropriate elevation in immunosuppressive therapy. Although half of the patients described by Glass et al received organs from living donors, the functional graft survival rate was only 52%.

The intestinal conduit method requires either a preparatory procedure several weeks prior to transplantation or an enterotomy at the time of engrafting. The former is preferred to avoid contamination by bowel soilage in an immunosuppressed patient. Even when constructed in advance, this method has technical factors that frequently lead to complications. Glass et al[8] reported that six complications were associated just with the creation of the stoma or the restoration of intestinal continuity. Ureteral stenosis with some degree of upper urinary tract obstruction and dilation and frequent ureteral reflux are recalcitrant problems, while the risk of peritoneal soilage has led to the recommendation that the anastomoses between the ureter and bowel segment be done and left in the extraperitoneal space if technically feasible.

An attractive alternative to intestinal diversion in some patients who simply have a neurogenic bladder is the procedure of chronic intermittent catheterization. Since its introduction by Guttman and Frankel[9] for the management of patients following spinal cord trauma, this technique has been used with varying success in the management of patients with a neurogenic bladder requiring kidney transplantation. However, the introduction of bacteria into the bladder of a transplant recipient is of concern for transplant surgeons, especially in their patients who have neurogenic bladder dysfunction where reflux occurs frequently. In a group of patients managed with clean intermittent catheterization followed up for a variable period, Barnett and associates[10] reported that about half had experienced bacteriuria or clinical urinary tract infections. This incidence compared favorably to the almost 100% incidence of bacteriuria in patients with intestinal conduits. Overall graft loss, renal dysfunction, or urosepsis could not be attributed to the intermittent catheter technique of bladder drainage. Despite the fact that some of these patients had only asymptomatic bacteriuria, Barnett and associates were concerned that a fatal infection could occur and cautioned that careful patient selection and instruction was necessary for this method to be useful.

Intermittent catheterization could have been utilized in several of our patients who were operated on earlier. In fact, in two recent transplant recipients, one, a diabetic patient with a neurogenic bladder who underwent a renal graft, and the other, a similar diabetic patient who received a combined renal and pancreas allograft with bladder drainage, the intermittent clean catheter technique has been used successfully by our service. Neither intermittent catheterization nor cutaneous drainage should be utilized to the exclusion of the other. Patient concerns, convenience, the medical status, and the social care aspects of each recipient must be considered when choosing the procedure for urinary drainage.

We currently consider those patients with neurogenic bladder who have a demonstrated inability or aversion to learn the intermittent self-catheter technique to be candidates for cutaneous ureterostomy drainage. Similarly, a patient with a disability that prevents him or her from undergoing the intermittent catheter procedure in a clean and safe manner is considered a candidate for cutaneous ureterostomy. Clearly, when the bladder is not available due to a congenital or traumatic abnormality, cutaneous drainage is the only option that will allow a successful transplant.

From previously described experiences, it would appear that no single method for urinary drainage of a transplanted kidney has proved ideal when a dysfunctional bladder is present. A successful cutaneous ureterostomy, where there is simplicity, an immediate availability for function, a low incidence of reflux, and no need to involve the intestinal tract, would have many advantages. Stomal complications and urosepsis are thought to be the major drawbacks of using a terminal cutaneous ureterostomy in a transplant recipient. A normal-caliber ureter removed from the donor has a tenuous blood supply, and this fact alone is thought to be the primary reason for stomal stenosis. However, Amin and associates,[11] in an experimental study in dogs and in a clinical series, reported that neovascularization of an isolated ureter occurred from the surrounding tissue when a terminal loop was used to construct the cutaneous ureterostomy. In this study, only one of 20 patients who required urinary diversion for a variety of reasons suffered a stomal stenosis requiring intubation.

Terminal loop cutaneous ureterostomy as described by Amin et al[11] and outlined herein has been used by our service for over 20 years with good results in both transplant recipients and in other patients requiring urinary drainage by the cutaneous route. In the present report, this technique has been utilized in six cadaveric kidney transplant recipients with moderate success. Four long-term graft survivors experienced no short- or long-term complications with the surgical procedure. There has been no stomal stenosis, and no stomal revisions have been needed. Encrustations requiring simple débridement occurred in the longest functional graft recipient, and only one invasive infection associated with ureteral obstruction from a lymphocele that required internal drainage has been documented. Similarly, the two early graft losses were not related to the type of urinary drainage used.

All patients continue to receive long-term urinary antisepsis medication since they do have constant bacteriuria, and the risk of urosepsis is always present and real. In these patients, the differential evaluation between urosepsis and rejection would appear to be simplified. Retrograde urography of the transplanted kidney is an easy procedure in those cases of renal dysfunction and, in our experience, invasive infection only occurs in the setting of urinary obstruction. The ureterostomy stoma does appear to reflect various changes within the graft after an initial period of edema and can be used as an indication of rejection. In two of our cases, marked edema of the stoma coincided with acute allograft rejection, and in one case, a small biopsy of the stoma showed lymphocytic infiltration at the time of the rejection episode. Stoma edema reversed in both instances with treatment and control of the rejection.

Terminal loop cutaneous ureterostomy appears, from the data reported herein, to be a safe and effective means for urinary drainage in selected renal transplant recipients. It is feasible if the ischemic, normal-caliber ureters provided with all renal donor grafts are utilized, and it remains viable and patent, secondary to the neovascularity that develops in the distal nonfunctional loop. Our experience with this procedure in six cadaveric transplant recipients makes it the procedure of choice, as opposed to the use of an intestinal conduit, for urinary drainage of a transplanted kidney when the bladder is not available. It avoids the necessity of preparatory bowel surgery that has its attendant risk of peritoneal contamination and leak in an immunocompromised patient. The presence of chronic bacteriuria and the subsequent risk of urosepsis do not appear to detract from its usefulness.

References

1. Stenzel KH, Stubenbond WT, Whitsell JC, et al: Kidney transplantation: Use of intestinal conduits. *JAMA* 1974;229:534-537.
2. Kogan SJ, Weis R, Hanna M, et al: Successful renal transplantation in a patient with a neurogenic bladder managed by clean intermittent catheterization. *J Urol* 1986;135:563-565.
3. Hume DM, Merrill JP, Miller BF: Homologous transplantation of human kidneys. *J Clin Invest* 1952;31:640-653.
4. Kuss R, Teinturier J, Milliez P: Quelques essais de greffe de rein chez l'homme. *Mem Acad Chir* 1951;77:755-764.
5. Martin DC, Mims MM, Kaufman TJ, et al: The ureter in renal transplantation. *J Urol* 1969;101:680-687.
6. Amin M, Howerton LW, Lich R: Terminal loop cutaneous ureterostomy: A method of urinary drainage in kidney transplantations. *J Urol* 1977;118:379-382.
7. Kelley WD, Merkel FK, Markland C: Ileal urinary diversion in conjunction with renal homotransplantation. *Lancet* 1966;1:222.
8. Glass NR, Uehling D, Sollinger H, et al: Renal transplantation using ileal conduits in five cases. *J Urol* 1985;133:666-668.
9. Guttman L, Frankel H: The value of intermittent catheterization in the early management of traumatic paraplegia and tetraplegia. *Paraplegia* 1966;4:63-67.
10. Barnett M, Bruskewetz R, Glass N, et al: Long-term clean intermittent self-catheterization in renal transplant recipients. *J Urol* 1985;134:654-657.
11. Amin M, Clark R, Howerton LW, et al: Terminal loop cutaneous ureterostomy: An experimental study and its clinical application. *J Urol* 1977;118:383-385.

Pentagastrin Stimulation of Human Colon Carcinoma

D. Byron McGregor, MD; Laura L. Morriss, PhD; Pacita B. Manalo, MD; Richard A. Bomberger, MD; Ronald S. Pardini, PhD

• This study examines the trophic effects of pentagastrin administration on the growth of transplanted human colon carcinoma in mice. Three different human colon carcinomas were implanted into dorsal subcutaneous pouches of BALB-C athymic mice—tumor A, COLO 320 DM undifferentiated carcinoma; tumor B, WiDr epithelial carcinoma; and tumor C, mucus-producing signet-ring cell adenocarcinoma from a patient volunteer. Tumors grew for four to six weeks and then groups were randomly assigned to receive either saline injections or pentagastrin, 2.0 mg/kg three times a day for 14 days before harvest. Tumors were homogenized and analyzed for DNA, RNA, and protein contents. Each tumor type showed a different biochemical pattern of response to pentagastrin stimulation. The data confirm that pentagastrin is trophic to human colon carcinoma and suggest a possible clinical role for hormonal manipulation.

(*Arch Surg* 1989;124:470-472)

Carcinoma of the colon remains the most prevalent and second most lethal internal malignancy of this society. Discouragingly, our therapeutic approaches have remained the same in substance and outcome for decades. While some other solid tumors, notably breast, thyroid, and prostate, have all been shown to respond to hormonal manipulation, no hormone or system of hormones has yet been demonstrated to be of therapeutic benefit in the treatment of this common neoplasm.

Over the last 15 years, the antral hormone, gastrin, has increasingly been shown to be a participant in the regulation of metabolic activities of the gut. In a series of articles[1-3] beginning in 1973, Johnson[2] demonstrated that gastrin is a trophic hormone to the mucosa of the colon as well as other sites along the gastrointestinal tract. In 1982, we demonstrated a stimulatory effect of both exogenous and endogenous gastrin on chemically induced colon tumors in rats.[4] Winsett et al[5] demonstrated a similar effect in transplantable murine tumors and demonstrated that the gastrin receptor antagonist, proglumide, was able to inhibit the growth of gastrin-responsive colon cancers.[6] Stimulation of growth of a human colon cancer has been performed in cell culture[7] but has yet to be applied clinically. Our project was designed to extend this physiology one step closer to the eventual clinical arena by studying the effects of the synthetic C-terminal pentapeptide, pentagastrin, on solid in vivo tumors of human origin.

MATERIALS AND METHODS

Three different human colon carcinomas were implanted into dorsal subcutaneous pouches of BALB-C athymic mice using methods previously described.[8] COLO 320 DM and WiDr human adenocarcinoma cell lines were used. The COLO 320 DM cells were maintained in RPMI 1640 medium with 10% fetal bovine serum, and the WiDr cells were maintained in Eagle's minimum essential medium with nonessential amino acids and 90% Earle's balanced salt solution with 10% fetal bovine serum. Approximately 10^6 cells from the fourth passage of each line were inoculated as single-cell suspensions into a subcutaneous pouch created 1 cm caudad to the scapula of each mouse using a 15-gauge needle. A third tumor, histologically classified as a mucinous adenocarcinoma, was harvested directly from a patient volunteer at the time of sigmoid resection. It was transported in iced buffered Hank's solution, sectioned into 1-mm cubes, and similarly implanted. Solid tumors were transferred a minimum of three times to assure sterility and viability of the tumor line.

Solid tumors from each of the three tumor lines were harvested, divided into 1-mm segments, and again implanted subcutaneously in 12 mice. The tumors were allowed to grow four to six weeks, at which time the animals were randomly assigned to control or experimental groups. Experimental animals received pentagastrin, 2.0 mg/kg subcutaneously at 12-hour intervals for 14 days. Control animals received similarly timed saline injections. Tumors were excised and stored in liquid nitrogen.

Tumors were homogenized in normal saline and assayed for DNA, RNA, and protein contents. The DNA and RNA were extracted and assayed according to the diphenylamine and orcinol methods of Schneider[9] using calf thymus DNA and calf liver RNA as standards. Protein was determined by the modified Lowry method of Ohnishi and Barr[10] using bovine serum albumin standard.

Accepted for publication Oct 4, 1988.

From the Departments of Surgery (Drs McGregor, Morriss, and Bomberger), Biochemistry (Dr Pardini), and Pathology (Dr Manalo), University of Nevada School of Medicine and Veterans Administration Medical Center, Reno, Nev.

Read before the 12th Annual Surgical Symposium of the Association of Veterans Administration Surgeons, Minneapolis, May 14, 1988.

Reprint requests to Department of Surgery, VAMC, 1000 Locust St, Reno, NV 89520 (Dr McGregor).

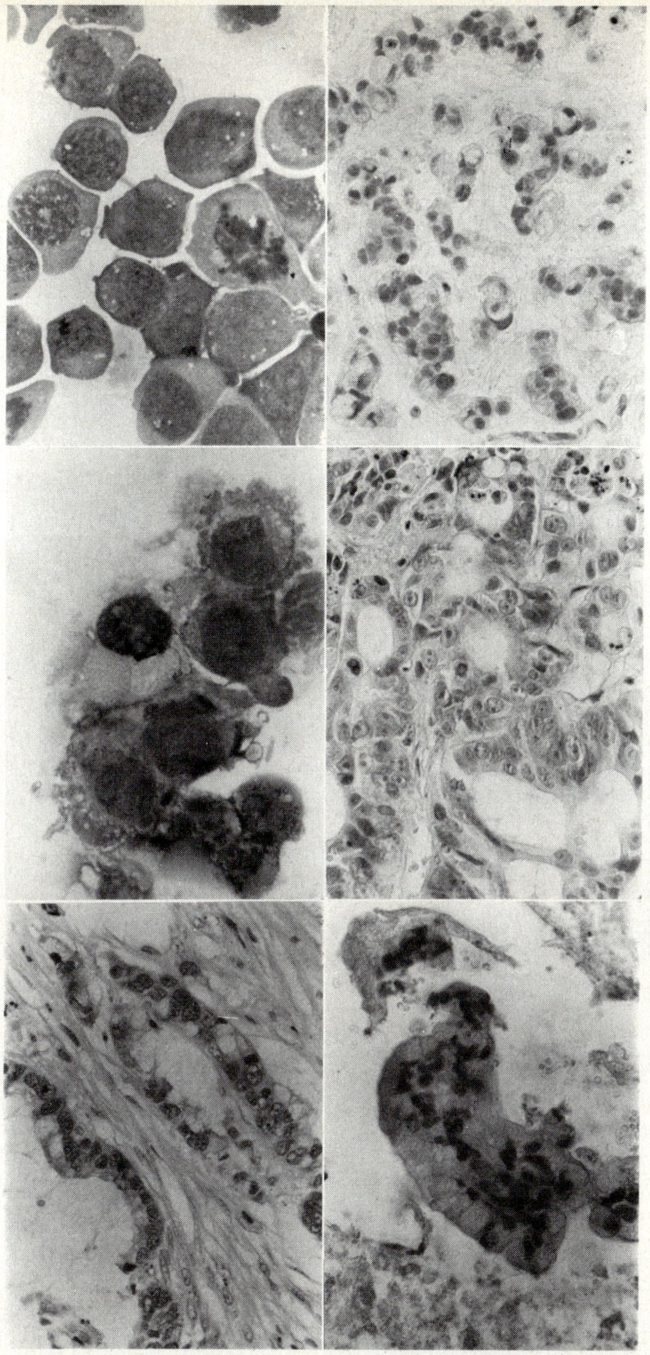

Fig 1.—Photomicrographic comparisons before and after transplantation. Top, COLO cytologic and histologic findings. Center, WiDr cytologic and histologic findings. Bottom, Volunteer xenograft from patient and after implantation. All histologic specimens stained with hematoxylin-eosin. Both cytologic specimens stained with Wright's stain.

DNA, RNA, and Protein Contents of Solid Transplanted Tumors With and Without Pentagastrin Pretreatment

Tumor	DNA, μg/mg	RNA, μg/mg	Protein, mg/mg
COLO cell line			
Control	293.8	767.2	54.6
Treated	560.6	1394.0	112.8
% increase	90*	82†	107*
No.	7	6	7
WiDr cell line			
Control	68.4	410.2	188.5
Treated	831.8	552.2	193.7
% increase	1116*	35*	...
No.	6	6	5
Xenograft			
Control	96.7	776.3	45.0
Treated	85.1	935.0	64.4
% increase	...	20‡	43*
No.	11	10	9

*$P<.001$.
†$P<.01$.
‡$P<.02$.

Statistical differences between group means for DNA, RNA, and protein were analyzed by Student's t test for small sample populations.[11] $P<.02$ was considered significant.

RESULTS

Each inoculation resulted in the formation of a solid tumor. Photomicrographs of harvested tumors (Fig 1) document the success of xenograft transfer. The COLO cell line is a moderately differentiated, highly secretory adenocarcinoma, originally obtained from the sigmoid colon of a 55-year-old woman and known to produce serotonin, norepinephrine, epinephrine, corticotropin, and parathormone. After transfer, the COLO (Fig 1, top) cell line retained its pleomorphic nuclei and abundant vacuolated cytoplasm demonstrating secretory activity. The WiDr cell line is a poorly differentiated epithelial adenocarcinoma known to produce carcinoembryonic antigen. With transplantation, the WiDr (Fig 1, center) cell line retained its epithelial homogeneity and nuclear hyperchromasia and pleomorphism. Its overlapping cells (cytologic feature) and occasionally irregular anaplastic lobulated nuclei (histologic feature) each confirm its rapid growth. Finally, after transplantation of the mucinous adenocarcinoma (Fig 1, bottom), it retained its morphologic features of eccentric nuclei, vacuolated cytoplasm, and high percentage of signet-ring–type cells consistent with slow growth and mucus production.

The results of biochemical analyses and the percentage increase in respective measurements of the pentagastrin-treated group are shown in the Table. Analyzed for DNA content, both epithelial cell types showed striking changes of from nearly double in the COLO cell line to nearly 12-fold in the WiDr cell line. The slow-growing mucinous xenograft showed no change. Likewise, analysis for RNA content showed considerably greater increases in the poorly differentiated tumors than in the signet-ring cell tumor. Analysis for protein content showed the nonsecretory WiDr to exhibit no change, while the mucus-secreting signet-ring cell xenograft and the highly secretory COLO cell line demonstrated significant increases.

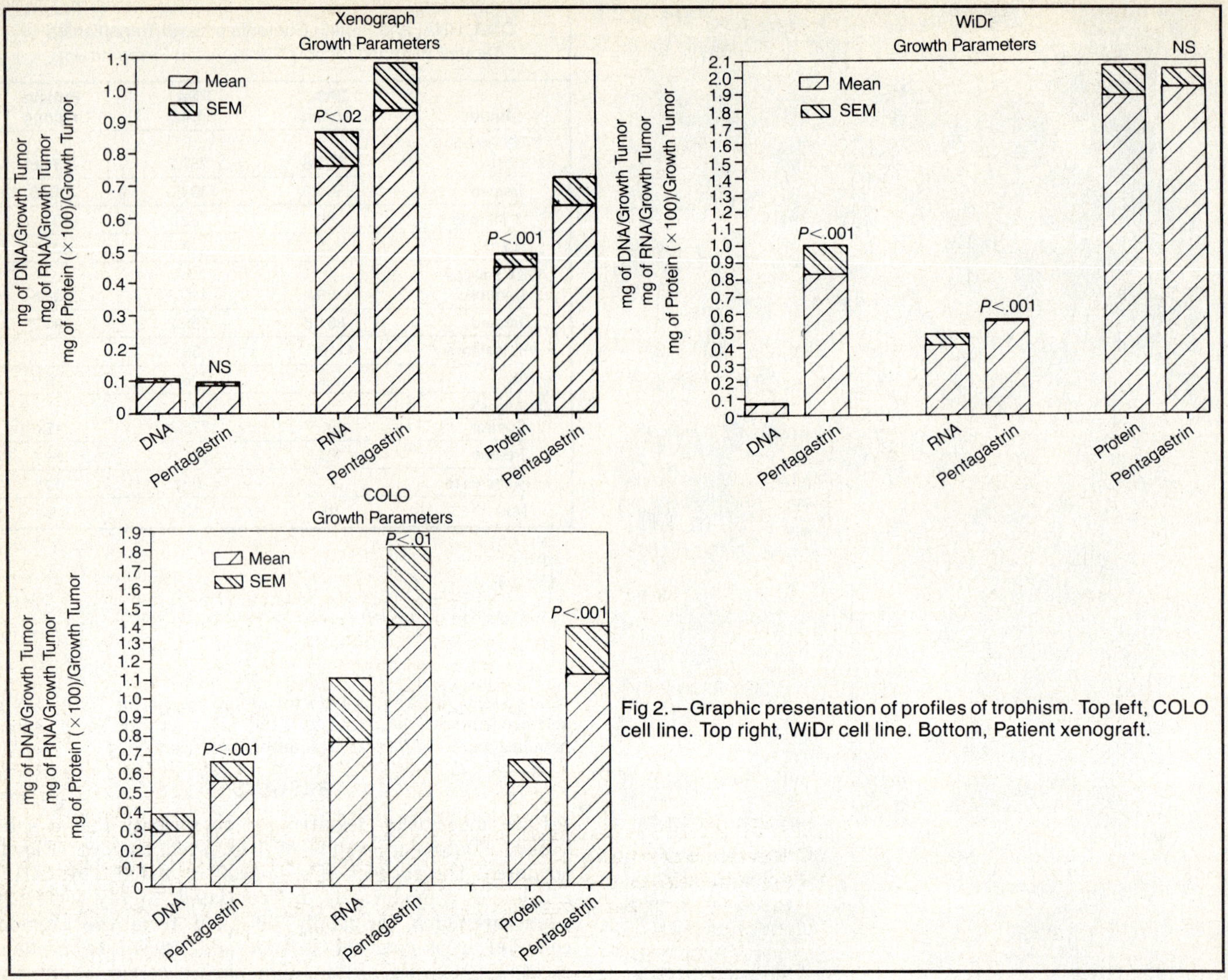

Fig 2.—Graphic presentation of profiles of trophism. Top left, COLO cell line. Top right, WiDr cell line. Bottom, Patient xenograft.

COMMENT

Although vastly different in their responses, each cell line displays a profile of stimulated activity as characteristic as its histologic features (Fig 2). The COLO cell line (Fig 2, top left) seems to exhibit a more classic model of trophism—increased DNA production stimulating increased RNA production which stimulates increased protein production. The WiDr cell line (Fig 2, top right) displays an equally stimulated system of nucleotides that does not seem to result in increased protein production. Finally, the mucinous signet-ring cell xenograft (Fig 2, bottom) shows no change in its nucleotide contents but nevertheless mounts a significant increase in synthetic activity at least of protein.

These data generate as many questions as they answer. The nature and function of gastrin receptors that must control the enzymatic activity resulting in these changes have not been adequately delineated. The observation that different tumor lines display unique patterns of biochemical responses suggests that pentagastrin must act at multiple sites to control synthesis, degradation, or both. Furthermore, any clinical role for such stimulatory activity, even if predictable, remains speculative. We are, however, able to conclude that pentagastrin does exert a stimulatory effect on solid human colon cancers at least as described in this model. Finally, the response of different cancers is not uniform, but, rather, each tumor seems to respond biochemically in ways consistent with its biologic behavior and histologic features.

This work was supported by a grant from the Reno (Nev) Cancer Center.

References

1. Lichtenberger L, Miller LR, Erwin DN, et al: Effect of pentagastrin on adult rat duodenal cells in culture. *Gastroenterology* 1973;65:242-251.
2. Johnson LR: Gastrointestinal hormones and their functions. *Ann Rev Physiol* 1977;39:135-148.
3. Takeuchi K, Speir GR, Johnson LR: Mucosal gastrin receptor: III. Regulation by gastrin. *Am J Physiol* 1980;238:G135-G140.
4. McGregor DB, Jones RD, Karlin DA, et al: Trophic effects of gastrin on colorectal neoplasms in the rat. *Ann Surg* 1982;195:219-223.
5. Winsett OE, Townsend CM, Glass EJ, et al: Gastrin stimulates growth of colon cancer. *Surgery* 1986;99:302-307.
6. Beauchamp RD, Townsend CM, Singh MD, et al: Proglumide, a gastrin receptor antagonist, inhibits growth of colon cancer and enhances survival in mice. *Ann Surg* 1985;202:303-309.
7. Kusyk CJ, McNeil NO, Johnson LR: Stimulation of growth of a colon cancer cell line. *Am J Physiol* 1986;251:G597-G601.
8. Pardini LL, Aaronson LM, Hering PL, et al: Heterotransplantation of equine carcinoma cells in athymic (nude) mice. *Am J Vet Res* 1986;47:610-614.
9. Schneider WC: Determination of nucleic acids in tissues by pentose analysis. *Meth Enzymol* 1957;3:680-684.
10. Ohnishi ST, Barr JK: A simplified method of quantitating proteins using the biuret phenol reagents. *Analyt Biochem* 1978;86:193-200.
11. Blaedel WJ, Meloche VW: *Elementary Quantitative Analysis,* ed 2. New York, Harper & Row Publishers Inc, 1963.

Inhibition of the Stimulated Canine Exocrine Pancreas by Amino Acids and Fat

Richard S. Stubbs, MB, ChB, MD, FRCS, FRACS, Bruce E. Stabile, MD

• **To investigate the possible exocrine pancreatic inhibitory actions of amino acids and fat, pancreatic fistula outputs and plasma concentrations of glucagon, somatostatin, and pancreatic polypeptide were measured in response to intravenous (IV) and intraduodenal nutrient administration in six dogs submaximally stimulated with cholecystokinin. Intravenous amino acids caused abrupt and significant 45% to 73% reductions in stimulated pancreatic protein, bicarbonate, and volume outputs. There were no significant associated changes in plasma hormone concentrations and no similar immediate pancreatic inhibition with IV mannitol, thus suggesting a possible direct inhibitory effect of amino acids. Intraduodenal amino acids and IV fat evoked no significant pancreatic output suppression. Intraduodenal fat rapidly caused significant 40% to 62% reductions in stimulated outputs that were associated with an 81% rise in plasma pancreatic polypeptide concentration, suggesting a gut-mediated inhibition. We conclude that IV amino acids and intraduodenal fat both inhibited stimulated pancreatic secretion but probably by different mechanisms.**

(*Arch Surg* 1989;124:473-478)

Intraluminal amino acids and fat are known to be potent stimulators of exocrine pancreatic secretion through a complex mechanism presumed to involve the release of cholecystokinin.[1-3] These nutrients have also been shown to release significant quantities of glucagon, somatostatin, and pancreatic polypeptide—peptide hormones known to have pancreatic inhibitory capability—from the pancreas and gut.[4-6] If release of these peptides by amino acids and fat has relevance to regulation of pancreatic secretion, then some degree of pancreatic inhibition by intraduodenal (ID) administration of the nutrients would be expected. Although largely untested, this hypothesis is suggested by the finding that the maximal pancreatic enzyme response to ID amino acids or fat is only 50% to 70% of that to exogenous cholecystokinin.[2,3,7]

While the exocrine pancreatic response to intravenous (IV) amino acids is incompletely understood, the response to IV fat has scarcely been investigated. The 1979 report by Konturek et al[8] contending that both IV amino acids and fat stimulated pancreatic secretion has largely been contradicted.[9,10] Still other investigations have suggested an inhibitory influence of IV nutrients on the human and canine pancreas stimulated with secretin and cholecystokinin.[11,12]

To further clarify the inhibitory effects of amino acids and fat on the stimulated pancreas and to elucidate the mechanisms involved, we administered these nutrients IV or ID to dogs during submaximal stimulation with cholecystokinin. Pancreatic outputs together with plasma concentrations of glucagon, pancreatic polypeptide, and somatostatin were measured before, during, and after the period of IV or ID nutrient delivery.

MATERIALS AND METHODS

Experimental Protocols

Six adult mongrel dogs weighing between 16 and 23 kg were prepared with chronic gastric and pancreatic fistulas by a modification of the method of Herrera et al.[13] Experiments were commenced no sooner than three weeks following operation and were performed at intervals of not less than 48 hours. Food but not water was withheld for 18 hours prior to each test. Experiments were performed in duplicate in each dog. At the beginning of each experiment, the gastric cannula was opened and the stomach gently flushed with water. If food residue was encountered, the study was cancelled. If the stomach was empty, the gastric fistula was left open to drain freely for the duration of the study. Using a hind limb vein, the tip of a long polyethylene catheter (PE 50) was advanced to lie in the inferior vena cava for central IV infusion of nutrients or 0.15 mol/L of sodium chloride. Perfusion of ID nutrients or saline was accomplished via the hollow obturator of the Herrera cannula. Using peristaltic pumps (Harvard), IV and ID administration rates were kept constant at 100 mL/h.

In the control studies, cholecystokinin octapeptide (CCK-OP, Bachem Fine Chemicals, Torrance, Calif) was infused IV at 250 ng/kg per hour for three hours after an initial 30-minute basal period. This submaximally stimulating dose of cholecystokinin octapeptide was chosen after preliminary dose-response studies

Accepted for publication Oct 4, 1988.

From the Department of Surgery, Wellington (New Zealand) Clinical School of Medicine (Dr Stubbs); and the Surgical Service, Veterans Administration Medical Center San Diego and the Department of Surgery, University of California at San Diego School of Medicine (Dr Stabile).

Read before the 12th Annual Surgical Symposium of the Association of Veterans Administration Surgeons, Minneapolis, May 13, 1988.

Reprint requests to Surgical Service (112) VA Medical Center, 3350 La Jolla Village Dr, San Diego, CA 92161 (Dr Stabile).

consistently revealed failure to sustain pancreatic secretion at a constant output for three hours in response to a maximal stimulating dose of 500 ng/kg per hour. Cholecystokinin octapeptide was dissolved in 0.5% bovine serum albumin solution and delivered via a Y-shaped connector into the central venous catheter at 30 mL/h. Experiments were then repeated with the addition of an IV infusion or ID perfusion of either mixed amino acid solution (10% Aminosyn, Abbott Laboratories, North Chicago, Ill) at 10 g/h or fat emulsion (20% Liposyn, Abbott Laboratories, North Chicago, Ill) at 20 g/h during the second hour of cholecystokinin octapeptide infusion. The composition of the mixed amino acid test solution is given below:

Amino Acid	mg/dL
Alanine	1280
Arginine	980
Histidine	300
Isoleucine	720
Leucine	940
Lysine	720
Methionine	400
Phenylalanine	440
Proline	860
Serine	420
Threonine	520
Tryptophan	160
Tyrosine	44
Valine	800
Glycine	1280

The composition of the fat emulsion test solution was as follows:

Fatty Acid	mg/dL
Linoleic	15400
Oleic	2600
Palmitic	1400
Stearic	500

Saline was infused IV during ID nutrient perfusion and vice versa. Blood samples were drawn at 30-minute intervals for somatostatin, pancreatic polypeptide, and glucagon determinations by specific radioimmunoassays (RIAs) and for measurements of plasma-free amino acids or serum triglyceride concentrations. For this purpose, a heparinized venous access needle was maintained in a limb other than that used for the IV infusion.

Because of the high osmolarity of the amino acid solution infused IV (1000 mOsm/L), an additional control study was performed to determine the effect of a hyperosmolar solution on the stimulated pancreas. For this purpose, the same experimental protocol was followed but with the substitution of IV mannitol (1000 mOsm/L) at 100 mL/h during the second hour of cholecystokinin octapeptide infusion.

Measurements

Pancreatic juice was collected continuously and divided into ten-minute samples. The volume of each sample was determined to the nearest 0.1 mL. Bicarbonate concentration was measured by adding 1 mL of 0.1 mol/L of hydrochloric acid to 0.5 mL of each sample and back-titrating to a pH of 7.0 with 0.2 mol/L of sodium hydroxide. Total protein concentration, as a measure of total enzyme concentration, was estimated by measuring absorbance at 280 nm, using an autoanalyzer with a spectrophotometer (Beckman DM) and employing bovine serum albumin as standard. The outputs of bicarbonate and protein were calculated by multiplying volume by concentration.

For peptide RIA, blood was collected in edetic acid tubes to which aprotinin (Trasylol [FBA Pharmaceuticals, New York]) 500 Kallikrein inhibitor units/mL of whole blood was added. Samples were immediately centrifuged at 4°C for ten minutes at 2500 rpm. The plasma sample was then divided into thirds and stored at −20°C for future RIA. The glucagon, somatostatin, and pancreatic polypeptide assays were performed by methods previously described.[14-16] For determination of plasma amino acid concentration, blood was collected in dry heparinized tubes and immediately centrifuged at 4°C for ten minutes at 2500 rpm. One milliliter of plasma was then added to 1 mL of a solution containing 45 mg of sulfosalicylic acid, vortexed, and recentrifuged at 4°C for a further 20 minutes at 2500 rpm. The supernatant was stored at −70°C for subsequent amino acid measurement by an amino acid analyzer (Beckman). For serum triglyceride measurement, blood was collected into plain tubes and centrifuged for ten minutes at 2500 rpm. The serum was stored at −20°C for subsequent analysis by an enzymatic method.

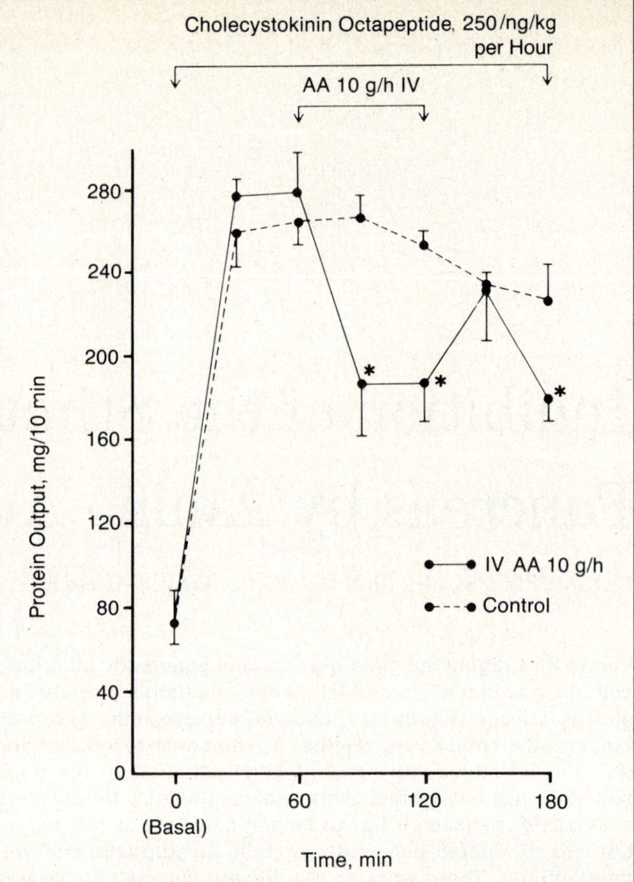

Fig 1.—Pancreatic protein output of six dogs with chronic pancreatic fistulas in response to three-hour intravenous (IV) infusion of cholecystokinin octapeptide, 250 ng/kg per hour, without (control) and with simultaneous IV infusion of mixed amino acids (AA), 10 g/h, during second hour. In this and subsequent figures, each point represents mean and each vertical line represents SEM. Asterisk indicates significant difference from control value.

Data Analysis

Pancreatic secretion has been expressed as the mean ten-minute response for the 30-minute interval preceding the designated time. This was calculated from two studies per dog. The pancreatic secretion obtained during each 30-minute interval of the IV amino acid or fat (or mannitol) infusion study or the ID amino acid or fat perfusion study was compared with the secretion during the same 30-minute interval in the control study by an analysis of variance. The plasma concentrations of somatostatin, pancreatic polypeptide, and glucagon measured at the midpoint and end of the 60-minute IV infusion or ID perfusion of amino acids or fat were compared with the corresponding concentrations at the same times in the control study using analysis of variance. The number of dogs (five or six) was used for calculation. *P* value of less than .05 was taken to indicate a significant difference.

RESULTS

Control Study

Infusion of cholecystokinin octapeptide, 250 ng/kg per hour, caused significant pancreatic stimulation of protein,

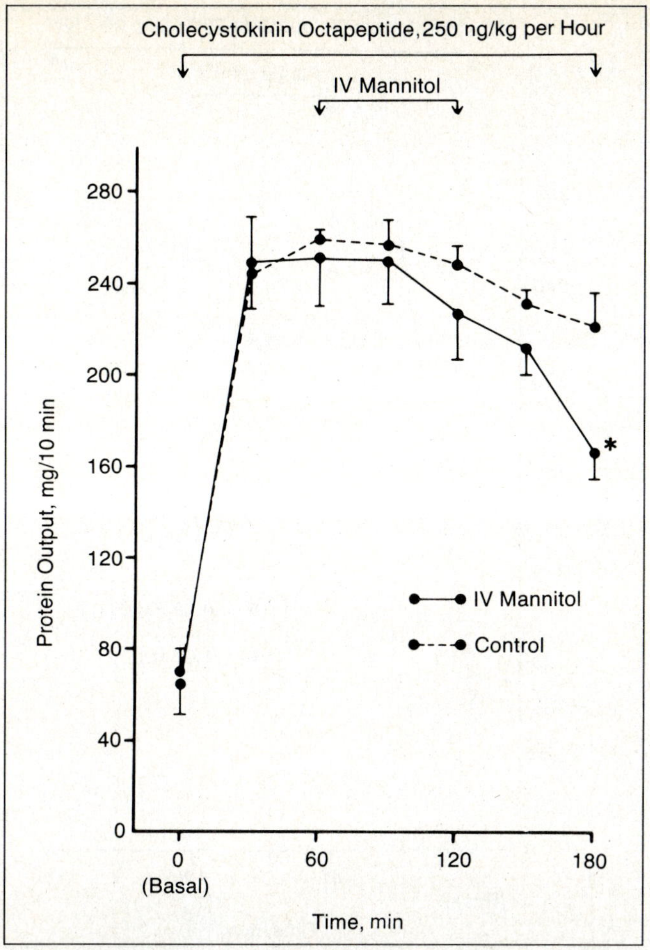

Fig 2.—Pancreatic protein output of five dogs in response to three-hour intravenous (IV) infusion of cholecystokinin octapeptide, 250 ng/kg per hour, without (control) and with IV mannitol (1000 mOsm/L) at 100 mL/h during second hour.

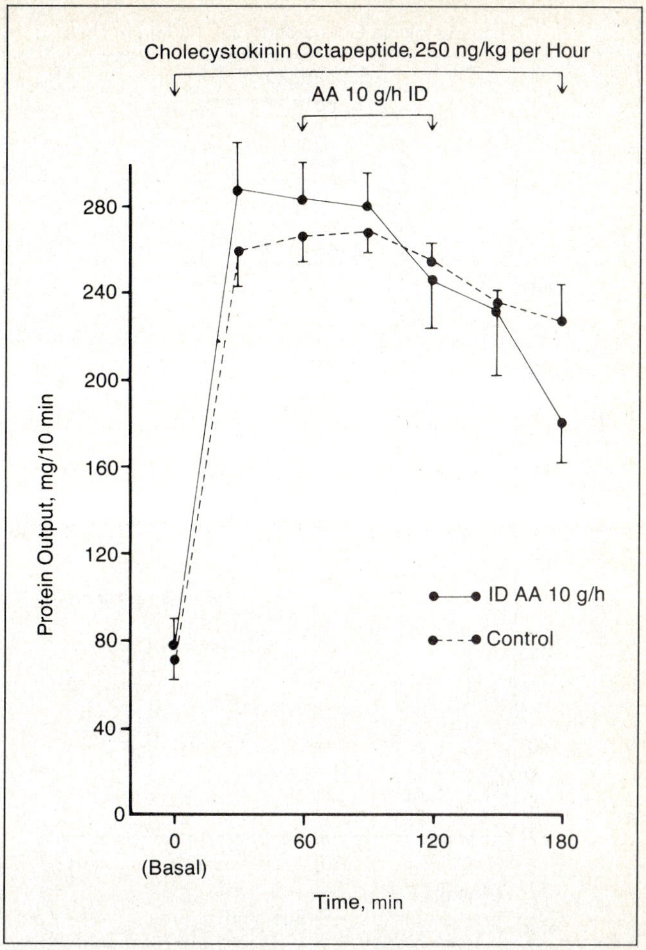

Fig 3.—Pancreatic protein output of six dogs in response to three-hour intravenous infusion of cholecystokinin octapeptide, 250 ng/kg per hour, without (control) and with simultaneous intraduodenal (ID) perfusion of mixed amino acids (AA), 10 g/h, during second hour.

volume, and bicarbonate outputs. The control protein responses are shown in Figs 1 through 5. Despite a minimal and insignificant decline in the level of secretion over the three-hour study period, a high level of stimulation was maintained. Parallel responses were noted for bicarbonate and volume outputs. The infusion of cholecystokinin octapeptide caused progressive and significant rises in plasma pancreatic polypeptide and glucagon levels. In contrast, the modest rise in plasma somatostatin levels was not significant. These control responses are shown in Fig 6.

IV Amino Acid Study

The infusion of IV mixed amino acids resulted in significant inhibition of the cholecystokinin octapeptide–stimulated pancreatic protein output (Fig 1). Parallel results were also noted for outputs of bicarbonate and volume. Stimulated protein secretion was reduced by 45% after 30 minutes of the amino acid infusion ($P<.05$). Stimulated bicarbonate secretion was reduced by 73% and stimulated volume output was reduced by 60% during the same period ($P<.05$). At this point, the plasma amino acid concentration had risen 70% above the preinfusion concentration (from 2.06 ± 0.15 mmol/L to 3.51 ± 0.08 mmol/L). Within 60 minutes of stopping the infusion, plasma amino acid concentration returned almost to basal (2.23 ± 17 mmol/L) while pancreatic protein secretion partially recovered and subsequently declined again (Fig 1). Despite minimal rises in plasma glucagon, pancreatic polypeptide, and somatostatin concentrations during the amino acid infusion, there were no significant increases over the levels in the control study, including at 90 and 120 minutes, when pancreatic inhibition was maximal.

IV Mannitol Study

No inhibition of cholecystokinin octapeptide–stimulated pancreatic secretion was observed over the period of the mannitol infusion (60 to 120 minutes). However, a significant decline in protein output was noted during the final 30 minutes of the experiment (Fig 2).

ID Amino Acid Study

Introduction of ID amino acids caused no significant inhibition of the cholecystokinin octapeptide–stimulated pancreatic outputs of protein, bicarbonate, or volume compared with controls. However, pancreatic secretion did decline during the second 30 minutes of the perfusion and, in the case of protein, continued to decline after cessation of the perfusion (Fig 3). Plasma-free amino acid concentration rose throughout the period of ID perfusion and peaked at the termination of the perfusion (from 2.02 ± 0.21 mmol/L to 2.78 ± 0.25 mmol/L). Plasma somatostatin levels were essentially unchanged by the cholecystokinin octapeptide

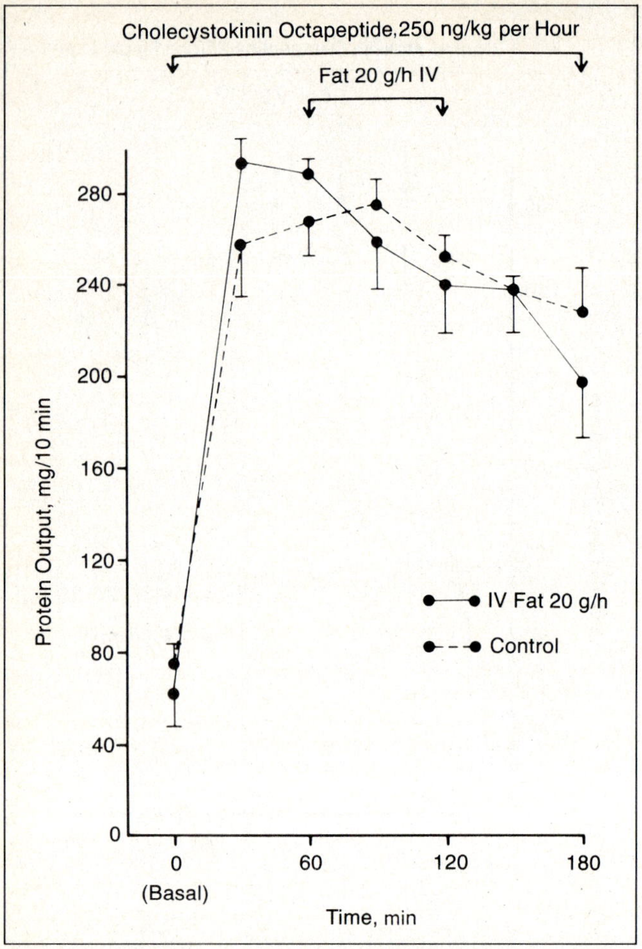

Fig 4.—Pancreatic protein output of five dogs in response to three-hour intravenous (IV) infusion of cholecystokinin octapeptide, 250 ng/kg per hour, without (control) and with IV infusion of fat emulsion, 20 g/h, during second hour.

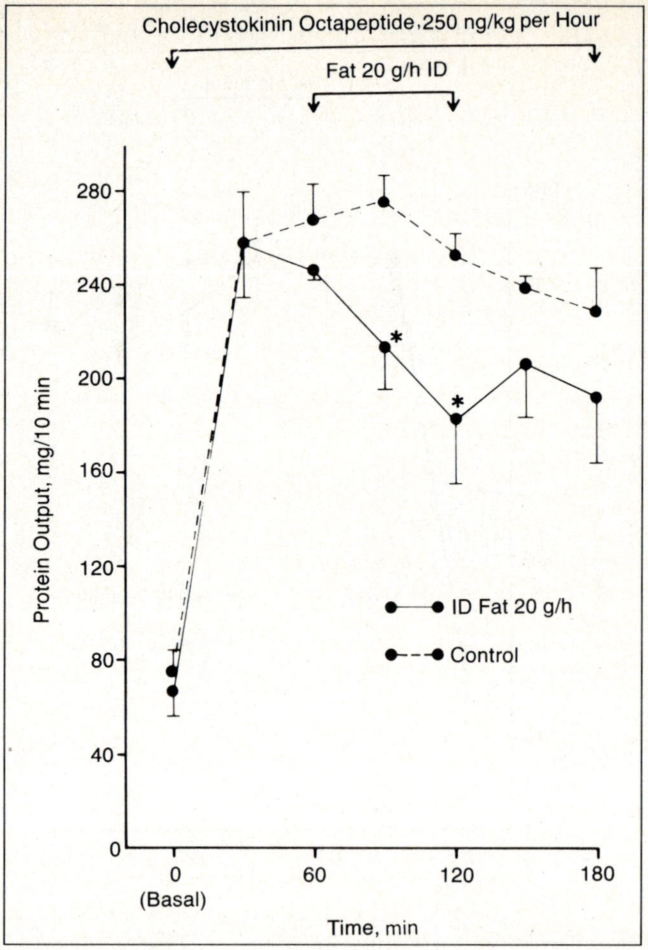

Fig 5.—Pancreatic protein output of five dogs in response to three-hour intravenous infusion of cholecystokinin octapeptide, 250 ng/kg per hour, without (control) and with intraduodenal (ID) perfusion of fat emulsion, 20 g/h, during second hour.

infusion alone or by the addition of ID amino acids. Plasma glucagon levels rose gradually throughout the study but were not significantly different from those at the corresponding time points in the control study. Plasma pancreatic polypeptide levels rose slightly but insignificantly above the control level at the conclusion of the ID perfusion with amino acids and subsequently returned to control levels.

IV Fat Study

No inhibition of pancreatic secretion was observed following IV infusion of fat emulsion (Fig 4) despite a dramatic rise in the level of circulating serum triglycerides (from 0.32±0.02 mmol/L to 6.74±0.62 mmol/L) in response to the infusion. Minimal rises were noted in plasma somatostatin, pancreatic polypeptide, and glucagon concentrations, but these were not statistically different from those observed in the control study with cholecystokinin octapeptide alone.

ID Fat Study

Perfusion of ID fat resulted in a 40% inhibition of the stimulated protein output from the cholecystokinin octapeptide–stimulated pancreas ($P<.05$) (Fig 5). Similar patterns of inhibition were noted for the stimulated bicarbonate and volume outputs with 52% and 62% reductions, respectively. The inhibition of pancreatic output began immediately after commencement of the ID fat perfusion, reached maximal degree at the end of the perfusion, and persisted with only minimal recovery throughout the remainder of the study. Serum triglyceride levels rose minimally and insignificantly only late in the study (from 0.26±0.02 mmol/L to 0.34±0.04 mmol/L). Intraduodenal fat perfusion did not alter plasma levels of somatostatin or glucagon in comparison to control values. In contrast, plasma pancreatic polypeptide concentrations rose after 30 minutes of ID fat perfusion, increased to 81% above control level after 60 minutes, and remained persistently elevated to the end of the study (Fig 6). While the mean pancreatic polypeptide responses above controls were large, the differences were not significant due to large variances.

COMMENT

The findings of the present study suggest that both mixed amino acids and fat are capable of exerting inhibitory as well as stimulatory effects on exocrine pancreatic secretion. However, while both nutrients caused significant 40% to 73% reductions in cholecystokinin octapeptide–stimulated outputs of protein, bicarbonate, and volume, the mechanisms of inhibition appear disparate.

The results for infusion of IV amino acids are in accor-

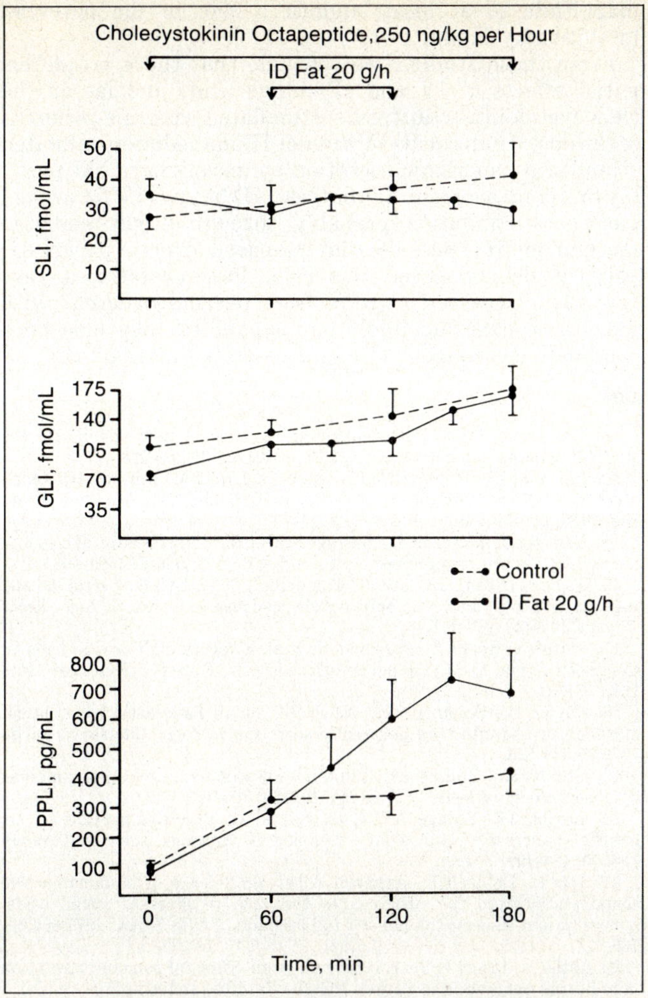

Fig 6.—Plasma levels of somatostatin (SLI), glucagon (GLI), and pancreatic polypeptidelike immunoreactivities (PPLI) in five dogs in response to three-hour intravenous infusion of cholecystokinin octapeptide, 250 ng/kg per hour, without (control) and with intraduodenal (ID) fat perfusion, 20 g/h, during second hour.

dance with the findings of DiMagno et al[11] and Saitoh et al.[12,17] Both the study of DiMagno et al and the present study demonstrate pancreatic inhibition paralleling the level of hyperaminoacidemia. It appears, however, that the degree of inhibition possible through this mechanism is limited. The maximal inhibition in the present study was noted after 30 minutes of amino acid infusion, notwithstanding a further rise in plasma amino acid concentration after 60 minutes. Only a slightly greater degree of inhibition was noted by Saitoh et al[12] following infusion of more than twice the load of amino acids. Similarly, DiMagno et al[11] infused protein hydrolysate IV into four volunteers at 24 g/h and observed only a 40% to 50% reduction in trypsin output evoked by the relatively weaker pancreatic stimulus of ID amino acids. The inhibition of protein output observed by us in response to IV amino acid infusion was biphasic. After cessation of the infusion and the subsequent fall in plasma amino acid concentration, there was a corresponding recovery of protein secretion. The subsequent decline in secretion at the end of the experiment may have been caused by fluid shifts resulting from the hyperosmolar infusate (1000 mOsm/L). This is suggested by the similar late inhibition imparted by infusion of mannitol (1000 mOsm/L) in the absence of significant inhibition during the actual infusion period.

While others[11,12] have suggested that glucagon release in response to hyperaminoacidemia was responsible for observed pancreatic inhibition, our results do not support this hypothesis. That glucagon is released in this experimental setting cannot be disputed, but the plasma levels achieved appear incapable of producing the degree of inhibition seen. DiMagno et al[11] found that after exogenous glucagon administration, the minimum plasma level that exerted pancreatic inhibition was 410 ng/L (approximately 117 fmol/mL), a level significantly higher than that detected in their study or in ours. Furthermore, our study for the first time has included an appropriate control study that indicates that cholecystokinin octapeptide infusion alone produces glucagon levels comparable to those caused by hyperaminoacidemia but without accompanying pancreatic inhibition. Although plasma pancreatic polypeptide and somatostatin levels also rose minimally in response to IV amino acid infusion, the changes were not different from those seen during the control study with cholecystokinin octapeptide alone. Thus, it would appear that the immediate inhibition of the cholecystokinin octapeptide–stimulated pancreas by IV amino acid infusion is not mediated by circulating glucagon, pancreatic polypeptide, or somatostatin nor is it related to the hyperosmolar nature of the infusate.

The present studies have failed to demonstrate a significant early inhibitory action of ID mixed amino acids on the stimulated exocrine pancreas. While confirmation of a modest release of pancreatic polypeptide by intraluminal amino acids coinciding with a slight decline in pancreatic secretion has been provided, little support for a modulating role of the circulating peptide in this setting can be offered. This is contrary to earlier findings in dogs given exogenous pancreatic polypeptide in doses producing smaller plasma increases than those evoked by a meal, which caused significant inhibition of pancreatic secretion stimulated by secretin plus cerulein.[18] The small decline in pancreatic secretion after 30 minutes of ID amino acid perfusion also coincided temporally with a significant hyperaminoacidemia and may reflect an effect of absorbed amino acids. We have presented evidence that minor inhibition of pancreatic secretion does follow absorption of intraluminal amino acids.[19] The more marked late decline in protein secretion 60 minutes after termination of the ID perfusion may represent inhibition imparted by release of a distal gut hormone such as peptide YY that is known to exert suppressive effects on pancreatic secretion.[20] While our studies showed no increases in circulating levels of glucagon or somatostatin following ID amino acid perfusion, previous reports employing selective visceral venous sampling or isolated perfused pancreatic preparations have documented somatostatin release under similar stimulation.[5,21] In eight human subjects, however, somatostatin administration at a dose producing levels similar to those measured after a meal did not affect pancreatic secretion stimulated by secretin and cerulein.[22]

The results of this study suggest that IV infusion of fat has no effect on stimulated pancreatic exocrine output. Despite a greater than 20-fold increase in serum triglyceride values, there were no differences from control levels of plasma glucagon, pancreatic polypeptide, or somatostatin. This lack of effect of IV fat is consistent with the findings of Matsuno et al[23] who studied five dogs and five postoperative patients with pancreatic fistulas. In both dogs and patients, IV infusion of a fat emulsion superimposed on pancreatic stimulation by combined secretin and cholecystokinin infusion exerted no consistent effects and no suggestion of significant inhibition.

Unlike amino acids, ID fat perfusion clearly did produce a significant degree of pancreatic inhibition. As this effect was evident immediately on initiation of the perfusion, a gut-mediated mechanism is suggested. Persistence of the inhibition after termination of the perfusion may reflect slow absorption of fat from the gut lumen. While there were no changes in plasma levels of glucagon or somatostatin relative to controls, there was a progressive though not quite significant rise above control levels of pancreatic polypeptide during and after ID fat perfusion. However, the level and duration of this increase was of sufficient magnitude to at least suggest a role in the observed inhibition by ID fat.

From these studies, we conclude that there are differential effects of IV and ID amino acids and fat on the cholecystokinin octapeptide–stimulated exocrine pancreas of the dog. Amino acids IV but not ID immediately inhibited stimulated pancreatic secretion by an unknown but possibly direct mechanism. In contrast, ID but not IV fat evoked pancreatic inhibition probably through a gut-mediated mechanism. It is possible that increased levels of pancreatic polypeptide subserved this role. Pancreastatin, a very recently discovered peptide from porcine pancreas with pancreatic exocrine inhibitory capability, may also be a candidate messenger in the gut-mediated mechanism.[24]

References

1. Wang CC, Grossman MI: Physiological determination of release of secretin and pancreozymin from intestine of dogs with transplanted pancreas. *Am J Physiol* 1951;164:527-545.
2. Meyer JH, Jones RS: Canine pancreatic responses to intestinally perfused fat and products of fat digestion. *Am J Physiol* 1974;226:1178-1187.
3. Meyer JH, Kelly GA: Canine pancreatic responses to intestinally perfused proteins and protein digest. *Am J Physiol* 1976;231:682-691.
4. Ohneda A, Yaube A, Maruhana Y, et al: Characterization of circulating immunoreactive glucagon in response to intraduodenal administration of fat in dogs. *Gastroenterology* 1975;68:715-721.
5. Schusdziarra V, Harris V, Conlon JM, et al: Pancreatic and gastric somatostatin release in response to intragastric and intraduodenal nutrients and HCl in the dog. *J Clin Invest* 1978;62:509-518.
6. Wilson RM, Boden G, Owen OE: Pancreatic polypeptide responses to a meal and to intraduodenal amino acids and sodium oleate. *Endocrinology* 1978;102:859-863.
7. Debas HT, Grossman MI: Pure cholecystokinin: Pancreatic protein and bicarbonate response. *Digestion* 1973;9:469-481.
8. Konturek SJ, Tasler J, Cieszkowski M, et al: Intravenous amino acids and fat stimulate pancreatic secretion. *Am J Physiol* 1979;236:E678-E684.
9. Stabile BE, Borzatta M, Stubbs RS, et al: Intravenous mixed amino acids and fats do not stimulate exocrine pancreatic secretion. *Am J Physiol* 1984;246:G274-G280.
10. Fried GM, Ogden WD, Rhea A, et al: Pancreatic protein secretion and gastrointestinal hormone release in response to parenteral amino acids and lipid in dogs. *Surgery* 1982;92:902-905.
11. DiMagno EP, Go VLW, Summerskill WHJ: Intraluminal and postabsorptive effects of amino acids on pancreatic enzyme secretion. *J Lab Clin Med* 1973;82:241-248.
12. Saitoh Y, Tokutake K, Matsuno S, et al: Effect of hypertonic glucose and amino acid infusion on pancreatic exocrine function. *Tohoku J Exp Med* 1978;124:99-115.
13. Herrera F, Kemp DR, Tsukamoto M, et al: A new cannula for the study of pancreatic function. *J Appl Physiol* 1968;25:207-209.
14. Faloona GR, Unger RH: Glucagon, in Jaffe BM, Berman HR (eds): *Methods of Hormone Radioimmunoassay*. Orlando, Fla, Academic Press Inc, 1974, pp 317-330.
15. Yamada T, Marshak D, Basinger S, et al: Somatostatin-like immunoreactivity in the retina. *Proc Natl Acad Sci USA* 1980;77:1691-1695.
16. Taylor IL, Impicciatore M, Carter DC, et al: Effect of atropine and vagotomy on the pancreatic polypeptide response to a meal in dogs. *Am J Physiol* 1978;235:E443-E447.
17. Saitoh Y, Honda T, Matasuno S, et al: Effect of eight amino acids on the exocrine and endocrine pancreatic function. *Tohoku J Exp Med* 1979; 129:257-272.
18. Taylor IL, Solomon TE, Walsh JH, et al: Pancreatic polypeptide: Metabolism and effect on pancreatic secretion in dogs. *Gastroenterology* 1979;76:524-528.
19. Stubbs RS, Stabile BE: Inhibition of stimulated exocrine pancreas by absorbed amino acids. *J Surg Res* 1984;36:395-400.
20. Adrian TE, Savage AP, Allen JM, et al: Effect of peptide YY on gastric, pancreatic, and biliary function in humans. *Gastroenterology* 1985;89:494-499.
21. Ipp E, Dobbs RE, Arimura A, et al: Release of immunoreactive somatostatin from the pancreas in response to glucose, amino acids, pancreozymin-cholecystokinin and tolbutamide. *J Clin Invest* 1977;60:760-765.
22. Gullo L, Priori P, Scarpignato C, et al: Effect of somatostatin 14 on pure human pancreatic secretion. *Dig Dis Sci* 1987;32:1065-1070.
23. Matsuno S, Miyashita E, Sasaki K, et al: Effects of intravenous fat emulsion administration on exocrine and endocrine pancreatic function. *Jpn J Surg* 1981;11:323-329.
24. Funakoshi A, Miyasaka K, Nakamura R, et al: Inhibitory effect of pancreastatin on pancreatic exocrine secretion in the conscious rat, abstracted. *Gastroenterology* 1988;94:138.

In Other AMA Journals

ARCHIVES OF OTOLARYNGOLOGY—HEAD & NECK SURGERY

Surgical Care of Submental Gunshot Wounds

Karen H. Calhoun, MD; Spencer Li, MD; William D. Clark, DDS, MD; Charles M. Stiernberg, MD; Francis B. Quinn, Jr, MD

The care of patients with self-inflicted facial gunshot wounds is complex and challenging. The magnitude and self-inflicted nature of the injuries naturally give rise to questions about potential for successful rehabilitation. The surgical care and rehabilitation of ten such patients are described. The initial grotesque disfiguration belies the reasonable chances for functional restoration. Patients in this series who completed reconstruction swallow well enough to maintain body weight, speak understandably, breathe without tracheostomy, and have an appearance sufficiently normal that they can interact socially without embarrassment. Guidelines are proposed for multidisciplinary medical care leading to satisfactory functional, aesthetic, social, and psychiatric rehabilitation (*Arch Otolaryngol Head Neck Surg* 1988;114:513-519).

From the Department of Otolaryngology, University of Texas Medical Branch, Galveston (Drs Calhoun, Clark, Stiernberg, and Quinn), and the Department of Internal Medicine, Baylor College of Medicine, Houston (Dr Li). Dr Clark is now in private practice in Las Cruces, NM.

Reprints not available.

Detection of the Cancer-Prone Colon, Using Transepithelial Impedance Analysis

Richard J. Davies, MD; Renah Joseph; Horacio Asbun, MD; Marc Sedwitz, MD

• Alterations in ionic conductance may represent an early mitogenic signal; therefore, impedance analysis was used to examine differences in the electrical properties of the distal colon in a cancer-susceptible (CF_1) and a cancer-resistant (DBA) strain of mouse following administration of the carcinogen dimethylhydrazine. The electrical conductance of the surface colonic epithelium increased in CF_1 mice from a mean (±SEM) of 41.1±3.0 milliSiemens•cm^{-2} (mS•cm^{-2}) in controls to 52.6±3.1 mS•cm^{-2} following dimethylhydrazine treatment. The conductance decreased in the cancer-resistant DBA group from 154.6±44.1 mS•cm^{-2} in controls to 35.1±17.2 mS•cm^{-2} following dimethylhydrazine treatment. This difference in response to the carcinogen may partly explain differences in susceptibility noted between these two species. Epithelial impedance analysis may be of use in the early detection of the colon at risk for subsequent cancer development.

(*Arch Surg* 1989;124:480-484)

Despite improvements in surgical and radiation therapy, the mortality from large-bowel cancer has remained virtually unaltered during the past 50 years. Adjuvant chemotherapy has also failed to make a significant impact on survival so that approximately 58% of patients die of this neoplasm during the five years from the time of initial diagnosis.[1-4] Consequently, this neoplasm is the second most common cause of death from cancer in the United States and many Western countries.[4] These dismal survival statistics have led to renewed interest in primary and secondary prevention. Primary prevention of colorectal cancer would require the identification of etiologic factors and their removal from the environment. Secondary prevention using screening techniques to identify early cancers or their precursors such as polyps is neither cost-effective nor has the sensitivity or specificity to gain widespread acceptance.[5-9]

Although it is not clear when initiation occurs, many authorities agree that it may take decades before the malignant phenotype is expressed.[10,11] During this period promoting events influence the large-bowel mucosa and eventually result in the malignant transformation of one cell or a few cells that develop into a neoplasm. Although the existence of synchronous or metachronous cancers is a well-recognized phenomenon, it is difficult to understand why multiple tumors do not develop more frequently since there are billions of cells exposed to similar environmental and genetic influences.[12] A field defect probably exists in patients with large-bowel cancer indicating that the mucosa at risk is different from mucosa derived from patients not at increased risk for the development of cancer. Most of the studies demonstrating a field defect involve cell proliferation studies using in vitro labeling techniques.[13-19] These studies have been done in patients with a genetic predisposition to develop colorectal cancer, such as patients with familial polyposis or nonpolyposis familial colon cancer syndromes. However, even in sporadically developing colorectal cancer (the most common variety), histologic changes have been observed in the mucosa at sites distant to the cancer suggesting that a field defect exists.[20] An increase in DNA synthesis and tritiated-thymidine labeling has been demonstrated in the normal-appearing mucosa derived from patients with sporadic large-bowel cancer compared with mucosa derived from patients without the disease.[21] These differences are relatively slight and subject to the errors of observer interpretation. In addition, the techniques are labor intensive, probably precluding these methods as a screening tool, which could be used to identify the mucosa at risk for cancer development in the nongenetically predisposed patient.[20,21]

Multiple changes occur at the cell surface during growth stimulation and transformation,[22,23] such as alterations in cell surface glycoproteins, altered cell membrane permeability, altered ion fluxes, changes in cell-to-cell coupling, and alterations in the epithelial tight junctions.[24-29] These changes may occur in the mucosa at risk for subsequent transformation before the malignant phenotype has been expressed. Since the large-bowel mucosa mainly consists of an epithelial cell layer interspersed with occasional goblet cells, its electrical properties are primarily determined by the ionic permeability of the tight junctions and the surface epithelial cells. When the resistance is coupled with the capacitance properties of the surface epithelium, it forms a parallel resistor-capacitor circuit with a characteristic time constant equal to the product of R (resistor) and C (capacitor). The equivalent circuit in its simplest form has an additional resistor in series with the parallel resistor-capacitor to represent the electrical barrier provided by the underlying subepithelial layer and muscle. This equivalent circuit may be termed a *lumped model*, although more complex circuits representing the electrical properties of the bowel wall can be constructed as depicted in Fig 1. Therefore, it is possible to construct an electrical equivalent circuit analog of the epithelium made up of resistors and capacitors. The characterization of the electrical circuit may be accomplished by measuring the electrical impedance, which is the ratio of the measured voltage to a constant applied sinusoidal current at a given frequency. At each frequency two quantities are measured: the ratio of the magnitudes of the applied voltage to the measured voltage, and the normalized time delay of the voltage sinusoid compared with the current sinusoid (the phase angle ø). This relationship can be represented as a Nyquist plot and the impedance characteristics of the epithelium may be measured.[30,31]

We have used epithelial impedance analysis to examine the electrical properties of the distal colon taken from a susceptible mouse strain (CF_1) after administration of saline or the carcinogen dimethylhydrazine, which produces large-bowel cancer. The changes in impedance were compared with those occurring in a resistant strain of mouse (DBA) following identical treatment. It is suggested

Accepted for publication Dec 12, 1988.

From the University of California Medical Center and the Veterans Administration Medical Center, San Diego.

Read before the 12th Annual Surgical Symposium of the Association of Veterans Administration Surgeons, Minneapolis, May 13, 1988.

Reprint requests to Division of Surgical Oncology, Department of Surgery, H891B, University of California Medical Center, 225 Dickinson St, San Diego, CA 92103 (Dr Davies).

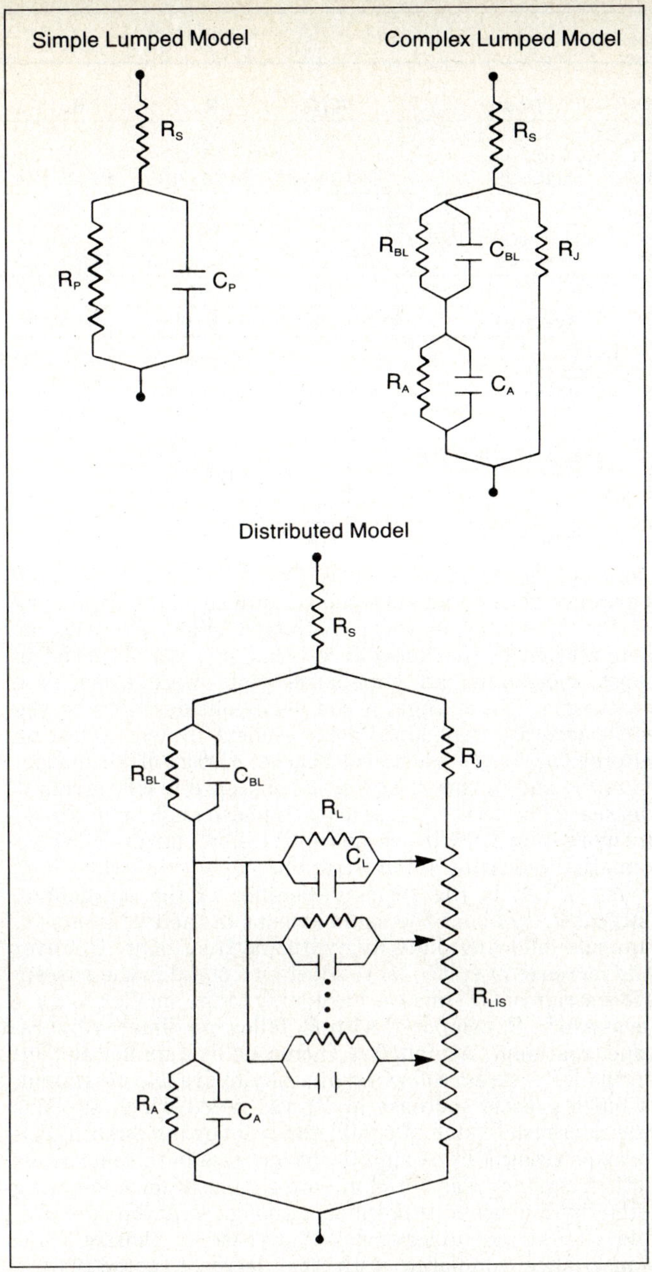

Fig 1.—Resistor-capacitor analogs representing electrical characteristics of large bowel. Simple Lumped Model: R_p and C_p represent resistance and capacitance of surface epithelium, respectively; R_s, series resistance due to underlying nonepithelial layers and chamber resistance. Complex Lumped Model: Subscripts A, BL, J, and S denote apical, baso-lateral, tight-junctional, and series, respectively. Distributed Model: Subscripts L and LIS denote lateral cell membrane and lateral intercellular space, respectively. Otherwise subscripts are same as in complex lumped model (from Davies et al[33]).

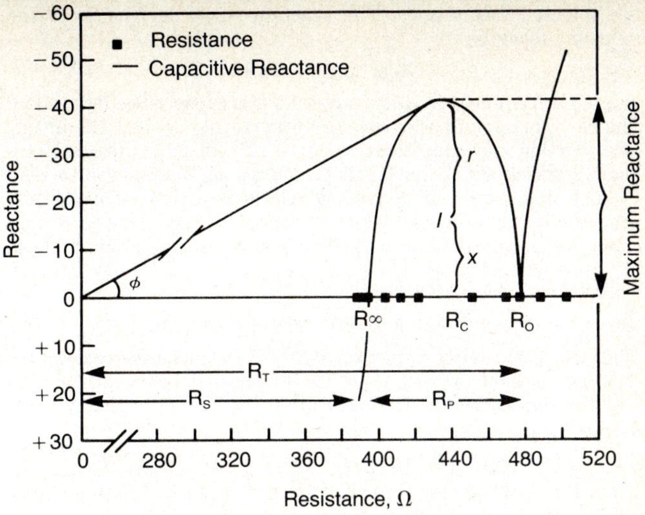

Fig 2.—Derivation of impedance profile. Abbreviations, terms, and their derivations are explained in "Materials and Methods" section. ø indicates phase angle at maximum reactance; *l*, center of impedance locus with *x* equal to displacement of locus from *x*-axis; and *r*, radius of impedance plot (from Davies et al[33]).

that this technique, which measures the electrical characteristics of the surface epithelium, may be useful in the detection of the cancer-prone colon or rectum.

MATERIALS AND METHODS

Nonfasting adult female CF_1 or DBA/2 mice weighing between 18 and 22 g were used in all experiments and were maintained under identical conditions of cyclic 12 hours of light and dark. Regular chow (Ralston Purina Co, St Louis) and water were allowed ad libitum. The carcinogen dimethylhydrazine (Aldrich Chemical Co Inc, Milwaukee) was freshly prepared on the day of injection and dissolved in 0.9% saline and injected subcutaneously into the groin in a dosage of 20 mg/kg weekly for four weeks. Following each weekly injection animals were kept in a negative flow hood for 12 hours to prevent atmospheric contamination. Control animals were subcutaneously injected with an identical volume of 0.9% saline.

One week after the fourth injection animals were killed using cervical dislocation and the colon was removed and rinsed with iced sodium-free Ringer's solution. Because preliminary studies have failed to demonstrate any difference in stability of the tissue whether the seromuscular layer was stripped, all experiments were performed on pieces of colon containing all layers, including the mucosa. Each distal segment of the colon was mounted within ten minutes in an acrylic chamber (area, 0.28 cm^2) and bathed on the mucosal and serosal side with equal volumes of sodium-free Ringer's solution at 37°C continuously oxygenated with 95% O_2 and 5% CO_2, maintained at a pH of 7.4, and circulated using a bubble-lift mechanism. The sodium-free Ringer's solution contained choline (which replaced Na), 140 mmol/L; K, 5.2 mmol/L; Ca, 1.2 mmol/L; Mg, 1.2 mmol/L; HCO_3, 25 mmol/L; HPO_4, 2.4 mmol/L; H_2PO_4, 0.4 mmol/L; Cl, 119.8 mmol/L; and glucose, 10 mmol/L. Sodium-free Ringer's solution was used because of previous observations that differences in the impedance profile were more evident in this solution following dimethylhydrazine treatment.[32,33]

Impedance measurements were made using two silver-silver chloride (Ag-AgCl) working electrodes and two Ag-AgCl measuring electrodes with one of each positioned on either side of the membrane. This configuration was chosen to avoid electrode polarization. A signal generator was used to excite the mucosa with a sine wave signal of adjustable frequency. The resultant voltage drop due to the bowel sample was compared with the voltage drop across an external adjustable load consisting of a parallel combination of a resistor and capacitor. When the comparison of these two signals yielded a "zero error," the tissue impedance was considered to be that of the external load. A constant driving voltage of 40 mV was used and the applied current varied between 30 and 60 μA. Pilot experiments confirmed that an identical Nyquist plot was obtained by measuring the impedance at 40 or 12 frequencies between 10 and 20 000 Hz, and therefore 12 frequencies were selected at 20, 50, 70, 100, 200, 500, 700, 1000, 2000, 5000, 7000, and 10 000 Hz. The resistance and capacitance were measured at each of these frequencies. Electrical stability of the tissue was noted for at least three hours, although a gradual decay of resistance and capacitance was observed during this period so that all experiments were performed at the same time to reduce temporally related errors. Further details of the methodology employed have been previously described.[32,33]

Values of resistance and capacitance were obtained at each of the selected frequencies. The reactance was derived from the following formula:

(1) $$\text{Reactance} = 1/2\pi fC$$

where f is frequency in Hertz units and C is capacitance in farads.[30] The real portion of impedance (Z) was plotted against the imaginary portion using an iterative curve fit routine (Labtech Notebook, Laboratory Technologies Corporation, Wilmington, Mass). Using a simple lumped model in which the resistive and capacitive components of the bowel wall are represented as a resistor and capacitor in parallel and a further resistor in series with these two components (Fig 1), the impedance (Z) can be written in complex notation as follows:

(2) $$Z = R_s + (R_p/j\omega C_p)/(R_p + 1/j\omega C_p)$$

where j is the complex operator $(1)^{1/2}$, R_s is the series resistance, R_p is the epithelial resistance, C_p is the epithelial capacitance, and ω is the angular frequency. Separating real from imaginary parts is shown as follows:

(3) $$Z = R_s + (R_p)/(1+\omega^2 C^2_p R^2_p) - j(\omega C_p R^2_p)/(1+\omega^2 C^2_p R^2_p)$$

From Fig 2, which demonstrates the derivation of the impedance profile, it can be seen that

(4) $$R_0 = R_p + R_s = R_t$$

and

(5) $$R_\infty = R_s$$

where R_0 and R_∞ are the resistance of the tissue at zero and infinite frequency, respectively, R_t is the total resistance of the tissue and $R_p C_p$ may be represented as the time constant T. Equation 3 may be rewritten as follows:

(6) $$Z = [R_\infty + (R_0 - R_\infty)/(1+\omega^2 T^2)] - j\{[\omega T(R_0 - R_\infty)(1+\omega^2 T^2)]\}$$

In this equation the first part of the equation is the real component R (resistance) of the colon impedance and the second part of the equation represents the reactance (reactive capacitance) in the xy plane. The reactive and real terms are functions of Z and ω. When the frequency was varied between zero and infinity, Z changed continually along the curve in the xy plane of the graph (Fig 2). This curve is almost a perfect semicircle although for the purpose of illustrating the derivation of the impedance profile, it has been distorted in the figure and is known as an impedance plot. Elimination of ω and T from equation 6 yields the expression for the impedance plot in the xy plane of Fig 2.

(7) $$\text{Reactance} = (R_0 - R_\infty)\,[R_0 - R)/(R_c - R_\infty)^{1/2}]\,[(R_0 - R_\infty)/(R - R_\infty)]$$

Equation 7 was used in the curve fitting program to determine R_0 and R_∞. The highest point on the curve is the maximum capacitive reactance of the tissue. This analytic expression for the impedance plot derived the impedance measurements for each piece of tissue and are summarized in the Table. The other impedance characteristics such as phase angle ø, characteristic frequency, characteristic capacitance, and resistance were calculated from these values using the planar trigonometry outlined in Fig 2.

An F test was used to examine the variance of each set of measurements derived from the impedance profiles obtained in each experimental group. Dimethylhydrazine-treated animals were compared with saline-treated controls using an unpaired Student t test as appropriate.[34] Two-tailed t tests were used in all instances. A statistically significant difference was considered probable when $P<.05$.

RESULTS

Bowel resistance and capacitance were measured at different frequencies to develop an impedance profile then plotted as a Nyquist plot for each tissue, from which the impedance characteristics were derived for each piece of colon. The Table summarizes the impedance characteristics of four groups of animals. The electrical conductance of the surface colonic epithelium increased in CF_1 mice from a mean ($\pm$SEM) of 41.1.$\pm$3.0 milliSiemens·cm^{-2} (mS·cm^{-2}) in controls to 52.6$\pm$3.1 mS·cm^{-2} ($P<.02$) following dimethylhydrazine treatment. Conductance decreased in the cancer-resistant DBA group from 154.6$\pm$44.1 mS·cm^{-2} in controls to 35.1$\pm$17.2 mS·cm^{-2} ($P<.001$) following dimethylhydrazine treatment.

The Nyquist plots of the colons demonstrated the dependence of the reactance and resistance on the frequency of the applied sine wave. Although slight elevation or suppression of the impedance locus "x" was observed in most specimens, all impedance plots were close to a semicircle. Phase angle ø has been considered to be the most accurate impedance measurement in demonstrating alterations in the electrical characteristics of an epithelium,[35,36] and in this study in the susceptible CF_1 strain it decreased by 28%. Conversely the phase angle ø increased by more than 280% in the susceptible DBA strain following dimethylhydrazine administration.

Mouse	R_0, Ω	R_∞, Ω	R_c, Ω
CF_1			
Control			
Mean ± SE	592.8 ± 8.6	515.8 ± 9.0	559.2 ± 10.4
n	11	12	12
With dimethylhydrazine			
Mean ± SE	639.0 ± 9.1	564.9 ± 11.9	598.8 ± 10.9
n	11	12	12
P value	<.005	<.005	<.02
DBA			
Control			
Mean ± SE	521.6 ± 15.1	498.5 ± 13.8	510.0 ± 14.1
n	11	11	11
With dimethylhydrazine			
Mean ± SE	642.3 ± 28.3	540.6 ± 21.8	591.4 ± 23.7
n	10	10	10
P value	<.005	NS	<.01

R_∞, which is the series resistance of the epithelium, increased by about the same amount in the two groups of animals following dimethylhydrazine treatment. However the increase in epithelial conductance noted in the susceptible strain of CF_1 mice is due mainly to the smaller relative increase in R_0 compared with R_∞ following dimethylhydrazine treatment. Although R_∞ increased by a similar amount in the DBA strain following dimethylhydrazine treatment, a much greater increase in R_0 was noted which explains the decreased value of conductance following dimethylhydrazine treatment. A significant increase in the characteristic frequency was noted in both strains of mice following dimethylhydrazine treatment, although only the susceptible CF_1 strain underwent an increase in characteristic capacitance compared with the decrease noted in the resistant DBA strain.

COMMENT

In this study we have demonstrated differences in the electrical properties of the bowel wall induced by a colonic carcinogen dimethylhydrazine in a susceptible (CF_1) and resistant (DBA) strain of mouse, both of which have been extensively studied as animal models of large-bowel cancer.[37,38] To our knowledge, the reason for the differential susceptibility noted between these two species is unknown. It was thought that resistant strains might be unable to metabolize the carcinogen dimethylhydrazine to its active form methylazoxymethanol, although recent experiments have demonstrated that direct administration of the active metabolite methylazoxymethanol failed to produce proliferative changes or cancers in DBA mice.[39]

These experiments were performed in a sodium-free Ringer's solution and therefore changes in sodium transport or permeability cannot explain these carcinogen-induced changes in impedance. We have previously reported that dimethylhydrazine induces an increase in Na^+/H^+ exchange in CF_1 but not DBA mice.[40] This has

Impedance Profile of a Susceptible and Resistant Strain of Mouse*

Reactance, Ω	G, mS·cm⁻²	Phase ø, Radians	x	r	F_c, Hz	T, s	W, Radians·s⁻¹	Cap_c, Microfarad·cm²
43.5±3.1	41.1±3.0	0.077±0.005	−21.2±1.6	22.2±1.6	561.0±10.5	0.000285±0.000005	3525±66	11.8±1.1
12	12	12	12	12	12	12	12	11
34.0±2.0	52.6±3.1	0.057±0.004	−16.5±1.0	17.5±1.0	599.8±10.9	0.000266±0.000005	3769±68	14.6±0.7
12	12	12	12	12	12	12	12	12
<.02	<.02	<.005	<.02	<.02	<.02	<.02	<.01	<.05
11.6±3.3	154.6±44.1	0.022±0.006	−5.3±1.7	6.3±1.7	510.3±14.1	0.000314±0.000008	3206±89	85.4±12.8
11	11	11	11	11	11	12	11	10
50.8±8.6	35.1±17.2	0.084±0.014	−24.9±4.3	25.9±4.3	594.2±24.0	0.000272±0.000010	3733±151	11.8±3.2
10	10	10	10	10	10	12	10	9
<.001	<.001	<.001	<.001	<.001	<.01	<.005	<.01	<.001

**P* value is derived from the unpaired Student *t* test comparing dimethylhydrazine-treated animals with controls; NS indicates not significant; n, number of animals; R_0, resistance at zero frequency; R_∞, resistance at infinite frequency; R_c, characteristic resistance of the tissue (these three values are non–area corrected); reactance, capacitive reactance of the tissue at the characteristic resistance; G, epithelial conductance corrected for area in milliSiemens·cm⁻²; Phase ø, phase angle; x, deviation of the impedance locus from the *x*-axis with a positive value indicating elevation and a negative value indicating suppression; r, radius of the impedance profile; F_c, characteristic frequency; T, time constant; W, time constant; and Cap_c, capacitance at the characteristic frequency and resistance.

also been recently demonstrated in rat colonic brush-border vesicles following dimethylhydrazine adminstration.[41] The impedance changes noted in the present study may represent changes in the tight junctions between cells or alterations in membrane fluidity.[41] One of the earliest changes induced by mitogens is an increase in cell membrane conductance[24]; this may represent a mitogenic signal leading to increases in cell proliferation.[22] Malignant transformation has been associated with loss of tight junction integrity[23,24] so that cells lose contact inhibition and pile up on one another. An increase in membrane ionic permeability or loss of tight junctional integrity would cause an increase in transepithelial conductance observed in the CF_1 mice in these experiments. Alternately, down regulation of membrane conductance or increased cell-to-cell adherence would be expected to produce the type of impedance changes noted in the DBA mice in these experiments. Further experiments using intracellular measurements will be required to separate the relative contributions of the cell membrane or the tight junctions to this phenomenon. It is of interest that the resistant DBA strain was not unresponsive to the dimethylhydrazine but underwent considerable changes in impedance in an opposite manner to the changes induced in the CF_1 mice; this suggests an adaptive response rather than unresponsiveness.

Preliminary studies from our laboratory have demonstrated that the impedance profile of large bowel from patients with a cancer is different when compared with bowel from patients without evidence of a malignant neoplasm (data not shown). Although it may be thought that the "normal" bowel at a distance from a bowel cancer is histologically normal, several studies have suggested alterations in crypt cell kinetics and structure even in the mucosa at a site remote from the primary malignant neoplasm.[20,21] This is especially true in patients with familial polyposis and familial colon cancer syndrome[13-16]; however, major differences in the uninvolved mucosa from patients with sporadic colon cancer have yet to be identified to our knowledge. It was noted that the conductance properties of the mucosa taken at least 5 cm from the index cancer were lower than in controls. The reduction in conductance was somewhere intermediate between the increase seen in the CF_1 mouse and the decrease seen in the DBA mouse. This may suggest that human colonic mucosa is of intermediate susceptibility when compared with a susceptible and resistant animal model of large-bowel cancer.

Although one must exercise caution before extrapolating animal data to humans, alterations in impedance may help diagnose susceptible individuals who have undergone initiation and are likely to develop cancer under the right promoting influences. It is possible that the normal-appearing mucosa has been exposed to the same carcinogenic or genetic influences as the mucosa giving rise to the index cancer although it has not yet undergone malignant transformation. The multistep hypothesis of carcinogenesis would suggest several events in the development of cancer with perhaps a lead time of several decades before a cancer actually develops.[10-12] If the initiating and early promotional events affect the entire mucosa, then alterations in the characteristics of the mucosa in the cancer-prone colon would have important screening and therapeutic implications.[42]

Whether altered impedance represents alteration in cell surface signaling within the epithelial layer or changes in the cytoskeletal structure cannot be determined. The capacitance properties of a complex layer of cells such as the bowel wall are thought to reside in the true epithelial layer.[36] We have not observed alterations in the capacitance properties by stripping away the underlying serosa and muscle layers. Therefore, it can be concluded that since the observed alterations take place in the frequency domain, these differences are epithelial in origin. Although we have previously noted alterations in sodium transport and transmural depolarization in a murine model of colon cancer, we have failed to observe an increase in the resistance of the bowel wall.[40,43,44] This may be because the previously employed methodologies using voltage clamp techniques have not been able to separate the resistance of the surface epithelial cells from the underlying layers. As can be seen from the Table, the resistance of the true epithelial layer only constitutes about 10% to 20% of the total resistance of the bowel wall. Therefore, it may not be possible to identify alterations in the resistance of the epithelial layer using these other techniques not employing capacitance measurements. These changes begin even before histologic evidence of dysplasia occurs and are progressive with increased doses of the carcinogen administered over a longer period of time.[32]

Since an alteration in ionic flux has been proposed as an early mitogenic signal[22,45,46] during growth stimulation or transformation, the alteration in epithelial impedance characteristics identified in this study may represent changes in ionic conductance following initiation. Whether altered ionic permeability represents a mitogenic signal or a nonobligatory event in the malignant process cannot be determined; however, the need for better screening methods for large-bowel cancer is apparent.[47-49] Present methods are plagued with insensitivity and nonspecificity.[5-9] Currently it is impossible to identify which patients should undergo frequent colonoscopy or contrast studies because of difficulty in assessing risk and identifying groups of patients who have already undergone initiation. Earlier diagnosis would appear to be of key importance in preventing death from this common malignant neoplasm.[50-52] Identification of the mucosa at risk before the malignant phenotype is fully expressed may be possible using epithelial impedance analysis to identify the cancer-prone large bowel. Whether this biophysical approach has a role toward this goal remains to be determined from more extensive studies.

This investigation was supported in part by the Research Services of the Veterans Administration and by a gift from American Mediscan Inc, Los Angeles.

The mice used in this investigation were provided by Charles River Breeding Laboratories Inc, Wilmington, Mass.

References

1. Olson RM, Perenevich NP, Malcolm AW, et al: Patterns of recurrence following curative resection of adenocarcinoma of the colon and rectum. *Cancer* 1980;45:2969-2974.

2. Evans JT, Vana J, Aronoff BL, et al: Management and survival of carcinoma of the colon: Results of a national survey by the American College of Surgeons. *Ann Surg* 1978;188:176-220.

3. Copeland EM, Miller LD, Jones RS: Prognostic factors in carcinoma of the colon and rectum. *Am J Surg* 1968;116:875-881.

4. Statistics of the American Cancer Society. *CA* 1987;37:2-19.

5. Eklund G, Carlsson U, Janzon L: The feasibility of large scale population screening. *Br J Surg* 1985;72(suppl):71-72.

6. Simon JB: Occult blood screening for colorectal carcinoma: A critical review. *Gastroenterology* 1985;88:820-837.

7. Frank JW: Occult blood screening for colorectal carcinoma: The risks. *Am J Prev Med* 1985;1:25-32.

8. Walsh TH, Spiro M: How accurately do we diagnose tumors at the rectosigmoid junction? *Practitioner* 1981;225:1317-1320.

9. Winawer SJ, Miller DG, Sherlock P: *Risk and Screening for Colorectal Cancer.* Chicago, Year Book Medical Publishers Inc, 1984, pp 471-496.

10. Lipkin M: Phase 1 and phase 2 proliferative lesions of colonic epithelial cells in diseases leading to colonic cancer. *Cancer* 1974;34:878-888.

11. Muto T, Bussey HJ, Morson BC: The evolution of cancer of the colon and rectum. *Cancer* 1975;36:2251-2270.

12. Nowell PC: The clonal evolution of tumor cell populations. *Science* 1976;194:23-28.

13. Kanemitsu T, Koike A, Yamamoto S: Study of the cell proliferation kinetics in ulcerative colitis, adenomatous polyps, and cancer. *Cancer* 1985;56:1094-1098.

14. Lipkin M, Blattner WE, Fraumeni JF Jr, et al: Tritiated thymidine ($ø_p$,$ø_n$) labeling distribution in the identification of hereditary predisposition to colon cancer. *Cancer Res* 1983;43:1899-1904.

15. Lipkin M, Blattner WA, Gardner EJ, et al: Classification and risk assessment of individuals with familial polyposis, Gardner's syndrome, and familial non-polyposis colon cancer from [^{3}H]thymidine labeling patterns in colonic epithelial cells. *Cancer Res* 1984;44:4201-4207.

16. Deschner EE, Lipkin M: Proliferative patterns in colonic mucosa in familial polyposis. *Cancer* 1975;35:413-418.

17. Iwama T, Utzunomiya J, Sasaki J: Epithelial cell kinetics in the crypts of familial polyposis of colon. *Jpn J Surg* 1977;7:230-234.

18. Lipkin M, Newmark H: Effect of added dietary calcium on colonic epithelial cell proliferation in subjects at high risk for familial colonic cancer. *N Engl J Med* 1985;313:1381-1384.

19. Lipkin M, Uehara K, Winawer S, et al: Seventh-Day Adventist vegetarians have quiescent proliferative activity in colonic mucosa. *Cancer Lett* 1985;26:139-144.

20. Shamsuddin AKM, Weiss L, Phelps PC, et al: Colonic epithelium: IV. Human colonic carcinogenesis: Changes in human colon mucosa adjacent to and remote from carcinomas of the colon. *JNCI* 1981;66:413-419.

21. Bleiberg H, Buyse M, Galand P: Cell kinetic indicators of premalignant stages of colorectal cancer. *Cancer* 1985;56:124-129.

22. Rozengurt E: Early signals in the mitogenic response. *Science* 1986;234:161-166.

23. Singer SJ: On the transduction of signals at the cell surface, in Galeotti T (ed): *Cell Membranes and Cancer.* New York, Elsevier Science Publishing Co Inc, 1985, pp 1-10.

24. Oplatka A, Friedman JE, Rosenheck K: Reorganization of the cytoskeleton in transformed and tumor cells may be intimately coupled with changes in ion transport through the plasma membrane, in Galeotti T (ed): *Cell Membranes and Cancer.* New York, Elsevier Science Publishing Co Inc, 1985, pp 117-123.

25. Filipe MI: Mucous secretions in rat colonic mucosa during carcinogenesis induced by dimethylhydrazine: A morphological and histochemical study. *Br J Cancer* 1975;32:60-77.

26. Schlessinger J: The mechanism and role of hormone induced clustering of membrane receptors. *Trends Biol Sci* 1980;5:210-214.

27. Moolenaar WH, Tertoolen LGJ, Tsien RY, et al: Na^+/H^+ exchange: Cytoplasmic pH and the action of growth factors in human fibroblasts. *J Biol Chem* 1983;259:8066-8069.

28. Paris S, Pouyssegur J: Growth factors activate the Na^+/H^+ antiporter in quiescent fibroblasts by increasing its affinity for intracellular H^+. *J Biol Chem* 1984;259:10989-10994.

29. Shamsuddin AKM, Trump BF: Colonic epithelium: II. In vivo studies of colonic carcinogenesis: Light microscopic, histochemical and ultrastructural studies of histogenesis of azoxymethane induced colonic carcinomas in Fischer 344 rats. *JNCI* 1981;66:389-401.

30. Schanne OF, P-Ceretti ER: Technical and theoretical aspects of biological impedance measurements, in *Impedance Measurements in Biological Cells.* New York, John Wiley & Sons Inc, 1978, pp 1-69.

31. Diamond JM, Machen TE: Impedance analysis in epithelia and the problem of gastric acid secretion. *J Membr Biol* 1983;72:17-41.

32. Davies RJ, Juncosa RD, Kaplan D, et al: Colonic epithelial impedance analysis in a murine model of large-bowel cancer. *Arch Surg* 1986;121:1253-1258.

33. Davies RJ, Joseph R, Kaplan D, et al: Epithelial impedance analysis in experimentally induced colon cancer. *Biophys J* 1987;52:783-790.

34. Snedecor GW, Cochran WG: *Statistical Methods,* ed 6. Ames, Iowa, Iowa State University Press, 1967, pp 549-550.

35. Valdiosera R, Clausen C, Eisenberg RS: Circuit models of the passive electrical properties of frog skeletal muscle fibers. *J Gen Physiol* 1974;63:432-459.

36. Clausen C, Lewis SA, Diamond JM: Impedance analysis of a tight epithelium using a distributed resistance model. *Biophys J* 1979;26:291-317.

37. Thurnherr N, Deschner EE, Stonehill EH, et al: Induction of adenocarcinomas of the colon in mice by weekly injections of 1,2-dimethylhydrazine. *Cancer Res* 1973;33:940-945.

38. Diwan BA, Meier H, Blackman KE: Genetic differences in the induction of colorectal tumors by 1,2-dimethylhydrazine in inbred mice. *JNCI* 1977;59:455-458.

39. Deschner EE, Long FC, Hakissian M, et al: Differential susceptibility of inbred mouse strains forecast by acute proliferative response to methylazoxymethanol. *JNCI* 1984;72:195-198.

40. Davies RJ, Weidema WF, Sandle GI, et al: Sodium transport in a mouse model of colonic cancer. *Cancer Res* 1987;47:4646-4650.

41. Brasitus TA, Dudeja PK, Foster ES: 1,2-dimethylhydrazine-induced alterations in Na^+-H^+ exchange in rat colonic brush-border vesicles. *Biochim Biophys Acta* 1988;938:483-488.

42. Sherlock P, Winawer SJ: Are there markers for the risk of colorectal cancer? *N Engl J Med* 1984;311:118-119.

43. Goller DA, Weidema WF, Davies RJ: Transmural electrical potential difference as an early marker in colon cancer. *Arch Surg* 1986;121:345-350.

44. Davies RJ, Weidema WF, Palmer L, et al: Increased sodium absorption by the distal colon in 1,2-dimethylhydrazine-treated Sprague-Dawley rat. *Surg Forum* 1983;34:183-185.

45. Leffert HL, Koch KS: Monovalent cations and the control of hepatocyte proliferation in chemically defined medium, in Boynton AL, McKeehan WL, Whittfield JF (eds): *Ions Cell Proliferation and Cancer.* Orlando, Fla, Academic Press Inc, 1982, pp 103-130.

46. Leffert HL, Koch KS: Growth regulation by sodium ion influxes, in Boynton AL, Leffert HL (eds): *Control of Animal Cell Proliferation.* Orlando, Fla, Academic Press Inc, 1985, vol 1, pp 367-413.

47. Winawer SJ, Sherlock P, Schottenfeld D, et al: Screening for colorectal cancer. *Gastroenterology* 1976;70:783-789.

48. Winawer SJ, Poleski MH, Sherlock P: Susceptibility for colorectal cancer: Current concepts of screening, diagnosis, and risk, in Berk J (ed): *Developments in Digestive Diseases.* Philadelphia, Lea & Febiger, 1979, pp 73-88.

49. Winchester DP, Sylvester J, Maker ML: Risks and benefits of mass screening for colonic neoplasia with the stool guaiac test. *Cancer* 1983;33:333-343.

50. Hertz RE, Deddesh MR, Day E: Value of periodic examinations in detecting cancer of the rectum and colon. *Postgrad Med* 1960;27:290-294.

51. Gilbertson VA: Proctosigmoidoscopy and polypectomy in reducing the incidence of rectal cancer. *Cancer* 1974;34:936-939.

52. DeCosse JJ: Are we doing better with large bowel cancer? *N Engl J Med* 1984;310:782-783.

Recent Trends in the Management of Incisional Herniation

Raymond C. Read, MD, PhD, Gordon Yoder, PAC

• There is a high incidence of risk factors for incisional herniation in hospitalized veterans. Almost half the defects appear more than 12 months after celiotomy. "Buttonholing" of the rectus sheath by a sawing motion of the continuous nonabsorbable suture may be responsible for this later herniation. Suturing with synthetic, slowly absorbed monofilament may reduce delayed herniation. The recurrence rate after primary repair was 24.8% (n=206), and after a second repair the recurrence rate was 41.7% (n=36). Plastic prostheses, used only in difficult cases (18% of the sample), were associated with a recurrence rate similar to that associated with sutures because of protrusion around the edge. The use of larger and better fixed ("sandwich") polypropylene mesh (Marlex) is indicated. Subxiphoid epigastric hernias following sternotomy do not require prosthetic herniorrhaphy.

(*Arch Surg* 1989;124:485-488)

Over the past decade, there has been a renewed appreciation of the seriousness of wound breakdown after closure of abdominal incisions. Since 2 million celiotomies are performed annually in the United States, the potential problem is considerable. Catgut had been shown to be associated with an unacceptably high rate of dehiscence.[1] This is not surprising, since healing takes three to four months and since these stitches have lost most of their tensile strength by two weeks. Concern over this experience has delayed the acceptance of new synthetic sutures that are more slowly absorbed through hydrolysis unaffected by sepsis. Norris[2] (1939) and Jones et al[3] (1941) found that evisceration and dehiscence could be reduced from 11% to 1% without the need for tension sutures, if mass "near-to-far" suturing was used rather than layered repair. To avoid suture granulomas, incisional pain, and wound sinuses, the use of "man-made" monofilament (nonabsorbable) continuous sutures has become widely accepted because of speed and the fact that tension is more evenly distributed.[4] The peritoneum does not need to be closed as a separate layer.[5]

Unfortunately, although dehiscence has been all but eliminated, incisional herniation has not, occurring in up to 44% of cases.[6] Whereas suture breakage, knot slippage, and protrusion between stitches no longer play important roles, extrusion of sutures due to excessive tension does. To reduce this hazard, replacement of large defects with a prosthesis has been used increasingly since the introduction of woven polyethylene in 1958[7] and knitted autoclavable nonfraying polypropylene mesh (Marlex) in 1962.[8] Despite these advances, incisional herniation continues to be seen, sometimes years after the scar should have stabilized.[9] A new type (subxiphoid) has been described following heart surgery.[10] To study the present dimensions of this problem, a retrospective analysis of an unselected consecutive experience over the past decade was carried out.

Accepted for publication Oct 4, 1988.

From the Departments of Surgery, John L. McClellan Memorial Veterans Hospital and the University of Arkansas for Medical Sciences, Little Rock.

Read in part before the 12th Annual Surgical Symposium of the Association of Veterans Administration Surgeons, Minneapolis, May 13, 1988.

Reprints not available.

METHODS

The records of patients undergoing an incisional hernia repair in the John L. McClellan Memorial Veterans Hospital, Little Rock, Ark, between 1977 and 1987 were gathered and reviewed. Some patients had their original celiotomy or incisional herniorrhaphy at other hospitals. Efforts were made to obtain pertinent information from these referring institutions. For each individual, data were arranged into five categories: personal details (eg, age and weight), the operation preceding herniation (site and type of incision), the incisional hernia, the repair, and follow-up. *Wound infection* was defined as discharge of pus up to one month postoperatively. Assessment of wounds was carried out in the clinic at intervals of 1, 3, and 6 months, or one year. Palpable knots, defects, protrusions, and pain were documented. An attempt was made to contact all living patients. *Incisional herniation* was defined as a palpable defect or defects greater than 1 cm in diameter and in close proximity to the scar, through which bulging was either palpable or visible when patients coughed or raised their legs from the examination couch. Patients who were aware of their hernias were asked when they had first been noticed. These data, along with information obtained at physical examination, defined the *appearance time*.

A consecutive series of 232 patients were operated on for incisional hernia. Twenty died (none within 30 days of their repair), and six were unavailable for follow-up. The remaining 206 comprised the study population. One hundred thirty-two patients continued to live locally and were seen in clinic. Seventy-four had to be contacted by telephone and questionnaire. There was only one woman in the group.

Mass closure with either interrupted or, more recently, continuous, nonabsorbable No. 1 monofilament (Prolene [far-to-near stitches]) was the basic technique used for laparotomies over the ten-year period. A similar repair was performed for incisional herniation (sutured); relaxing incisions in the rectus sheaths were sometimes added. If the surgeon considered the defects too large or too numerous for stitches, a single plastic prosthesis (almost always Marlex) was inserted either as an inlay or, more frequently, as an onlay. An attempt was made to cover the bowels with peritoneum or omentum, and the remaining abdominal wall was treated as a single layer after the peritoneal sac had been removed where indicated. The peritoneum was opened and adhesions were removed if the hernia was incarcerated or loculated or if there had been a history of abdominal colic; occasionally, inadvertent entry into the peritoneal cavity or the bowel occurred. Intraperitoneal placement of a Marlex graft was used if necessary because other workers had found it to be eminently satisfactory.[11] Operations were performed by residents under staff supervision. Suction

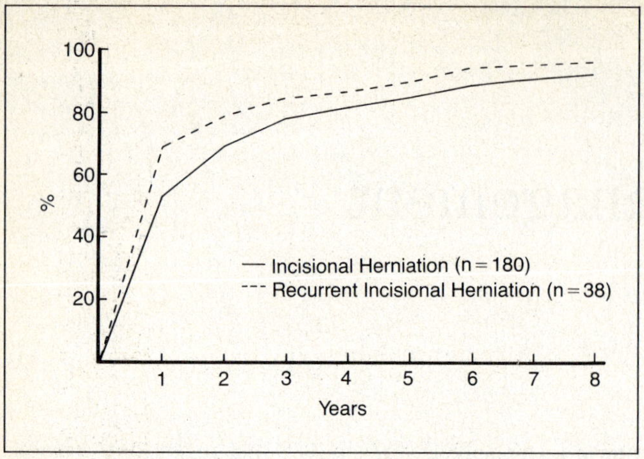

Fig 1.—Appearance time of incisional and recurrent incisional hernias.

drainage was used in a minority (12%), mainly if a large prosthesis had been inserted. Patients received prophylactic intraoperative and short-term postoperative treatment with antibiotics (usually a cephalosporin or a penicillin, unless some other drug was indicated).

RESULTS

Two hundred six patients aged 26 to 90 years (average, 58.3 years) underwent a primary incisional hernia repair; 169 (82%) were sutured, and in 37 (18%) a plastic prosthesis was also used. The appearance time for the incisional hernia subsequent to the initial laparotomy was one to 332 months (median, 28.3 months). At one year 56.1% were present, at two years 71.1% were present, at three years 79.4% were present, and at five years 86% were present (Fig 1). Overall, 41 (19.9%) of 206 patients had wounds that were infected after the initial operation; the incidence varied with the site from zero (left upper quadrant) to 50% (left lower quadrant) (Table). Only eight repairs were grossly infected; in three of these the Marlex had to be removed. Even though the bowel was entered to remove adhesions in 11 cases (5.0%), the overall infection rate was only 3.9%, which is about twice our rate for elective, noncontaminated abdominal surgery and much below the rate at initial laparotomy (19.9%). Most of the patients were overweight (87% to 159% of ideal body weight [average, 117.8%]). Seventy-one (34.4%) of these individuals had had multiple abdominal operations before herniation. The procedure leading to herniation had been an emergency operation in 64 (31.1%); trauma was a precipitating event in 18 (8.7%). Six patients had had a gastric bypass procedure for morbid obesity. Forty-six patients had had cholecystectomy (25 in the right upper quadrant and 21 epigastric). Twenty-one patients had had operations on the aorta. In eight, the original operation was for ventral herniation (umbilical). There were 30 instances of incarceration (14.6%) and five cases of strangulation (2.4%). Eleven of the 206 patients had suffered major dehiscence requiring reoperation, secondary closure, or skin grafting after the original laparotomy. Hernia size averaged 4.1×6.2 cm². The defect tended to be larger in midline herniation and after recurrence. The average size of Marlex graft was 7×10 cm². There were 51 recurrences (24.8%), including three dehiscences. The recurrence rate in the sutured group was 24.3% (41/169), and the recurrence rate with a plastic prosthesis was 27% (10/32).

The most common site of the incisional hernias was midline (153 of 206 [74.3%]). Twenty-six of these 153 followed wound infection as follows (Fig 1): subxiphoid, ten (6.5%); epigastric, 89 (58.2%); periumbilical, 40 (26.1%); and hypogastric, 14 (9.2%). The original operation usually was on the stomach, colon, aorta, gallbladder, pancreas, or spleen (Fig 2). Sixty-four (31.1%) were emergency procedures. Of the epigastric and periumbilical hernias, 24 of 131 were multiple; most of them were buttonhole hernias[12] (58%), ie, multiple, small, eccentric hernias, in the rectus sheaths. All the patients with subxiphoid hernias had had cardiopulmonary bypass and open heart surgery, usually for coronary artery disease.[9,10] They had been repaired with interrupted, nonabsorbable synthetic sutures. The

Incidence of Wound Infection Preceding Incisional Herniation

Site of Incision	n	No. (%) With Wound Infection
Linea alba		
Subxiphoid	10	1 (10.0)
Epigastric	89	18 (20.2)
Periumbilical	40	6 (15.0)
Hypogastric	14	1 (7.1)
Total	**153**	**26** (17.0)
R upper quadrant	25	5 (20.0)
L upper quadrant	1	0
R flank	5	1 (20.0)
L flank	5	2 (40.0)
R lower quadrant	13	5 (38.5)
L lower quadrant	4	2 (50.0)
Total	**206**	**41** (19.9)

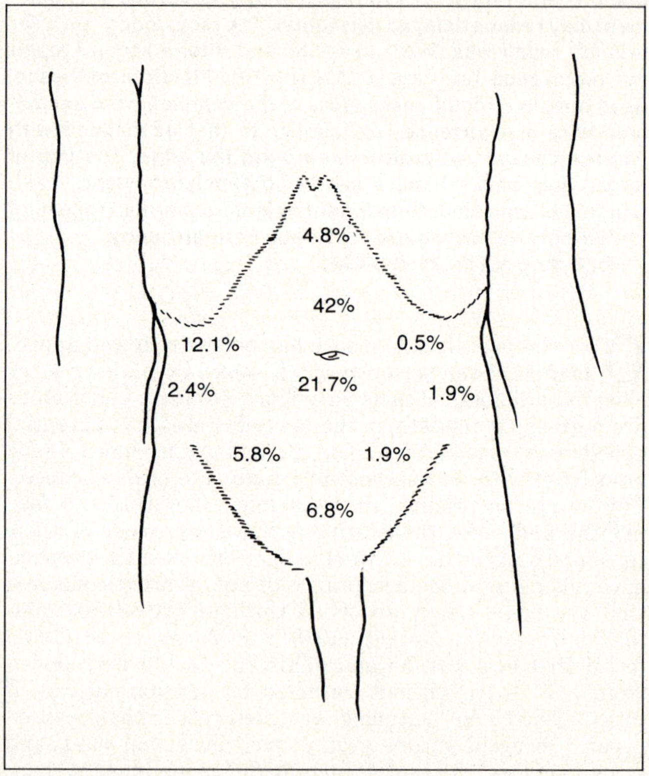

Fig 2.—Distribution of original surgical procedures.

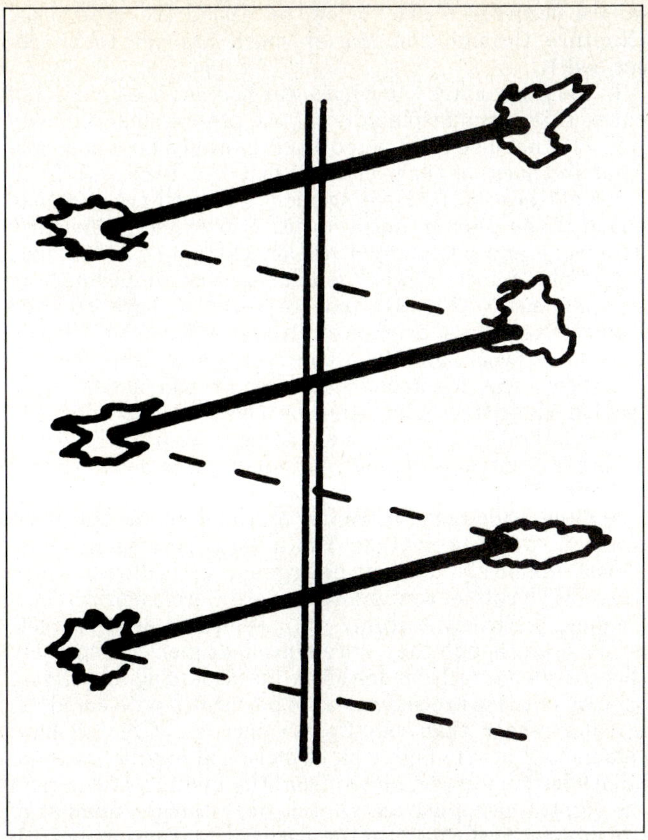

Fig 3.—Gradual sawing through ("buttonholing") of myofascial defects by continuous nonabsorbable monofilament suture.

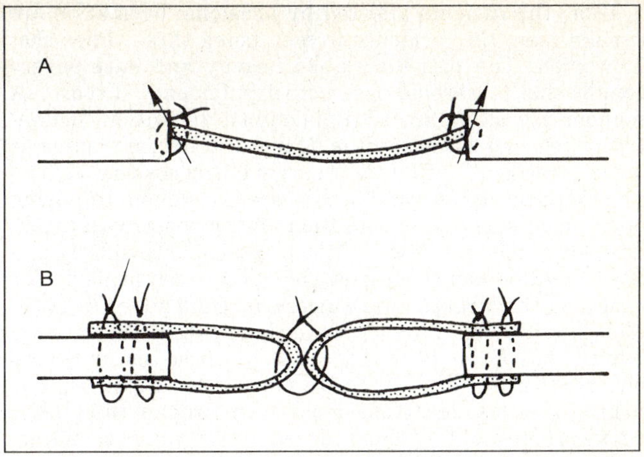

Fig 4.—A, Limited fixation of knitted polypropylene mesh (Marlex) to edge of defect. B, Sandwich repair giving good lateral fixation.

second most common site of herniation was the right upper quadrant, with lesions occurring in 25 (12.1%). Almost all of these hernias followed cholecystectomies, most of which were emergency procedures. Thirteen hernias in the right lower quadrant (6.3%) followed urgent appendectomy. Five hernias in the right flank (2.4%) and five in the left flank (2.4%) followed operations on the kidney or aorta or for trauma. (A few were at drain sites, sometimes coupled with right-upper-quadrant or midline hernias.) Hernias in the left lower quadrant were seen after sigmoid colostomy or retroperitoneal approaches to the iliac vessels. The one lesion in the left upper quadrant followed a splenectomy.

Of the 51 patients whose incisional hernia recurred, 36 were reoperated on: 16 were sutured, and 20 received Marlex grafts (55.6%). Their body weight was 93% to 159% of ideal weight (mean, 125.6%). Fifteen (41.7%) of these 36 reoperations failed: seven with sutures (43.8%) and eight with Marlex (40%). Ten of 15 patients had a second operation for recurrent incisional herniation; three (30%) failed. Two of six were sutured and one of four received Marlex. All three with failed procedures had a third operation for recurrence. They were sutured, and none recurred. Recurrent incisional herniation appeared earlier than primary (Fig 1). At one year 68.4% were present, at two years 78.9% were present, at three years 84.2% were present, and at five years 89.4% were present.

COMMENT

There are only a few long-term studies of large unselected series of patients with this common but neglected problem. Until recently, follow-up was terminated at one year, as the scar was considered to be stable by six months. However, Akman[13] reported in 1962 that only 68% of incisional hernias were noted by one year. Ponka[14] reported 77%. Prospective data from Europe in the past five years have documented[15,16] that only a little more than half of incisional hernial defects can be identified within 12 months. Further, a significant number, albeit mainly small and asymptomatic, continue to appear even after five years. A similar delayed manifestation of such defects was observed in the present study. Recurrent incisional herniation appeared sooner than primary. The lag in manifestation of these protrusions was originally blamed on observer error because of the masking effect of obesity, along with a lack of symptoms. Preplaced radio-opaque clips[17] or computed tomographic scanning[18] have been shown to assist in the diagnosis of small protrusions. However, Ellis et al[16] did not find a relationship between obesity and delayed herniation. They also could not confirm another hypothesis, ie, deep-seated infection.[19] An alternative, more plausible mechanism was suggested by the observation of buttonholes in the rectus sheath caused by a sawing motion of the nonabsorbable sutures[12] (Fig 3). This suggestion is consistent with our results in that many of these late defects were small, multiple, and eccentric to the midline scar. Now that longer-lasting synthetic sutures of proved absorbability are available,[4] it may be that their use will reduce late buttonholing. However, Ellis et al[16] reported delayed herniation after procedures with both kinds of sutures. More information is needed.

Incisional herniation is common in a population of hospitalized veterans because they have almost all the known risk factors for this entity. These risk factors and their incidence in our population of veterans are as follows:

Risk Factor	Incidence, %
Male sex	99.5
Age>60 y	47
Obesity	118-126 ideal body weight
Smoking	96
Alcoholism	20
Multiple laparoscopies	34
Incisions>18 cm	48
Trauma	18
Other emergencies	31
Cancer	19
Wound sepsis	20
Surgeons in training	100
Midline incision	74
Diabetes	10

Thus, the patients affected by incisional herniation are usually men, the incidence in men being three times that in women. The patients smoke heavily and have severe coughs due to chronic obstructive pulmonary disease. A number are alcoholics with abdominal distention, malnutrition, cirrhosis, and ascites. Many suffer from trauma or delay treatment until urgent surgery is necessary. Atherosclerotic cardiac or vascular disease is common, requiring open heart surgery or operation on the aorta with attendant long incisions. Many of these patients are elderly and have had abdominal surgery for cancer (particularly for cancer of the larger bowel), ulcers, or gallbladder disease. Most are overweight, some to such an extent that gastric bypass has been required. Finally, these patients are operated on by surgeons in training whose supervision is many times lax, since incisional hernia repair (like other herniorrhaphies) is often regarded as a trivial procedure.

An important risk factor common to all series of incisional herniation is wound sepsis. The infection rate following celiotomy has been reported as high as 80%.[20] Pollock et al[21] believed that this predisposing cause could be reduced to great effect. Our infection rate of slightly less than 20% is considerably lower than that in many reports. Particularly gratifying is the low infection rate of 3.5% after repair, even though a few wounds were contaminated with bowel contents and a plastic prosthesis was inserted in a minority. Short-course antibiotic coverage may well have contributed. Lewis[22] made a similar comment after finding an infection rate of 4% in difficult cases treated with Marlex, his rate being almost identical to ours.

As in other series, every attempt was made to repair these defects without inserting a large foreign body (ie, a plastic prosthesis). The fairly high recurrence rate after simple suturing (24%) could argue in favor of the use of Marlex. Instead of using Marlex in one fifth of our cases, perhaps a third should have had this material inserted. The use of Marlex was associated with an initial recurrence rate of 27%, which is higher than the rate after simple suturing. However, the rate after suturing likely would have been higher had we continued to use sutures since failure rates of 44% have been reported under these circumstances.[6] As in other reports, we also found that failure occurred above, below, or beside the prosthesis. (Rupture through the Marlex mesh has yet to be described.)

In too many cases the whole scar had not been dissected out to rule out multiple or eccentric protrusions, the body wall had not been dissected back laterally far enough in front and back, or the prosthesis had been too small. Even when all these pitfalls are avoided, a critical problem may ensue if the Marlex mesh is not overlapped sufficiently externally and internally at its attachment to the cleared rim of the defect. Usher[23] emphasized the importance of this maneuver (Fig 4), and we recently have adopted Rubio's[24] technique originating from the same city (Houston). Thirty years ago the problem of lateral fixation of the prosthesis was identified.[7] It remains and needs to be tackled vigorously. Since tension necrosis is avoided and better lateral fixation can be obtained, we prefer inlay (if necessary, intraperitoneal) to onlay placement, as did Usher and more recent investigators.[25]

Midline abdominal incisions continue to be the most common site of herniation. The incision is popular and is almost uniformly used in emergency procedures, which have a high rate of contamination. We were surprised how frequently cholecystectomy was performed on these veterans, even though they were almost all men. Presumably this prevalence reflects one of the diseases of aging. Almost one half of these procedures were performed with a midline incision rather than the Kocher incision. Others[26] have commented on the high risk of incisional herniation when biliary surgery is conducted from the midline rather than the right upper quadrant. Aortic operations, a number of which were performed on the patients in our sample with vascular disease, require long xiphoid to pubis exposure, adding to the risk of herniation. Vascular disease affecting the coronary arteries has brought on a new type of epigastric hernia: the subxiphoid. This hernia occurs despite interrupted sutures of nonabsorbable monofilament and an absence of infection. An eccentric abdominal component of the sternal split has been recommended to avoid this sequela. Our experience differs in that plastic prosthesis was unnecessary for successful repair.[10]

References

1. Goligher LC, Irvin TT, Johnston D, et al: A controlled clinical trial of three methods of closure of laparotomy wounds. *Br J Surg* 1975;62:823-829.
2. Norris JD: A review of wound healing and the mechanics of dehiscence. *Surgery* 1939;5:775-786.
3. Jones TE, Newell ET, Brubaker RE: The use of alloy steel wire in the closure of abdominal wounds. *Surg Gynecol Obstet* 1941;72:1056-1059.
4. Schoetz DJ, Coller JA, Veidenheimer MC: Closure of abdominal wounds with polydioxanone: A prospective study. *Arch Surg* 1988;123:72-74.
5. Ellis H, Heddle R: Does the peritoneum need to be closed at laparotomy. *Br J Surg* 1977;64:733-736.
6. George CD, Ellis H: The results of incisional hernia repair: A 12 year review. *Ann R Coll Surg Engl* 1986;68:185-187.
7. Usher FC, Oschsner J, Tuttle LL Jr: Use of Marlex mesh in the repair of incisional hernias. *Am Surg* 1958;24:969-974.
8. Usher FC, Allen JE Jr, Crosthwait RW, et al: Polypropylene monofilament: A new biologically inert suture for closing contaminated wounds. *JAMA* 1962;179:780-782.
9. Harding KG, Mudge M, Leinster SJ, et al: Late development of incisional hernia: An unrecognised problem. *Br Med J* 1983;286:519-520.
10. Cohen MJ, Starling JR: Repair of subxiphoid incisional hernias with Marlex mesh after median sternotomy. *Arch Surg* 1985;120:1270-1271.
11. Adloff M, Arnaud J-P: Surgical management of large incisional hernias by an intraperitoneal mersilene mesh and an aponeurotic graft. *Surg Gynecol Obstet* 1987;165:204-206.
12. Krukowski ZH, Matheson NA: 'Button hole' incisional hernia: A late complication of abdominal wound closure with continuous non-absorbable sutures. *Br J Surg* 1987;74:824-825.
13. Akman PC: A study of five hundred incisional hernias. *J Int Coll Surg* 1962;37:125-142.
14. Ponka JL: Hernias of the abdominal wall, in Ponka JL (ed): *Incisional Hernias.* Philadelphia, WB Saunders Co, 1980, pp 369-396.
15. Mudge M, Hughes LE: Incisional hernia: A 10 year prospective study of incidence and attitudes. *Br J Surg* 1985;72:70-71.
16. Ellis H, Gajraj H, George CD: Incisional hernias: When do they occur. *Br J Surg* 1983;70:290-291.
17. Playforth MJ, Sauven PD, Evans M, et al: The prediction of incisional hernias by radio-opaque markers. *Ann R Coll Surg Engl* 1986;68:82-84.
18. Ghahremani GG, Jimenez MA, Rosenfeld M, et al: CT diagnosis of occult incisional hernias. *AJR* 1987;148:139-142.
19. Bucknall TE, Ellis H: Abdominal wound closure: A comparison of monofilament nylon and polyglycolic acid. *Surgery* 1981;89:672-677.
20. Fischer JD, Turner FW: Abdominal incisional hernias: A ten-year review. *Can J Surg* 1974;17:202-204.
21. Pollock AV, Greenall MJ, Evans M: Single-layer mass closure of major laparotomies by continuous suturing. *J R Soc Med* 1979;72:889-893.
22. Lewis RT: Knitted polypropylene (Marlex) mesh in the repair of incisional hernias. *Can J Surg* 1984;27:155-157.
23. Usher FC: New technique for repairing incisional hernias with Marlex mesh. *Am J Surg* 1979;138:740-741.
24. Rubio PA: New technique for repairing large ventral incisional hernias with marlex mesh. *Surg Gynecol Obstet* 1986;162:275-276.
25. Larson GM, Vandertoll DJ: Approaches to repair of ventral hernia and full-thickness losses of the abdominal wall. *Surg Clin North Am* 1984;64:335-349.
26. Blomstedt B, Welin-Berger T: Incisional hernias. *Acta Chir Scand* 1972;138:275-278.

Biochemical Adaptation of Venous Patches Placed in the Carotid Circulation

Dean M. Govostis, MD; Dennis F. Bandyk, MD; Thomas M. Bergamini, MD; Jonathan B. Towne, MD

• The influence of venous patching on luminal prostacyclin (PGI_2) and thromboxane A_2 (TBX) production of endarterectomized arteries was studied in a canine model. Fifteen dogs underwent bilateral common carotid endarterectomies. In each dog, one artery was closed primarily and the contralateral artery was closed by vein-patch angioplasty. At six and 12 weeks after operation, luminal prostanoid production from the venous patch, adjacent endarterectomized artery, and control artery and vein was measured by radioimmunoassay for 6-keto-prostaglandin $F_{1\alpha}$ and thromboxane B_2. Venous patches underwent "incomplete" biochemical adaptation with decreased luminal production of PGI_2 compared with control and endarterectomized arteries. Thromboxane production from venous patches was increased compared with normal vein but similar to control and endarterectomized arteries. At six weeks, PGI_2 production of vein-patched arterial segments was increased compared with arteries closed primarily. These data indicate that vein-patch angioplasty favorably influences surface thrombogenicity of healing, endarterectomized arteries and support its use in reparative carotid surgery.

(*Arch Surg* 1989;124:490-493)

The routine use of vein-patch angioplasty during carotid endarterectomy has been recommended by a number of authors to reduce the incidence of restenosis and minimize thrombogenicity of the endarterectomized segment.[1-3] Preference for this method of vessel closure following endarterectomy is based on concepts that, compared with primary closure, suture stricture is less likely to occur with vein-patch closure, vessel enlargement minimizes restenosis produced by the predictable circumferential myointimal hyperplasia that develops after operation, and the vein-patch endothelium may favorably influence healing of the endarterectomized artery. Whether these characteristics of vein-patch angioplasty are applicable in improving the functional patency of carotid endarterectomy in humans is unknown, since the mechanisms are based on limited experimental evidence in animals.

Placement of autologous vein grafts in the arterial circulation results in predictable changes in morphology and luminal prostanoid production termed "arterialization."[4-6] In a canine model of carotid artery healing following endarterectomy, we found venous patching did not influence patency or the rate and pattern of endothelial regeneration.[7] In both vein-patched and primarily closed arteries, endothelial regeneration was incomplete at two to three weeks after operation and complete by four to five weeks. An interesting observation of the study was that less severe intimal thickening was observed to develop in the vein patches compared with the healing endarterectomized artery wall. These findings suggested that the fate of venous patches in the arterial circulation may differ from that of vein grafts. A varied adaptation to "arterialization" can result from differences in surgical trauma and hemodynamics of vein-patch arterial segments compared by venoarterial grafting.[8-10]

Although the precise mechanisms by which vascular endothelium resists thrombus formation remain largely unknown, the production and luminal release of prostacyclin (PGI_2) by endothelial cells result in potent inhibition of platelet aggregation, an important initial step in arterial thrombus formation. Arterialized vein grafts demonstrate functional (biochemical) adaptation, which includes an increase in luminal PGI_2 production in addition to the well-known morphologic changes of thickening, fibrosis, and subendothelial myointimal cell proliferation.[6,11] The purpose of this study was to examine the biochemical adaptation of venous patches placed in the carotid circulation. Using our previously described canine model of carotid endarterectomy,[7] we serially measured luminal production of PGI_2 and thromboxane A_2 (TBX) from vein patches, adjacent healing endarterectomized artery wall, and normal carotid artery and external jugular vein after operation. In addition, the influence of venous patching on the biochemical recovery of endarterectomized carotid arteries was studied by comparing luminal prostanoid production in vein-patched artery segments with arteries closed by continuous suture.

Accepted for publication Nov 7, 1988.

From the Surgical Service, Veterans Administration Medical Center (Drs Bandyk, Bergamini, and Towne), and the Department of Surgery, Medical College of Wisconsin (Drs Govostis, Bandyk, and Towne), Milwaukee.

Read before the 12th Annual Surgical Symposium of the Association of Veterans Administration Surgeons, Minneapolis, May 13, 1988.

Reprint requests to Department of Surgery, MCMC, 8700 W Wisconsin Ave, Milwaukee, WI 53226 (Dr Bandyk).

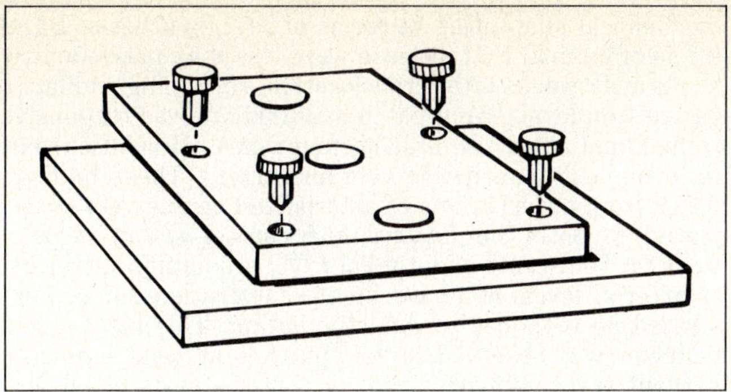

Fig 1.—Template incubation chamber designed for measurement of vein patch and vessel luminal surface production of prostacyclin and thromboxane A_2; 4×10-mm elliptical hole exposes 36 mm^2 of luminal surface for assay.

MATERIALS AND METHODS

Canine Model

Fifteen adult mongrel dogs of either sex (weighing 24 to 30 kg) underwent bilateral common carotid endarterectomies. The dogs were anesthetized with 30 to 40 mg/kg of intravenous pentobarbital sodium, intubated, and placed on mechanical ventilation. On induction of anesthesia, cefazolin sodium (25 mg/kg) was given intravenously. Using sterile technique and ×2.5 optical magnification, the left external jugular vein and bilateral common carotid arteries were carefully dissected over a distance of 8 cm. The external jugular vein was excised using "no touch" technique and placed in a cold, heparinized lactated Ringer's solution (100 U/mL). Following systemic heparinization (100 U/kg), the common carotid arteries were occluded with vascular clamps and an endarterectomy was performed on each, over a 3-cm segment of the artery through a 4-cm arteriotomy. A cleavage plane was developed in the media using a scalpel, allowing excision of the entire intimal layer and inner attached media. The arteriotomy of the left carotid artery was closed with a continuous monofilament of 7-0 polypropylene suture. The right carotid artery was closed with a 4-mm–wide external jugular vein patch using continuous 7-0 suture. Intraoperative pulsed Doppler spectrum analysis was used to assess the operative site for technical errors based on changes in the center-stream blood flow patterns.[12,13]

At two time intervals following endarterectomy (six and 12 weeks), the common carotid arteries were excised and patency was determined. These periods after operation were selected based on reports demonstrating that canine vein graft arterialization, in terms of increased PGI_2 production, occurs ten weeks following placement in the arterial circulation.[6,11] Luminal surface production of PGI_2 and TBX was measured only in patent arteries. Nine dogs were reoperated on after six weeks and the remaining six dogs after 12 weeks. No heparin was administered before vessel excision. Assays for control native vein prostanoid production were performed at both time intervals after operation by excision of the previously unoperated-on right external jugular vein. Control native artery levels were determined from proximal segments of previously undissected common carotid artery. Luminal prostanoid production was also measured from two sites (midpoint and end point) of the vein-patch itself, and healing endarterectomized carotid arteries were closed by continuous suture or vein-patch angioplasty. All dogs received humane care in compliance with the *Guide for the Care and Use of Laboratory Animals*.[14]

Radioimmunoassay Preparation and Methods

Excised external jugular vein and common carotid artery segments for radioimmunoassay of 6-keto-prostaglandin $F_{1\alpha}$ (6-keto-$PGF_{1\alpha}$) and thromboxane B_2, the stable metabolites for PGI_2 and TBX, were immediately rinsed with Hepes buffered saline (25 mmol/L, pH 7.5) to remove adherent blood elements and opened longitudinally. Vein-patched arterial segments were transected at the midpoint of the patched segment before opening the vessel along its longitudinal axis to permit exposure of both the venous patch and the endarterectomized artery lumen for prostanoid production measurements. Specimens were placed in a custom-designed template incubation chamber apparatus (Fig 1). Each 4×10-mm elliptical hole in the upper plate formed an incubation chamber that exposed 0.36 cm^2 of lumen surface for assay of 6-keto-$PGF_{1\alpha}$ and thromboxane B_2 production according to the method of Weksler et al.[15] A 0.25-mL aliquot of TRIS–sodium chloride buffer (15 mmol/L, pH 8.6) was pipetted into the incubation well for two minutes, quickly transferred to a polypropylene centrifugation tube, and then frozen at −20°C. A second incubation was then performed using TRIS buffer containing 20 μmol/L of arachidonic acid (AA) for stimulated PGI_2 measurements.

Luminal surface synthesis of PGI_2 was measured for both basal and AA-stimulated conditions by radioimmunoassay of tritiated

Prostacyclin and Thromboxane Production for External Jugular Vein, Carotid Artery, and Venous Patches*

Condition	Control: Vein (n=9/6)	Control: Artery (n=7/4)	Vein Patch (n=18/12)	Endarterectomized Artery: Patch Closure (n=9/6)	Endarterectomized Artery: Primary Closure (n=14/8)
6-Keto-$PGF_{1\alpha}$ Production					
Basal	11±2	39±5	. . .	. . .	. . .
6 wk	. . .	. . .	16±2†	37±10	17±4‡
12 wk	. . .	. . .	15±3†	25±7	23±8
Stimulated	60±5	88±9	. . .	. . .	. . .
6 wk	. . .	. . .	24±5§	78±15	43±6‖
12 wk	. . .	. . .	37±7§	87±13	102±13
Thromboxane B_2 Production					
Basal	2±0.5	5±1	. . .	. . .	. . .
6 wk	. . .	. . .	8±1¶	9±3	4±1
12 wk	. . .	. . .	8±2¶	8±3	4±1

*6-Keto-$PGF_{1\alpha}$ indicates 6-keto-prostaglandin $F_{1\alpha}$. Values are nanograms per two minutes per 0.36 cm^2, mean±SEM. *P* values are derived from Mann-Whitney *U* test. Group numbers are six week/12 week.

†$P<.005$ compared with control artery.

‡$P<.01$ compared with vein-patch closure and control artery.

§$P<.02$ compared with control vein.

‖$P<.002$ compared with normal artery, 12-week primary closure.

¶$P<.005$ compared with control vein.

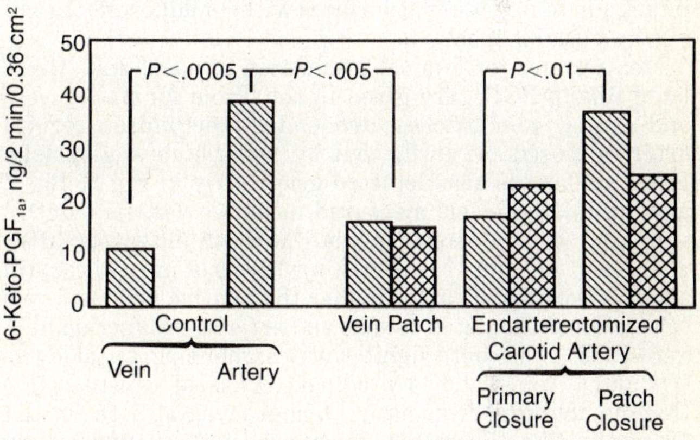

Fig 2.—Histogram of mean basal 6-keto-prostaglandin $F_{1\alpha}$ (6-keto-$PGF_{1\alpha}$) production at six weeks (diagonally striped bars) and 12 weeks (cross-hatched bars) after endarterectomy from control vein and artery (six- and 12-week measurements combined), vein patch, and endarterectomized arteries closed primarily or by vein-patch angioplasty. Values for *P* derived from Mann-Whitney *U* test for continuous data.

6-keto-$PGF_{1\alpha}$. Thromboxane B_2, the stable metabolite of TBX, was similarly determined by radioimmunoassay of tritiated thromboxane B_2. Standard curves were constructed for each assay using known amounts of labeled 6-keto-$PGF_{1\alpha}$ and thromboxane B_2, respectively. Prostanoid release values are expressed as nanograms per two minutes per 0.36 cm^2 of lumen surface.

Data Analysis

All data are expressed as mean±1 SEM. Differences in prostanoid levels between the various vessel segments were analyzed by the Mann-Whitney *U* test to avoid assumptions regarding the distribution of the data. A *P* value below .05 was considered significant.

RESULTS

Eleven (73%) of 15 common carotid arteries closed primarily were patent at the time of excision compared with all 15 arteries closed with vein-patch angioplasty ($P<.05$; χ^2 with $df=4.6$). Occluded carotid arteries were found in two of the study dogs undergoing reoperation at both the six- and 12-week follow-up intervals. Doppler flow analysis of center-stream blood flow patterns did not demonstrate severe flow disturbance proximal to, in the midpoint of, or distal to endarterectomized segments. Decreased blood flow velocity compared with primarily closed arteries and regions of flow separation (spectral broadening during late systole with flow reversal in early diastole) were identified in vein-patched arterial segments both at the primary operation and before excision. All patent carotid arteries after opening longitudinally had intact, glistening luminal surfaces without adherent thrombus by visual inspection.

Mean values for luminal production of basal and stimulated 6-keto-$PGF_{1\alpha}$ are given in the Table for native vein and artery, vein patches, and endarterectomized carotid arteries closed primarily and by vein-patch angioplasty. Basal values are also depicted graphically in Fig 2. Basal and stimulated levels measured in native vessels (control vein and artery) were similar at both intervals after operation. Assay of basal PGI_2 synthesis of normal carotid arteries was significantly higher than native venous levels ($P<.0005$). Stimulated venous and arterial production of 6-keto-$PGF_{1\alpha}$ were both significantly higher than basal levels ($P<.001$). Vein patches produced levels of 6-keto-$PGF_{1\alpha}$ that did not differ from native venous levels at both six and 12 weeks after operation. Compared with native artery levels, vein patches produced significantly less PGI_2 ($P<.005$). Endarterectomized arteries closed by vein-patch angioplasty produced basal levels of 6-keto-$PGF_{1\alpha}$ similar to native artery levels at both intervals after operation. In contrast, endarterectomized carotid arteries closed primarily had significantly less PGI_2 than control and vein-patched arteries at six weeks under both basal and stimulated conditions ($P<.01$). By 12 weeks, PGI_2 levels produced by primarily closed arteries were increased compared with levels measured in native and vein-patched arteries.

The mean basal levels of thromboxane B_2 synthesis measured from identical vessel segments used in the PGI_2 measurements are given in the Table. Normal and healing endarterectomized carotid arteries produced more thromboxane B_2 than normal veins ($P<.05$). At both six and 12 weeks after operation, vein patches placed in the carotid circulation produced increased thromboxane B_2 levels compared with native veins ($P<.005$).

COMMENT

Venous patches when placed in the carotid circulation as a vein-patch angioplasty appear to undergo "incomplete" biochemical adaptation in terms of PGI_2 synthesis. Basal levels of luminal PGI_2 release were less than native artery levels at 12 weeks after translocation, remaining similar to native vein levels. Vein-patch endothelium was responsive to maximal substrate enhancement (AA stimulation) but to levels less than native vein and artery. These findings differ from observations of arterialized canine vein grafts placed in both the femoral and carotid artery circulations.[6,11] Vein graft endothelial PGI_2 production increased to arterial levels at 12 weeks after operation but demonstrated no response to AA stimulation. This biochemical behavior was observed in vein-patched arterial segments without severe abnormalities in center-stream blood flow pattern. We had previously observed that if vein-patch endothelium was preserved and medial necrosis was minimized following transposition into arterial circulation, early (four- to five-week) intimal thickening of the venous transplant was avoided. The less severe morphologic changes observed in venous patches compared with venoarterial grafts in canine models suggest severity of vein harvest trauma may play a more important role than exposure to arterial pressure and hemodynamics in the biochemical adaptation involving prostanoid metabolism.

Our finding of decreased PGI_2 production from arterialized venous patches agrees with the observations of Bush et al[8,16] for in situ vein grafts and Eldor et al[9] for jugular veins placed in the carotid circulation after six weeks. The in situ grafting technique, which is associated with minimal vein wall surgical trauma, resulted in chronically arterialized vein grafts that produced PGI_2 levels lower than native artery produced, higher TBX levels compared with native veins, and less severe morphologic abnormalities of the flow surface than in excised, reversed venoarterial grafts. It is unknown whether the increased prostanoid production (PGI_2 and TBX) of arteries compared with veins, observed in this study and by other investigators,[6,9,11] represents intrinsic differences in biochemical capability of the endothelial cells or adaptation to the difference in hemodynamic environments (pressure, wall tension, shear stress, oxygen tension) to which the endothelial cells are exposed. Further study of healed endarterectomized segments closed by vein-patch angioplasty using techniques that localize and quantitate endothelial cell proliferation (tritiated thymidine labeling with autoradiography) is necessary to correlate biochemical adaptation of venous transplants with acute and chronic endothelial cell injury. It is unknown whether the increased PGI_2 production of arterialized vein grafts reflects or retards the development of myointimal hyperplasia universally observed in these substitute arterial conduits.

The presence of an intact and functionally normal endothelium is important in resisting platelet–vessel wall interaction and thrombus formation. This study and patency data pooled from our prior report document increased patency with vein-patch closure (96%) in this canine model of carotid endarterectomy compared with primary closure (71%) of the endarterectomized arterial segment ($P<.01$; χ^2 with $df=6.5$). It should be noted that endarterectomy site patency in this model was very sensitive to technical factors, including avoidance of deep media cleavage plane with exposure of adventitial elements, meticulous closure of the arteriotomy to minimize suture stenosis, and intravenous administration of heparin.[17]

In this canine model, endothelialization of the endarterectomized segment occurred by migration from the endarterectomy end points and suture line, with the rate and pattern similar in patched and unpatched vessels.[7] Endothelial regeneration was completed by five weeks, although scattered areas void of endothelial cells were commonly found by scanning electron microscopy in arteries closed by either method. The present study confirmed that return of normal luminal PGI_2 synthesis lags behind reendothelialization of the endarterectomized segment. Despite endothelial coverage by four to five weeks after operation, basal and stimulated levels of PGI_2 similar to native arteries were not produced until 12 weeks after operation. At six weeks, PGI_2 production of arteries closed primarily was less compared with arteries closed by vein-patch angioplasty ($P<.01$). This delay in return of normal biochemical function was probably related to variation in the extent or stability of endothelium regeneration in primarily closed arteries. Blood flow patterns recorded both in primarily closed and vein-patched arteries at six and 12 weeks after operation did not vary appreciably from those observed at the primary operation. Blood flow velocity was increased in primarily closed arteries compared with vein-patched arteries and not associated with regions of boundary layer separation and flow reversal uniformly observed in dilated portions of the vein-patch angioplasty. These differences in blood flow between patched and unpatched vessels may influence the biochemical recovery of regenerated endothelium.

The patency and luminal prostanoid synthesis data of this study suggest that vein-patching angioplasty favorably influences surface thrombogenicity of healing endarterectomized arterial segment. Venous patches provide an endothelial cell–lined flow surface that resists thrombus formation and has a luminal PGI_2 synthesis capability similar to native veins. In addition, vein-patch angioplasty, by altering anatomy, hemodynamics, and the biochemical arterial environment, promotes earlier return of normal PGI_2 synthesis by the endarterectomized artery wall. These benefits of venous patching are probably most important in the immediate postoperative period, when thrombogenicity of the endarterectomized wall is highest. The biochemical benefit of vein-patch angioplasty may be blunted by the increased TBX released observed from vein-patch luminal surfaces. Thromboxane A_2 is one of the most potent stimulators of platelet aggregation and release action and is also a strong vasoconstrictor. Platelet activation initiates the coagulation cascade as well as the release of smooth-muscle cell mitogens that facilitates cellular proliferation.[18,19] Since all blood elements, especially platelets, produce TBX, the increased synthesis observed from the luminal surface of arterialized venous patches may have been related to platelet aggregation on the endothelium rather than release by perturbed endothelial or modified endothelial structures such as smooth-muscle cells or fibroblasts. The increased TBX levels of venous patches combined with platelet aggregation on traumatized endothelium support the use of antiplatelet therapy in the perioperative period to inhibit platelet aggregation and release mechanisms.

The decision to use venous patches in carotid surgery is commonly based on the intraoperative appearance of a small-diameter internal carotid artery or operative attempts to prevent stenosis in vessel repair. Prior investigation has documented that vein-patch angioplasty will increase vessel diameter and prevent the development of early circumferential intimal thickening.[7] Whether these benefits also occur when venous patches are used in peripheral graft revision or anastomotic stenosis due to intimal hyperplasia has not been examined. This study suggests that despite incomplete biochemical adaptation of venous patches placed in the carotid circulation, in terms of PGI_2 production, vein-patch angioplasty does favorably influence the arterial environment with regard to patency and normalization of PGI_2 synthesis by regenerated endothelium. These attributes support an increased role for venous patching in carotid endarterectomy to improve the functional patency of this arterial reconstruction.

References

1. Deru GP, Ballotta E, Bonvina L, et al: The rationale for patch-graft angioplasty after carotid endarterectomy: Early and long-term follow-up. *Stroke* 1984;15:972-979.
2. Archie JP: Prevention of early restenosis and thrombosis occlusion after carotid endarterectomy by saphenous vein patch angioplasty. *Stroke* 1986;17:901-905.
3. Eikelboom BC, Ackerstaff RG, Hoeneveld H, et al: Benefits of carotid patching: A randomized study. *J Vasc Surg* 1988;7:240-247.
4. Carrel A, Guthrie CC: Results of the biterminal transplantation of veins. *Am J Med Sci* 1906;10:415-422.
5. Fonkalsrud EW, Sanchez M, Zerubavel R: Morphological evaluation of canine autologous grafts in the arterial circulation. *Surgery* 1978;84:253-264.
6. Henderson VJ, Cohen RG, Mitchell RS, et al: Biochemical (functional) adaptation of 'arterialized' vein grafts. *Ann Surg* 1986;203:339-345.
7. Stewart GW, Bandyk DF, Kaebnick HW, et al: Influence of vein patch angioplasty on carotid endarterectomy healing. *Arch Surg* 1987;122:364-371.
8. Bush HL, Hong SI, Deykin D, et al: The effect of surgical trauma on prostacyclin production by vein grafts. *Surg Forum* 1982;33:463-465.
9. Eldor A, Hoover EL, Pett SB, et al: Prostacyclin production by arterial autogenous vein grafts in dogs. *Prostaglandins* 1981;22:485-498.
10. Bush HL Jr, Jakubowski JA, Curl GR, et al: The natural history of endothelial structure and function in arterialized vein grafts. *J Vasc Surg* 1984;3:204-215.
11. Cahill PD, Brown BA, Handen CE, et al: Incomplete biochemical adaptation of vein grafts to the arterial environment in terms of prostacyclin production. *J Vasc Surg* 1987;6:496-503.
12. Bandyk DF, Zierler RE, Thiele BL: Detection of technical error during arterial surgery by pulsed Doppler spectral analysis. *Arch Surg* 1984;119:421-428.
13. Bandyk DF, Kaebnick HW, Adams MB, et al: Turbulence occurring after carotid bifurcation endarterectomy: A harbinger of residual and recurrent carotid stenosis. *J Vasc Surg* 1988;7:261-274.
14. *Guide for the Care and Use of Laboratory Animals*, US Dept of Health and Human Services publication 80-23. National Institutes of Health, 1978.
15. Weksler BB, Marcus AJ, Jaffe EA: Synthesis of prostaglandins I_2 (prostacyclin) by cultured human and bovine endothelial cells. *Proc Natl Acad Sci USA* 1977;74;3922-3926.
16. Bush HL Jr, Graber JN, Jakubowski JA, et al: Favorable balance of prostacyclin and thromboxane A_2 improves early patency of human in situ vein grafts. *J Vasc Surg* 1984;1:149-159.
17. Dirrenberger RA, Sundt TM: Carotid endarterectomy: Temporal profile of the healing process and effects of anticoagulation therapy. *J Neurosurg* 1978;48:201-219.
18. Ross R, Vogel A: The platelet-derived growth factor. *Cell* 1978;14:203-210.
19. Clowes AW, Adams MC: Smooth muscle cell proliferation and arterial graft failure, in Bergan JJ, Yao JST (eds): *Reoperative Arterial Surgery.* New York, Grune & Stratton, 1986, pp 3-13.

Limitations to Donating Adequate Autologous Blood Prior to Elective Orthopedic Surgery

Lawrence T. Goodnough, MD; J. Wasman; Kathleen Corlucci; Ann Chernosky

• We reviewed 175 patients who predeposited autologous blood prior to elective orthopedic surgery to define potential limitations of procuring adequate autologous blood. These potential limitations include physician underordering, storage interval, and erythropoietic response. We found that a continuing medical education intervention increased the amount of autologous blood requested by physicians for storage: from 121 U for 50 patients (mean = 2.4) before CME to 195 U for 65 patients (mean = 3.0) afterward; eight (16%) of 50 patients had 4 U or more requested before CME vs 25 (38%) of 65 patients afterward. Continuing medical education had no impact on mean (± SD) effective storage interval, 22.6 ± 9.0 vs 21.6 ± 9.4 days. Thirty (17%) of 175 patients were deferred (hematocrit ≤0.34) and were unable to donate units of blood requested; of these, 13 (43%) received homologous blood compared with 19 (13%) of 145 not deferred. We conclude that a significant percentage of patients are deferred from autologous donation because of hematocrit limitations and receive homologous blood. This problem is not related to physician underordering or inappropriate physician transfusion behavior, but rather to the erythropoietic response to serial phlebotomy over a limited storage interval. Future studies should focus on mechanisms to maximize autologous blood procurement.

(*Arch Surg* 1989;124:494-496)

Preoperative autologous blood donation (ABD) before elective surgery is a desirable clinical practice encouraged by a number of organizations such as the American Medical Association,[1] the American Association of Blood Banks,[2] the National Institutes of Health Consensus Conference on Acquired Immunodeficiency Syndrome,[3] and the American Red Cross.[4] Potential benefits of transfusion with autologous blood have been cited that include the following: it is the "safest" form of blood transfusion[5]; it represents a potential source of blood for both the national blood inventory and hospital-scheduled elective surgical procedures[6,7]; and it has a salutary effect on physician transfusion behavior.[8] We have previously shown that an ABD program can be an effective method of improving physician transfusion behavior. This salutary effect, however, was accompanied by insufficient procurement of autologous blood to minimize subsequent homologous blood transfusion.[8] In this study, we evaluated our ABD program to define the potential limitations of procuring adequate autologous blood and to assess the impact of a continuing medical education (CME) program on these limitations.

Accepted for publication Aug 29, 1988.

From the Department of Medicine, Case Western Reserve University and University Hospitals of Cleveland.

Reprint requests to Department of Medicine, University Hospitals of Cleveland, 2074 Abington Rd, Cleveland, OH 44106 (Dr Goodnough).

METHODS

Autologous Preoperative Blood Deposit Program

The University Hospitals of Cleveland Component Therapy Unit currently procures approximately 1000 U of blood from 400 elective surgical patients yearly. Approximately 70% of these patients undergo elective orthopedic procedures.[8] Guidelines established by the American Association of Blood Banks (AABB) for autologous blood storage[9] are followed. The number of units to be procured is determined by each patient's surgeon. Ferrous sulfate, 325 mg to be taken three times daily by mouth, is prescribed for every patient. Units are stored as whole blood in citrate-phosphate-dextrose-adenine with a 35-day outdate.

Audit

One hundred seventy-five consecutive patients who predeposited autologous blood and who were scheduled for elective orthopedic procedures from July 1, 1985, to Aug 15, 1987, were studied. Fifty consecutive patients in the ABD program scheduled for elective orthopedic procedures before (series 1, July 1, 1985, to June 30, 1986), 65 consecutive such patients after (series 2, Feb 26, 1987, to May 31, 1987) a CME intervention (below), and 60 such patients seen subsequently (series 3, June 1, 1987, to Aug 15, 1987) were audited by reviewing blood bank, component therapy, and medical records. The following data were recorded: units of autologous blood requested for storage; blood units stored; storage interval; recorded hematocrits (HCT); deferrals for inadequate HCT (≤0.34)[9] or other reasons; and transfusions subsequently received (units of autologous and homologous blood). The distribution of orthopedic procedures in the 175 patients is shown in Table 1. The three series of patients in this study were not different when analyzed for patient age, sex, and surgical procedure.

CME Intervention

One of us (L.T.G.) gave a 50-minute lecture presentation, "To Transfuse or Not to Transfuse," the content of which included risks of homologous blood exposure,[10-12] benefits of preoperative autologous blood storage,[13] issues of informed consent and quality assurance relevant to red blood cell transfusion,[14,15] acceptance of intraoperative and postoperative normovolemic anemia,[16] effect of our ABD program on physician transfusion behavior,[8] potential

Table 1.—Distribution of Elective Orthopedic Procedures in Patients With Predeposited Autologous Blood

	Series, No. (%)			
	1 (N=50)	2 (N=65)	3 (N=60)	Total (N=175)
Laminectomy	6 (14)	11 (17)	15 (25)	**32** (18)
Total hip	16 (32)	19 (29)	18 (30)	**53** (30)
Total knee	8 (16)	12 (19)	10 (25)	**30** (17)
Spine fusion	12 (24)	13 (20)	12 (20)	**37** (21)
Miscellaneous	8 (18)	10 (16)	5 (21)	**23** (13)

limitations that result in inadequate storage of autologous blood with special emphasis on the desirability of storing as much blood as possible during our 35-day storage interval[9]; and the logistics of arranging autologous storage for patients at our institution. The CME program consisted of seven presentations: Surgery Grand Rounds (Sept 13, 1986), Medicine Grand Rounds (Sept 29, 1986), Anesthesia Grand Rounds (Oct 29, 1986), Gynecology Grand Rounds (Feb 13, 1986), Orthopedic Grand Rounds (Feb 14, 1987), Plastic Surgery Grand Rounds (Feb 14, 1987), and Head and Neck Surgery Grand Rounds (Feb 28, 1987).

Statistics

Differences in means were evaluated by the Student t test for data of parabolic distribution. The Mann-Whitney U test was used to compare data of nonparabolic distribution.

RESULTS OF THE CME INTERVENTION

Storage Intervals

Evaluation of 50 consecutive orthopedic patients in the ABD program before (series 1) and 65 consecutive patients after (series 2) the CME intervention revealed no impact on mean (±SD) storage intervals (time from first unit drawn to surgical date): 22.6±9.0 days vs 21.6±9.4 days. The time from last unit donated to surgical date also was not different: 8.7±5.5 days vs 7.5±4.0 days. Storage intervals were not related to whether patients had an HCT[10] deferral from phlebotomy in either series 1 patients (24.6±8.2 days [deferred] vs 22.1±9.3 days [nondeferred] or series 2 patients (24.9±12.8 days vs 20.8±8.4 days).

Autologous Blood Units Requested

The number of autologous units requested by surgeons for storage significantly increased after the CME intervention. One hundred twenty-six units were requested for 50 patients (series 1, mean=2.4) before CME intervention compared with 195 U for 65 patients after CME intervention (series 2, mean=3.0); eight (16%) of 50 patients were requested to store 4 U or more prior to CME compared with 25 (38%) of 65 after CME (P<.05).

Homologous Blood Transfused

As shown in Table 2, units of homologous blood transfused to patients able to predonate the requested number of autologous units declined significantly: from 12 (28%) of 42 in series 1, to six (11%) of 52 in series 2, to one (2%) of 51 in series 3 (P<.05). There was no such decline in homologous blood exposure in patients unable to donate the amount of autologous blood requested: five of eight patients in series 1, four of 13 patients in series 2, and four of nine patients in series 3. Thus, CME intervention toward physician transfusion practice significantly affected subsequent homologous blood exposure in patients who were able to predonate the amount of autologous blood requested by their physicians, but not in patients unsuccessful in

Table 2.—Homologous Blood Exposure in Patients Undergoing Elective Orthopedic Surgery

	7/85-6/86 Series 1 (N=50)	2/87-5/87 Series 2 (N=65)	6/87-9/87 Series 3 (N=60)	Total (N=175)
Patients able to donate requested units	42	52	51	**145**
Subsequent homologous exposure	12	6	1	**19** (13%)*
Patients unable to donate requested units	8	13	9	**30**
Subsequent homologous exposure	5	4	4	**13** (43%)*

*P<.05.

Table 3.—Subsequent Homologous Exposure Is Not Related to Physician Underordering

	No. of Patients	Subsequent Homologous Exposure, No. (%)
Patients able to donate requested units	**145**	19 (13)*
≤3 U requested	110	16 (14)
≥4 U requested	35	3 (8.6)
Patients unable to donate requested units	**30**	13 (43)*
≤3 U requested	7	4 (57)
≥4 U requested	23	9 (39)

*P<.05.

predonating adequate autologous blood. The consequences of understoring autologous blood in patients undergoing elective orthopedic surgery are also shown in Table 2. Of 30 patients who were deferred and unable to store the requested units of autologous blood, 13 patients (43%) subsequently received homologous blood; this is compared with 145 patients who successfully predonated the requested amount of autologous blood, of whom 19 (13%) received homologous blood (P<.05). Chart audit of patients receiving homologous blood indicated that transfusion in almost all circumstances (16 of 17 patients) was appropriate.

Autologous Patients Deferred From Phlebotomy

Six of 175 patients were deferred from phlebotomy for reasons other than HCT limitation; none of these patients subsequently received homologous blood transfusion. Thirty (17%) of 175 patients in the combined series were unable to store the units requested because of low HCT (≤0.34) by AABB standards.[9] The initial HCT at first phlebotomy was significantly lower in these patients than in those not deferred: 0.38±0.03 vs 0.43±0.03 (P<.001). Twenty of the 30 deferred patients were female. Deferral was related to the number of autologous units requested (Table 3): seven (6%) of 117 patients in whom 3 U or less were requested were deferred compared with 23 (39%) of 58 patients in whom 4 U or more were requested (P<.05). Of 30 patients who were deferred and unable to store the requested units of autologous blood, seven patients were asked to predonate 3 U or less; four of seven patients subsequently received homologous blood. Twenty-three patients were asked to predonate 4 U or more; nine of 23 received homologous blood (no different). In 145 patients able to donate the requested units of autologous blood, 110 were asked to give 3 U or less; 16 (14%) of 110 patients subsequently received homologous blood. Thirty-five patients were asked to give 4 U or more; three of 35 received homologous blood (no different). Thus, subsequent homologous blood exposure was related to whether patients successfully stored the requested number of autologous units and was not related to the number of autologous units requested for storage (ie, physician underordering).

COMMENT

Autologous preoperative blood deposit programs have received widespread support from the medical community[1-4] because of the potential benefits for patients, blood inventory, and physician transfusion behavior.[5-8] A previous multicenter study has shown that ABD is underutilized[13]; this underutilization can be improved with a coordinated program involving hospital blood banks, information services, and physicians.[6] Nevertheless, we have previously shown that patients predeposit insufficient autologous blood to minimize or eliminate their subsequent exposure to homologous blood.[8] Potential problems limiting sufficient autologous blood procurement include physician underordering, limitations of the storage interval, and erythropoietic response to phlebotomy.

Continuing medical education is perhaps the most traditional approach toward altering physician practice. In this study, we have shown that CME can correct the problem of physician underordering and profoundly reduce subsequent homologous blood exposure in patients who successfully store the amount of autologous blood requested by their physicians, from 12 (28%) of 42 in series 1, to six (11%) of 52 in series 2, and to one (2%) of 51 in series 3. Continuing medical education had no impact on the effective storage interval during which blood can be collected and inventoried for elective surgery. The consistency of the limitation of the erythropoietic response to serial phlebotomy over an effective storage interval is seen in Table 2, where the percent of patients deferred and unable to donate the requested units remains unchanged in each series of patients: eight (16%) of 50, 13 (20%) of 65, and nine (15%) of 60, respectively.

Table 3 illustrates that homologous blood exposure is not related to physician underordering. Fifty-eight patients were asked to donate 4 U or more; 23 (40%) were deferred and nine (39%) of 23 subsequently received homologous blood. This is compared with seven (6%) of 117 patients deferred when asked to donate 3 U or less with four (57%) of seven subsequently receiving homologous blood. We have thus demonstrated that when an autologous predeposit program is accompanied by an intervention, homologous blood exposure is related to donor deferral rate rather than physician underordering or inappropriate transfusion behavior.

The erythropoietic response to mild anemia (HCT $\geq$0.34) is clearly inadequate to avoid autologous donation deferral in 30 of 175 patients overall and in 23 of 58 patients asked to store 4 U or more. Thus, future studies of autologous predeposit programs should focus on the erythropoietic response as a limitation to procuring adequate autologous blood. Erythropoietic response to phlebotomy is a third limiting factor in procuring sufficient autologous blood to minimize the need for homologous blood exposure. The AABB standards have guidelines for elective autologous blood preoperative deposit that include a hemoglobin value of no less than 110 g/L or a packed cell volume of no less than 34%, and phlebotomy no more frequently than every three days and not within 72 hours of surgery.[10]

Erythropoietic response to serial phlebotomy is limited by functional iron availability and bone marrow response to erythropoietin. In our series, 20 of 30 deferred patients were female (compared with 83 of 145 of the nondeferred patients); this supports a role for iron availability and/or circulating blood volume as limitations. Others have shown that a significant number of normal community blood donors, especially women, are iron deficient and respond to iron therapy.[17] Even though patients in our ABD program are asked to take iron, noncompliance with ferrous sulfate has been well described[18] and the possibility of a functional iron limitation must be considered in some of these patients. Endogenous erythropoietin-induced bone marrow response as a limitation in procuring adequate autologous blood prior to elective orthopedic surgery is the focus of a current multi-institutional study.[19]

In conclusion, we have shown that (1) a significant percentage of patients are deferred because of HCT limitations and they subsequently receive homologous blood; (2) CME corrects physician underordering and reduces homologous exposure in patients who are able to store the amount of blood requested; and (3) storage interval remains a limitation for procuring adequate autologous blood before elective surgery. Future studies in ABD programs should focus on mechanisms to maximize blood procurement.

Dr Goodnough is the recipient of transfusion medicine academic award K-07-HLO-1625 from the National Institutes of Health, Bethesda, Md.

References

1. Council on Scientific Affairs: Autologous blood transfusions. *JAMA* 1986;256:2378-2380.
2. AABB establishes national autologous resource center. *Am Assoc Blood Banks Newsbriefs*, May 1987, vol 10, No. 5.
3. Consensus Conference (National Institutes of Health): The impact of routine HTLV III antibody testing of blood and plasma donors on public health. *JAMA* 1986;256:1778-1783.
4. Mintz P: Autologous transfusion endorsed. *JAMA* 1985;254:507.
5. Newman MM, Hamstra R, Block M: Use of banked autologous blood in elective surgery. *JAMA* 1971;218:861-863.
6. Kruskall MS, Glazer EE, Leonard SS, et al: Utilization and effectiveness of a hospital autologous preoperative blood donor program. *Transfusion* 1986;26:335-340.
7. FDA Blood Products Advisory Committee. *Blood Bank Week*, Feb 12, 1987, pp 1-2.
8. Wasman J, Goodnough LT: Effect of autologous blood donation for elective surgery on physician transfusion behavior: A matched control study. *JAMA* 1987;258:3135-3137.
9. Holland PV, Schmidt PH (eds): *Standards for Blood Banks and Transfusion Services*, ed 12. Arlington, Va, American Association of Blood Banks, 1987, p 39.
10. Aach RD, Kahn RD, Kahn RA: Post-transfusion hepatitis—current perspectives. *Ann Intern Med* 1980;92:539-546.
11. Curran JW, Lawrence DN, Jaffe H, et al: Acquired immunodeficiency syndrome associated with transfusions. *N Engl J Med* 1984;310:69-75.
12. Myhre BA: Fatalities from blood transfusion. *JAMA* 1980;244:1333-1335.
13. Toy PT, Strauss RG, Stehling LC, et al: Predeposit autologous blood for elective surgery: A multicenter study. *N Engl J Med* 1987;316:517-520.
14. AABB issues recommendations on informed consent for transfusion. *Am Assoc Blood Banks Newsbriefs*, July 1986, vol 9, No. 7.
15. Grindon AJ, Tomasulo PS, Gergin JJ, et al: The hospital transfusion committee. *JAMA* 1985;253:540-543.
16. Cosgrove DM, Coop FD, Lutze BW, et al: Determinants of blood utilization during myocardial revascularization. *Ann Thorac Surg* 1985;40: 380-384.
17. Gordeuk VR, Brittenham GM, Bravo J, et al: Replacement of iron in female blood donors with low-dose, short-term carbonyl iron, abstracted. *Clin Res* 1987;35:850A.
18. Hallberg L, Ryttinger L, Solvell C: Side effects of oral iron therapy: A double-blind study of different compounds in tablet form. *Acta Med Scand* 1966;459(suppl):3-10.
19. Goodnough LT, Rudnick S, Price T, et al: A randomized clinical trial of recombinant erythropoietin in autologous blood donors, abstracted. *Blood*, in press.

Adenocarcinoma Arising in an Ileostomy

Report of Two Cases and Review of the Literature

Patricia L. Roberts, MD; Malcolm C. Veidenheimer, MD;
Sharon Cassidy, RN, ET; Mark L. Silverman, MD

• Adenocarcinoma arising in an ileostomy is rare. Two cases are reported, one of a 58-year-old woman and the other of a 54-year-old man who had each undergone a colectomy for chronic ulcerative colitis. Seven other cases previously reported in the literature are reviewed. Though the exact pathogenesis is uncertain, several possibilities, particularly with regard to antecedent dysplasia and backwash ileitis, are discussed. Routine yearly follow-up and examination of the stoma by a physician or enterostomal therapist may lead to earlier detection of this rare complication.

(*Arch Surg* 1989;124:497-499)

Stomal complications have been reported in 30% to 86% of patients undergoing conventional ileostomy.[1,2] These include necrosis, retraction, prolapse, parastomal herniation, obstruction, fistula, skin irritation, improper construction, and poor location. A rarely reported complication is adenocarcinoma arising in the ileostomy. We describe two such cases and review the seven cases previously reported in the literature.

REPORT OF CASES

Case 1.—A 58-year-old woman presented to the Lahey Clinic Medical Center, Burlington, Mass, in late 1986 with an ulcerated area along the inferior pole of the ileostomy. At the age of 13 years, she had experienced bloody diarrhea and weight loss and was diagnosed as having ulcerative colitis. Six years later, in 1947, a proctoscopic biopsy of a sigmoid polyp revealed adenocarcinoma, and she underwent left hemicolectomy and proctectomy. Pathologic studies at the time revealed chronic ulcerative colitis as well as adenocarcinoma arising in a polyp with no evidence of involvement in any lymph nodes. She did well until the age of 24 years, when she had a flare-up of ulcerative colitis and underwent right hemicolectomy and Brooke ileostomy. Review of the microsections of the resected specimen of colon by one of us (M.L.S.) confirmed the presence of chronic ulcerative colitis and backwash ileitis with no evidence of dysplasia. However, review of the resected specimen of polyp was thought to indicate severe dysplasia and not invasive cancer.

Accepted for publication Jan 29, 1988.

From the Departments of Colon and Rectal Surgery (Drs Roberts and Veidenheimer and Ms Cassidy), and Pathology (Dr Silverman), Lahey Clinic Medical Center, Burlington, Mass.

Reprint requests to Department of Colon and Rectal Surgery, Lahey Clinic Medical Center, 41 Mall Rd, Burlington, MA 01805 (Dr Roberts).

No further complications were apparent until one month before admission, when she began to have difficulty with adherence of the ileostomy appliance. On examination, she was a well-nourished woman. Abdominal examination revealed no masses or hepatomegaly. A large ulcerated area was observed on the inferior portion of the ileostomy, and a biopsy revealed adenocarcinoma. Results of laboratory studies were normal, including a hematocrit level of 0.39, normal serum electrolyte levels, and a serum carcinoembryonic antigen value of 1 ng/mL (normal, 0 to 5 ng/mL).

The patient subsequently underwent en bloc excision of the ileostomy and anterior abdominal wall and transposition of the stoma to the left lower quadrant. The abdominal wall defect was closed with synthetic (Marlex) mesh. Recovery was uneventful. Final pathologic studies revealed a moderately differentiated primary small-bowel adenocarcinoma with extension into the muscularis propria, invasion into the dermis with clear margins, and negative nodes with no evidence of dysplasia (Fig 1).

Case 2.—A 54-year-old man with a history of ulcerative colitis presented to Lahey Clinic Medical Center in early 1987 because of difficulty with adherence of the ileostomy appliance. In 1951 he had experienced bloody diarrhea and was diagnosed as having ulcerative colitis. He did well for 13 years but then had a flare-up of disease and underwent total abdominal colectomy and ileostomy. Pathologic studies revealed chronic ulcerative colitis with backwash ileitis. Interval proctectomy was performed one year later. The final pathologic diagnosis was chronic ulcerative colitis with no evidence of dysplasia.

He did well for 12 years. About one year before the present admission he began to have progressive difficulty with adherence of the appliance. On examination, a bluish, comedolike ridge surrounded the stoma, which essentially was floating free in a 4- to 5-cm ulcer (Fig 2). Biopsy revealed invasive adenocarcinoma. Results of preoperative laboratory studies were normal, including a hematocrit level of 0.35 and a serum carcinoembryonic antigen value of 1 ng/mL.

The patient subsequently underwent an en bloc excision of the ileostomy and anterior abdominal wall and transposition of the stoma to the left side. The abdominal wall defect was repaired with synthetic mesh, and the wound was left open to granulate for subsequent skin grafts. At operation, a synchronous small-bowel cancer was located approximately 15 cm proximal to the ileostomy cancer. Pathologic studies revealed two distinct small-bowel cancers. The ileostomy cancer was a poorly to moderately differentiated adenocarcinoma, and the more proximal cancer was a mucin-producing adenocarcinoma (Fig 3). Dysplasia was not evident. Metastases were found in three of five lymph nodes. Each involved lymph node contained metastatic disease representing

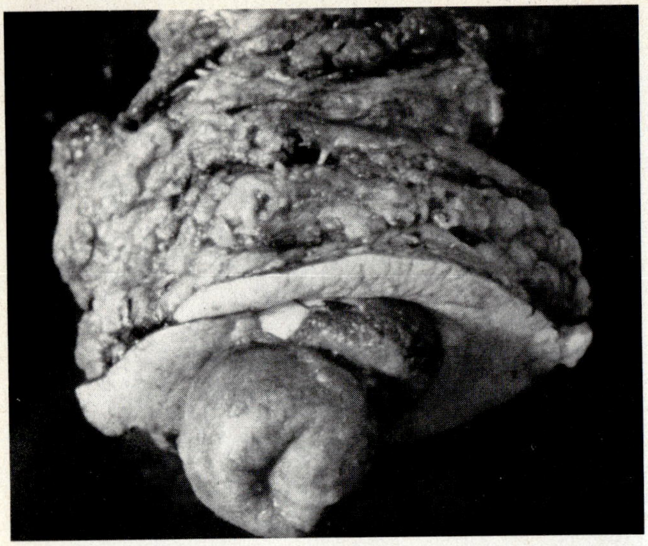

Fig 1.—En bloc specimen of ileostomy with attached ileum and anterior abdominal wall.

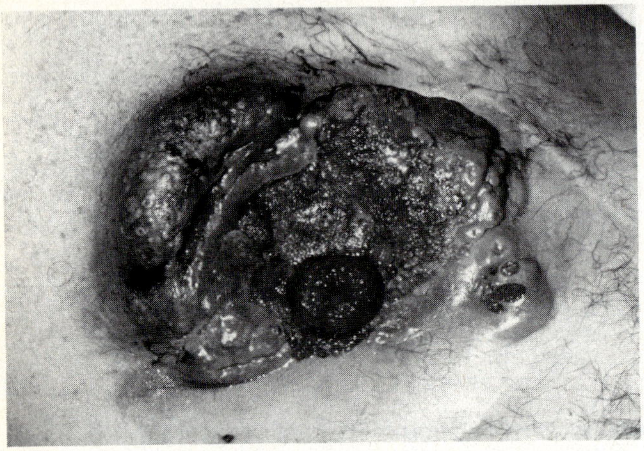

Fig 2.—Preoperative photograph demonstrating large comedolike ridge with free-floating stoma.

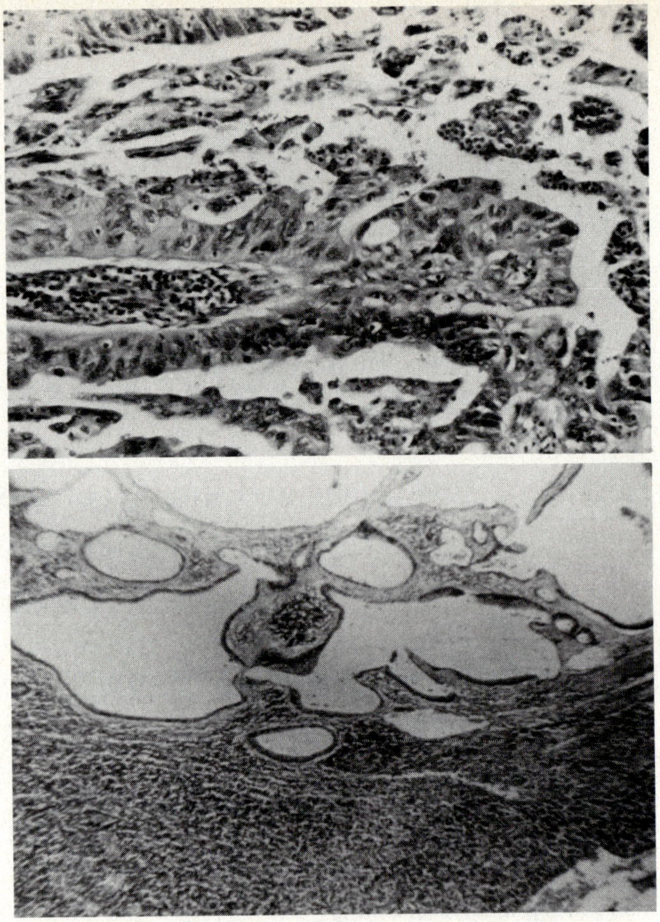

Fig 3.—Two distinct small-bowel cancers in same patient. Top, Cancer arising in ileostomy was poorly to moderately differentiated adenocarcinoma (hematoxylin-eosin, ×400). Bottom, More proximal ileal cancer was mucin-producing cancer (hematoxylin-eosin, ×100).

both primary histologic types. At present, the wound is almost completely healed by secondary intention, and the patient has not required skin grafting.

COMMENT

Since the original description in 1969 by Sigler and Jedd,[3] six more cases of adenocarcinoma arising in an ileostomy have been reported.[4-9] Our two patients bring the total number to nine. The majority of patients had a previous proctocolectomy performed for ulcerative colitis.[3-6,8,9] One case has been reported of a patient with familial polyposis in whom an adenocarcinoma developed in the ileostomy. This patient was believed to have an adenocarcinoma arising in a previous villous adenoma.[7] One patient with an ileostomy cancer is not included herein as this was thought to represent contiguous spread of a rectal cancer after resection of an ileorectal anastomosis and subsequent conversion to a Brooke ileostomy.[10]

Both of our patients had a previous diagnosis of chronic ulcerative colitis. Both also had backwash ileitis, which was confirmed by review of original microsections by one of us (M.L.S.). Furthermore, although the first patient was originally diagnosed as having sigmoid cancer, our review demonstrated high-grade dysplasia and not frank invasive cancer, thereby excluding contiguous spread even though the temporal sequence strongly suggested the impossibility.

Reports of Carcinoma in an Ileostomy*

Source, y	Patient Age, y/Sex	Years After Colectomy	Follow-up
Sigler and Jedd,[3] 1969	56/F	19	Liver metastases, dead at 10 mo
Cuesta and Donner,[6] 1976	60/M	6	Well at 9 mo
Roth and Logio,[7] 1982	44/M	9	...
Baciewicz et al,[4] 1983	45/F	19	...
Stryker,[8] 1983	66/F	13	Well at 7 y
Bedetti and DeRisio,[5] 1986	45/M	23	Liver metastases, dead at 4 mo
Vasilevsky and Gordon,[9] 1986	69/M	30	...
Present study, 1986	58/F	33	Well at 10 mo
Present study, 1987	54/M	23	Well at 5 mo

*All patients had wide local excision of the carcinoma.

The rarity of small-bowel cancer is well known.[11] The paucity of case reports attests to the fact that carcinoma arising in an ileostomy is even rarer. Some have speculated, therefore, that the presence of chronic inflammation (backwash ileitis), epithelial regeneration, or dysplasia places patients at an increased risk for malignant transformation of the ileum.[3-6,8,12,13] The majority of previous case reports have described the presence of either antecedent backwash ileitis or dysplasia.[3,4,6,8] In addition, others have described patients with ulcerative colitis in whom ileal cancers developed, which suggests that the ileum itself, if involved with backwash ileitis or dysplasia, may have malignant potential.[12-14] Though we have never seen dysplasia in an ileostomy, both of our patients had backwash ileitis noted at their original colectomy.

The pathogenesis of cancers arising in an ileostomy is largely speculative. Thus, review of additional cases will be necessary before patients at high risk for the development of these cancers can be identified. One cannot discount the fact that, with one exception, all patients had chronic ulcerative colitis as their underlying disease, and all patients had antecedent backwash ileitis or dysplasia. These concomitants of colitis may have placed them at higher risk for the development of ileostomy cancer. If backwash ileitis and dysplasia in the ileal mucosa place patients at a higher risk for the development of small-bowel cancer, routine ileoscopy with biopsy of the mucosa may be necessary for surveillance. At present, however, ileostomy cancers are so rare that the cost of a widespead program of surveillance cannot be justified. Instead, regular yearly inspection of the stoma by an enterostomal therapist or physician may be sufficient.

As in our two patients, all reported instances of carcinoma in an ileostomy occurred many years after the patient's colectomy (Table). Although biopsy established the diagnosis in our two patients, others have pointed out that biopsies are frequently unreliable and often reveal either atypia or inflammation.[9] One must therefore have a high index of suspicion and undertake aggressive biopsy of any unusual or ulcerated-appearing area. Though a normal biopsy finding does not rule out a malignant neoplasm, the presence of atypia or dysplasia warrants further close follow-up and biopsy.

All patients should be treated with wide local excision and transposition of the stoma to the opposite side. As with other malignant bowel neoplasms, survival appears to be related to the stage of the tumor at the time of the original resection. However, the small number of patients and a lack of follow-up in many preclude any conclusions with respect to long-term survival. Greater awareness of this entity as well as routine yearly follow-up and examination of the stoma by a physician or enterostomal therapist may lead to earlier detection of this rare condition.

References

1. Cassidy S, Veidenheimer MC: Complications of intestinal stomas. *Probl Gen Surg* 1985;2:545-560.
2. Pearl RK, Prasad L, Orsay CP, et al: Complications of intestinal stomas. *Contemp Surg* 1984;24:17-22.
3. Sigler L, Jedd FL: Adenocarcinoma of the ileostomy occurring after colectomy for ulcerative colitis: Report of a case. *Dis Colon Rectum* 1969;12:45-48.
4. Baciewicz F, Sparberg M, Lawrence JB, et al: Adenocarcinoma of an ileostomy site with skin invasion: A case report. *Gastroenterology* 1983;84:168-170.
5. Bedetti CD, DeRisio VJ: Primary adenocarcinoma arising at an ileostomy site: An unsual complication after colectomy for ulcerative colitis. *Dis Colon Rectum* 1986;29:572-575.
6. Cuesta MA, Donner R: Adenocarcinoma arising at an ileostomy site: Report of a case. *Cancer* 1976;37:949-952.
7. Roth JA, Logio T: Carcinoma arising in an ileostomy stoma: An unusual complication of adenomatous polyposis coli. *Cancer* 1982;49:2180-2184.
8. Stryker SJ: Primary stomal adenocarcinoma: An unusual complication of ileostomy. *Dis Colon Rectum* 1983;26:47-49.
9. Vasilevsky C-A, Gordon PH: Adenocarcinoma arising at the ileocutaneous junction occurring after proctocolectomy for ulcerative colitis. *Br J Surg* 1986;73:378.
10. Johnson WR, McDermott FL, Pihl E, et al: Adenocarcinoma of an ileostomy in a patient with ulcerative colitis. *Dis Colon Rectum* 1980;23:351-352.
11. Mason GR: Tumors of the duodenum and small intestine, in Sabiston DC Jr (ed): *Textbook of Surgery: The Biological Basis of Modern Surgical Practice*, ed 13. Philadelphia, WB Saunders Co, 1986, vol 1, pp 868-873.
12. Brown CH, Diaz RJ, Michener WM: Carcinoma of the colon and ileum in chronic ulcerative colitis with reflux ileitis: Report of a case of a 16-year-old boy. *Gastroenterology* 1964;47:306-312.
13. Schlippert W, Mitros F, Schulze K: Multiple adenocarcinomas and premalignant changes in 'backwash' ileitis. *Am J Med* 1979;66:879-882.
14. Jalan KN, MacLean N, Path MC, et al: Carcinoma of the terminal ileum and sarcoidosis in a case of ulcerative colitis. *Gastroenterology* 1969;56:583-588.

In Other AMA Journals

AJDC

Appendicitis in Children: Accuracy of the Barium Enema

Cristian Garcia, MD; Nancy S. Rosenfield, MD; Richard I. Markowitz, MD; John H. Seashore, MD; Robert J. Touloukian, MD; Domenic V. Cicchetti, PhD

The barium enema (BE) may be useful in the diagnosis of atypical appendicitis in children. We analyzed our experience with 18 children in whom appendicitis was suspected and BE was performed. All of the children underwent surgical exploration. Nonfilling of the appendix with cecal indentation, extravasation of barium from the appendix, or both, were considered positive signs of an inflamed appendix on BE. Using these criteria, 12 of 14 cases of proved appendicitis were true positive and two were equivocal. Four children were proved not to have appendicitis; one of these patients had a true-negative BE, two had equivocal BEs, and there was one false-positive BE (Schönlein-Henoch purpura). Extravasation of barium into the peritoneal cavity was noted in one patient; this was a rare complication (*AJDC* 1987;141:1309-1312).

Reprint requests to Department of Diagnostic Imaging, Yale University School of Medicine, 333 Cedar St, New Haven, CT 06510 (Dr Rosenfield).

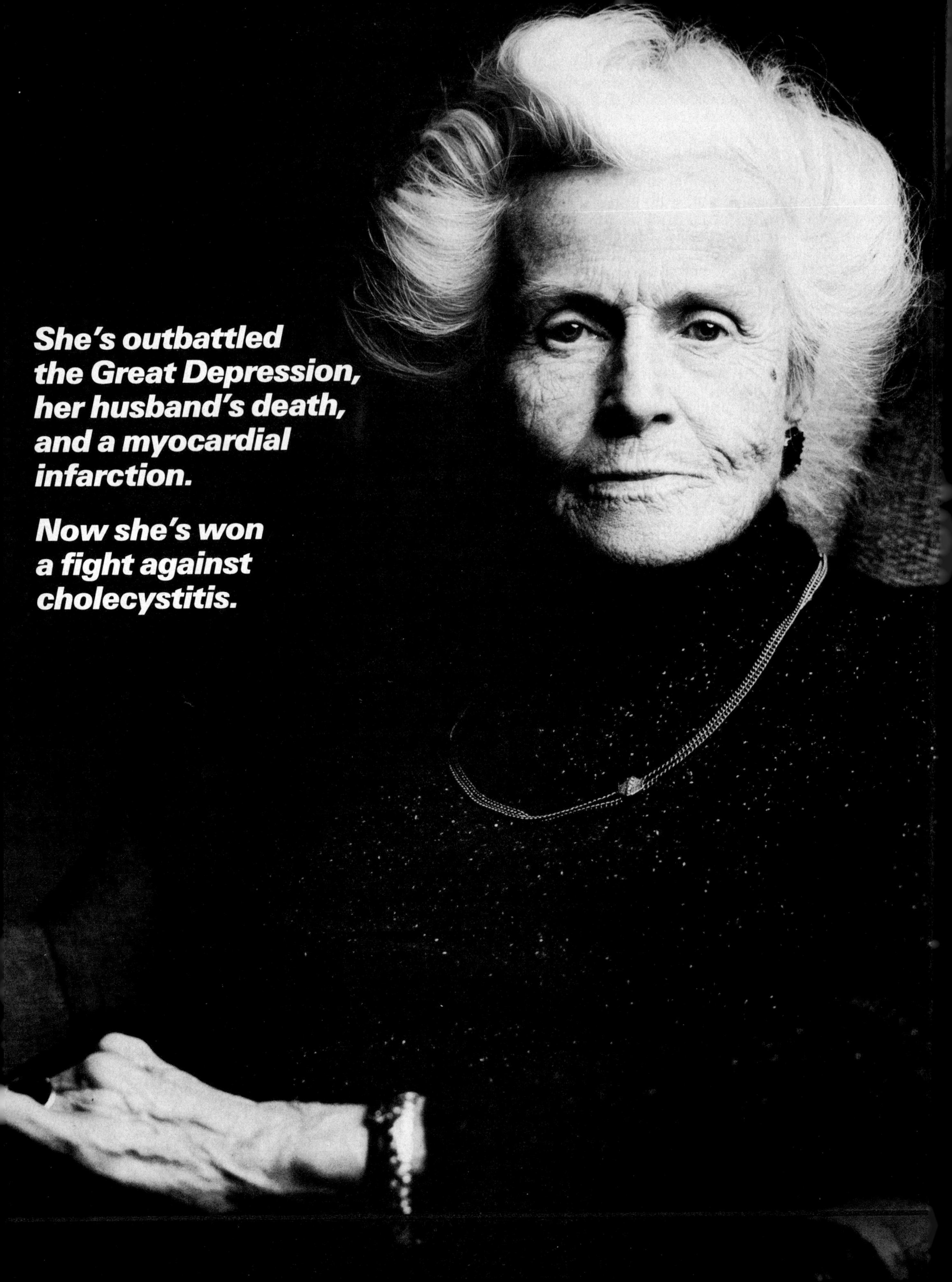
She's outbattled
the Great Depression,
her husband's death,
and a myocardial
infarction.
Now she's won
a fight against
cholecystitis.

Successful Reconstruction of Late Portal Vein Stenosis After Hepatic Transplantation

Velma P. Scantlebury, MD; Albert B. Zajko, MD; Carlos O. Esquivel, MD, PhD; Ignazio R. Marino, MD; Thomas E. Starzl, MD, PhD

• Stenosis of the portal vein anastomosis occurred in three pediatric patients seven to 42 months after transplantation. Dominant symptoms were those of portal hypertension and hypersplenism. Diagnosis was made by angiography. Successful surgical reconstruction was possible in all three patients.

(*Arch Surg* 1989;124:503-505)

Biliary tract complications and thrombosis of the hepatic artery are the most common technical problems observed following orthotopic liver transplantation (OLT).[1,2] In contrast, portal vein (PV) complications are unusual; however, they are associated with high morbidity and mortality.[3-6] Three pediatric patients presented 7, 10, and 42 months after OLT with PV stenoses that were successfully treated by excision of the stenotic segment and reanastomosis.

PATIENTS AND METHODS

The condition of the PV, hepatic artery, and vena cava is determined routinely with ultrasonography in all liver transplant recipients. Between March 1980 and January 1986, three of 184 children who survived more than three months after transplantation had evidence of PV stenosis. The diagnosis was confirmed by selective angiography. In one patient (case 3), venous pressures were measured across the stenosis after transhepatic catheterization of the PV. The following parameters were reviewed: age, indication for transplantation, time interval between OLT and diagnosis of PV stenosis, symptoms, physical and laboratory findings at the time of diagnosis, angiograms, the type of technique for secondary reconstruction, and clinical outcome. The technique for liver transplantation has been previously reported.[7]

RESULTS

The Table summarizes the profile of these three patients and their clinical features at the time PV stenosis was diagnosed. Two of the three patients were symptomatic. The other patient (case 2) had no overt symptoms, although she had mild hepatic dysfunction. On further evaluation, she was found to have splenomegaly and sonographic findings of hepatofugal flow. Because of this, she underwent angiographic evaluation. The cause of hepatic dysfunction was from a stricture of the common bile duct.

Angiographic Findings

All three patients underwent selective celiac and superior mesenteric angiography. In each case, stenosis of the PV anastomosis was identified (Fig 1, left).

Two patients (cases 1 and 3) underwent further evaluation by transhepatic catheterization of the PV to determine if there was a significant pressure gradient across the anastomotic stenosis. Successful catheterization of the PV was possible in both cases. However, in only one patient could the catheter be advanced across the stenosis to measure a gradient (Fig 2). In the other patient, transhepatic portal venography clearly demonstrated a marked stricture even though a gradient could not be measured (Fig 3).

In two patients (cases 1 and 3), evidence of portal hypertension was found as manifested by gastroesophageal varices (Fig 2). In the third patient (case 2), no varices were seen despite the presence of a severe stenosis (Fig 1, left). This last patient underwent follow-up angiography after operative revision of the PV anastomosis, documenting a widely patent PV (Fig 1, right).

Operative Findings

Operation was performed through the same subcostal incision that had been used for the transplantation. In one patient (case 3), the choledochojejunostomy was not taken down because mobilization of the Roux-en-Y allowed adequate exposure of the PV. In the other two cases, the choledochojejunostomy was taken down to facilitate the exposure. Both of these patients (cases 1 and 2) had biliary strictures.

Stenosis of the PV in all three patients was at the anastomoses. The gross pathologic findings were similar in each case. The veins were phlebosclerotic, with focal calcification and foreign-body reaction at the site of the

Accepted for publication July 15, 1988.

From the Departments of Surgery (Drs Scantlebury, Esquival, Marino, and Starzl) and Radiology (Dr Zajko), University Health Center of Pittsburgh, University of Pittsburgh, and the Veterans Administration Medical Center, Pittsburgh (Dr Starzl).

Reprint requests to Department of Surgery, 3601 Fifth Ave, Falk Clinic 4 West, Pittsburgh, PA 15213 (Dr Scantlebury).

Case No./Age, y	Indication for Orthotopic Liver Transplantation	Time From Orthotopic Liver Transplantation, mo	Clinical Symptoms	Physical Findings	Laboratory Findings
1/10	Familial cholestasis	7	Variceal hemorrhage	Splenomegaly and ascites	Pancytopenia
2/6	Biliary atresia	10	Asymptomatic	Splenomegaly	Leukopenia
3/6	Biliary hypoplasia	42	Fatigue	Splenomegaly	Thrombocytopenia and leukopenia

Summary of Profile and Clinical Features at Time of Diagnosis of Portal Vein Stenosis

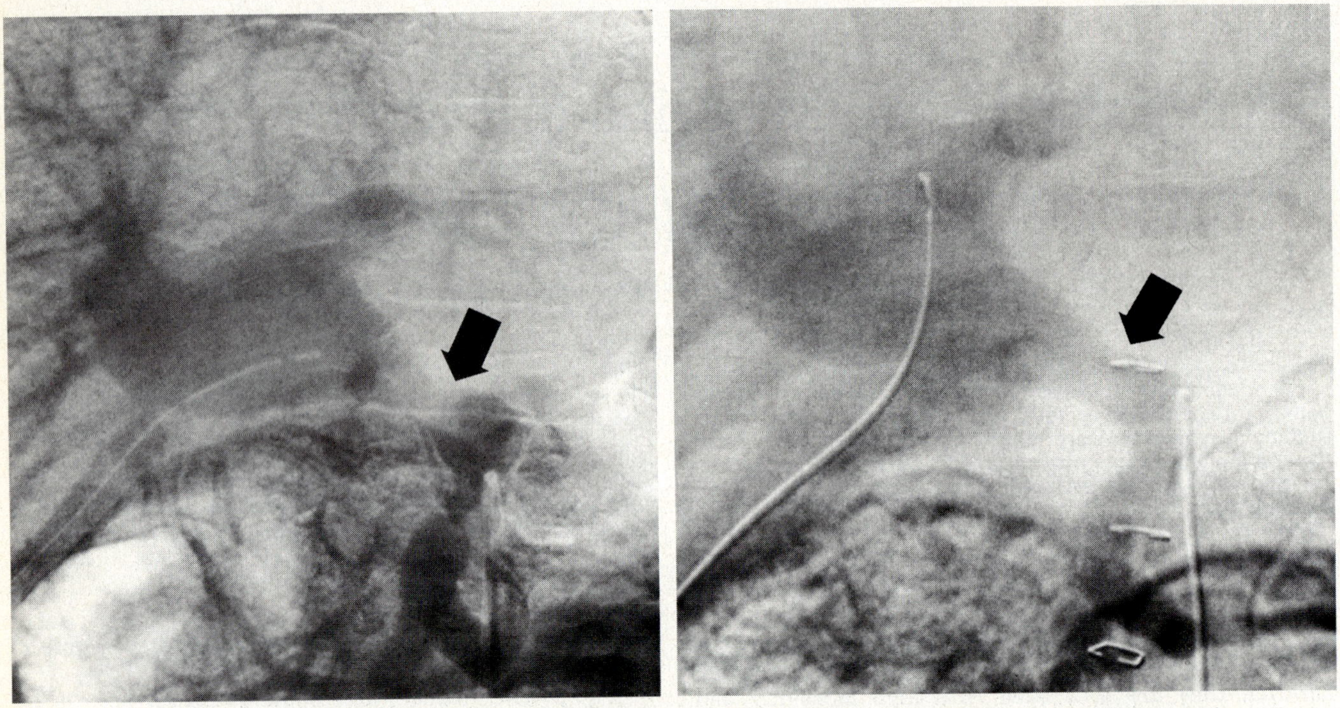

Fig 1.—Case 2. Left, Portal vein anastomotic stenosis (arrow) demonstrated on venous phase of superior mesenteric arteriogram. Poststenotic dilatation of portal vein is evident. Right, Widely patent portal vein anastomosis (arrow) demonstrated on venous phase of superior mesenteric arteriogram performed six days after portal vein revision. Decrease in previously seen poststenotic dilatation is shown.

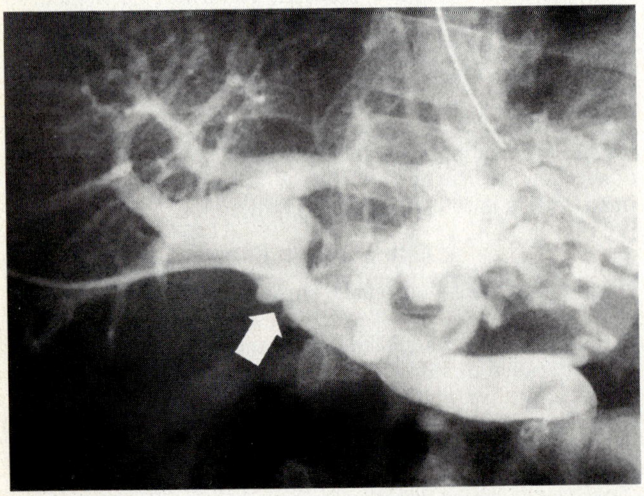

Fig 2.—Case 3. Portal vein anastomotic stenosis (arrow) demonstrated on transhepatic portogram. Prominent gastric varices are seen. Pressure in splenic vein was 29 mm Hg, and pressure in intrahepatic portal vein was 12 mm Hg.

anastomoses. In one patient (case 1), a recent clot was found in the donor side of the PV that extended into the hilum. Histologic examination of this specimen showed mural thrombosis with recanalization. Thrombectomy was performed.

In each case the anastomosis was excised by removing a ring of vein measuring 1 to 2 cm long after obtaining proximal and distal vascular control. In all three cases the length of the vein was adequate for allowing reapproximation of the two ends without tension. The anastomoses were performed end-to-end with 7-0 polypropylene suture. Systemic heparinization was not used. All patients recovered successfully and were discharged in excellent condition. The spleen in all three patients was noted to have decreased in size at the time of last follow-up.

COMMENT

Portal vein thrombosis after OLT occurs more frequently in pediatric patients. Symptoms of portal hypertension are the primary manifestations. Lerut et al[3] reported seven cases of PV thrombosis following OLT, with an overall incidence of 1.8%. Five of the seven patients developed variceal hemorrhage.

Previous portosystemic shunt and partial or complete thrombosis of the portal system requiring thrombectomy

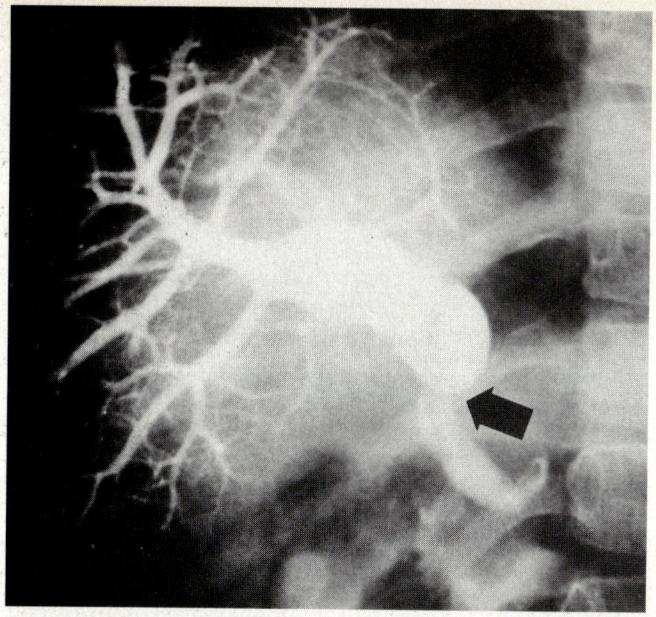

Fig 3.—Case 1. Marked stenosis of portal vein anastomosis demonstrated on transhepatic portogram (arrow). Catheter could not be advanced across stenosis to measure pressure gradient.

at the time of transplantation are thought to be contributing factors to the development of postoperative PV complications. However, not all patients demonstrate an obvious cause. Of the seven cases reported by Lerut, only three had contributing factors. One patient had a portacaval shunt, one had a thrombosed PV, and one had hypoplasia of the PV. None of the three patients described herein had any contributing cause for the development of PV stenosis following transplantation. However, dense scarring in the portal area may have contributed; two of the three recipients also had a stricture at the site of bile duct anastomosis. The best possibility is that technical errors were made at the time of the original transplantation. The fact that secondary repair was possible without vein grafts might suggest that the cuffs were originally made too long, which consequently caused kinking or distortion.

In all three cases, the diagnosis was suspected by physical examination and confirmed by angiography. Evidence of a recent clot in the portal vein extending into the hilum of the liver was found in one patient (case 1). This clot was not demonstrated by angiographic studies performed three and eight days before revision and may have been contributed to by the instrumentation. Pathologic findings of focal calcification, thickening, and fibrosis in the area of the anastomotic suture line were common to all cases.

The status of the extrahepatic PV should be evaluated in patients after transplantation with recurring symptoms of portal hypertension, hypersplenism, or both. Ultrasonography can be performed for screening, but definitive diagnosis requires angiography. Successful surgical correction of PV anastomotic stenosis can be achieved with little morbidity. The possibility of balloon dilatation of the strictures after transhepatic PV catheterization was not seriously considered for these patients, but this may be a viable nonoperative option for the future.

This study was supported in part by research grants from the Veterans Administration, Pittsburgh, and grant AM 29961 from the National Institutes of Health, Bethesda, Md.

References

1. Tzakis AG, Gordon RD, Shaw BW Jr, et al: Clinical presentation of hepatic artery thrombosis after liver transplantation in the cyclosporine era. *Transplantation* 1985;4:667-671.
2. Iwatsuki S, Shaw BW Jr, Starzl TE: Biliary tract complications in liver transplantation under cyclosporine steroid therapy. *Transplant Proc* 1983;15:1288-1291.
3. Lerut J, Tzakis AG, Bron K, et al: Complications of venous reconstruction in human orthotopic liver transplantation. *Ann Surg* 1987;205:404-414.
4. Wozney P, Zajko AB, Bron KM, et al: Vascular complications after liver transplantation: A five-year experience. *AJR* 1986;147:657-663.
5. Cardella JF, Castaneda-Zuniga WR, Hunter D, et al: Angiographic and interventional radiologic considerations in liver transplantation. *AJR* 1986;147:143-153.
6. Zajko AB, Bron KM: Hepatopetal collaterals after portal vein thrombosis following liver transplantation. *Cardiovasc Intervent Radiol* 1986;9:46-48.
7. Starzl TE, Iwatsuki S, Esquivel CO, et al: Refinements in the surgical technique of liver transplantation. *Semin Liver Dis* 1985;5:349-356.

In Other AMA Journals

ARCHIVES OF INTERNAL MEDICINE

Frequency of Isolated Proximal Colonic Polyps Among Patients Referred for Colonoscopy

David A. Lieberman, MD, Frederic W. Smith, MD

The American Cancer Society now advocates screening asymptomatic populations over the age of 40 to 50 years for colonic malignancy. It is possible, however, that fecal occult blood testing and sigmoidoscopy to 60 cm would fail to identify patients with adenomatous polyps located only in the proximal colon. The purpose of this study was to determine how many patients without polyps in the distal 60 cm of the colon would have more proximal lesions. Ninety-eight consecutive patients with positive fecal blood test results or suspicious barium enema results were studied, using the assumption that if they had been seen six months earlier, when asymptomatic, they would have been candidates for screening examination. Forty-one (42%) of 98 patients had adenomatous polyps or cancer, and 15 (37%) of these patients had isolated proximal lesions. The polyp detection rate from 0 to 60 cm was significantly less than the detection rate for a full colonoscopy (27% vs 42%). We conclude that isolated proximal colonic polyps may be common (*Arch Intern Med* 1988;148:473-475).

Reprint requests to Department of Medicine, Division of Gastroenterology, Portland Veterans Administration Medical Center, 3710 SW US Veterans Hospital Rd, PO Box 1034, Portland, OR 97207 (Dr Lieberman).

Cardiac Contusion

The Effect on Operative Management of the Patient With Trauma Injuries

Patrick Ross, Jr, MD, PhD; Linda Degutis, MSN; Christopher C. Baker, MD

• Sixty-four patients with cardiac contusion documented by electrocardiographic changes and creatine kinase MB fraction assay following blunt chest injury were reviewed to assess the impact of cardiac contusion on subsequent management. Fifty-eight patients had elevated creatine kinase MB levels; 35 patients had electrocardiographic abnormalities, including ST-segment and T-wave changes (25), premature ventricular contraction (ten), right bundle-branch block (nine), atrioventricular block (three), atrial fibrillation (three), and premature atrial contraction (two). Thirty patients underwent general anesthesia. There were only four perioperative complications: ventricular ectopy, ventricular fibrillation, nodal rhythm, and pulmonary edema. There were no deaths attributable to cardiac contusion. In summary, patients with blunt trauma who have sustained a cardiac contusion can undergo elective operation with a low incidence of complication. In the emergency setting, however, hemodynamic monitoring for early detection of arrhythmias is indicated.

(*Arch Surg* 1989;124:506-507)

Cardiac injury as a consequence of blunt chest trauma is being recognized with increasing frequency. Cardiac contusion represents a major category within the spectrum of cardiac injuries, with an estimated 17% to 20% of patients sustaining blunt chest trauma.[1-3] Since cardiac contusion was first described,[4,5] efforts have been directed toward delineating criteria that allow precise documentation of this injury.[6-14] Specifics of management have been limited to patients developing complications. Thus, patients with cardiac contusion have been treated with protocols developed for patients with recent myocardial ischemia. Several clinical reports and animal experiments have documented significant cardiac dysfunction following blunt injury, including arrhythmias and ventricular dysfunction.[7,9,15,16]

Since cardiac morbidity may be severe, cardiac contusion could be expected to influence the course of the multiply injured patient. Therefore, this study was initiated to address the impact of the presence of cardiac contusion on the management of the patient with multiple trauma, with specific reference to subsequent operative management for other injuries.

PATIENTS AND METHODS

The records of 100 patients admitted to Yale–New Haven (Conn) Hospital between January 1984 and July 1985 with the diagnosis of cardiac contusion were reviewed. Data were extracted on initial presentation, hospital course, operations, and medical history. Cardiac contusion was diagnosed either by electrocardiogram (ECG) or creatine kinase MB fraction (CK-MB) assay based on results obtained during the first 72 hours of hospitalization. The ECG criteria included arrhythmias, atrial or ventricular ectopy, conduction defects, and ischemic changes. Elevation of the CK-MB percentage over 2.5% constituted a positive test.

Accepted for publication May 5, 1988.

From the Department of Surgery, Yale University School of Medicine, New Haven, Conn. Dr. Ross is now with Hospital of the University of Pennsylvania, Philadelphia.

Reprint requests to Department of Surgery, Yale University School of Medicine, 333 Cedar St, New Haven, CT 06510 (Dr Ross).

RESULTS

Patient Characteristics

Sixty-four patients sustained cardiac contusion by the criteria outlined above. Forty-five were male patients and 19 were female patients. The age distribution ranged from 7 to 89 years. The mean age was 37 years. The majority of the patients were injured in motor vehicle or motorcycle accidents (85%), with the remainder sustaining injury as pedestrians (6%) and from falls or industrial accidents (9%).

Associated Injuries

Forty patients (63%) had additional chest injuries and 18% of the patients were hypotensive (systolic pressure, 90 mm Hg) at the scene or on arrival in the emergency room. Concomitant chest injuries included rib fractures (n = 25), pneumothorax and hemothorax (n = 12), pulmonary contusion (n = 11), sternal fracture (n = 5), clavicle fracture (n = 3), and aortic tear (n = 1). The mean number of organ systems injuries exclusive of the chest was two.

Diagnostic Method

Fifty-eight patients (91% of the study population) had elevated levels of the CK-MB fraction: 29 patients (45%) had CK-MB elevation alone and 29 patients had elevated CK-MB levels and ECG abnormalities (Table). The mean CK-MB rise was 0.04, with a range from 0.03 to 0.12. The peak serum CK-MB level occurred at admission in 21 patients and at eight hours after injury in an additional 29 patients. Fifty-seven of 58 patients with elevated levels of CK-MB fractions exhibited a maximal CK-MB level by 16 hours after admission.

Thirty-five patients (55%) manifested ECG abnormalities; six of these 35 patients had ECG changes without an accompanying CK-MB release. Electrocardiographic abnormalities were as follows: ST-segment alteration (n = 12), T-wave changes (n = 13), premature ventricular contractions (n = 10), right bundle-branch block (n = 9), atrioventricular block (n = 3), atrial fibrillation (n = 3), and premature atrial contraction (n = 2).

Operative Complications

Thirty patients underwent general anesthesia for exploratory laparotomy, repair of complex lacerations, or open reduction and internal fixation of fractures. Only four of these patients had perioperative complications, and there

Method of Diagnosis*

	No. (%) With Elevated CK-MB Level	No. (%) With Normal CK-MB Level	Total No. (%)
Normal ECG	29 (45.3)	0	**29** (45.3)
Abnormal ECG	29 (45.3)	6 (9.4)	**35** (54.7)
Total	**58** (90.6)	**6** (9.4)	**64** (100)

*ECG indicates electrocardiogram; CK-MB, creatine kinase MB isoenzyme.

were no deaths attributable to cardiac contusion. The complications included ventricular ectopy, ventricular fibrillation, nodal rhythm, and pulmonary edema; each event occurred in a single patient. The complications appeared to be unrelated to older age, a history of cardiac disease, level of CK-MB, or total number of systems injured.

COMMENT

Cardiac contusion is a frequent and significant sequela of blunt chest trauma, and efforts should be made to document this lesion when it is suspected. Historical features, including symptoms and mechanism of injury, suggest the diagnosis, which can be confirmed by serial ECGs and measurement of specific cardiac enzyme levels. Additionally, recent reports suggest that two-dimensional echocardiography and radionuclide angiography may be sensitive indicators of myocardial injury.[12,14] Both tests assess ventricular function; abnormalities in ventricular wall motion may correlate with injury. These reports, however, did not address the impact of the injury on the patient's hospital course. In the current study, two-dimensional echocardiography and radionuclide angiography were not used primarily because the tests were cumbersome to perform in the patient with multiple injuries. The role of either modality in the diagnosis of cardiac contusion will require further evaluation.

Previous studies have documented right and left ventricular dysfunction, persistent arrhythmias, and malignant arrhythmias in both clinical reports and experimental models.[9,17-19] These earlier data suggested that patients who had sustained cardiac contusion were at high risk for perioperative cardiac complications. The results reported here, however, demonstrate that patients with injuries with cardiac contusion can be operated on with a low risk (13%) of complications. The complications were easily managed and significantly there was no associated mortality. It is important to note that preoperative evaluation does not allow detection of the population at risk for development of these complications, since complications were not associated with patient age, extent of other injuries, or history of cardiac disease. Thus, all patients with this diagnosis should have perioperative cardiac monitoring.

The findings in this study carry substantial clinical relevance. Frequently, the patient with multiple trauma injuries undergoes delayed operation (particularly for fractures or reconstruction) because of fear of complications associated with cardiac contusion. Conversely, it has become increasingly clear[20] that early definitive fixation of fractures is critical to achieving an optimal outcome in the multiply injured patients. The findings in this study show that patients with cardiac contusion may undergo surgery with a surprisingly low risk of complications.

We conclude several points from this study on cardiac contusion. First, cardiac contusion is a common problem in the patient with trauma injuries, but ECG manifestations of injury may be absent initially in up to 45% of patients. Second, hemodynamic monitoring is indicated in patients requiring emergency operation for trauma injuries in whom cardiac contusion is suspected. Third, preparations for early detection and treatment of arrhythmias must be made in patients undergoing semielective surgery, since preoperative factors do not identify patients at risk. Finally, multiply injured patients who have sustained a cardiac contusion can undergo elective operation with a low incidence of complications.

References

1. Parmley LF, Manion WC, Mattingly TW: Nonpenetrating traumatic injury of the heart. *Circulation* 1958;18:371-396.
2. Symbas PN: Cardiac trauma. *Am Heart J* 1976;92:387-396.
3. Saunders CR, Doty SB: Myocardial contusion. *Surg Gynecol Obstet* 1977;144:595-603.
4. Beck CS: Contusions of the heart. *JAMA* 1935;104:109-114.
5. Bright EF, Beck CS: Nonpenetrating wounds of the heart. *Am Heart J* 1935;10:293-321.
6. Lindsey D, Navin TR, Finley PR: Transient elevation of serum activity of MB isoenzyme of creatinine phosphokinase in drivers involved in automobile accidents. *Chest* 1978;74:15-18.
7. Viano DC, Artinian CG: Myocardial conducting system dysfunctions from thoracic impact. *J Trauma* 1978;18:452-459.
8. Michelson WB: CPK-MB isoenzyme determinations: Diagnostic and prognostic value in elevation of blunt chest trauma. *Ann Emerg Med* 1980; 9:562-567.
9. Sutherland GR, Calvin JE, Driedger AA, et al: Anatomic and cardiopulmonary responses to trauma with associated blunt chest injury. *J Trauma* 1981;21:1-22.
10. Miller FA, Seward JB, Gersh BJ, et al: Two-dimensional echocardiographic findings in cardiac trauma. *Am J Cardiol* 1982;50:1022-1027.
11. Rodriguez A, Shatney C: The value of technetium^{99m} pyrophosphate scanning in the diagnosis of myocardial contusion. *Ann Surg* 1982;48:472-474.
12. King RM, Mucha P, Seward JB, et al: Cardiac contusion: A new diagnostic approach utilizing two dimensional echocardiography. *J Trauma* 1983;23:610-614.
13. Kumar SA, Puri VK, Mittal VK, et al: Myocardial contusion following nonfatal blunt chest trauma. *J Trauma* 1983;23:327-333.
14. Harley DP, Mena I, Narahara KA, et al: Traumatic myocardial dysfunction. *J Thorac Cardiovasc Surg* 1984;87:386-393.
15. Cane RD, Schamroth L: Prolongation of the Q-T interval with myocardial contusion. *Heart Lung* 1975;7:652-656.
16. Liedtke AJ, Allen RP, Nellis SH: Effects of blunt cardiac trauma on coronary vasomotion, perfusion, myocardial mechanics and metabolism. *J Trauma* 1980;20:777-785.
17. Stein PD, Sabah HN, Viano DC, et al: Response of the heart to nonpenetrating cardiac trauma. *J Trauma* 1982;22:364-373.
18. DeGroot M, Prewitt RM: Right ventricular contusion: Experimental pathophysiology and treatment in an open heart canine preparation. *J Trauma* 1984;24:721-727.
19. Potkin RT, Werner JA, Trobaugh GB, et al: Evaluation of noninvasive tests of cardiac damage in suspected cardiac contusion. *Circulation* 1982; 66:627-631.
20. Lozman J, Sero SC, Feastel PJ, et al: Pulmonary and cardiovascular consequences of immediate fixation or conservative management of long bone failures. *Arch Surg* 1986;121:992-999.

Invited Editorial Comment

The article by Ross and colleagues again points out that cardiac contusion is a common problem in the population with blunt trauma and that these patients may undergo operation with an expected low rate of cardiac complications.

It remains difficult to know just how often cardiac contusion occurs. All studies (even prospective analyses) are hampered by the lack of an accepted "gold standard" against which to measure any diagnostic test (eg, CK-MB level and ECG). The more sophisticated the test (echocardiogram, multiple-gated acquisition [MUGA] scan), the more frequently the diagnosis of cardiac contusion is made.

The investigators have relied on elevated CK-MB isoenzyme levels and abnormal ECG to define cardiac contusion. It is certainly possible that they are underestimating the true incidence. It is well documented that cardiac contusion can exist at surgery or autopsy with no preoperative or antemortem ECG evidence. Similarly, it has been demonstrated that myocardial biopsy specimens from ventricles of young victims may contain almost no MB isoenzyme content.

Although all would agree with Ross and coworkers that preparations for early detection and treatment of arrhythmias is necessary, some would disagree with their point that preoperative factors do not identify patients at risk. One group has documented an incidence of dysrhythmia that is 13 times greater when two-dimensional echocardiographic findings are abnormal. In most institutions, however, it remains difficult to obtain such studies at odd hours; therefore, one must be prepared to treat arrhythmias in every patient with blunt chest trauma.

Most important, it is pointed out by Ross et al that patients who have sustained "cardiac contusion" can undergo operation safely. One should not forego the substantial benefits of early fixation of skeletal fractures because of concern for dysrhythmia or pump failure.

D. Ian Soutter, MD, FRCSC
Toronto

Endorectal Ileal Pullthrough

To the Editor.—The article by Fonkalsrud et al[1] in the September 1988 issue of the ARCHIVES[1] presents the progression of technical improvements in endorectal ileal pullthrough with better end results. The operation can still present problems. The terminal ileum has specific absorptive capability and mechanism to slow the intestinal stream.[2] It would be interesting to have noted how much of the terminal ileum is retained. The distal ileal 4 cm is a zone of elevated pressure. Its resting pressure is 20 mm Hg greater than colonic pressure.[3] It does not permit reflux, even with distal obstruction to the point of cecal rupture. Bacterial colonization proximal to the junction is rare. This may be an important factor in preventing reflux enteritis, especially in an ileal reservoir.

The ileal mucosa extends to 1 cm of the apex of the protuberance, and a transitional mucosa extends to the apex.[4] Retention of the ileocecal junction musculature may eliminate or modify the need of an ileal reservoir. Professor David Johnston (Department of Surgery, Leeds University, England, oral communication, Oct 5, 1988) has so far done ten such procedures with good initial results in eight of them. It will be interesting to follow up his progress. This may be an initial effort in a new direction.

LAWRENCE BRASLOW, MD
Riverside, Calif

1. Fonkalsrud EW, Stelzner M, McDonald N: Experience with the endorectal ileal pullthrough with lateral reservoir for ulcerative colitis and polyposis. *Arch Surg* 1988;123:1053-1058.
2. Braslow L: Ileocecal valve: Misconceptions. *Arch Surg* 1982;117:249.
3. Davenport HW: *Physiology of the Digestive Tract*, ed 5. Chicago, Year Book Medical Publishers Inc, 1982, p 80.
4. Braslow L: Ileocecostomy. *Arch Surg* 1988;123:782.

In Reply.—We appreciate Dr Braslow's suggestions and recommendations regarding the endorectal ileal pullthrough procedure. As indicated in our article, the ileum is divided approximately 1 to 2 cm from the ileocecal valve unless there is active disease in the terminal ileum, in which case a small amount of ileum is resected. After mobilizing the superior mesenteric artery up to its origin from the aorta, the terminal ileum is divided approximately 15 cm from the end, but preserving the blood supply to the distal segment. The reservoir is constructed in a side-to-side manner over a distance of approximately 12 to 13 cm, which leaves an ileal "spout" distal to the lower end of the reservoir of approximately 1.5 to 2 cm.

With regard to preserving the ileocecal valve and a portion of ileum for the pullthrough segment, it has been our experience that almost all patients with ulcerative colitis will have involvement of the entire colon, including the cecum. In most patients, however, the cecum is the least involved segment, although it is quite likely to develop a flare-up if it is preserved after the colon and rectum are removed. In addition, the blood supply to the cecum is largely dependent on the ileocolic artery, which is not sufficiently long to permit the cecum to extend to the anus. We question the feasibility of placing the cecum in the rectal canal for anastomosis to the anus, considering the high likelihood of recurrent colitis and the tenuous blood supply. Nonetheless, we are very interested in Dr Braslow's clinical experience and look forward to hearing more about his results over the course of time.

Lastly, we are unclear about the term *reflux enteritis* in an ileal reservoir after a pullthrough procedure. Reservoir inflammation or pouchitis is almost invariably related to fecal stasis in the ileal pouch. This is often due to rectal stricture or a long ileal spout.

ERIC W. FONKALSRUD, MD
Los Angeles

Hepatic Packing in Major Hepatic Trauma

To the Editor.—I read with great interest the recent article of Stain et al[1] in the October 1988 issue of the ARCHIVES. Although I certainly agree with their major conclusion, ie, that hemorrhage is the major cause of mortality in patients with severe liver injury, I must take issue with their relative condemnation of hepatic packing with planned reexploration for obtaining hemostasis in such patients. I submit a report of a recent case that supports the practice of hepatic packing in major hepatic trauma, including juxtahepatic venous injury.

Report of a Case.—A 17-year-old healthy male patient was involved in a motor vehicle accident May 18, 1988. He was admitted while in shock to a community hospital in rural Georgia. After a brief attempt at resuscitation he underwent celiotomy and was found to have exsanguinating hemorrhage from the liver. Due to the limited resources in this small hospital, no attempt was made to repair this injury, and the liver was packed and the abdomen closed. He was transferred by helicopter to Crawford Long Hospital of Emory University, Atlanta, Ga, a distance of 160 km, having received 6 U of packed red blood cells during surgery and transport.

On arrival at Crawford Long Hospital he was in hemodynamically stable condition. He was admitted to the intensive care unit and underwent transfusion with fresh-frozen plasma to correct coagulopathy. Complete evaluation at that time revealed a fracture of the right humerus and right iliac wing but no other injuries. There was no evidence of ongoing hemorrhage.

After a 36-hour period of stabilization, the site was reexplored on May 20, 1988, at which time he was found to have a massive stellate laceration of the right lobe of the liver, a tear of the right hepatic vein, and a tear of the retrohepatic vena cava, which had decompressed through the liver laceration. The right hepatic vein was ligated and the retrohepatic vena caval injury repaired using an atriocaval shunt. During this operative procedure there was significant blood loss and subsequent hypothermia, resulting in coagulopathy. Thus, no attempt was made at débridement of devitalized liver. The abdomen was again packed and he was returned to the intensive care unit for stabilization and correction of coagulopathy and hypothermia. The site was reexplored on May 23, 1988, and devitalized liver tissue was débrided. After this final procedure he required ventilator support for 5 days due to adult respiratory distress syndrome and required percutaneous computed tomographic scan–directed drainage of a right subphrenic abscess on the 14th postoperative day. Otherwise, his postoperative course was unremarkable.

Comment.—I feel that this case illustrates the value of hepatic packing in providing temporary hemostasis. During this period of temporary hemostasis, coagulopathy and hypothermia can be reversed and resources amassed to care for these devastating injuries. As noted above, packing can control even major juxtahepatic venous injuries, allowing temporary hemostasis. Hepatic packing clearly has a place in the management of liver injuries, as already noted.[2]

CHARLES M. FERGUSON, MD, FACS
Atlanta, Ga

1. Stain SC, Yellin AE, Donovan AJ. Hepatic trauma. *Arch Surg.* 1988;123:1251-1255.
2. Feliciano DV, Mattox KL, Jordan GL. Intra-abdominal packing for control of hepatic hemorrhage: a reappraisal. *J Trauma.* 1981;21:285-290.
3. Cogbill TH, Moore EE, Jurkovich GJ, Feliciano DV, Morris JA, Mucha P. Severe hepatic trauma: a multi-center experience with 1335 liver injuries. *J Trauma.* 1988;28:1433-1438.

In Reply.—Dr Ferguson's well-documented case demonstrates the value of packing a major hepatic and juxtahepatic venous injury in two clinical situations. The first indication was as a temporary expedient to permit transfer of the patient to a site more suitable for definitive treatment. We cited Blumgart and colleagues' report[1] in this regard; this clearly is a useful expedient. The second was to permit correction of hypothermia that develops intraoperatively with concurrent coagulopathy. Both Feliciano and associates[2] and Cogbill and associates[3] have reported favorable results with packing of the hepatic wound after repair of major venous injury with ensuing coagulopathy. The survival rates of their patients were 34% and 59%, respectively. We have recently had a favorable experience in a similar circumstance.

Both Feliciano et al[2] and Cogbill et al[3] and their respective associates also reported that packing was ineffective when undertaken as a desperation measure for continuing hemorrhage. This would be consistent with the experience that we reported. Perhaps the decision to pack should be made earlier in the course of the operation. Our report was not intended to condemn packing. The five patients that we treated with packing all died because of continuing hemorrhage. We stated, "This should not be interpreted as a condemnation of the technique and may reflect patient selection."

Additional reports that precisely document the nature of the hepatic injuries treated with packing will be important. Such reports, though relatively rare in the recent literature, should provide guidance for the selection of patients most likely to benefit from packing and for evaluation of results. This evaluation should include documentation regarding the value of packing in controlling hemorrhage from major exposed and unrepaired juxtahepatic venous and hepatic vein injuries.

Steven C. Stain, MD
Albert E. Yellin, MD
Arthur J. Donovan, MD
Los Angeles, Calif

1. Blumgart LH, Drury JK, Wood CB. Hepatic resection for trauma, tumor and biliary obstruction. *Br J Surg.* 1979;66:762-769.
2. Feliciano DV, Mattox KL, Burch JM, Bitondo CG, Jordan GL. Packing for control of hepatic hemorrhage. *J Trauma.* 1986;26:738-743.
3. Cogbill TH, Moore EE, Jurkovich GJ, Feliciano DV, Morris JA, Mucha P. Severe hepatic trauma: a multi-center experience with 1335 liver injuries. *J Trauma.* 1988;28:1433-1438.

Intestinal Malrotation and Midgut Volvulus With Intussusception: An Unusual Association

To the Editor.—Intestinal malrotation with midgut volvulus is an important surgical emergency in pediatric practice. Successful outcome of this clinical condition depends on prompt diagnosis and timely surgical intervention. Delay in diagnosis can lead to an increase in mortality and morbidity. Malrotation volvulus is associated with other anomalies of the gastrointestinal tract in 15% to 31% of cases,[1-3] but its association with intussusception is very rare. Two such cases of malrotation volvulus associated with intussusception are reported herein, and the literature is reviewed briefly.

Report of Cases.—Case 1.—An 8-month-old girl presented with a two-day history of bloody diarrhea, irritability, and green vomiting. Examination of the abdomen disclosed a mobile tender mass in the left iliac fossa with exaggerated bowel sounds but no distention. A rectal examination disclosed bright red blood. A plain abdominal roentgenogram demonstrated a dilated stomach and duodenal loop with a paucity of gas distally.

At surgery, an ileocolic intussusception was found and was reduced manually. After reduction of the intussusception it was seen that proximal gut loops were collapsed and twisted clockwise. The duodenojejunal junction was found to be on the right of the midline and a well-defined band of Ladd was seen. The small gut was derotated, a Ladd's procedure was performed, and an appendectomy was done. The postoperative period was uneventful.

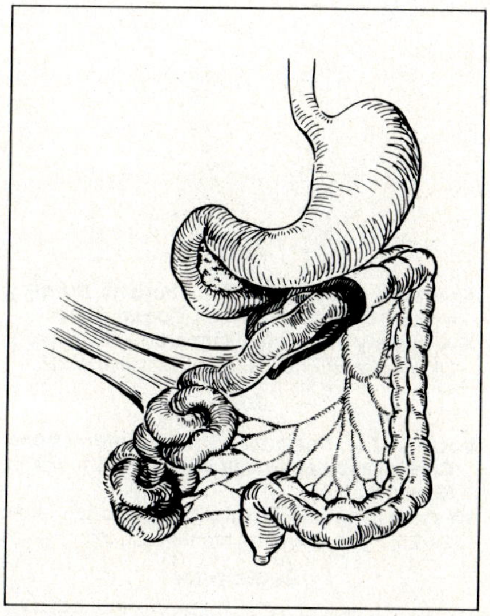

Diagram showing simultaneous ileocolic intussusception, volvulus of midgut, and band of Ladd.

Case 2.—A 1½-year-old boy presented with a seven-day history of green vomiting and a four-day history of blood passed through the rectum. Examination showed the patient to be moderately dehydrated. Examination of the abdomen disclosed a mobile tender mass in the left iliac fossa with exaggerated bowel sounds, without any distention. During a rectal examination the apex of an intussusception was felt. A plain roentgenogram of the abdomen disclosed a dilated stomach with no gas distally. At laparotomy an ileocolic intussusception reaching up to the rectum along with the band of Ladd and volvulus of the midgut were seen (Figure). Reduction of the intussusception, untwisting of the volvulus, Ladd's procedure, and an appendectomy were performed. The postoperative period was uneventful.

Comment.—Sporadic cases of intestinal malrotation associated with intussusception have been cited from time to time in many series.[1-4] Brereton et al[5] described malrotation of the gut in 40% of cases of intussusception, but the incidence of malrotation and midgut volvulus with intussusception is extremely rare; to my knowledge, only one case has been reported (by Ornstein et al[6]). Association of malrotation volvulus with intussusception can complicate management by causing gangrene of the gut if the volvulus goes unrecognized. Patients with intussusception with associated malrotation of the gut may present a confusing picture on hydrostatic reduction.[3] An absence of abdominal distention and a paucity of gas distally on an abdominal roentgenogram are two possible indicators that may point toward associated intestinal malrotation and midgut volvulus in a case of intussusception. If such an association is suspected, the case should be treated surgically instead of with hydrostatic reduction to avoid serious complications such as vascular compromise of the gut due to associated volvulus.

Sudhir Kumar Jain, MBBS, MS
Delhi, India

1. Stewart DR, Colodny AL, Daggett WC: Malrotation of the bowel in infants and children: A 15-year review. *Surgery* 1976;79:716-720.
2. Kiesewetter WB, Smith JW: Malrotation of the mid gut in infancy and childhood. *Arch Surg* 1958;77:483-491.
3. Filston HC, Kirks DR: Malrotation: The ubiquitous anomaly. *J Pediatr Surg* 1981;16:614-620.
4. Welch GH, Azmy AF, Ziervogel MA: The surgery of malrotation and midgut volvulus: A nine year experience in neonates. *Ann R Coll Surg Engl* 1983;65:243-247.
5. Brereton RJ, Taylor B, Hall CH: Intussusception and intestinal malrotation in infants: Waugh's syndrome *Br J Surg.* 1986;73:55-57.
6. Ornstein MH, Lund RJ: Simultaneous occurrence of malrotation volvulus and intussusception in an infant. *Br J Surg* 1981;68:440-441.

Fine-Needle Aspiration for Breast Masses

To the Editor.—If fine-needle aspiration is to make an economic impact on medical care, it must do so by eliminating surgery for benign lesions. This has been accomplished in the management of thyroid lesions, as documented in numerous studies.[1-3]

In the recent report from Seattle, Wash, published in the January 1988 issue of the ARCHIVES, this point was not made for breast fine-needle aspiration.[4] In fact, there were errors in the calculations presented in Table 2 of that report. If one defines "positive" as any result requiring biopsy and "negative" as indicating conservative close follow-up only, then the calculations are as appear in the accompanying Table.

Despite these adjustments, the persistent flaw of the study lies in the five fine-needle aspiration negative results that were biopsy positive. Other studies have shown better results.[5-7] One wonders whether increased proficiency with the technique of fine-needle aspiration could have reduced these. For this reason, many authorities have recommended that the pathologist collect the specimen, smear it, read it, and interpret it.[8] Only then will the goals of high specificity and, thereby, high negative predictive value be achieved, so as to impact maximally on the medical care system.

HOWARD GOLDMAN, MD
Martinez, Calif

Decision Analysis Values

Value	Definition (No. of Cases)	%
Sensitivity	True positives (93) / [True positives (93) + false negatives (5)]	95
Specificity	True negatives (23) / [True negatives (23) + false positives (19)]	55
Positive predictive value	True positives (93) / [True positives (93) + false positives (19)]	83
Negative predictive value	True negatives (23) / [True negatives (23) + false negatives (28)]	82

	Biopsy Positive	Biopsy Negative
FNA Positive	TP: 70 + 19 + 4	FP: 7 + 12
FNA Negative	FN: 5	TN: 23

FNA indicates fine-needle aspiration; TP, true positive; FP, false positive; FN, false negative; and TN true negative.

1. Miller TR, Abele IS, Greenspan FS. Fine-needle aspiration biopsy in the management of thyroid nodules. *West J Med.* 1981;134:198-205.
2. Hamberger B, Gharib H, Melton LJ, Goellner JR, Zinsmeister AR. Fine-needle aspiration biopsy of thyroid nodules: impact on thyroid practice and cost of care. *Am J Med.* 1982;73:381-384.
3. Van Herle AJ, Rich P, Jung B-ME, Ashcraft MW, Solomon DH, Keeler EB. The thyroid nodule. *Ann Intern Med.* 1982;6:221-232.
4. Adye B, Jolly PC, Bauermeister DE. The role of fine-needle aspiration in the management of solid breast masses. *Arch Surg.* 1988;123:37-39.
5. Frable WJ. Needle aspiration of the breast. *Cancer.* 1984;53:671-676.
6. Wanebo HJ, Feldman PS, Wilhelm MC, Covell JL, Birns RL. Fine-needle aspiration cytology in lieu of open biopsy in management of primary breast cancer. *Ann Surg.* 1984;199:569-579.
7. Gen HJ, Sprenger E, Dowlatshahi K. Stereotaxic needle localization and cytological diagnosis of occult breast lesions. *Ann Surg.* 1986;204:580-584.
8. Bottles K, Cohen MB, Sacks ST. Clinician perception of fine needle aspiration of cytology. *Diagn Cytopathol.* 1985;1:249-254.

Calendar of Events

April

Association College of Surgeons, (Spring), April 2-6, Boston, Mass.

Association for Surgical Education, April 5-8, Tampa, Fla. Local Coordinator: Dr Charles Cox, University of South Florida.

Society for Clinical Vascular Surgery, April 5-9, Innisbrook, Tarpon Springs, Fla.

Association for Surgical Education, April 6-8, Harbour Island Hotel, Tampa, Fla.

American Surgical Association, April 10-12, Broadmoor, Colorado Springs, Colo.

Surgical Infection Society, April 13-14, The Broadmoor, Denver, Colo.

Southwestern Surgical Congress 41st Annual Meeting, April 23-26, Hyatt Regency, Monterey, Calif.

May

American Association for Thoracic Surgery, May 8-10, Sheraton/Hynes, Boston, Mass.

The Society of Surgical Oncology Inc, May 21-24, Westin St Francis, San Francisco, Calif.

June

Society for Vascular Surgery/International Cardiovascular Society, June 18-21, Hilton, New York, NY.

Western Thoracic Surgical Association, June 21-25, Hyatt Regency, Monterey, Calif.

September

Society of Thoracic Surgeons, September 10-13, Convention Center, Baltimore, Md.

33rd World Congress of Surgery, September 10-16, Toronto, Canada. Contact: Congress Canada, 73 Richmond St W, Suite 300, Toronto, Ontario, Canada M5H 1Z4.

October

American Association for the Surgery of Trauma, October 5-7, Chicago, Ill.

American Society of Anesthesiologists, October 14-16, New Orleans, La.

American College of Surgeons (Congress), October 15-20, World Congress Center, Atlanta, Ga.

American College of Chest Physicians, October 30-November 3, Boston, Mass.

November

Western Surgical Association, November 11-14, St Louis, Mo.

American Heart Association, November 13-16, New Orleans, La.

Color Atlas of Head and Neck Surgery: Face, Skull and Neck, by Jatin Shah, 256 pp, with illus, $149.50, Orlando, Fla, Grune & Stratton Inc, 1987.

Head and neck surgery has become an increasingly complex field. Since it incorporates techniques in such fields as neurosurgery, maxillofacial surgery, oral surgery, and microvascular surgery, the practicing head and neck surgical oncologist needs to refine existing technical skills and constantly learn new ones. This volume, designed for the aspiring head and neck surgeon, attempts to fill that information gap; unfortunately, it only partly succeeds.

The volume is a photographic atlas of head and neck surgical procedures categorized by anatomic regions. It begins with some perfunctory chapters on operating room setup, anesthetic considerations, and basic surgical techniques.

The remaining chapters show intraoperative photographs of commonly performed operations, supplemented by a clearly written text. For the most part, the photographs, taken by the author, nicely document the procedure and take the reader through a clear description of how he does it. Where the anatomy or the procedure is particularly complex, simple line drawings are used to assist the reader. Unfortunately, none of the photographs is labeled, and several of the images would have been improved by one larger F stop or a closer, faster lens. For experienced surgeons, these deficiencies are not major. For the novice, however, it would be difficult to use this book as a guide to the cervicofacial landscape. I found the chapters on neck dissection and skull-base surgery to be particularly informative.

At a time when we have high-quality videotape, videodisc, and computer imaging, the surgical atlas still has a place. It is a convenient, readily accessible reference and does not require sophisticated viewing equipment. However, learning to perform an operation from still pictures is like understanding a movie by looking at the still shots on a marquee. Only by watching the flow of the action and the interrelationship of the anatomic characters in three dimensions can you appreciate the content and complexity of the surgery.

Despite its drawbacks, I would recommend this book for reference libraries and for the libraries of experienced surgeons. As the author acknowledges, the single-author approach has its advantages and disadvantages. Fortunately, for the reader, this atlas gives us the advantage of the many things Dr Shah has to teach us.

Arlen D. Meyers, MD
Denver

Limb Salvage and Amputation for Vascular Disease, R. M. Gleenhalgh, C. W. Jamieson, and A. N. Nicolaides, 459 pp, $125, Philadelphia, WB Saunders Co, 1988.

Amputation is the profession's equivalent to Chapter 11 for vascular surgeons; an admission of failure and occasionally the result of poor judgment. This book, edited by three distinguished British vascular surgeons, is an in-depth study of such disease progression and management failure.

Eighty authors from ten countries provide chapters on subjects ranging from the epidemiology of disease and anticipated clinical course following amputation to the need to use a multidisciplinary team in the management of amputee rehabilitation. It is interesting to note that despite the obvious enthusiasm for the team approach, no hard numbers are provided to prove its advantages. Obviously, it is logical to use all the help one can get from such ancillary services, but future studies should try to quantitate the advantages.

I suspect that this book in no way resembles what Professor McColl's Blue Ribbon Governmental Committee had in mind when it asked Gleenhalgh to review artificial limb and rehabilitation centers in the United Kingdom. This aside, the committee received full credit in the resulting publication. It contains a solid and supportive 92-page section involving the rehabilitation team and a compact 189-page critique of diagnostic and operating techniques valuable in managing patients with advanced arteriosclerosis and threatened with limb loss. Those who perform vascular surgery will of course benefit from this part of the book. The clinical setting results in many situations where the slightest mistake in judgment or flaw in technique may mean the difference between limb salvage and amputation.

The book addresses the classic problem of deciding what level of amputation should be performed or whether revascularization is worth a try. As has been the case so often in the past, the critical reader emerges from the discussions with admiration for the scientific ingenuity of the investigators, but also with a vague sense that such new techniques as magnetic resonance imaging, pedal arch arteriography, and transcutaneous oxygen measurement will probably be of no more value than have many other promising techniques that were touted during the past 20 years.

Faced with impending amputation, the vascular surgeon understandably grasps at even the most flexible straws. Mountaineers call such unimpressive support "vegetable belays." This book provides appropriate critical reviews of such adjunct topics as antiplatelet drugs, lumbar sympathectomy, and various forms of chemical vasodilators. If the vascular surgeon chooses to use these techniques, he should at least know the database of their performance.

It is interesting that only the last five pages of *Limb Salvage and Amputation for Vascular Disease* address the comparative cost-effectiveness of amputation and revascularization. This is a subject that primarily interests those who pay for health care. I believe that we surgeons are going to be forced to alter our focus on simple limb survival or graft patency and consider whether patients are more satisfied with repeated hospitalizations and operations or the alternative of amputation. Such redirection of our postrevascularization accounting system, I suspect, will bear out the advantages of attempts to save a limb. We should preempt the obvious criticism with additional reports analyzing the question.

Numerous texts have appeared during the past ten years pertaining to many aspects of peripheral vascular surgery. This is one of the better ones, concentrating as it does on vascular reconstruction and amputation.

B. Eiseman, MD
Denver

2V MEDTECH INTERNATIONAL CORP.

DIAGNOSIS 2V STAT™ TREATMENT

PRESENTS

2V STAT Medical Decision Support Software Covering 69 Specialties—Algorithms and Text.

PLUS

COMPUTER 80286/12 MHz Turbo CPU, 80 MB HD, EGA Color Monitor, Color Graphic Card, 40 MB Back-up Drive, and Printer.

$5962
(for complete system)

ORDER NOW!
1•800•228•STAT
Technical Support Call 1•404•956•1855

2480 Windy Hill Road, Suite 201 • Marietta, Georgia 30067
Fax 404•956•7068 Telex 551341 MedVideo EasyLink 622779660

FLORIDA, OKLAHOMA

General Surgery Opportunities

FLORIDA: Gainesville-based regional multi-hospital Healthcare System has immediate need for BE/BC general surgeons. Paid malpractice, salary guarantee, office space, moving expenses, others.

OKLAHOMA: BE/BC general surgeon needed to join multi-specialty group. Fee-for-service practice. Progressive, thriving, family oriented community. Excellent income potential and relocation package.

Contact:
Leonard Graivier, M.D. or
Tony C. Rasberry
1-800-336-2575
Physician Network of America, Inc.
8505 Freeport Parkway, Suite 130
Irving, Texas 75063
FAX 214/929-4568

Me Retire?

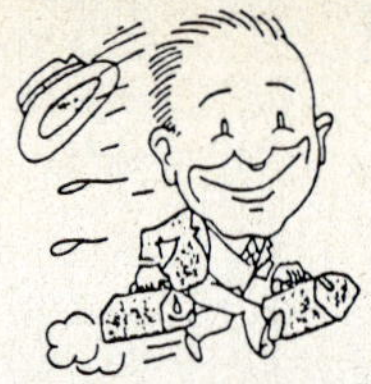

NEVER!

BUT RETIREMENT ULTIMATELY REACHES OUT TO ALL OF US

When should I retire, how do I retire, where should I retire, what does it "cost," have I saved enough, what will inflation do to me, what can I do in my spare time, what do others do in retirement, can my spouse "stand" me in retirement, can my spouse "retire" also?

DON'T TURN YOUR BACK ON THESE QUESTIONS . . . someday they will have to be answered.

THE AMERICAN ASSOCIATION OF SENIOR PHYSICIANS can help you get more out of your later years—medical retirement is our specialty, our ONLY specialty.

Get practical, authoritative, knowledgeable information to assist you in YOUR retirement.

- Bimonthly Newsletter
- Retirement Planning Seminars
- Literature Resource Center
- Part-time work or volunteer ideas
- Interesting travel opportunities
- Health Insurance
- Various medical magazines, auto rental & hotel discounts
- Guidelines for disposing of a practice

For a membership application and more details, write or call:

AASP
American Association of Senior Physicians
One East Erie Street
Suite 240
Chicago, IL 60611
312-280-7260

NON CARDIAC THORACIC-VASCULAR, ONCOLOGIC SURGEONS:

Board eligible/certified required for large multispecialty group in the San Francisco Bay Area. Competitive salary, excellent benefits and pleasant working conditions. Send CV with all inquiries to:

S. Ramachandra, M.D.,
Chief of Surgery
Permanente Medical Group
27400 Hesperian Boulevard
Hayward, California 94545

CHAIRMAN DEPARTMENT OF SURGERY

A 271 bed community hospital, located in a residential area of South Philadelphia, has a position available for Chairman of the Department of Surgery. We are a preferred affiliate of one of the major teaching institutions in Philadelphia with residents on rotation in Medicine, Surgery, Obstetrics and Gynecology, ENT and Emergency Medicine.

Located in close proximity to the Sports Complex, Philadelphia International Airport, major bridges and the interstate highway system, the Emergency Room is active in treating trauma and admits 60% of those patients to the Hospital.

Six newly constructed operating rooms provide the physicians with adequate space to perform in excess of 6000 surgical procedures per year. A very active Obstetrics Service delivers over 1700 babies per year.

Interested individuals should forward their CV to:

Frank A. Bove, M.D.
Chairman, Search Committee
Methodist Hospital
2301 South Broad Street
Philadelphia, Pennsylvania
19148

The New England Surgical Society

The surgical investigator must be a bridge tender, channeling knowledge from biologic science to the patient's bedside and back again. He traces his origin from both ends of the bridge. He is thus a bastard, and is called this by everybody. Those at one end of the bridge say that he is not a very good scientist and those at the other end say he does not spend enough time in the Operating Room.[1]

FRANCIS D. MOORE
1958

This issue of the ARCHIVES carries articles presented at the 69th Annual Scientific Meeting of the New England Surgical Society (NESS). Founded on February 5, 1916, at the Harvard Club in Boston, Mass, this society has a long and distinguished history in American surgery. Their indoctrination memorandum to new members states that

> the original members were not only leaders in New England in the art and science of surgery, but were also New England gentlemen. Further, the Society developed an ever-awareness that its chief concern was not what benefits may be conferred on its individual members but rather what the individual members working as a unit can accomplish for surgical practice in New England and particularly what they can do for the surgical welfare of the community at large.

The NESS has been blessed with distinguished leadership since the election of its original president, Samuel J. Mixter of Boston, and has included such stalwarts as Frank H. Lahey, Leland S. McKittrick, Francis A. Sutherland, Marshall K. Bartlett, Richard Warren (a former editor of the ARCHIVES, 1970-1976), John J. Byrne (current member of the ARCHIVES Editorial Board), Joseph Murray, Clement A. Hiebert, and its current president, James Foster. The most recent editor of the ARCHIVES, Arthur E. Baue, is a member of the NESS.

The presidency of this regional surgical organization is a distinguished and prestigious appointment for senior surgeons. Sixty percent of the NESS presidents were graduates of the Harvard Medical School, not a surprisingly high figure. Two former presidents of the NESS have been elected to the presidency of the American Surgical Association. Two have served as chairman and vice-chairman of the American Board of Surgery and nine as directors. Five former NESS presidents have been regents of the college, and two were elected to the presidency of the American College of Surgeons. In addition, eight were members of the Residency Review Committee (Surgery), and two were editors of major surgical journals. The ARCHIVES is pleased to publish the proceedings of the NESS for its readers and looks forward to a continuing, productive professional relationship.

CLAUDE H. ORGAN, JR, MD
Editor

1. Moore FD. The university in American surgery. *Surgery.* 1958;44:1-10.

Seldom Come By

The Worthwhileness of a Career in Surgery

Clement A. Hiebert, MD

The title of my essay is the name of a town a long way Down East, and my subject is the joy of surgery, the magic stuff, the grail that once moved every doctor in this room to become a surgeon and that even now beckons through the jading mists of tedium and time. Strip away the corrupting dullness and look afresh at our profession. I contend it to be the most splendiferous of all professions and will argue this: first, with a distant mirror on medical adventuring in a remote island setting and, second, with a hand lens applied to three wonders of the surgeon's world, wonders of the body, mind, and spirit.

THE SURGEON'S CHARMED LIFE IN A REMOTE SETTING

Come with me to Newfoundland, where, during the summer between the third and fourth years at Harvard Medical School, classmates, Jerry Foster and Arnold Nevis, and I first fulfilled our dreams to be real doctors. The time: 4 AM. The place: a rocky path in front of a fisherman's cottage on Twillingate, an island off the northeast coast. Icebergs loomed in the bay, and I shivered, partly from the chill of the night and partly at the prospect of my first home delivery. My doctor's bag had been carried by my father on innumerable house calls in the North End of Boston before I was born and, now more than two decades later, its cracked leather interior still smelled of ether and iodoform. The bag had been tested aplenty. Not so the new hands that carried it. As I walked up the rocky path, I hoped the baby would arrive before I did.

Minutes later, the child was born in an upstairs room that was illuminated by a faltering flashlight. Anxiety gave way to relief, but it was short lived. I lay the flashlight down, rummaged in the shadows for the cord, and was startled to grasp instead a tiny foot. For an instant, I thought it belonged to the child just delivered but whose presence at the foot of the bed I confirmed. "Twins!" I announced soberly. "Oh, dear," responded Mrs Pardy, "Do I have to go through all this again?" And with heart and soul I thought, "Oh, dear, do *I* have to go through all this again?" Why hadn't I paid attention to Duncan Reid's lecture on difficult obstetric presentations? Was the critical maneuver in the delivery of a footling breech flexion of the neck or extension? And what if I guessed wrong? Would this child die for my falling asleep during a third-year lecture? Mrs Pardy decided the issue by squeezing her baby straight out. Again, relief. And again, embarrassment. As I set about the details of tying off and wrapping up, Mrs Pardy asked me about "grease" for the babies. I was new to the Newfoundland dialect and innocent of the local practice of oiling the skin of newborns; I interpreted the word "grease" as a request to say *grace* for the twins. After that got sorted out, I tucked a baby under each arm and retreated down narrow stairs to the kitchen where children and relatives had gathered around the stove, that is, all but the father who was outside, operating in the predawn light on a pile of codfish. Ecstatically I called over, "You have *two*!" He barely looked up as he asked, "Are these your first?"

I learned three things from this experience: (1) a measure of self-reliance, (2) chance favors even the unprepared mind, and (3) the purpose of boiling water at a home delivery is so everyone can sit around afterward with a cup of hot tea.

Two weeks later, I gave open-drop ether anesthesia to the father during an operation for a strangulated hernia. I do not recall his asking me then, "Is this your first?"

Such was the stuff of an intensely memorable summer in an unspoiled land peopled by the sturdy followers of John and Sebastian Cabot who made their landfall in 1497. The struggle of Cabots' followers to survive and the loneliness of their lives in communities that were joined only by boat in the summer and dogsled in the winter are reflected in the names that they gave their settlements: Hell's Mouth, Wreck Cove, Come By Chance, Friday's Bay, and Seldom Come By.

Our hero teacher and near deity to the people of Notre Dame Bay was John Olds who first came to Newfoundland as a medical student from Johns Hopkins. On graduation, he returned to Twillingate where he founded a 150-bed hospital, trained nurses, a pharmacist-technician, made his own surgical instruments, and established a contract with the people of Notre Dame Bay for full hospital and

Accepted for publication December 14, 1988.
From the Department of Surgery, Maine Medical Center, Portland.
Presented as the Presidential Address at the 69th Annual Meeting of the New England Surgical Society, Montreal, Canada, September 17, 1988.
Reprint requests to Department of Surgery, Maine Medical Center, 22 Bramhall St, Portland, ME 04102 (Dr Hiebert).

home care for less than $10 per family per year. All of this took place 50 years before the idea of health maintenance organizations surfaced in the imagination of health planners in the United States.

The hospital cared for the medical needs of approximately 25 000 people scattered over 400 miles of coastline. The *Bonnie Nell*, a 60-ft floating outpatient department, was equipped with an x-ray machine, cook, skipper, nurse, and doctor, and plied the coast to care for the accumulated ailments of patients who lived beyond the daily working radius of the hospital. In the winter, this contracted to 20 miles, the distance a dog team could cover. As for Jerry, Arnie, and myself, we ordinarily made our house calls by open fishing boat, evading icebergs on the way. Standing in the bow, *Merck Manual* in hand, icy spray stinging our exposed cheeks and hands, we would shout our questions to the helmsman who more often than not was the patient's next of kin. In this way, we hoped that we might anticipate both the diagnosis and the remedy and be spared the embarrassment of surreptitious bedside research later.

One learned never to ask, "What is the matter?" For that would surely bring the rejoinder, "That is for ye to find out." Instead it was, "What does she find?" "Oh, doctor, she 'as a wonderful hake in 'er stomach." We encountered rickets, scurvy, and much tuberculosis. Tuberculosis was the dreaded word then much as cancer is now. Virtually every household had seen it. The best discoveries were something to be operated on. We became ambulance drivers, dentists, family physicians, pharmacists, x-ray technicians, anesthetists, and public health officers. Most of all, we were surgeons. Think of it! As third-year students, we did appendectomies, cesarean sections, and tonsillectomies, and we extracted countless teeth besides. Holding a retractor for an intern's first appendectomy during our fourth year at Harvard Medical School seemed pretty dull after that.

Before embarking on an operation, Dr Olds insisted that we affirm our diagnosis by dropping a quarter in a box that he called the "education fund." Only if that diagnosis were correct, was the coin returned. The box filled altogether too quickly. One day I asked Dr Olds to what purpose the fund was to be put. "That's for your education, son. So you will remember never to make that damn fool diagnosis again!"

Always a man of few words, Dr Olds was once the featured speaker at the dedication of the new Twillingate dock. His turn on the program came after numerous individuals from clergy to local businessmen had waxed long and eloquently on the multiple blessings that the new dock would confer on this fishing community. When Dr Olds' turn came, he stepped to the podium and said, "I really believe that everything that needs to be said about this dock has already been said," and he sat down.

THE THREE DIMENSIONS OF SURGERY

Now, let us put aside the distant mirror on this unforgettable excursion to the land of Seldom Come By, pick up the hand lens, and explore, in detail, the magic of the surgeon's life, the charmed life, which knows neither time nor geography, the life of the *body, mind*, and *spirit*.

The Body

We shall begin with physical activity—projects in the operating room. Our very name derives from the Greek meaning "to work with the hands," an activity that as long ago as Hippocrates was equated with success. Four centuries later, the down-to-earth Roman, Celsus, noted that there are three ways to treat a patient: diet, medicine, and surgery, but only surgery works.[1]

Surgery works, and we aspire to be part of things that work. We thrive on it and are nourished by it; operating restores the surgeon even as he or she restores the patient. A surgeon would rather work at his project in the operating room than eat, drink, or sleep.

There are *five attributes of a project*. First, it has a *beginning and an end*. It is something that you can look back on, as well as ahead to. Contrast working with organs to working with organizations. Bureaucratic undertakings have beginnings but seldom well-defined ends. Two exceptions are construction projects and crises, each of which, when completed or resolved, gives to administrators a satisfaction otherwise denied them in their endless swamp of committees and conferences.

Second, *the surgeon's project can be completed within a few hours*. Can you think of anything half so worthwhile, so durable, and so satisfying that one human being can achieve in the short span of "skin to skin?" Surgeons become impatient when the operation takes too long. A former third-year medical student named Larry Barrows once told me that he had just spent a steamy Saturday in the operating room watching a neurosurgical operation on a patient whose history and physical examination he had done. He had no other responsibilities for the case that proved unexpectedly difficult; usual courtesies were forgotten, the operation dragged on, and by the end of the 12th hour, our medical student was just about the only person who had escaped chastening by the surgeon. Unmasked at the end with his swarthy complexion showing, my friend heard the surgeon thunder, "And furthermore young man, the next time you come in to watch me operate, I want you to be clean shaven." "Sir," replied Barrows, "when I came in here, I *was* clean shaven."

A project has a third attribute of *stress to be overcome*, ie, a problem to be resolved. Two centuries ago, John Collins Warren wrote, from London, England, a letter to his father on this aspect of operating:

> Once, I remember you asked whether I intended to become a surgeon. . . . At that time, I had seen enough to have an idea of the difficulties of an operation, but none of its pleasures: now I see a good operation with the pleasure I used to feel at the successful solution of Euclid's problems, –a pleasure greater than almost any I know.[2]

A fourth dimension of a project is that it is *focused activity*, an attribute of all joyful times from climbing a mountain to playing a musical instrument. Surgeons take on one patient at a time, one organ at a time, and one bleeder at a time. Extraneous stimuli are excluded. Discipline and focus are dimensions of the surgeon's world of projects. Three examples: I once worked in a tropical hospital where the Bovie cord short-circuited and set afire the smock of the British registrar opposite me. I watched in amazement as he stolidly clung to the Deaver retractor while flames rose almost to his chin. Only then did he back off from the table, flapping at the fire with his gloved hands. At this point, the theatre sister admonished, "Jones, you are contaminating yourself. You will have to change!"

I recall watching Philip Allison, the regius professor of surgery at Oxford, operate with one foot on a switch that, when depressed, would illuminate a large sign in the gallery marked, "SILENCE!" Bombs could fall outside and, while any surgeon might crave silence, he would continue to operate without regard for anything but the project at hand.

Bombs did fall outside during the North African Campaign of World War II when the late Prof Ian Aird was operating in a field hospital in Gasr el Abid. No-man's-land was poorly defined, and at any given time, the hospital tent might be on one side of the line or the other. Professor Aird was operating on a wounded German commander when into the operating tent strode none other than Field Marshall Rommel. Aird's words:

> It was a strange and perhaps unparalleled scene—British doctors in captivity, German officers no longer arrogant, British blood flowing in, German blood flowing out, British shells falling on German tanks. . . .[3]

The surgeon asked if it might be possible to move the tanks a bit farther from the tent to reduce the ruckus, and Field Marshall Rommel, the Desert Fox, passed the order to move the panzer column 200 yd along.

The fifth and final dimension of the surgeon's relationship to his project is the quality of *in-chargeness.* For all the talk of team effort, operating is a solo activity, all the more so when speedy action is required. In any emergency setting, confusion is a function of the cube (N^3) of the number of people involved. (C.A.H., unpublished data, 1969). In his book, *Mortal Lessons,* Seltzer[4] makes the following observation:

> And he is *alone.* No matter how many others crowd about the mouth of the wound, no matter their admiration and encouragement, it is *he* that rappels this crevasse, dangles in this dreadful place, and he is afraid—for he knows well the worth of this belly, that it is priceless and irreplaceable.

We are the ones who are enfranchised to make this legal assault. We are the ones who make the responsible decisions. We are the ones who explain to the relatives operations that go well, and we are the ones who hold the relatives' hands when they do not. We are accustomed to success. Our colleagues know it and, from time to time, urge us to challenge an unbeatable enemy. But we know what we can do and what we can not do. The lines from Horatio at the Bridge by Macaulay remind us to be cautious: "Those behind cried '*Forward!*' and those in front cried '*Back!*'." "Spoken with all the courage of a noncombatant," Lamar Soutter would say.

Winston Churchill surely understood and identified with the *in-chargeness* requirement of the surgeon's life; on July 10, 1951, he proclaimed before an obvious audience:

> I can practice in an honorary fashion the arts of surgery and medicine. Unless there is a very marked shortage of capable men in both these professions, I shall not press myself upon you. No doubt in these difficult times, it will be a comfort, not only to the profession, but to the nation at large if you have me in reserve. I have not yet taken any final decision as to which of these beneficial branches I should give priority in case an emergency arises. Being temperamentally inclined to precision and a sharp edge, it might be thought that I should choose the surgeon's role.[5]

The Surgeon's Mind

Surgery is not a trivial pursuit. Close by the motor area of the brain that oversees hand function is the vastly larger region reserved for thinking. The surgeon's cerebral cortex has two zones: The first area is for clinical reasoning, and the second is for inventing. One locus discerns. The other discovers. The first unveils disease. The second unmasks illusions. The cortex for clinical stuff plods, ponders, and is purposeful. Its circuits hum away and, in the end, enables the surgeon to sing, "I do believe she'll make it!"

The cortex for inventing, on the other hand, is intuitive, unconventional, and less predictable. Its molecules toss, turn, wander, and wonder, while the inventor, himself slumbers and dreams until, at last, he or she awakens with the eruptive cry, "EUREKA!"

Koestler[6] believes that artistic creation has two poles that were epitomized by George Bernard Shaw's "90% perspiration, 10% inspiration" on the one hand and by Picasso's *Je ne cherche pas, je trouve* ("I do not seek—I find") on the other.

The New England Surgical Society is resplendent with the company of both kinds of discoverers. Our Picassos include the likes of Joe Murray who, before transplanting the first kidney, drew a mental picture of a man with three kidneys, and Jack Burke who can drape the human figure with artificial skin. Before transplanting these organs, both Murray and Burke transported their minds. We have other Picassos in our midst, and their "Eurekas" transport all our minds. We would rub elbows with them more often if we could.

Most members of this society are Shaw's 90% "perspirers." Our "eurekas" are spelled with a small *e,* and our reasoning is less conspicuous than the creative eruption of the inventor.

The *clinical* cortex has only once worn the Nobel crown, and that was in 1909, when the Swiss surgeon, Emil Kocher, received the Olympian honor. All the same, discoveries, problem solving, and our rewards happen everyday; the restored patient crowns us with joy and fulfillment beyond compare. On our intellectual activity hinge matters of life and death. The brain work is endless and involves us at home, at the desk, by the bedside, and in the operating theatre. We listen, look, probe, and peek. We ponder, diagnose, and test our hypothesis in a floodlit field where layer by layer we uncover and approach the moment of truth.

As Cassell[7] notes,

> Surgeons are rarely allowed the luxury of second thoughts; they cannot try a treatment, see if it works, augment or alter it, and then, if their first attempt is unsuccessful, try another approach. At the operating table, the surgeon must manifest decisiveness, certitude, control; emergencies must be resolved, unexpected findings anticipated, small advantages exploited.

The spleen, which hours ago had been proclaimed "enlarged," is found instead to be tiny and tucked away. Appendicitis turns out to be ileitis. The hypochondriacal neighbor has inoperable cancer. We are chastened, saddened, and wiser. The legal world has mistrials and processes of appeals. In sports, errors are expected, the second serve in tennis, four downs in football, and the "mulligan" in golf. Baseball parks proclaim errors on the scoreboard. Miscalculations of the surgeon are chiseled in the granite of graveyards, and the remembrance of them lingers in the solar plexus.

As a resident, I recall a young woman greeting me with the words, "Hello, Dr Hiebert," and then after a pause, "You don't remember me, do you? You took care of my baby." I remembered her but not in the proper context and replied, "Yes, of course I remember you. How is your baby doing?" Her response, "Don't you remember, doctor? He died."

Our balm is time and the cleansing agony of open confession before our peers. When he was a resident, George Richardson once began his report on the week's deaths and complications with a quotation from the second book of the *Aeneid* where Aeneas is asked by Queen Dido to give an account of himself after being washed up on the shore following a tumultuous voyage. Aeneas responded, *Infandum regina iubes renovare dolorem!* ("Unspeakable O Queen the grief thou bidst me retell!")

Whether in academia or "practicemia," all of us are involved in observing and thinking. Discovering means the uncovering of truths that have always been there but have been obscured by our clinging to comfortable but illusory ideas. As we add to knowledge, we also subtract from knowledge, knowledge overtaken by new certainties. How can we trust our senses? Does the left gastroepiploic artery really exist? (I have never seen it, at least as depicted in any standard textbook.) Where are the phleboliths of yesteryear? What ever happened to the "congenitally short" esophagus? Whither gastric freezing, uterine suspension, ligation of the internal mammary artery for angina, or excision of the carotid body for asthma? *Skepticism and curiosity.* Now there is a credo for surgeons!

We are the custodians of a tradition. Knowledge was handed to us, and we must pass it on, scrubbed clean, so as to leave the place better and brighter than we found it. The surgeon father of Gordon Scannell taught my father many years ago. Gordon helped me as a student and resident. My son, Timothy, in another discipline, was briefly the teacher of Gordon's only son. Three generations teaching one another! Can there be a keener joy than to overhear a resident use a phrase, pass on advice, or ask a question of an intern that we once taught the resident and that once was taught to us by Frannie Moore, Dr Churchill, Leland McKittrick, George Nardi, or Earle Wilkins? Taking time to pass it on is the rent that we pay for the privilege of being here. It is a fulfillment of the very title we wear; doctor (*docere*), after all, means to teach.

The Spiritual Bond

The final and finest offering of a career in surgery has spiritual dimensions. Like mountain climbers, bonded by fearful obstacles overcome, surgeons at their core are one. "Man is a knot, a web, a mesh into which relationships are tied. Only those relationships matter," wrote Antoine de Saint-Exupéry[8] in 1942. The fellowship of surgeons extends to all lands and to all ages. It is unique, and it delights and nourishes the soul.

The bonds that I speak of today are the ties with our patients. "Surgery is an irrevocably invasive remedy which links patient and surgeon more clearly than in other areas of medicine," notes Borsk[9] in his book, *Forgive and Remember.* Albert Schweitzer[10] spoke of the fellowship of pain, the invisible bond that unites all "those who bear the mark of pain," to which we might add, "and those who love and care for them." The exultation of pain relieved, life prolonged, and body restored is a celebration that goes on and on and is multiplied both by the quality of new life and its duration. Decades later, a patient may recall the very date of the event, especially if the surgeon has added caring to the curing. The prescription filled, the diet proposed, and the advice given less of an imprint.

Every person in this room could tell of innumerable instances where the poignancy of the relationship overshadowed the operation. Herewith are four illustrations.

One of the first patients to receive a permanent pacemaker at the Maine Medical Center was a woman who sailed through the modest procedure but who afterward came close to dying of totally unexplained coma. She required prolonged intubation and, eventually, a tracheostomy. Months later, she came to the office to confess that she had been jilted as a teenager and had resolved to hate men all her life, even to the point of not allowing those who attended her in the hospital to succeed. She had been overwhelmed by the care given, repented, and rejoined society, even to the extent of doing volunteer work in the hospital.

On a lighter note, a woman from Rumford rambled on through a similar procedure while she was under local anesthesia. She told one Maine story after another. At the end, I indicated that her operation was over and that her new pacemaker was working just fine. To which she responded, "Well, even if it isn't, we had a nice time didn't we!"

My career has included operating in a variety of faraway settings, including the Republic of Guinea in West Africa on the first of two tours with Project HOPE.

Two months after my return from Guinea, I was disembarking from a Boston-to-Portland flight and, by sheer chance, glanced around to discover that a former patient from Africa had been on the same plane. Traore Kabine, a 19-year-old schoolteacher, had somehow obtained an air ticket to America and traveled 7000 miles to search for the surgeon who had failed to correct his massive aortic insufficiency while in Africa. He spoke Sousou, Malenke, Foula, and French, and he had $25 in his pocket. It was apparent that he fully expected to be met, even though I had no inkling that he was on the way.

It was 1965, and our single, aging heart-lung machine was in diastole. Gordon Scannell, who also had been to West Africa on the HOPE ship, generously came to Traore's rescue and replaced his aortic valve at the Massachusetts General Hospital. The patient returned to Portland and remained with us for 5 months. We took him camping, which he regarded as the best part of his trip because it was "just like home!" I asked him one time, "What would you have done had I not been at the airport when you arrived?" He replied, "That could not have happened because my mother was at home praying we would meet!"

Some years ago, a frail couple in their 80s came to the office because the wife was concerned over her husband's newly acquired habit of belching. As it turned out, he had esophageal cancer. They were a dear and devoted pair; I remember their leaving the office, holding hands.

A year following an uncomplicated esophagogastrectomy, the patient's physician in Blue Hill, telephoned news of recurrent cancer. I thought about the socked-in mediastinum, the couple in their 80s, and the 300-mile round-trip required merely to repeat the sober news. I told the family physician to say that everything that could be done for the patient had already been done and that Blue Hill, Me, was the place to be. . . . The deaths of both patient and wife were reported in the news on the following morning. Somewhere in a bureau of Maine statistics are two death certificates, one listing the cause of death as murder and the other as suicide. Missing are the words: "abandoned and unconsoled."

EPILOGUE

We are nearly at the end of our quest for the essential truths of the surgeon's world. Our search began with a nostalgic look at a long-ago adventure in a Newfoundland fishing village where the only battle was with disease. There, in the springtime of life, in the land of Seldom Come By, we found joy and enchantment beyond compare.

From the seasoned vantage of later life, we have looked beyond the clutter of daily concerns at the three dimensions of surgery, projects of the hands, head, and heart. I have argued these to be the essence of the fulfillment that we seek.

Is the grail beyond our reach? Are we fettered forever by the mundane and the material? Can we recapture the sense of wonder and worthwhileness of surgery? Can we go home again?

Eight years ago, I returned to Twillingate. One of the twins, from my first home delivery, had died at 6 months, but his surviving brother heard that I was on the island and searched me out. He is a handsome fisherman. His parents had named him after me: not "Clement," but

"Hiebert"—in a land where *h*'s are not pronounced. The island has changed, thanks to a causeway that now connects it to the mainland. Dr Olds was then living, still at work, cussedly original, and independent as ever. The dusty hospital lane had been paved, and his old hospital replaced and taken over by the Canadian government. (Although the new hospital has an annual budget of $2 million, fewer patients are cared for now than in 1950, when Dr Olds was the sole practitioner with a total budget of $50 000!) The chief surgeon is a woman. "Did you train her?" I asked. "No, but I delivered her," was not unsurprising answer.

A tribute in the Newfoundland press on the occasion of Dr Olds' 75th birthday recalled an encounter with the surgeon who was riding horseback over the frozen Twillingate bright: "It was snowing at the time, he was holding a compass in one hand, and the reins in the other. He was traveling over the ice to visit a patient on New World Island."

"Excellence is a strange bargain," said John Mason Brown[11]; "Life owes us little; we owe it everything. The only true happiness come from squandering ourselves for a purpose."

The best kept secret in surgery is that to find fulfillment, you must lose yourself in something larger than the operative field and the luxury that it brings. The enchantment of the surgeon's life, the good practice, the bon practice is still there. Disease, pain, and suffering are the enemy; we fight back with hands, head, and heart.

I sit in the nurses' station where the resident makes signout rounds by touching each chart as he recites to his replacement, "The gallbladder in 308 is okay. Check the -lytes and the cardiac indices on the cabbage in 310." Stethoscope slung about the doctor's neck has displaced the staff of Aesculapius as the authenticating symbol, and Brownian movement around computer terminals has replaced the doctor's lonely walk up the path to the fisherman's cottage. I think of Dr Olds sitting on his horse in a snowstorm, compass in hand, making his way across the frozen bay to see his patient. And I recall that summer under the northern lights with Jerry and Arnie. And most of all, I remember the dawn when Mrs Pardy got twins, Twillingate two new citizens, and a fledgling surgeon a cup of black tea.

References

1. Majno G. *The Healing Hand, Man and Wound in the Ancient World.* Cambridge, Mass: Harvard University Press; 1975:253.
2. Churchill ED. *To Work in the Vineyard of Surgery, the Reminiscences of J. Collins Warren (1842-1927).* Cambridge, Mass: Harvard University Press; 1958:13.
3. McLeave H. *The Life of Ian Aird, the Surgeon.* London, England: Heinemann Medical Books Ltd; 1964:98-105.
4. Seltzer R. *Mortal Lessons, Notes on the Art of Surgery.* New York, NY: Simon & Schuster Inc Publishers; 1987:38.
5. Churchill W. *Never Give In, the Challenging Words of Winston Churchill.* Kansas City, Mo: Hallmark Publishers; 1967.
6. Koestler A. *The Act of Creation.* New York, NY: Dell Publishing Co Inc; 1967:120.
7. Cassell J. *On Control, Certitude, and the 'Paranoia' of Surgeons.* Dordrecht, the Netherlands: D Reidel Publishing Co; 1987:231.
8. De Saint-Exupéry A. *Flight to Arras.* New York, NY: Harcourt Brace Jovanovich Publishers; 1942:chap 19.
9. Borsk CL. *Forgive and Remember, Managing Medical Failure.* Chicago, Ill: University of Chicago Press; 1979:29.
10. Schweitzer A. *Out of My Life and Thought.* New York, NY: Holt Rinehart & Winston; 1949:268.
11. Brown JM. Quoted by: Gardner JW. *Excellence, Can We Be Excellent and Equal Too?* New York, NY: Harper & Row Publishers Inc; 1962:149.

In Other AMA Journals

ARCHIVES OF INTERNAL MEDICINE

Major Upper Gastrointestinal Tract Bleeding: Relation to the Use of Aspirin and Other Nonnarcotic Analgesics

Micha Levy, MD; Donald R. Miller, MS; David W. Kaufman, ScD; Victor Siskind, PhD; Pamela Schwingl, MS; Lynn Rosenberg, ScD; Brian Strom, MD; Samuel Shapiro, MB, FRCP(E)

In a hospital-based case-control study, the risk of a first episode of major upper gastrointestinal tract bleeding in subjects now known to be predisposed was assessed in relation to the use of nonnarcotic analgesics. For aspirin use within the week before the onset of symptoms, the rate ratio estimates, adjusted for potential confounding, were 15 (95% confidence interval, 6.4 to 34) for regular use (at least four days a week) and 5.6 (confidence interval, 2.7 to 12) for occasional use. For aspirin use discontinued at least one week earlier, the estimate was 1.6 (confidence interval, 0.6 to 4.2). There was no evidence that acetaminophen use increased the risk. For the regular use of other analgesics in the week before onset, the adjusted rate ratio estimate was 9.1 (confidence interval, 2.7 to 31); there were insufficient data to evaluate occasional use. The findings suggest that the risk of bleeding is increased substantially by aspirin, even when used occasionally. With the exception of acetaminophen, other nonnarcotic analgesics may also increase the risk, but they remain to be evaluated individually (*Arch Intern Med* 1988;148:281-285).

Reprint requests to Drug Epidemiology Unit, 1371 Beacon St, Brookline, MA 02146 (Dr Shapiro).

Lung Transplantation

Samuel Jason Mixter Lecture

F. Griffith Pearson, MD, FRCSC

In 1963, James Hardy and associates[1] of Jackson, Miss, published their report of the first human single lung transplant. Twenty years elapsed before the first long-term success with single lung transplantation was realized. In November 1983, a 58-year-old man with idiopathic pulmonary fibrosis received a right lung transplant,[2] and this patient has remained well. Since this first case, the Toronto (Canada) Lung Transplant Group has accumulated significant experience and achieved considerable success with both single and double lung transplantation in humans with end-stage lung disease. This presentation summarizes our effort and represents the work of a large number of individuals participating in a well-coordinated, multidisciplinary program. Joel D. Cooper, MD, has played a key role in the development and coordination of the present Toronto Lung Transplant Group.

HISTORICAL BACKGROUND

Using a canine model, Metras[3] in France and Hardin and Kittle[4] in the United States demonstrated the feasibility of single lung homotransplantation, and they defined operative approaches for this procedure that differ little from those in current clinical use. Our experimental studies in Toronto began in 1963 with the use of a canine model for single lung transplantation that addressed the issues of operative technique, posttransplant pulmonary function, and the fate of the interrupted bronchial circulation.[5-7] In 1978, we performed a transplant on our first human patient, a 19-year-old man who was ventilator dependent following an inhalation burn injury.[8] This young man died on the 19th postoperative day owing to necrosis and dehiscence of the transplanted bronchus.

Ours was the 31st patient undergoing single lung transplantation since the original patient of Hardy et al[1] in 1963. It was discouraging that only 1 of these 31 patients was discharged from the hospital and survived for 10 months following right lung transplantation.[9] Twenty of these 31 patients survived beyond the first postoperative week, and in 16 of these 20 survivors, significant airway complications were documented. These included mucosal ulceration, bronchial stenosis, massive necrosis, and dehiscence.

Impaired bronchial healing apparently was a major cause of failure in these patients. After our initial unsuccessful effort, Joel D. Cooper, MD, Toronto Lung Transplant Group, initiated a laboratory program to evaluate those factors potentially responsible for defective bronchial healing: rejection, immunosuppressive therapy, and bronchial ischemia. Initial experiments were done using a canine model of single lung autotransplantation that obviates any effects of rejection. Animals were randomized to a treatment group receiving the standard immunosuppressive therapy of that time (azathioprine and prednisone) and a control group that received no immunosuppression. Treated animals had significant bronchial complications, including ischemia, necrosis, and disruption of the bronchial anastomosis.[10] Later experiments showed that it was prednisone and not azathioprine that was responsible for the defective healing; also, cyclosporine did not have any adverse effect on healing at the bronchial anastomosis.[11] Further studies were undertaken to evaluate the role of ischemia that results from interruption of the systemic bronchial arterial supply in this experimental transplant model. It is important to note that the lung transplant is the only organ transplant in which systemic circulation (bronchial arteries) is not immediately restored at the time of implantation. Canine models for both autotransplantation and homotransplantation showed that enveloping the bronchial anastomosis with a pedicle of greater omentum resulted in an early and vigorous augmentation of the systemic bronchial circulation to the donor bronchus and significantly improved anastomotic healing.[12,13]

Encouraged by these laboratory observations, the advent of improved immunosuppression with cyclosporine, and reports of successful heart/lung transplantation,[14] our Toronto group cautiously reactivated the clinical program. In September 1982, a right lung transplantation was done in a young man with ventilator-dependent insufficiency due to herbicide (paraquat) poisoning.[15] This patient survived for 10 weeks, during which time a left lung transplantation was done because of herbicide damage to the transplanted right lung. At the time of death, both transplanted lungs were functioning well and the bronchial anastomoses had healed satisfactorily. Omentopexy was used to augment the bronchial circulation on the right side, and a pericardial pedicle was used on the left. This patient's death was primarily due to multiple effects of the herbicide poisoning that included widespread loss of skeletal muscle function. Failure was not due to complications in the transplanted lung, but rather to the underlying disorder and inappropriate patient selection.

CLINICAL EXPERIENCE: SINGLE LUNG TRANSPLANTATION

A review of past failures clearly identifies poor patient selection as a frequent contributing cause. Patients with pulmonary sepsis or emphysema are unsuitable for single lung transplantation since the remaining, diseased native lung may prejudice function in the transplant. Further exclusions include patients who are ventilator dependent, or cannot be maintained without continuing steroid therapy, and patients with multiorgan failure.

Patients with end-stage pulmonary fibrosis were considered the most suitable candidates for unilateral transplantation. Reduced compliance and increased vascular resistance in the native lung promotes preferential ventilation and perfusion on the side of transplantation, and there is usually no significant sepsis. Between November 1983 and September 1988, 16 patients with pulmonary fibrosis have undergone single lung transplantation. Ages range from 15 to 58 years. All but 3 patients had idiopathic pulmonary fibrosis. The exceptions had familial pulmonary fibrosis (1 patient), eosinophilic granuloma (1 patient), and sarcoidosis (1 patient). Use of conventional therapy, including corticosteroids, had failed in all patients; patients had a declining

Accepted for publication December 14, 1988.

From the Department of Surgery, University of Toronto and Toronto General Hospital, Canada.

Read before the 69th Annual Meeting of the New England Surgical Society, Montreal, Canada, September 17, 1988.

Reprint requests to Bell Wing 1-636, Toronto General Hospital, 200 Elizabeth St, Toronto, Ontario, Canada M5G 2C4 (Dr Pearson).

exercise tolerance and were increasingly oxygen dependent; and disease progression was judged to preclude survival beyond 12 months.

DONOR SELECTION AND PRESERVATION

The donor lung was considered suitable if the chest roentgenogram was normal, arterial oxygen tension exceeded 300 mm Hg on 100% inspired oxygen and 5 cm of end-expiratory pressure, and there was no evidence of airway sepsis at bronchoscopy. The recipient was matched for ABO compatibility but not for other histocompatibility factors. Suitable lung size was determined from a consideration of body weight, height, chest circumference, and vertical and transverse measurements of the thorax as determined from chest roentgenograms. In patients with pulmonary fibrosis, the diseased lungs are contracted and "undersized." It is therefore desirable to select a donor lung that is relatively larger than that of the recipient. Left lung transplantation was favored because the left hemidiaphragm will descend more freely than the right following implantation of an oversized lung. Preparation of an adequate atrial cuff on both donor and recipient organs is easier on the left than on the right side.

Preservation of the donor lung was achieved in all cases by simple immersion of the collapsed lung in Eurocollins solution at 4°C. Ischemic periods varied from 2 to 4 hours. We anticipate that improved preservation will be achieved in the future using the technique of flushing the pulmonary circulation with cold electrolyte solution in combination with vasodilator agents.

All recipients for single lung transplantation were prepared for possible assisted circulation during the operative procedure. In each case, the groin was prepared and draped in the operative field to permit access to the femoral vessels. In only 4 of the 16 patients, however, was it necessary to use partial venoarterial bypass for temporary circulatory support. Details of the operative techniques, immunosuppressive regimen, and the recognition and management of rejection have been described in previous reports.[16,17] Omentopexy was used to enhance the circulation at the bronchial anastomosis in all patients, and routine steroid therapy was withheld for 2 to 3 weeks following transplantation and was only administered in pulse doses for the management of rejection episodes.

RESULTS

Between November 1983 and September 1988, 16 patients underwent unilateral lung transplantation. The left lung was transplanted in 14 of the 16 patients. There were 4 postoperative deaths: 2 of the early deaths were due to selection of unsatisfactory donor lungs, 1 was the result of accidental venous air embolism on the 10th postoperative day, and the fourth was due to viral pneumonia with death between the third and fourth weeks. There were 2 late deaths: 1 patient died of chronic rejection and sepsis after 6 months, and another died of a B-cell lymphoma after 8 months.

None of the 6 deaths that occurred in these 16 patients was due to failure of healing at the bronchial anastomosis. A significant bronchial stricture did develop in 2 of the 10 long-term survivors, and in each of these patients, an area of necrosis and partial separation just beyond the anastomosis developed in the donor bronchus. In 1 patient, the dehiscence was noted at bronchoscopy on the 14th postoperative day and appeared to heal without functional obstruction during the next 4 weeks. Ten weeks following transplantation, however, the patient was readmitted to the hospital with fibrous stricture in the left main bronchus and an adequate airway could not be established by a combination of repetitive dilation and laser resection. The stricture was ultimately managed by insertion of an endobronchial silicone stent 8 months after left lung transplantation. This stent has remained in place and has provided a satisfactory airway for the past 3 years. In the second patient, necrosis and partial dehiscence at the anastomosis was identified at bronchoscopy on the 23rd postoperative day. A computed tomographic scan on day 34 demonstrated the dehiscence as well as a small abscess cavity on the outside of the bronchus at the level of the anastomosis. This space was well contained by the omental wrap and appeared to heal by secondary intention during the next 2 weeks. At 51 days after transplantation, however, there was an obvious stenosis due to granulation tissue. A silicone stent was used to bridge this defect as well, and a satisfactory airway has been maintained during the year that has elapsed since the stent was introduced.

FUNCTIONAL RESULTS

Pulmonary function, perfusion, and exercise performance data were obtained on all 12 patients surviving for more than 1 month. Pulmonary function studies included lung volumes, flow rates, diffusing capacity, and quantitative VQ scans. Exercise tolerance was measured by a modified Bruce protocol and by a 6-minute walk test. These studies were done before operation and at regular intervals following transplantation: every 3 months during the first year, every 6 months during the second year, and annually thereafter. Total lung capacity, forced vital capacity, and forced expiratory volume in the first second all improved rapidly during the first postoperative month. Continued improvement was observed thereafter throughout the period of follow-up. Lung volumes and flow rates returned to near-normal levels, and 80% of the improvement had been achieved at the end of the first postoperative month.

Quantitative ventilation perfusion scans demonstrated equal perfusion for the right and left lungs before operation in all but 1 patient. Within 1 to 4 days of transplantation, flow to the donor lung was either equal to or greater than that in the native diseased lung. Thereafter, there was a progressive increase in the relative flow to the donor lung: 75% donor lung perfusion after 1 month (7 patients), 78% after 3 months (10 patients), and 85% in 4 patients studied more than 18 months after operation.

Exercise tolerance improved dramatically in all patients. Before operation, six patients were quite unable to complete even stage 0 of a modified Bruce protocol, and all required supplemental oxygen in the range of 1 to 6 L/min. Eight patients were tested within the first month and again at 3 months, with performance ranging between stage 1 and stage 3 of the Bruce protocol. Maximal aerobic capacity was achieved within 6 months in most patients, although a few continue to demonstrate further improvement. Results of the 6-minute walk test were similar to those observed with the modified Bruce protocol. Supplemental oxygen was not required for any of the patients after transplantation during these exercise tolerance tests.

Diffusing capacity (DLCO-single breath method) averaged 36% of predicted normal before operation, improved rapidly within the first month, and increased to an average of 70% of predicted normal by the end of the first year. With the exception of one patient who suffers from chronic rejection, none of the function test results have deteriorated with the passage of time and sequential testing. More importantly, all patients have been able to resume a relatively normal and active life-style.

DOUBLE LUNG TRANSPLANTATION: BACKGROUND AND CLINICAL EXPERIENCE

Patients with bilateral pulmonary sepsis or emphysema are presently considered unsuitable for unilateral lung transplantation. A small number of patients with these conditions have been treated with combined heart/lung transplantation in a number of centers throughout the world. Many of these patients with chronic sepsis or emphysema have normal or recoverable cardiac function, and one can logically speculate that such patients would be best treated by replacement of both lungs without removal of a normal heart. It is known that rejection may occur independently and asynchronously in the heart and lungs of a patient who has undergone a combined heart/lung transplantation.[18] Coronary atherosclerosis may develop in the patient who underwent cardiac transplantation following either heart or heart/lung transplantation.[19] Furthermore, most donor hearts are used for the proliferating number of successful cardiac transplantation programs and this severely limits the donor pool for combined heart/lung transplantation. Isolated transplantation of one or both lungs obviously provides a donor heart that may be used in a separate recipient.

HISTORICAL BACKGROUND

In 1972, Vanderhoeft et al[20] in Belgium described a technique for en bloc simultaneous transplantation of both lungs in dogs. Dark et al[21] (including two physicians in our Toronto group) developed a successful model for simultaneous, bilateral pulmonary transplantation.[21] In November 1986, we performed our first human double lung transplantation in a 41-year-old woman with emphysema and α_1-antitrypsin deficiency.[22] This first patient is living and well as of September 1988, and an additional 12 patients have undergone double lung transplantation since this first effort.

PATIENTS AND METHODS

Between November 1986 and September 1988, 13 patients have undergone double lung transplantation. The underlying abnormality was emphysema in 8 patients (α_1-antitrypsin deficiency, 6 patients; bronchiolitis obliterans, 1 patient; idiopathic, 1 patient), bronchiectasis in 2 patients, cystic fibrosis in 1 patient, eosinophilic granuloma in 1 patient, and primary pulmonary hypertension in 1 patient. All patients suffered from progressive disability, were oxygen dependent or had experienced life-threatening episodes of respiratory failure within the preceding 12 months, and had an anticipated life expectancy of no more than 12 to 18 months. None were receiving corticosteroids at the time of transplantation and their conditions had been evaluated with extensive preoperative studies of pulmonary, cardiac, hepatic, and renal function, as well as a psychosocial evaluation. All patients were considered to have normal or recoverable cardiac function. Right ventricular function was evaluated noninvasively with echocardiography and nuclear angiography, and all patients selected for transplantation had a right ventricular ejection fraction greater than 20% using the first-pass method of nuclear angiography.

All patients selected for transplantation were entered in a rehabilitation and exercise program that included treadmill walking, cycling, weight training, and light calisthenics. Potential recipients from other communities established temporary residence in Toronto and participated in this rehabilitation program. Significant improvements in exercise tolerance were achieved in most patients.

DONOR SELECTION

Donors were less than 50 years of age and had no history of heavy smoking. Both lung fields were clear in the chest roentgenogram and there was no evidence of airway sepsis or purulent secretions identified by bronchoscopy. At bronchoscopy, specimens were obtained for Gram's stain and culture and served as a potential future guide for antibiotic management of the recipient. Satisfactory gas exchange required that the arterial oxygen pressure be greater than 300 mm Hg during ventilation with 100% oxygen and 5 cm of end-expiratory pressure. Donors were ABO compatible, but further histocompatibility crossmatching was not performed.

Because the emphysematous recipient lungs are grossly hyperinflated, it is desirable to obtain donor lungs of a size estimated to be appropriate for the height and ideal weight of the recipient.

In 5 of the 13 patients, the double lung block was harvested from a donor in an adjacent operating room. In the remaining 8 patients, the double lung block was harvested remotely from another center. Simple immersion of the donor lungs in cold Eurocollins solution (4°C) was our standard method for preservation, and ischemic times ranged between 2 and 5 hours. Eight of the 13 donor hearts were successfully harvested for cardiac transplantation in other recipients. The technique for separate extraction of the heart and the double lung block is described in a recent publication.[23]

OPERATIVE TECHNIQUE

Details of the operative technique were reported in a recent publication.[24] Exposure in the recipient is obtained by full median sternotomy with extension into the upper abdomen for mobilization of an omental pedicle that is used to envelop the tracheal anastomosis. The procedure requires full cardiopulmonary bypass with bicaval and aortic cannulation. Three anastomoses are required and are done in the following sequence: distal trachea, left atrium, and common pulmonary artery.

IMMUNOSUPPRESSION

Cyclosporine, 300 mg orally, and azathioprine, 2 mg/kg intravenously, are administered preoperatively. Initial postoperative immunosuppression consists of cyclosporine, Minnesota antilymphoblast globulin, and azathioprine. Cyclosporine is administered orally to obtain plasma trough levels of 150 to 200 ng/L using a radioimmunoassay method. Azathioprine is administered as a daily oral dose of 1 to 2 mg/kg per day, and antilymphoblast globulin is given in a continuous intravenous infusion, 10 to 20 mg/kg daily for 1 to 2 weeks, until adequate plasma levels of cyclosporine are achieved. Treatment with oral prednisone is withheld during the first 2 to 3 weeks and is then initiated at a dosage of 0.5 mg/kg per day. Suspected episodes of rejection are treated with three daily pulse doses of intravenous methylprednisolone, 500 to 1000 mg.

Maintenance immunosuppression consists of cyclosporine, prednisone, and azathioprine. Cyclosporine is gradually reduced during the first 6 months until plasma trough levels of 75 to 125 ng/L are obtained. Oral prednisone is reduced to a level of 12.5 mg/d.

RESULTS

Three of the 13 patients with double lung transplants have died, and all 3 deaths were directly attributable to major ischemia and necrosis of the proximal donor airway. All 10 surviving patients have been discharged from the hospital and are functioning well. All have achieved near-normal levels of pulmonary function, which was evaluated by sequential postoperative studies of lung volumes and flow rates, arterial blood gas analysis, diffusing capacity, and exercise tolerance tests (Bruce protocol and 6-minute walk test). To date, evidence of bronchiolitis obliterans has not developed in any patient and the improvements in pulmonary function and exercise tolerance have been sustained. The length of follow-up in many of these patients, however, is very short, and it is premature to make judgments regarding long-term performance and late complications.

AIRWAY COMPLICATIONS

In contrast to the good bronchial healing observed in most patients undergoing unilateral transplantation, a serious impairment of airway healing has occurred in 7 of the 13 patients with double lung transplants. In 3 patients, this complication was the primary cause of failure and death. In each of these 3 patients, there was evidence of marked ischemia of the donor trachea, carina, and left main bronchus within the first postoperative week. Separation at the tracheal anastomosis and distal airway necrosis ensued. One patient died after 22 days of hemoptysis due to erosion of a major vessel. In a second patient, retransplantation was performed on the 14th postoperative day, and the patient died 2 days later of graft failure. The third patient was considered a candidate for retransplantation, but a suitable donor was not found and the patient died of chronic pulmonary sepsis on the 72nd day.

Four of the 10 surviving patients had defective healing at the tracheal anastomosis. In 1 of these 4, a posterior defect in the membranous trachea at the level of the anastomosis was apparent during the first postoperative week. This defect appeared to heal spontaneously by the end of the first month, and the airway has remained healthy and patent since. The other 3 surviving patients, however, have all had strictures develop in the donor airway that involve the proximal left main bronchus, the carina, and tracheal anastomosis. The development of stenosis was quite delayed in these patients and was not recognized until 2½, 3, and 4 months, respectively. All three of these strictures proved unmanageable by bronchoscopic dilation and have required insertion of a silicone tracheobronchial Y-shaped stent. A detailed report of these airway complications will be provided in a forthcoming publication.

COMMENT

It is apparent that some patients with end-stage lung disease can be effectively treated by lung transplantation. Factors critical to success include strict selection criteria for both donors and recipients, attention to technical details, improved immunosuppression, and avoidance of perioperative corticosteroids. A comprehensive transplant program will include the capability of single lung, double lung, and combined heart/lung transplantation.

Unilateral transplantation is effective treatment for patients with end-stage pulmonary fibrosis. In patients followed up for longer than 4 years, near-normal pulmonary function has been sustained, and the late complication of bronchiolitis obliterans has yet to be documented in any of our survivors. The use of omentopexy and the withholding of perioperative corticosteroids has resulted in good bronchial healing in most patients. In two patients in whom ischemic strictures in the donor bronchus did develop, the complication has been managed effectively with bronchoscopic dilation and insertion of an endobronchial silicone stent.

During the relatively short period of follow-up since the first double lung transplant was done in November 1986, good functional results have been obtained and the complication of bronchiolitis obliterans has not been documented. Donor airway ischemia, however, remains a major problem with the current model of double lung replacement. Seven of 13 patients suffered complications of proximal airway ischemia that proved fatal in 3 of the 7 patients. Omentopexy alone seems insufficient to reliably augment the blood supply to the short segment of donor trachea and the proximal main bronchi. Alternative models are desirable to resolve this problem in the future. Although technically difficult, it is possible to carry the systemic bronchial arterial circulation with the double lung transplant. If successful, this would ensure circulation at system pressures to the proximal donor airway. Another option is preservation of the entire recipient trachea and carina and reconstruction of the airway with two separate bronchial anastomoses. With this model, the resultant ischemic defect should be comparable to that observed in single lung transplantation.

Heart/lung transplantation is the appropriate operation for patients with irreversible cardiac and pulmonary disease. There is, however, clinical and experimental evidence that suggests that the adverse effects of pulmonary hypertension on the right ventricle may be reversible in some patients following restoration of normal pulmonary vascular resistance. In such patients with primary pulmonary hypertension and reversible cardiac disease, either single or double lung transplantation may offer a promising alternative.

This report provides a summary of the current experience in Toronto with lung transplantation. As stated in the introduction, this work has been accomplished by a large and well-coordinated multidisciplinary group of physicians, nurses, and other health care workers. The members of the Toronto Lung Transplant Group are as follows: *Surgery:* Joel D. Cooper, MD, Bernard S. Goldman, MD, Melvyn Goldberg, MD, Robert J. Ginsberg, MD, F. Griffith Pearson, MD, G. Alexander Patterson, MD, Hugh E. Scully, MD, Thomas R. J. Todd, MD, Paul Waters, MD; *Immunology:* Phillip Halloran, MD; *Anesthesia:* Wilfred DeMajo, MD, Vite Zulys, MD; *Hematology:* Michael F. Glynn, MD; *Infectious Disease:* Hiller Velland, MD; *Pathology:* Dean Chamberlain, MD; *Physiotherapy:* Cheryl Dear, Anne Kuus; *Psychiatry:* J. Craven, MD, Jane Bright, MSW; *Organ Donor Coordinator:* Judy Boychuk, RN; *Transplant Coordinator:* Kandy Rogers, RN.

References

1. Hardy JD, Webb WR, Dalton ML, Walker GR. Lung homotransplantation in man. *JAMA.* 1963;186:1065-1074.
2. Cooper JD, Pearson FG, Patterson GA, et al. Technique of successful lung transplantation in humans. *J Thorac Cardiovasc Surg.* 1987;93:173-181.
3. Metras H. Note preliminaire sur la graffe totale du poumon chez le chien. *Fr Acad Sci.* 1950;230:1176-1177.
4. Hardin CA, Kittle F. Experiences with transplantation of the lung. *Science.* 1954;119:97-98.
5. Stone RM, Ginsberg RJ, Colapinto FM, Pearson FG. Bronchial artery regeneration after radical hilar stripping. *Surg Forum.* 1966;17:109-110.
6. Pearson FG, Goldberg M, Stone RM, Colapinto RF. Bronchial arterial circulation restored after reimplantation of canine lung. *Can J Surg.* 1970; 13:243-250.
7. Andrews MJ, Pearson FG. The relation of bronchial arterial circulation and other factors to the transient defect in oxygen uptake following autotransplantation of the canine lung. *Can J Surg.* 1973;16:1-33.
8. Nelems JM, Rebuck AS, Cooper JD, Goldberg M, Halloran PF, Vellen H. Human lung transplantation. *Chest.* 1980;78:569-573.
9. Derom F, Barbier F, Ringoir S, et al. Ten-month survival after lung homotransplantation in man. *J Thorac Cardiovasc Surg.* 1971;61:835-846.
10. Lima O, Cooper JD, Peters WJ, et al. Effects of methylprednisolone and azathioprine on bronchial healing following lung autotransplantation. *J Thorac Cardiovasc Surg.* 1981;82:211-215.
11. Goldberg M, Lima O, Morgan E, et al. A comparison between cyclosporin A and methylprednisolone plus azathioprine on bronchial healing following canine lung allotransplantation. *J Thorac Cardiovasc Surg.* 1983;85:821-826.
12. Dubois P, Choiniere L, Cooper JD. Bronchial omentopexy in canine lung allotransplantation. *Ann Thorac Surg.* 1984;38:211-214.
13. Morgan WE, Lima O, Goldberg M, Ayabe H, Ferdman A, Cooper JD. Improved bronchial healing in canine left lung reimplantation using omental pedicle wrap. *J Thorac Cardiovasc Surg.* 1983;85:134-139.
14. Reitz DA, Wallwork JL, Hunt SA, et al. Heart-lung transplantation: successful therapy for patients with pulmonary vascular disease. *N Engl J Med.* 1982;306:557-564.
15. Toronto Lung Transplant Group. Sequential bilateral lung transplantation for paraquat poisoning. *J Thorac Cardiovasc Surg.* 1985;89:734-742.
16. Toronto Lung Transplant Group. Unilateral lung transplantation for pulmonary fibrosis. *N Engl J Med.* 1986;314:1140-1145.
17. Toronto Lung Transplant Group. Experience with single lung transplantation for pulmonary fibrosis. *JAMA.* 1988;259:2258-2262.
18. Griffith BP, Hardesty RL, Trento A, Bahnson HT. Asynchronous rejection of heart and lungs following cardiopulmonary transplantation. *Ann Thorac Surg.* 1985;40:488-493.
19. Dawkins KD, Jamieson SW, Hunt SA, et al. Long-term results, hemodynamics and complications after combined heart-lung transplantation. *Circulation.* 1985;71:919-926.
20. Vanderhoeft P, Dubois A, Lauvan N, et al. Bloc allotransplantation of both lungs with pulmonary trunk and left atrium in dogs. *Thorax.* 1972; 27:415-419.
21. Dark JH, Patterson GA, Al-Jilaihawi AN, Hsu H, Cooper JD. Experimental en bloc double-lung transplantation. *Ann Thorac Surg.* 1986; 42:394-398.
22. Patterson GA, Cooper JD, Dark JH, Jones MT, and the Toronto Lung Transplant Group. Experimental and clinical double-lung transplantation. *J Thorac Cardiovasc Surg.* 1988;95:70-74.
23. Todd TR, Goldberg M, Kosajl A, et al. Separate extraction of cardiac and pulmonary grafts from a single organ donor. *Ann Thorac Surg.* 1988; 46:356-359.
24. Patterson GA, Cooper JD, Goldman B, et al. Technique of successful clinical double-lung transplantation. *Ann Thorac Surg.* 1988;45:626-633.

Papers Read Before the 69th Annual Meeting of the New England Surgical Society, Montreal, Canada, Sept 15 to Sept 17, 1988

Management of General Surgical Complications Following Cardiac Transplantation

Verdi J. DiSesa, MD; Robert L. Kirkman, MD; Nicholas L. Tilney, MD; Gilbert H. Mudge, MD; John J. Collins, Jr, MD; Lawrence H. Cohn, MD

• Between February 1984 and May 1988, 55 patients underwent orthotopic cardiac transplantation at the Brigham and Women's Hospital, Boston, Mass. Basic immunosuppression was accomplished with steroid and cyclosporine therapies. Twelve patients suffered 14 major complications, including perforated ulcer in 3 patients; pancreatitis in 3 patients; pneumatosis coli in 2 patients; and cholecystitis, colonic necrosis, appendicitis, incarcerated umbilical hernia, pancreatic abscess, and toxic epidermal necrolysis in 1 patient each. Aggressive management of the patients included laparotomy in all but 2 patients with mild pancreatitis and the patient with toxic epidermal necrolysis, who was treated as a patient with a severe burn. In all of the patients, there was a resolution of these complications, except in one 59-year-old man with fatal hemorrhagic pancreatitis. Eleven of the 14 complications occurred during the initial hospitalization. The fatal case of pancreatitis was 1 of 5 (9%) operative mortalities in the entire series. Fifty operative survivors have been followed up for an average of 19 months, with four late deaths (8%) related to rejection. The actuarial probability of survival in patients discharged from the hospital was 90% at 12, 24, and 48 months.

(*Arch Surg.* 1989;124:539-541)

General surgical complications following kidney transplantation have been well documented.[1-8] Patients undergoing cardiac transplantation also may be prone to significant complications, requiring the care of a general surgeon, especially in the early postoperative period.[9-12] All patients undergoing cardiac transplantation have end-stage heart failure prior to their surgery. The resulting preoperative catabolic state may predispose these patients to postoperative complications. In addition, all patients undergoing cardiac transplantation are given high doses of immunosuppressive drugs, which have been associated with potential surgical problems. Other drugs commonly given to these patients may also have substantial toxicity. Patients undergoing heart transplantation also are exposed to potential complications of cardiopulmonary bypass and may have underlying atherosclerotic cardiovascular disease that contributes to postoperative difficulties.

Accepted for publication December 13, 1988.

From the Departments of Surgery (Drs DiSesa, Kirkman, Tilney, Collins, and Cohn) and Medicine (Dr Mudge), Brigham and Women's Hospital, Boston, Mass.

Read before the 69th Annual Meeting of the New England Surgical Society, Montreal, Canada, September 17, 1988.

Reprint requests to Brigham and Women's Hospital, 75 Francis St, Boston, MA 02115 (Dr DiSesa).

When potentially catastrophic complications do occur following cardiac transplantation, management is made more difficult by the patient's catabolic state and the need for immunosuppressive drugs. These conditions may retard postoperative healing and may predispose the patient to infectious complications if general surgical intervention is required.

We reviewed the successful management of general surgical complications during the first 4 years of our experience at the Brigham and Women's Hospital, Boston, Mass, caring for patients having cardiac transplantations.

PATIENTS AND METHODS

The charts of all patients undergoing cardiac transplantation who had surgery between February 1984 (when our program was initiated) and May 1988 were reviewed. Particular attention was directed to the management of complications that would require patients to consult with a general surgeon. The outcome in this subset of patients and in all patients who had cardiac transplantation were analyzed.

RESULTS

Fifty-five patients underwent orthotopic cardiac transplantation during this period. There were 43 men and 12 women with a mean age of 40 years (range, 14 to 61 years). A preoperative diagnosis to determine the cause of heart failure indicated idiopathic cardiomyopathy in 30 patients, coronary artery disease in 22 patients, and other conditions, including valvular heart disease and congenital heart disease, in 3 patients. Immunosuppression was achieved with cyclosporine therapy, with the dosage adjusted to maintain serum levels between 100 and 200 ng/mL, and prednisone, initially administered at 1 mg/kg and tapered to 0.5 mg/kg at the time of hospital discharge. In patients with persistent rejection despite this therapy, or in patients who developed azotemia related to cyclosporine use, azathioprine was added to the regimen. Episodes of rejection documented histologically on endomyocardial biopsy were initially treated with a 3-day steroid pulse. Steroid-resistant rejection episodes were treated with either rabbit polyclonal antithymocyte (ATG) or commercially available murine monoclonal antithymocyte (OKT3).

Twelve patients had 14 major complications requiring general surgical intervention. Eleven of the 14 complications occurred during the initial hospitalization within 30 days of the transplantation procedure, 1 occurred after 90

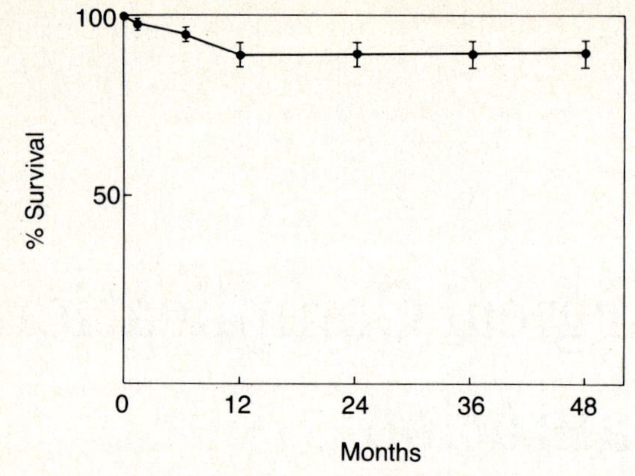

Actuarial probability of survival following cardiac transplantation in 50 patients discharged from the hospital.

days, another after 8 months, and the other after 14 months. Complications included perforated ulcer in 3 patients; pancreatitis in 3 patients; colonic pneumatosis in 2 patients, 1 of whom had cytomegalovirus infection of the colon; and cholecystitis, colonic necrosis, appendicitis, incarcerated umbilical hernia, pancreatic abscess, and toxic epidermal necrolysis (TEN) in 1 patient each. Ten patients had abdominal pain with mild to moderate distention as their presenting manifestation of intra-abdominal disease. One patient with colonic pneumatosis was asymptomatic. Free intraperitoneal air was detected on a chest roentgenogram obtained when this patient was admitted for treatment of rejection. Roentgenographic findings in other patients were nonspecific. The patient with TEN presented with a 70% second-degree burn and rapidly developed burn-wound sepsis. Only 2 patients had an initial body temperature greater than 37.8°C and white blood cell counts ranged from 8.2 to 27.1×10^9/L, with a mean of 16.4×10^9/L.

Surgical intervention included laparotomy in 11 patients with intra-abdominal complications. The surgical procedure employed included oversewing of ulcer in 3 patients; pancreatic drainage in 2 patients; colectomy in 3 patients; and appendectomy, repair of umbilical hernia, and cholecystectomy in 1 patient each. All patients requiring laparotomy had intensive antibiotic and nutritional support. Immunosuppressive drugs were given parenterally with adjusted dosages until patients could resume oral intake. The patient with cytomegalovirus infection and colonic pneumatosis also underwent systemic antiviral therapy. Temporary ileostomy or colostomy was performed when the bowel was resected. Two patients with milder pancreatitis were treated with nasogastric suction and parenteral nutrition. The patient with TEN had intensive burn therapy with occlusive dressings, including heterograft skin, antibiotic therapy, and intensive nutritional support.

Eleven of the 12 patients survived and are alive without sequelae 3 to 36 months postoperatively. All have normal gastrointestinal function. One patient with severe hemorrhagic pancreatitis died 27 days after transplantation due to unremitting intra-abdominal sepsis and hemorrhage.

The overall operative mortality in the 55 patients who had heart transplantation during this period was 9% (5/55), including the 1 patient who died of complications from hemorrhagic pancreatitis. The incidence of late death was 8% (4/50). All late deaths were in patients with severe recurrent rejection episodes, 1 of whom also had substantial graft atherosclerosis. Mean follow-up for 50 operative survivors was 19 months (range, 1 to 51 months). The actuarial survival of patients discharged from the hospital was 90% at 12, 24, and 48 months (Figure).

COMMENT

In 1968, Penn and colleagues[1] reviewed surgically correctable intra-abdominal complications following renal transplantation. These authors documented the significant incidence of these complications and advocated an early and aggressive approach to their therapy. Early recognition and vigorous intervention were also seen to be the keys to improved results in a review by Hau and associates[13] from the University of Minnesota, Minneapolis. Notably, they observed a mortality rate of 78.5% in patients undergoing renal transplantation with peritoneal infections. As noted previously, upper and lower intestinal complications have been observed following kidney transplantation.[2-8]

Pancreatitis and intestinal complications have also been seen after heart and heart-lung transplantation.[9-12,14] The causes of these complications are not well understood. The use of immunosuppressive drugs, both in the context of transplantation and in other settings, has been associated with pancreatitis, intestinal necrosis, and perforation.[15-17] Not only may immunosuppressive drugs render patients receiving transplants prone to these types of complications, but they clearly increase the hazards of surgical intervention when complications do arise. The high mortality rates observed in other series may reflect the impaired inflammatory response associated with high-dose steroids, cyclosporine, and other immunosuppressive agents.

Other factors that may contribute to the incidence of intestinal perforation and necrosis and the development of pancreatitis include the patients' debilitated preoperative condition. All patients undergoing cardiac transplantation have end-stage heart failure preoperatively. The associated circulatory and nutritional deficits may make patients more susceptible to intra-abdominal complications after the stress of a major operation. Cardiopulmonary bypass may also contribute to the development of these complications. In the past, pancreatitis was thought to be a complication of cardiopulmonary bypass, although today this complication is rare after routine cardiac operations. Finally, many patients undergoing cardiac transplantation have underlying atherosclerotic cardiovascular disease. Based on this, intestinal ischemia may contribute to the development of intra-abdominal complications.

In addition to immunosuppressive drugs, patients receiving transplants are exposed to a variety of other pharmacologic agents, including antibiotics used for long-term suppression of opportunistic infections. These, particularly trimethoprim-sulfamethoxazole, have been associated with the development of TEN.[18,19] Trimethoprim-sulfamethoxazole is used routinely for prophylaxis in patients receiving transplants, and our patient with TEN was taking this drug when the syndrome developed. Toxic epidermal necrolysis has also been associated with the use of anticonvulsant drugs, agents to which these patients may be exposed. Aggressive burn therapy with vigorous nutritional support and rapid wound coverage are recommended for treatment of this devastating problem.[20-22] These measures were successful in our immunosuppressed patient who had a 70% partial-thickness skin loss.

The diagnosis of these complications requires a high index of suspicion. As noted, immunosuppressive drugs may blunt the response to major catastrophes, particularly intra-abdominal inflammatory disease. When these occur in the early postoperative period after cardiac transplantation, they must be differentiated from the functional gastrointestinal disturbances that often accompany cardiac surgery. This is especially important since many of these patients are relatively immobilized preoperatively and may not have normal gastrointestinal function before the transplant procedure.

Our experience documents that an aggressive approach to countering major general surgical complications following cardiac transplantation can lead to a high degree of success with resolution of the complications and resumption of normal life. Aggressive intervention and early general surgical consultation is crucial for prompt recognition of these complications when they occur. Systemic signs may be few despite substantial inflammatory disease. Multiple factors may contribute to the development of these complications, including the immunosuppressive and other drugs that are required after cardiac transplantation. The preoperative catabolic state of many of the patients combined with the stress of cardiopulmonary bypass and open cardiac surgery may further predispose these individuals to substantial complications.

When conservative measures fail, early operative intervention, including laparotomy when intra-abdominal disease is suspected, can be lifesaving. Meticulous attention to surgical technique and postoperative nutritional support can minimize secondary complications. Immunosuppressive drug therapy must be continued to preserve the graft, but often the dosages have to be adjusted, especially when medication must be given parenterally. Similar aggressive wound and nutritional support has been effective in treating major losses of dermal integrity. Our patients with appendicitis and spontaneous pneumatosis occurring months after transplantation emphasize that patients postoperatively remain susceptible to other major illnesses despite adequate rehabilitation. Persistent and meticulous surgical care can lead to a successful outcome in immunosuppressed patients in whom potentially catastrophic general surgical complications occur following cardiac transplantation.

References

1. Penn I, Groth CG, Brettschneider L, Martin AJ Jr, Maarchioro TL, Starzl TE. Surgically correctable intra-abdominal complications before and after renal homotransplantation. *Ann Surg.* 1968;168:865-870.
2. Archibald ST, Jirsch DW, Bear RA. Gastrointestinal complications of renal transplantation, I: the upper gastrointestinal tract. *CMA Journal.* 1978;119:1291-1296.
3. Archibald SD, Jirsch DW, Bear RA. Gastrointestinal complications of renal transplantation, II: the colon. *CMA Journal.* 1978;119:1301-1314.
4. Powis SJA, Barnes AD, Dawson-Edwards P, Thompson H. Ileocolonic problems after cadaveric renal transplantation. *Br Med J.* 1972;1:99-101.
5. Thompson WM, Seigler HF, Rice RP. A complication following renal transplantation. *AJR.* 1975;125:723-730.
6. Guice K, Rattazzi LC, Marchioro TL. Colon perforation in renal transplant patients. *Am J Surg.* 1979;138:43-48.
7. Demling RH, Salvatierra O Jr, Belzer FO. Intestinal necrosis and perforation after renal transplant. *Arch Surg.* 1975;110:251-253.
8. Hadjiyannakis EJ, Samellie WAB, Evans DB, Calne RY. Gastrointestinal complications after renal transplantation. *Lancet.* 1971;2:781-784.
9. Adiseshiah M, Wells RC, Cory-Pearce R, Wallwork J, English TA. Acute pancreatitis after cardiac transplantation. *World J Surg.* 1983;7:519-521.
10. Oaks TE, Pennock JL, Myers JL, Wisman CB. Survival following a pancreatic abscess in a heart transplant recipient. *J Heart Transplant.* 1986;5:148-153.
11. Steed DL, Brown B, Reilly JJ, et al. General surgical complications in heart and heart-lung transplantation. *Surgery.* 1985;98:739-745.
12. Colon R, Frazier OH, Kahan BD, et al. Complications in cardiac transplant patients requiring general surgery. *Surgery.* 1988;103:32-38.
13. Hau T, VanHook EJ, Simmons RL, Najarian JS. Prognostic factors of peritoneal infections in transplant patients. *Surgery.* 1978;84:403-416.
14. Aziz S, Bergdahl L, Baldwin JC, et al. Pancreatitis after cardiac cardiopulmonary transplantation. *Surgery.* 1985;97:653-661.
15. Matolo NM, Garfinkle SE, Wolfman EF. Intestinal necrosis and perforation in patients receiving immunosuppressive drug. *Am J Surg.* 1976;132:753-754.
16. Warshaw AL. Acute perforation of the colon associated with chronic corticosteroid therapy. *Am J Surg.* 1976;131:442-446.
17. ReMine SG, McIlrath DC. Bowel perforation in steroid-treated patients. *Ann Surg.* 1980;192:581-586.
18. Guillaume JC, Roujeau JC, Revuz J, Penso D, Touraine R. The culprit drugs in 87 cases of toxic epidermal necrolysis (Lyell's syndrome). *Arch Dermatol.* 1987;123:1166-1170.
19. Nwokolo C, Byrne L, Misch KJ. Toxic epidermal necrolysis occurring during treatment with trimethoprim alone. *Br Med J.* 1988;296:970.
20. Revuz J, Penso D, Roujeau JC, et al. Toxic epidermal necrolysis. Clinical findings and prognosis factors in 87 patients. *Arch Dermatol.* 1987;123:1160-1165.
21. Birchall N, Langdon R, Cuono C, Maguire J. Toxic epidermal necrolysis: an approach to management using cryopreserved allograft skin. *J Am Acad Dermatol.* 1987;16:368-372.
22. Heimbach DM, Engrav LH, Marvin JA, Harnar TJ, Grube BJ. Toxic epidermal necrolysis: a step forward in treatment. *JAMA.* 1987;257:2171-2175.

Discussion

ROBERT T. SCHWEIZER, MD, Hartford, Conn: My colleagues and I have also seen general surgical complications in heart transplant recipients. We have had 4 in a series of 49 recipients, and 3 of these required laparotomy. There were no operative deaths from those procedures. Also, in the 49 patients there was 1 hospital death within the first 40 postoperative days; of the 48 remaining patients, 42 of them are alive.

We agree with the authors that these patients with surgical complications need very aggressive postoperative care. One of the most important aspects in the management of patients is what to do with their immunosuppression. Obviously, if we reduce it too much, the patients may develop an irreversible rejection episode. How did you manage that aspect of their care?

MENELAOS ALIAPOULIOS, MD, Boston, Mass: The actuarial probability of survival at 4 years following cardiac surgery in their hands of 90% and the overall operative mortality of 9% despite a not-unexpected complication rate of 22% are truly remarkable. The general surgical complications listed are familiar to us as those that typically follow complex procedures, especially in sick patients who are immunosuppressed. The point is once again emphasized that a high index of suspicion and aggressive intervention with early meticulous surgical involvement are crucial, especially since systemic signs and symptoms are few.

Since perforated ulcers were significant complications, do these patients routinely receive histamine receptor–blocking agents? What role do diagnostic techniques, such as magnetic resonance imaging and laparoscopy, play to assist in the early diagnosis?

DR DISESA: I appreciate the comments of Drs Aliapoulios and Schweizer. All of our patients do receive both histamine receptor–blocking antacids and oral antacids; despite this, we did see a significant incidence of loss of mucosal integrity that goes along with the severity of the patients' preoperative illness and the magnitude of their surgery. We have actually found sophisticated diagnostic techniques such as magnetic resonance imaging not particularly useful, and it is bedside examination that is done repeatedly and meticulously that is the most helpful in making the decision for surgical intervention. Many of these patients had abnormal gastrointestinal function preoperatively because they were at bed rest, so that many of them have some degree of intestinal dysfunction postoperatively. Only by repeated examination can you tell what is normal from what is truly pathological. We have not used laparoscopy at all.

Obviously, when these patients have abdominal surgery they are not able to take their immunosuppressive drugs orally and so we have given them intravenously. When you give cyclosporine intravenously, you have to reduce the dosage. We have not had any significant incidence of rejection associated with making that transition. Obviously, it is crucial to maintain immunosuppression to preserve the graft.

Ibuprofen Causes Reduced Toxic Effects of Interleukin 2 Administration in Patients With Metastatic Cancer

Timothy J. Eberlein, MD; Deric D. Schoof, PhD; Hamish R. Michie, FRCS; Anthony F. Massaro; Ulrike Burger; Douglas W. Wilmore, MD; Richard E. Wilson, MD

• Metastatic cancer was treated with interleukin 2 and lymphokine-activated killer cells with the addition of the cyclooxygenase inhibitor ibuprofen in an attempt to reduce side effects in 13 patients (eight male and five female). Twenty-six patients treated with only interleukin 2 and lymphokine-activated killer cells formed the control group. After interleukin 2 administration, a significantly increased number of lymphokine-activated killer cells were transfused in ibuprofen-treated patients. Cytotoxic effects were not significantly different in the treated and untreated groups. With regard to cell phenotype, both groups of patients manifested significant activation of the immune system as measured by T10 and OK1a. Symptom scores were dramatically reduced in patients treated with ibuprofen. Temperatures above 37°C were rare. Ibuprofen did not significantly alter rate of response in this immunotherapy trial (38% vs 42%). Ibuprofen is now routinely used in all of our current immunotherapy trials.

(*Arch Surg.* 1989;124:542-547)

Interleukin 2 (IL-2)[1] causes the activation and proliferation of several lymphocyte subpopulations, including cytotoxic T cells, helper T lymphocytes, T-suppressor cells, natural killer cells, and B cells.[2-4] Coculture of lymphocytes with high concentrations of IL-2 also results in the acquisition of tumor nonspecific cytotoxic effects, and these cells have become known as lymphokine-activated killer (LAK) cells.[5] Animal models have been developed that show regression of primary and metastatic tumors after systemic administration of IL-2 in combination with the adoptive transfer of IL-2–activated splenocytes.[6,7] Rosenberg et al[8] first reported efficacy of IL-2 and LAK cells against certain human malignant neoplasms refractory to conventional therapy. More recent reports have documented the high toxic effects of these protocols, often requiring admission to an intensive care unit; these effects include hypotension, pulmonary distress, central nervous system changes, and even death.[9,10]

In October 1986, the Brigham & Women's Hospital (Boston, Mass) began an IL-2/LAK cell immunotherapy trial that incorporated three important changes from earlier trials: (1) a different recombinant IL-2 (rIL-2) was used, (2) a commitment was made to a low-dose bolus infusion, and (3) IL-2 was administered for a prolonged period after LAK cell infusion to compensate partially for the low dose of IL-2 used. This protocol[11] demonstrated marked reduction in serious toxic effects, with only one patient requiring admission to the intensive care unit. There was no hypotension, respiratory distress, mental status change, or death. This reduction in toxic effects was accompanied by a 42% response rate. However, virtually all of the patients suffered from fever, chills, myalgias, nausea, vomiting, diarrhea, stomatitis, and rashes, which in some cases limited the administration of rIL-2. This report describes the addition of ibuprofen to the original protocol, which has significantly reduced the toxic effects associated with IL-2/LAK cell therapy.

PATIENTS AND METHODS

Patient Population

Patients who had failed all standard therapy, as well as patients for whom no standard therapy was available, were eligible for this protocol. In addition, patients could not have received chemotherapy, radiation therapy, or hormonal therapy within 1 month of entry into the trial. Previous therapy with nitrosoureas or mitomycin within 6 weeks was also an exclusion criterion, as was major surgery within the past month.

Twenty-six patients consecutively admitted to the protocol formed the control population that did not receive ibuprofen therapy. Nine of those patients had metastatic renal cell carcinoma, eight had metastatic melanoma, four had metastatic colorectal tumors, three had diffuse lymphoma, one had metastatic ovarian

Accepted for publication December 12, 1988.

From the Division of Surgical Oncology, Brigham & Women's Hospital, and the Department of Surgery, Harvard Medical School, Boston, Mass.

Read before the 69th Annual Meeting of the New England Surgical Society, Montreal, Canada, September 18, 1988.

Reprint requests to Brigham & Women's Hospital, 75 Francis St, Boston, MA 02115 (Dr Eberlein).

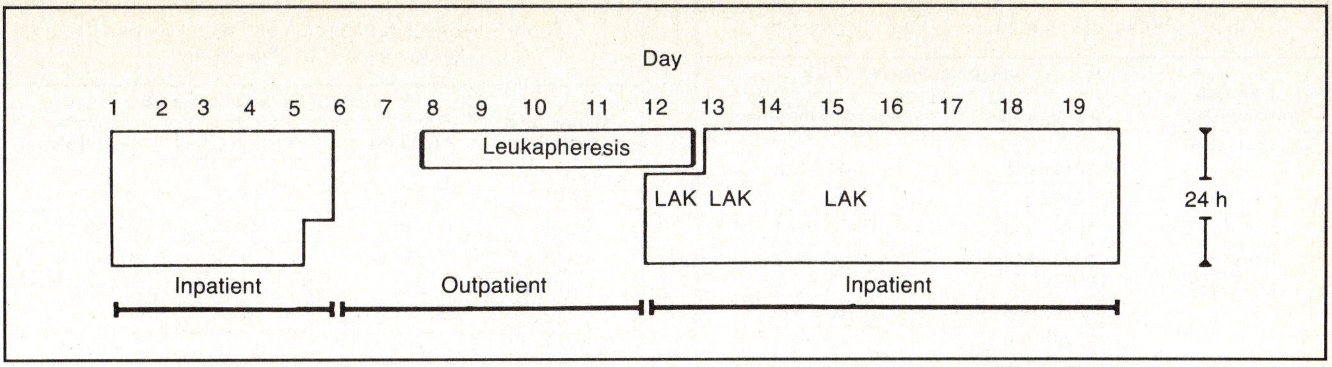

Fig 1.—Treatment protocol. During the first and third treatment periods, the patients received recombinant human interleukin 2 intravenously every eight hours. LAK indicates infusion of lymphokine-activated killer cells.

carcinoma, and one had metastatic uterine sarcoma. There were 19 men and seven women.

A second group of 13 patients, again consecutive and prospective, comprised the ibuprofen-treated patients. Three patients had metastatic renal cell carcinoma, seven had metastatic melanoma, one had diffuse lymphoma, one had metastatic ovarian carcinoma, and one had metastatic sarcoma. There were eight men and five women.

All but one of the patients in each group had received previous treatment. Many received multiple regimens of chemotherapy or combinations of radiotherapy and immunotherapy. One patient in the group that did not receive ibuprofen had an autologous bone marrow transplant, and one patient in the same group received no previous therapeutic intervention.

Source of IL-2

The IL-2 used in these trials was recombinant methionyl human IL-2 (ala-125) (made by Amgen Corp, Thousand Oaks, Calif). This material contains no detectable pyrogen and has been shown to be highly effective in activation of human peripheral blood mononuclear cells (PBMCs) in vitro.

Clinical Protocol

All patients were treated at the Brigham & Women's Hospital Clinical Research Center after they gave informed consent. Patients were entered on a three-part, 19-day protocol (Fig 1). The first portion of the protocol consisted of intravenous bolus infusion of 30 000 units/kg of body weight of rIL-2 (Ortho Pharmaceutical Corp, Raritan, NJ) every 8 hours for a total of 14 doses over a period of 5 days. After a 2-day rest, the patients begin the second part of the protocol, which consisted of five consecutive leukaphereses over 5 days. During this time, IL-2 was not administered, and the patient was treated on an outpatient basis. The third portion of the protocol included three infusions of rIL-2–activated PBMCs over a 4-day period and up to 22 doses of intravenous rIL-2. Patients were commonly discharged from the hospital within 48 hours after the last dose of rIL-2.

All assessable tumor was measured before and 2 and 6 weeks after completion of the protocol. A partial response to the treatment was registered if the sum of the products of the longest perpendicular diameters of all measurable lesions decreased by more than 50%. A complete response was recorded if all measurable tumor disappeared.

In this study, the first 26 consecutive patients who did not receive any ibuprofen comprised the control population. The next consecutive 13 patients comprised the treatment group. Each of these patients received ibuprofen (Motrin; Upjohn Co, Kalamazoo, Mich), 600 mg orally every 6 hours, beginning the evening before the first IL-2 administration on day 1 of the protocol. Ibuprofen administration was restarted on the evening of day 11, again before IL-2 administration.

Effector Cell Generation

Patients' PBMCs were obtained by leukapheresis as described previously[12] and suspended to a concentration of 3×10^6 cells per milliliter in RPMI 1640 (Whittaker, MA Bioproducts Inc, Walkersville, Md) supplemented with 2% group AB serum, 50 U/mL of penicillin, 50 mg/L of streptomycin, 2 mmol/L of 1-glutamine, and 1000 U/mL of rIL-2. The PBMCs were cultured in plastic culture bags (PL732 tissue culture flask; Fenwal Laboratories, Deerfield, Ill) placed into a 37°C, 5% carbon dioxide incubator. Cells were harvested from tissue culture bags and washed with saline by means of the CS3000 blood cell separator (Fenwal, Fenwal Laboratories, Deerfield, Ill).[12]

Peripheral blood for in vitro studies was collected by antecubital venipuncture into heparinized syringes (heparin; Elkin-Sinn Inc, Cherry Hill, NJ) and separated into mononuclear populations on Ficoll gradients (Lymphocyte Separation Medium; Litton Bionetics, Charleston, SC). The cells were washed three times before use and LAK and mitogen assays or cell phenotype analysis. Peripheral blood was collected into edetic acid for complete blood cell counts.

Table 1.—Effect of Ibuprofen on Cell Number*

	Mean No. of Cells $\times 10^{10} \pm$ SE	
	No Ibuprofen	**Ibuprofen Treatment**
PBMCs cultured, harvest day		
1	1.78 ± 0.28	1.86 ± 0.20
2	1.39 ± 0.17	1.66 ± 0.19
3	1.19 ± 0.14	1.25 ± 0.11
4	0.99 ± 0.09	1.32 ± 0.15
5	0.80 ± 0.08	1.10 ± 0.09
Total†	6.32 ± 0.66	7.28 ± 0.49
LAK cells infused, infusion day		
1	2.26 ± 0.34	2.64 ± 0.30
2	0.73 ± 0.08	0.95 ± 0.08
3	1.18 ± 0.12	1.92 ± 0.19
Total‡	4.16 ± 0.49	5.63 ± 0.42

*PBMCs indicates peripheral blood mononuclear cells; LAK, lymphokine-activated killer.
†Not significantly different between treatment groups ($P > .05$, two sided).
‡Significantly different between treatment groups ($P < .05$, two sided).

In Vitro Cytotoxicity

Activated PBMCs were assessed for in vitro cytotoxicity to Daudi and K562 (American Type Culture Collection, Rockville, Md). Target cells were labeled with 200 μCi of chromium 51 (Dupont NEN Medical Products, North Billerica, Mass) at 37°C for 60 minutes. The cells were washed with RPMI 1640 plus 10% fetal calf serum (Gibco Laboratories, Grand Island, NY) and distributed into round-bottom plates (5×10^3 cells per well). Effectors were added at a ratio of 40:1 and incubated at 37°C. Four hours later, the supernatants were collected (Skatron Inc, Sterling, Va) and counted in the gamma counter (Gamma Track 1191; TM

Table 2.—Effect of Ibuprofen on In Vitro Cytotoxicity

LAK Cell Infusion Day*	Lytic Units Infused × 10³†	
	No Ibuprofen	Ibuprofen Treatment
Daudi targets		
1	2950 ± 485	1599 ± 378
2	525 ± 80	329 ± 100
3	1030 ± 203	939 ± 267
Total‡	4905 ± 614	3065 ± 697
K562 targets		
1	3919 ± 665	3193 ± 660
2	822 ± 116	843 ± 133
3	3050 ± 1532	1850 ± 207
Total‡	8092 ± 2066	6214 ± 830

*LAK indicates lymphokine-activated killer.
†Average lytic unit (40%) ± SE.
‡Not significantly different between treatment groups (*P*>.05, two sided).

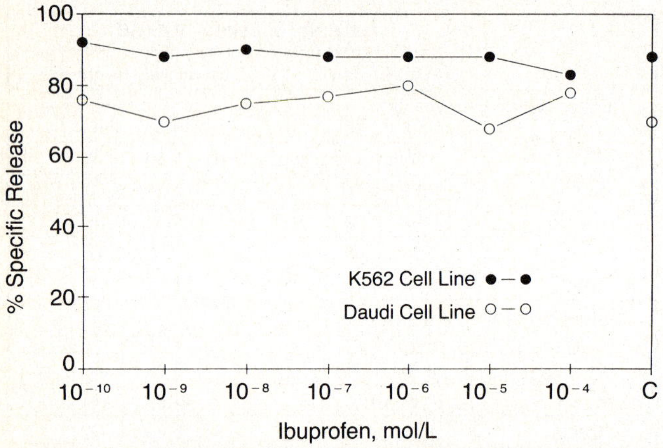

Fig 2.—Lymphokine-activated killer cell activity of peripheral blood mononuclear cells cocultured with 1000 U/mL of recombinant interleukin 2 for 4 days in the presence of various concentrations of ibuprofen. Lymphokine-activated killer cell activity was measured in a 4-hour chromium release assay. C indicates control.

Analytic, Elk Grove Village, Ill). Results were converted to percentage specific release. Chromium release data expressed as lytic units describe the number of effector cells required to cause 40% lysis of the target cell population.

Flow Cytometry

The PBMC phenotypes were assessed by flow microfluorometry. Fluoresceinated monoclonal antibodies OKT3, OKT4, OKT8, OKT10, OKB7, OKM1, and OKIa were used. The IL-2 receptor expression was monitored with fluoresceinated anti–IL-2 receptor antibodies (Bectin Dickinson Immunocytometry Systems, Mountain View, Calif). Cells were analyzed on a flow cytometer (Coulter Epic C; Coulter Electronics, Hialeah, Fla). Each conjugate was incubated with approximately 10^6 PBMCs for 45 minutes at 4°C. Cells were washed with Hanks' balanced salt solution plus 5% fetal calf serum (Gibco) and 0.1% sodium azide and then fixed in 1% paraformaldehyde.

Symptom Score

Fevers, chills, headache, rigors, myalgias, tachycardia, nausea, vomiting, diarrhea, rash, stomatitis, and hypotension (not requiring vasopressors) were measured prospectively in every patient every day of the protocol. They were prospectively recorded in each patient's case record form. The total number of symptoms from this list was then recorded for each patient every day of the protocol. The mean numbers of symptoms for all of the patients were then totaled and divided by the number of patients in each group. To avoid subjectivity, no attempt was made to score degree of symptoms. Symptom scores for the ibuprofen-treated group and the nontreated group were compared by means of the Wilcoxon two-sample test.

Table 3.—Effect of Ibuprofen on Peripheral Blood Mononuclear Cell Phenotype

Monoclonal Antibody	% of Cells Stained ± SE		
	All Patients	No Ibuprofen	Ibuprofen
Day 1*			
OKT3	47 ± 4	44 ± 5	55 ± 4
OKT4	44 ± 3	43 ± 5	45 ± 3
OKT8	13 ± 2	10 ± 2	19 ± 2
OKT10†	25 ± 3	19 ± 3	36 ± 4
OKB7	11 ± 2	9 ± 3	15 ± 3
OKIa†	17 ± 2	13 ± 2	23 ± 5
OKM1	17 ± 3	18 ± 3	16 ± 5
IL2R	10 ± 3	8 ± 5	13 ± 4
Day 8			
OKT3	51 ± 3	47 ± 4	58 ± 5
OKT4	38 ± 3	36 ± 3	42 ± 4
OKT8	20 ± 2	17 ± 3	24 ± 4
OKT10	43 ± 4	42 ± 6	46 ± 5
OKB7	8 ± 1	8 ± 2	8 ± 2
OKIa	27 ± 3	25 ± 3	29 ± 5
OKM1	20 ± 3	23 ± 4	18 ± 4
IL2R	13 ± 2	9 ± 2	20 ± 4
Day 19			
OKT3	47 ± 4	41 ± 5	60 ± 3
OKT4	30 ± 3	27 ± 4	37 ± 4
OKT8	24 ± 3	20 ± 4	30 ± 5
OKT10	48 ± 4	43 ± 5	59 ± 6
OKB7	10 ± 2	12 ± 3	6 ± 1
OKIa	39 ± 4	32 ± 5	50 ± 5
OKM1	26 ± 4	27 ± 3	25 ± 7
IL2R	18 ± 2	16 ± 3	21 ± 3

*Day of protocol.
†Comparison of activation markers OKT10 and OKIa between day 1 and day 19 for both nontreated and ibuprofen-treated groups is significant (*P*<.05). However, comparison of the increase in OKT10 and OKIa expression between both treatment groups is not significantly different (*P*>.05).

In Vitro Effects of Ibuprofen on Generation of LAK Cells

Ibuprofen (Sigma Chemical Co, St Louis, Mo) stock solutions prepared in ethyl alcohol were diluted with RPMI-1640. Diluted ibuprofen was added at various concentrations to cultures of PBMCs at the beginning of LAK cell activation. The PBMCs were cultured at 2×10^6 cells per milliliter in RPMI-1640 supplemented with 1000 U/mL of rIL-2 for 4 days at 37°C. Cytotoxicity against chromium-labeled target was measured, with an effector-target cell ratio of 40:1.

RESULTS

Cell Yield

Detailed comparisons of white blood cell count and lymphocytosis after IL-2 administration showed no significant differences between patients treated with ibuprofen and those not treated with ibuprofen (data not shown). Table 1 shows a detailed analysis of the total number of cells cultured from each pheresis day for all of the patients in each group. The number of cells harvested from patients and cultured in plastic bags was greater for each pheresis day in the group of patients treated with ibuprofen. This is reflected in the total number of PBMCs cultured. The ibuprofen-treated group had 7.28×10^{10} lymphocytes cul-

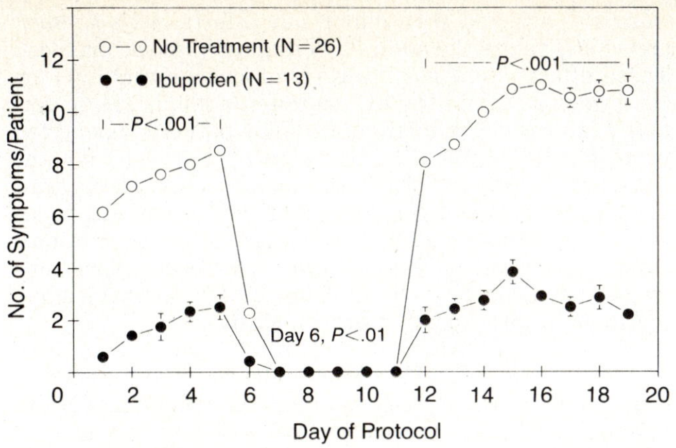

Fig 3.—Symptoms of toxic effects in the two treatment groups. Symptoms were recorded prospectively for each patient (mean ± SE) each day of the protocol and were retrospectively enumerated in a quantal fashion. No attempt was made to assess qualitatively the degree of an individual symptom.

tured compared with 6.32×10^{10} cells for the group not treated with ibuprofen. This was not statistically significant ($P>.05$); however, the number of PBMCs infused into ibuprofen-treated patients after coculture with rIL-2 was significantly greater than in the group not receiving ibuprofen ($P<.05$). Once again, for each LAK cell infusion day, the group receiving ibuprofen tended to have more LAK cells infused, and this group averaged 5.63×10^{10} LAK cells compared with 4.16×10^{10} cells for the patients not treated with ibuprofen.

In Vitro Cytotoxicity

Table 2 shows in vitro cytotoxicity against the natural killer–resistant cell line Daudi and the natural killer–sensitive cell line K562 for each LAK cell infusion day for all of the patients. The number of Daudi lytic units infused (3065) was lower for the ibuprofen-treated patients than for the untreated patients (4905). However, this difference was not statistically significant ($P>.05$). This same trend was seen against K562 targets, with an average of 6214 lytic units infused for the ibuprofen-treated patients vs 8092 for the untreated population. Again, this is not statistically significant.

Figure 2 shows one of four separate experiments that demonstrate that varying doses of ibuprofen added exogenously to human PBMCs do not alter the ability of these cells to become activated killer cells (LAK cells) when cocultured with recombinant IL-2. Concentrations of ibuprofen from 10^{-10} mol/L up to 10^{-4} mol/L did not significantly diminish cytotoxicity to Daudi or K562 in vitro. Addition of ibuprofen to these in vitro cultures of human PBMCs did not change cytotoxicity from control populations that had no ibuprofen in vitro; thus, ibuprofen appeared not to have an inhibitory effect on the generation of LAK cells in vitro.

Cell Phenotype

The PBMC phenotype did not differ between the group of patients treated with ibuprofen and the patients not treated. Table 3 shows that the percentages of T3, T4, and T8 populations were comparable in each of the groups of patients. As a group, the ibuprofen-treated population recorded changes in OKT10 and OKIa from day 1 to day 19 that were not significantly different from those of the untreated group. Thus, ibuprofen did not change cell phenotype, nor did it diminish the ability of the patient to demonstrate activated lymphocytes at the completion of the protocol.

Table 4.—Response Rates*

	No Ibuprofen			Ibuprofen		
Tumor	**N**	**CR, No.**	**PR, No.**	**N**	**CR, No.**	**PR, No.**
Renal	9	0	4	3	0	1
Melanoma	8	1	3	7	1	3
Colon	4	0	0	0	0	0
Lymphoma	3	1	1	1	0	0
Ovarian	1	1	0	1	0	0
Sarcoma	1	0	0	1	0	0
Total†	**26**	**3**	**8**	**13**	**1**	**4**

*CR indicates complete response; PR, partial response.
†No significant difference in response rates between treatment groups ($P>.05$).

Toxic Reactions

Toxic effects were measured for each patient for 12 different symptoms. If the patient manifested the symptom once for that particular day of the protocol, it was recorded as positive. No attempt was made to evaluate subjectively the severity of the symptom; in general, however, symptoms of patients treated with ibuprofen were much milder than symptoms manifested in patients not treated with ibuprofen. A comparison of the average symptom score for patients treated with ibuprofen and those not treated with ibuprofen is shown in Fig 3. The reduction in toxic effects for the 12 variables measured was dramatic. On day 6 of the protocol, the day the symptoms scores were closest, treatment with ibuprofen offered statistically significant benefit ($P<.01$). Comparisons for all other days between the two groups were even more highly statistically significant.

Response Rates

Table 4 shows the response rates for both treatment groups. The overall response rate in ibuprofen-treated patients was 38% compared with 42% in the control group ($P>.05$). Assessment of the numbers of complete responders and partial responders in the two groups also showed similar results. For the most common diagnosis in the study, malignant melanoma, there was one complete response and three partial responses among seven ibuprofen-treated patients, and also one complete response and three partial responses among eight patients with melanoma in the control group.

COMMENT

While the original Brigham & Women's Hospital protocol demonstrated a reduction in toxic effects from that of previous protocols, it was still desirable and necessary to investigate further and reduce the causes of toxic effects. Although fever, chills, nausea, and vomiting are not necessarily life-threatening toxic effects, these symptoms did cause premature cessation of the protocol in patients not treated with ibuprofen.

One hypothesis as to the cause of the toxic effects secondary to IL-2 administration was that it was caused by endotoxin contamination, since IL-2 is produced from bacteria. In data presented elsewhere,[13] IL-2 administration was associated with fever, neurohormonal symptoms, and acute-phase responses that were similar to those that occur after endotoxin administration. However, endotoxin contamination was ruled out in this protocol because (1) the toxic reaction was predictably delayed in onset from the time course of responses after endotoxin administration, (2) circulating tumor necrosis factor was not detected after IL-2 administration, as it was after endotoxin administration,[14] and (3) increased circulating γ-interferon concentrations were always detected 4 to 6 hours after IL-2 administration, whereas this cytokine was never detected in plasma after endotoxin administration. Thus, the metabolic responses resulting from IL-2 administration may represent combined responses to both tumor necrosis factors and γ-interferon acting in synergy. The tumor necrosis factors may still be secreted and circulate below the limits of existing assays.

Activation of cyclooxygenase may be the final common pathway mediating many of the metabolic responses after IL-2 administration, as it is after administration of endotoxin,[15] tumor necrosis factor,[16] and interleukin.[17] The pivotal role of cyclooxygenase in these responses to various cytokines has considerable implications for the development of strategies to modify the course of critical illness.

In data from this laboratory presented elsewhere,[13] when cortisol, corticotropin, and epinephrine levels were determined at exactly the same times after IL-2 administration with or without ibuprofen, plasma cortisol level was markedly attenuated by ibuprofen, and plasma corticotropin concentration and epinephrine levels were also lower. In the 13 patients treated with ibuprofen in the current protocol, plasma cortisol and corticotropin levels remained at baseline throughout the duration of the study.

With regard to the total number of cells cultured and number of LAK cells infused, ibuprofen had a significantly positive effect. Despite the relatively low doses of IL-2 used in the first week compared with other protocols, thus producing a smaller degree of lymphocytosis, the number of LAK cells infused with ibuprofen was comparable with those in previously reported series with much larger priming doses of IL-2.[8,10] Cytotoxic effects were not significantly different between the group treated with ibuprofen and the group of patients not so treated. In fact, Fig 2 shows that a wide range of exogenous ibuprofen did not inhibit the generation of LAK activity in in vitro cytotoxicity assays. Thus, cyclooxygenase inhibitors did not appear to inhibit the development of LAK activity in vitro and, if anything, augmented the number of cells adoptively transferred. With regard to the phenotype, again there were no significant differences between the group of patients treated with ibuprofen and those who were not. There was substantial activation in the ibuprofen-treated patients, as measured by the activation markers of T10 and OKIa. Thus, significant activation of the immune system was accomplished throughout the course of the protocol, despite cyclooxygenase inhibition.

Ibuprofen administration demonstrated a marked reduction in the number of toxic symptoms throughout the entire protocol. This was especially true with regard to fever, chills, rigors, myalgias, and nausea and vomiting. The reduction in these toxic side effects was in turn manifested by an increase in oral intake, energy count, and albumin (data not shown). Diarrhea, rash, and stomatitis were generally not much affected by ibuprofen administration, except indirectly. That is, it appeared that the better the patient was able to maintain an oral diet, the less likely that the patient would have significant diarrhea.

Thus, while life-threatening side effects were markedly reduced by the earlier protocol modifications to lower the dose and prolong administration of IL-2, most patients were still afflicted with minor side effects, such as fever and chills, before the addition of ibuprofen to the protocol. These effects were not always protocol limiting, but cyclooxygenase inhibition by ibuprofen administration certainly improved the quality of life for patients during the protocol. In addition to being more tolerable for the patients, the protocol was less time consuming and easier to manage from the perspective of the nurses and house staff. The patients still required a great deal of emotional support; however, with toxic effects reduced, more time was able to be devoted to psychosocial effort, thus leading to further improvement in patient care.

Of course, a further reduction in toxic effects from previous studies would not be significant without a concurrent maintenance of response rate. Although the patient numbers were small, response rates were almost identical between the two groups. It is difficult to compare directly the duration of response, since by definition the sequential accrual of patients makes the ibuprofen-treated patients have an overall shorter follow-up period. Response rates in both groups were not only comparable, but also favorable in comparison with previously reported series.[9,10,18]

Finally, ibuprofen administration did not in itself appear to cause significant side effects. Several patients had slight gastrointestinal tract upset and nausea (which was counted as an IL-2 toxic effect), but it was temporally related to doses of ibuprofen taken on an empty stomach. There were no episodes of gastrointestinal tract hemorrhage as manifested by hematemesis, hematochezia, or melena. Similarly, no significant effects of fluid retention were observed in patients who received ibuprofen. In fact, because of their better oral intake, fluid management in these patients was made easier. Most of the patients did not require exogenous fluid administration during the first week of the protocol, and several patients required fluid boluses to increase urine output during the last week of IL-2 administration.

In conclusion, the use of a low-dose bolus IL-2 infusion for prolonged periods and the addition of ibuprofen have caused a significant decrease in the toxic effects associated with this immunotherapeutic approach. This leaves the possibility open for increasing the dose of IL-2, or combining it with other biologic response modifiers that may increase effectiveness without increasing toxic effects. This same approach is planned for a trial about to begin at the Brigham & Women's Hospital with a combination of low-dose IL-2, low-dose cyclophosphamide, and tumor-infiltrating lymphocytes.

This study was supported by an American Cancer Society Career Development Award (Dr Eberlein) and by grant CA 40555 and Clinical Research Center Grant 20-9299 from the National Institutes of Health, Bethesda, Md.

The IL-2 and the monoclonal antibodies used in this study were generously provided by Ortho Pharmaceutical Corp, Raritan, NJ.

References

1. Morgan DA, Ruscetti FW, Gallo RC. Selective in vitro growth of T-lymphocytes from normal human bone marrows. *Science*. 1976;193:1007-1008.

2. Gillis S, Smith KA. Long-term culture of tumor-specific cytotoxic T-cells. *Nature (Lond)*. 1977;268:154-156.

3. Watson J. Continuous proliferation of murine antigen-specific helper T-lymphocytes in culture. *J Exp Med*. 1979;150:1510-1519.

4. Farrar JJ, Benjamin WR, Hilfiker ML, Howard M, Farrar WL, Fuller-Farrar J. The biochemistry, biology and role of interleukin 2 in the induction of cytotoxic T-cell and antibody-forming B cell responses. *Immunol Rev*. 1982;63:129-166.

5. Grimm EA, Mazumder A, Zhang HZ, Rosenberg SA. The lymphokine-activated killer cell phenomenon: lysis of NK resistant fresh solid tumor cells by IL-2 activated autologous human peripheral blood lymphocytes. *J Exp Med*. 1982;155:1823-1841.

6. Cheever MA, Greenberg PD, Fefer A. Specificity of adoptive chemoim-

munotherapy of established syngeneic tumors. *J Immunol.* 1980;125:711-714.

7. Eberlein TJ, Rosenstein M, Rosenberg SA. Regression of a disseminated syngeneic solid tumor by systemic transfer of lymphoid cells expanded in interleukin-2. *J Exp Med.* 1982;156:385-397.

8. Rosenberg SA, Lotze MT, Muul LM, et al. Observations on the systemic administration of autologous lymphokine-activated killer cells and recombinant interleukin-2 to patients with metastatic cancer. *N Engl J Med.* 1985;313:1485-1492.

9. Rosenberg SA, Lotze MT, Muul LM, Chang AE, Avis FP, Leitman S, et al. A progress report on the treatment of 157 patients with advanced cancer using lymphokine-activated killer cells and interleukin-2 or high-dose interleukin-2 alone. *N Engl J Med.* 1987;316:889-897.

10. Boldt DH, Mills BJ, Gemlo BT, et al. Laboratory correlates of adoptive immunotherapy with recombinant interleukin-2 and lymphokine-activated killer cells in humans. *Cancer Res.* 1988;48:4409-4416.

11. Eberlein TJ, Schoof DD, Jung S, et al. A new regimen of interleukin-2 and lymphokine-activated killer cells: efficacy without significant toxicity. *Arch Intern Med.* In press.

12. Schoof DD, Gramolini B, Davidson D, Massaro A, Wilson RE, Eberlein TJ. Adoptive immunotherapy of human cancer using low-dose recombinant interleukin-2 and lymphokine-activated killer cells. *Cancer Res.* 1988;48:5007-5010.

13. Michie HR, Eberlein TJ, Spriggs DR, Manogue KR, Cerami A, Wilmore DW. Interleukin-2 initiates metabolic responses associated with critical illness in humans. *Surgery.* 1988;208:493-503.

14. Michie HR, Manogue KR, Spriggs DR, et al. Detection of circulating tumor necrosis factor after endotoxin administration. *N Engl J Med.* 1988;318:1481-1486.

15. Revhaug A, Michie HR, Manson JM, et al. Inhibition of cyclooxygenase attenuates the metabolic response to endotoxin in humans. *Arch Surg.* 1988;123:162-170.

16. Kettlehut IC, Fiers W, Goldberg AL. The toxic effects of tumor necrosis factor in vivo and their preparation by cyclooxygenase inhibitors. *Proc Natl Acad Sci USA.* 1987;84:4273-4277.

17. Okusawa S, Gelfand JA, Ikejima T, Connolly RJ, Dinarello CA. Interleukin-1 induces a shock like state in rabbits. *J Clin Invest.* 1988;81:1162-1172.

18. West WH, Tauer KW, Yannelli JR, Marshall GD, Orr DW, Thurman GB, et al. Constant-infusion recombinant interleukin-2 in adoptive immunotherapy of advanced cancer. *N Engl J Med.* 1987;316:898-905.

Discussion

Roger S. Foster, Jr, MD, Burlington, Vt: Dr Eberlein's presentation of the Brigham group's experience with IL-2 and LAK cell therapy I think provides a glimpse of the future. Many of us feel that biologic response modifier therapy, which is really in its infancy, will in the not too distant future play a major role, along with surgery and radiotherapy and chemotherapy, in the management of cancer patients. In a small percentage of the patients in whom there is a complete response to IL-2 and LAK cell therapy, the response can truly be dramatic. Our own experience confirms that.

We have also found that cyclooxygenase inhibitors can reduce toxic effects, and we have used indomethacin. We agree that the first priority is to have a more effective therapy. The toxic effects in the past have been enough to limit treatment to very vigorous patients; therefore, it was difficult to contemplate using this therapy for patients not in a vigorous condition or to use it in an adjuvant setting.

I have one question for the authors. I think they have made a step in the right direction by showing maintenance of therapeutic effect and reduction of toxic effects, but both indomethacin and ibuprofen can, under certain circumstances, precipitate acute renal failure, particularly in patients with reduced renal blood flow. Patients treated with IL-2 and LAK cells have a loss of intravascular volume and therefore a potential for reduced renal blood flow. Dr Sondel's group at the University of Wisconsin has shown a greater degree of renal dysfunction in their IL-2-treated patients who have been treated with indomethacin. My question is, do the authors have a comparison for their two groups as to before and after institution of the ibuprofen protocol?

Dr Eberlein: Actually, we do have data on the comparison of renal failure. The renal dysfunction as measured by serum urea nitrogen and creatinine levels is actually substantially less in the patients treated with ibuprofen. I suppose that as we administer ibuprofen to more and more patients, we probably will see a patient who develops acute renal failure solely on that basis. But in fact, we find that the fluid balance that is such an integral part of this protocol is much easier to manage with the ibuprofen administration. The patients maintain an oral diet, as reflected by energy counts, and their albumin levels are much better with ibuprofen administration. This obviously makes management of their general fluid status, as well as their renal status, much easier.

In Other AMA Journals

ARCHIVES OF INTERNAL MEDICINE

Preoperative Pulmonary Evaluation

Maj Cary V. Jackson, MC, USAF

Factors related to risk of perioperative pulmonary complications include site of incision, obstructive lung disease, prolonged anesthesia time, smoking history with productive cough, and obesity. Hypercapnia is a consistent indicator of high risk. There is no difference between spinal and general anesthesia with regard to risk of pulmonary complications. In patients being evaluated for lung resection, high-risk indicators include predicted postoperative forced expiratory volume in one second of less than 1000 mL, hypercapnia, severe dyspnea on exertion, or advanced age when it is associated with advanced cardiopulmonary disease. Newer methods of assessing cardiopulmonary reserve may prove useful in identifying which patients with one or more of these risk factors are suitable operative candidates. Prevention of postoperative complications in chronic obstructive pulmonary disease patients should begin in the preoperative period with discontinuation of smoking at least eight weeks before surgery and vigorous pulmonary toilet in the 48 to 72 hours before surgery. Prophylactic lung expansion maneuvers can be effective in decreasing the incidence of postoperative atelectasis in high-risk patients undergoing high-risk operations (*Arch Intern Med* 1988;148:2120-2127).

Reprint requests to SGHM, US Air Force Hospital Keesler, Keesler AFB, MS 39534 (Dr Jackson).

Tamoxifen as an Alternative to Surgical Resection for Selected Geriatric Patients With Primary Breast Cancer

Richard G. Margolese, MD, Roger S. Foster, Jr, MD

• Thirty elderly patients with primary operable breast cancer were treated initially, because of refusal of surgery or because of infirmity, only with the antiestrogen tamoxifen citrate. Nineteen patients had regression of the primary tumor (complete in five and partial in 14). Eight patients were stable with no change, and three had measurable increases in the size of their primary tumors. Nine of the 30 eventually required locoregional treatment with surgery or radiotherapy for progression or recrudescence of their tumors after initial regression. No patient developed uncontrollable locoregional disease. For selected geriatric patients, treatment with tamoxifen alone permits a delay of surgery, which for some exceeds life expectancy.
(*Arch Surg.* 1989;124:548-551)

Elderly patients with primary breast cancer may be reluctant to undergo surgery or to accept the attendant hospitalization. The reluctance may be related to infirmity or to their perception as to the best quality for their remaining life. Since elderly patients tend to have breast cancers that are well differentiated and are commonly positive for estrogen and progesterone receptors, their cancers are likely to be responsive to antiestrogens such as tamoxifen citrate. We report herein on a series of selected older patients with primary operable breast cancer who, after diagnosis by needle biopsy, were treated with tamoxifen only.

PATIENTS AND METHODS

Since 1980 we have treated 30 women with primary operable breast cancer with tamoxifen citrate, 10 mg twice daily, after cytologic diagnosis by fine-needle aspiration (25 patients) or core-cutting needle biopsy (five patients). The patients in this retrospective review were selected for nonoperative treatment because they either refused surgical treatment or were judged to be relatively poor surgical candidates, and the alternative approach was suggested to them by their surgeon. The mean age at initiation of treatment was 82 years (range, 73 to 92 years). The mean longest diameter of the breast tumors was 3.2 cm (range, 1 to 10 cm). Three had clinically palpable axillary nodes that were judged to contain metastases. None of the patients had clinical evidence of systemic metastases at diagnosis. None of the patients were lost to follow-up.

RESULTS

Eighteen of the 30 patients had a measurable reduction in the diameter of the primary tumor (Figure). Five of these had complete regression. Fourteen patients were judged to have partial regression (greater than 50% reduction in diameter of the tumor). Eight patients had minimal change in their tumor size and were labeled stable. In three of the 30 patients, the breast cancer measurably increased in size despite the tamoxifen therapy. Six other patients had recrudescence of disease after an initial partial response that had lasted for a mean of 35 months. Thus, nine patients required either surgical resection or radiotherapy for local disease. No patient developed uncontrollable locoregional disease. The mean follow-up time after surgery or radiotherapy was 24 months (range, 3 to 43 months), with two of the nine dying at 33 and 29 months.

Twenty patients were still alive after a mean interval of 33 months after initiation of treatment (range, 6 to 81 months) (Table). The average survival time of the ten patients who died was 52 months (range, 25 to 90 months); one death was due to breast cancer and nine were due to competing causes. Only two of the ten patients who died had required surgery for local disease. Of the nine patients eventually requiring locoregional treatment (mean total follow-up, 62 months), one died of metastatic breast cancer and one died of unrelated causes. Eight of the 21 patients not requiring locoregional therapy died.

COMMENT

It has long been recognized that some breast cancers are dependent on estrogens. Tamoxifen is a synthetic nonste-

Accepted for publication December 9, 1988.
From the Department of Surgery, McGill University, McGill Cancer Center, and The Sir Mortimer B. Davis Jewish General Hospital, Montreal, Canada (Dr Margolese); and Department of Surgery, Vermont Regional Cancer Center, University of Vermont, Burlington (Dr Foster).
Read before the 69th Annual Meeting of the New England Surgical Society, Montreal, Canada, September 16, 1988.
Reprint requests to Department of Surgery, The Sir Mortimer B. Davis Jewish General Hospital, 3755 Chemin de la Cote, Ste Catherine, Montreal, Quebec, Canada H3T 1E2 (Dr Margolese).

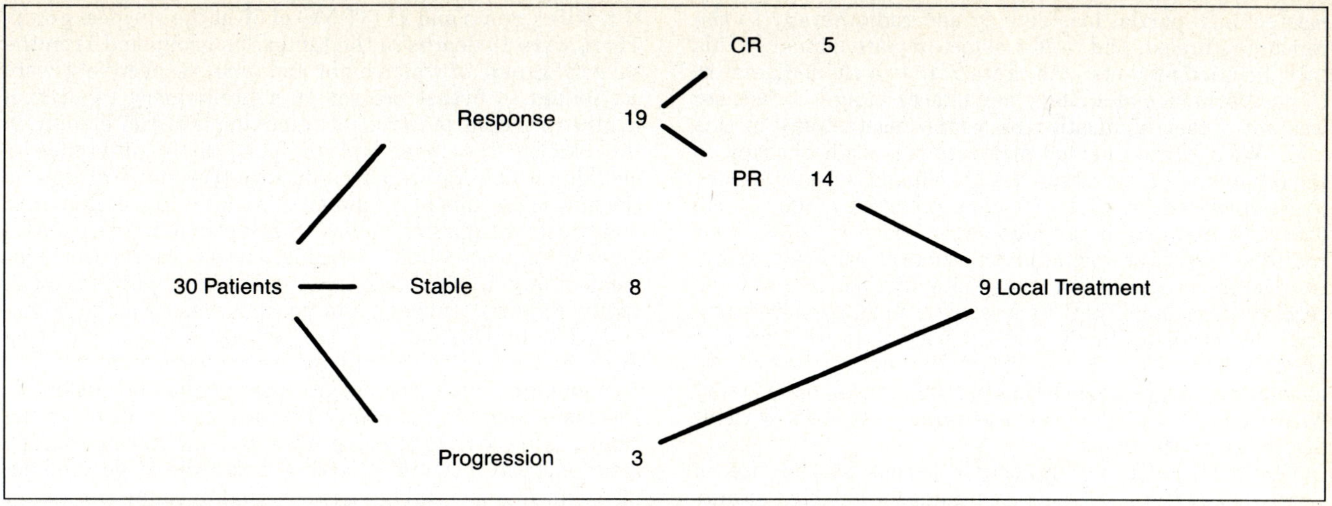

Locoregional disease outcome in 30 patients with primary operable breast cancer who were initially treated solely with tamoxifen. CR indicates complete response; PR, partial response with greater than 50% reduction in longest diameter.

roidal antiestrogen that has become the endocrine treatment currently most widely used for patients with advanced breast cancer.[1] Adjuvant therapy with tamoxifen has also proved to be effective for some patients with primary operable breast cancer after surgical resection either with or without radiotherapy.

The United States National Cancer Institute (Bethesda, Md) Consensus Conference[2] recommended tamoxifen as adjuvant therapy for postmenopausal patients with axillary node metastases who are not on research protocols. Although the early clinical trials and the consensus conference suggested that tamoxifen be used for 1 to 2 years, recent results suggest that long-term therapy (eg, 5 years) or even indefinite tamoxifen therapy is more effective in reducing recurrence and improving survival.[3,4] Recent results have suggested that tamoxifen is also of benefit in reducing recurrences when used as adjuvant therapy for axillary node–negative patients whose primary tumors are estrogen receptor positive.[4,5]

Tamoxifen and its major metabolites are antiestrogens that inhibit estradiol binding to estrogen receptors and block breast cancer cells at the G1 phase of the cell cycle.[6-8] There has, however, been a lack of complete correlation between the beneficial effects of tamoxifen and the estrogen or progesterone content of the primary tumor. It is quite possible that tamoxifen has therapeutic effects in addition to its antiestrogen effects, as it has been shown to increase natural killer cells.[9]

Tamoxifen is a remarkably nontoxic agent. Minor side effects that may occur with initiation of treatment and usually then disappear include hot flashes, nausea, and occasionally vomiting. Moderate thrombocytopenia and leukopenia occur in 10% to 15% of patients given tamoxifen but rarely require dose adjustment.[10] Less frequent side effects that usually do not require discontinuation of treatment include vaginal discharge and vaginal bleeding.

The biologic behavior and management of breast cancer in the elderly have recently been reviewed.[11] Unfortunately, there are few data from randomized clinical trials, as most breast cancer trials have systematically excluded patients over the age of 70 or 75 years. In general, the breast cancers of older patients tend to have somewhat greater histologic differentiation, lower proliferative rates, and higher estrogen receptor content. In older patients under treatment for breast cancer, there will be deaths due to competing causes; however, the relative rate of death due to cancer in most large studies is only slightly different among the various age groups.

Outcome and Follow-up

Outcome	n	Mean Follow-up, mo (Range)
Local progression	9	62 (35-90)
No local progression	21	46 (25-71)
Dead	10	52 (25-90)
Surviving	20	33 (6-81)

Age alone is not generally considered a contraindication to general anesthesia, and reports indicate a surgical mortality of 1% to 2% for mastectomy in the elderly. Medicare recipients, who are mostly over the age of 65 years, have a reported postoperative mortality after mastectomy of 1.2%.[12] The appropriate surgical treatment of primary operable breast cancer is probably best determined by extrapolation from the randomized clinical trials carried out mostly on patients under the age of 75 years. Axillary dissection in the management of breast cancer provides both staging information and control of regional disease. The results of the National Surgical Adjuvant Breast Project randomized trial (B-04) have shown that prophylactic removal of clinically normal nodes provides no survival benefit over a "watch and wait" policy of therapeutic dissection for the 20% of patients who eventually develop clinical evidence of progression of axillary disease.[13] If a decision relative to the use of systemic therapy is going to be made on the basis of the information from an axillary dissection, then that is a definite indication for axillary dissection. If, in an elderly patient, a decision as to the type of systemic adjuvant therapy is not going to be based on the pathologic status of the axillary nodes, then the management of the axillary nodes is elective. Prophylactic axillary dissection, radiotherapy to the axilla, and careful observation and therapeutic dissection result in similar survival.

The results of the National Surgical Adjuvant Breast Project trial B-06 show that the survival after partial mastectomy, partial mastectomy and radiotherapy to the remaining breast, and total mastectomy are similar.[14] This trial included patients with cancers up to 4 cm in diameter. Clinical evidence of axillary metastases (stage II disease) was not a contraindication to partial mastectomy in this trial. With limited partial mastectomies, radiotherapy to the remaining breast tissue has been found to be necessary to decrease the chance of tumor recurrence within the breast, which may be as high as 40% at 5 years without radiotherapy. Systemic adjuvant therapy with either cytotoxic chemotherapy or tamoxifen further reduces the recurrence of tumor in the breast after partial mastectomy and radiotherapy. In the elderly patients with clinically negative axillas for whom surgical treatment is elected, we most commonly perform either partial or total mastectomy with the patient under local or general anesthesia, without dissection of the axillas.

The results we are reporting herein of the use of tamoxifen as the sole initial treatment for elderly patients with primary operable breast cancer are consistent with the results of nonrandomized trials reported by several other authors.[15-18] In our experience and in the experience of others, approximately two thirds of the patients with localized breast cancer who have been treated initially with tamoxifen only have had an objective regression of their disease.

A recent report[19] presented the early results of a prospective randomized trial of tamoxifen vs surgery in 116 elderly patients with breast cancer. Patients in the surgical arm were treated with either wide local resection or total mastectomy. At a median follow-up of 3 years, local relapse or progression was seen in 15 (25%) of 60 patients in the tamoxifen group and 21 (37.5%) of 56 in the surgical group. There were 13 deaths in the tamoxifen group and 11 in the surgical group, of which eight and nine, respectively, were attributed to breast cancer. In a preliminary report[20] of another randomized trial of tamoxifen vs mastectomy in the elderly, the investigators found little difference in overall survival but a better disease-free survival time in the surgical arm when compared with the tamoxifen arm, and the investigators believe that optimum treatment of elderly patients with operable breast cancer includes mastectomy. In our study, nine (30%) of 30 patients eventually required surgery, but local disease was well controlled in all. One fourth of the patients died of competing diseases without ever requiring locoregional treatment.

Tamoxifen, which has been valuable when used alone in the management of advanced breast cancer in older patients, is increasingly being used as an adjuvant therapy after surgical resection. Further data from large randomized clinical trials will be needed to define more completely the conditions under which tamoxifen alone can be used as the treatment of primary operable breast cancer. Until that time, we believe that for most vigorous older patients with primary operable breast cancer, the principles of locoregional management either by mastectomy or by partial mastectomy and radiotherapy are similar to those for younger women. As we have reported, tamoxifen as sole treatment definitely provides an alternative treatment. In selected geriatric patients in whom avoidance of hospitalization and/or avoidance of a surgical procedure are an important part of quality of life considerations, treatment with tamoxifen alone permits a delay of surgery, which for some exceeds their life expectancy.

References

1. Furr BJA, Jordan VC. The pharmacology and clinical uses of tamoxifen. *Pharmacol Ther.* 1984;25:127-205.
2. National Institutes of Health consensus development panel on adjuvant chemotherapy and endocrine therapy for breast cancer: introduction and conclusions. *NCI Monogr.* 1986;1:1-14.
3. Fisher B, Brown A, Wolmark N, et al. Prolonging tamoxifen therapy for primary breast cancer. *Ann Intern Med.* 1987;106:649-654.
4. Report from the Breast Cancer Trials Committee. Adjuvant tamoxifen in the management of operable breast cancer: the Scottish Trial Report from the Breast Cancer Trial Committee. *Lancet.* 1987;2:171-175.
5. Fisher B, Costantino J, Redmond C, et al. A randomized clinical trial evaluating methotrexate and fluorouracil in the treatment of patients with node-negative breast cancer who have estrogen-receptor–negative tumor. *N Engl J Med.* 1989;320:473-478, 479-484.
6. Jordan VC, Bain RR, Brown RR, et al. Determination and pharmacology of a new hydroxylated metabolite of tamoxifen observed in patient sera during therapy for advanced breast cancer. *Cancer Res.* 1983;43:1446-1450.
7. Kemp JV, Adam HK, Wakeling AE, et al. Identification and biological activity of tamoxifen metabolites in human serum. *Biochem Pharmacol.* 1983;32:2045-2052.
8. Osborne CK, Boldt DH, Clark GM, et al. Effects of tamoxifen on human breast cancer cell cycle kinetics: accumulation of cells in early G_1 phase. *Cancer Res.* 1983;43:3583-3585.
9. Berry J, Green BJ, Matheson DS. Modulation of natural killer cell activity by tamoxifen in stage I post-menopausal breast cancer. *Eur J Clin Oncol.* 1987;23:517-520.
10. Tormey DC, Lippman ME, Edwards BK, et al. Evaluation of tamoxifen doses with and without fluoxymesterone in advanced breast cancer. *Ann Intern Med.* 1983;98:139-144.
11. Stewart JA, Foster RS Jr. Breast cancer and aging. *Semin Oncol.* 1989;16:41.
12. Shortell SM, Hughes FXE. The effects of regulation, competition and ownership on mortality rates among hospital inpatients. *N Engl J Med.* 1988;318:1100-1107.
13. Fisher B, Redmond C, Fisher ER, et al. Ten year results of a randomized clinical trial comparing radical mastectomy and total mastectomy with or without radiation. *N Engl J Med.* 1985;312:674-681.
14. Fisher B, Bauer M, Margolese R, et al. Five-year results of a randomized clinical trial comparing total mastectomy and segmental mastectomy with or without radiation in the treatment of breast cancer. *N Engl J Med.* 1985;312:665-673.
15. Preece PE, Wood RAB, Mackie CR, et al. Tamoxifen as initial sole treatment of localized breast cancer in elderly women: a pilot study. *Br Med J.* 1982;284:869-870.
16. Hellenberg A, Lundgren B, Norin T, et al. Treatment of early localized breast cancer in elderly patients by tamoxifen. *Br J Radiol.* 1982;55:511-515.
17. Allan SG, Rodger A, Smyth JF, et al. Tamoxifen as primary treatment of breast cancer in elderly or frail patients: a practical management. *Br Med J.* 1985;290:358.
18. Bradbeer JW, Kyngdon J. Primary treatment of breast cancer in elderly women with tamoxifen. *Clin Oncol.* 1983;9:31-34.
19. Gazet J-C, Ford HT, Bland JM, et al. Prospective randomized trial of tamoxifen versus surgery in elderly patients with breast cancer. *Lancet.* 1988;1:679-681.
20. Robertson JFR, Blamey RW. Breast cancer, tamoxifen, and surgery. *Lancet.* 1988;1:1044.

Discussion

W. Bradford Patterson, MD, Brookline, Mass: Dr Margolese and Dr Foster have made independent contributions before in the field of breast cancer, through the National Surgical Adjuvant Breast Project, and I am glad they are continuing to present their results. I wonder whether or not they think this drug is ready for use in all operable patients.

I have one comment about tamoxifen. I used to think that ethylalcohol was God's gift to the cancer patient, because no matter what you did with it, it would help. One could take it by mouth in a dilute solution, and it would help the appetite; one could rub it on the skin, and it would reduce a fever; one could inject it along nerve roots, and it would relieve pain. But it appears that tamoxifen is becoming even more important as a great gift to the breast cancer patient. As was pointed out, it is effective in advanced disease and has now been shown to be effective in "operable" disease. At a recent chemoprevention conference in Washington, there was discussion about several ongoing clinical trials that suggest strongly that tamoxifen may prevent breast cancer. Were it not for the liability that the manufacturer worries about in terms of the tiny risk of using this drug in a very large trial, it probably would soon be introduced in a national trial as a breast cancer preventative. Tamoxifen is an important and effective drug in breast cancer management.

Peter Deckers, MD, Hartford, Conn: These studies serve to reinforce a central thesis of the National Surgical Adjuvant Breast Project, specifically the heterogeneity of breast cancer. It should not be considered unusual that in different subsets of women very different therapies might have competitive results, both locoregionally and systemically.

I reviewed my personal experience during the past eight years with primary breast cancer in women over 80 years old. Eight patients over 80 years old, all considered at prohibitive risk with general anesthesia, were treated as outpatients by segmentectomy with local anesthesia and then with tamoxifen indefinitely. Seven of eight have died, but none died of cancer, none developed any recurrence in the breast, and none developed systemic metastases. The one patient still alive was free of disease for 3 years after I thought she was at prohibitive risk for any kind of major surgery. Her family and the patient believe she has had a very sensible approach to her particular problem.

The challenge of the data presented today is their potential use in even younger women. If tamoxifen can be used in some without tumor removal and in others after segmentectomy alone without an adverse effect on survival and locoregional recurrence, and if tamoxifen is advocated for selected women with positive as well as negative nodes, why is such therapy limited only to the very elderly or very infirmed? Is there a difference in the menopausal state of a 60-year-old woman and an 80-year-old woman? While it may be nihilistic to suggest tamoxifen alone without tumor removal for younger, more viable patients, it does seem reasonable to define that subset of patients who are appropriate candidates for segmentectomy and adjuvant tamoxifen without chemotherapy, radiotherapy, or axillary dissection. Multiple different treatment options, appropriately selected for individual patient subsets, is not heretical, but merely consistent with the heterogeneity characteristic of breast cancer biology.

Dr Margolese: Both discussants asked how widely we should think of applying these results. The National Surgical Adjuvant Breast Project has designed a new study that will involve preoperative chemotherapy. This means that patients will have the diagnosis made by needle biopsy and then will be randomized to receive preoperative chemotherapy for four cycles followed by surgery, or have routine primary surgery followed by four cycles of chemotherapy. Other experience suggests that many of the presurgery patients will have the tumor disappear and will have to have a blind surgical procedure done. This might be a little difficult if the trend continues toward the segmental type of operation, and the tumor has disappeared clinically, as our results with tamoxifen have demonstrated in some patients.

I began my career in the days of radical surgery and have seen the changes that Dr Deckers described. If we think about it, we are going from an era where radical surgery was aimed at cure to the present era where surgery is seen as an initial treatment, with chemotherapy as backup to control micrometastases. We are now beginning a phase in which the primary therapy may well be nonsurgical, and surgery may be seen as an adjunct. Now, that's a big jump from the paper I presented, and I have said it very blithely. It would take probably about an hour to trace the biology behind those thoughts, but I could produce a pretty reasonable case for evaluating this change from our classic paradigm. I also think that the chemotherapies that we have used probably have worked as far as they can go. As we understand a little more about growth factors and the control of normal cell division and cancer cell growth, we will get compounds that will interfere much more precisely with the growth of cancers. I think tamoxifen should be thought of in this context, and not only as an antiestrogen or antihormone. So, I think there will be changes; I think that the observations that Dr Foster and I have made point us in the direction of some considerations that, in time, may become very important to us as surgeons treating breast cancer.

In Other AMA Journals

ARCHIVES OF DERMATOLOGY

Verrucous Malignant Melanoma

Andreas Steiner, MD; Klaus Konrad, MD; Hubert Pehamberger, MD; Klaus Wolff, MD

Five cases of verrucous malignant melanoma—a rare variant of melanoma that was described in 1967, but is rarely mentioned today—are presented and the clinical and histopathologic criteria defining this variant are discussed. The importance of this rare entity in the differential diagnosis of verrucous pigmented skin lesions is emphasized (*Arch Dermatol* 1988;124:1534-1537).

Reprint requests to Department of Dermatology I, University of Vienna, Alser Strasse 4, A-1090 Vienna, Austria (Dr Steiner).

Primary Cancer of the Liver

Evaluation, Treatment, and Prognosis

William V. McDermott, MD; Blake Cady, MD; Basil Georgi, MD; Glenn Steele, Jr, MD; Urmila Khettry, MD

• Between 1970 and 1985, a diagnosis of primary hepatocellular carcinoma was established in 98 patients. Sixty-one cases developed in the presence of chronic liver disease, and only six of these were considered resectable. Of these, the median survival was 19 months. There was one perioperative death. Of the 98 tumors, 37 arose in normal livers. Of the 16 patients with tumors in normal livers that were resected, all survived operation. The long-term median survival was 32 months. Two subsets of the fibrolamellar and clear-cell variants appeared to carry a more favorable prognosis.
(*Arch Surg.* 1989;124:552-555)

The literature of the past 2 to 3 decades provides an excellent view of the relative occurrence of primary hepatocellular carcinoma (HCC) throughout the world and an analysis of the epidemiology, cause, and treatment of this tumor, which has been classified as the most commonly occurring cancer in the world, excluding superficial malignant lesions of the skin.

While relatively uncommon in the United States[1-3] and Canada,[4] HCC is certainly the most frequent malignant tumor and most common cause of death from cancer in Africa,[5] China,[6] Hong Kong,[7,8] Malaysia,[9] and other parts of the Orient.[10] Although the incidence is high in Japan,[11] the results of surgical therapy have been much better there than elsewhere[12-14] and may indicate a different basic cause and prognosis.[15]

The cause of this particular cancer relates both to the hepatitis B virus[5,8] and to aflatoxins[5] originating from contamination of grain supplies by the fungus *Aspergillus flavus*, as well as to many other undetermined factors. In Western countries, the incidence is much lower[1-3,16] and the cause less clear.[16]

Survival rates in general have been dismal,[5,6] ranging from 1 to 2 months in Africa and Asia to 4 months in the United States.

Accepted for publication December 7, 1988.
From the Departments of Surgery, Harvard Medical School, and New England Deaconess Hospital, Boston, Mass.
Read before the 69th Annual Meeting of the New England Surgical Society, Montreal, Canada, September 18, 1988.
Reprint requests to Department of Surgery, New England Deaconess Hospital, 110 Francis St, 3A, Boston, MA 02215 (Dr McDermott).

PATIENTS AND METHODS

During a 15-year period (1970 to 1985), the diagnosis of primary HCC was established histologically in 98 cases. Of these, 37 arose in otherwise histologically normal livers, while a background of cirrhosis existed in 61. Twenty-two tumors were resected, and the results of these cases were analyzed in this study (Fig 1).

Of the 22 tumors resected, six were in cirrhotic patients. These were all male, with a median age of 62 years (range, 39 to 71 years). The 16 patients without cirrhosis were equally divided in sex; their median age was 48 years (range, 18 to 73 years).

The tumor pathologic type in the cirrhotic group was a straightforward HCC in all patients. This tumor was found in the majority of the group with normal livers, but there were two distinct subsets (fibrolamellar [three cases] and clear-cell [two cases] variants), which seemed, in this small series, to carry a better prognosis.

In addition, 13 cases of cholangiocarcinoma (nine in normal and four in cirrhotic livers) were identified. These were excluded from this study since they were thought to represent a biologically different type of tumor.

Of the 61 patients with HCC and demonstrable cirrhosis in the hepatic parenchyma, 8 had liver findings characteristic of alcoholic cirrhosis. Of the remainder, 3 livers were classified as having hemochromatosis and 50 as having micronodular or macronodular cirrhosis, mostly classifiable as posthepatitic. Less than half underwent measurement of surface antigens for hepatitis B, and of these 57% were positive.

Less than half of the patients in whom α-fetoprotein levels were measured showed an elevation at any time.

Diagnosis

The clinical presentation varied widely. Pain in the right subcostal area or on top of the shoulder from phrenic radiation was common, as were symptoms of fatigue, anorexia, and weight loss. Unexplained fever was not uncommon. The enlarged liver and palpable mass sometimes made the diagnosis obvious. Hemorrhage into the peritoneal cavity is a propensity of this tumor and may be massive and fatal. Any sudden deterioration in a patient with known liver disease raised suspicions of HCC, as did positive test for hepatitis B surface antigen or an elevated α-fetoprotein level.

Various radiologic studies were used to confirm or negate suspicion. The liver-spleen scan has now been almost replaced by ultrasound and computed tomography in liver scanning for hepatoma. After scanning, more specific definition was achieved by celiac and superior mesenteric arteriograms.

We believe that percutaneous liver biopsy carries a high risk of hemorrhage and has little role in the workup.

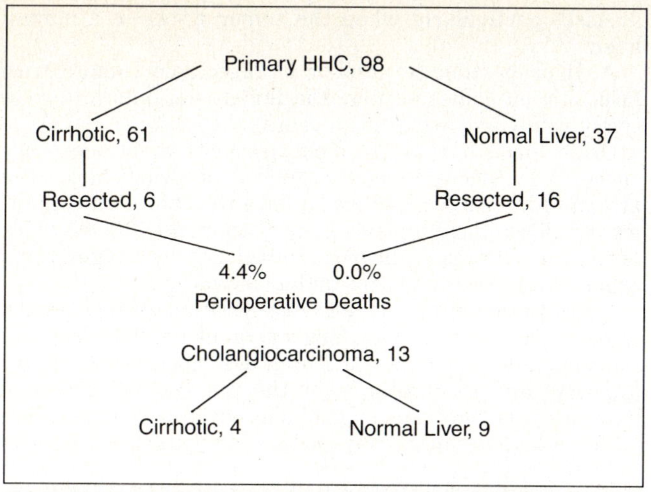

Fig 1.—Primary hepatocellular carcinoma (HCC) and cholangiocarcinoma at New England Deaconess Hospital, Boston, Mass, 1970 to 1985.

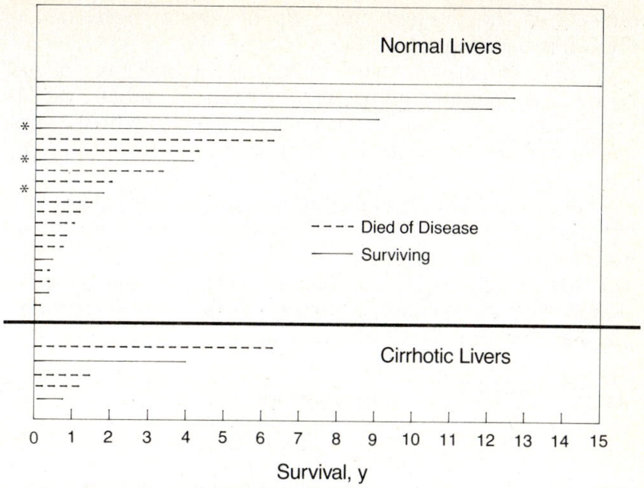

Fig 2.—Individual survivals of patients with resection for hepatocellular carcinoma. Asterisks indicate fibrolamellar variant.

Results of Resection for Primary Hepatocellular Carcinoma in 22 Patients*

		Survival		
	No.	Range	Median, mo	Mean, mo
Survivors	**21**	2 mo–15 y	22	48
With cirrhotic livers	5	5 mo–6 y	19	33
With normal livers	16	2 mo–15 y	32	53

*There was one perioperative death.

Resection

A total of 22 of the 98 patients with HHC were considered suitable for primary hepatic resection. One patient died in the perioperative period (a cirrhotic patient whose death was attributable to an intractable coagulopathy), giving an overall operative mortality of 4.4%.

The advisability of hepatic resection for HCC with liver disease is dubious. Joishy and Balsageram[9] in Malaysia, Ong and Chan[8] in Hong Kong, and Fortner et al[17] in the United States concluded that, except in the most favorable cases where a limited resection is feasible, cirrhosis is a contraindication to operation. This is consistent with our own experience, in which the multifocal nature or location of the tumor, the degree of liver dysfunction, or extrahepatic spread precluded operative removal in all but 6 of 61 patients.

Of the nine patients who survived more than 4 years, seven had normal hepatic parenchyma and two had hemochromatosis rather than alcohol or hepatitis as a cause of their cirrhotic process.

RESULTS

In the six patients whose tumors arose in cirrhotic livers, two had hemochromatosis as the primary diagnosis and the other four were classified as having posthepatitic cirrhosis (three of whom were positive for hepatitis B surface antigen). One patient died of a coagulopathy in the perioperative period after right hepatic lobectomy (Table). Three other patients with cirrhosis died of recurrent disease at 15, 18, and 75 months. Of the remaining two patients, both treated with wedge resections, one died of recurrent disease at 75 months and the other was living, free of disease, 4 years after surgery. Interestingly, the two long-term survivors both had hemochromatosis as the underlying disease.

In the noncirrhotic group there were no perioperative deaths. Total median survival was 32 months (Table). Eight patients were alive and well 5 months to 15 years postoperatively, with a median survival to date of 11 years. Of the eight patients who ultimately died of their disease, the median survival was 17 months, with a range of 2 months to 6 years.

Operations in both groups ranged from extensive anatomic procedures to limited wedge resections, and there was no direct relationship between survival and extent of operation except in the small group of cirrhotic patients, where the two longest survivors had peripheral lesions treated by wedge resection.

All patients who had margins less than 1 cm, venous invasion, or capsular rupture died of recurrent disease in less than 15 months. No evident regression or prolongation of life could be defined in the five patients treated with chemotherapy.

Perioperative morbidity was significantly higher in the cirrhotic group; complications included subphrenic abscess (two), pneumothorax (one), infected central line (one), upper gastrointestinal tract hemorrhage (one), and subhepatic abscess (one). In the noncirrhotic group, there were fewer complications; they included wound infection (two), subhepatic abscess (one), and pulmonary embolus (one), and none was critical. Survival data for both groups (cirrhotic and normal livers) are shown in Fig 2.

Only one patient ultimately died of disease after surviving for more than 4 years. Otherwise, there were no recurrences in the long-term survivors.

In the patients who developed HCC in normal livers, there were some points of particular interest. Three patients, all young and female (age range, 15 to 40 years), who survived from 22 to 77 months to date without recurrence had a histologic diagnosis of the fibrolamellar variant, which has been recognized by others[17-23] as occurring in young women and carrying a relatively favorable prognosis.

Two patients with clear-cell HCC had long survivals. Although one developed recurrent disease and died 30 months after resection, the other, a young woman, had resection of a huge primary at age 19 years and was living and well 15 years later despite the presence of multiple small, histologically proved metastases in the remaining lobe. She has had no treatment and has no demonstrable disease at the present time. Spontaneous regression of HCC has been reported.[24]

Of the 22 patients who underwent resection, 18 had lymph nodes submitted with the specimen, and of these 16 were negative for cancer. The two patients in whom lymph nodes showed metastatic malignant disease both died within 2 years.

The size of the tumor did not appear to affect the prognosis if there was an adequate margin (>1 cm) of hepatic parenchyma and no satellite nodules.

There is little evidence that any form of therapy other than resection, including dearterialization and chemotherapy, has any significant effect on survival.[25]

COMMENT

The favorable results of liver resection in the treatment of HCC in this and other series reported from Western countries,[1-4,26,27] as compared with Asian and African data, suggest either a different biologic tumor or earlier diagnosis and treatment. The experiences reported from Japan[11-13,28] are still different inasmuch as the great majority of tumors seem to arise in cirrhotic patients with relatively mild liver dysfunction. Operability and survival are much higher in Western series than series reported from Asia and Africa.[5-10]

The low perioperative mortality in this series and the number of long survivals (eight more than 5 years) reflect a high degree of selectivity (22 resections from a total of 98 cases), but they do indicate that HCC is not a hopeless disease, particularly when the tumor arises in a normal liver.

A disproportionate number of resectable tumors with favorable outcomes occurred in female patients in a relatively young age group (<40 years).

Other forms of therapy in our series have not been very successful. Various chemotherapeutic programs have been attempted, with a consistent failure to achieve any significant palliation. A review by Lee[25] confirms this evidence of failure. Efforts at thromboembolism, cryosurgery, and other esoteric methods are under evaluation.

A brief comment on hepatic regeneration after resection is perhaps relevant. The surgeon relies on this dramatic phenomenon, which has been well described in laboratory animals[29] and in humans,[30] for the restoration of normal liver function and the physiologic basis of regeneration, which was described many years ago by Bucher.[31,32] Probably one of the reasons for the poor results of resection of cirrhotic livers for HCC relates to the inability of these diseased organs to regenerate properly.

Since the initiation of our liver transplant program in 1983, five transplantations have been carried out for HCC. These were not included or analyzed in this report; it is too early and the numbers are too small for adequate evaluation. A survey by Schaarschmidt[33] provided preliminary data from four centers. Some hepatocellular tumors were included in the report by Iwatsuki et al[34] on liver resection for tumors. Calne[35] provided encouraging reports on a few cases. In all probability, there will be a role for liver transplantation in the treatment of HCC, but the application should be selective and critical.

References

1. Crutcher HP, Terz JJ, Kay S, Lawrence W Jr. Primary liver cancer. *Surgery.* 1971;70:467-479.
2. Malt RA. Surgery for hepatic neoplasms. *N Engl J Med.* 1985;25:1591-1596.
3. Stehlin JS Jr, Ipolyi PD, Greeff PJ, McGaff CJ Jr, Davis BR, McNary L. Treatment of cancer of the liver: 20 years' experience with infusion and resection in 414 patients. *Ann Surg.* 1988;208:23-35.
4. Scudamore CH, Ragaz J, Dluftinger AM, Owen DA. Hepatocellular carcinoma: a comparison of oriental and caucasian patients. *Am J Surg.* 1988;155:659-662.
5. McDermott WV. Surgical disease in East Africa. *Arch Surg.* 1987;122:397-402.
6. Lee Y-TN. Primary carcinoma of the liver: diagnosis, prognosis, and management. *J Surg Oncol.* 1983;22:17-25.
7. Lai ECS, Choi TK, Tong SW, Ong GB, Wong J. Treatment of unresectable hepatocellular carcinoma: results of a randomized controlled trial. *World J Surg.* 1986;10:501-509.
8. Ong GB, Chan WKW. Primary carcinoma of the liver. *Surg Gynecol Obstet.* 1976;143:31-38.
9. Joishy SK, Balsageram M. Hepatic resection for malignant tumors of the liver: essentials for a unified surgical approach. *Am J Surg.* 1980;139:360-369.
10. Lee CS, Sung JL, Hwang JY, et al. Surgical treatment of 109 patients with asymptomatic hepatocellular carcinoma. *Surgery.* 1986;99:481-490.
11. Nagasue N, Yukaya H, Ogawa Y, Yukiharu S, Chang TC, Tiimi K. Clinical experience with 188 hepatic resections for hepatocellular carcinoma. *Surgery.* 1986;99:694-702.
12. Kinami Y, Takashima S, Miyazaki I. Hepatic resection for hepatocellular carcinoma associated with liver cirrhosis. *World J Surg.* 1986;10:294-301.
13. Nagao T, Inoue S, Goto S, et al. Hepatic resection for hepatocellular carcinoma: clinical features and long-term prognosis. *Ann Surg.* 1987;205:33-40.
14. Okamoto E, Tanaka N, Yamanaka N, Toyosaka A. Results of surgical treatments of primary hepatocellular carcinoma: some aspects of improved long-term survival. *World J Surg.* 1984;8:360-366.
15. Agasua N, Yukawa S, Amada T, Hirose S, Kanashima R, Inokudir K. The natural history of hepatocellular carcinoma: a study of 100 untreated cases. *Cancer.* 1984;56:1461-1465.
16. Bengmark S, Hafstrom L, Jeppsson B, Sundqvist K. Primary carcinoma of the liver: improvement in sight? *World J Surg.* 1982;6:54-60.
17. Fortner JG, Kim DK, MacLean BJ, et al. Major hepatic resection for neoplasia: personal experience in 108 patients. *Ann Surg.* 1978;188:363-371.
18. Case records of the Massachusetts General Hospital: weekly clinicopathological exercises. *N Engl J Med.* 1987;317:556-564. Case 35-1987.
19. Teitelbaum DH, Tuttle S, Carey LC, Clausen KP. Fibrolamellar carcinoma of the liver: review of three cases and the presentation of a characteristic set of tumor markers defining this tumor. *Ann Surg.* 1985;202:36-41.
20. Wood WJ, Rawlings M, Evans H, Lim CNH. Hepatocellular carcinoma: importance of histologic classification as a prognostic factor. *Am J Surg.* 1988;155:663-666.
21. Nagorney DM, Adson MA, Welland LH, Knight CD, Smalley Sr, Zinsmeister AR. Fibrolamellar hepatoma. *Am J Surg.* 1985;149:113-119.
22. Starzl TE, Iwatsuki S, Shaw BW, Nalesnik MA, Farhi DC, Van Thiel DH. Treatment of fibrolamellar hepatoma with partial or total hepatectomy and transplantation of the liver. *Surg Gynecol Obstet.* 1986;162:145-147.
23. Basile RM, Ross JS, Spector JI, Zimbler H. Fibrolamellar oncocytic hepatoma: a surgical disease. *Contemp Surg.* 1988;32:26-29.
24. Lam KC, Ho JCI, Yeung RTT. Spontaneous regression of hepatocellular carcinoma. *Cancer.* 1982;50:332-336.
25. Lee TND. Systemic and regional treatment of primary carcinoma of the liver. *Cancer Treat Rev.* 1977;4:195-212.
26. Luna G, Florence L, Johnsen J. Hepatocellular carcinoma: a 5 year institutional experience. *Am J Surg.* 1985;149:591-594.
27. Nagao T, Inone S, Mizuta T, Saito H, Sawan H, Movioka Y. One hundred hepatic resections: incisions and operative results: 1985. *Ann Surg.* 1985;202:22-29.
28. Tsuzuki T, Toshiro O, Shuhei I, Shimazu M. Hepatic resection in 125 patients. *Arch Surg.* 1984;119:1025-1032.
29. Islami AH, Pack GT, Hubbard JC. The humoral factor in regeneration of the liver in parabiotic rats. *Surg Gynecol Obstet.* 1959;108:549-554.
30. McDermott WV Jr, Greenberger NJ, Isselbacher KJ, Weber AL. Major hepatic resection: diagnostic techniques and metabolic problems. *Surgery.* 1963;54:56-66.
31. Bucher NLR. Regeneration of the mammalian liver. *Int Rev Cytol.* 1963;15:245-300.
32. Bucher NLR. Experimental aspects of hepatic regeneration. *N Engl J Med.* 1967;277:686-696.
33. Schaarschmidt BF. Human liver transplantation: analysis of data on 540 patients from four centers. *Hepatology.* 1984;4(suppl):95-101.
34. Iwatsuki S, Gordon RO, Shaw BW, et al. Role of liver transplantation in cancer therapy. *Ann Surg.* 1985;202:401-407.
35. Calne RY. Liver transplantation for liver cancer. *World J Surg.* 1982;6:81-85.

DISCUSSION

JOHN W. BRAASCH, MD, Burlington, Mass: I would like to ask about the place of segmental resection or minimal resection in patients who have a background of cirrhosis. Does this influence the authors' judgment? They turned down a lot of patients; on what basis were they turned down?

IRVIN M. MODLIN, MD, New Haven, Conn: I wonder if the authors would consider excluding the fibrolamellar hepatomas from this group. They secrete large amounts of neurotensin and are clearly neuroendocrine tumors. In fact, the tumors can be diagnosed by measurement of the plasma neurotensin and immunocytochemical localization of neurotensin to the tumor cells. They are amenable to both early diagnosis and long-term therapy with the appropriate antiendocrine cytotoxic agents. Furthermore, their clinical behavior is quite different from that of carcinoma of the liver. I wonder, therefore, if they might not be excluded from the standard management profile of hepatomas.

JAMES FOSTER, MD, Hartford, Conn: My own experience encompasses 22 adults and six children who had liver resection for primary cancer. The overall results were similar. There was one operative death and a 36% 5-year survival (actual, not actuarial). Careful analysis showed that most of the long-term survivors either were young or had unusual pathologic variants. One patient had cirrhosis, and a small primary cancer discovered with α-fetoprotein testing was resected by wedge technique. Fifteen months later he was dead with recurrent disease. This experience strengthened my continuing bias that resection of primary cancer of the liver in *Western* patients is not warranted except to control hemorrhage.

Six of eight 5-year survivors had something other than primary HCC. Two were infants with hepatoblastomas, three (two of whom were less than 25 years of age) had fibrolamellar carcinoma, and the last had a primary low-grade sarcoma of the liver. We should continue to be aggressive about resecting localized primary liver cancer in patients without cirrhosis, but we should be quite selective in adults with HCC and cholangiocarcinoma.

Although major liver resection can be done with simple tools, it is not a simple operation. Between us, we have done less than 50 cases for primary liver cancer in 15 years. Should these patients all be referred to the few centers with significant experience, or should any well-trained surgeon tackle these fortunately rare problems?

MAUREEN F. MARTIN, MD, Burlington, Mass: I would like to ask Dr McDermott what he thinks the place of liver transplantation is in the face of a hepatocellular malignant neoplasm.

DR MCDERMOTT: In its broadest sense, primary cancer of the liver would include a number of subgroups, including cholangiocarcinoma, HCC, tumors of mixed histologic pattern, and the clear-cell and fibrolamellar variants. This last subgroup is of particular interest since some of them have been shown to have neuroendocrine secretory activity. We did eliminate the cholangiocarcinomas, which might fit better with tumors of biliary tract origins, but finally decided to include the others.

Dr Foster's question about palliative resection was particularly pertinent since there was one patient in the series, a young woman with a large clear-cell carcinoma, who had histologically demonstrable metastases in the liver remaining after a left hepatic lobectomy. No further treatment was given, and she was still alive and well without demonstrable disease 15 years after operation.

In answer to Dr Braasch's question regarding the extent of resection, the existing data would indicate that a margin of 1.0 cm is adequate, and further extension does not improve survival.

Dr Martin raised the advisability of liver transplantation as treatment for primary cancer of the liver. There have been five hepatomas in our hospital in the past few years, but Dr Jenkins and I both agreed that the series and the follow-ups were too limited to include in this series. Dr Starzl's initial experience was dismal, but in recent years they have had long survivals in a number of patients who were found to have incidental carcinomas in cirrhotic livers. Professor Calne has also reported some success in this area.

In Other AMA Journals

ARCHIVES OF INTERNAL MEDICINE

Selective Screening for Abdominal Aortic Aneurysms With Physical Examination and Ultrasound

Frank A. Lederle, MD; Janine M. Walker, RN; Donovan B. Reinke, MD

Abdominal aortic aneurysm (AAA) is an important cause of preventable death in older persons. Persistently high rupture mortality rates indicate that these deaths can be prevented only by early detection and treatment of AAA. In an effort to develop an effective and efficient program of AAA detection, we selectively screened a high-risk population. Men aged 60 to 75 years with hypertension and/or coronary artery disease were randomly selected from a general medicine clinic and screened with physical examination and ultrasound. Eighteen previously unsuspected aneurysms, 3.6 to 5.9 cm in size (mean, 4.4 cm), were detected in 201 patients, for a prevalence of 9% (95% confidence interval: 4.7% to 13.3%). The specificity and positive predictive value of ultrasound were each 100%. Abdominal palpation detected only half of these aneurysms, but missed none in patients with an abdominal girth less than 100 cm (n = 6). This degree of sensitivity did not occur with "routine" examinations and requires that the examination be directed specifically toward AAA detection. We conclude that undiagnosed AAAs are common in this large subgroup of the clinic population, that ultrasound is an excellent screening test for AAAs, and that physical examination may be adequate for screening thin patients. We recommend that every two or three years persons over the age of 50 years undergo careful abdominal palpation aimed at detecting AAAs, as part of the periodic health examination. We further recommend that obese older men at high risk for AAA have at least one-time screening with abdominal ultrasound, regardless of findings on physical examination (*Arch Intern Med* 1988;148:1753-1756).

Reprint requests to Department of Medicine III-0, Minneapolis Veterans Administration Medical Center, 54th Street and 48th Avenue S, Minneapolis, MN 55417 (Dr Lederle).

Management of Biliary Obstruction

A Comparison of Percutaneous, Endoscopic, and Operative Techniques

Janice G. Rothschild, MD; Marshall M. Kaplan, MD; Victor G. Millan, MD; Randolph B. Reinhold, MD

• Surgery for obstructive jaundice is being challenged by endoscopic and percutaneous techniques. To compare their safety and efficacy, the courses of 157 patients treated for biliary obstruction were examined. Outcome was judged by mortality, complications, and need for further intervention. Forty-eight patients underwent endoscopic papillotomy (43 [90%] had stone disease) with two deaths and 11 cases of (23% incidence) of cholangitis. Pancreatitis developed in 9 (19%). Twenty-seven patients (56%) required further endoscopic, percutaneous, or surgical intervention. Sixty-five patients underwent transhepatic drainage (58 [89%] had malignant neoplasms) with a 28% (n = 18) mortality rate. Cholangitis developed in 26 (40%), and 50 (77%) required further transhepatic or surgical intervention. Forty-four patients underwent surgery (22 [50%] had stone disease and 12 [27%] had malignant neoplasms) with a 4.5% (n = 2) mortality rate. Cholangitis developed in 3 (7%), pancreatitis developed in 2 (4.5%), and bleeding developed in 1 (2%). Eight (18%) required further intervention. While endoscopic papillotomy provides efficacious treatment for stone disease, surgery provides a more expeditious, less morbid relief for malignant obstruction.

(*Arch Surg.* 1989;124:556-560)

The last decade has seen marked changes in the evaluation and management of biliary tract disease. Options have broadened from the historical standard of cholecystectomy with surgical common duct exploration or bypass to include endoscopic, percutaneous transhepatic, and lithotriptic techniques. While the treatment of patients presenting with primary common duct stones is still evolving,[1,2] multiple operations for the treatment of retained common bile duct stones can be avoided with endoscopic papillotomy.[1,3] Biliary lithotriptic techniques have increased options further.[4] Similarly, the last decade has seen safer and more sophisticated access to the biliary tree using percutaneous transhepatic techniques allowing visualization and diagnosis of a wide range of biliary abnormalities.[5,6] Commensurate with this progress in access, the indications for percutaneous treatment have been expanded. To assess and compare the safety and efficacy of these techniques and how they might best interface in the treatment of the patient with obstructive jaundice, we reviewed our experience in the surgical, endoscopic, and percutaneous treatment of biliary obstruction.

Accepted for publication December 28, 1988.

From the Department of Surgery, New England Medical Center, Boston, Mass.

Read before the 69th Annual Meeting of the New England Surgical Society, Montreal, Canada, September 16, 1988.

Reprint requests to Department of Surgery, New England Medical Center, 750 Washington St, Boston, MA 02111 (Dr Rothschild).

PATIENTS AND METHODS

Two hundred thirty-three patients were admitted to the New England Medical Center, Boston, Mass, with obstructive jaundice between 1980 and 1986. All available charts were reviewed. The patients included for evaluation underwent treatment for biliary obstruction as defined by a bilirubin value of more than 34 μmol/L and/or an alkaline phosphatase value of more than 200 U/L. The study group consisted of 157 patients, including 90 men and 67 women. The average age at presentation was 66 years (range, 22 to 98 years). The cause of obstruction was malignant neoplasm in 72 (46%) and stone disease in 67 (43%). Other causes included inflammatory disease (7 [4%]), postoperative changes (2 [1%]), pancreatitis (1 [1%]), and those of an idiopathic nature (4 [2.5%]) (Table 1).

The choice of initial mode of treatment was made by the primary physician caring for the patient. The physician group included all staff surgeons and gastroenterologists at the New England Medical Center. All medical charts with a complete database were reviewed to evaluate the primary form of therapy. Outcome was judged by subjective and objective relief of signs and symptoms, the incidence of early mortality and complications, as well as a need for further intervention.

Presenting complaints included jaundice in 76% and pain in 69%. Nausea/vomiting and weight loss were the next most common complaints present in 71 (45%) and 61 (39%), respectively. Fever and pruritus were present in 55 (35%) and 42 (27%), respectively. Mean duration of symptoms prior to presentation was 4.8 months (range, 0 to 60 months). The average bilirubin value at the time of presentation was 180 μmol/L and the average alkaline phosphatase value was 526 U/L (Table 2). Ninety-five patients (61%) had 97 previous operations. These included exploratory laparotomy in 14, cholecystectomy in 61, surgical common bile duct exploration in 18, and gastrectomy in 4 patients.

RESULTS

The most common diagnostic procedure was ultrasonography undertaken in 86 (55%) of patients. This was diagnostic of biliary dilatation in 67% of studies and suggested the cause in 47 (55%). Computed tomographic scans were done in 58 (37%), were diagnostic of dilatation in 35 (60%), and suggested the cause in 39 (67%). Endoscopic retrograde

Table 1.—Causes of Obstruction

Cause	ERCP*	PTC*	Surgery	Overall
Malignant neoplasm	2	58	12	**72**
Stones	43	2	22	**67**
Inflammatory	0	1	4	**5**
Postoperative	0	0	2	**2**
Sclerosing cholangitis	1	1	0	**2**
Pancreatitis	0	0	1	**1**
Combination	1	1	2	**4**
Unknown	1	2	1	**4**
Total	**48**	**65**	**44**	**157**

*ERCP indicates endoscopic retrograde cholangiopancreatography; PTC, percutaneous transhepatic cholangiography.

Table 2.—Laboratory Values at Presentation

Value	ERCP*	PTC*	Surgery	Overall
Bilirubin, µmol/L	82	279	140	180
Alkaline phosphatase, U/L	464	700	337	526
Albumin <30 g/L, %	25	22	20	22

*ERCP indicates endoscopic retrograde cholangiopancreatography; PTC, percutaneous transhepatic cholangiography.

cholangiopancreatography and percutaneous transhepatic cholangiography were common diagnostic procedures as well, done in 80 (51%) and 46 (48%), respectively. These diagnostic procedures provided information regarding the cause of obstruction in 62 (78%) and in 73 (96%), respectively. Percutaneous or endoscopic biopsies and cytologic studies were done in 44 (28%) of patients. Pathologic findings were diagnostic of the cause in 25 (49%) of the biopsies done.

ENDOSCOPY

Of the 157 patients, 48 underwent endoscopic papillotomy as their initial form of therapy. These 48 patients comprised 21 men and 27 women with an average age of 72 years (range, 22 to 98 years). Endoscopic papillotomy was done in 43 (90%) of these for stone disease, 2 (4%) for malignant neoplasms, and 1 (2%) for inflammatory disease. Diagnosis was not clarified in 1 (2%) (Table 1). The average bilirubin value of the patients undergoing endoscopic drainage was 82 µmol/L and the alkaline phosphatase value was 464 U/L (Table 2). The average duration of symptoms prior to treatment was 9 months.

There was a 4% (n=2) 30-day mortality rate and 33 (69%) of the patients had complications develop. While preprocedure antibiotic therapy is standard, cholangitis, as defined by fever and chills in a jaundiced patient, developed in 11 (23%) of the patients. Septicemia was documented by positive blood cultures in 2 (4%) of the patients who required transfer to an intensive care unit. Pancreatitis developed in 9 (19%) and bleeding developed in 4 (8%). Perforation occurred in 1 patient (Tables 3 and 4). Of the patients undergoing papillotomy, 27 (56%) required further intervention. This included 20 (42%) of the patients who required repeated endoscopy with or without repeated papillotomy. Two (4%) required transhepatic cholangiographic drainage and 5 (10%) went on to surgery for failure of adequate drainage. Over the 6 months following hospital discharge an additional 5 (50%) of the patients followed up required further intervention, including repeated endoscopy with enlargement of the papillotomy in 1 patient, percutaneous drainage in 1 patient, and surgery in 2 patients.

Table 3.—Complications (Episodes)*

Complications	ERCP (n=48)	PTC (n=65)	Surgery (n=44)
Cholangitis	11	26	3
Septicemia	2	13	1
Abscess	0	1	0
Bile leak	0	2	2
Fistula	0	1	2
Perforation	1	1	1
Pancreatitis	9	1	2
Bleeding	4	8	1
Transfer to ICU	2	5	2
Catheter dislodgment	0	7	1
Need for further procedure			
ERCP	20	1	3
PTC	2	25	4
Surgery	5	24	1
Other, related to procedure	5	3	6
Other, unrelated to procedure	3	8	5
None	15	9	25

*ERCP indicates endoscopic retrograde cholangiopancreatography; PTC, percutaneous transhepatic cholangiography; and ICU, intensive care unit.

Table 4.—Mortality Rates

	ERCP* (n=48)	PTC* (n=65)	Surgery (n=44)	Overall (n=157)
Sepsis	1	4	0	5
Hemorrhage	0	3	0	3
Liver failure	0	3	1	4
Inanition	0	1	0	1
Other, related	0	0	0	0
Other, unrelated	1	2	0	3
Unknown	0	5	1	6
Total	**2**	**18**	**2**	**22**

*ERCP indicates endoscopic retrograde cholangiopancreatography; PTC, percutaneous transhepatic cholangiography.

PERCUTANEOUS TRANSHEPATIC CHOLANGIOGRAPHY

Sixty-five patients underwent percutaneous transhepatic drainage as the primary mode of therapy. There were 44 men and 21 women with an average age of 66 years (range, 22 to 91 years). Causes included malignant neoplasms in 58 (89%) and stone disease in 2 (3%). Other causes included inflammatory disease in 2 (3%); the diagnosis was unknown in 2 (3%) (Table 1). The average bilirubin value was 279 µmol/L and the alkaline phosphatase value was 700 U/L (Table 2). The average duration of symptoms prior to treatment was 2.4 months.

Common diagnostic procedures included ultrasound, done in 42 (65%) of the patients, and computed tomographic scan, done in 40 (62%). These were diagnostic in 13 (31%) and 28 (70%), respectively. Thirty-six (55%) of the patients underwent a biopsy procedure with their cholangiogram, including cytologic study and brush biopsy. This was diagnostic in 18 (50%) of the biopsy specimens.

There was a 28% (n = 18) 30-day mortality rate and 56 (86%) of the patients had complications develop. These included cholangitis in 26 (40%) and septicemia in 13 (20%). Other complications included bleeding in 8 (12%) and bile leakage in 2 (3%). Transfer to an intensive care unit was required in 5 (8%) of these patients. Early catheter dislodgment occurred in 7 (11%). Abscess formation, perforation, and pancreatitis occurred in 1 patient each (Tables 3 and 4).

While only nine (14%) of the procedures were considered preoperative at the outset, 24 (37%) of the patients went on to surgery during the same hospitalization. Twenty-five (38%) required early repeated cholangiography or catheter adjustment. One patient required a further endoscopic procedure. Thirteen (50%) of the patients discharged from the hospital required further intervention within the next 6 months, including repeated cholangiogram with tube replacement in 9 patients and surgery in 4 patients.

SURGERY

Forty-four patients underwent surgery as their primary form of therapy. There were 25 men and 19 women with an average age of 58 years (range, 25 to 92 years). Twenty-two (50%) of the patients were found to have stone disease as the cause of their obstruction and 12 (27%) had neoplasms. Two (5%) of the patients underwent surgical exploration for postoperative complications and the remainder underwent surgical exploration for inflammatory conditions (Table 1). The average bilirubin value on presentation was 140 μmol/L and the alkaline phosphatase value was 337 U/L (Table 2). The average duration of symptoms was 3.8 months.

The most common diagnostic procedures preoperatively were ultrasound, done in 28 (64%) of the patients, and computed tomographic scan, done in 13 (30%). These examinations were diagnostic in 25 (89%) and 7 (54%) of the patients, respectively. Six (14%) of the patients had a preoperative attempt at biopsy and in 2 (33%), those biopsy specimens provided a diagnosis. Surgical procedures included the following: cholecystectomy (29 operations); surgical common duct exploration (30 operations); biliary enteric anastomosis (19 operations); resection of malignant neoplasm (pancreas [6 operations], biliary [2 operations], and hepatic [1 operation]); repair of strictures (2 operations); and tube drainage (2 operations).

The postoperative mortality rate was 4.5% (n = 2) and the morbidity rate was 43% (n = 19). Complications included cholangitis in three (7%) and septicemia in one (2%). Other complications included anastomotic leakage in two patients, with fistula formation in two patients. Pancreatitis developed in two patients, bleeding in one patient, and a gastrointestinal leak in one patient (Tables 3 and 4).

One (2%) of the patients required reoperation during the same hospitalization. Four (9%) needed percutaneous drainage and three (7%) required endoscopy. Two (8%) of the patients required further intervention over the first 6 months following hospital discharge; one patient required percutaneous drainage and one required repeated surgical exploration.

COMMENT

While the advancement of technology has placed a wide range of diagnostic and therapeutic options at the hands of the physician, the mere capacity to intervene does not always imply the best course of treatment for the patient. In the patient presenting with jaundice, it is necessary to determine that the jaundice is "surgical," ie, obstructive, rather than "medical," ie, cholestatic. Further diagnostic procedures should be continued only as long as they may alter the ultimate choice of treatment. Using ultrasound examination alone, Eyre-Brook et al[7] determined that 80 of 132 patients could be treated surgically with the appropriate procedure without needing further diagnostic tests. Lewis et al[8] reported that not only was percutaneous drainage not therapeutically helpful in the preoperative patient but the diagnostic information elicited did not alter the treatment plan. Ultrasonography was the most common examination undertaken in our patients. This confirmed the presence of obstruction in the majority. Computed tomographic scan was equally sensitive for the diagnosis of ductal dilatation and was slightly more likely to reveal the cause of this dilatation.

A large volume of literature has confirmed the ability of the endoscopist to treat retained or recurrent bile duct stones with a morbidity similar to that of the surgeon.[2,3] In the patient presenting with retained common bile duct stones, the duct can be cleared of these stones in up to 90% of patients.[1,3] The role of sphincterotomy preoperatively in the group with gallbladders in situ is still undetermined, but the group at highest risk for emergency surgery after papillotomy is that group with their gallbladders in situ.[1,9] In the elderly and infirm patients, sphincterotomy alone may help to avoid surgery in up to 87% of patients.[1,2,9,10] In younger and healthy patients who are likely to have recurrent biliary symptoms develop, surgery is probably indicated.

The optimal treatment of malignant obstruction of the biliary tree is more controversial. In the patient who is a reasonable surgical risk, surgical exploration is warranted in the absence of documented metastatic disease in hopes of offering a curative resection.[8,11,12] It is in the patient with symptomatic unresectable malignant obstruction suffering from pruritus and cholangitis that the optimal form of palliation needs to be elucidated. Many would argue that percutaneous drainage with prosthesis, internal or external catheter placement, offers adequate and reasonable palliation. Leung et al,[11] Berquist et al,[5] and Ferucci et al,[6,13] reported achievement of internal drainage in 87%, 42%, and 74% of attempts, respectively. Recent reports abound on the ability of interventional radiographic techniques to achieve placement of percutaneous catheters into the duodenum.

This palliation has a cost, however, with a reported mortality rate of 2.5% to 31.5% and a morbidity rate of 24% to 87.5%.[5,6,11,13] In early series, hemorrhage was the most common complication, followed by cholangitis. Our series bears out the significant morbidity and mortality rates associated with transhepatic palliation.

The incidence of complications, which in recent reports, including ours, is most frequently cholangitis, seems to relate most strongly with multiple obstructions and inadequate drainage.[13-15] While enteric organisms from bile, possibly related to retrograde duodenal reflux, grow in cultures from most patients, only those with an element of persistent obstruction have cholangitis develop, which, in turn, contributes to a decreased survival rate.

In addition, the "success" of palliation needs to be questioned when further intervention with tube manipulation, replacement, or surgery is required in 19% to 47% of patients.[5,11] Ferucci et al[6] confirmed the need for tube adjustments in up to 76% of patients. This is supported by a recent prospective controlled series reported by Bornman et al.[16] Patients were randomized to receive either cholecystojejunostomy with or without gastrojejunostomy vs percutaneous drainage. The success rate in palliation was similar among the two groups, 84% vs 76%, as was the complication rate and survival. An initial advantage in decreased hospital stay for percutaneous transhepatic cholangiography was ultimately blunted by the need for hospital readmissions for tube manipulations. We believe that the rate of catheter obstruction remained as low as it did only because of the dismal prognosis in this patient group. Similar discouraging data are reported for preoperative percutaneous drainage, with no survival or morbidity advantage for a course of preoperative drainage.[8,17]

Endoscopic placement of prostheses is another option for the treatment of malignant obstruction. Successful placement of prostheses is reported in 83% to 89% of patients.[11,18,19] While the technique-related complications of percutaneous transhepatic cholangiography are obviated, the difficulties of cholangitis related to clogging of the prosthesis and inadequate drainage result in mortality rates of 14% to 16% and hospital readmissions for catheter adjustment in a similar percentage.

Surgical series of the treatment of biliary obstruction can be better evaluated in this light. As already noted, cholecystectomy with surgical common duct exploration offers a reasonable treatment for young or healthy patients with common bile duct stones[1,3,20] with respect to morbidity and the need for future surgery.

In a large series McSherry and Glenn[21] confirmed that elective biliary tract surgery can be done with a mortality rate of less than 2%. As in reports on endoscopic drainage, morbidity and mortality are related to age and cardiovascular disease rather than to any discreet surgical risk.

Similarly, success rates for the surgical treatment of benign biliary tract disease provide a time-tested standard for comparison. Long-term success in the treatment of biliary stricture or stone disease should exceed rates of 86% to 93% as reported by Bismuth et al[22] and Genest et al.[23]

While patient selection makes it difficult to compare series of patients treated operatively and nonoperatively for malignant disease, surgical series are clear with respect to the results that can be expected from operative palliation. Many agree that surgical exploration with an eye toward resection is warranted in the absence of obvious metastatic disease as it offers the only clear hope of cure.[8,11,12] Once at celiotomy "operative biliary enteric bypass is a better means of palliation [than stent placement]."[24] Mortality rates in this population range from 7% to 18% with survivals generally less than 1 year.[12,24] However, laparotomy alone with no discreet treatment carries a mortality rate in excess of 25%, reflecting a selection bias. Our mortality rate of 8% in patients operated on for malignant disease is consistent with this range. Cholangitis is reported to occur in 0% to 10% of patients treated with internal surgical drainage, depending on the type of bilioenteric bypass employed. Our series, reporting the lowest need for further intervention following surgical treatment, both immediately and over 6 months, confirms the satisfactory level of palliation. The advantage of surgical treatment is not only in immediate morbidity, mortality, or survival, but also in the absence of long-term instrumentation of the biliary tree with its attendant morbidity and effect on quality of life. We conclude, therefore, that in the patient with malignant obstruction, early initial surgical decompression is warranted, even in the face of unresectable disease.

The avoidance of surgery is often the unstated goal of many practitioners presented with the patient with obstructive jaundice. We find that endoscopy is efficacious and safe for the treatment of obstructive stone disease. It is in the patient with malignant obstruction of the biliary tract that we need be most critical regarding treatment. Overall, survival is so dismal that the best we can do for our patient is offer a safe, comfortable palliation that will serve over the limited life expectancy. Compared with percutaneous transhepatic drainage, surgery is a more expeditious and less morbid route to the relief of obstruction.

References

1. Neoptolemos JP, Carr-Locke DL, Fossard DP. Prospective randomised study of preoperative endoscopic sphincterotomy versus surgery alone for common bile duct stones. *Br Med J.* 1987;294:470-474.
2. Cotton PB. Endoscopic management of bile duct stones (apples and oranges). *Gut.* 1984;25:587-597.
3. Miller BM, Kozarek RA, Ryan JA, Ball TJ, Traverso LW. Surgical versus endoscopic management of common bile duct stones. *Ann Surg.* 1988;207:135-141.
4. Sackmann M, Delius M, Sauerbruch T, et al. Shock-wave lithotripsy of gallbladder stones. *N Engl J Med.* 1988;318:393-397.
5. Berquist T, May G, Johnson CM, Adson MA, Thistle JL. Percutaneous biliary decompression: internal and external drainage in 50 patients. *AJR.* 1981;136:901-906.
6. Ferucci JT Jr, Mueller PR, Harbin WP. Percutaneous transhepatic biliary drainage technique, results and applications. *Diagn Radiol.* 1980;135:1-13.
7. Eyre-Brook IA, Ross B, Johnson AG. Should surgeons operate on the evidence of ultrasound alone in jaundiced patients? *Br J Surg.* 1983;70:587-589.
8. Lewis WD, Cady B, Rohrer RJ, Jenkins RL, Benotti PN, McDermott WV. Avoidance of transhepatic drainage prior to hepaticojejunostomy for obstruction of the biliary tract. *Surg Gynecol Obstet.* 1987;165:381-386.
9. Escourrou J, Cordova JA, Lazorthes F, Frexinos J, Ribet A. Early and late complications after endoscopic sphincterotomy for biliary lithiasis with and without the gallbladder 'in situ.' *Gut.* 1984;25:598-602.
10. Summerfield J. Biliary obstruction is best managed by endoscopists. *Gut.* 1988;29:741-745.
11. Leung JWC, Emery R, Cotton PB, Russell RCG, Vallon AG, Mason RR. Management of malignant obstructive jaundice at the Middlesex Hospital. *Br J Surg.* 1983;70:584-586.
12. Langer JC, Langer B, Taylor BR, Zeldin R, Cummings B. Carcinoma of the extrahepatic bile ducts: results of an aggressive surgical approach. *Surgery.* 1985;98:752-759.
13. Mueller PR, Van Sonnenberg E, Ferucci JT Jr. Percutaneous biliary drainage: technical and catheter-related problems in 200 procedures. *AJR.* 1982;138:17-23.
14. Audisio RA, Bozzetti F, Severini A, et al. The occurrence of cholangitis after percutaneous biliary drainage: evaluation of some risk factors. *Surgery.* 1988;103:507-512.
15. Clouse ME, Evans D, Costello P, Alday M, Edwards S, McDermott WV. Percutaneous transhepatic biliary drainage: complications due to multiple duct obstructions. *Ann Surg.* 1983;198:25-29.
16. Bornman PC, Harries-Jones EP, Tobias R, Van Stiegmann G, Terblanche J. Prospective controlled trial of transhepatic biliary endoprosthesis versus bypass surgery for incurable carcinoma of head of pancreas. *Lancet.* 1986;1:69-71.
17. McPherson GAD, Benjamin IS, Hodgson HJF, Bowley NB, Allison DJ, Blumgart LH. Preoperative percutaneous transhepatic biliary drainage: the results of a controlled trial. *Br J Surg.* 1984;71:371-375.
18. Cotton PB. Endoscopic methods for relief of malignant obstructive jaundice. *World J Surg.* 1984;8:854-861.
19. Huibregtse K, Tytgat GN. Palliative treatment of obstructive jaundice by transpapillary introduction of large bore bile duct endoprosthesis. *Gut.* 1982;23:371-375.
20. Crumplin MKH, Jenkinson LR, Kassab JY, Whitaker CM, Al-Boutiahi FH. Management of gallstones in a district general hospital. *Br J Surg.* 1985;72:428-432.
21. McSherry CK, Glenn F. The incidence and causes of death following surgery for nonmalignant biliary tract disease. *Ann Surg.* 1980;191:271-275.
22. Bismuth H, Franco D, Corlette MB, Hepp J. Long-term results of Roux-en-y hepaticojejunostomy. *Surg Gynecol Obstet.* 1978;146:161-167.
23. Genest JF, Nanos E, Broniatowski SG, Vogt D, Hermann RE. Benign biliary strictures: an analytic review (1970 to 1984). *Surgery.* 1986;99:409-413.
24. Sarr MG, Cameron JL. Surgical palliation of unresectable carcinoma of the pancreas. *World J Surg.* 1984;8:906-918.

Discussion

Warren W. Francis, MD, Providence, RI: I wonder if anybody can explain why a papillotomy stays open, and why when we used to do sphincterotomies surgically, they did not stay open.

Ricardo L. Rossi, MD, Burlington, Mass: In this retrospective study the patients treated with endoscopic, percutaneous, and surgical techniques differed in regard to age, and type and severity of disease. Dr Rothschild has pointed out the limitations of percutaneous and endoscopic measures and has emphasized the benefits of surgery. We would agree that surgery is preferable in patients judged to have resectable tumors by imaging techniques, in good surgical-risk patients judged to have unresectable lesions, and in patients with duodenal obstruction; that endoscopy is best in patients with retained common duct stones; and that patients judged to have unresectable tumors and who are unfit for surgery should be considered for stenting techniques, preferably through an endoscopic route. However, the necessary information to resolve the controversial role of these different evolving modalities of therapy will probably come from prospective trials. Factors that should be considered include the nature and extent of the underlying disease, its location, associated conditions, life expectancy, early and late mortality and morbidity associated with each procedure, the survival and quality of palliation of each technique, and the relative comparative costs. Speer et al (*Lancet.* 1987;2:57-62), in a prospective randomized trial, demonstrate the superiority of endoscopic drainage over percutaneous techniques. Shepherd showed minimal difference on the relative benefits of retrograde stenting over bypass operations in patients believed to have unresectable disease. Both percutaneous and endoscopic procedures are evolving, and better results could be obtained from improvement in techniques.

I would like to ask Dr Rothschild, first, can you advise us on the proper workup of these patients? Second, what are the results of the different therapeutic methods on patients with malignant neoplasms? Third, with regard to the 19% incidence of pancreatitis, was this a laboratory finding or clinically apparent? Fourth, you accounted for only 157 of the 233 patients who presented with obstructive jaundice at your institution; what happened to the remainder?

Dr Rothschild: Let me first account for the number of patients. There were nearly 250 patients admitted to the hospital for treatment of obstructive jaundice. Only 157 patients whose cases were reported were documented to have a bilirubin value of more than 34 μmol/L or an alkaline phosphatase value of more than 200 U/L (usually both). In an attempt to try to standardize the group, we counted only those patients.

With respect to the pancreatitis following papillotomy, the majority of the cases of pancreatitis occurred earlier in the series and included both chemical and clinical pancreatitis. If patients were documented as having hyperamylasemia, they were kept in the hospital longer for observation, affecting the outcome.

With respect to diagnostic procedures, Eyre-Brook and coworkers[7] have done a study showing the effect of operating based on ultrasound examination alone. In 80 of 132 patients, a proper surgical operation could be planned and carried through based on ultrasound examination alone without the need for any further diagnostic techniques. If the decision is made not to go ahead with percutaneous drainage, and the level of obstruction can be documented by ultrasound, that probably is sufficient and no further information is needed if one is willing to undertake resection if found and palliation if unresectable.

It was of interest that the patient group was self-selected in terms of treatment. The majority of the patients who underwent endoscopy did so for benign disease; our facility does not have a lot of experience with endoscopic stent placement for malignant disease. There were a few attempts at stent placement, one of which resulted in a mortality following a need for percutaneous and then surgical treatment. The surgical group, as I said, was more evenly distributed with malignant neoplasms and can be compared with the percutaneous group. Overall, we could not find any difference in terms of nutrition, laboratory values, and overall degree of illness between the two groups, and the results were as discussed.

In Other AMA Journals

ARCHIVES OF PATHOLOGY & LABORATORY MEDICINE

New Techniques for Compatibility Testing

Fred V. Plapp, MD, PhD

Hospital transfusion services and blood centers have continued to use manual hemagglutination methods for most of their pretransfusion compatibility testing. Automation with continuous-flow and batch analyzers has been practical only for the largest blood-processing centers. During the past 20 years, other methods of streamlining compatibility testing have evolved. Two of the most successful approaches have employed microplates to perform either liquid agglutination tests or solid-phase red blood cell adherence tests. Increasing numbers of automated systems for compatibility testing, based on these technologies, have become commercially available. These systems were optimally designed for batch processing. More recently, dipsticks for ABO grouping and direct antiglobulin testing have been developed, which were ideally suited for individual testing (*Arch Pathol Lab Med.* 1989;113:262-269).

Reprint requests to Department of Laboratory Medicine, St Luke's Hospital, 44th Street and Wornall Road, Kansas City, MO 64111 (Dr Plapp).

Liver Abscess

The Need for Complete Gastrointestinal Evaluation

Jeffrey L. Cohen, MD; F. Maureen Martin, MD; Ricardo L. Rossi, MD; David J. Schoetz, Jr, MD

• The cause of liver abscess is frequently obscure at initial presentation. We reviewed the medical records of 20 patients with pyogenic liver abscess over a 6-year period from 1981 to 1987. Liver abscess was suspected in only 3 patients on admission; the most common initial diagnosis was fever of unknown origin. Subsequently, the origin of the abscess was found to be intestinal in 7 patients, pancreatobiliary in 11 patients, and cryptogenic in 2 patients. Eleven patients underwent percutaneous transhepatic drainage of the abscess as the initial treatment, while open operation was the initial treatment in 9 patients. Percutaneous transhepatic drainage was ultimately successful in only 4 patients (36%). In the absence of an obvious pathologic condition of the biliary tract, all patients should undergo full gastrointestinal evaluation.

(*Arch Surg.* 1989;124:561-564)

During the past several years there has been a proliferation of articles on liver abscess. Although liver abscess was once regarded as an almost uniformly fatal disease, advances in antimicrobial chemotherapy and in diagnostic and therapeutic modalities have altered the prognosis for patients with this problem.[1-3] Recently, emphasis has been placed on the changing epidemiology of hepatic abscesses, with the majority of abscesses noted to be the result of a pathologic condition of the biliary tract.[1,2,4-7] Because of this, along with the trend toward attempts at percutaneous transhepatic drainage of these abscesses, fewer patients are investigated for evidence of pathologic involvement of the gastrointestinal tract. We reviewed a 6-year experience with pyogenic liver abscess to assess the role of the gastrointestinal tract in causing liver abscesses and to determine the best role for percutaneous transhepatic drainage in the treatment of this problem.

PATIENTS AND METHODS

A retrospective medical record review was conducted of all patients admitted to the Lahey Clinic, Burlington, Mass, from 1981 to 1987 who underwent drainage of a liver abscess. Criteria for inclusion in the study were age greater than 18 years, documentation of purulence within the abscess cavity, a pyogenic cause of the liver abscess, and either a surgical or roentgenographic attempt at treatment of the abscess. Data collected included patient demographics; admitting and final diagnoses; onset, duration, and type of symptoms referable to both the liver abscess and underlying cause; pertinent laboratory data; roentgenographic investigations, including number and location of liver abscesses; microbiologic studies; and treatment with outcome and subsequent follow-up. All patients were followed up to this writing. Most follow-up information was obtained from patients' medical records. When necessary, telephone interviews were conducted.

The cause of the liver abscess was determined to be pancreatobiliary when evidence of pathologic involvement of the gallbladder, pancreatic or biliary tumor, or extrahepatic biliary obstruction was present. For the liver abscess to be considered as occurring secondary to an intestinal source, a pathologic gastrointestinal condition must have been documented at the time of operation or clear roentgenographic evidence must have been present during investigations initiated because of the liver abscess.

When percutaneous transhepatic drainage was used in the treatment of patients with liver abscess, either computed tomographic scan or ultrasound guidance was used to place an 8F to 14F catheter by the modified Seldinger technique. Percutaneous transhepatic drainage was considered to have failed when the patient's condition remained toxic despite what was considered to be adequate drainage, when residual abscess was noted on serial follow-up computed tomographic scans, or when a surgical procedure was required to treat patients for the abscess or underlying pathologic disease.

RESULTS

Twenty patients were identified who fulfilled the criteria for inclusion in this study. Sixteen patients were men and four were women, with a median age of 56 years (range, 21 to 81 years). The median duration of symptoms before patients were admitted to the hospital was 21 days (range, 3 to 60 days). The most common signs and symptoms on admission were fever (85%), malaise (70%), abdominal pain (50%), night sweats (40%), and weight loss (40%). Jaundice was present in four patients (20%), all of whom had a pancreatobiliary source of their liver abscess. Four patients (20%) had symptoms specifically related to the intestinal tract.

The cause of the liver abscess was pancreatobiliary in 11 patients (55%), intestinal in 7 patients (35%), and cryptogenic in 2 patients (10%). Specific disease processes are listed in the tabulation below.

Cause	No. of Patients
Pancreatobiliary	
Pancreatic carcinoma	2
Bile duct carcinoma	2
Cholelithiasis	2
Bile duct stricture	2
Bile duct fistula	1
Zollinger-Ellison syndrome	1
Pancreatic abscess	1
Intestinal	
Diverticulitis	3
Crohn's disease	2
Appendicitis	1
Carcinoma of the colon	1
Cryptogenic	2

A comparison of patients with intestinal vs pancreatobiliary sources of abscess demonstrated several differences (Table 1). Patients with an intestinal source tended to be younger, had a longer duration of symptoms before presentation, and

Accepted for publication February 11, 1989.

From the Departments of General Surgery (Dr Rossi) and Colon and Rectal Surgery (Dr Schoetz), Lahey Clinic Medical Center, Burlington, Mass. Dr Cohen is now in private practice in Hartford, Conn. Dr Martin is now with the Department of Surgery, New England Deaconess Hospital, Boston, Mass.

Winner of the Resident's Prize at the 69th Annual Meeting of the New England Surgical Society, Montreal, Canada, September 16, 1988.

Reprint requests to Department of Colon and Rectal Surgery, Lahey Clinic Medical Center, 41 Mall Rd, Burlington, MA 01805 (Dr Shoetz).

had more gastrointestinal symptoms. Furthermore, although the patients with intestinal sources had a higher white blood cell count, those with pancreatobiliary sources had more abnormal results of liver function tests. Notably, 6 (86%) of 7 patients with intestinal causes of the liver abscess presented with fever of unknown origin. This was in contrast to 8 (72%) of 11 patients with pancreatobiliary causes who presented with the underlying condition already known. Ten patients presented with a single abscess cavity, while the remaining 10 patients had multiple abscesses. The majority of the abscesses were located in the right lobe (60%), with 20% in the left lobe and 20% in both lobes.

Nineteen of 20 patients had positive results of blood or abscess cultures, with 7 patients having positive results of both. Eleven patients (55%) had one organism isolated from their cultures, with the remaining patients' cultures yielding multiple organisms. Twelve different organisms were isolated from the 20 patients' cultures, with *Escherichia coli* being present in 40% of the cultures. Comparison of patients with intestinal and pancreatobiliary sources disclosed a predominance of gram-negative rods in the pancreatobiliary group, as shown in the following tabulation.

Organism	No. of Patients
Intestinal	
α-Hemolytic streptococcus	2
E coli	1
Streptococcus viridans	1
Fusobacterium nucleatum	1
Anaerobic gram-positive rods	1
Anaerobic gram-negative rods	1
Staphylococcus	1
Pancreatobiliary	
E coli	6
α-Hemolytic streptococcus	2
Enterococcus	2
Morganella	2
Enterobacter	1
Klebsiella	1
Bacillus fragilis	1

All patients were treated with broad-spectrum parenteral antibiotics during the course of their disease.

The initial treatment of patients with an abscess cavity was percutaneous drainage in 11 patients (55%) and operation in 9 patients (45%). No difference in age or sex ratio was distinguishable between the two groups, although the duration of symptoms was longer (28 days vs 18 days) in the group undergoing operation as the initial treatment (Table 2). No difference was noted between the two groups with respect to the underlying cause of the abscess or the number and location of liver lesions. Furthermore, no difference was observed between patients undergoing percutaneous transhepatic drainage and patients undergoing operation when presenting symptoms, temperature, or laboratory data, including liver function test results, were compared.

Percutaneous transhepatic drainage was successful as sole treatment in four patients (36%). Two of these patients required a second roentgenographic drainage procedure to effect a cure. The other seven patients were considered to have failed percutaneous transhepatic drainage because of inability to drain the abscess successfully (one patient) or because surgical intervention was ultimately required to eradicate the abscess or address the underlying cause (six patients), as shown in the following tabulation.

Treatment	No. of Patients
Operative drainage	2
Operative drainage and treatment of underlying problem	2
Treatment of underlying problem	2
Technical problem	1

Table 1.—Patients With Intestinal vs Pancreatobiliary Involvement

Factor	Intestinal (n=7)	Pancreatobiliary (n=11)
Median age, y	51	65
Duration of symptoms, d	25	14
Gastrointestinal symptoms, % of patients	43	18
Median white blood cell count, $\times 10^9$/L	20.1	13.5
Median sedimentation rate, mm/h	106	95
Median alkaline phosphatase, U/L	155	420
Median aspartate aminotransferase, U/L	53	54
Total bilirubin, μmol/L	22.23	35.9

Table 2.—Percutaneous Transhepatic Drainage vs Surgery

Factor	Percutaneous Transhepatic Drainage	Surgical Drainage
Median age, y	60	56
Sex, No. M/No. F	9/2	7/2
Duration of symptoms, d	18	28
Hospital stay, d	23	28
Origin, No. of patients		
Pancreatobiliary	6	5
Intestinal	4	3
Cryptogenic	1	1
Distribution of liver lesions, No. of patients		
Single	6	4
Multiple	5	5

Two patients had episodes of sepsis related to percutaneous transhepatic drainage, with one patient requiring brief ventilatory support. No patients in this group died while in the hospital. The median follow-up period was 5 months, during which time two patients died of the underlying disease and a third patient died of unrelated causes.

Eight of the nine patients undergoing operation as their initial treatment were ultimately cured. However, two patients required a second operation to achieve success. Both of these patients had ongoing sepsis despite initial operative drainage. Posttransfusion hepatitis developed in one patient, and a self-limited and disseminated intravascular coagulation that was drug-induced developed in another patient. No patients in this group died while in the hospital. The median follow-up period was 6 months, during which time three patients died. One patient died of a myocardial infarction, and one died of an underlying pancreatic cancer. The third death was of the patient whose follow-up computed tomographic scan demonstrated residual abscess. Postmortem examination was not permitted, and the source of the abscess and the cause of death were never ascertained.

COMMENT

During the preantibiotic era, portal sources, especially appendicitis, were the leading causes of pyogenic liver abscess.[8] With the advent of effective antimicrobial therapy, the source of hepatic abscess has undergone an important change.

Although portal sources are still a factor, pathologic conditions of the biliary tract now produce between 31% and 51% of all liver abscesses.[1,2,4-6] Because of the emphasis being placed on a biliary source, the gastrointestinal tract may be overlooked in the investigation of these patients. Nevertheless, these same series have reported an incidence of portal causes of 14% to 26%, and our own series demonstrated a 35% incidence of gastrointestinal sources. Furthermore, the majority of our patients had pathologic gastrointestinal disease that was unsuspected at presentation, with a diagnosis on admission of fever of unknown origin noted in 86% of patients. An attempt was made to identify characteristics of the presentation that would alert the clinician to initiate an intensive gastrointestinal investigation. Although the patients who were eventually shown to have an intestinal source were younger and presented with a longer duration of symptoms, these findings must be considered nonspecific. Certainly, when the patient presents with gastrointestinal complaints, as was the case in 43% of patients with an intestinal source, the need for a comprehensive intestinal evaluation is indicated. At a minimum, barium enema and proctosigmoidoscopy are indicated. Examination by barium enema was performed in five of the seven patients who eventually had confirmation of intestinal sources. Evidence of resolving diverticulitis was found in two patients, and Crohn's colitis and sigmoid carcinoma were found in one patient each. The fifth patient undergoing examination by barium enema had diverticulosis but no evidence of diverticulitis, which was only identified at operation. Gyorffy et al[1] also found examination by barium enema to be useful in detecting occult colonic disease, and they identified three patients with pathologic conditions as a result of six examinations that they performed.

Consideration of laboratory data revealed much higher alkaline phosphatase and bilirubin levels in patients with a pancreatobiliary source of liver lesions. Although these indexes are generally a measurement of extrahepatic biliary obstruction, the alkaline phosphatase level was still found to be at least mildly elevated in all of the patients with intestinal sources. These abnormalities in liver function tests have been noted previously[1,4,5]; however, none of these authors attempted to correlate laboratory values with the cause of the abscess.

Finally, a comparison of the bacteriologic studies of the two groups demonstrated a predominance of gram-negative rods, especially *E coli*, in the pancreatobiliary group. Although other studies have compiled comprehensive lists of the organisms isolated from abscess or blood cultures, the only analysis of these data was performed with respect to mortality rates.[4,6,7] Gyorffy et al[1] suggested that multiple anaerobic isolates implicate a colonic source, while pure cultures of *E coli* should direct attention toward the biliary tree. Our data confirm this observation.

The value of determining the cause of the liver abscess relates to the ability to direct therapeutic intervention. For the majority of liver abscesses caused by intestinal pathologic disease, drainage of the abscess is not enough. Four of seven patients with an intestinal source of disease required surgical treatment in our series. Two patients had severe Crohn's disease, one patient had a diverticular abscess, and one patient had sigmoid carcinoma. All four of these patients were admitted to the hospital with a diagnosis of fever of unknown origin. Although he reported the first percutaneous drainage of a hepatic abscess caused by Crohn's disease, Crass[9] noted that the patient still required surgical treatment for the underlying problem. He reviewed the literature on liver abscess secondary to Crohn's disease and noted that in six of seven patients for whom follow-up data were available, operation was necessary to manage extensive pathologic disease outside the liver.

This raises the issue of how best to treat patients with liver abscess. In an analysis of factors influencing the mortality rate in patients with pyogenic liver abscesses, Pitt and Zuidema[6] reported that 27 of 28 patients treated with antibiotics alone died. This was contrasted with a 66% survival rate when antimicrobial therapy was combined with surgical drainage. Although reports have been made of successful treatment with antibiotics alone,[10,11] the preponderance of accumulated evidence supports some form of drainage combined with antibiotics in the management of pyogenic liver abscesses.[1,3-6,12,13]

Substantial controversy remains as to whether percutaneous transhepatic drainage or surgical procedure is the preferred method of drainage for liver abscess. Although percutaneous transhepatic drainage is not a new concept,[14] refinements in technique and equipment have markedly increased its usefulness.[15-17] In the past decade, numerous reports have been made of successful management of liver abscesses by percutaneous transhepatic drainage, with survival rates comparable to those for surgical drainage.[2,3,5,16-18] Unfortunately, a substantial shortcoming of percutaneous transhepatic drainage not addressed by most of these studies is its inability to eradicate the underlying problem. This issue cannot be separated from that of drainage itself. When the underlying cause is not addressed as part of the total treatment regimen, not only may the abscess recur but also the patient will suffer from progression of the precipitating state of disease.

When viewed in this regard, it is not surprising that, despite equivalent groups, we found surgical drainage to be superior to percutaneous transhepatic drainage. The overall success rate for operation was 89% compared with 36% for percutaneous transhepatic drainage. Among our seven patients in whom percutaneous transhepatic drainage failed, four required operative intervention to address the underlying state of disease. For this reason, we concur with Gyorffy et al[1] and Miedema and Dineen[4] that the role for percutaneous transhepatic drainage is best thought of as palliative. Percutaneous transhepatic drainage may enable a critically ill patient to experience a resolution of the septic state, thereby decreasing his or her surgical risk. However, surgical intervention will still be required in the majority of patients with pyogenic liver abscesses, if not to effect complete drainage of the abscess then to treat patients for the underlying disease. The current attitude that the treatment of patients with liver abscess has become the domain of internists and radiologists, with minimization of the role of surgery, is incorrect.

References

1. Gyorffy EJ, Frey CF, Silva J Jr, McGahan J. Pyogenic liver abscess: diagnostic and therapeutic strategies. *Ann Surg.* 1987;206:699-705.

2. Bertel CK, van Heerden JA, Sheedy PF II. Treatment of pyogenic hepatic abscesses: surgical vs percutaneous drainage. *Arch Surg.* 1986;121:554-558.

3. Falk KA, Angerås UJ, Friman VZ, Gamklov GR, Lukes PJ. Pyogenic liver abscesses: have changes in management improved the outcome? *Acta Chir Scand.* 1987;153:661-664.

4. Miedema BW, Dineen P. The diagnosis and treatment of pyogenic liver abscesses. *Ann Surg.* 1984;200:328-335.

5. McDonald MI, Corey GR, Gallis HA, Durack DT. Single and multiple pyogenic liver abscesses: natural history, diagnosis and treatment, with emphasis on percutaneous drainage. *Medicine.* 1984;63:291-302.

6. Pitt HA, Zuidema GD. Factors influencing mortality in the treatment of pyogenic hepatic abscess. *Surg Gynecol Obstet.* 1975;140:228-234.

7. Kandel G, Marcon NE. Pyogenic liver abscess: new concepts of an old disease. *Am J Gastroenterol.* 1984;79:65-71.

8. Ochsner A, DeBakey M, Murray S. Pyogenic abscess of the liver: analysis of 47 cases with review of literature. *Am J Surg.* 1938;40:292-319.

9. Crass JR. Liver abscess as a complication of regional enteritis: interventional considerations. *Am J Gastroenterol.* 1983;78:747-749.

10. Herbert DA, Fogel DA, Rothman J, Wilson S, Simmons F, Ruskin J.

Pyogenic liver abscesses: successful non-surgical therapy. *Lancet*. 1982;16:134-136.

11. Maher JA Jr, Reynolds TB, Yellin AE. Successful medical treatment of pyogenic liver abscess. *Gastroenterology*. 1979;77:618-622.

12. Bergamini TM, Larson GM, Malangoni MA, Richardson JD. Liver abscess: review of a 12-year experience. *Am Surg*. 1987;53:596-599.

13. Cheung NK, Malfitan RC, Najem AZ, Rush BF Jr. Pyogenic liver abscess. *Am Surg*. 1978;44:272-278.

14. McFadzean AJS, Chang KPS, Wong CC. Solitary pyogenic abscess of liver treated by closed aspiration and antibiotics: a report of 14 consecutive cases with recovery. *Br J Surg*. 1953;41:141-152.

15. Karlson KB, Martin EC, Fankuchen EI, Schultz RW, Casarella WJ. Percutaneous abscess drainage. *Surg Gynecol Obstet*. 1982;154:44-48.

16. Johnson RD, Mueller PR, Ferrucci JT Jr, et al. Percutaneous drainage of pyogenic liver abscesses. *AJR*. 1985;144:463-467.

17. Gerzof SG, Johnson WC, Robbins AH, Nasbeth DC. Intrahepatic pyogenic abscesses: treatment by percutaneous drainage. *Am J Surg*. 1985;149:487-494.

18. Gray R, Leekam R, Mackenzie R, St Lovis EL, Grosman H. Percutaneous abscess drainage. *Gastrointest Radiol*. 1985;10:79-84.

Discussion

JAMES FOSTER, MD: I can look at these same data and reach an opposite conclusion. One's biases do shade one's understandings, and my bias is that percutaneous drainage of most liver abscesses should be attempted before laparotomy.

That bias is based on several factors. First, an acutely infected abscess, even one well defined by a computed tomographic scan, can be hard to find at operation. The wall may be soft and difficult to distinguish by palpation. Second, the infected mushy liver parenchyma can bleed profusely when broken into, and that hemorrhage may be very difficult to control. Third, percutaneous drainage will relieve pressure and it is pressure that promotes systemic sepsis. A more deliberate approach can be made to both the diagnosis and treatment of any extrahepatic primary lesion if sepsis can be controlled first with a percutaneous catheter. Finally, percutaneous drainage works in most patients in my own experience and that of many others.

Liver abscess remains a "surgical" disease, and the radiologist who attempts percutaneous drainage without a surgeon close by is foolish. However, it is not necessarily an "operative" disease and we and our patients should be grateful that there is another option available.

BLAKE CADY, MD, Boston, Mass: Another reason for using the percutaneous catheter is that it acts as a highway for later surgical drainage, if needed. The preliminary placement of the percutaneous catheter obtains material for culture so that selective antibiotics can be used. At formal exploration, the previously placed catheter can be followed directly down to the abscess cavity, simplifying the entire process of open surgical drainage of these lesions.

RICHARD E. WILSON, Boston: How many of the patients with a liver abscess of gastrointestinal origin required an operation for the gastrointestinal problem?

DR COHEN: Dr Foster, I think we are in partial agreement. I was prompted to do this study because the literature contains reports of percutaneous aspiration or antibiotic treatment with no discussion of the follow-up of these patients. The treatment of liver abscess is moving into the realm of medicine and away from surgery. I believe that a surgeon needs to be involved in the care of the patient along with the radiologist or the internist. If you look at our data, it can be interpreted in several ways. Actually, 3 of the 11 patients who underwent percutaneous drainage required surgery for drainage of the abscess because of failure; that is not an insignificant number.

Four years ago the Boston Veterans Administration group reported a 16% incidence of failure when draining the abscess percutaneously. Probably the major article is by the Massachusetts General Hospital group, who, along with physicians at the University of California, San Diego, reported a 25% incidence of failure at attempting to drain the liver abscess by percutaneous drainage and after multiple attempts. Therefore, surgical backup is a necessity. Surgical input is also needed to address the underlying disease state. In four of our patients who underwent percutaneous drainage, surgery was ultimately required at least to treat the underlying disease, if not to drain the abscess.

To answer Dr Wilson's question, of the patients who were found to have intestinal sources, two had acute diverticulitis with abscess that required resection, and one had Crohn's disease that required resection. The patient whom we treated most recently was found to have a colon carcinoma as a source of the abscess. If the gastrointestinal evaluation had not been conducted, we might have missed it. I think, therefore, that it is worthwhile to look for an intestinal source, as many times we will need to operate there.

In Other AMA Journals

ARCHIVES OF OTOLARYNGOLOGY–HEAD & NECK SURGERY

Leeches: Objective Monitoring of Altered Perfusion in Congested Flaps

Richard E. Hayden, MD, CM, FRCS; John G. Phillips, MD; Patrick W. McLear, MD

In plastic and reconstructive surgery, there has been new interest in the use of the medicinal leech (*Hirudo medicinalis*) for the treatment of venous congestion. To the best of our knowledge, no study has been performed to objectively demonstrate the benefits of leeching a congested flap. Doppler laser perfusion monitoring (DLPM) was used to record blood flow changes in pig rump flaps compromised by venous occlusion. With the application of leeches to nine congested pig rump flaps, significant increases in blood flow were demonstrated both clinically and by DLPM. It is concluded from this study that DLPM can demonstrate objective improvement in microcirculatory perfusion with leeching (*Arch Otolaryngol Head Neck Surg* 1988;114:1395-1399).

Reprints not available.

Intrahepatic Cholangiojejunostomy as a Palliative Procedure in Primary Sclerosing Cholangitis

James R. Goldenring, MD, PhD, C. Elton Cahow, MD

• Primary sclerosing cholangitis is an idiopathic disease characterized by progressive diffuse stricture of extrahepatic and intrahepatic bile ducts. Eighteen patients with end-stage symptoms of primary sclerosing cholangitis were evaluated during a 10-year period from 1976 to 1986. Nine patients presented with disease amenable to intrahepatic cholangiojejunostomy. All patients presented with elevated liver function test results, and six of nine patients had a history of ulcerative colitis. The mean survival after intrahepatic cholangiojejunostomy was 3.9 years (range, 4 months to 10 years). Two of three of the patients with biliary cirrhosis died within 1 year after surgery. Four of nine patients remain alive today, with a mean survival of 4.7 years. For patients with end-stage primary sclerosing cholangitis, intrahepatic cholangiojejunostomy provides effective surgical palliation in those without secondary biliary cirrhosis.

(*Arch Surg.* 1989;124:565-567)

Primary sclerosing cholangitis (PSC) is an idiopathic disease characterized by the progressive and multiple stricture of intrahepatic and extrahepatic bile ducts.[1] Primary sclerosing cholangitis predominantly affects middle-aged men and has been associated with a number of autoimmune syndromes[2,3] and inflammatory bowel disease, especially ulcerative colitis.[4,5] While a number of recent series have suggested that PSC may follow a benign and asymptomatic course,[6-8] the predominance of data indicates that symptomatic PSC follows an inevitable course that leads to the patient's early demise. Since no medical treatment has shown any demonstrable effect on the course of PSC,[9,10] surgery remains the only hope for patients with end-stage PSC. We present here the results of our series of patients with terminal PSC who underwent intrahepatic cholangiojejunostomy (IHCJ) for palliation of PSC.

PATIENTS AND METHODS

Eighteen patients with symptomatic PSC were evaluated by the surgical service during a 10-year period from 1976 to 1986. The diagnosis was established by an intraoperative cholangiogram in 5 patients and by endoscopic retrograde cholangiopancreatography in the other 13. Nine patients were deemed to be eligible for IHCJ. In five patients, the general physical condition precluded a major operative procedure. Three patients were not amenable to this procedure because the extent of disease would not allow adequate decompression. One patient, a 39-year-old woman with Crohn's disease, had undergone multiple small-bowel resections and a total proctocolectomy in the past. She received a choledochoduodenostomy for a predominant extrahepatic stricture in the common duct, and she remains alive 12 years after surgery.

Intrahepatic cholangiojejunostomy was performed by one of two methods. In two patients, IHCJ was performed with an anastomosis to the left hepatic duct by a simplification of the procedure of Longmire and Sanford[11] as reported previously by Cahow.[12] Briefly, a small probe was inserted into a dilated subcapsular bile ductule. The probe was advanced into the more proximal ducts, and an incision was made in the liver parenchyma over the probe to uncover the hepatic duct radical. The probe was advanced until a duct of at least 5 mm in diameter was encountered. Bleeding was controlled with electrocautery and fine silk sutures. The bile duct was incised longitudinally to a length of 4 to 5 cm. A Roux-en-Y loop of jejunum was then mobilized, and a side-to-side, two-layer, mucosa-to-mucosa anastomosis was carried out. The serosa of the jejunum was approximated with the liver capsule by utilizing interrupted silk sutures. In one patient, a Silastic stent was placed across the anastomosis at the time of the operation and removed 1 month following the operation. More recently, we have not utilized stents, without any significant alteration in results.

Seven of the nine patients received a central IHCJ, with the anastomosis performed at the proximal left hepatic duct similar to the technique described by Blumgart and Kelley.[13] For this approach, the left proximal portal triad was exposed with identification of the left hepatic artery and portal vein. The dissection then continued with exposure of the confluence of the left and right hepatic ducts. The left hepatic duct was then incised longitudinally, and where possible, the incision was carried across to the right duct to provide adequate decompression of both sides. A two-layer, side-to-side, mucosa-to-mucosa anastomosis was performed with a Roux-en-Y loop of jejunum.

Patients were followed up at 3- to 6-month intervals postoperatively. Five-year survival statistics were computed by using life-table analysis. Preoperative and postoperative liver function test results were compared with Student's *t* test for paired samples.

RESULTS

Composition of Study Group

The nine patients involved in the series underwent ten operations for construction of IHCJ. The group consisted of six men and three women. The mean age of the group was 47.9 years (median age, 48.0 years). Six (66.7%) of the

Accepted for publication December 7, 1988.
From the Department of Surgery, Yale University School of Medicine, New Haven, Conn.
Read before the 69th Annual Meeting of the New England Surgical Society, Montreal, Canada, September 16, 1988.
Reprint requests to Department of Surgery, Yale University School of Medicine, PO Box 3333, New Haven, CT 06510 (Dr Cahow).

Liver Function Test Results		
	Mean (±SD) Value	
Level	Preoperative	Postoperative
Total bilirubin, μmol/L	268 (154)	52 (34)*
Alkaline phosphatase, U/L	292 (112)	250 (167)
Aspartate aminotransferase, U/L	82 (35)	80 (40)

*$P<.05$, Student's *t* test.

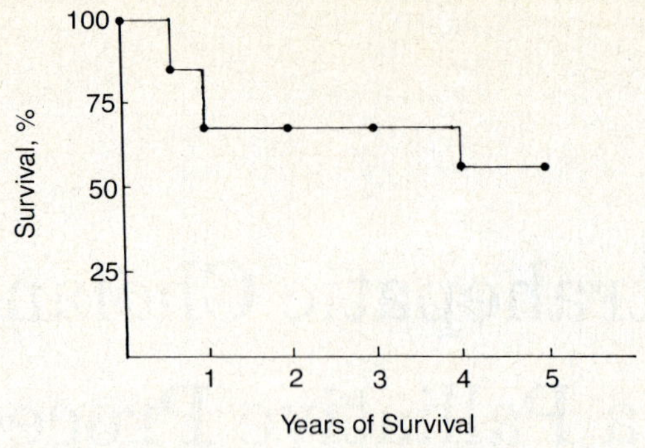

Survival statistics for nine patients following intrahepatic cholangiojejunostomy.

patients carried a diagnosis of ulcerative colitis for an average of 11.9 years before the onset of PSC. One patient developed ulcerative colitis 3 years following the diagnosis of PSC. Operative intervention was required an average of 2.8 years following the diagnosis of PSC (median, 2 years). Liver function test results on presentation are listed in the Table. All patients presented with elevations in their liver function test values, with a mean bilirubin level of 268 μmol/L, alkaline phosphatase level of 292 U/L, and aspartate aminotransferase level of 82 U/L.

Results of IHCJ

Following IHCJ, the nine patients have been observed for a mean follow-up period of 3.9 years (range, 4 months to 10 years; median follow-up of 3.75 years). Liver biopsy specimens, taken at the time of laparotomy, confirmed histology consistent with sclerosing cholangitis in all patients. Three patients displayed biliary cirrhosis on liver biopsy specimens.

Five patients died during the course of the study period. There was no operative mortality. One patient underwent an orthotopic liver transplantation 9 years after IHCJ for recurrent symptoms and was found to have cholangiocarcinoma at the time of the transplantation. A second patient died 4 months after successful IHCJ of carcinomatosis secondary to malignant cholangiocarcinoma. Two patients with secondary biliary cirrhosis died within 1 year following IHCJ secondary to complications from worsening hepatic failure. The IHCJ was revised in one patient for recurrence of jaundice, at which time an intraductal hepatic carcinoid tumor was found to be obstructing the previous anastomosis. One patient with cirrhosis remains alive today 3 years following IHCJ but continues to be jaundiced.

For the six long-term survivors (>1 year), IHCJ provided a significant decrease in the bilirubin level ($P<.05$, Student's *t* test). The aspartate aminotransferase and alkaline phosphatase levels were not significantly changed (Table). The overall mean survival for these nine patients was 3.9 years (range, 4 months to 10 years), with a median survival of 3.75 years. For the six noncirrhotic patients, the mean survival was 5.5 years (3 to 10 years). Life-table analysis results are depicted in the Figure and demonstrate an overall 53.6% 5-year survival rate. Four patients remain alive today, with a mean survival of 4.7 years. One patient has experienced two episodes of cholangitis that required hospitalization for intravenous antibiotic therapy. Six of the nine patients were able to return to their previous employment within 6 months following IHCJ.

COMMENT

Primary sclerosing cholangitis is an idiopathic disease of the biliary tree that often follows an insidious and inexorable course.[1,9] Recent investigations from three institutions have suggested that the majority of patients who present with PSC are asymptomatic.[6-8] These patients are usually found serendipitously when endoscopic retrograde cholangiopancreatography is performed to investigate an isolated elevation in the alkaline phosphatase level or as an incidental finding on intraoperative cholangiogram at the time of cholecystectomy. Indeed, Helzberg et al[7] found that none of their asymptomatic patients developed symptoms or jaundice during a mean 3-year follow-up. However, severely symptomatic patients show a much higher morbidity and mortality, generally following a spiraling course toward biliary obstruction and secondary biliary cirrhosis.[7,8] A number of medical interventions have been attempted, including the use of corticosteroids[9] and penicillamine,[10] all of which have yielded disappointing results. Balloon dilatation of strictures through percutaneous radiographic or endoscopic routes has yielded limited success.[14] However, these procedures are only effective in treating patients with single major strictures, a group that comprises only 10% of the total.[14] It is therefore clear that, for the patient with symptomatic PSC, surgical intervention holds the only clear hope of palliation.

Two major surgical options are available for the patient with symptomatic PSC: (1) biliary-enteric decompression or (2) orthotopic hepatic transplantation. Previous investigations have shown that T tube decompression of the extrahepatic biliary tree does not provide adequate palliation or improve survival.[15] The results described in this study demonstrate that biliary bypass via IHCJ can provide effective palliation in patients with end-stage PSC. In this study, IHCJ has achieved long-term survival in greater than 50% of patients. Cameron et al[16] have recently reported a mean 5-year survival of 63% in their series of 31 patients who received biliary decompression through resection of the hepatic duct bifurcation and bilateral stenting.

Two institutions have reported their results with orthotopic liver transplantation for patients with PSC. Busuttil et al[17] have reported a 71% 1-year mean survival in seven patients who underwent transplantations for PSC. More recently, Marsh et al[18] have reviewed their results with 55 transplantations performed for PSC, and they found a 57% 2-year actuarial survival. Their results with patients who had PSC are similar to those for the body of patients with liver transplants as a whole.

As noted previously by several authors, PSC is associated with an increased risk of cholangiocarcinoma.[19] In our study, two patients, only one of whom had ulcerative colitis, developed cholangiocarcinoma. In one of the patients, cholangiocarcinoma was detected in the liver transplant excision sample. Marsh et al[18] have reported a 9% incidence of cholangiocarcinoma in liver specimens at the time of liver transplantation. To our knowledge, we also report here the first instance of a carcinoid tumor in a patient with PSC. The relationship of this tumor with PSC is unclear.

While both intrahepatic biliary decompression and transplantation appear to produce acceptable results in symptomatic patients, each has a rational place in the armamentarium of treatment of this disease. First, the report from Marsh et al[18] notes that patients older than the age of 50 years did not undergo transplantations. Our own group had a higher median age and four of the nine patients were older than 50 years of age. Intrahepatic cholangiojejunostomy or intrahepatic biliary decompression may be an appropriate option for patients older than 50 years of age. Second, however, findings from our own study and that of Cameron et al,[16] confirm that patients with secondary biliary cirrhosis do not do well with biliary-enteric decompression. Indeed, on account of this finding, we believe that it is imperative that symptomatic patients with PSC undergo a liver biopsy as part of their preoperative evaluation. The results of such a biopsy to rule out cirrhosis, as well as cholangiocarcinoma, could markedly alter the choice of definitive therapy. Thus, patients with cirrhosis, who are acceptable candidates, should be treated with transplantation where possible. Finally, it is important to note that performance of IHCJ does not preclude subsequent liver transplantation. Marsh et al[18] performed liver transplantations on 15 patients who had previous IHCJs, with survival rates that were similar to those in patients without previous major surgical biliary decompression. Thus, in the younger patient, surgical biliary decompression may be offered as an intermediate-term palliation in anticipation of transplantation at a later date.

The results of our own work and those found by Cameron et al[16] and Marsh et al[18] underscore the impression that surgical management of end-stage PSC provides effective palliation of disease.

References

1. LaRusso NF, Wiesner RH, Ludwig J, MacCarty RL. Primary sclerosing cholangitis. *N Engl J Med.* 1984;310:899-903.
2. Whiteside TL, Lasky S, Si L, Thiel DHV. Immunological analysis of mononuclear liver tissues and blood of patients with primary sclerosing cholangitis. *Hepatology.* 1985;5:468-474.
3. Montefusco PP, Geiss AC, Bronzo RL, Randall S, Kahn E, McKinley MJ. Sclerosing cholangitis, chronic pancreatitis and Sjögren's syndrome: a syndrome complex. *Am J Surg.* 1984;147:822-826.
4. Schrumpf E, Fausa O, Kolmannskog F, Elgjo K, Ritland S, Gjone E. Sclerosing cholangitis in ulcerative colitis: a follow-up study. *Scand J Gastroenterol.* 1982;17:33-39.
5. Quigley EMM, LaRusso NF, Ludwig J, MacSween RNM, Birnie GG, Watkinson G. Familial occurrence of primary sclerosing cholangitis and ulcerative colitis. *Gastroenterology.* 1983;85:1160-1165.
6. Chapman RW, Burroughs AK, Bass NM, Sherlock S. Longstanding asymptomatic primary sclerosing cholangitis. *Dig Dis Sci.* 1981;26:778-782.
7. Helzberg JH, Petersen JM, Boyer JL. Improved survival with primary sclerosing cholangitis. *Gastroenterology.* 1987;92:1869-1875.
8. Wiesner RH, Beaver SJ, Ludwig J, LaRusso NF. The natural history of symptomatic and asymptomatic primary sclerosing cholangitis. *Gastroenterology.* 1987;90:1780.
9. Wiesner RH, LaRusso NF. Clinicopathologic features of the syndrome of primary sclerosing cholangitis. *Gastroenterology.* 1980;79:200-206.
10. LaRusso NF, Wiesner RH, Ludwig J, et al. Randomized trial of penicillamine in primary sclerosing cholangitis. *Hepatology.* 1986;6:1205.
11. Longmire WP, Sanford MC. Intrahepatic cholangiojejunostomy with partial hepatectomy for biliary obstruction. *Surgery.* 1948;128:330-347.
12. Cahow CE. Intrahepatic cholangiojejunostomy: a new simplified approach. *Am J Surg.* 1979;137:443-448.
13. Blumgart LH, Kelley CJ. Hepaticojejunostomy in benign and malignant high bile duct stricture: approaches to the left hepatic ducts. *Br J Surg.* 1984;71:257-261.
14. May GR, Bender CE, LaRusso NF, Wiesner RH. Nonoperative dilatation of dominant strictures in primary sclerosing cholangitis. *Am J Radiol.* 1985;145:1061-1064.
15. Pitt HA, Thompson HH, Tompkins RK, Longmire WP. Primary sclerosing cholangitis: results of an aggressive surgical approach. *Ann Surg.* 1982;196:259-266.
16. Cameron JL, Pitt HA, Zinner MJ, et al. Resection of hepatic duct bifurcation and transhepatic stenting for sclerosing cholangitis. *Ann Surg.* 1988;207:614-622.
17. Busuttil RW, Colonna JO, Hiatt JR, et al. The first 100 liver transplants at UCLA. *Ann Surg.* 1987;206:387-402.
18. Marsh JW, Iwatsuki S, Makowka L, et al. Orthotopic liver transplantation for primary sclerosing cholangitis. *Ann Surg.* 1988;207:21-25.
19. Wee A, Ludwig J, Coffey RJ, LaRusso NF, Wiesner RH. Hepatobiliary carcinoma associated with primary sclerosing cholangitis and chronic ulcerative colitis. *Hum Pathol.* 1985;16:719-726.

Discussion

John W. Braasch, MD, Burlington, Mass: This important contribution by Drs Goldenring and Cahow to the literature on sclerosing cholangitis defines a subgroup of patients in whom the relief of biliary obstruction has been obtained, and the possibility of increased longevity has been raised.

Sclerosing cholangitis is a difficult disease to get hard data on because it has such a wide range of presentations, all the way from its association with AIDS, as a distal biliary obstruction, as primarily intrahepatic disease, or presenting with a major stricture in the common hepatic duct.

It has been shown by Wiesner, using a large series at the Mayo Clinic, Rochester, Minn, that the chance of death in symptomatic patients is around 23%, and in asymptomatic patients, it is 2.6%. The follow-up period was 7 or 8 years in the first category and about 5 years in the second category. Patients in the present series are better off symptomatically, no doubt, but has improved survival been achieved? I ask Dr Goldenring to answer this point.

Relative to the preferred treatment, most surgeons with experience in dealing with the disease agree that with major obstruction, anastomosis is indicated. With cirrhosis and portal hypertension, liver transplantation should be carried out. The controversy centers about those patients without a major obstruction. At The Johns Hopkins Hospital, Baltimore, Md, a patient would get a resection of the bifurcation, a double anastomosis, and double transhepatic tubes. The evidence to support this procedure is equivocal, in my view.

Finally, may I ask Dr Goldenring why a common hepatic duct anastomosis is called an intrahepatic anastomosis? Also, how were the cases selected for this series?

Dr Goldenring: First, I will deal with the question of how the patients were selected. This is a very difficult group to control for since these patients are so ill when they present, often with bilirubin levels as high as 479 μmol/L. What you will also notice is that the time span from diagnosis to the time of surgical intervention was only 2.5 years. Thus, most of these patients have suffered an acute decompensation of their disease, rather than the indolent course that is prominently discussed in much of the literature. Basically, in these patients, surgery was performed because there was no other choice. These patients required some emergent palliative measure. A number of these patients were actually referred to Dr Cahow from Dr Gerald Klatskin who thought that something needed to be done other than just routine medical therapy.

Have we improved the survival? This is very difficult to say. Nevertheless, I think it is clear that we have certainly given them good palliation for their end-stage disease. What we may consider in the long term is a group of patients who will need hepatic transplantation to improve their survival, since the bypass will give them only palliation. The disease will continue to progress despite decompression. So, as I said before, the operation needs to be used selectively as either a prelude to transplantation, or as a definitive treatment in the older population.

I think it is important to note in this disease that we consider for operation only those patients who truly are symptomatic. Patients with primary sclerosing cholangitis need close follow-up, especially in the first 3 to 4 years after diagnosis. If they begin to deteriorate, biliary decompression in highly selected patients should be seriously considered.

Intrapleural Regional Analgesia for Pain Management in Cholecystectomy

Moustafa A. El-Naggar, MD; Frank J. Schaberg, Jr, MD; Martin R. Phillips, MD

• Fifty patients undergoing cholecystectomy either electively or urgently were treated in the postoperative period with the intrapleural injection of 30 mL of 0.75% bupivacaine hydrochloride with epinephrine (1:200 000). The frequency of narcotic administration and the postoperative stay were compared with those of 50 historical controls. The group receiving intrapleural regional analgesia had significant, prolonged pain relief requiring minimal narcotic analgesics in the first 24 hours postoperatively and had a significantly shortened hospital stay. There were no complications related to catheter insertion or bupivacaine toxic effects. This technique is safe and effective in controlling perioperative pain.

(*Arch Surg.* 1989;124:568-570)

Pain after abdominal surgery has been associated with a significant increase in pulmonary, circulatory, cardiac, and gastrointestinal tract complications and prolonged hospital stay.[1-6] Many methods to try to improve postoperative pain management have been reported.[5] Despite their side effects and inconsistent efficacy, the centrally acting narcotic analgesics remain the mainstay of postoperative pain relief. Epidural analgesics, infiltration of the surgical incision with local anesthetics, regional nerve blocks, and transcutaneous nerve stimulation have been used with variable success.[1-3,5]

Recently it has been shown[4,6] that the administration of local anesthetics into the pleural space provides satisfactory analgesia in the dermatomes innervating the upper part of the abdomen. The current study was designed to evaluate the efficacy of intrapleural regional analgesia in the management of postoperative pain after cholecystectomy.

PATIENTS AND METHODS

After institutional approval and informed consent were obtained, 50 patients scheduled for cholecystectomy were recruited. At the termination of their surgical procedures, the patients were turned to the left lateral decubitus position for insertion of the intrapleural catheter. The chest was prepared and draped under sterile conditions, the tip of the scapula was identified, and the skin was infiltrated with 1% lidocaine at the angle of the rib approximately 10 cm from the midline. A dual cannula system (MANCOA; Pajunk GMGH, Medizin-Technik, Havel's Inc, Cincinnati, Ohio) was advanced to the rib. The needle was slightly withdrawn, and a 17-gauge blunt-ended cannula was advanced and locked into position. The system was then redirected to the superior border of the identified rib and advanced off of the top of the rib until a distinct loss of resistance was encountered. The hub of the cannula was occluded with the operator's thumb and advanced slightly during the expiration. A 20-gauge epidural catheter was threaded into the inner cannula during the expiratory cycle and advanced approximately 5 cm through the side hole toward the midline. The stylet was then removed, the needle and cannula were withdrawn, the proximal adaptor was attached, and the catheter was fixed in position. The patient was then turned onto a stretcher and escorted to the postanesthesia care unit. A chest roentgenogram was taken to confirm the position of the catheter in the pleural space and the absence of a significant pneumothorax.

In the postanesthesia care unit, the patients were followed up according to the usual postanesthesia protocol. Humidified oxygen was applied by face mask, the electrocardiogram was monitored, and systemic blood pressure was measured frequently.

Thirty milliliters of 0.75% bupivacaine hydrochloride with epinephrine (1:200 000) was administered through the intrapleural catheter. In five patients, serial arterial blood levels of bupivacaine were measured 15, 30, 60, and 120 minutes after injection by means of gas chromatography.[7]

The frequency of narcotic administration in the first 24 hours postoperatively, the length of postoperative hospital stay, changes in blood pressure and pulse rate in the immediate postoperative period, and the prevalence of epidemiologic variables in the patients who received intrapleural regional analgesia (group 1) and 50 historical controls (group 2) were compared. The group 2 patients underwent similar surgical procedures performed by the same group of surgeons. None of the patients in group 1 received narcotics as premedicants or intraoperatively to supplement inhalation anesthetics. Nearly all of the patients in group 2 received narcotics preoperatively and intraoperatively.

RESULTS

There were no significant differences between the two groups in age, sex, body habitus, physical status, or operative findings (Table 1). The postoperative hospital stay was decreased by an average of 2.2 days, and the need for narcotic analgesics in the first 24 hours postoperatively was markedly diminished in the patients in group 1 (Table 2).

The intrapleural injection of 30 mL of 0.75% bupivacaine hydrochloride with epinephrine (1:200 000) resulted uniformly in prompt reduction in pain as judged by the patient, the physician, and the nurse. In patients in whom it was appropriate, early ambulation the night of surgery was

Accepted for publication December 7, 1988.

From the Departments of Anesthesiology (Dr El-Naggar) and Surgery (Drs Schaberg and Phillips), Memorial Hospital of Rhode Island, Pawtucket; and Department of Surgery, School of Medicine, Boston (Mass) University (Drs Schaberg and Phillips).

Read before the 69th Annual Meeting of the New England Surgical Society, Montreal, Canada, September 16, 1988.

Reprint requests to Memorial Hospital of Rhode Island, 111 Brewster St, Pawtucket, RI 02860 (Dr El-Naggar).

Table 1.—Distribution of Age, Sex, Weight, Height, Physical Status, Duration of Anesthesia, and Time in Postanesthesia Care Unit in Groups 1 and 2

	Pleural Catheter (Group 1)						Control (Group 2)							
		Range						Range						
	Mean	Minimum	Maximum	Difference	SE	SD	Mean	Minimum	Maximum	Difference	SE	SD	*t*	*P*
Age, y	54.6	16	91	75	2.85	19.98	58.2	16	92	76	3.17	21.31	1.16	.25
Sex, M/F	1.5	1	2	1	0.07	0.5	1.8	1	2	1	0.05	0.38	...	...
Weight, kg	73.0	45	108	63	2.31	16.19	69.3	45	123	78	2.58	17.12	0.79	.43
Height, cm	163.8	142	191	49	1.37	9.45	159.8	150	180	30	1.40	8.03	1.43	.16
Physical status*	2.2	1	4	3	0.11	0.79	2.0	1	4	3	0.15	0.91	...	...
Duration of anesthesia, min	133.6	57	320	263	7.26	50.83	128.0	45	255	210	7.78	51.64	0.51	.60
Time in postanesthesia care unit, min	186.5	60	480	420	12.25	85.8	212.7	62	530	468	15.78	103.51	1.63	.10

*Scored according to the American Society of Anesthesiologists' Classification System.

Table 2.—Hospital Stay and Narcotic Use in Groups 1 and 2

	Pleural Catheter (Group 1)						Control (Group 2)							
		Range						Range						
	Mean	Minimum	Maximum	Difference	SE	SD	Mean	Minimum	Maximum	Difference	SE	SD	*t*	*P*
Postoperative hospital stay, d	7.3	3	17	14	0.50	3.51	9.5	4	31	27	0.85	5.61	2.25	.02
Total narcotics, frequency	1.9	0	4	4	0.21	1.46	5.6	3	10	7	0.28	1.88	9.17	.00001
Narcotics in postanesthesia care unit, frequency	0.061	0	2	2	0.04	0.32	1.5	0	5	5	0.18	1.20	7.74	.00001

easily accomplished, and postoperative respiratory care was facilitated by the patient's comfort. Postoperative complications were no different in the two groups (Table 3).

The mean values of serum bupivacaine levels 15, 30, 60, and 120 minutes after intrapleural injection were 1.3, 1.6, 0.75, and 0.65 mg/L, respectively, all below the toxic level (0.4 mg/L). There was no significant pneumothorax and no evidence of bupivacaine toxic effects in any of the treated patients.

COMMENT

Intrapleural regional analgesia for pain management after cholecystectomy is safe and effective. The technique was first described by Kvalheim and Reistadt in 1984.[8] Since then, several investigators[9-16] have reported its use in a variety of clinical situations. As originally described, the technique used 20 mL of 0.5% bupivacaine hydrochloride. Early experience with this regimen produced inadequate pain relief of short duration.[6,12] We have shown that use of a larger volume of more concentrated bupivacaine with epinephrine produces significantly longer pain relief with no toxic effect.[6,9]

The longer duration of analgesia permitted fewer injections for patient comfort, administrator's convenience, and decreased risk of toxic effects. Because the cumulative effect of repeated intrapleural bupivacaine administration has not yet been studied, we used a single injection. In this study, pain control was supplemented by intramuscular narcotics as requested by the patient.

There was no significant pneumothorax in this group of patients or in the more than 300 intrapleural catheters inserted in our institution for a variety of indications. This favorable result is credited to the use of the blunt-ended dual lumen system. Reports of significant complications[17,18] of the procedure appear to be related to the introducer system.

Table 3.—Postoperative Complications*

	No. of Patients	
Complication	Group 1	Group 2
Postoperative death	2	2
Admission to intensive care unit	5	4
Respiratory failure	1	3
Congestive heart failure	0	1
Myocardial infarction	1	0
Pulmonary embolism	0	1
Deep vein thrombosis	1	1
Urinary retention	1	0
Wound infection	0	1

*Analysis of variance concluded that distribution of postoperative mortality and morbidity was statistically equal in both groups.

The mechanism of action of intrapleural regional analgesia is poorly understood. Many investigators[4,6] have presumed that the anesthetic agents diffuse through the pleura and create an intrathoracic intercostal nerve block. This is yet to be scientifically demonstrated. Although retrograde diffusion from the pleural space to the intrathoracic sympathetic chain has been hypothesized,[14] we have found no incidence of Horner's syndrome or bradyarrhythmias in any of our patients. Possible splanchnic nerve block has also been suggested.[15]

Our results show that, in comparable groups of patients, the intrapleural catheter group had a statistically significant decrease in the frequency of narcotics administered in the first 24 hours after surgery. This may well account for improved patient comfort, early ambulation, and shortened hospital stay.

There are few contraindications to the use of intrapleural regional analgesia. Anatomic abnormalities (bullous emphysema), previous thoracotomy, and severe chronic pulmonary disease would preclude the use of this technique. Other relative contraindications, such as coagulopathy and mechanical ventilation with positive end-expiratory pressure, can usually be overcome.

Since completion of this study, we have treated a second group of patients with intrapleural injections every 24 hours for the first 48 to 72 hours postoperatively. Combining this with patient-controlled analgesia, we have found remarkable improvements in patient comfort. The technique is applicable to other surgical situations in which an incision or painful condition is localized to one side of the abdomen. It has been used in patients with rib fractures, renal surgery, mastectomy, and unilateral thoracotomy, with excellent results. In midline incisions we have used bilateral intrapleural regional analgesia.[9] Further investigation of these areas is being undertaken.

References

1. Adisson NV, Bear FA, Budd K, Whittacker M. Epidural analgesia following cholecystectomy. *Br J Surg* 1974;61:850.
2. Sjogren S, Wright B. Circulation, respiration and lidocaine concentration during continuous epidural blockade. *Acta Anaesthesiol Scand Suppl.* 1972;16:5.
3. Murphy DF. Continuous intercostal nerve blockade for pain relief following cholecystectomy. *Br J Anaesth.* 1983;55:521-524.
4. Reistadt F, Stromskag KE. Intrapleural catheter in the management of post-operative pain: a preliminary report. *Reg Anaesth.* 1986;11:89-91.
5. Buckey FP, Simpson BR. Acute traumatic and post-operative pain management. In: Cousins MJ, Bridenbough PO, eds. *Neural Blockade.* Philadelphia, Pa: JB Lippincott; 1980:586-615.
6. El-Naggar M, Raad C, Yogaratnam G, Poritz A, Bennett B. Intrapleural intercostal nerve block using 0.75% bupivacaine. *Anesthesiology.* 1987;67:A258.
7. Park GB, Erdamsky PE, Brown RR, Kulberg MP, Edelson J. Analysis of mepivacaine, bupivacaine, etidocaine, lidocaine and tetracaine. *J Pharm Sci* 1980;69:603-605.
8. Kvalheim L, Reistadt F. Interpleural catheter in the management of post-operative pain. *Anesthesiology.* 1984;61:A231.
9. El-Naggar MA, Bennett B, Raad C, Yogaratnam G. Bilateral intrapleural intercostal nerve block. *Anesth Analg.* 1988;67:S57.
10. Kambam JR, Handte RE, Flanagan J, Fisher K, Lupinetti M, Hammon J. Intrapleural anesthesia for post-thoracotomy pain relief. *Anesth Analg.* 1987;66:S90.
11. Stromskag KE, Reistadt F, Holmquist ELO, Ogenstad S. Intrapleural administration of 0.25%, 0.375% and 0.5% bupivacaine with epinephrine after cholecystectomy. *Anesth Analg.* 1988;67:430-434.
12. Seltzer JL, Larigani GE, Goldberg ME, Marr AT. Intrapleural bupivacaine: a kinetic and dynamic evaluation. *Anesthesiology.* 1987;67:798-800.
13. Rosenberg PH, Scheminin BMA, Lepantalo MJ, Linfors O. Continuous intrapleural infusion of bupivacaine for analgesia after thoracotomy. *Anesthesiology.* 1987;67:811-813.
14. Durrani Z, Winnie AP, Ikuta P. Interpleural catheter for pancreatic pain. *Anesth Analg.* 1988;67:479-481.
15. Bruce DL, Gerken MV, Lyon GD. Post cholecystectomy pain relief by intrapleural bupivacaine in patients with cystic fibrosis. *Anesth Analg.* 1987;66:1187-1189.
16. Brismar B, Petterson N, Tokis L, Strandberg A, Hedenstierna G. Post-operative analgesia with intrapleural administration of bupivacaine-adrenaline. *Acta Anaesth Scand.* 1987;31:515-520.
17. El-Baz N, Faber PL, Tvankovich AD. Intrapleural infusion of local anesthetic: a word of caution. *Anesthesiology.* 1988;68:809-810.
18. Gomez MN, Symreng T, Johnson B, Ressi NP, Chiang CK. Intrapleural bupivacaine for intra-operative analgesia: a dangerous technique? *Anesth Analg.* 1988;67:S78.

Discussion

John W. Braasch, MD, Burlington, Mass: One of the end points of this study was the hospital stay. Our current hospital stay after cholecystectomy is around 4 days, and we don't use nerve blocks. I note that there are historical controls in this paper. Another survey of hospital stay without this intrapleural injection might be of interest. I wonder if the authors would comment on that.

Dr Schaberg: In reference to the hospital stay, I think that the important issue is that the average age of these people was 56 years, but they ranged from 19 to 92 years. We have a very elderly population and see many people who have already been in the hospital several days on the medical service for various reasons before they are operated on. This also addresses the mortality problem. I think that we have used the technique extensively in the sicker, older patients with concomitant disease, and we find that the ability to avoid giving them morphine has made a significant improvement in their early postoperative care. We originally had reservations about both safety and efficacy. It was the enthusiasm of Dr El-Naggar that really got us started on doing this. I think what we have basically found is what has been alluded to in the comments, that is, that there is a group of people who are undergoing purely elective cholecystectomies who are in their 20s, 30s, 40s, and 50s and are otherwise well, who are going to come in, have their operation as a same-day procedure, and go home in 3 or 4 days, no matter what you do. If you use this, they will be a little more comfortable those first couple of days, but it probably does not really affect their outcome. On the older, sicker people, we believe it makes a considerable difference.

Management of Pancreatic Fistulas

F. Maureen Martin, MD; Ricardo L. Rossi, MD; J. Lawrence Munson, MD;
Stephen G. ReMine, MD; John W. Braasch, MD

• **Conservative management of pancreatic fistulas resulting from trauma, operation for tumor, or operation for pancreatitis has met with variable success. To assess optimal management strategies and outcome, we reviewed the records of 35 patients with external pancreatic fistulas (26 patients), pancreatic ascites (6 patients), or pancreatic pleural effusion (3 patients). Treatment included no operation in 5 patients, oversewing of the fistula in 7 patients, internal drainage in 11 patients, and resection in 12 patients. One (3%) postoperative death occurred. The overall rate of operative success was 83% (25 patients). The incidence of recurrent fistulas was about the same regardless of the procedure. Patients treated successfully without operation did not have pancreatitis as an underlying disease. Patient selection is of great importance in the decision to resect or to drain and is based in part on imaging the pancreatic duct and fistula.**

(*Arch Surg.* 1989;124:571-573)

The pancreas is unpredictable and unforgiving in response to inflammation, injury, or surgical manipulation. Loss of integrity of the pancreatic duct results in the formation of a fistula, which may be external or internal, with pancreatic ascites or pleural effusion. The cause can be external trauma, operative trauma in a setting of neoplasm or pancreatitis, or the result of a primary inflammatory process of the pancreas.

Because only a few centers have collected data on a large enough number of patients to comment on optimal treatment strategies, management of pancreatic fistulas remains controversial with as many advocates for conservative therapy as for surgical treatment.[1-6] We reviewed the medical records of 35 patients with pancreatic fistulas to identify factors affecting treatment, morbidity, and outcome.

PATIENTS

The charts of patients with externally draining pancreatic fistulas, pancreatic ascites, or pancreatic pleural effusion who were seen at the Lahey Clinic, Burlington, Mass, in a 15-year period were reviewed. Inclusion criteria were the presence of pleural effusion characterized by a high pleural fluid amylase level and protein content with or without evidence of pancreatitis, ascites with an accompanying high peritoneal fluid amylase level and protein content, or an externally draining pancreatic fistula and elevated amylase level in fistula fluid. Minimal volume of drainage for inclusion in the study was 250 mL/d.

Patients were divided into groups based on pathogenesis and were classified as having fistulas resulting from trauma (4 patients), operation (12 patients), or pancreatitis (19 patients). The 19 men and 16 women with a median age of 51 years (range, 22 to 76 years) and a median hospital stay of 31 days (range, 10 to 360 days) were followed up from 1 month to 15 years.

Operative reports, hospital charts, and clinical courses were evaluated. Follow-up was obtained in all patients by letter, office visits, or physician contact.

Accepted for publication December 13, 1988.

From the Department of General Surgery, Lahey Clinic Medical Center, Burlington, Mass.

Read before the 69th Annual Meeting of the New England Surgical Society, Montreal, Canada, September 18, 1988.

Reprint requests to Department of General Surgery, Lahey Clinic Medical Center, 41 Mall Rd, Burlington, MA 01805 (Dr Braasch).

Fistulas From Trauma

Four patients with fistulas resulting from trauma underwent first operative procedures elsewhere. Three patients with blunt abdominal injury had draining skin fistulas after exploratory laparotomy elsewhere and drainage of the pancreatic bed (two patients) or suture ligation of the point of duct leakage (one patient). No attempt was made to resect the pancreas or to demonstrate ductal integrity at the first surgical exploration elsewhere. Successful closure of the fistula was achieved in all three patients by distal pancreatectomy and splenectomy at our institution.

The fourth patient sustained a gunshot injury. At celiotomy elsewhere, lacerations of the left renal vein and transverse mesocolon were sutured, and a disrupted pancreatic duct was ligated. The patient was transferred to the Lahey Clinic 1 month later with ongoing sepsis and a high-flow pancreatic fistula draining through the abdominal wound. He underwent urgent surgical exploration and drainage of a pancreatic abscess with removal of a necrotic distal segment of the pancreas with a resulting persistent low-flow draining fistula that closed spontaneously after 16 months. Despite prolonged attempts (from 1 to 12 months) at conservative and expectant treatment of patients with fistula after trauma, operation was ultimately required in all patients.

Fistulas After Operation in Patients Without Pancreatitis

Twelve patients were seen with fistulas after operation. Eight patients had undergone pancreatic resection for tumor (five Whipple operations and three distal pancreatectomies). One patient had a double bypass and pancreatic biopsy. Three patients had severe intra-abdominal complications after miscellaneous gastric and biliary operations with resulting pancreatic fistulas. In four of eight patients who had undergone resection for tumor, the fistulas closed with conservative management and total parenteral nutritional (TPN) support in our hospital from 7 to 90 days (median, 39 days).

Two patients who had fistulas resulting from operation for tumor required internal drainage by Roux-en-Y pancreaticojejunostomy to close the fistulas successfully after each patient had had 41 days of unsuccessful conservative management. One patient who had a Whipple operation required total pancreatectomy for a high-flow fistula from the pancreaticojejunal anastomosis. One patient with a fistula after distal pancreatectomy underwent resection after 32 days of failed conservative treatment. Both procedures were successful.

Two of three patients with fistulas complicating biliary tract or gastric surgery had closure of the fistula with internal drainage procedures after failed conservative management for 42 and 52 days, respectively. The third patient has a minimal persistent fistula after pancreaticojejunostomy following failed conservative management of intra-abdominal complications of gastrectomy.

In the patient who had exploratory laparotomy and biliary decompression with pancreatic biopsy, an internal pancreatic fistula and ascites developed that required Roux-en-Y pancreaticojejunostomy. The fistula closed after 23 days of conservative treatment had failed.

Fistulas in Patients With Pancreatitis

Six patients had pancreatic ascites, and three patients had pleural effusion. The three patients with effusion had elevated pleural fluid amylase levels and radiologic demonstration of fistulous tracts extending upward into the mediastinum. Two of the three patients who had radiologic evidence of chronic pancre-

Results of Treatment of Pancreatic Fistulas*									
		Internal Drainage		Resection		Over-sewing of Fistula		No Surgery	
	Total No.	S	F	S	F	S	F	S	F
Trauma	4	0	0	3	1	0	0	0	0
Postoperative	12	3	1	2	0	2	0	4	0
Pancreatitis	19	6	1	5	1†	4	1	0	1
Total	**35**	**9**	**2**	**10**	**2**	**6**	**1**	**4**	**1**

*S indicates success; F, failed, persistent fistula.
†Postoperative death.

atitis despite a paucity of abdominal complaints had been admitted to the hospital for evaluation of pleural effusion. Treatment consisted of thoracentesis followed by internal drainage of leaking pseudocysts in two patients (cystojejunostomy) while the third patient required distal pancreatectomy. Operation resulted in closure of the fistula in all patients. Resection of distal pancreas with leaking duct (one patient) or internal drainage pancreaticojejunostomy (four patients) was successful in five of six of the patients with ascites. These six patients had had 4 to 18 weeks of conservative treatment, including hyperalimentation without closure of the fistula. The only perioperative death in this series occurred in the group of patients who had long-standing chronic pancreatitis and ascites. Treatment (3 months) with home TPN failed to resolve the ascites and abdominal pain. Preoperative endoscopic retrograde cholangiopancreatography (ERCP) demonstrated a possible leakage in the neck of the pancreas. Exploratory laparotomy revealed extensive loculated ascites with inflammation and obliteration of tissue planes. The point of pancreatic duct leakage could not be located with certainty. Massive bleeding during a difficult distal pancreatectomy and splenectomy resulted in a prolonged and stormy postoperative course with multiorgan system failure, sepsis, and, ultimately, liver necrosis. The patient died 5 weeks later.

In the other 10 patients in this group, an external fistula developed after drainage of a pancreatic abscess in 4 patients, after drainage of a pseudocyst in 2 patients, and after pancreaticojejunostomy or distal pancreatectomy in 4 patients. All 10 patients had acute (5 patients) or chronic (5 patients) pancreatitis. These patients were operated on after 2 weeks to 6 months of conservative treatment. Oversewing of the fistula was employed in 5 patients whose pancreatic duct was not obstructed on ERCP. One of these procedures failed. Three patients had distal pancreatectomy, which was successful, and 1 patient had Roux-en-Y pancreaticojejunostomy, which failed. The 10th patient had a brief high-flow fistula but mostly a very low-flow fistula after pancreaticojejunostomy for chronic pancreatitis. This low-flow fistula persisted for 6 months in an indolent state without surgical intervention.

OVERALL RESULTS

A total of 40 major complications was seen in 18 patients, with the majority occurring in patients with pancreatitis. One fistula-related death occurred from infection and multiorgan system failure. Six patients required transfusions of at least 2 U of blood because of major hemorrhage and subsequent reoperations. Intra-abdominal abscesses were seen in 4 patients and required reoperation. Pneumonia in 5 patients necessitated ventilatory support in 2 patients. Multiorgan system failure, including respiratory and renal failure, was common in the patients with fistulas from pancreatitis and resulted in high morbidity and prolonged hospital stays.

Thirty of the 35 patients required operation in an attempt to close the fistula, to control ascites, or to resolve pleural effusion. Surgical treatment was successful in 25 patients (83%), and failures occurred in 1 patient with fistula from trauma, in 1 patient with fistula from operation for tumor, and in 3 patients with fistulas from pancreatitis (Table). Of the failures, 2 had minimal leakage, and 1 patient died.

Radiologic visualization revealed ductal integrity to be abnormal in 22 of 26 patients. Endoscopic retrograde cholangiopancreatography and fistulography were invaluable in planning the operative approach.

COMMENT

The approach to the management of pancreatic fistulas is best considered in light of the underlying cause of the fistula. Fistulas occurring after trauma are often associated with other intra-abdominal injuries. After initial stabilization of the patient's condition, celiotomy management of other injuries and careful surgical exploration of the pancreas should be carried out. Simple capsular tears can be handled with wide sump drainage, but as seen in three patients, ligation or oversewing of a disrupted duct will result in fistula formation. If the disruption is distal, resection offers definitive treatment although more proximal damage will require demonstration of ductal integrity with retrograde pancreatography performed preoperatively before more radical procedures can be employed. Although drainage alone is inadequate with proximal duct obstruction, a variety of rational alternatives may be employed, such as Roux-en-Y anastomosis, segmental resection of the pancreas with distal or proximal pancreaticojejunostomy, 95% distal pancreatectomy, or duodenal diverticularization.[7] Radical pancreatoduodenectomy is rarely indicated and should be reserved for extensive devitalization injuries of the pancreas and duodenum.

Postoperative fistulas after pancreatic resection for tumor are seen in 15% to 20% of patients and commonly occur when managing a soft gland and a small pancreatic duct. Leakages seen after distal pancreatectomy are, for the most part, well controlled by sump drainage. Complete dehiscence of the pancreaticojejunal anastomosis after the Whipple operation is a cause for reoperation and may require total pancreatectomy to prevent the devastating effects of free pancreatic juice in the abdominal cavity. Most patients, however, can be managed successfully using TPN alone and a minimum of interventional diagnostic procedures. The majority of nonsurgical successes were seen in this group of patients.

Although not used in our patients, nonrandomized reports of acceleration of fistula closure using somatostatin and other agents in addition to TPN should be considered, but caution should be exercised because of recurrences after cessation of therapy and subsequent reports of life-threatening water intoxication with the use of somatostatin.[8-10]

Fistulas associated with pancreatitis are the most heterogeneous and difficult to manage. The rare complications of ascites and pleural effusion are almost exclusively related to the sequelae of pancreatitis. Delayed diagnosis is the rule with effusion unless a high index of suspicion is maintained. Effusion treated by nutritional support and tube thoracostomy alone will rarely resolve the fistula without simultaneous internal drainage. The importance of radiologic intervention and demonstration of ductal integrity cannot be overemphasized in this group of patients as an aid in planning the surgical approach. When externally draining skin fistulas are present, fistulography will often reveal either a pseudocyst cavity or a direct communication with the pancreatic duct. Patients with ascites or pleural effusion should undergo ERCP, and if ductal disruption or fistulous tracts or both are identified and confined to the distal gland, resection will enable the diseased gland and the fistula to be managed successfully. The stable patient with an identifiable well-developed fistulous tract and a minimum of peripancreatic inflammation as seen in the chronic pancreatitis group can be managed successfully with an internal drainage procedure.

Our approach to pancreatic fistulas will continue to be individualized for each patient. Adequate preoperative nutritional support is mandatory along with extensive use of radiologic imaging to demonstrate ductal anatomy and to permit planning for resection or internal drainage in the majority of patients with fistulas resulting from pancreatitis or trauma. Postoperative fistulas can be managed with assurance with TPN and external sump drainage for a high degree of success.

References

1. Jordan GL Jr. Pancreatic fistula. *Am J Surg.* 1970;119:200-207.
2. Cameron JL, Kieffer RS, Anderson WJ, et al. Internal pancreatic fistulas: pancreatic ascites and pleural effusions. *Ann Surg.* 1976;184:587-593.
3. Smith RB III, Warren WD, Rivard AA Jr, et al. Pancreatic ascites: diagnosis and management with particular reference to surgical technics. *Ann Surg.* 1973;177:538-546.
4. Weaver DW, Walt AJ, Sugawa C, Bouwman DL. A continuing appraisal of pancreatic ascites. *Surg Gynecol Obstet.* 1982;154:845-848.
5. Cameron JL. Chronic pancreatic ascites and pancreatic pleural effusions. *Gastroenterology.* 1978;74:134-140.
6. Belli G, McPherson GA, Blumgart LH. Conservative management of pancreatic ascites. *J R Soc Med.* 1985;78:949-950.
7. Graham JM, Mattox KL, Jordan GL Jr. Traumatic injuries of the pancreas. *Am J Surg.* 1978;136:744-748.
8. Joehl RJ, Nahrwold DL. Inhibition of human pancreatic secretion by terbutaline as a potential agent for treating patients with pancreatic fistula. *Surg Gynecol Obstet.* 1985;160:109-114.
9. Prinz RA, Pickleman J, Hoffman JP. Treatment of pancreatic cutaneous fistulas with a somatostatin analog. *Am J Surg.* 1988;155:36-42.
10. Halma C, Jansen JB, Janssens AR, et al. Life-threatening water intoxication during somatostatin therapy. *Ann Intern Med.* 1987;107:518-520.

Discussion

David W. Butsch, MD, Montpelier, Vt: I wonder if there is any use for adjunctive measures? I heard once that acetazolamide (Diamox) might be helpful. Although the previous report suggested that H_2 antagonists would not be helpful, I wonder if you have ever tried them? Do you know of any medications that may diminish the output of a pancreatic fistula?

George L. Nardi, MD, Boston, Mass: This is such a complex aggregate of heterogeneous problems: fistulas with and without abscesses and fistulas in the special group of patients who have had transplants; it is hard to find a common denominator. Pancreatic fistula is alleged to be the most common complication of any pancreaticojejunal anastomosis. The fact that the Lahey Clinic could get together only 41 patients, including their special group of patients, over a 15-year period is a compliment to their management, particularly since they see a large group of patients with this type of problem.

I would agree completely with the authors that there are three important considerations in the management of any pancreatic fistula. First, every patient has to be individualized. Some may have a simple fistula, some may have an abscess, some may have subphrenic complications, and some may have all these enzymes going that have been spoken about; there are no two that are similar. The second consideration is the use of nutritional support, and the third is radiologic visualization of the fistula and pancreatic duct. I would be inclined to do the ERCP first whenever possible, because a sinogram may show you a communication with the pancreatic duct, but you do not know if that pancreatic duct is patent or not. That is where the ERCP may come in if complete filling is not seen. So, you certainly need the ERCP; sometimes you need both.

After you visualize the pancreatic duct, it is particularly important to decide what to do. Now, they reported three postoperative diabetic problems. The big choice is, do you do a distal resection or do you do an internal bypass (Roux-en-Y or pancreaticojejunostomy)? I have always attempted to preserve tissue, do the bypass, and take the chance that you will get a stricture. If you do, then do a resection.

One thing I did not understand was excision of the fistula. I can understand the other procedures, but how do you excise a fistula? Does that mean you just went down, dissected to the opening in the gland, and oversewed it? If that worked, would it not have probably healed spontaneously since the duct had to be patent to permit the repair to heal?

David M. Sensenig, Togus, Me: Dr Martin and her colleagues are to be congratulated on an interesting report on the management of pancreatic fistulas. I want to mention a method that resolved the problem of a continuing troublesome pancreatic fistula due to trauma.

A 23-year-old woman drove her car into a tree. She was brought to the Eastern Maine Medical Center, where she underwent operation on October 18, 1986, at which time an extensive laceration of the liver was sutured, the lesser sac and duodenum were surgically explored, and a laceration of the right knee was repaired. There was some ecchymosis around the pancreas and in the transverse mesocolon, but no visible pancreatic laceration. She was discharged from the hospital, but a symptomatic fluid collection in the pancreatic head and neck developed later that was drained percutaneously in late December. Large amounts of pancreatic juice continued to drain from the patient despite TPN, a low-fat diet, and propantheline bromide (Pro-Banthine) therapy. An ERCP revealed a pancreas divisum. An injection of the fistulous tract as an outpatient demonstrated the pancreatic duct with no connection to the duodenum.

On February 23, 1987, a laparotomy was performed with resection of 3 cm of the distal pancreas, preserving the spleen, and a retrograde pancreaticojejunostomy, Roux-en-Y. There were two ducts in the tail, both judged too small for direct mucosa-to-mucosa suturing. Polyethylene catheters (No. 50 and No. 90) were inserted into the ducts and then implanted through the mucosa into the jejunum. The drainage then rapidly reduced, and the fistula closed. The patient was doing well with a weight gain of 5.4 kg when seen at follow-up 9 months later; she has continued to do well. I mention this case to emphasize that this method can be of use in handling a persistent pancreatic fistula.

Dr Martin: Thank you, Dr Nardi, for your comments, and to the other commentators as well. The technique for excision of the fistula was what Dr Nardi suggested—excision of a fistulous tract that was well developed. Preoperative ERCP done on these patients revealed no communication between the main pancreatic duct and the external draining skin fistula.

Diabetes developed in three patients postoperatively; two of these patients had had distal pancreatic resections and one patient had had internal drainage. The majority have chronic pancreatitis, and regardless of what is done, diabetes ultimately develops in 60% to 70%. It is very difficult to know at what point one is dealing with progression of disease and development of diabetes or whether one accelerates this with a distal pancreatic resection. It is quite clear, though, that if the gland in a borderline patient with chronic pancreatitis is resected, the risk of the development of diabetes is much higher.

I agree with the approach of pancreaticojejunostomy to the distal limb. I think that that is an appropriate management of patients with these kinds of pancreatic fistulas.

Finally, there are a number of pharmacologic manipulations that can be done to inhibit pancreatic secretion. Perhaps the best studied and most reported is the use of somatostatin, although glucagon, acetazolamide, and various other agents have been used. Past studies are, for the most part, uncontrolled and nonrandomized. The Verona group has addressed the use of pharmacologic manipulation in the management of pancreatic fistulas.

In 45 patients studied who were receiving various agents, including somatostatin, there was no significant change in the rate of closure of the fistulas; however, somatostatin, when compared with the other agents, did diminish and accelerate the time during which these fistulas closed.

Cholecystokinin Augmentation of 'Surgical' Pancreatitis

Benefits of Receptor Blockade

Irvin M. Modlin, MD; Anton J. Bilchik, MD; Karl A. Zucker, MD;
Thomas E. Adrian, PhD, MRCPath; Jeffrey Sussman, MD; Scott M. Graham, MD

• The management of acute pancreatitis has not changed appreciably throughout several decades. Recent evidence has suggested that cholecystokinin (CCK) may play an important role in pancreatic disease. Investigations into the precise role of CCK in acute pancreatitis have been hampered by the lack of a specific CCK receptor antagonist. Using a newly described, highly potent and specific CCK receptor antagonist, L-364,718, the effect of CCK in two models of acute "surgical" pancreatitis was examined: (1) the bile salt ductal perfusion model in the rat and (2) a traumatic model in the guinea pig. At a suboptimal dose for pancreatic enzyme secretion (25 pmol/kg/h), CCK was found to potentiate the severity of the ensuing pancreatitis in both models. Continuous CCK receptor blockade with L-364,718 (25 nmol/kg/h) improved biochemical, morphologic, and survival indexes. This study suggests that physiologic levels of CCK play an important permissive role in the evolution of acute pancreatitis. The use of L-364,718 as an investigative probe or therapeutic tool for acute pancreatitis is worthy of further consideration.
(*Arch Surg.* 1989;124:574-578)

Acute pancreatitis remains one of the more difficult therapeutic challenges faced by the surgeon today. Treatment of this disease process has not changed appreciably in the past several decades, with supportive management remaining the mainstay of therapy. Development of specific and effective therapeutic modalities has undoubtedly been hampered by the lack of a clear understanding of the cause of this disease despite nearly a century of experimental and clinical investigation.

Along with the investigation of a large number of regulatory gut hormones, there has been an accumulation of evidence to suggest that cholecystokinin (CCK) may play a significant role in pancreatic pathophysiology. This regulatory peptide is released from the proximal small bowel following the ingestion of fats or proteins. Its primary biologic role appears to be as a stimulant of pancreatic enzyme secretion and gallbladder contraction.[1] The observation that supramaximal dosages of cerulein (a CCK analogue of amphibian origin) resulted in the rapid development of an interstitial form of edematous pancreatitis provided the initial evidence that CCK might play a role in pancreatic pathophysiology.[2] More recently, infusion of less toxic concentrations of CCK has been shown to increase dramatically the mortality of the acute, hemorrhagic pancreatitis of mice, consequent on the ingestion of a choline-deficient, ethionine-supplemented diet.[3] The ensuing hypothesis proposes that CCK may play an important permissive or contributory role in the pathogenesis of pancreatitis. The corollary of this postulate would suggest that blockade of the CCK receptor might be of benefit in the treatment of acute pancreatitis.

Until recently, a more detailed investigation into the role of CCK in pancreatic disease has been hampered by the lack of potent and specific antagonists. Previously available CCK antagonists, such as proglumide and benzotript, are relatively weak and nonspecific agents with numerous side effects. Recently, however, a number of highly specific and potent CCK receptor antagonists (ie, asperlicin, CR1409, and L-364,718) have been developed.[4-7] The utilization of these agents has allowed a more focused study of the role of CCK in the evolution of the pancreatitic process.

In this study, we examined the effect of CCK in two models of acute pancreatitis that involved direct injury to the gland: (1) the bile salt ductal perfusion model in the rat[8] and (2) a traumatic model of necrotizing pancreatitis in the guinea pig.[9] The potential therapeutic efficacy of continuous CCK receptor blockade, utilizing the CCK antagonist L-364,718, was examined in both models.

METHODS and MATERIALS

Ductal Perfusion Experiments

Male Wistar rats (Small Animal Section, National Cancer Institute, Bethesda, Md), weighing from 275 to 300 g, were fasted 18 to 24 hours before each experiment but allowed water ad libitum. Acute hemorrhagic pancreatitis was induced by a retrograde perfusion of the common pancreaticobiliary duct with a 3.5% taurocholate sodium solution (Sigma Chemical Co, St Louis, Mo) according to the method of Aho et al.[8] Briefly, animals were anesthetized by an intraperitoneal injection of pentobarbital sodium (25 mg/kg of body weight). A midline laparotomy was performed, the duodenum was mobilized medially, and the common bile duct was cannulated transduodenally with polyethylene tubing (PE = 20, Clay Adams, Parsippany, NJ). A noncrushing bulldog clamp (OmegaMed, Minneapolis, Minn) was applied at the hilum of the liver to exclude the hepatic ductal system from the perfusate. Bile salts were perfused at a rate of 100 μL/100 g of body weight during a 60-s interval with a Harvard infusion pump. Following the perfusion, the clamp and tubing were removed, and the abdominal incision was closed. Animals received a 1.0-mL saline solution bolus intraperitoneally at the time of closure to support perioperative fluid balance.

Cholecystokinin was administered as a continuous infusion (25 pmol/kg/h) via subcutaneously implanted osmotic minipumps (Model 2001, Alza Corp, Palo Alto, Calif). The CCK receptor antagonist, L-364,718 (Merck & Co, Inc, West Point, Pa), was infused via a separate osmotic pump at a rate of 25 nmol/kg/h. Control animals received vehicle solution alone (60% dimethyl sulfoxide and 0.154-mol/L sodium chloride saline solution) via osmotic pumps.

Animals were divided into five groups with 16 animals in each group as follows: (1) control animals receiving sham laparotomy, (2) bile salt ductal perfusion alone, (3) exogenous CCK beginning 12 hours before ductal perfusion, (4) exogenous CCK and L-364,718 both beginning 12 hours before ductal perfusion, (5) L-364,718 alone beginning 12 hours before ductal perfusion. Animal mortality was determined at 24, 48, and 72 hours after the operative procedure (onset of pancreatitis). Tissue for light microscopy was obtained from the gastric, splenic, and duodenal lobes of the pancreas and was evaluated by an experienced gastrointestinal pathologist in a blinded fashion. Serum for lipase

Accepted for publication December 12, 1988.
From the Gastrointestinal Surgical Research Group, Yale University School of Medicine and the Veterans Administration Medical Center, New Haven, Conn.
Read before the 69th Annual Meeting of the New England Surgical Society, Montreal, Canada, September 17, 1988.
Reprint requests to Department of Surgery, Yale University School of Medicine, 333 Cedar St, New Haven, CT 06510 (Dr Modlin).

Table 1.—Mortality of Rats (n = 16 in Each Group) 24, 48, and 72 Hours After Bile Duct Perfusion*

	Mortality, %		
	24 h	48 h	72 h
Sham laparotomy	0	0	0
Perfusion alone	37	75	75
Perfusion + CCK	56	88	88
Perfusion + L-364,718	12†	56‡	62
Perfusion + CCK + L-364,718	18‡	50‡	68

*Perfusion was performed with 3.5% taurocholate sodium. Cholecystokinin and L-364,718 were infused via osmotic minipumps 12 hours before bile duct cannulation. CCK indicates cholecystokinin.
†$P<.01$ (compared with perfusion + CCK).
‡$P<.05$ (compared with perfusion + CCK).

Table 2.—Comparison of Basal and 24-Hour Serum Amylase and Lipase Levels After Bile Salt Perfusion*

	Mean ± SEM	
	Amylase Level, μmol/L	Lipase Level, U/L
	Baseline/24 h	Baseline/24 h
Sham laparotomy	1420 ± 625/1589 ± 397	3.1 ± 1.1/3.0 ± 0.9
Perfusion alone	1306 ± 511/10 334 ± 2214	3.3 ± 1.3/11.3 ± 3.5
Perfusion + CCK	1192 ± 397/11 980 ± 1760	3.4 ± 1.1/14.3 ± 3.1
Perfusion + CCK + L-364,718	1646 ± 397/4599 ± 1249†	3.0 ± 0.9/5.1 ± 1.7‡

*CCK indicates cholecystokinin.
†$P<.05$ vs perfusion alone and perfusion + CCK.
‡$P<.05$ vs perfusion + CCK.

Table 3.—Serum Amylase Levels in Traumatic Pancreatitis*

	Mean ± SEM Amylase Level, μmol/L				
	−24 h	0 h	24 h	48 h	72 h
Sham laparotomy	1250 ± 170	1250 ± 170	1420 ± 227	1589 ± 227	1589 ± 227
Trauma alone	1022 ± 170	1078 ± 170	1533 ± 170	2044 ± 227	1816 ± 227
Trauma + CCK	1136 ± 113	1136 ± 113	1589 ± 170	1873 ± 113	2158 ± 227
Trauma + CCK + L-364,718	851 ± 57	851 ± 57	1022 ± 454	1136 ± 57†	1192 ± 113†

*Serum amylase concentrations in traumatic pancreatitis were taken 24 hours before pancreatic injury, at the time of injury (0 hours), and 24, 48, and 72 hours after insult. CCK indicates cholecystokinin.
†$P<.05$ vs trauma alone and trauma + CCK.

and amylase measurements was obtained from the tail vein before ductal perfusion and 24 hours later from surviving animals.

Traumatic Pancreatitis

In the second set of experiments, the effect of exogenous CCK administration and continuous CCK receptor blockade was examined in a traumatic model of pancreatitis, as previously described.[9] In brief, female guinea pigs (strain 2; weight range, 400 to 500 g) were fasted 24 hours before surgery but allowed free access to water. Animals were anesthetized with pentobarbital sodium (25 mg/kg intraperitoneally), and a 3.0-cm abdominal midline incision was made. The stomach and duodenum were mobilized cephalad to expose the gastric and splenic lobes of the pancreas. The exposed pancreas was cross-clamped with a modified Spencer-Wells noncrushing vascular clamp in three areas: (1) the distal splenic lobe, (2) the midsplenic lobe, and (3) the proximal gastric lobe, each for 15 s. Guinea pigs were divided into four groups with eight animals in each group as follows: (1) sham laparotomy alone, (2) pancreatic trauma alone, (3) pancreatic trauma with CCK infusion (25 pmol/kg/h) beginning 24 hours before surgery, and (4) pancreatic trauma with both CCK and L-364,718 (25 nmol/kg/h) beginning 24 hours before surgery. This dose of L364,718 has previously been shown in our laboratory to block the effects of even pharmacologic doses of cerulein (25 μg/kg).[10] Cholecystokinin and L-364,718 (60% dimethyl sulfoxide and 0.154-mol/L sodium chloride saline solution) were administered via miniosmotic pumps that were implanted subcutaneously. The sham laparotomy and the pancreatic trauma groups received the vehicle solution alone. Serial blood samples (1 mL) for pancreatic enzyme secretion were obtained from each animal by cardiac puncture as follows: 24 hours before laparotomy; at the time of surgery; and at 24, 48, and 72 hours postoperatively. Fluid was replaced by a 3-mL intraperitoneal bolus injection. Survivors were killed at 72 hours, and the pancreas were examined for areas of necrosis, inflammation, and saponification. The pancreas was carefully dissected out, and wet pancreatic weight was recorded as an indicator of acute edematous changes. The pancreas was sectioned at 10-μm intervals, and tissue from the entire gland was examined with light microscopy. The hematoxylin-eosin–stained slides were coded and examined in a blinded fashion. Areas of necrosis, hemorrhage, and saponification were quantified by morphometric analysis.[11]

Statistical Analysis

Comparisons between normally distributed data were made using the Student's t test, paired analysis was used for temporal within-group comparisons, and the unpaired t test was used for comparisons between groups. Comparison of mortality data were done using χ^2 analysis.

RESULTS

Bile Salt Ductal Perfusion

Mortality in those rats that underwent bile salt ductal perfusion is shown in Table 1. Twenty-four hours after bile salt perfusion, there was a 37% mortality in the animals that were treated with perfusion alone, and mortality was 0% in the control (sham laparotomy) group. In animals that received exogenous CCK, there was a 56% mortality. There was no significant difference between animals that were treated with perfusion alone and perfusion plus CCK at either 24 or 48 hours. However, in rats that received both CCK and L-364,718, there was only an 18% mortality ($P<.05$). A similar pattern was observed at 48 hours with a 75% mortality in the animals that were treated with perfusion alone and an 88% mortality in the CCK-treated animals compared with a 50% mortality in animals that were administered L-364,718 ($P<.05$).

Serum amylase and lipase measurement results are shown in Table 2. Twenty-four hours after ductal perfusion, the serum amylase level rose from a baseline mean (± SEM) value of 1306 ± 511 μmol/L to 10 334 ± 2214 μmol/L in the group that was treated with perfusion alone and 11 980 ± 1760 μmol/L in animals that received CCK before perfusion (both $P<.001$ as compared with control animals, 1420 ± 625 μmol/L). Administration of L-364,718 partially blocked this rise in the serum amylase level at 24 hours (4599 ± 1249 μmol/L; $P<.05$ as compared with the group that was treated with perfusion alone). Serum lipase values manifested a similar rise with perfusion and CCK, with L-364,718 also showing a protective effect (Table 2).

Histologic examination of the pancreas at 24 hours showed extensive fat necrosis, interstitial edema, patchy areas of hemorrhage, and acute inflammation. Widespread foci of necrosis were present in the acini, and surviving acini were vacuolated.

Traumatic Pancreatitis

Guinea pigs that underwent laparotomy alone or laparotomy with pancreatic trauma were killed 72 hours after surgery. At necropsy, gross surface anatomic changes in the traumatized, untreated group consisted of patchy areas of erythema and irregular stellate areas of yellow discoloration. These were most severe in the surrounding areas of direct trauma, although they were distributed throughout the gland. There were marked macroscopic changes in the group that was treated with CCK. The entire pancreas appeared to be saponified with minimal areas of normal pancreas. In contrast, the areas of hemorrhage and saponification were overtly smaller and more localized in the L-364,718-treated animals. The mean (±SEM) wet pancreatic weight was increased from 300±17 mg/100 g of body weight in the control group to 426.3±23.5 mg/100 g of body weight in the traumatized group alone and 485.6±41.7 mg/100 g of body weight in the traumatized group that was treated with CCK ($P<.05$, significantly different from the control group but not from the trauma alone group). The pancreatic weight of animals that received L-364,718 was significantly lower (369±22.3 mg/100 g of body weight) than that of the traumatized group that received CCK ($P<.05$). With pancreatic trauma alone, the serum amylase level rose from a preoperative value of 1022±170 to 1533±170 μmol/L at 24 hours and 2044±227 μmol/L at 48 hours (Table 3). Traumatized animals that received CCK showed a similar rise in the serum amylase level. This increase was not statistically different on an unpaired basis. The rise in the serum amylase level in both traumatized groups was blocked by the administration of L-364,718 ($P<.05$). The serum lipase level (Fig 1) showed a similar pattern with a ninefold increase (73±9 U/L) over the preoperative value (8±3 U/L) in the traumatized group and a 15-fold increase (137±19 U/L) in the traumatized animals that received CCK. Traumatized guinea pigs that received L-364,718 exhibited a substantial diminution of the serum lipase level at 24 hours (50±5 U/L) ($P<.05$ as compared with either the trauma alone or trauma plus CCK groups).

Histologic examination of control animals revealed normal pancreatic lobules with islets scattered throughout the parenchyma. In CCK-treated, traumatized animals, sharply demarcated areas of injury were evident, with areas of acute and chronic inflammation showing foci of coagulative and fat necrosis (Fig 2, left). A striking proliferation of cells that formed ductulelike spaces in a disordered or lobular pattern were present in the granulation tissue. These changes were most prominent in areas that had undergone previous direct clamp injury; however, areas of inflammation and necrosis were evident in areas distal to this. Smaller areas of coagulative and fat necrosis were seen in the L-364,718-treated group (Fig 2, right).

Morphometric analysis revealed an approximate twofold increase in coagulative necrosis with an approximately fourfold increase in fat necrosis in untreated animals as compared with animals that were pretreated with L-364,718. The CCK-treated animals manifested a threefold increase in coagulative necrosis with a sixfold greater increase in fat necrosis than in animals in the L-364,718-treated group.

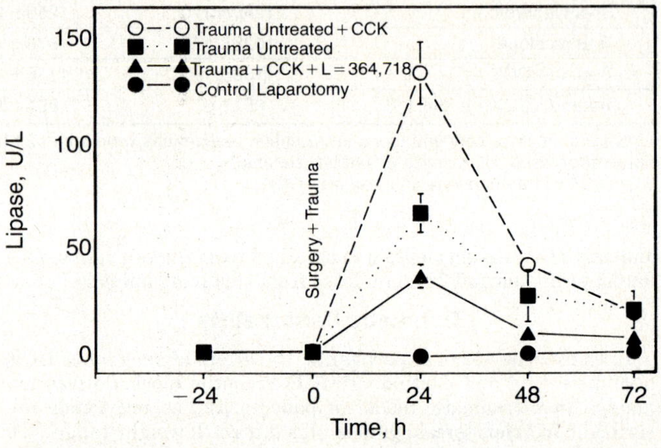

Fig 1.—Comparison of serum lipase levels in traumatized pancreas with and without cholecystokinin (CCK) and L-364,718. Change in lipase level from baseline value shows ninefold rise at 24 hours in untreated, traumatized group (closed square) without CCK and 15-fold rise in traumatized animals receiving CCK (open circles). This rise was significantly ameliorated in treated group (solid triangles) with only threefold to fourfold rise above control values ($P<.001$).

Fig 2.—Pancreas histologic characteristics. In untreated, traumatized group treated with cholecystokinin, foci of coagulative necrosis and saponification are evident (left) (hematoxylin-eosin, ×31). Group that was treated with L-364,718 shows evidence of minimal areas of necrosis and only occasional minor areas of fat necrosis (right) (hematoxylin-eosin, ×31).

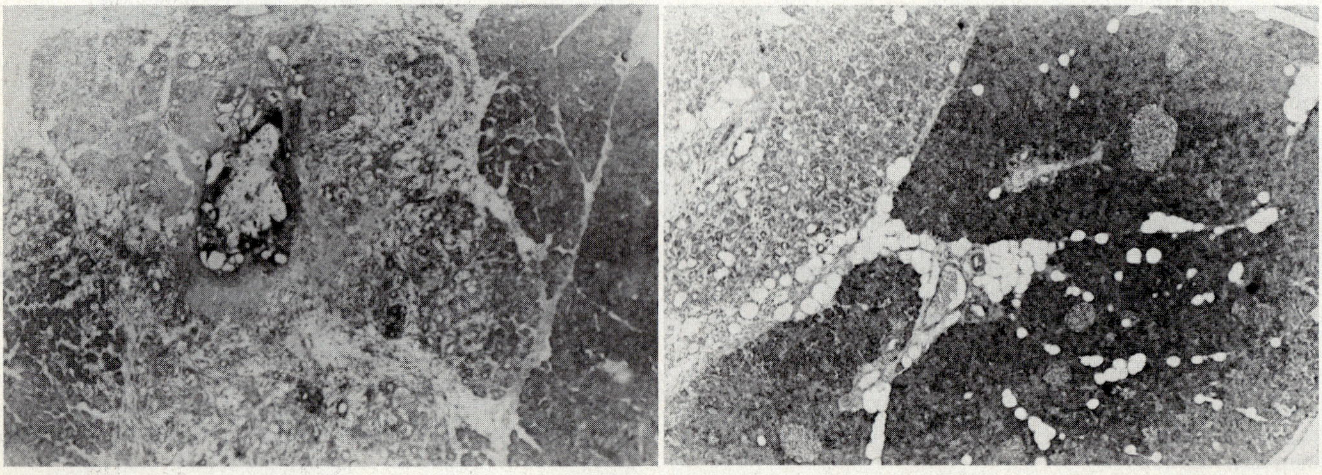

COMMENT

Acute pancreatitis often represents the final end-organ target of a number of diverse pathologic events, such as cholelithiasis, alcohol toxicity, lipid metabolic abnormalities, drugs, venoms, and direct blunt or penetrating trauma. Despite nearly a century of clinical and experimental investigation, little is known of the precise events involved in the pathogenesis of pancreatitis. Not surprisingly, there are few therapeutic regimens that appear to be of direct benefit. Currently, supportive management remains the mainstay of treatment. The failure to identify either the initiating agents or the cellular mechanisms of the disease has limited therapeutic options. The more recent identification of chemical messengers and regulators of pancreatic secretory function has allowed a better understanding of pancreatic physiology. The examination of the role of these various regulators in the initiation of pancreatitis and the evolution of its systemic sequelae is, therefore, of considerable pertinence. It is probable that the disease process involves a disturbance of regulatory function and that the numerous systemic effects of pancreatitis are consequent on the bioactivity of diverse peptides and amines that are released following cell damage by the potent proteolytic and lipolytic enzymes.

Cholecystokinin is a chemical regulator that has been demonstrated to have potent biologic effects not only as a neurotransmitter, but also as a pancreatic secretagogue and stimulant of gallbladder and smooth-muscle contractility. Its regulatory role as one of the most potent agonists of pancreatic zymogen secretion has suggested that it may be of considerable relevance in the genesis of acute pancreatitis. In this investigation, we have studied the role of CCK in two established models of pancreatitis that involved direct injury to the gland, both of a chemical and a mechanical nature. In both models, exogenous CCK was found to potentiate the severity of the ensuing pancreatitis. The dose of CCK used in these studies (25 pmol/kg/h) has been well characterized as that which results in submaximal pancreatic enzyme release when administered parenterally. It is thus reasonable to propose that the experimentally induced pancreatitic models are being exposed to plasma CCK levels that are consistent with those found under physiologic circumstances. The CCK itself, when administered in large amounts (5 μg/kg/h), has previously been shown to initiate pancreatitis.[12] This dose is many orders of magnitude greater than that employed in our study. It is thus unlikely that CCK itself (25 pmol/kg/h) could have generated pancreatitis in our model.

Of further relevance is the fact that in these experiments we also found that continuous CCK receptor blockade promoted a partial protective effect in both models of acute pancreatitis. Since L-364,718 has been demonstrated to be a potent and highly specific CCK receptor antagonist with virtually no cross-reactivity with brain CCK or peripheral gastrin receptors, it is likely that this is a specific anti-CCK effect. The dosages of L-364,718 used in this study (25 nmol/kg/h) have previously been demonstrated to block completely the effects of CCK concentrations several orders of magnitude greater than those used here.[10] The data are thus consistent with the interpretation that CCK plays a permissive role in the evolution of acute pancreatitis. Indeed, results of previous studies by Niederau et al,[3] who examined the effect of CCK receptor blockade in a hemorrhagic model of pancreatitis, produced by a choline-deficient ethionine-diet, are consistent with the results obtained in our studies. Taken together, these findings would support our proposal that physiologic levels of CCK may play a permissive and contributory role in the progression of acute pancreatitis.

In the bile salt ductal perfusion model, CCK was found to increase the severity of the inflammation and necrosis as evidenced by histologic changes and an increase of pancreatic enzymes in the systemic circulation. Similarly, in the traumatic model of pancreatitis, CCK had similar effects. The ability of the specific CCK receptor antagonist to ameliorate the morbidity and mortality of the disease process again supports the putative role of CCK in the augmentation of the pancreatitic process.

There are, however, a number of potential flaws in the interpretation of studies of this kind. Since the pathophysiology of acute pancreatitis is not clearly understood, the use of different models to study the process raises the question of relevance to the human disease process. The second issue, which is of particular importance, is the observation that the CCK antagonist, despite being administered in an optimal dosage known to obliterate zymogen secretion completely did not, in fact, produce a parallel decrease in mortality. This suggests strongly that other factors are at play and that blockade of a solitary (CCK) receptor site may not provide a complete resolution of the problem. It was somewhat disappointing to note that the addition of CCK in the bile salt model failed to elevate the mortality rate to a statistically significant level. At each time period, however, the CCK-augmented group exhibited a higher mortality rate. If we were to assume that this trend would have been maintained, then increasing the number of animals in each group from 16 to 20 would have resulted in statistical significance using either Fisher's Exact Test or χ^2 analysis. While this does not necessarily confirm the role of CCK in the evolution of acute pancreatitis, it is consistent with our argument.

Although plasma amylase levels are used in the clinical diagnosis of pancreatitis, their magnitude may be misleading as a predictor of severity or outcome of the disease process. Similarly, the use of amylase in the guinea pig poses certain interpretative difficulties. First, the level of plasma amylase in these animals is significantly higher under even normal circumstances since a considerable proportion of the plasma amylase is of nonpancreatic (salivary gland) origin. Second, repetitive anesthesia for guinea pigs raises plasma amylase levels (A.J.B., K.A.Z., I.M.M., et al, unpublished data, 1988). This observation has previously been reported in humans who undergo anesthesia.[13] Thus, the variability of basal amylase levels and the alterations in certain stimulated pancreatic-amylase levels may not be clearly apparent when the total plasma amylase level is measured. The amylase methodology that was employed in this study did not delineate pancreatic amylase as isozyme analysis was not used. We have thus focused our attention particularly on the lipase data as it is an enzyme that is predominantly pancreatic in origin. In both models, the plasma lipase level was significantly elevated. Similarly, CCK produced a further elevation that was significantly inhibited by the use of L-364,718. It is therefore clear that CCK influenced the release of a major membrane destabilizing agent (lipolytic) and that this deleterious effect could, to a significant extent, be inhibited by the CCK receptor antagonist.

It has been reported that free oxygen radicals may play a significant role in the genesis of acute pancreatitis.[14] Our vehicle for delivery of L-364,718 contained dimethyl sulfoxide, an agent that has been reported to be effective in the scavenging of oxygen-free radicals. Dimethyl sulfoxide alone did not ameliorate the inflammation in the traumatic group (control). It is possible, however, that it may have contributed to the effects exhibited by L-364,718.

Another fact that needs to be considered is the presence in the pancreatic acini of large quantities of preformed zymogen granules. Thus, blockade of the secretory process by antagonism at the receptor site may simply inhibit a further secretory stimulus and enzyme release. It probably cannot significantly alter the cellular synthesis of the destructive degradative enzymes (lipolytic/proteolytic) that are released when the pancreatitic process disrupts cell membranes and tight junctions. A complete understanding of the synthetic process of zymogens is urgently required for the development of an agent that will inhibit pancreatic protein synthesis. A rational therapeutic program would thus require probes that would block the receptor responsible for the initiation of secretion and simultaneously inhibit protein synthesis within the pancreatic acinus itself. However, these studies are of some value in that they illuminate a new area of study whereby the development of specific molecular probes may be used to switch off secretory cell function and, hence, impede the progress of a disease that is, in essence, fueled by itself.

The limited efficacy of a CCK receptor antagonist in these studies suggests an obvious need for a better understanding of the intracellular processes of pancreatic protein secretion. Not withstanding this however, it is possible that the use of such specific receptor antagonists may be important in situations where pancreatitis may be predictable. These would include pretreatment before pancreatic surgery or therapeutic procedures that involve the gastroduodenal area. In addition, in situations where pancreatic injury is detected early or of high probability, such as in blunt abdominal injury or inadvertent trauma during surgery, a reasonable protective role may be proposed.

In conclusion, our studies demonstrate that CCK has a permissive role in the evolution of pancreatitis. It is also highly probable that other regulatory or biologic agents play an important part in the genesis of this process. Blockade of the CCK receptor site may be a reasonable beginning in the attempt to discern the mechanisms necessary to switch off pancreatic function and, hence, ameliorate the development of pancreatitis.

References

1. Adler G, Kern HF, Steele GA. Experimental models and concepts in acute pancreatitis. In: Go VLW, DiMugo EP, Lebenthal E, Brooks FP, Gardner JD, Scheele GA, eds. *The Exocrine Pancreas' Biology, Pathobiology, and Diseases.* New York, NY: Raven Press; 1986:407-421.

2. Lampel M, Kern HF. Acute interstitial pancreatitis in the rat induced by excessive doses of a pancreatic secretagogue. *Virchows Arch A.* 1977; 373:97-117.

3. Niederau C, Liddle RA, Ferrell LA, Grendell JA. Beneficial effects of cholecystokinin-receptor blockade and inhibition of proteolytic enzyme activity in experimental acute hemorrhagic pancreatitis in mice. *J Clin Invest.* 1986;78:1056-1063.

4. Chang RSL, Lotti VJ, Monaghan RL, Birnbaum J, Stapley EO, Goetz MA, et al. A potent non-peptide cholecystokinin antagonist selective for peripheral tissues isolated from *Aspergillus alliaceus. Science.* 1985;230: 177-179.

5. Chang RSL, Lotti VJ. Biochemical and pharmacological characterization of an extremely potent and selective non-peptidal cholecystokinin antagonist. *Proc Natl Acad Sci USA.* 1986;83:4923-4926.

6. Lotti VJ, Pendleton RG, Gould RJ, Hansen HM, Chang RSL, Clineschmidt BV. In vivo pharmacology of L-364,718, a new nonpeptide peripheral cholecystokinin antagonist. *J Pharmacol Exp Ther.* 1987;241:103-109.

7. Makovec F, Christie R, Bani M, Pacini A, Setnikar I, Rovati AL. New glutaramic acid derivatives with potent competitive and specific cholecystokinin antagonists activity. *Arzneimittelforschung.* 1985;35:1048-1055.

8. Aho HJ, Koskensalo SML, Nevalainen TJ. Experimental pancreatitis in the rat sodium taurocholate induced acute hemorrhagic pancreatitis. *Scand J Gastroenterol.* 1980;15:411-416.

9. Bilchik AJ, Zucker KA, Adrian TE, Modlin IM. Amelioration of traumatic pancreatitis by a new specific CCK receptor antagonist. *Gastroenterology.* 1988;94:A35. Abstracted.

10. Zucker KA, Adrian TE, Zdon MJ, Ballantyne GH, Modlin IM. New potent CCK antagonist block caerulein induced pancreatitis. *Surg Forum.* 1987;38:142-144.

11. Bahr GF, Mikel UV. Mass, volume and dimensional distributions in biology with special reference to cells. *Anal Quant Cytol Histol.* 1987;9: 341-354.

12. Watanabe O, Baccino FM, Steer ML, Meldolesi J. Supramaximal caerulein stimulation and ultrastructure of rat pancreatic acinar cell: early morphological changes during development of experimental pancreatitis. *Am J Physiol.* 1984;246:457-467.

13. Mcmahon MJ. Amylase and the diagnosis of pancreatic disease. In: Mitchell CJ, Kelleher J, eds. *Pancreatic Disease in Clinical Practice.* London, England: Pitman Books Ltd; 1981:173-192.

14. Sanfey H, Bulkley GB, Cameron JL. The pathogenesis of acute pancreatitis: the source and role of oxygen-derived free radicals in three different experimental models. *Ann Surg.* 1985;201:633-638.

Discussion

John C. Russell, MD, Hartford, Conn: Dr Modlin and his colleagues have shown us, using two different experimental models, that cholecystokinin (CCK) acts as a promoter, although probably not an initiator, of pancreatitis, and that specific inhibitory agents (L-364,718) can diminish the inflammatory response as measured by histologic features, gross appearance, and serum amylase and lipase determinations. In at least one of the models, it did seem to have a beneficial effect on long-term animal survival.

In experimental pancreatitis, it has been well known that there must be both stimulation and obstruction to cause pancreatitis: either process alone will not predictably cause life-threatening pancreatitis. Only when given in truly pharmacologic doses, not in the doses that are given in the present study's data, does CCK cause pancreatitis. The dosage used here acts only as a stimulator. The unanswered question is, what causes the process of activation to be initiated within the parenchyma of the gland? Several years ago, crinophagy or the linkage of zymogen granules with lysosomes within pancreatic acinar cells was described by Michael Steer, MD, and colleagues, but we still do not know if that is the cause or merely an epiphenomenon.

Aprotinin, a specific trypsin inhibitor, has been previously studied in a very much similar set of experiments. Pretreatment with aprotinin dramatically reduces the severity of experimentally induced pancreatitis. However, when given after the initiation of pancreatitis, it does not seem to have much effect. When used clinically as a prophylaxis against pancreatitis by Skinner's group, aprotinin again was not shown to be efficacious.

I have several questions. Have Dr Modlin and his coworkers looked at the efficacy of specific CCK inhibition after the initiation of pancreatitis? Did it in any way affect the subsequent course? Finally, would Dr Modlin care to speculate on what he thinks is the mechanism of initiation of clinical pancreatitis?

Dr Modlin: In response to Dr Russell's question of CCK receptor blockade and its efficacy when administered after introduction of the injury. We have, in experiments not presented in this study, demonstrated that 4 hours after the initiation of pancreatitis, the ameliorative effect of receptor blockade is, in fact, the same as when administered either 12 or 24 hours before the insult. However, when one moves out beyond 12 hours, this protective effect appears to wane at an exponential rate. This is predictable given the nature of the cascade of biochemical effects that then are taking place within the pancreatic cell system. The institution of receptor blockade at this juncture appears to have little effect on the escalation of the process once established.

Dr Russell's second question addresses the nature of the cellular events occurring within the pancreatic cell that result in the explosive biochemical process that is clinically recognized as acute pancreatitis. This area has been extensively studied by a number of authors, including Frederick Gorelick, MD, and Steven Leach, MD, of our own group. Basically, it is believed that there is a disorder of traffic regulation within the pancreatic acinar cell that culminates in the clinical disease of acute pancreatitis. The peptides that are sequenced into the digestive enzymes by the endoplasmic reticulum and the Golgi apparatus may have an abnormality in their coding message. This message is responsible for the direction of the lysosomal enzymes to the lysosomes and of the digestive enzymes to the condensing vacuoles. In the circumstances that generate acute pancreatitis, there appears to be evidence that sequencing of the signal message may be disordered. Thus, granules of digestive enzymes, instead of progressing normally to the cell surface and then into the lumen, are inappropriately conveyed toward the lysosomes. Under these circumstances, the lysosomes that contain cathepsins and other acid proteases may fuse with enzyme granules and inappropriately activate the digestive enzymes within the pancreatic cell. The bioactivity of these potent proteolytic and lipolytic enzymes that are activated within the pancreatic cell leads to the destruction of cell membranes and subsequent cascade of biochemical events that manifests as acute pancreatitis.

Selective Nonoperative Management of Blunt Splenic Trauma in Adults

James R. Elmore, MD; David E. Clark, MD; Robert J. Isler, MD; William R. Horner, MD

• **The use of selective nonoperative management of blunt splenic trauma in adults is based on the undeniable benefits of this approach in children. Proper patient selection requires hemodynamic stability, lack of generalized peritoneal irritation, and minimal blood transfusion needs. Computed tomography is now used to make the diagnosis, but the decision for laparotomy is based on clinical grounds. Forty-one (87%) of 47 patients selected for nonoperative management were treated successfully without laparotomy, while the remaining 6 patients underwent delayed operations for persistent splenic bleeding. Blood transfusion requirements were significantly less in the observed group than in the operative group for patients with isolated trauma and for patients with polytrauma. There were no known missed intra-abdominal injuries and no deaths with the nonoperative approach. Analysis of our results has confirmed that nonoperative management is a safe and effective alternative to immediate laparotomy in properly selected patients and it can result in splenic salvage without the need for an operation.**

(*Arch Surg.* 1989;124:581-586)

Controversy surrounds the use of a selective nonoperative approach for the treatment of blunt splenic trauma in adults. Concerns have been raised over the potential of increased blood transfusions and the possibility of missing other associated intra-abdominal injuries. The controversy continues owing to small patient groups and variably reported success rates in the literature.

Historically, splenic rupture treated nonoperatively was first reported in the early 1900s with mortality rates ranging from 77% to 100%.[1] This prompted surgeons to recommend splenectomy routinely. Splenectomy continued as the gold standard until 1968, when the Hospital for Sick Children in Toronto, Canada, first published its outstanding results using a nonoperative approach in children.[2] The undeniable benefits of selective nonoperative management of blunt splenic trauma in children prompted the use of this approach in adults in the 1970s. Since that time there has been an increasing body of literature dealing with this topic.

Successful nonoperative management preserves splenic function and alleviates the need for a laparotomy. It is also our contention that this approach, when used selectively, has a minimal risk of missing other abdominal injuries and does not result in increased blood transfusion requirements. This report analyzes our results with the use of nonoperative management of blunt splenic trauma during the past 8 years, and it was undertaken to determine if this is a safe and efficacious form of therapy.

PATIENTS AND METHODS

There were 143 consecutive adult patients treated at the Maine Medical Center, Portland, for documented blunt splenic trauma from January 1980 to July 1988. During this period, a selective approach to the treatment of splenic trauma was employed with some minor variation among the individual surgeons. Initially 47 of these patients were treated nonoperatively. A retrospective review of their charts was carried out to identify the characteristics of each subgroup of patients. Special attention was given to those patients who were treated with nonoperative management, but all charts were reviewed to provide comprehensive information on the remaining patients. Patients were separated into categories based on age, sex, mechanism of injury, diagnostic modality employed, and treatment option employed. The patients were further divided into categories based on the injury severity score (ISS)[3]: the first group of patients had isolated trauma (ISS≤20) and the second group of patients had polytrauma (ISS>20). Adult patients in this study were considered to be those aged 16 years or older. Penetrating and iatrogenic splenic injuries were not included. The average age was 33 years (range, 16 to 70 years) and 67% of the patients were male.

Nonoperative management was employed only in patients who were hemodynamically stable and without generalized peritoneal irritation. Patients requiring immediate surgical intervention for other abdominal injuries or who were hemodynamically unstable were treated with operative repair or splenectomy. Hemodynamically stable patients underwent diagnostic imaging with radionuclide liver-spleen scans or more recently with computed tomographic (CT) scans. Diagnostic peritoneal lavage was used for hemodynamically unstable patients or those with generalized peritoneal irritation. Nonoperatively treated patients were closely observed at bed rest in an intensive care or intermediate care unit. Hematocrits were checked every 6 hours for 24 to 48 hours along with frequent physician visits. Patients were initially treated with nasogastric tube decompression until the expected ileus resolved, and then they were generally discharged from the hospital on the ninth hospital day. Until follow-up scans were obtained at 6 to 8 weeks, physical activity was limited.

A statistician performed statistical analysis using χ^2 analysis and Kruskal-Wallis nonparametric comparisons.

RESULTS

Over the 8-year period, 143 adult patients were treated selectively: 96 patients underwent immediate surgery, resulting in splenectomy in 69 patients and splenic salvage in 27 patients. Of the 47 patients chosen for nonoperative treatment, 41 patients (87%) were treated successfully while 6 required a delayed laparotomy for persistent bleeding or hypotension and underwent splenectomy. Use of this selective approach resulted in splenic preservation (including splenorrhaphy and successful nonoperative

Accepted for publication December 7, 1988.
From the Departments of Surgery (Drs Elmore, Clark, and Horner) and Radiology (Dr Isler), Maine Medical Center, Portland.
Read before the 69th Annual Meeting of the New England Surgical Society, Montreal, Canada, September 17, 1988.
Reprint requests to Department of Surgery, Maine Medical Center, 22 Bramhall St, Portland, ME 04102 (Dr Elmore).

management) in 78% of the patients with isolated injuries and in 29% of the patients with polytrauma. This represents a statistically significant difference in outcome based on degree of trauma ($P<.005$). Overall splenic preservation was possible in 48% of all 143 adults (Fig 1).

Nonoperative treatment was used for 47 adults, with 6 patients eventually requiring a delayed laparotomy. The multitrauma group accounted for 5 of the 6 patients requiring a delayed operation, resulting in a 64% (9/14) success rate for the polytrauma patients. The remaining 33 patients with isolated injuries were treated nonoperatively and only 1 of these patients ultimately required operation (Fig 2). This represents a 97% success rate and is significantly better than the results obtained with multiply injured patients ($P<.005$). The mechanisms of injury are listed in Fig 3. The nonoperative group had a greater percentage of injuries due to falls, sporting injuries, and assaults, whereas the cause in the primary operative group was primarily motor vehicle accidents ($P<.005$). As expected, diagnosis was made most often with either CT scans or liver-spleen scans in the nonoperative group and with peritoneal lavage in the operative group ($P<.005$).

There were no deaths in patients treated with a nonoperative approach. The entire series of 143 patients had an overall mortality rate of 11%; 63% of these patients died within 24 hours of hospital admission. All deaths occurred in patients with an ISS of at least 50. Complications occurred in 15% of the patients with isolated injuries treated nonoperatively and included 3 urinary tract infections and 2 cases of pneumonia. Comparatively, complications in 43% of the polytrauma patients treated nonoperatively included 3 urinary tract infections, 3 cases of pneumonia, and 2 patients with jaundice.

Associated intra-abdominal injuries requiring surgery occurred in 22% of the 96 patients undergoing immediate operation. None of the patients selected for nonoperative treatment were identified to have other associated intra-abdominal injuries requiring surgery, including the 6 patients who underwent delayed laparotomy after a failed nonoperative approach.

Blood transfusion requirements were significantly less in the nonoperative groups. The isolated trauma patients treated nonoperatively (including delayed laparotomy) required 1.1 U per patient as opposed to 3.6 U per patient in the operative group ($P<.001$). Of particular note is the fact that, in the isolated group treated nonoperatively, 20 of 33 patients required no blood transfusions at all. In similar fashion, the polytrauma patients required 5.7 U per patient if treated nonoperatively (including delayed laparotomy) as compared with 10.9 U per patient in the immediate laparotomy group (Fig 4). Only 13 patients in the nonoperative group required more than 2 U of blood with 5 (39%) of these 13 undergoing delayed laparotomy. This compares with 34 patients in the nonoperative group who required no more than 2 U of blood, of whom only 1 (3%) required delayed laparotomy. This trend of increased failure with an increased amount of blood transfusions is not unexpected given our treatment approach and is statistically significant ($P<.005$). The 1 patient who underwent delayed laparotomy with minimal transfusion requirements was a patient who refused blood for religious reasons.

Age does appear to be a complicating factor in those aged 65 years or older. Two (50%) of the 4 older patients (aged ≥65 years) required delayed operation, while only 4 (99%) of 43 younger patients (aged <65 years) did. Based on statistical analysis this is a significant difference ($P<.005$). Theories concerning the elasticity of splenic tissue may play a role in the poorer outcome in the older patients.

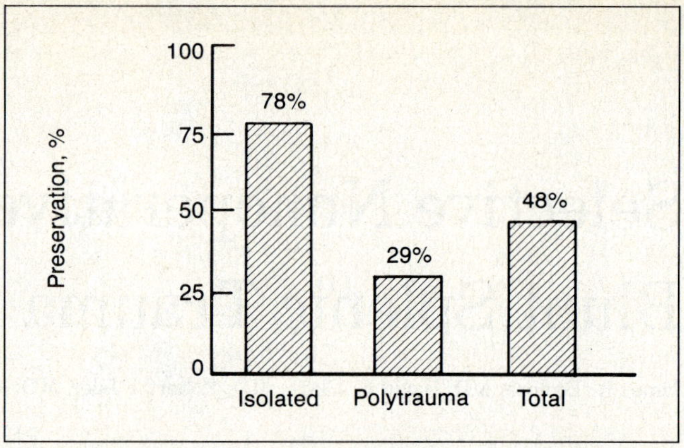

Fig 1.—Splenic preservation. Includes patients with splenorrhaphy or successful nonoperative treatment. Statistically significant difference in outcome between isolated trauma and polytrauma patients ($P<.005$).

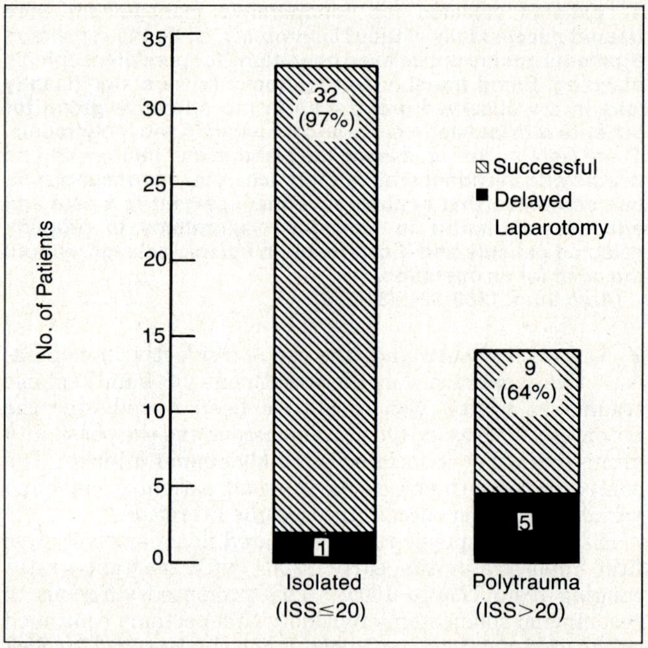

Fig 2.—Nonoperative treatment in 47 patients. Statistically significantly improved results in isolated trauma patients ($P<.005$). ISS indicates injury severity score.

Computed tomographic scanning was used in 18 patients treated nonoperatively (Fig 5). Classification of the degree of splenic injury based on CT was performed by the radiologist. Using the system developed by Buntain et al,[4] this group included 1 patient (5.5%) with type 1, localized capsular disruption; 11 patients (61%) with type 2, parenchymal injury; 5 patients (28%) with type 3, deep fracture extending to the hilum; and 1 patient (5.5%) with type 4, fragmented spleen. We also retrospectively graded each CT examination according to the scoring system proposed by Resciniti et al.[5] Six of our 18 patients had scores less than 2.5; none of these required delayed surgery. Of the remaining 12 patients who had scores equal to or greater

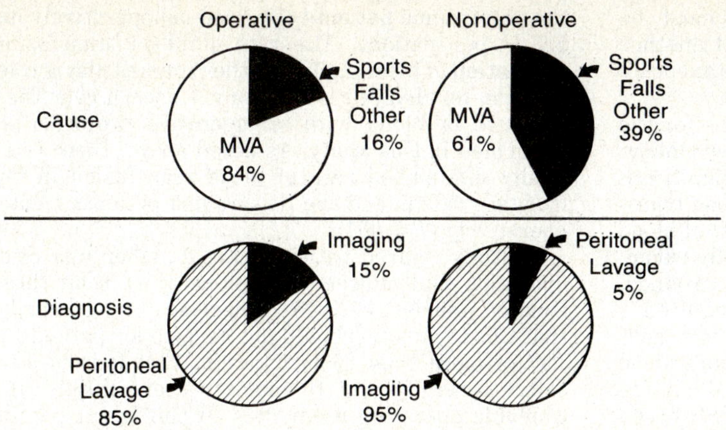

Fig 3.—Cause and diagnosis of injury. Statistically significant difference between operative and nonoperative groups ($P<.005$). MVA indicates motor vehicle accidents.

than 2.5, only 1 of these (score = 4) required delayed laparotomy and splenectomy.

COMMENT

In 1952, King and Shumacker[6] first reported on an overwhelming postsplenectomy infection syndrome in 5 children with congenital spherocytosis, which was fatal in 2. The classic literature review in 1973 by Singer[7] revealed that there were 4 deaths secondary to overwhelming sepsis in 688 pediatric and adult patients following splenectomy for trauma. This yielded a mortality rate of 0.58%. He estimated that the mortality rate from sepsis in the general population was 0.01% and therefore concluded that, in this group of patients, their risk of death was increased 58 times over the general population. This overwhelming postsplenectomy infection syndrome is now a well-recognized entity in children and has prompted pediatric surgeons to advocate splenic preservation whenever possible.

In 1984, Malangoni et al[8] reviewed the trauma literature on adults and combined data from five series to analyze a total of 604 patients who had undergone splenectomy. In this group of patients, there were 10 serious infections and no deaths. A recent 10-year review with a 10-year follow-up by the Massachusetts General Hospital[9] of its experience with 77 adults who underwent splenectomy for trauma had no documented episodes of the overwhelming postsplenectomy infection syndrome. Up to 1984,[10] there were 47 case reports in the literature describing the overwhelming postsplenectomy infection syndrome in adults after splenectomy for trauma. In these 47 patients, death occurred in 28 and disseminated intravascular coagulopathy occurred in 23. There were 39 episodes that took place within 10 years of the splenectomy. These studies support the concept that in adults who have undergone splenectomy for trauma, there is a small but definite risk of late sepsis.

In 1968, Upadhyaya and Simpson,[2] from the Toronto Hospital for Sick Children, first reported on nonoperative management of splenic trauma. There were 52 children with splenic injuries of whom 12 were treated nonoperatively. Since this first publication, the Hospital for Sick Children has been a strong advocate of nonoperative management in pediatric patients. In the most recently published article by Wesson et al,[11] 44 children were treated nonoperatively, and only one patient required late surgical exploration for a pseudocyst. The conclusion was that nonoperative treatment of splenic injuries is safe and effective. In their opinion, operative intervention is indicated when blood loss requirements exceed 40 mL/kg or approximately one half the child's total blood volume.

In 1981, Lutzker and Chun[12] published the first relatively large series that included reports of nine adult patients who were successfully treated nonoperatively. The Table lists the more recent series[4,5,12-24] that have data on this form of treatment in adults. Excluded are reports that did not separate data between pediatric and adult patients. The majority of these series have had good results, but there are four exceptions, and it is not clear why these four centers had less success with this form of treatment. Overall, our 87% success rate compares favorably with the 66% success rate in the literature. Our excellent success rate is most likely due to our selection process. Although a strict protocol was not followed, general principles were adhered to in all of these patients. Patients selected for nonoperative treatment had to be hemodynamically stable, lack generalized peritoneal signs, and require minimal blood transfusions for the splenic injury. Hemodynamic stability was present in all patients selected for nonoperative treatment. Transient hypotension (systolic blood pressure <100 mm Hg) easily reversed with only crystalloid infusion on arrival was believed to represent relative hemodynamic stability and seven of such patients were treated nonoperatively. No patients were treated nonoperatively who required large-volume fluid resuscitation (>2 L) or blood transfusions on hospital arrival to raise the systolic blood pressure above 100 mm Hg. This represents a departure from the classic approach in children where up to 50% of the blood volume may be used to stabilize the patient's condition.

Lack of generalized peritoneal irritation was also a necessary component in the selection process. None of the nonoperatively treated patients had generalized irritation. If this were present, it would indicate either significant intra-abdominal bleeding or other associated injury and in our hands would prompt diagnostic peritoneal lavage and subsequent surgical exploration. No missed intra-abdominal injuries were identified in those patients selected for nonoperative treatment, including the 6 who underwent delayed laparotomy. In the remaining 96 patients, there was a 22% incidence of other associated intra-abdominal injuries requiring surgery. For nonoperative treatment of blunt splenic trauma to be successful, a certain subgroup of patients must be identified who do not have serious associated intra-abdominal injuries requiring surgery and we base that decision on these guidelines. Of course, all patients selected for nonoperative treatment must be monitored closely to rule out the possibility that another significant intra-abdominal injury might simultaneously exist with the splenic injury.

The requirement of minimal blood transfusions for the patient with a splenic injury is the last guideline we follow. As noted in the "Results" section, there was a significant difference in outcome based on the amount of blood transfused. Patients receiving less than or equal to 2 U of blood were successfully treated 97% of the time; the only exception was a patient who refused blood on religious grounds. Patients receiving more than 2 U of blood required a delayed laparotomy in 39% of the cases. This is a self-fulfilling prophecy as those patients receiving more blood were often taken to the operating room based on the amount of blood and this decision was not necessarily based on hypotension or other symptoms. For isolated splenic trauma, a guideline of 2 U per patient is appropriate given the fact that, from our data, 20 of the 33 patients in this group required no blood at all. Of the remaining isolated trauma patients, only 4 required more than 2 U of blood (which includes one of the failures). The Mayo Clinic (Rochester, Minn)[25] analyzed 19 failures of nonoperative management in a group of pediatric and adult patients and recommended a maximal transfusion of 2 U per patient prior to laparotomy. In multiply injured patients, the decision about the need for delayed laparotomy based on the number of transfusions is more difficult given the other potential bleeding sites. The average blood transfusion in the polytrauma patients observed nonoperatively has been 5.7 U per patient. The rate of blood transfusions and estimation of bleeding from other sources play a role in the decision for delayed laparotomy. Concern over the excessive use of blood with nonoperative protocols was not confirmed in this study. As noted above, there is a statistically diminished rate of blood transfusion in both the isolated trauma and the polytrauma patients treated nonoperatively ($P<.001$).

Multiply injured patients have a higher rate of delayed operation and subsequent splenectomy than those with isolated injuries ($P<.005$). This does not necessarily imply that this technique should not be used for patients with an ISS of more than 20 but, rather, that it is necessary to select carefully and to monitor them closely and have available operating room staff. If this is not possible in a given institution, then nonoperative management should not be used in these higher-risk patients. These polytrauma patients must still fit the basic criteria of hemodynamic stability, lack of generalized peritoneal irritation, and minimal blood transfusions for the splenic injury, taking into account other sources of blood loss. This is not a technique that should be widely used in these more injured patients. Only 16% of the polytrauma patients were treated nonoperatively as compared with 61% of the isolated trauma patients. In our institution, we still have been successful in 64% of the polytrauma patients treated nonoperatively.

Computed tomography offers a noninvasive method to detect and classify solid-organ injuries. As compared with the more nonspecific diagnostic peritoneal lavage, a specific injury diagnosis is achievable by CT; the retroperitoneum can be evaluated, and the amount of intra-abdominal fluid can be quantified. The less common hollow viscus injuries continue to be difficult to diagnose by CT. Recent attempts have been made to estimate the risk of nonoperative management based on CT grading of traumatic injuries. Buntain et al[4] recommended early operation for CT-graded type 2, 3, and 4 splenic injuries to improve splenic salvage. Resciniti et al[5] proposed a CT scoring system for splenic injury and suggested that a score of less than 2.5 had a very low probability of requiring delayed operation. In the series of Resciniti et al, there were 15 patients with scores of 2.5 or greater and 8 of these patients required delayed splenectomy. In our series of 18 patients evaluated by CT, no patient with a score below 2.5 required surgery, confirming the suggestion of Resciniti et al that CT scans may be

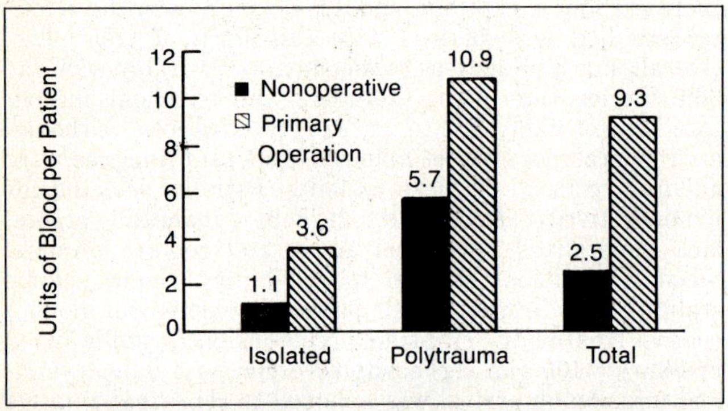

Fig 4.—Blood transfusions. Statistically significantly decreased amount of transfusions in patients treated nonoperatively ($P<.001$). Nonoperative statistics include those with delayed laparotomy.

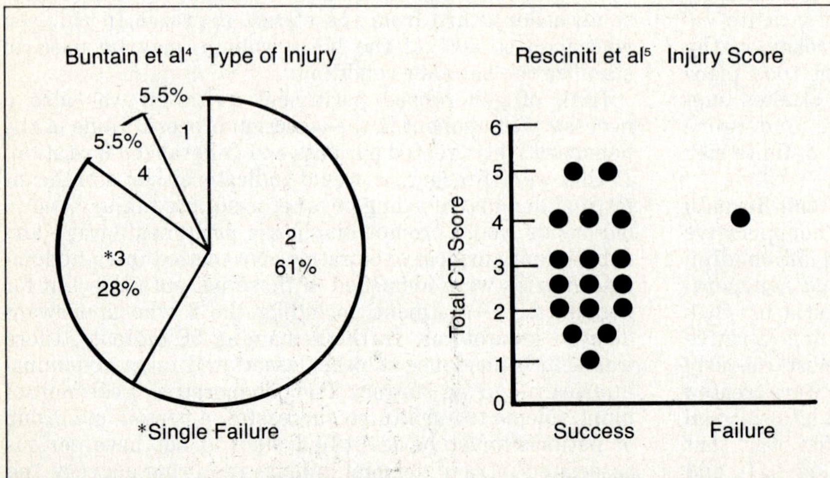

Fig 5.—Computed tomographic (CT) scan data from 18 most recent patients.

Nonoperative Management			
Source, y	**Institution**	**Success Rate**	**% of Success**
Lutzker and Chun,[12] 1981	Albert Einstein, Bronx, NY	9/9	0
Morgenstern and Uyeda,[13] 1983	Cedars Sinai, Los Angeles, Calif	17/17	100
Malangoni et al,[14] 1984	Medical College of Wisconsin, Milwaukee	3/10	30
Bitseff and Adkins,[15] 1984	Vanderbilt University, Nashville, Tenn	9/30	30
Mahon and Sutton,[16] 1985	Dartmouth, Hanover, NH	3/11	27
Tom et al,[17] 1985	William Beaumont, Royal Oak, Mich	17/19	89
Tibi et al,[18] 1985	University of Rochester, Rochester, NY	10/12	83
Oakes and Sherck,[19] 1985	Stanford University, Stanford, Calif	10/17	59
Andersson et al,[20] 1986	University of Lund, Lund, Sweden	13/13	100
Johnson and Shatney,[21] 1986	University of Florida at Jacksonville	8/11	73
Moss and Hopkins,[22] 1987	Christ Community Hospital, Oak Lawn, Ill	5/7	71
Wiebke et al,[23] 1987	Johns Hopkins, Baltimore, Md	7/10	70
Buntain et al,[4] 1988	University of Tennessee, Knoxville	10/10	100
Nallathambi et al,[24] 1988	New York Medical College, Bronx	3/10	30
Resciniti et al,[5] 1988	University of Massachusetts, Worcester	17/27	63
Total Success Rate	...	**141/213**	66
Present series	...	41/47	87

predictive of minimal splenic injuries not requiring surgery. However, 12 of our 18 patients had scores of 2.5 or greater and only 1 of these (score = 4) required delayed surgery. Our successful nonoperative management of grade 2, 3, and 4 injuries, and spleens with scores of greater than 2.5, lead us to conclude that CT scan findings alone need not lead to immediate laparotomy in the more severely injured spleen. It has been our practice to use CT to establish the diagnosis of splenic injury and to base a decision on the need for laparotomy on clinical grounds.

Analysis of our results has confirmed that nonoperative management is a safe and effective alternative to immediate laparotomy. Proper patient selection requires hemodynamic stability, lack of generalized peritoneal irritation, and minimal blood transfusion requirements. The multiple trauma patients carefully selected for nonoperative management have had a statistically higher increase in delayed laparotomy as compared with those with isolated injuries. Therefore, these patients must be followed up closely or undergo immediate operation at the time of initial presentation. Patients who are over the age of 64 years or who have received more than 2 U of blood are also at increased risk of needing a laparotomy. Patients who do not fit the criteria for nonoperative management should undergo an attempted splenic salvage procedure or splenectomy depending on the degree of splenic damage and the severity of associated injuries. This series has demonstrated that nonoperative management in the appropriate clinical setting can result in splenic salvage without the need for an operation. Splenic preservation in the properly selected patient has now become an accepted approach for both pediatric and adult trauma patients.

References

1. Zabinski EJ, Harkins HN. Delayed splenic rupture: a clinical syndrome following trauma. *Arch Surg.* 1943;46:186-213.
2. Upadhyaya P, Simpson JS. Splenic trauma in children. *Surg Gynecol Obstet.* 1968;126:781-790.
3. Greenspan L, McLellan BA, Greig H. Abbreviated injury scale and injury severity score: a scoring chart. *J Trauma.* 1985;25:60-64.
4. Buntain WL, Gould HR, Maull KI. Predictability of splenic salvage by computed tomography. *J Trauma.* 1988;28:24-34.
5. Resciniti A, Fink MP, Raptopoulous V, et al. Nonoperative treatment of adult splenic trauma: development of a computed tomographic scoring system that detects appropriate candidates for expectant management. *J Trauma.* 1988;128:828-831.
6. King H, Shumacker HB. Splenic studies, I: susceptibility to infection after splenectomy performed in infancy. *Ann Surg.* 1952;136:239-242.
7. Singer DB. Postsplenectomy sepsis. In: Rosenberg HS, Bolande RP, eds. *Perspectives in Pediatric Pathology.* Chicago, Ill: Year Book Medical Publishers Inc; 1973;1:285-311.
8. Malangoni MA, Dillon LD, Klamer TW, et al. Factors influencing the risk of early and late serious infection in adults after splenectomy for trauma. *Surgery.* 1984;96:775-782.
9. Chaikof EL, McCabe CJ. Fatal overwhelming postsplenectomy infection. *Am J Surg.* 1985;149:534-539.
10. Zarrabi MH, Rosner F. Serious infections in adults following splenectomy for trauma. *Arch Intern Med.* 1984;144:1421-1424.
11. Wesson DE, Filler RM, Shandlng B, et al. Ruptured spleen: when to operate? *J Pediatr Surg.* 1981;16:324-326.
12. Lutzker LG, Chun KJ. Radionuclide imaging in the nonsurgical treatment of liver and spleen trauma. *J Trauma.* 1981;21:382-387.
13. Morgenstern L, Uyeda RY. Nonoperative management of injuries of the spleen in adults. *Surg Gynecol Obstet.* 1983;157:513-518.
14. Malangoni MA, Levine AW, Droege EA, et al. Management of injury to the spleen in adults. *Ann Surg.* 1984;200:702-705.
15. Bitseff EL, Adkins RB. Splenic trauma: a trial at selective management. *South Med J.* 1984;77:1286-1290.
16. Mahon PA, Sutton JE. Nonoperative management of adult splenic injury due to blunt trauma: a warning. *Am J Surg.* 1985;149:716-721.
17. Tom WW, Howells GA, Bree RL, et al. A nonoperative approach to the adult ruptured spleen sustained from blunt trauma. *Am Surg.* 1985;5:367-371.
18. Tibi P, Ouriel K, Schwartz SI. Splenic injury in the adult: splenectomy, splenorrhaphy, or nonoperative management. *Contemp Surg.* 1985;26:73-76.
19. Oakes DD, Sherck JP. Successful expectant management of splenic injury in adults. *J Trauma.* 1985;25:706.
20. Andersson R, Alwmark A, Gullstrand P, et al. Nonoperative treatment of blunt trauma to liver and spleen. *Acta Chir Scand.* 1986;152:739-741.
21. Johnson H, Shatney CH. Splenic injuries in adults: selective nonoperative management. *South Med J* 1986;79:5-8.
22. Moss JF, Hopkins WM. Nonoperative management of blunt splenic trauma in the adult: a community hospital's experience. *J Trauma.* 1987;27:315-318.
23. Wiebke EA, Sarr MG, Fishman EK, Ratych RE. Nonoperative management of splenic injuries in adults: an alternative in selected patients. *Am Surg.* 1987;53:547-552.
24. Nallathambi MN, Ivatury RR, Wapnir I, et al. Nonoperative management versus early operation for blunt splenic trauma in adults. *Surg Gynecol Obstet.* 1988;166:252-258.
25. Mucha P, Daly RC, Farnell MB. Selective management of blunt splenic trauma. *J Trauma.* 1986;26:970-979.

Discussion

Eugene W. Grabowski, MD, Bennington, Vt: Donald Trunkey recently stated that this nonoperative management of splenic injury in adults required further evaluation in academic centers before it could be applied in a community hospital setting. In fact, 10 years ago, Gerry Strauch, MD, now trauma director at the American College of Surgeons and a member of this group, presented a report on methods of splenic preservation in nine patients and decried the premeditated nonoperative management of splenic trauma in the adult as being too dangerous. Two of the patients in Dr Strauch's report were treated nonoperatively, but only because of delayed recognition in very stable patients. The authors have indicated from their choice of discussant and from the details of their fine clinical study, that nonoperative splenic conservation in the adult may be ready for the common man.

If the community surgeon plans to observe and not operate on adults with ruptured spleens, several important caveats must be observed, however. If the physician is not in the hospital with that patient, as perhaps he should be during the first 24 to 48 hours, he must live around the corner from the hospital, just a few minutes away. He is not an academic trauma surgeon in the suburbs far from a city hospital. His monitoring personnel must be experienced and dedicated trauma or critical care nurses with the same degree of sophistication as more senior surgical residents, not junior or first-year residents in July or August of their initial year. Finally, he must have a ready, quality CT scanner, blood bank, and operating room on call at all times.

I am again pleased to see that the authors show us in this report that sound clinical judgment is sufficient to determine the need for surgery once the CT scan has established the diagnosis of injury. The CT grading system can remain, then, as a useful tool in the academic study of such patients. Such a grading system might be helpful in deciphering a special or specific type of splenic injury that might alert us to a higher probability of that rare, yet late, splenic hemorrhage that we all still rightly fear. Many of our patients in Bennington, Vt, with splenic injury are the self-proclaimed indestructible, stunt-skiing, young studs who want to know when they can tempt fate again with that next back scratcher or helicopter. Many simply want to know when it would be safe to travel to remote areas or engage in less risky, but still vigorous, physical activity. Many want to know if they should wear a Medical Alert bracelet. I hope the authors plan to extend their excellent study and help us answer these questions. We should have the wisdom to see that just as careful, long-term, large-volume statistical analyses reveal the rare cases of postsplenectomy sepsis and profoundly influence our management of splenic injury, so might similar long-term, large-volume statistical studies uncover the equally rare, but equally lethal, delayed splenic hemorrhage that we all still must studiously avoid. I propose this as a top-priority item on a clinical study agenda.

I have two questions of Dr Elmore. Has the CT scan completely replaced the liver-spleen scan in your institution for noninvasive evaluation of splenic injury? I note that all of your patients and six of the seven patients in Milwaukee, Wis, who failed nonoperative observation required splenectomy. How many of your patients required splenectomy because of late laparotomy and higher blood loss, making visualization more difficult and time for splenorrhaphy less available? In other words, is there any benefit to getting in there early to achieve early hemostasis and save more spleens? Some authors point out that the process of spleen localization at surgery causes more damage and hence results in more spleens being removed. What are your conclusions on this?

Charles P. Shoemaker, Jr, MD, Newport, RI: Two questions. One has to do with the subset of the polytrauma patient. I am unclear as to whether you did a peritoneal lavage in all those patients. If so, what was your cutoff? If the results of the tap were abnormal, did you go ahead? Or was there a group of patients with polytrauma who did not get tapped and whom you followed up?

This question is sort of a follow-up to Dr Grabowski's question. What do you tell the patient? How many days in the hospital are you going to watch these people? The ones I have seen have become pain free in a couple of days and begin to eat, but when can you really feel comfortable about sending them home? Another question: if they are skiers or football players, when do you tell them that they can go back to full activity?

Christopher C. Baker, New Haven, Conn: There is not as much difference between academic and community surgeons who take care of critically injured patients as one might think, just the resources and the amount of time that one has at the bedside. I enjoyed Dr Elmore's article and I would compliment him and his colleagues on their results.

We have had similar experiences at Yale (New Haven, Conn), and I would agree with almost everything the authors have said. There are a couple of questions that I would like to raise. First of all, in the delayed operation (you have one patient in the isolated group who had delayed operation), did the need for surgery occur in the hospital or after hospital discharge? Have you had any patients who have subsequently had ruptures requiring operation after hospital discharge? We had one patient who had a rupture during toileting 2 weeks after hospital discharge and it was only an astute resident who remembered the patient when he called about this and who then told him to get to the nearest hospital in a hurry that saved his life. It is rare, but I think it does happen.

The other question I had was related to missed injuries. Robert Buckman, MD, last year at the American Association of Surgery of Trauma meeting presented a report from Baltimore, Md, on his group's series of noninvasive diagnostic imaging in trauma patients. Dr Buckman found that patients who underwent operation had a 5% incidence of occult injury, such as diaphragmatic rupture and retroperitoneal injuries, that might be missed by peritoneal lavage. You mention that you did not have any missed injuries, but I wonder if you have seen any missed injuries subsequently? I think diaphragmatic injuries are a risk in these patients and that this is something we have to remember.

Frederick W. Ackroyd, MD, Boston, Mass: How do you deal with the multitrauma patient who is going to the operating room for a lengthy head or orthopedic surgical exploration whom you suspect may have an injury to the spleen?

Dr Elmore: I would like to thank Dr Grabowski for his comments. We would agree that it is now time for this technique to be used more widely in the community but only in selected patients with isolated injuries. We would not recommend this for higher-risk patients in smaller hospitals.

We included CT scoring for academic purposes. We wanted other investigators to be able to compare their results with ours. We also document with CT scores that these were not trivial splenic injuries but that there were significant injuries to the spleens.

Computed tomographic scanning has replaced liver-spleen scans at our institution for the stable trauma patient. There are many articles that support liver-spleen scans in making the diagnosis of a splenic injury; however, CT scanning can provide more information about other structures and injuries. In answer to Dr Shoemaker, peritoneal lavage is now used in those patients who are hemodynamically unstable or do not fit the other criteria for nonoperative management.

The late splenectomy in the six patients was carried out due to significant splenic injury and adjacent hematoma. We believe that a nonoperative approach saves more spleens than by operating on these patients early and this is confirmed by our high splenic salvage rate of 78% in the isolated injury group and an overall salvage rate of 48% in all patients.

Dr Baker asked about the possibility of a delayed rupture in those treated nonoperatively. None of our patients has had a delayed rupture. It is a potential problem and patients must be instructed to limit their activity after discharge from the hospital.

The possibility of a missed intra-abdominal injury is something that makes us select these patients very carefully. As we observe these patients with nonoperative management, we look for signs of peritonitis or unexplained fevers, at which point we would perform a diagnostic peritoneal tap to rule out a hollow viscus injury. A diaphragmatic injury in any blunt trauma patient is difficult to diagnose and continues to be a problem.

Dr Ackroyd asked about multitrauma patients. The vast majority of patients multiply injured did not fit the criteria for nonoperative management. If a patient were undergoing a long orthopedic or neurosurgical procedure, the splenic injury would be treated operatively. Only a select group of multitrauma patients is treated nonoperatively, and they are followed up very closely.

Progress in Experimental Porcine Small-Bowel Transplantation

Hironori Kaneko, MD; Wayne Hancock, MD, PhD; Robert T. Schweizer, MD

• Studies in large animals are needed to overcome technical complications, allograft rejection, and graft-vs-host disease, which are major problems that prevent clinical application of small-bowel transplantation. The small bowel was allografted heterotopically or orthotopically into 30 pigs with the use of cyclosporine, prednisone, and azathioprine. When cyclosporine was given orally to heterotopically transplantation recipients, rejection was frequent, and graft-vs-host disease caused one death. After 30 days of intravenous cyclosporine followed by oral administration, no rejection occurred. Graft-vs-host disease was mild or absent, and there were some long-term survivors. Technical failures were relatively infrequent, but death from sepsis, eg, intra-abdominal abscess, occurred in 17% (5/30). Anastomoses of donor superior mesenteric vein to recipient portal vein offered no advantages over systemic venous drainage. Although the high cyclosporine levels used would be intolerable in humans, these results indicate that successful small-bowel transplantation can be achieved with adequate immunosuppression in a large animal.

(*Arch Surg.* 1989;124:587-592)

The small bowel remains one of the last clinically important organs that has not yet been transplanted with long-term success. In addition to technical difficulties and the allograft rejection process, the large number of immunocompetent lymphocytes in Peyer's patches and mesenteric lymph nodes can induce graft-vs-host disease (GVHD). Attempts at allotransplantation of the small intestine without immunosuppression invariably have resulted in rejection and the death of the recipient. Prevention of rejection with azathioprine and prednisone proved to be difficult before the cyclosporine era, although survival was occasionally prolonged.[1-3] The effective immunosuppressive activity of cyclosporine in kidney, heart, and liver transplantation has rekindled interest in small-bowel transplantation. Recent studies have shown that cyclosporine can inhibit rejection episodes of small-bowel transplants.[4-6] However, despite improved results, irreversible rejection remains the major obstacle, with GVHD apparently contributing to mortality. More consistent and greater prolongation of survival in a large animal model is needed.

We began using cyclosporine and prednisone, along with azathioprine, in our heart and cadaver kidney transplant recipients in 1984 and demonstrated that this triple-drug regimen remarkably improved graft survival.[7] Therefore, we evaluated the effects of cyclosporine, plus prednisone and azathioprine, on the survival of heterotopic and orthotopic small-bowel transplants in pigs.

Accepted for publication December 9, 1988.

From the Surgical Research Laboratory (Drs Kaneko, Hancock, and Schweizer) and Transplantation Service (Drs Kaneko, Hancock, and Schweizer), Department of Surgery, Hartford (Conn) Hospital, and the University of Connecticut School of Medicine (Drs Hancock and Schweizer), Farmington.

Read before the 69th Annual Meeting of the New England Surgical Society, Montreal, Canada, September 16, 1988.

Reprint requests to Transplantation Service, Department of Surgery, Hartford Hospital, Hartford, CT 06115 (Dr Kaneko).

MATERIALS AND METHODS

Nonlittermate female Yorkshire pigs that weighed 15 to 20 kg were used. General endotracheal anesthesia was administered with the use of halothane and air inhalation. Donor small bowel from the proximal jejunum to the terminal ileum (80% to 90% of the small intestine) was removed on a vascular pedicle that consisted of the superior mesenteric artery and portal vein. The small bowel was cooled in situ by perfusion through the superior mesenteric artery with 2000 mL of Ringer's solution at 4°C. The first three small-bowel transplants used Euro-Collins solution for this cooling. The small-bowel lumen was washed with 5% neomycin sulfate solution and stored at 4°C for 1 to 2 hours, while the recipient was prepared.

The small-bowel allografts were revascularized by an end-to-end anastomosis between the donor superior mesenteric artery and the recipient iliac artery, or by an end-to-side anastomosis between the donor superior mesenteric vein and recipient inferior vena cava, or end to end between the donor superior mesenteric vein and recipient superior mesenteric vein, with the use of 7-0 polypropylene suture. Mannitol (6.25 g) and methylprednisolone sodium succinate (40 mg) were given intravenously (IV) before reperfusion. Heterotopic transplants had cutaneous stomas at both ends (Thiry-Vella loops), which permitted intestinal mucosal biopsies to be done. In orthotopic transplants, a small segment of the bowel with an intact mesentery and a cutaneous stoma was placed subcutaneously.

Prednisone (40 mg/d) and azathioprine (50 mg/d) were given from the first postoperative day. All recipients received 1000 mL of Ringer's or 5% dextrose and water solution with 20 mEq of potassium chloride, 150 mg of cimetidine hydrochloride, 1 g of cephalothin sodium, and 20 mg of gentamicin sulfate daily, until a standard pig chow diet was begun on the third to sixth postoperative day.

Experimental groups are summarized in Table 1. Group 1 (n=6) recipients received heterotopic small-bowel transplants, with the host's native bowel being left in place at the transplant procedure. All recipients in group 1 received oral cyclosporine (15 mg/kg or 30 mg/kg) from postoperative day 2. Group 2 (n=3) recipients received heterotopic small-bowel transplants and the same immunosuppressive regimen as group 1. In addition, donor mesenteric lymph nodes were removed. Group 3 (n=3) recipients received heterotopic small-bowel transplants, and cyclosporine was administered IV (15 mg/kg) for 30 days, followed by oral cyclosporine (30 mg/kg). In group 4 (n=7), the recipient's jejunum and ileum were resected at the time of the transplantation, leaving 5 to 10 cm at each end for anastomosis. All recipients received continuous IV cyclosporine (15 mg/kg) and prednisone and azathioprine, as in group 3. In group 5 (n=3), orthotopic small-bowel transplantation was performed as in group 4, but the anastomosis of the donor superior mesenteric vein was to the recipient's superior mesenteric vein. The immunosuppression was the same as in group 3.

The animal's general condition, weight, output and consistency of the stool, and appearance of the mucosa of the intestinal stoma were observed. Hematologic and serum chemistry findings, vitamin B_{12} levels, and whole blood radioimmunoassay results for cyclosporine were monitored. Sequential biopsy specimens were taken from the stoma by biopsy forceps, and autopsies were performed on all animals. Group 3 animals were killed on postoperative day 60 if they were still alive. All animals that had technical failure of the transplant within 7 days of surgery were excluded from the tabulation of data. Statistical analysis of data was made using the Student's t test.

Table 1.—Experimental Groups*

	Group 1	Group 2	Group 3	Group 4	Group 5
Cyclosporine	Oral, 15 mg/kg (n=3) and 30 mg/kg (n=3)	Oral, 30 mg/kg	IV, 15 mg/kg for 30 d; oral, 30 mg/kg	IV, 15 mg/kg for 30 d; oral, 30 mg/kg	IV, 15 mg/kg for 30 d; oral, 30 mg/kg
Transplants	Heterotopic	Heterotopic with removal of donor mesenteric lymph nodes	Heterotopic	Orthotopic	Orthotopic
Venous drainage	IVC	IVC	IVC	IVC	SMV

*IV indicates intravenous; IVC, inferior vena cava; SMV, superior mesenteric vein.

Table 2.—Postoperative Survival and Cause of Death

Group 1 (n=6)		Group 2 (n=3)		Group 3 (n=3)		Group 4 (n=7)		Group 5 (n=3)	
Survival, d	Cause of Death	Survival, d	Cause of Death	Survival, d	Cause of Death	Survival, d	Cause of Death	Survival, d	Cause of Death
10*	Rejection	9	Rejection	48	Sepsis	21	Sepsis	18	Intra-abdominal abscess
	Rejection	22	Rejection	60	Killed	...	...		
15*	Rejection	53	Rejection	60	Killed	39	Sepsis	23	Intussusception
22*	Rejection	...	...	...	...	45	Obstruction	42	Sepsis
27	GVHD†	...	...	...	...	50	Perforated small bowel at autopsy	...	Obstruction
38	Rejection	...	...	...	...	60	Unknown	...	...
						100	Alive and well	...	...
						260	Alive and well	...	...

*Oral cyclosporine, 15 mg/kg.
†GVHD indicates graft-vs-host disease.

RESULTS

In the heterotopic small-bowel transplantations, all pigs in groups 1 and 2 that received oral cyclosporine died primarily of rejection within 60 days. In contrast, animals in group 3 that received IV cyclosporine for 30 days had no rejection episodes detected. One animal died of pneumonia on postoperative day 48, and two animals were surviving well when they were killed at postoperative day 60. In pigs that received orthotopic small-bowel transplants, ie, groups 4 and 5, all pigs received IV cyclosporine induction, and there were no episodes of rejection detected. Also, no clinical evidence of GVHD was seen. Deaths were usually due to sepsis or intestinal obstruction (Table 2).

The technical failure rate within postoperative day 7 was 20% (3/15) in heterotopic transplantation groups 1, 2, and 3 (Table 3). Three pigs in group 1 died intraoperatively at the time of reperfusion of the graft. These deaths appeared to be due to hyperkalemia from the Euro-Collins solution, despite flushing of the graft immediately before revascularization with Ringer's solution. Serum potassium ion levels in two of these pigs at the time of death were greater than 7.0 mmol/L. In orthotopic transplantation, the technical failure rate was 22% (2/9) in group 4, and 50% (3/6) in group 5 for an average technical failure of 36% (5/14).

Hematologic and serum chemistry study values for survivors in all groups at 2 to 5 weeks after transplantation were not significantly different. All animals were slightly anemic and had a leukocytosis and slight hypoalbuminemia. Serum creatinine levels were within normal ranges in all animals. Liver enzyme levels were normal in most animals. Serum ammonia and triglyceride levels in animals with venous drainage into the systemic circulation (group 4) were not significantly different when compared with those drained into the portal system (group 5). Vitamin B_{12} levels in groups 4 and 5 were slightly decreased at 1 week but equaled or exceeded preoperative levels thereafter (Fig 1).

Table 3.—Technical Complication Within Postoperative Day 7

	n	% of Total
Heterotopic transplantation	3/15	20
Anesthesia? (hyperkalemia?)	3	
Orthotopic transplantation	5/15	33
Group 4		
Arterial thrombosis	1	22
Gastric volvulus	1	
Group 5		
Anesthesia?	2	50
Arterial thrombosis	1	...

Cyclosporine levels are shown in Fig 2. Pigs with no rejection episodes had high cyclosporine levels. In contrast, cyclosporine levels of pigs with rejection were low. Pigs without rejection resumed normal growth after 4 postoperative weeks, and the stools in those pigs were normal in appearance and consistency.

Histologic examination of biopsy specimens revealed rejection activity at generally the same intensity as that found with the more complete histologic studies of the intestine (Fig 3). The findings in the biopsy specimens taken from the subcutaneous segments in groups 4 and 5

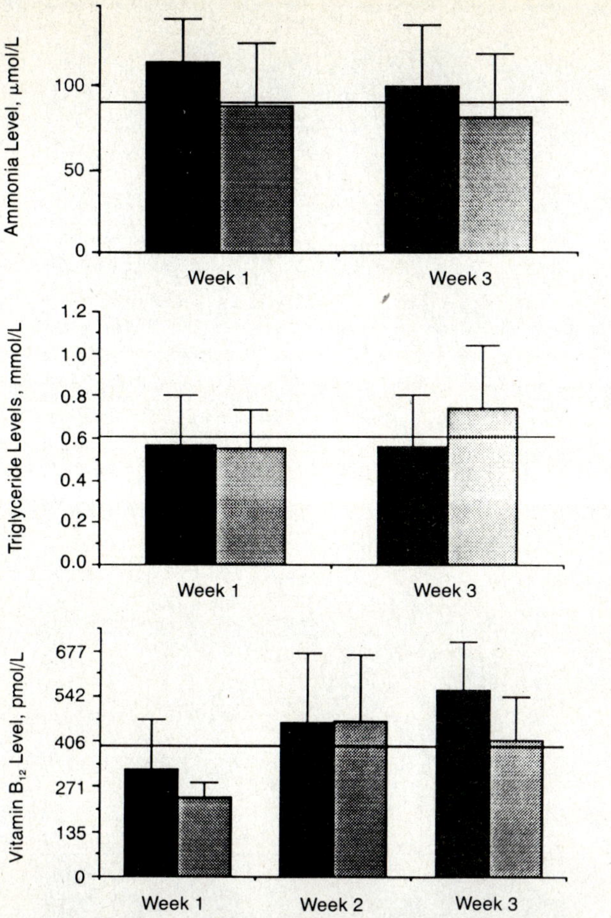

Fig 1.—Ammonia, triglyceride, and vitamin B_{12} levels in group 4 and 5 animals. There was no significant difference between those animals with portal venous drainage into systemic circulation (group 4, closed bars) and those drained into portal system (group 5, shaded bars).

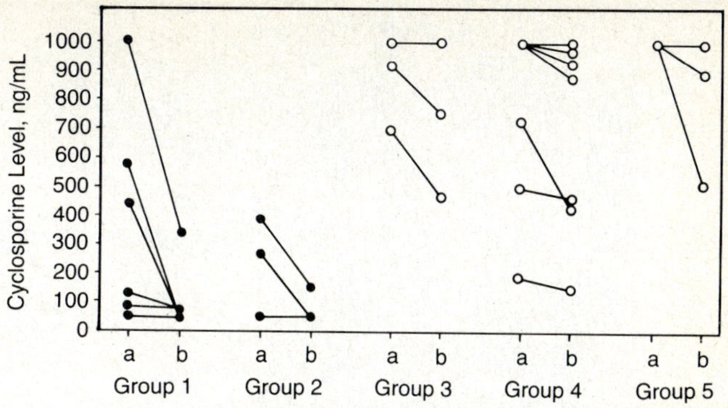

Fig 2.—Cyclosporine levels 8 hours after dose of oral or intravenous cyclosporine. a indicates highest levels for individual animal; b, levels before rejection, death, or most current level. Most pigs with no rejection episodes were maintained at high cyclosporine levels (>400 ng/mL). In contrast, cyclosporine levels of most pigs with rejection fell considerably.

revealed no rejection activity. In only one animal in group 1 were the findings of GVHD severe enough to have contributed to death. In three other animals, one in group 4 and two in group 5, some evidence of GVHD was found (Fig 4). This was manifested by plasma cell and immunoblast infiltrates in recipient lymph nodes, native intestine, and, occasionally, spleen or liver. However, these findings of GVHD were focal and limited, eg, not occurring in all organs, and, thus, did not appear to have been involved with the cause of death in those animals.

COMMENT

Although several groups have shown that treatment with oral cyclosporine prevents small-bowel allograft rejection, both in orthotopic and heterotopic transplants,[4-6,8,9] its benefit has been less consistent in comparison with kidney, liver, and heart transplantation. It has been demonstrated that oral cyclosporine is absorbed through the small bowel via lymphatic vessels.[10] Fat absorption is severely disturbed in small-bowel transplantation because of total lymphatic disruption. In a report by Ricour et al,[11] it was not until 2 to 8 weeks after transplantation that intestinal lipid absorption became normal. This was probably concomitant with resumption of lymphatic function.[12] Thus, cyclosporine must be administered IV during the malabsorption period of implanted small bowel when the recipient has no functional small bowel.

Intravenous cyclosporine has been used for small-bowel transplantation in pigs.[5,11] The recent report by Grant et al[13] studied different doses of IV cyclosporine in small intestinal allografts. In our studies, IV cyclosporine appeared to be the most important factor in the prevention of small-bowel allograft rejection. Although, in one study, prednisone was added to cyclosporine to control allograft rejection better, no increase in recipient survival occurred.[5] To our knowledge, our use of the triple immunosuppressive regimen, cyclosporine, azathioprine, and prednisone, has not been previously reported in experimental studies of small-bowel transplantation. The results demonstrated that despite the use of azathioprine and prednisone, the initial IV administration of cyclosporine was most important in preventing rejection activity (groups 3, 4, and 5). The combined use of IV cyclosporine administration for 4 weeks with prednisone and azathioprine, followed by oral cyclosporine to maintain high cyclosporine levels, consistently prevented small-bowel allograft rejection in our studies.

Technical failures and sepsis are also frequent and serious problems in small-bowel transplantation. The technical complication rate in large animals was 50% to 60% in two reports,[14,15] with vessel thrombosis occurring frequently. Although the technical complication rate of heterotopic and orthotopic small-bowel transplantation in our experiments was less, it still remained a problem. However, only 2 of our 30 transplants had vessel thrombosis.

Although there is little information about flush preservation solutions for small-bowel transplantation, three pigs early in our experiment probably suffered intraoperative cardiac arrests from hyperkalemia due to Euro-Collins solution despite a Ringer's solution flush.

A high infection rate also occurred, despite antibiotic therapy and intraluminal irrigation with neomycin. Raju et al[16] suggested that pretreatment of the donor with antibiotics, as well as extensive intraluminal irrigation of the small bowel, are important measures. Lower doses of prednisone, or a delayed use, might also help prevent intra-abdominal abscess formation.

There has been concern whether the venous drainage from small-bowel allografts would be better into the portal system than into the systemic circulation. For example, it has been shown that serum ammonia levels were significantly elevated with a portacaval anastomosis with modest prolongation of graft survival in rats.[17] Our results did not

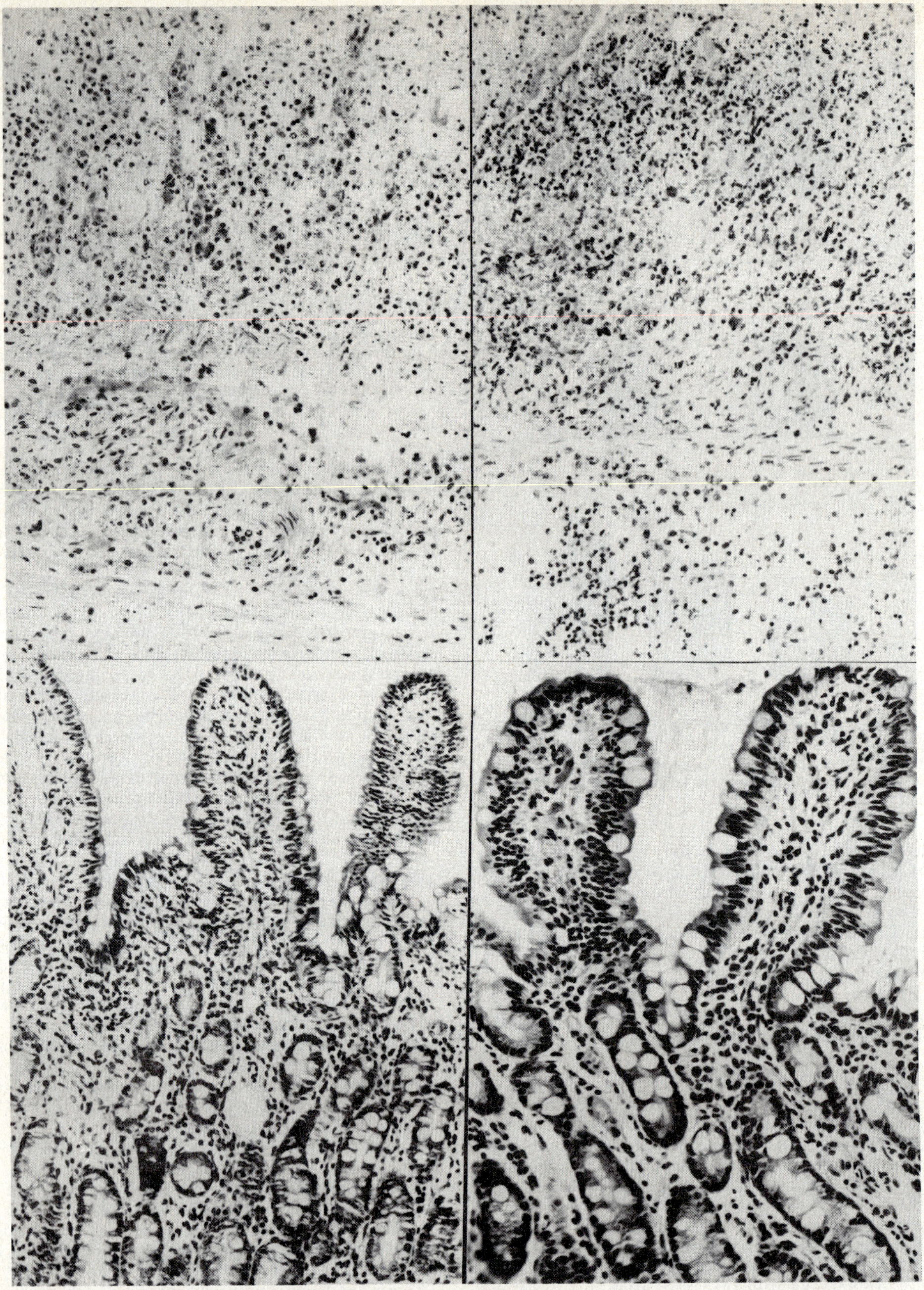

Fig 3.—Utility of stomal biopsy specimens in monitoring small-bowel graft survival is shown by comparison of stomal biopsy specimens and intra-abdominal small-bowel tissues collected post mortem at 30 days after transplantation. Both stomal (top left) and postmortem (top right) specimens from group 1 pig that received oral cyclosporine show full-thickness necrosis, with sloughing of mucosa as result of acute rejection. Beneficial effects of intravenous cyclosporine treatment are seen in normal appearance of stomal (bottom left) and postmortem (bottom right) tissues collected when a group 4 pig was killed (paraffin sections, hematoxylin-eosin, all magnifications ×250).

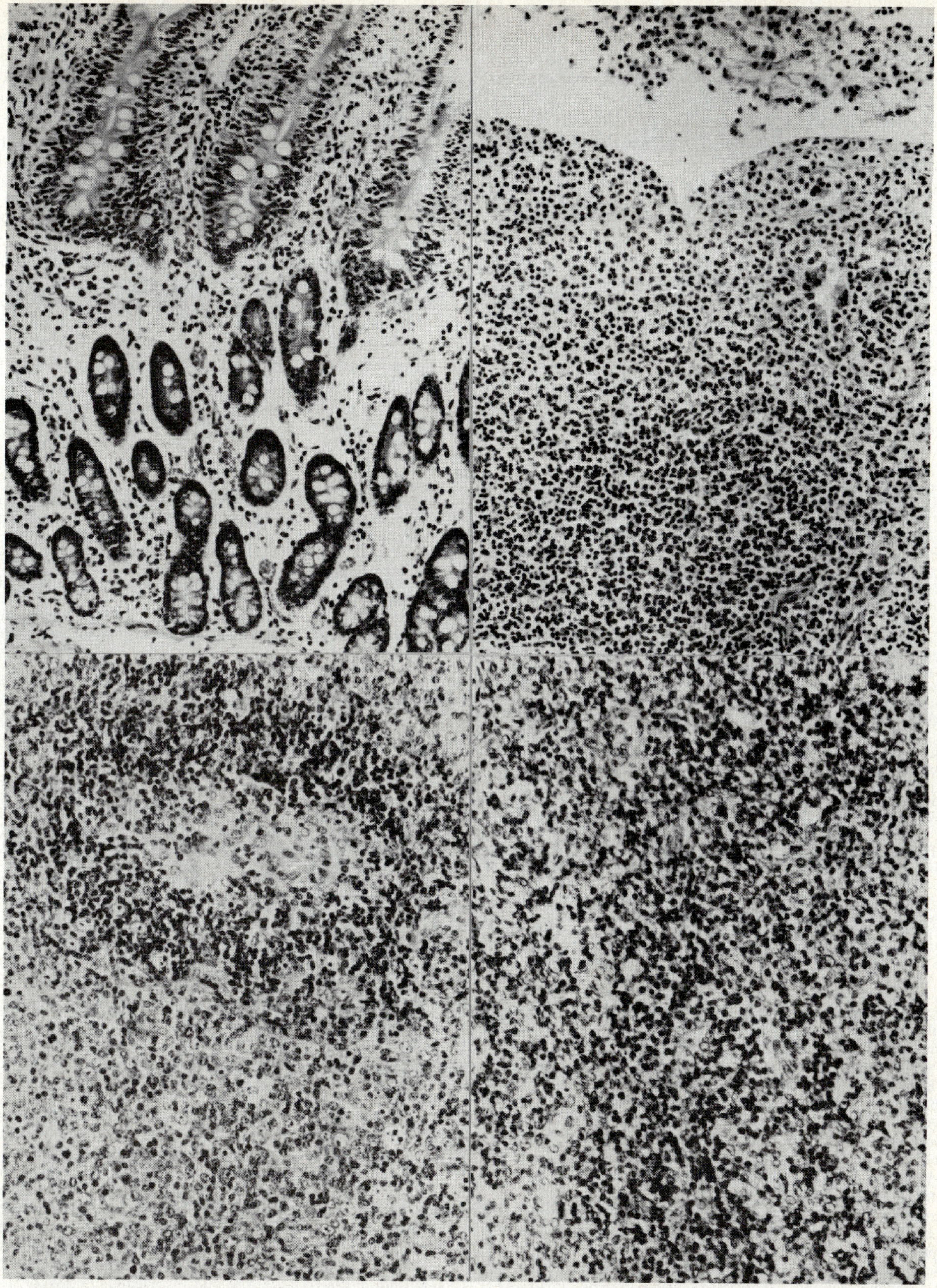

Fig 4.—Histologic evidence of graft-vs-host disease in group 4 pig is shown in these photomicrographs. Top left, Donor-transplanted small bowel has normal appearance, in contrast with necrotic recipient small bowel (top right), which is grossly infiltrated by plasma cells. Bottom left, Examination of *donor* lymph node shows preservation of lymphoid architecture; note follicle in upper half of this field. Bottom right, By contrast, this *recipient* lymph node shows destruction of normal architecture and extensive infiltration by plasma cells and pyroninophilic immunoblasts (paraffin sections, hematoxylin-eosin, all magnifications ×250).

show any advantage in graft survival or ammonia levels with a portaportal anastomosis. It was also technically more difficult, and we encountered considerable intraoperative acid-base imbalance. However, additional studies are needed to clarify this point. In human small-bowel transplantation, venous drainage should probably be directed into the systemic circulation because it is technically easier and safer.

Although gross inspection of the small-bowel segment was unreliable, histologic study of the isolated small-bowel segment was useful in monitoring intra-abdominal small-bowel rejection activity. Several investigators[4,18] have cautioned against biopsies as an index of rejection activity because histologic alterations that were seen during rejection were sometimes variable in both distribution and intensity. It is therefore suggested that random biopsies should be supplemented by serial functional tests, such as D-xylose, glucose tagged with carbon 14, and lauric acid absorption. Other and perhaps more specific tests may serve as markers of rejection, eg, monocyte procoagulant activity[19] or *N*-acetyl hexosaminidase.[20]

Graft-vs-host disease is another major concern in small-bowel transplantation. Kirkman[21] suggested that the development of severe GVHD in large animals following small-bowel transplantation may not occur, and that allograft rejection rather than GVHD plays the major role in graft loss. We observed GVHD histologically in our study, but this was not a serious systemic problem in animals that received IV cyclosporine induction. These results indicate that GVHD might not be a clinically important problem in intestinal transplantation, but further study is needed.

Intravenous cyclosporine induction resulted in high serum cyclosporine levels, and it permitted normal growth and longer survival by preventing allograft rejection and serious GVHD. While these findings are encouraging for small-bowel transplantation in humans, very high-dose IV cyclosporine was needed. Such doses cannot be used in humans because of toxic side effects. However, these studies demonstrate a successful model of small-bowel transplantation in a large animal that may allow development of more clinically relevant immunosuppressive protocols.

References

1. Alican F, Hardy JD, Caryiri M, et al. Intestinal transplantation: laboratory experience and report of a clinical case. *Am J Surg.* 1971;121:150-159.
2. Ruiz JO, Vchida H, Schultz LS, Lillehei RC. Problems in absorption and immunosuppression after internal allotransplantation. *Am J Surg.* 1972;123:297-303.
3. Hardy MA, Quint J, State D. Effect of antilymphocyte serum and other immunosuppressive agents on canine jejunal allografts. *Ann Surg.* 1970;171:51-60.
4. Craddock GN, Nordgrem SR, Reznick RK, et al. Small bowel transplantation in the dog using cyclosporine. *Transplantation.* 1983;35:284-288.
5. Raju S, Didlake RH, Cayiri M, Turner MD, Grogan JB, Achord J. Experimental small bowel transplantation utilizing cyclosporine. *Transplantation.* 1984;38:561-566.
6. Kirkman RL, Madara JL, Lear PA, Ythier A. The utility of cyclosporine in small bowel transplantation. *Transplant Proc.* 1985;17:1401-1402.
7. Schweizer RT, Rovelli M, Roper L, Bartus S. A flexible immunosuppression protocol for organ transplantation using cyclosporine, azathioprine and prednisone. *Transplant Proc.* 1987;19:1944-1946.
8. Diliz-Perez HS, McClure J, Bedetti C, et al. Successful small bowel allotransplantation in dogs with cyclosporine and prednisone. *Transplantation.* 1984;37:126-129.
9. Hatcher PA, Deaton DH, Bollinger RR. Transplantation of the entire small bowel in inbred rats using cyclosporine. *Transplantation.* 1987;43:478-484.
10. Wassef R, Cohen Z, Nordgreen S, Langer B. Cyclosporine absorption in intestinal transplantation. *Transplantation.* 1985;39:496-499.
11. Ricour C, Revillon Y, Arnaud-Battandier D, et al. Successful small bowel allografts in piglets using cyclosporine. *Transplant Proc.* 1983;15: 3019-3026.
12. Chomette G, Cerf M, Hay JM, et al. Experimental autotransplantation of the small intestine in the pig: histologic, enzymatic and ultrastructural studies. *Ann Anat Pathol (Paris).* 1975;20:343-356.
13. Grant D, Duff J, Zhong R, et al. Successful intestinal transplantation in pigs treated with cyclosporine. *Transplantation.* 1988;45:279-284.
14. Pritchard TJ, Kirkman RL. Small bowel transplantation. *World J Surg.* 1985;9:860-867.
15. Roznick RK, Craddock GN, Langer B, Gilas T, Cullen JB. Structure and function of small bowel allografts in the dog. *Can J Surg.* 1982;25:51-55.
16. Raju S, Fujiwara H, Lewin JR, Grogan JB. Twelve-hour and twenty four-hour preservation of small bowel allografts by simple hypothermia. *Transplantation.* 1988;45:290-293.
17. Schrant WH, Abraham VS, Lee KKW. Portal versus caval venous drainage of small bowel allografts: technical and metabolic consequences. *Surgery.* 1986;99:193-198.
18. Rosemurgy AS, Schrant WH. Small bowel allografts: sequence of histologic changes in acute and chronic rejection. *Am J Surg.* 1986;151:470-475.
19. Silverman R, Cohen Z, Levy G, Craig M, Cullen J, Langer B. Immune responses in small intestinal transplantation in the rat: correlation of histopathology and monocyte procoagulant activity. *Surgery.* 1987;102:395-402.
20. Maeda K, Schwartz MZ, Bamberger MH, Daniller A. A possible serum marker for rejection after small intestine transplantation. *Am J Surg.* 1987;153:68-74.
21. Kirkman RL. *Small Bowel Transplantation: Progress in Transplantation.* New York, NY: Churchill Livingstone Inc; 1986;3:175-198.

Discussion

Robert L. Kirkman, MD, Boston, Mass: I thought it might be useful to the members of this society to try to put this study in perspective with the other work that has been done in this field, as it is not widely known.

This is, to my knowledge, the fourth paper that has looked extensively at a pig small-bowel transplantation model, with an equivalent number of such studies using dogs. The results in all of those experiments are quite similar to those reported here, namely, a fairly high technical complication rate, but an occasional long-term survivor. The problem in all of the studies is that the amount of immunosuppression required is, as in this study, much higher than is possible in humans. The cyclosporine doses used here are five times those that would be acceptable in any current clinical transplantation program.

That, however, has not stopped human experimentation in small-bowel transplantations. There were seven human small-bowel transplantations before the availability of cyclosporine; none were successful. Since the availability of cyclosporine, and following these studies in animal models, there have been about 10 human small-bowel transplantations using cyclosporine. Of those, only one graft has survived longer than a few months, and none has provided substantial nutrition; about half of the patients are dead. It seems clear that improvements in immunosuppressive therapy are required before extensive human experimentation.

One question that I would like to ask has to do with the issue of graft-vs-host disease (GVHD). Most large animal models of small-bowel transplantations have not seen this; this is the second study where there is good evidence of GVHD. To see it, one may have to give so much immunosuppression that one may overcome rejection and leave the graft-vs-host response possible. Does Dr Kaneko think that is occurring in this circumstance?

Dr Kaneko: Graft-vs-host disease is another major concern in small-bowel transplantation, and we observed GVHD histologically in 4 of 30 pigs in our study. This was not a serious systemic problem in three pigs in the intravenous cyclosporine induction group, and GVHD did not cause their death. These results indicate that GVHD might not have been a clinically important problem in small-bowel transplantation, and intravenous cyclosporine might have prevented the development of severe GVHD.

As Dr Kirkman has suggested, the development of severe GVHD in large animals following small-bowel transplantation may not occur, and graft rejection rather than GVHD plays the major role in graft loss. However, further study is needed.

Use of the Triplex Scanner in Diagnosis of Deep Venous Thrombosis

Alfred V. Persson, MD; Catherine Jones; Russell Zide; Edward R. Jewell, MD

• **We report our experience with 264 patients who underwent triplex scans for venous occlusive disease over a 10-month period. Venography was obtained in 30 of these patients. Correlation between the two procedures was 100%. The anatomic location of thrombosis and the extent of disease were identical in both studies. The presence of intraluminal clot by angiodynography is detected by looking for changes in the venous color-flow patterns and in the B-mode image. Newer clots have low echogenicity and are seen as large black areas in the gray-scale image. Older clots are more echogenic. The presence of enlarged venous collateral veins as well as absence of color flow and inability to compress the veins confirm the diagnosis of acute deep venous thrombosis. The results of angiodynography alone can be used safely in diagnosing acute deep venous thrombosis in patients. Equally important, treatment can be withheld safely in a patient with normal results.**

(*Arch Surg.* 1989;124:593-596)

Deep venous thrombosis is a common clinical problem. Approximately 10 million cases occur each year, and a pulmonary embolus will develop in as many as 10% of patients with acute deep venous thrombosis.[1,2] This potentially lethal complication is a concern to all clinicians.

Many patients with extensive deep venous thrombosis will have few if any symptoms. Some patients with pain and swelling suggestive of deep venous thrombosis will have other causes of the symptoms. Clinical signs and symptoms are only 50% accurate in the diagnosis of deep venous thrombosis. Although venography using contrast material has long been considered the "gold standard" for the diagnosis of deep venous thrombosis,[3] it is expensive and causes discomfort, and results are often difficult to obtain. These and other problems have led to the development of many noninvasive tests over the last two decades[4,5] that have added greatly to the treatment and the diagnosis of patients suspected of having acute deep venous thrombosis. Although these noninvasive techniques correlate well with venography using contrast material, they do not define the anatomic extent of the disease.[6]

For the last 2 years, we have been using the triplex scanner (Angiodynograph, Quantum Medical Systems, Issaquah, Wash) to aid in the diagnosis of deep venous thrombosis. Our experience from September 1987 through July 1988 is reported herein.

PATIENTS, MATERIALS, AND METHODS

Over a 10-month period, 264 patients suspected of having deep venous thrombosis were studied in the noninvasive vascular laboratory at the Lahey Clinic Medical Center, Burlington, Mass, using angiodynography (the triplex scanner).[7,8] The majority of the patients (236) underwent study of the leg veins (134 normal results, 102 abnormal results), and 28 patients underwent angiodynographic scans of the arm veins (18 normal results, 10 abnormal results).

Accepted for publication December 7, 1988.

From the Section of Peripheral Vascular Surgery, Lahey Clinic Medical Center, Burlington, Mass.

Read before the 69th Annual Meeting of the New England Surgical Society, Montreal, Canada, September 17, 1988.

Reprint requests to Section of Peripheral Vascular Surgery, Lahey Clinic Medical Center, 41 Mall Rd, Burlington, MA 01805 (Dr Persson).

Venography using contrast material was performed in 30 patients. Comparisons were made as to presence or absence of disease and the anatomic location of the abnormality in the venous system. Angiodynographic scans and venograms were interpreted independently and without knowledge of the results of the other study. The angiodynographic scans were performed first in all patients. The venograms were interpreted by a radiologist using criteria reported by Rabinov and Paulin.[9]

The criteria used for making the diagnosis of deep venous thrombosis by angiodynographic scan were absence of spontaneous or augmented color flow in the affected vein (Color Fig 1); incompressibility of the vein with external pressure from a probe; visualization of the thrombus within the lumen of the vein (ie, an increased echogenic area with no color flow) (Color Fig 2); distention of the affected vein; and increased velocity in collateral veins, especially the greater saphenous vein.

Patients were selected for angiodynography based on the results of noninvasive screening tests.[10] Patients with clearly abnormal results on Doppler ultrasonography were referred for angiodynography for confirmation and better identification of the extent of disease. Triplex scans were also used in patients who had equivocal results on continuous-wave Doppler examination. Furthermore, patients with clinical symptoms (ie, severe swelling and pain) and normal results on continuous-wave Doppler examination underwent scanning studies to rule out partial thrombosis. Phlebography and impedance plethysmography are used extensively in our laboratory as well. When the results of either of these tests were equivocal, the patients were examined by angiodynography. All patients suspected of having deep venous thrombosis involving the upper extremities also underwent angiodynography.

SCANNING TECHNIQUE

The veins in the lower extremities are scanned with the patient lying in the reverse Trendelenburg position. The feet are placed approximately 30 cm below the head. The entire venous system is imaged systematically using a 7.5- or 5.0-MHz transducer. Scanning begins with a longitudinal projection at the level of the right common femoral vein below the inguinal ligament (Figure). The vein is identified medial to the artery. The scan proceeds distally and medially, identifying the junction of the saphenous and femoral veins and the origin of the deep femoral vein. Usually, the superficial femoral vein can be followed to its entrance to the adductor canal. The 5.0-MHz probe is usually used to examine the distal thigh, particularly in obese patients. The proximal popliteal vein is examined from the posterior position by placing the probe of the transducer in the popliteal fossa while the patient is in the prone position. The popliteal vein is visualized in its entirety down to the tibiofibular trunk in the calf. In most patients, the tibial veins can be viewed to midcalf. The entire scan is then repeated in a transverse projection, beginning again in the common femoral vein at the inguinal ligament and scanning distally. Visualization of the entire vein in both longitudinal and transverse projections is important to confirm a normal venous system.

The lumen of the vessel is defined in the image by color flow within the gray-scale boundaries (Color Fig 3). The examiner looks for spontaneous as well as augmented flow, obtained by squeezing the calf or the thigh. The distinction and superiority of angiodynography compared with previous methods are apparent in the observation of flow patterns in real time. The size of the lumen of the vein is compared with the corresponding vein in the contralateral leg or with the adjacent artery.

The veins in the upper extremities are scanned using a 7.5-MHz probe, except in very obese patients. The arm is abducted to approximately 90°. Scanning begins in the distal subclavian vein with a longitudinal projection just below the clavicle. The examination proceeds distally, identifying the junction of the cephalic and axillary veins. The examination proceeds along the medial aspect of the arm to the antecubital fossa. As in the legs, the scan is repeated in a transverse projection beginning again at the clavicle and moving distally. In some patients, visualization of the proximal subclavian vein above the clavicle is possible.

RESULTS

During the 10-month period from September 1987 to July 1988, 264 patients were studied because of a clinical suspicion of deep venous thrombosis. Of these patients, 236 underwent angiodynography of the leg and 28 underwent angiodynography of the arm, with 1 patient undergoing study of both arms and legs. Of the patients who underwent study of the lower extremities, 134 had normal results and 102 had abnormal results. Results of bilateral studies were abnormal in 24 patients, for a total of 126 studies of the leg with abnormal results. No distinction was made between chronic and acute deep venous thrombosis. Triplex scans of the arms were performed in 28 patients, of whom 18 had normal results and 10 had abnormal results. One patient had bilateral thrombosis of the subclavian vein, for a total of 11 studies of the arm with abnormal results.

The anatomic locations of the thrombosis for patients who underwent triplex scans of the legs are listed below.

Location	No. of Patients
Proximal superficial femoral	41
Proximal common femoral	26
Distal superficial femoral	18
Distal common femoral	16
Distal popliteal	15
Isolated proximal common femoral	5
Miscellaneous	5

Patients were classified by the upper extent of the occlusion. Most of the patients had occlusions from this point distally to include the popliteal vein. Five patients had thrombosis isolated to the proximal common femoral vein only, with the popliteal and superficial femoral veins free of disease.

The miscellaneous category included five patients with an unusual location for the thrombosis. One patient had thrombosis of the saphenous vein that had extended into the common femoral vein. The rest of the venous system was normal. One patient had a thrombosis of the deep femoral vein with partial extension into the common femoral vein. This patient had normal venous hemodynamics with normal results on impedance plethysmography and continuous-wave Doppler ultrasonography. Two patients had thrombosis of the distal femoral vein between the origin of the deep femoral vein and the origin of the saphenous vein. In addition, these patients had thrombosis of the popliteal vein with a normal vein in between. One patient had a clot in the lower calf only. These clots were confirmed on venography.

Venography was obtained in 30 of the 264 patients. Venography of the leg was performed in 24 patients, of whom 8 had normal results and 16 had abnormal results. Fifteen patients had clots in the popliteal vein and above and 1 patient had a clot in the veins of the calf only. Six patients underwent venography of the arms. One patient had normal results, and 5 had abnormal results. Three of the 5 abnormal studies occurred in patients with a subclavian catheter in place, and 1 occurred in a patient with an effort thrombosis syndrome associated with thoracic outlet syndrome. The fifth patient was receiving long-term hyperalimentation and underwent fibrinolytic therapy. Postfibrinolytic studies indicated partial recanalization of the subclavian vein.

The anatomic locations of the thrombi using venography are listed below.

Location	No. of Patients
Veins of the leg	
Proximal superficial femoral	6
Distal superficial femoral	3
Distal popliteal	3
Proximal common femoral	2
Isolated common femoral	1
Distal tibial	1
Veins of the arm	
Proximal subclavian	4
Distal subclavian	1

Most occlusions seemed to end just proximal to a major collateral branch. One patient had a thrombus in an isolated common femoral vein, and one patient had occlusion of the distal tibial vein only.

A correlation of 100% was revealed when the results of venography and angiodynography were compared. Also, both studies agreed with regard to the anatomic location and extent of the thrombosis.

COMMENT

As a method of diagnosing deep venous thrombosis, duplex ultrasonic imaging of the veins has been used for several years. Correlation, when compared with venography using contrast material, has been good. Investigators[11,12] have reported sensitivities ranging from 89% to 95% and specificities ranging from 97% to 100%.

Angiodynography displays Doppler information in color superimposed within the B-mode image. This image of color flow adds a new dimension to venous sonography because it permits physiologic and anatomic interrogation of the venous system in real time. Normal and abnormal flow patterns can be visualized easily.

The criteria for the diagnosis of deep venous thrombosis using the duplex scanner have been developed over the last few years.[13] When a vein is not compressible and a Doppler signal cannot be obtained, a clot is suspected.[8] The so-called wink sign, a term used to describe a normal vein when it is compressed and quickly released, is absent. The vein appears to be winking, particularly when it is visualized in the transverse projection.

One group of investigators[6] found compressibility to be accurate when used as the sole criterion for a normal venous system. We do not rely on compressibility as the sole criterion for the diagnosis of acute deep venous thrombosis. In approximately 10% of our patients, partially occluding clots would have been missed had we relied on this factor as the sole criterion. Some patients would have been diagnosed as having normal findings, and in others, the extent of the disease would have been underestimated.

Intraluminal venous thrombosis can be diagnosed by ultrasonography based on visualization of a thrombus. A clot in the venous lumen appears as a few echoes and an absence of color flow (Color Fig 4). The presence of intraluminal hyperechogenic areas is associated with chronic deep venous thrombosis. A clear distinction between chronic deep venous thrombosis and acute deep venous thrombosis has not been possible solely on the basis of clot echogenicity. On several occasions, a hypoechogenic thrombus has been found in patients with a history of deep venous thrombosis of longer than 30 days, but patients with a large echolucent (black) clot usually have a history of deep venous thrombosis of less than 1 week's duration.

The presence or absence of a Doppler signal is the third criterion commonly used for the diagnosis of deep venous thrombosis by ultrasonography. The absence of spontaneous or augmented color flow in a vein using angiodynogra-

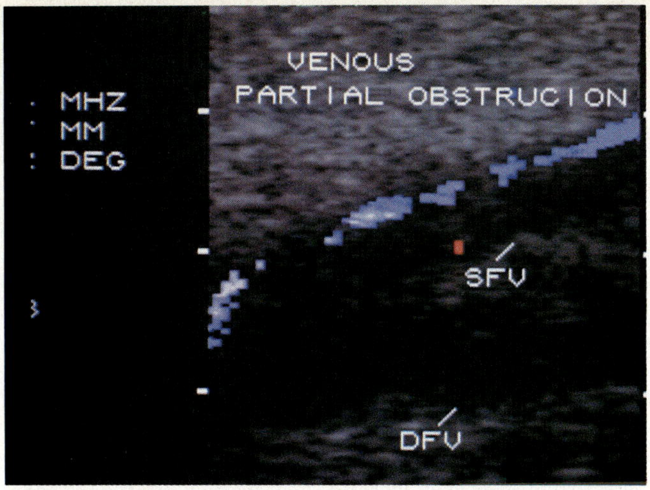

Color Fig 1.—Clot in the superficial femoral vein (SFV) and deep femoral vein (DFV).

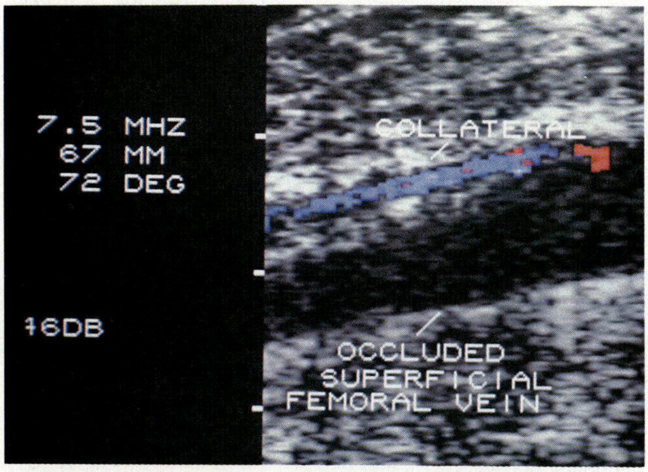

Color Fig 2.—Old clot in the superficial femoral vein.

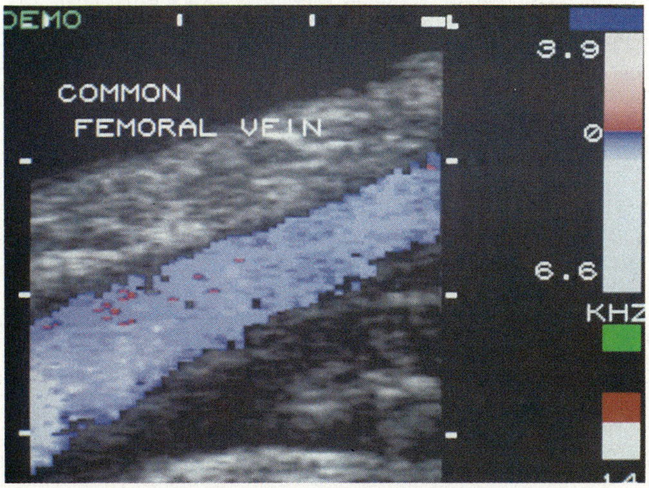

Color Fig 3.—Triplex scan of the common femoral vein.

phy is analogous to the absence of a Doppler signal with the standard duplex examination. However, real-time color analysis is quicker and more convincing, particularly with partial occlusion and in small veins.

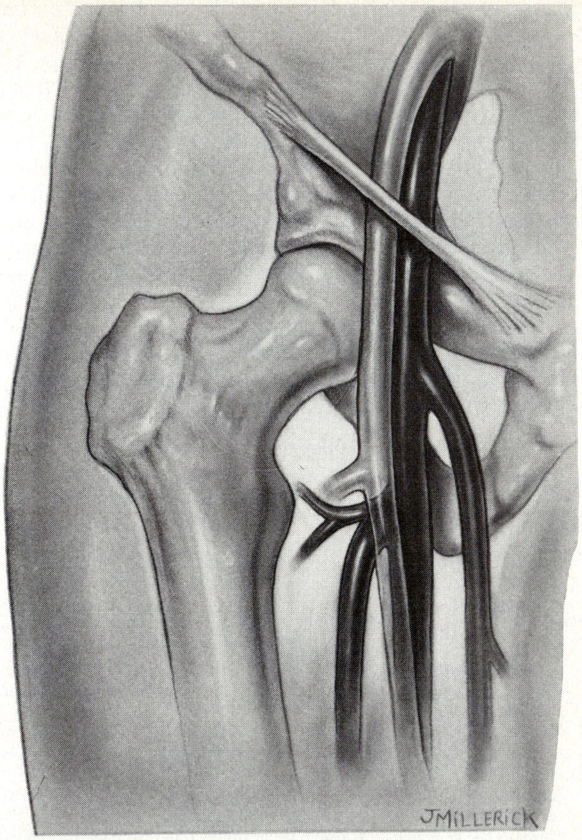

Right inguinal region showing relationship of the femoral artery to the femoral vein (by permission of Lahey Clinic).

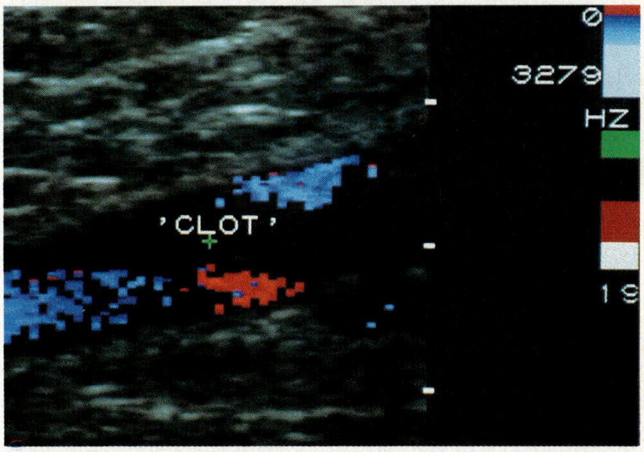

Color Fig 4.—Triplex scan of superficial femoral vein reveals intraluminal clot.

In addition to the established criteria used for the diagnosis of deep venous thrombosis with the duplex scanner, enlargement of the affected vein and increase in collateral flow were added factors. An increase in the diameter of the affected vein and an increase in both the size and flow in collateral veins have been noted in the majority of patients with acute deep venous thrombosis. In many patients, these vessels enlarge to twice the size of the corresponding artery or normal collateral vein. This criterion cannot be used alone because veins with valvular incompetence can be dilated considerably. Increased flow in collateral veins is also common in extremities of patients with cellulitis, in patients who have had recent surgery, and in patients who have experienced recent trauma. Why the vein is larger is uncertain because the clot is thought to start in the calf and proceed upward. On serial examinations, these large veins will become smaller over time.

This prospective study is biased in that patients selected for venography that uses contrast material were patients whose clinical situation was less suggestive of deep venous thrombosis. Despite this, the results of angiodynography and venography were identical in the 30 patients who underwent both studies. No false-positive and no false-negative results were recorded. The anatomic extent of the disease was identical in both procedures. In the remaining 234 patients, treatment was based solely on results obtained with angiodynography.

References

1. Roberts HJ. Controversies and enigmas in thrombophlebitis and pulmonary embolism: perspectives on alleged overdiagnosis. *Angiology.* 1980;31:686-699.

2. Atik M. Venous thromboembolic disease. In: Moore WS, ed. *Vascular Surgery: A Comprehensive Review.* New York, NY: Grune & Stratton; 1983:821-866.

3. Kakkar VV, Corrigan TP. Detection of deep vein thrombosis: survey and current status. In: Sasahara AA, Sonnenblick EH, Lesch M, eds. *Pulmonary Emboli.* New York, NY: Grune & Stratton; 1975:45-55.

4. Cranley JJ, Canos AJ, Sull WJ, et al. Phleborheographic technique for diagnosing deep venous thrombosis of the lower extremities. *Surg Gynecol Obstet.* 1975;141:331-339.

5. Mullick SC, Wheeler HB, Songster GF. Diagnosis of deep venous thrombosis by measurement of electrical impedance. *Am J Surg.* 1970;119:417-422.

6. Appelman PT, De Jong TE, Lampmann LE. Deep venous thrombosis of the leg: US findings. *Radiology.* 1987;163:743-746.

7. Persson AV, Powis RL. Recent advances in imaging and evaluation of blood flow using ultrasound. *Med Clin North Am.* 1986;70:1241-1252.

8. Persson AV. Use of ultrasonic colour imaging in the evaluation of the vascular system. In: Nicolaides A, Salmasi A-M, eds. *Cardiovascular Applications of Doppler Ultrasound.* New York, NY: Churchill Livingstone Inc; 1988:357-364.

9. Rabinov K, Paulin S. Roentgen diagnosis of venous thrombosis in the leg. *Arch Surg.* 1972;104:134-144.

10. Barnes RW. Doppler techniques for lower extremity venous disease. In: Zwiebel WJ, ed. *Introduction to Vascular Ultrasonography.* New York, NY: Grune & Stratton; 1982:333-350.

11. Vogel P, Laing FC, Jeffrey RB, Wing VW. Deep venous thrombosis of the lower extremity: US evaluation. *Radiology.* 1987;163:747-751.

12. Dosick SM, Blakemore WS. The role of Doppler ultrasound in acute deep vein thrombosis. *Am J Surg.* 1978;136:265-268.

13. Sullivan ED, Peter DJ, Cranley JJ. Real-time B-mode venous ultrasound. *J Vasc Surg.* 1984;1:465-471.

Discussion

William W. Babson, Jr, MD, Plymouth, Mass: One of the problems we have found in our noninvasive vascular laboratory is the proximal clot in the iliac veins. B-mode image resolution of veins deeper than 4 cm is not very good because of the lower frequency probe required, as reported by Talbot (In: Zwiebel WJ, ed. *Introduction to Vascular Ultrasonography.* 2nd ed. New York, NY: Grune & Stratton; 1986:352). We have missed the diagnosis in two patients with deep vein thrombophlebitis involving the iliac veins. One patient, who was 6 months pregnant, developed pain and edema involving the left calf and thigh. Diagnosis could not be made with initial continuous-wave Doppler, duplex Doppler, and conventional venography. On the third day of hospitalization, the continuous-wave Doppler examination findings became abnormal, and a repeated venogram showed extensive thrombus formation in the common and superficial femoral veins and the popliteal veins. I would like Dr Persson to comment on the use of the triplex scanner to evaluate the proximal iliac thrombus.

Edwin W. Salzman, MD, Boston, Mass: I think it is important to point out that the usual experience with this procedure is that it is effective in the diagnosis of thrombi in the thigh but almost totally insensitive in the calf. It would appear that none of Dr Persson and colleagues' patients had distal thrombi, as they presented them to us, since they claimed 100% sensitivity. That would be unprecedented in a patient population referred for suspicion of deep vein thrombosis in whom one would expect to find a substantial fraction with thrombi limited to the calf. Not only is the claimed sensitivity of 100% remarkable, but the sensitivity of the referring physicians must have been 100% also, since they missed no cases of deep venous thrombosis below the knee. Could Dr Persson tell us about his experience with distal thrombi?

Lenworth M. Jacobs, Jr, MD, Hartford, Conn: I wondered if there was any concern, risk, or danger in directly manipulating a clot, and was there any evidence of embolization?

H. Brownell Wheeler, MD, Worcester, Mass: The color flow images we have seen are indeed impressive, as is Dr Persson and colleagues' accuracy of 100%. This remarkable sensitivity and specificity are based on a relatively small and highly selected series, but one could argue that the selection bias might actually be expected to decrease the accuracy. Of note is the fact that Dr Persson and colleagues' laboratory took a year to define the diagnostic criteria and to become familiar with the instrument before they undertook the study they have reported. My concern, therefore, is not so much about the impressive accuracy in Dr Persson and colleagues' laboratory but instead involves the accuracy we might expect in our own laboratories, particularly at first.

I was interested in the impact of duplex scanning and, more recently, "triplex" scanning on the usage of other diagnostic tests in our hospital. The increase in B-mode scanning has been remarkable. It does not involve taking the patient down to the radiology department, one does not have to inject contrast material, the procedure is repeatable, and it is cheaper than venography. On the other hand, the use of impedance plethysmography, our principal screening technique, has actually increased at the same time that there has been a modest falloff in venograms. We apparently still need a simple, objective, and inexpensive screening technique at the bedside, even in this era of more sophisticated diagnostic modalities.

I have some quick questions for Dr Persson. First, do you use triplex scanning for all preliminary screening or do you still rely on more conventional noninvasive tests? Second, what is the approximate cost of this color-coded Doppler instrument, and what is the cost of the procedure? Finally, what is required to achieve the remarkable accuracy you report in terms of the training and experience required for a new technician?

Dr Persson: To answer the question regarding training, it takes about 6 months for me to train a technician or for an experienced technician to train another technician. This is not a simple procedure.

We use impedance plethysmography and the hand-held Doppler routinely in our laboratory and very few patients go to the triplex scanner first. We use the other screening tests a great deal. The reason for this is that it takes an hour to do a triplex scan. In the best of circumstances, we will therefore do only eight in a day. If you have an institution like ours where the scanner is used for other indications, it is simply not feasible to scan all patients suspected of having deep venous thrombosis. We have found that the number of venograms has gone down since we started using the scanner.

The instrument, I think, costs between $160 000 and $175 000. There are several of them on the market and you would have to quibble with the various companies. Presently, the cost of the examination is $450, which includes the reading fee.

We had no problems with pushing clots or clots embolizing during the examination. We have not had any problem nor has anyone else reported this using the duplex scanner that has been around for years.

I purposely have avoided reporting on calf clots because we do not have enough corresponding venograms to know the accuracy of the instrument. We do see clots in the tibial veins but I am not sure how accurate we are because we do not have a standard. We cannot visualize the iliac veins with this instrument. Those few patients who have isolated iliac clots only will be missed. Most clots, however, start in the popliteal or tibial vein and progress upward. We must also remember that venograms have the same weakness; if you put the needle in the foot and there are no clots until the inguinal ligament, you will not visualize clots in the iliac veins. If you are suspicious of iliac-only thrombosis, then you must put the needle in the common femoral vein. I have twice seen such clots go undetected until the second venogram was done.

The Impact of an Ambulatory Surgical Service in a Community Hospital

Horace A. Laffaye, MD

• The purpose of this study was to quantify the savings accrued from shifting surgical cases from an inpatient to an outpatient setting. There was an increase in the total number of operations from 7952 in 1973 to 10 250 in 1987. The percentage of ambulatory procedures showed a continuous increase from 17.9% to 56.3%. The 15-year experience accumulated at this institution now exceeds 43 000 cases, with no mortality. The study closely examined hospital charges, not costs, for 2 months, which were then annualized. The calculated average savings per case was $2000 and 3.07 hospital days. The estimated savings for fiscal 1987 were $11.5 million and 17 726 hospital days. Based on this experience, the operation of an in-hospital ambulatory surgical unit is recommended as a cost-saving, safe, and efficient method of performing many surgical procedures.

(*Arch Surg.* 1989;124:601-603)

Norwalk (Conn) Hospital, a 427-bed acute care facility, established an ambulatory surgical unit in 1973.[1] This event occurred before the advent of Public Law 93-641, also known as the Health Planning Resources Act, which promoted ambulatory care. This law, in conjunction with a change in reimbursement policies by Blue Cross and other insurers, brought about a great increase in the number of ambulatory surgical facilities throughout the country.[2] The 1987 American Hospital Association annual survey indicated that 83.4% of US hospitals provided ambulatory surgical services.[3]

During the first year of operation, 1423 cases were treated in our Ambulatory Surgical Unit, 17.9% of all operations performed that year at Norwalk Hospital. There has been an increase in the total number of procedures, from 7952 in 1973 to 10 250 in 1987 (Fig 1). However, there has been a significant increase in the ambulatory cases, from 1423 in our first year of operation to 5774 in fiscal 1987. The percentage of ambulatory procedures to total cases is shown in Fig 2. It rose from 17.9% in 1973 to 56.3% in 1987. The curve shows a continuous increase in the percentage of ambulatory surgery with a significant climb in the last 2 years, during which period the 50% mark for ambulatory surgery was exceeded. This indicates a continuous increase in the percentage of ambulatory surgery, after a steady but perhaps tentative utilization during the first 6 years of operation. The 15-year experience at our institution includes 43 322 cases, with no mortality.

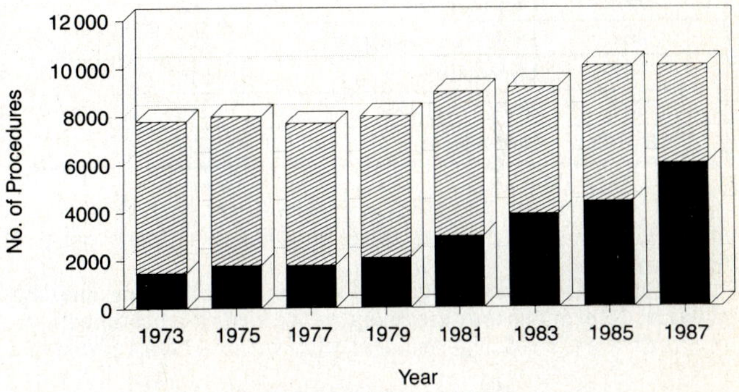

Fig 1.—Numbers of ambulatory procedures (black bars) and surgical procedures (hatched bars) by year.

MATERIALS AND METHODS

Criteria for Patient Selection and Procedures

The time limit per procedure has arbitrarily been set at 90 minutes, although in practice it is not enforced. No emergency operations are allowed. There is no age limit, except to exclude newborns. Premature infants are not operated on if they are under 3 months of age. Patients with an anesthetic risk of American Society of Anesthesiologists classes I and II are accepted, although occasionally a class III patient has been operated on.

Before surgery, the patient is checked by his or her personal physician; a medical history and physical examination are done within 48 hours before admission and recorded in a short-form admission record. This record must include the laboratory and electrocardiogram reports, of which the minimum requirement is a hematology profile; the current trend in preoperative screening is followed in that, in the absence of specific indications, routine laboratory tests can reasonably be eliminated.[4] Tests performed by outside laboratories are acceptable if performed within 7 days of surgery. Chest roentgenograms are not done on the day of

Accepted for publication December 9, 1988.

From the Departments of Surgery, Yale University School of Medicine, New Haven, Conn, and Norwalk (Conn) Hospital.

Read before the 69th Annual Meeting of the New England Surgical Society, Montreal, Canada, September 16, 1988.

Reprint requests to Department of Surgery, Norwalk Hospital, Norwalk, CT 06856 (Dr Laffaye).

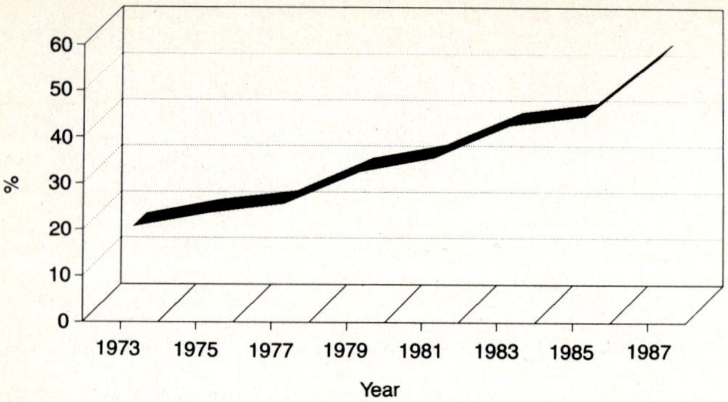

Fig 2.—Percentage of total cases performed as ambulatory procedures. There was an increase from 17.9% in 1973 to 56.3% in 1987.

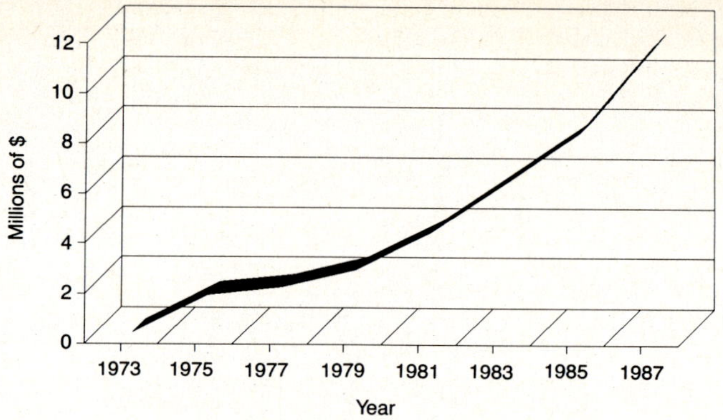

Fig 3.—Ambulatory surgery program savings. Savings increased from $139 409 in 1973 to $11 500 000 in 1987.

The Six Most Common Ambulatory Procedures

Diagnosis Related Group No.	Procedure	No. of Patients	Average Charge, $	Annual Savings, $	Total Days Saved	Average Days Saved/Patient
39	Intraocular lens insertion	300	1426.12	368 919.78	630.0	2.1
262	Breast biopsy	258	817.38	340 936.20	593.4	2.3
364	Dilation and curettage	234	493.55	324 503.04	514.8	2.2
62	Myringotomy	216	333.68	242 804.94	280.8	1.3
222	Knee procedures	216	939.36	773 950.98	756.0	3.5
161-163	Hernia repair	204	676.87	380 231.58	712.8	3.5

surgery, since such practice tends to delay the timely onset of operations.

The patients are discharged as soon as the attending anesthesiologist determines they are ready, on the basis of a postanesthetic recovery score. Discharge usually occurs within 4 hours of surgery.

Purpose and Methods

The purpose of this study was to quantify the savings accrued from shifting surgical cases from an inpatient to an outpatient setting. No attempt was made to account for presumed savings to society at large or to the individual in terms of time and earnings. Also, the study does not take into consideration the dollar value of home care contributed by family members. The study closely examined charges, not costs, for the randomly selected months of May and June 1987, which were then annualized.

All ambulatory admissions for May and June of 1987 were listed. Those patients admitted to the inpatient service for "same-day surgery," ie, patients electively admitted for at least one night, were then deleted. The diagnosis related group charge was determined, assuming inpatient care, and the dollar difference and inpatient days saved per case were then calculated. Finally, statistical outliers were deleted. For example, if the patient's diagnosis related group charge was greater than five times the actual ambulatory charge, it was discarded.

RESULTS

The calculated average savings per case was $2000 and 3.07 hospital days. Taken one step further, with 5774 ambulatory cases treated in fiscal 1987, the estimated savings were $11.5 million and 17 726 days. The study also took into consideration inflation by adjusting the savings per case to the medical component of the Consumer Price Index. The adjusted savings per case was $694 in 1974, $1227 in 1980, and $2000 in 1987. The savings growth is indicated in Fig 3. It shows a very close relationship to the percentage of ambulatory cases (Fig 2). The cumulative savings accrued from the program from its inception was calculated to be $62 966 700.

The study also examined the six most commonly performed ambulatory procedures for fiscal 1987: insertion of intraocular lenses; breast biopsy and local excision; dilation and curettage and conization; myringotomy in patients under 17 years old; knee procedures up to age 69 years, without complications; and inguinal and femoral hernias (Table). All of these operations indicated significant savings in both charges and hospital days when compared with similar inpatient diagnosis related groups.

COMMENT

The purpose of this study was to investigate the savings derived from performing operations on an outpatient basis rather than an inpatient setting. The study did not address the issue of potential savings to society and families, such as the one by Stanwick and his associates,[5] indicating that the ambulatory setting was cost-effective for families whose children underwent surgery. They found that the outpatient surgery group incurred an average total time cost of 16.1 hours, compared with 37.1 hours for the inpatient group. Parents in the outpatient group spent an average of $63.91, against $84.21 incurred by the parents of the inpatient cohort.

Savings

Karpman[6] examined the savings associated with converting six different surgical procedures from inpatient to outpatient surgery. The operations selected were dilation and curettage; laparoscopy; nonrecurrent inguinal hernia; breast biopsy; cataracts; and hemorrhoids. Of the total of 1397 inpatient and 195 day surgery charts, 151 and 26 records, respectively, were sampled. The final conclusion was a 0.3% savings in the hospital's yearly operating expense.

The data from Temple University in Philadelphia, Pa, indicate a 19% differential in savings for ambulatory procedures.[7] In a careful study of patients undergoing plastic surgery, Muñoz and his coworkers[8] found that ambulatory procedures had lower total hospital costs and a greater profit per patient under diagnosis related group methods than did inpatient procedures. They also found that hospital cost per patient rose with age for both inpatients and outpatients. Underscoring the difference between treating the elderly and the young, another Canadian study, by Evans and Robinson,[9] indicated that the expense of pediatric ambulatory surgery was 70% that of the same inpatient procedure, largely due to reduction in direct patient care expenses and in the overhead associated with hospital beds.

In a recent symposium on ambulatory surgery, Davis[10] wrote, "Major ambulatory surgery is possibly the clearest and most evident example of economy in the health care system. By avoiding hospitalization the one greatest factor in health care savings is effected. Egdahl[11] pointed out the wide range of procedures that can safely and efficiently be performed on an ambulatory basis.

In a randomized clinical trial, Pineault and coworkers[12] concluded that 1-day surgery can be a cost-efficient arrangement for performing certain types of surgery. All of these studies are in general agreement with the current one regarding the substantial savings that can be effected by transferring procedures from an inpatient to an outpatient setting.

Decrease in Length of Surgical Waiting Lists

Lakhani et al[13] reported on the effect of an ambulatory unit on the inpatient waiting lists of a busy district general hospital over a 4-year period. During this time, 15% of the general surgical beds were closed. During the period covered by the study, the total number of operations remained the same while the number of patients on the waiting list showed a progressive decrease from approximately 1750 to 1100.

In another report from the same institution, the authors indicated that waiting lists for hernia surgery dropped from 2 years to 6 weeks.[14] They also examined recurrences and reported the same rates from outpatient, short-stay, and inpatient series.

Safety

There has been no mortality in our Ambulatory Surgical Unit. During the last fiscal year, 35 patients had to be admitted to the hospital because of complications in our ambulatory unit, a 0.6% rate. Complications numbered 156 (2.7%).

Pineault and colleagues[12] reported a complication rate of 5.3% for 1-day surgery and 7.8% for inpatients. None of the complications were considered to be life threatening. Natof[15] recorded a total of 17 deaths, 11 related to anesthesia, in all types of ambulatory surgery facilities from 1970 to 1985.

It can be concluded that the safety component of ambulatory surgery is proved, provided that patients are selected adequately, types and length of operations are carefully monitored, and anesthetic management is safe. We favor a hospital-based unit for the simple reason that if complications occur, there is ample medical and technological support in place and immediately available without the potential risk of a crosstown ambulance ride.

Conclusion

On the basis of this experience with over 43 000 patients in 15 years, the operation of an in-hospital ambulatory surgery unit is recommended as a cost-saving, safe, and efficient method of performing many surgical procedures.

I wish to acknowledge Lee Ludwig, vice president for planning, Norwalk Hospital, for performing the statistical analysis and also the contributions of the following persons in the preparation of this study: Jo-Ann DiPanni, Dave Discenza, Sharon Duda, Mark Gentilozzi, Ken Lalime, Linda Moffat, Anita Oestreich, Pat Percy, Marianne Starrett, and Deidre VanCollie.

References

1. Hughes WF. An ambulatory surgical service by Norwalk Hospital department of surgery. *Conn Med.* 1976;40:592-596.

2. Detmer DE, Buchanan-Davidson DJ. Ambulatory surgery. *Surg Clin North Am.* 1982;62:685-704.

3. *Hospital Statistics.* Chicago: American Hospital Association; 1987:207.

4. Kaplan EB, Sheiner LB, Boeckmann AJ, et al. The usefulness of preoperative laboratory screening. *JAMA.* 1985;253:3576-3581.

5. Stanwick RS, Horne JM, Peabody DM, et al. Day-care versus inpatient pediatric surgery: a comparison of costs incurred by parents. *Can Med Assoc J.* 1988;137:21-26.

6. Karpman S. Day surgery versus inpatient surgery: a cost comparison. *Health Manage Forum.* 1983;4:54-63.

7. Stein H. Ambulatory surgery: evolution, organization, cost efficiency. *Med Health.* 1986;1:113-119.

8. Muñoz E, Angus G, Calabro S, et al. DRGs, costs, and outcome for plastic surgical patients. *Surgery.* 1988;82:116-124.

9. Evans RG, Robinson GC. Surgical day care: measurements of the economic payoff. *Can Med Assoc J.* 1980;123:873-880.

10. Davis JE. The future of major ambulatory surgery. *Surg Clin North Am.* 1987;67:893-901.

11. Egdahl RH. Ways for surgeons to increase the efficiency of their use of hospitals. *N Engl J Med.* 1983;309:1184-1187.

12. Pineault R, Contandriopoulos A-P, Valois M, et al. Randomized clinical trial of 1-day surgery. *Med Care.* 1985;23:171-182.

13. Lakhani S, Leach RD, Jarrett PEM. Effect of a surgical day unit on waiting lists. *J R Soc Med.* 1987;80:628-692.

14. Morris GE, Jarrett PEM. Recurrence rate following local anesthetic day care inguinal hernia repair by junior surgeons in a district general hospital. *Ann R Coll Surg Engl.* 1987;69:97-99.

15. Natof HE. Complications. In: Wetchler BV, ed. *Anesthesia for Ambulatory Surgery.* Philadelphia, Pa: JB Lippincott; 1985:321-356.

Routine Intraoperative Angioscopy in Lower Extremity Revascularization

Arnold Miller, MB, ChB; David R. Campbell, MD; Gary W. Gibbons, MD; Frank B. Pomposelli, Jr, MD; Dorothy V. Freeman, MD; Stephen J. Jepsen, MD; Robert S. Lees, MD; Jonathan L. Isaacsohn, MD; David Purcell, MD; Mark Bolduc, MD; Frank W. LoGerfo, MD

• The inability to see through blood remains the main obstacle to the widespread and routine use of angioscopy. Local irrigation with a balanced salt solution is presently the most widely used method to clear the blood. By applying basic principles of irrigation and using a unique, dedicated, irrigation pump, we found that routine angioscopy during lower extremity revascularization that yields consistent high-quality studies is feasible, clinically useful, and safe. Between May 1, 1987, and July 31, 1988, 136 intraoperative angioscopies were performed during 112 peripheral bypass procedures, 15 thrombectomies, 2 embolectomies, and 7 miscellaneous revascularization procedures. Mean total irrigation fluid used in the peripheral bypasses was 398 mL (range, 0 to 1400 mL). Good visual quality was obtained in more than 80% of angioscopies and the failure rate was only 1.8%. On the basis of the findings in 71 of the 136 angioscopies, 78 clinical or surgical decisions were made. No complications were directly attributable to the insertion of the angioscope or use of the pump.

(*Arch Surg.* 1989;124:604-608)

Endoscopy of the blood vessels, or intraoperative angioscopy, is being used with increasing frequency during lower extremity revascularization.[1-9] It allows the immediate detection and correction of technical errors and deficiencies during surgery and has been shown to be a safe, effective alternative or adjunct to intraoperative angiography.[6-8] Angioscopy may also facilitate intraluminal therapeutic procedures, such as thrombectomy and embolectomy,[9] and may play an important role in the development and application of the newer therapeutic ablative therapies for occlusive arteriosclerosis. Furthermore, the ability to see the intraluminal pathologic changes directly and in vivo, which has already made a significant impact on the understanding of the pathogenesis and management of occlusive coronary artery disease,[10,11] may make a similar contribution to the study of occlusive peripheral vascular disease, particularly with regard to problems of late graft failure and restenosis.

Despite advances in fiberoptic technology and the availability of flexible angioscopes as small as a millimeter or less, which allow access to most blood vessels of the body, the inability to see through blood and the necessity of complete removal of blood from the visual field remain the primary obstacles to the widespread and routine use of angioscopy during lower extremity revascularization. Local irrigation with a balanced salt solution is presently the most widely used method to clear the blood.

This study was undertaken to determine whether applying the principles of irrigation and using a dedicated irrigation pump described in a previous in vitro and in vivo study[12] would make routine intraoperative angioscopy feasible during lower extremity revascularization. The study was also undertaken to establish the irrigation fluid requirements and pump flow settings as well as the clinical usefulness and safety of the procedure.

MATERIALS AND METHODS

Angioscopic Equipment

In these studies we used five prototype angioscopes with outer diameters of 0.8, 1.4, 2.2, 2.8, and 3 mm (Olympus Corp, Lake Success, NY). The 2.2- and 3-mm angioscopes were steerable 120° in two directions, but in a single plane. The 2.8- and 3-mm angioscopes had in addition a built-in irrigation channel. All the other devices were solid, with no irrigation channel; they consisted of a central imaging fiber bundle surrounded by a concentric ring of illumination fibers and were sheathed in a polyvinyl chloride jacket.

The angioscope was connected to a 300-W xenon light source (Olympus CLV-10). The eyepiece was connected to a videocamera (MIC-6/MIC-7; MP Video Inc, Hopkinton, Mass), allowing continuous monitoring on a high-resolution television monitor (AM-1401R, Mitsubishi, Electronic Sales America Inc, Torrance, Calif), and recording on 3/4-in videotape (KCA-60 BRS, Sony Corp of America, San Diego, Calif) with a videocassette recorder (VD 5600, Sony).

Irrigation

Collateral irrigation, through a separate irrigation catheter, was used almost exclusively. Four types of irrigation catheters were used: a standard, commercially available, 16-gauge, 20-cm catheter (Intracath, Deseret Medical Inc, Parke Davis & Co, Salt Lake City, Utah); an intravenous 18-gauge Teflon catheter (Catholon IV, Critikon, Tampa, Fla); and an 18-gauge Mark's needle and prototype single-channel polyurethane catheters 300×2.5 mm and 300×3.5 mm in outer diameter, respectively, allowing simultaneous irrigation and passage of the angioscope (Olympus Corp).

Irrigation fluid was saline, a balanced salt solution (Ringer's lactate), or a balanced salt solution with a normalized pH (Normosol, Abbott Laboratories, Chicago, Ill). No heparin or other drugs were added. All patients were systemically heparinized for the vascular procedure in a dosage of 0.5 to 1.5 mg/kg, according to the preference of the individual surgeon. In our initial 18 patients, irrigation fluid was provided by a pressure-cuff device (C-Fusor 500, Medex Inc, Teaneck, NJ) placed around a liter of saline or balanced salt solution in a plastic container and inflated to a pressure between 400 and 450 mm Hg. In the remaining 118 cases, we used a prototype dedicated angioscopy pump.[12] This peristaltic pump was designed to provide flow rates between 10 and 400 mL/min and has the unique ability to provide both a high-volume high-flow rate to rapidly clear the blood vessel of all blood and establish a clear column of fluid and a low-volume low-flow rate to maintain the clear fluid column and prolong the endoscopic visualization, all under the control of a single, double-action foot switch.

Method of Study

A standard method of angioscopic examination was developed for each application and varied according to the operative procedure and the nature of the region of interest. In the in situ vein or nonreversed vein bypass, angioscopy was performed at the completion of the procedure in lieu of or as an adjunct to the

Accepted for publication December 9, 1988.

From the Division of Vascular Surgery, Department of Surgery (Drs Miller, Campbell, Gibbons, Pomposelli, Freeman, Jepsen, Purcell, Bolduc, and LoGerfo), and the Department of Medicine (Drs Lees and Isaacsohn), New England Deaconess Hospital, Boston, Mass.

Read before the 69th Annual Meeting of the New England Surgical Society, Montreal, Canada, September 16, 1988.

Reprint requests to Department of Surgery, New England Deaconess Hospital, 110 Francis St, Suite 3B, Boston, MA 02215 (Dr Miller).

intraoperative angiogram. In the reversed vein graft or synthetic graft, angioscopy was performed on completion of the distal anastomosis after blood flow had been reconstituted, either prior to or after tunneling the graft. Where the information was of critical importance, such as the siting of an anastomosis or determining the adequacy of thrombectomy, angioscopy was performed prior to or during the revascularization procedure.

In general, for bypass surgery, only the distal artery, the distal anastomosis, and the graft were examined. Retrograde or upstream angioscopy, to examine the proximal artery and anastomosis, was performed in only a few selected cases where inflow problems were encountered.

In this study, angioscopy was always performed by a separate team consisting of a surgeon and technician or operating room nurse, in cooperation with the primary surgeon. Each study was recorded in its entirety on videotape. Following each procedure the tape was reviewed and interpreted, and a standardized data collection sheet was completed. A report of each study was included in the patient's hospital record, and the data were entered and stored in a dedicated computer database system (Cyberex Inc, Denville, NJ).

Case Material

Case selection was dependent on the availability of the angioscopy team and equipment, as well as the clinical findings and the inclination of the primary surgeon to do the study.

One hundred thirty-six intraoperative angioscopies were performed during lower extremity revascularization procedures between May 1, 1987, and July 31, 1988. These included 112 peripheral bypass procedures, 15 thrombectomies, 2 embolectomies, and 7 miscellaneous procedures. Angioscopy was not done during all lower extremity procedures performed over the same period.

Peripheral Bypass Procedures

The clinical profile, indications for surgery, and bypass procedures performed are shown in Tables 1 through 3. Autogenous vein, greater saphenous vein in 100 bypasses and arm vein in 5 bypasses, was the material most commonly used (105 of 112 bypasses) and included 52 in situ, 31 nonreversed, and 22 reversed bypasses. ePTFE 5- or 6-mm grafts alone were used only seven times. For irrigation, the pressure-cuff device was used in the first 16 patients, and the dedicated pump was used in the subsequent 96 intraoperative angioscopies.

Thrombectomy/Embolectomy

Angioscopy was performed in 15 graft thrombectomies and 2 embolectomies and included 8 femoropopliteal, 3 axillofemoral, 3 femorodistal (2 femorotibial and 1 femoro–dorsalis pedis), and 1 popliteal–dorsalis pedis bypass grafts. The thrombectomies were performed from a few hours to 5 months following the primary graft procedure. The 2 embolectomies were of the superficial femoral and popliteal arteries in the one patient and of the common, superficial, and profunda femoris arteries in another.

Miscellaneous

The miscellaneous group of seven bypasses included an aortobifemoral graft, an iliofemoral graft, an ilio–profunda femoral graft, an axillobifemoral graft, a femorofemoral graft, a common femoral endarterectomy, and a below-knee femoropopliteal in situ vein bypass graft performed elsewhere 3 months previously (the patient was referred for ligation of multiple, large, residual arteriovenous fistulas). Angioscopy was used to assess the distal anastomoses and distal native vessels in all these cases. In addition, in the femoropopliteal graft, both proximal and distal arteries, both anastomoses, and the entire graft were examined.

RESULTS

Peripheral Bypass Procedures

Details of irrigation are shown in Table 2. The mean total volume of irrigation fluid used for all the peripheral bypasses was 398 mL (range, 0 to 1400 mL). Mean pump settings for the various bypass procedures ranged from a mean of 243 to 315 mL/min for the high-volume high-flow rate, or "bolus" fluid, and 44 to 75 mL/min for the low-volume low-flow rate, or "maintenance" fluid.

In Table 4, the visual quality of the studies in the peripheral bypass group is shown, comparing the ability of the pressure-cuff device with the pump, to achieve a good visual study. Overall, 84.8% (95/112) of the studies were of good quality, 7.1% (8/112) were of fair quality, and 6.2% (7/112) were of poor quality. There were two (1.8%) failures, one due to a mechanical pump failure and the other due to choice of an angioscope too rigid to be inserted into the graft within the popliteal fossa.

Visualization of the distal artery, distal anastomosis, and

Table 1.—Clinical Data and Indications for Surgery in 112 Peripheral Bypass Procedures*

	Clinical Data			Indications for Surgery		
Bypass Procedure	No.	Mean Age, y	Sex, M:F	DM	Threatened Limb	Claudication
Femoral-Pop						
AK	18	64	6:12	14	16	2
BK	24	58	13:11	14	21	3
Femoral-tibial						
AT	13	68	6:7	9	13	...
PT	21	61	13:8	14	20	1
Peroneal	12	64	9:3	9	11	1
Femoral-DP	14	67	9:5	11	14	...
Pop-DP	7	63	5:2	6	7	...
Pop-PT	3	78	3:0	3	3	...
Total	**112**	...†	**64:48**	**80‡**	**105**	**7**

*Pop indicates popliteal; AK, above knee; BK, below knee; AT, anterior tibial; PT, posterior tibial; DP, dorsalis pedis; and DM, diabetes mellitus.
†Mean age, 65 years; range, 41 to 86 years.
‡71.4%.

Table 2.—Method of Irrigation, Pump Settings, and Volume of Irrigation Fluid Used in 112 Peripheral Bypass Procedures

			Pump Settings, mL/min		
Procedure*	Pressure-Cuff Device	Irrigation Pump	High (Range)	Low (Range)	Total Irrigation Fluid Volume, mL (Range)
Femoral-Pop					
AK	3	15	315 (250-400)	68 (50-90)	436 (0-1400)
BK	2	22	291 (250-300)	62 (50-85)	478 (150-900)
Femoral-tibial	8	38	266 (150-300)	66 (50-85)	518 (100-1000)
Femoral-DP	3	11	276 (250-300)	44 (0-80)	439 (100-800)
Pop-DP	...	7	243 (150-285)	75 (50-100)	250 (50-500)
Pop-PT	1	2	248 (220-275)	63 (50-75)	267 (150-450)
Total	**17**	**95**	...	...	398 (0-1400)

*Pop indicates popliteal; AK, above knee; BK, below knee; DP, dorsalis pedis; and PT, posterior tibial.

Table 3.—Intraoperative Angiograms in 112 Peripheral Bypass Procedures That Included Intraoperative Angioscopy

Procedure*	Intraoperative Angiogram		
	None	Control	Runoff
Femoral–Pop AK	40	2	...
Femoral-tibial	38	4	4
Femoral-DP	12	1	1
Pop-DP	7	...	...
Pop-PT	3	...	...
Total	**100**	**7**	**5**

*Pop indicates popliteal; AK, above knee; DP, dorsalis pedis; and PT, posterior tibial.

Table 4.—Visual Quality of Angioscopic Studies Performed During 112 Peripheral Bypass Procedures Compared With Results With Pressure-Cuff Device and Irrigation Pump

		No. (%)			
	No.	Good Quality	Fair Quality	Poor Quality	Failed
Pressure-cuff device	16	7 (43.7)	3 (18.8)	5 (31.3)	1 (6.3)
Irrigation pump	96	88 (91.7)	5 (5.2)	2 (2.1)	1 (1.0)
Total	**112**	**95** (84.8)	**8** (7.1)	**7** (6.2)	**2** (1.8)

Table 5.—Clinical or Surgical Decisions Based on Angioscopic Findings in 136 Lower Extremity Revascularizations

	No. of Decisions	No. of Angioscopies
Bypass procedures (n=112)	...	54
Competent valves/leaflets	14	...
Unligated tributaries	31	...
Siting of anastomosis	2	...
Assess distal popliteal artery	2	...
Evaluate proximal intimal flap	1	...
Redo anastomosis	1	...
Identify graft torsion	1	...
Identify vein sclerosis	2	...
Assess valvulotome injury	3	...
Thrombectomy/embolectomy (n=17)	...	17
Assess completeness of procedure	17	...
Identify cause of graft occlusion		
Posterior plaque	1	...
Residual competent leaflet	1	...
Incorrect tunneling	1	...
Total	**3**	...
Unsuspected distal stenosis requiring bypass	1	...
Miscellaneous (n=7)	...	0
Total	**78**	**71**

graft was achieved in 80.4% (90/112), 84.8% (95/112), and 89.3% (97/112), respectively, of the 112 bypass grafts. Only 12 intraoperative angiograms were obtained in these 112 peripheral bypasses, 7 as controls for the angioscopic findings and 5 for distal runoff (Table 3). Of the 95 patients in whom angioscopy alone was performed, the serum creatinine level in 14 patients was above 150 µmol/L, and 9 of these patients were receiving dialysis.

Fifty-seven clinical or surgical decisions were made in 54 of the 112 bypasses based on angioscopic findings and are summarized in Table 5. In 12 (23.1%) of 52 in situ and 2 (6.5%) of 31 nonreversed bypasses, residual competent valves or valve leaflets were detected and subsequently lysed. In 31 (60%) of 52 in situ bypasses, even though Doppler examination for the detection of residual arteriovenous fistula was routinely performed, one to five unligated tributaries were detected and subsequently ligated. Assessment of the distal artery and siting of the distal anastomosis were made following angioscopy in four cases. A stenosis in the popliteal artery just distal to the completed and technically adequate distal anastomosis of a femoropopliteal above-knee graft necessitated a reanastomosis. In one femorotibial bypass graft, a 360° torsion of the vein graft was detected and corrected. Poor inflow in a distal superficial femoral artery–tibial bypass was shown to be due to a large obstructing intimal flap in the proximal portion of the superficial femoral artery, necessitating a proximal inflow procedure. Local vein sclerosis was noted in two cases and assessment of segmental vein injury by the valvulotome was made in three cases.

Five (4.4%) of the 112 bypass grafts occluded and required reexploration in less than 8 days. There were 2 below-knee femoropopliteal nonreversed vein bypass grafts: 1 done 5 days after surgery had been incorrectly tunneled and 1 done 8 days after surgery had a partially cut but still competent valve leaflet not noted on the original angioscopy detected at the time of reoperation and thrombectomy. There were 2 popliteal–dorsalis pedis bypass grafts: 1 done 5 days after surgery was a nonreversed saphenous vein graft, and 1 done 4 days after surgery was a reversed cephalic vein graft, where the underlying problem was not detected even at thrombectomy. However, at the original completion angioscopy, a 1- and 1.4-mm angioscope could not be inserted through the anastomosis and into the dorsalis pedis artery in either case. Finally, a femoro–anterior tibial in situ saphenous vein bypass where organized thrombus obstructing the distal end of the anterior tibial artery was seen on angioscopy, and the finding was "disregarded" because of a lack of angioscopy experience and reliance placed on the preoperative and intraoperative angiograms in which the obstruction was interpreted as atherosclerotic disease. At reoperation less than 24 hours later, the thrombus was easily located by the light of the angioscope shining through the skin on the dorsum of the foot in a darkened operating room. The thrombus was removed through a separate small incision and the bypass graft was salvaged.

Thrombectomy/Embolectomy

The volumes of irrigation fluid used ranged from 150 to 1300 mL. The mean bolus pump settings were all above 300 mL/min and ranged from 300 to 360 mL/min. The maintenance pump settings ranged from 50 to 85. The visual quality was good in 16 (94%) of these 17 studies. After embolectomy or thrombectomy, intraoperative angiograms were obtained in only 3 of the 17 cases. In all 3 cases, there were no new findings, but the angiograms significantly underestimated the volume of residual thrombus in all cases.

Twenty-one clinical decisions were made in 17 thrombectomy or embolectomy cases and are summarized in Table 5.

Complications

No complications directly attributable to the insertion of the angioscope or use of the pump were noted during this study. Mild spasm induced in the vein graft was noted on a few occasions but was always easily overcome and not a cause for abandonment of any procedure. Intraluminally, no significant damage attributable to the passage of the angioscope was seen. No perforations, disruptions of anastomoses, or elevation of plaques or intimal flaps occurred in any of the cases.

The use of the irrigation pump with the high flow rates resulted in distention of some vein grafts, but no disruption of any anastomoses or vein graft was seen. No episode of acute cardiac decompensation occurred intraoperatively or in the immediate postoperative period, although two patients did develop acute cardiac failure on the first and fourth postoperative days.

COMMENT

Our results show that with the use of the prototype angioscopic pump, the principles and techniques of irrigation for angioscopy developed in the animal laboratory,[12] and our clinical experience, we were able to perform routine intraoperative angioscopy during surgical revascularization of lower extremities with consistently high-quality studies. Our results confirm the experience of others[1-9] and suggest that intraoperative angioscopy may be a useful and safe addition to the practice of modern vascular surgery, refining and extending the possibilities of therapeutic interventions. They show that angioscopy, as a method of monitoring the surgical procedure intraoperatively, may play a role in the improvement of graft patency by avoiding both technical and judgmental errors that may result in early graft occlusion when direct inspection of the native vessels, the bypass graft, or anastomoses cannot be achieved. Our results suggest that intraoperative angioscopy is a good alternative to intraoperative angiography in most cases and a useful adjunct in others. The three-dimensional in vivo visualization of the endovascular abnormality may have significant implications in furthering our understanding and appreciation of the pathogenesis of the underlying atherosclerotic disease and graft failure.

Currently, the optical systems of all the angioscopes used in this study, from as small as 0.8 to 3 mm, together with the chip videocameras and high-resolution monitors, are now of such high quality that if the visual field can be cleared of blood, consistently good angioscopic studies may be obtained. Subtle adjustments of the video and electronic equipment, including the "white and color balance," focusing, and light intensity, can affect the overall quality of the study. Nevertheless, the ability to establish and maintain a clear column of fluid in the vessel or graft to be examined is the essence of successful angioscopy. Because blood is opaque, it must be removed completely from the vessel before angioscopy. Even a small volume of blood produces blurring of the visual field and produces a video image that appears to be "out of focus." Any more blood prevents any meaningful visualization.

With the pressure-cuff device alone, the ability to achieve a high-quality study was 43.7% (Table 4), and the studies were limited to only segments of the bypass graft or performed in a bloodless field, before removal of the vascular clamps and reestablishment of blood flow. With the dedicated pump, the overall quality of the study was good in more than 80% of studies, and we were consistently able to visualize the distal artery, anastomosis, and graft in more than 80% of the peripheral bypass procedures. No study failed completely because of inability to obtain adequate flushing with the irrigation pump. However, some studies were limited in their extent to avoid fluid overload. This is in contrast to other reported angioscopic series, where the failure rate was 15% and almost always due to inability to completely clear the blood from the visual field.[13] Furthermore, these latter angioscopies were more limited in their extent, with the distal anastomosis being visualized in less than 50% of bypasses. In fact, with our pump, the only limitations to visualization of the entire procedure, including the graft, distal anastomosis, and distal artery, was the availability of the correct-sized angioscope and the amount of irrigation fluid that could be safely used in that patient.

Our studies define the fluid requirements for angioscopy in the various peripheral bypass procedures and also establish the most commonly used pump settings for these procedures (Table 2). Our clinical findings confirmed our experimental studies[12] and showed that rapidly establishing the initial clear column of fluid diminishes the total volume of irrigation fluid used. We accordingly gradually increased the pump settings as the study proceeded. Nevertheless, the overall mean volume of irrigation fluid used per study was only 398 mL. By aggressive intraoperative hemodynamic monitoring and coordination of the patient's total fluid requirements during surgery with the anesthetist, few patients were excluded from this study for fear of inducing fluid overload. No patient experienced acute, uncompensated cardiac failure during angioscopy or during the immediate postoperative period, although acute cardiac decompensation developed in two patients at 24 hours and 4 days postoperatively, respectively.

Intraoperative angioscopy as the sole monitoring procedure proved to be an effective alternative to intraoperative angiography in 100 of the 112 peripheral bypasses in our high-risk group of peripheral bypass cases, where 70% of the patients were diabetic and 62.5% of the bypasses performed were distal to the popliteal artery. The intraoperative angiogram has always been the "gold standard" for monitoring of bypass grafts, particularly the distal bypasses and although extremely specific, has only a moderate sensitivity.[14] In our study no new findings were noted on the control angiograms, but as previously reported,[6,9,10] the angiogram always grossly underestimated the amount of residual thrombus in the native artery or graft, did not differentiate between atherosclerotic disease and organized thrombus, and did not delineate subtle findings, such as small regions of intimal denudation or thrombus in a vein graft, small intimal flaps, or irregularities of the suture line in an anastomosis or different patterns of atherosclerotic disease in the native vessels. These endovascular pathologic findings, when correlated with long-term graft patency and clinical outcome, may have significant implications in our understanding of late graft failure as well as the pathogenesis and progression of occlusive peripheral atherosclerotic disease. Performing intraoperative angioscopy with a separate "angioscopy" team had the advantage of concentrating the learning experience and facilitating the establishment and implementation of techniques that minimized disruption of the ongoing surgery and delay in the operating room. Unlike intraoperative angiography, angioscopy requires no precautions for radiation hazard. The ability to view any findings and corrective procedures in real time, avoiding the inevitable delay of repeating angiography or the reliance on "clinical judgment" alone, significantly reduced operating time and enhanced the quality of surgery. Angioscopy also avoided the problems of contrast-induced renal failure,[15] which constituted a significant problem in our high-risk group of patients, 14 of whom underwent bypass (12.5%) and had a raised serum creatinine level. Some change in the surgical procedure or clinical decision was made in more than half of the angioscopic cases (78 of 136) (Table 5). Although the angioscopic study in the peripheral bypasses was not randomized and the cases were selected, the early (<30 days) reocclusion rate of only 5 (4.4%) of 112 peripheral bypass grafts, particularly in our high-risk patient population, is low. In our hands, angioscopy avoided obvious undetected errors that may have increased our incidence of early occlusion. It proved particularly useful in the in situ and nonreversed saphenous vein bypass grafts, not only localizing and allowing complete lysis of residual competent valves or valve leaflets, which potentially may result in graft failure, but also in detecting arteriovenous fistula not found even after using the standard Doppler technique.

Our follow-up was too short to comment on the impact of angioscopy on graft patency after more than 30 days. We are still in the learning phase in interpreting findings in the graft, anastomosis, and native vessels. We have only a few documented cases of "subtle" findings, such as vein sclerosis or residual thrombus in grafts, that resulted in late graft failure. With time and meticulous follow-up of all these patients, this knowledge may modify our surgical approach and improve our future results.

References

1. Vollmar JF, Storz LW. Vascular endoscopy. *Surg Clin North Am.* 1974; 54:111-122.
2. Towne JR, Bernhard VM. Vascular endoscopy: useful tool or interesting toy? *Surgery.* 1977;82:415-419.
3. Tanabe T, Yokota A, Sugie S. Cardiovascular fiberoptic endoscopy: development and clinical application. *Surgery.* 1980;87:375-379.
4. Itoh T, Hori M. Vascular endoscopy for major vascular reconstruction: experimental and clinical studies. *Surgery.* 1983;93:391-396.
5. Litvack F, Grundfest WS, Lee ME, et al. Angioscopic visualization of blood vessel interior in animals and humans. *Clin Cardiol.* 1985;8:65-70.
6. Mehigan JT, Olcott C. Video-angioscopy as an alternative to intraoperative arteriography. *Am J Surg.* 1986;152:139-145.
7. Seeger JM, Abela GS. Angioscopy as an adjunct to arterial reconstructive surgery: a preliminary report. *J Vasc Surg.* 1986;4:315-320.
8. Olcott C. Clinical applications of video angioscopy. *J Vasc Surg.* 1987; 5:664-666.
9. White GH, White RA, Kopchok BS, Wilson SE. Angioscopic thrombectomy: preliminary observations in a recent technique. *J Vasc Surg.* 1988; 7:318-325.
10. Sherman TC, Litvack F, Grundfest WS, et al. Coronary angioscopy in patients with unstable angina pectoris. *N Engl J Med.* 1986;315:913-919.
11. Forrester JS, Litvack F, Grundfest WS, Hickey A. A perspective of coronary disease seen through the arteries of living man. *Circulation.* 1987; 75:505-513.
12. Miller A, Lipson WE, Isaacsohn JL, Schoen FJ, Lees RS. Intraoperative angioscopy: principles of irrigation and description of a new dedicated irrigation pump. *Am Heart J.* In press.
13. Grundfest WS, Litvak F, Glick D, et al. Intraoperative decisions based on angioscopy in peripheral vascular surgery. *Circulation.* 1988; 78(suppl 1):1-113–1-17.
14. Stept LL, Flinn WR, McCarthy WJ III, Bartlett ST, Bergan JJ, Yao JST. Technical defects as a cause of early graft failure after femorodistal bypass. *Arch Surg.* 1987;22:599-604.
15. Cruz C, Hriac H, Sambouri F, Smith RF, Eyler WR, Levin NW. Contrast media for angiography: effect on renal failure. *Radiology.* 1986; 158:109-112.

Discussion

Nathan P. Couch, West Roxbury, Mass: I am uncertain as to how this mechanism is designed. How are the pressure cuffs used? Specifically, where do you introduce the angioscope, and how do you use the constant-flow method? How do you manage to keep the vessel clear of blood?

I am impressed that the operating team includes many members, but how do you "concentrate the experience," as stated in the report? This brings up another question. Insurance companies use the term *team surgery.* If an operation is performed with more than one surgeon when a single surgeon could do the whole procedure, the fee for that single surgeon will be all that the insurance company will pay. Could individual surgeons be easily trained to do this procedure so they would not have to call in a second team?

This is a challenging but extremely promising technique that deserves a much wider application than it has had so far, but these questions need to be answered.

Martha D. McDaniel, MD, Hanover, NH: We have all been interested in ensuring optimal results in these extremely delicate operations. Early in our experience with the in situ bypass, when we had questions about the patency or amount of disease in the recipient tibial artery vessel, we were in the habit of probing gently with a small Fogarty catheter whose balloon was not inflated. We have been impressed over the years that this produced a fair amount of spasm in the recipient vessel.

I would like to ask Dr Miller and his colleagues whether they have recognized either the short-term complication of spasm with this technique or the long-term complication of neointimal hyperplasia either related to endothelial damage from the saline infusion or to the mechanical presence of the angioscope within the vessel.

R. Clement Darling, MD, Boston, Mass: My 30-year experience with femoropopliteal grafting started about the time that arterial homografts were abandoned and the Linton technique of reversed autogenous saphenous vein became accepted. One can look back and see four fairly distinctive periods. The early nonreversed grafting was carried out with meticulous technique using multifilament suture and took many pioneer surgeons perhaps 6 hours to obtain a satisfactory operative result. In the early 1970s, a new era using fine polypropylene suture, optical magnification, and coaxial fiberoptic illumination made the procedure easier and faster and gave better results. A third era developed with the reintroduction of in situ vein grafting, particularly for limb salvage, to small vessels below the knee. The early failure rate more than 20 years ago was about 10% to 15%, and even today return rates to the operating room are in the 5% range. Angioscopy opens up a new era. I have reviewed Dr Miller's excellent audiovisual setup, and it is absolutely amazing how miserable these incompetent valves look when seen directly, as are the imperfections of many of the anastomoses and the persistence of arteriovenous communications. Angiograms and Doppler monitoring are imperfect, at best. Dr Miller and his group have demonstrated how cost-effective this procedure can be. The surgeon, however, needs a special team, nonbiased and with authoritative and dependable credentials. The learning curve is incredibly high, and I think the angioscopist may have to be an entirely separate individual from the immediate operating team.

A. David Drezner, MD, Hartford, Conn: My question concerns the cost-effectiveness of this procedure. To be cost-effective, the additional time spent in the operating room would have to be less than the time that would have been spent had angioscopy not been done and the patient had been returned to the operating room as the need dictated. Dr Miller and coworkers had a quite respectable 4.4% failure rate within 30 days, but what was their failure rate at 30 days before angioscopy was performed?

Dr Miller: The experience was "concentrated" in the sense that I headed the team that did almost all the angioscopies. The purpose of this study was to investigate whether intraoperative angioscopy was a useful procedure for the vascular surgeon and whether, with previously developed techniques and a dedicated irrigation pump, angioscopy could be performed routinely during lower extremity revascularization.

Angioscopy was extremely useful in the in situ and nonreversed bypass, where the incidence of retained valves was 17% and the incidence of unligated tributaries was 60%, but many of our most dramatic findings were noted in the so-called simple femoropopliteal bypass grafts.

It is well known that irreversible spasm has been caused by inserting a large angioscope into a blood vessel. It has been one of the reasons that many have previously abandoned angioscopy. In our own series, spasm was not a problem, and we have never abandoned a case because of irreversible spasm. There are two reasons for this. First, the angioscopes we are now using are much smaller than what was previously available, and second, we do not pass the angioscope unless there is flowing blood within the blood vessel or the vessel has been gently distended with irrigation fluid.

As far as cost-effectiveness is concerned, time is saved in the operating room when angioscopy is performed in lieu of intraoperative angiography and, in our experience, routine angioscopy has decreased the incidence of reoperation within the first 30 postoperative days.

Limb Salvage Despite Extensive Tissue Loss

Free Tissue Transfer Combined With Distal Revascularization

Jack L. Cronenwett, MD; Martha D. McDaniel, MD; Robert M. Zwolak, MD, PhD;
Daniel B. Walsh, MD; Joseph R. Schneider, MD; William F. Reus, MD; Lawrence B. Colen, MD

• Extensive lower-extremity tissue loss may preclude limb salvage despite successful arterial reconstruction. We attempted to avoid limb loss in such patients by combining arterial bypass with microvascular free tissue transfer. Fourteen patient (12 diabetic), 33 to 74 years of age, presented with extensive tissue loss in 15 lower extremities, exposing bone or tendon on the heel, ankle, lower part of the leg, or hindfoot. Mean ulcer size was 5 × 8 cm. Four patients had had previous contralateral below-knee amputations. Femorodistal (seven), popliteal-distal (three), or femoropopliteal (four) bypass, or tibial angioplasty (one), was perfomed to provide sufficient inflow for free tissue tranfer. Serratus anterior, scapular, latissimus dorsi, rectus abdominis, gracilis, ulnar, or temporalis free flaps were used. One free flap failed due to venous thrombosis and was corrected with a second flap. Limb salvage was achieved in 14 (93%) of 15 limbs during a mean follow-up of 24 months. The single amputation occurred due to severe foot ischemia in a patient whose femorodistal bypass remained patent only to the viable free flap. The remaining 13 patients (14 limbs) became ambulatory, including those with free flaps to weight-bearing regions.

(*Arch Surg.* 1989;124:609-615)

Advances in vascular surgery have led to improved limb salvage despite severe lower-extremity ischemia. Distal tibial and pedal artery revascularizations have particularly benefited diabetic patients, with their predominance of infrapopliteal occlusive disease. Despite these successes, there remains a group of patients in whom extensive tissue loss at the time of presentation precludes limb salvage by conventional techniques. These patients are often diabetic, with large hindfoot or ankle ulcers that expose tendon and bone and are accompanied by chronic infection. They have traditionally required below-knee amputation even though a distal arterial bypass might be technically possible.

Accepted for publication December 20, 1988.

From the Sections of Vascular (Drs Cronenwett, McDaniel, Zwolak, Walsh, and Schneider) and Plastic (Drs Reus and Colen) Surgery, Department of Surgery, Dartmouth-Hitchcock Medical Center, Hanover, NH, and Veterans Administration Medical Center, White River Junction, Vt.

Read before the 69th Annual Meeting of the New England Surgical Society, Montreal, Canada, September 16, 1988.

Reprint requests to Section of Vascular Surgery, Dartmouth-Hitchcock Medical Center, Hanover, NH 03756 (Dr Cronenwett).

The advent of microsurgery and the successful use of free tissue transfer have provided an additional technique for potential limb salvage in these patients. Since the first successful report of free flap transfer to the leg with the use of microvascular anastomoses in 1973, this techniqe has been used by plastic surgeons to close many soft-tissue defects that were previously unreconstructible.[1-4] Free tissue transfer has usually been done, however, when normal arterial inflow was available, such as in association with trauma, extirpative surgery, or soft-tissue/bone infection.[3-6]

The convergence of distal arterial reconstruction and free tissue transfer has afforded an opportunity to obtain limb salvage in patients with extensive ischemic tissue loss of the distal part of the leg. Neither technique alone would suffice in this subgroup of patients, since healing of large soft-tissue defects would not occur despite adequate revascularization, and free tissue transfer would not be possible without adequate arterial inflow. This report describes our experience with patients who required arterial reconstruction combined with free tissue transfer to obtain limb salvage in the presence of extensive tissue loss.

PATIENTS AND METHODS

From 1983 to 1988, 14 patients who presented with extensive tissue loss in 15 lower extremities were selected for leg revascularization followed by free tissue transfer to achieve limb salvage. All patients had chronic ischemic ulcers that would traditionally have been impossible to heal despite revascularization, because of their large size (usually >5 cm in diameter), exposure of tendon or bone, underlying osteomyelitis, or location on weight-bearing areas. Patients with smaller or more superficial ulcers, or forefoot lesions, were treated with revascularization plus local procedures and were not considered for free flap transfer. Similarly, patients with adequate arterial circulation who required free tissue coverage were excluded from this review.

Of the 14 patients so treated, there were 11 men and 3 women, aged 33 to 74 years (mean, 59 years) (Table). Twelve (86%) were diabetic; 7 required insulin (type I) and 5 used oral hypoglycemic agents (type II). Most patients had associated ischemic heart disease, and many had complications of advanced diabetes, such as renal failure. A total of 16 separate ulcers were treated in 15 lower extremities (Table). One patient (patient 2) had bilateral heel ulcers, while another patient (patient 1) developed a second ulcer in the same location (heel) in a successful weight-bearing

Data Summary for 14 Patients Who Underwent Lower-Extremity Revascularization and

Patient/ Age, y/Sex	DM*	Ulcer Location	Size, cm	Cause†	Arterial Procedures (Date)‡	Free Flap (Date)§	Outcome‖ Arterial	Flap	Status
1/74/M	II	R heel	5×8	N	Pop-DP RSVG (5/82); angioplasty pop anastomosis (2/83)	Gracilis+STSG (8/83)	P-R	H	Ambulatory
		R heel	4×6	N	...	Scapular (6/85)	...	H	Ambulatory
2/60/M	I	R heel	5×9	N	R fem-pop (PTFE) (4/84); thromb fem-pop (8/85)	Scapular (4/84)	P (2°)	H	Ambulatory
		L heel	5×6	N	Aortobifem (6/78); L fem-pop (PTFE) (6/82); thromb fem-pop (11/83); L pop-AT (PTFE) (11/83); thromb L AFB limb (2/84)	Scapular (5/84)	P-R	H	Ambulatory
3/52/M	N	R ankle	5×6	O	Fem-PT RSVG (6/84)	Serratus anterior +STSG (3/85)	P	H	Ambulatory
4/52/M	I	R heel	5×7	N	Fem-pop ISSVG (5/85)	Scapular (6/85)	P	H	Ambulatory
5/47/M	I	L heel	5×5	T	Pop-DP ISSVG (6/85)	Serratus anterior +STSG (7/85)	P	H-R	Ambulatory
6/64/M	N	L ankle	4×4	T	Aortobifem (1/86); profundaplasty (1/86); fem-pop ISSVG (1/86)	Temporalis fascia +STSG (2/86)	P	H	Ambulatory
7/72/F	II	L ankle	7×10	T	Pop PTLA (3/86); pop-PT ISSVG (3/86)	Latissimus dorsi +STSG (3/86)	P	H	Ambulatory
8/71/M	II	R anterior lateral lower leg	7×12	S	Fem embolectomy (7/86); fem-AT ISSVG (8/86)	Scapular (8/86)	P	F	...
						Latissimus dorsi +STSG (8/86)	...	H	Ambulatory
9/34/M	I	L heel	6×8	T	AT PTLA (9/86)	Serratus anterior +STSG (12/86)	P	H-R	Ambulatory
10/49/F	I	L heel	2×3	N	Fem-AT ISSVG (4/87)	Rectus abdominis +STSG (4/87)	P	H	Ambulatory
11/62/F	I	R lateral foot	6×10	B	Fem-PT ISSVG (4/87)	Serratus anterior +STSG (4/87)	P	H	Ambulatory
12/72/M	II	L heel	4×4	N	Fem-peroneal ISSVG with branch to flap (4/87)	Serratus anterior +STSG (4/87)	P¶	F	Below-knee amputation
13/65/M	II	L pretibial	6×25	O	Fem-PT ISSVG (9/87)	Rectus abdominis +STSG (9/87)	P	H	Ambulatory
14/58/M	II	R heel	5×7	N	Iliac PTLA (2/88); Fem-pop ISSVG (5/88)	Ulnar+STSG (6/88)	P	H-R	Ambulatory

*I indicates type I (insulin dependent); II, type II (non–insulin dependent); and N, nondiabetic.
†N indicates neurotrophic; T, specific trauma; B, burn; O, chronic osteomyelitis; and S, unhealed surgical incision.
‡Pop indicates popliteal; DP, dorsal pedal; fem, femoral; AT, anterior tibial; PT, posterior tibial; RSVG, reversed saphenous vein graft; ISSVG, in situ saphenous vein graft; PTLA, percutaneous transluminal angiolasty; PTFE, polytef; AFB, aortobifemoral bypass; and thromb, thrombectomy.
§STSG indicates split-thickness skin graft.
‖P indicates patent (primary); P (2°), patent, secondary (after thrombectomy); P-R, patency maintained with later revision to prevent thrombosis; H, healed; H-R, healed after minor surgical revision; and F, failed.
¶Graft branch to peroneal artery occluded; graft branch to free flap patent.

flap placed 22 months previously. Ulcers had been present from 3 to 15 months, except in one site of tibial osteomyelitis, present for 58 years. Many had undergone previous unsuccessful attempts at closure with local flaps or split-thickness skin grafts (STSGs). Although all ulcers were associated with significant ischemia, the underlying cause was considered to be neuropathy in eight, direct trauma in four, chronic osteomyelitis in two, burn in one, and previous fasciotomy incision in one case. The heel was the most common location affected (10), followed by the ankle (three), anterior lower part of the leg (two), and lateral hindfoot (one). The smallest ulcer was 2×3 cm on the weight-bearing heel, while the largest ulcer measured 6×25 cm on the pretibial region at the site of chronic osteomyelitis. Mean (±SD) ulcer size was $5.1 \pm 1.2 \times 8.1 \pm 5.1$ cm (N=16).

Preoperative evaluation disclosed significant arterial insufficiency in all patients. Ankle-brachial indexes were routinely measured, but only four patients had compressible tibial arteries, with a mean ankle-brachial index of 0.34. All patients had poor monophasic or aphasic Doppler ankle waveforms and skin trophic changes consistent with advanced arterial disease. Four patients had previously undergone contralateral below-knee amputation but were ambulatory with a prosthesis.

Bypass grafts to the tibial or peroneal arteries were usually required to achieve adequate revascularization in these patients. Femorotibial/peroneal bypass was performed in seven limbs (five in situ saphenous vein grafts [ISSVGs], one reversed saphenous vein graft, and one polytef [PTFE] graft); popliteal-distal bypass in three limbs (two ISSVGs and one reversed saphenous vein graft); femoropopliteal bypass in four limbs (three ISSVGs and one polytef); and anterior tibial percutaneous transluminal angioplasty in one limb. Thus, of the 15 limbs in 14 patients, 11 (73%) required reconstruction at the infrapopliteal level. In addition to the principal arterial reconstruction done before the free flap transfer, six patients had undergone nine previous vascular interventions, including four proximal arterial reconstructions, two proximal percutaneous transluminal angioplasties, two proximal graft thrombectomies, and one previous embolectomy.

Muscular or fascial free flaps combined with STSGs, or fasciocutaneous free flaps, were used to obtain soft-tissue coverage in these patients. A separate surgical procedure for débridement of

Free Tissue Transfer

Follow-up Since Flap, mo	Final Outcome
22	Developed new ulcer in healed, weight-bearing flap; required 2nd flap procedure
37	Died 8/87 (sepsis, chronic renal failure)
22	...
21	Died 2/86 (myocardial infarction)
41	Current
38	Current (required interval contralateral below-knee amputation)
37	Current
30	Current
29	Current
...	Graft necrosis due to venous outflow thrombosis; required 2nd flap procedure
24	Current
20	Current
16	Current
4	Died 8/87 (stroke)
...	Flap viable but foot ischemic
11	Current
2	Current

the chronic ulcer and associated necrotic tendon or bone usually preceded free flap coverage. In only two cases were the free flap and arterial reconstructive procedures performed during the same operation. The mean interval between arterial reconstruction and free flap coverage was 13 days (median, 8 days) in our more recent (last 11) cases. This interval was used to establish the adequacy of arterial reconstruction and allow débridement and local care of the ulcer before free flap placement.

A total of 17 free flaps were placed in these patients. The scapular fasciocutaneous flap and the serratus anterior muscular flap combined with STSGs were used most frequently (five cases each), followed by the latissimus dorsi and rectus abdominis flaps (two cases each), and the gracilis muscle, ulnar fasciocutaneous, and temporalis fascia flaps in one case each. A two-team approach was used simultaneously to dissect the flap, débride the wound, and expose the recipient artery and vein. Microvascular anastomoses were performed with an operating microscope with the use of interrupted 9-0 polypropylene suture. Of the 17 free flaps, 8 were anastomosed to tibial arteries distal to the arterial reconstruction, while 9 were anastomosed directly to the saphenous vein bypass graft. Arterial anastomoses were end to side, while venous anastomoses were usually end to end to a deep system vein. Low-molecular-weight dextran was used perioperatively and aspirin was used postoperatively in an attempt to improve graft pedicle patency. Postoperatively, patients were usually kept at bed rest with extremity elevation for 2 weeks, then gradually allowed to increase extremity dependency, progressing to ambulation during the third and fourth weeks. Compressive elastic wrapping and heat-molded shoe inserts were used to protect the operative site from unnecessary trauma.

RESULTS

Of the 15 primary arterial reconstructions (including one percutaneous transluminal angioplasty), 14 (93%) remained patent to date (or until death), while 1 bifurcated femoroperoneal graft partially occluded, resulting in the only amputation in this review (patient 12, described in detail below). Of the 13 patent bypass grafts, 1 required a subsequent vein patch angioplasty of the popliteal anastomosis to prevent thrombosis (patient 1). One femoropopliteal PTFE graft occluded and required thrombectomy with PTFE graft extension to the infrageniculate popliteal artery to maintain secondary patency (patient 2). The mean ($\pm$SD) duration of graft patency to date was 26 ± 17 months. Duplex ultrasonography was useful for monitoring graft flow and velocity during follow-up, particularly when the free flap procedure precluded direct measurement of ankle or foot pressures. In each case, it was possible to image the arterial anastomosis of the free flap and to measure pedicle flow, which was 1 to 20 mL/min, with peak velocities of 21 to 127 cm/s (Fig 1, top).

Of the 17 free flaps, 12 (71%) healed primarily without further surgical intervention and 3 healed after minor surgical revision of the wound edges, for an 88% success rate. One scapular flap (patient 8) failed early due to venous outflow obstruction secondary to preexisting anterior tibial vein thrombosis that was initially unrecognized. Revision of this flap with a latissimus dorsi free flap with the use of the posterior tibial venous outflow resulted in primary flap healing. The only free flap that did not result in limb salvage was associated with severe, progressive ischemia of the surrounding part of the foot that required below-knee amputation despite a viable free flap and patent arterial graft (patient 12; see below). Of the 16 ulcers treated in 14 patients, 15 (94%) healed completely, resulting in limb salvage during follow-up of 4 to 38 months (mean$\pm$SD, 24 ± 12 months) after free flap transfer. Weight-bearing ambulation was achieved in 13 (93%) of 14 patients 1 to 6 weeks after free flap coverage, although several patients required continued assistance (eg, use of a walker) due to underlying health problems.

There were no postoperative deaths after the vascular or plastic surgical procedures. Three patients experienced uncomplicated myocardial infarction after their free flap procedures. These infarcts did not delay ambulation, since the mobilization regimen after free tissue transfer coincided with normal cardiac rehabilitation. During follow-up, one patient (7%) required a below-knee amputation of the contralateral leg due to severe distal ischemia. Three of the 14 patients died a mean interval of 21 months after free flap placement due to complications of diabetes or cardiac disease. All were ambulatory with patent bypass grafts and healed free flaps at the time of death.

REPORT OF CASES

Case 7.—A 72-year-old, ambulatory, diabetic woman sustained an avulsion injury to the left ankle in a motor vehicle accident. This resulted in a 7×10-cm nonhealing ulcer over the lateral malleolus with osteomyelitis of the distal fibula (Fig 2, top left). An attempt to obtain skin coverage with an STSG failed at another hospital. Four months after her initial injury, she was referred to our institution, where arteriography demonstrated localized stenoses of the midsuperficial femoral and popliteal arteries, occlusion of the proximal tibial and peroneal arteries, and reconstitution of a distal posterior tibial artery.

She underwent percutaneous transluminal angioplasty of the

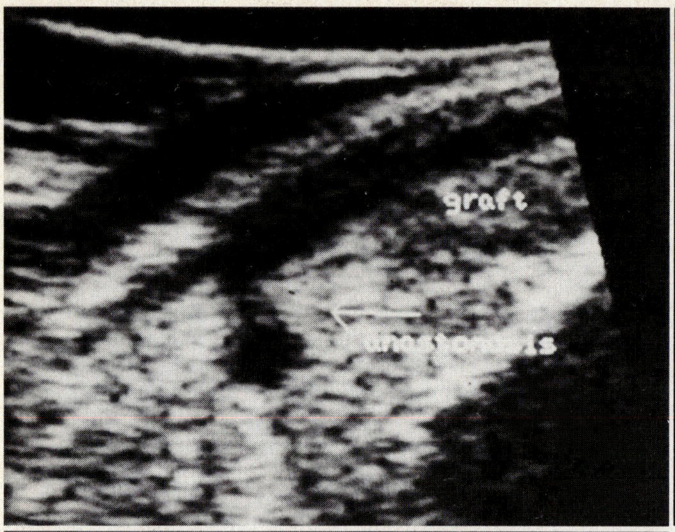

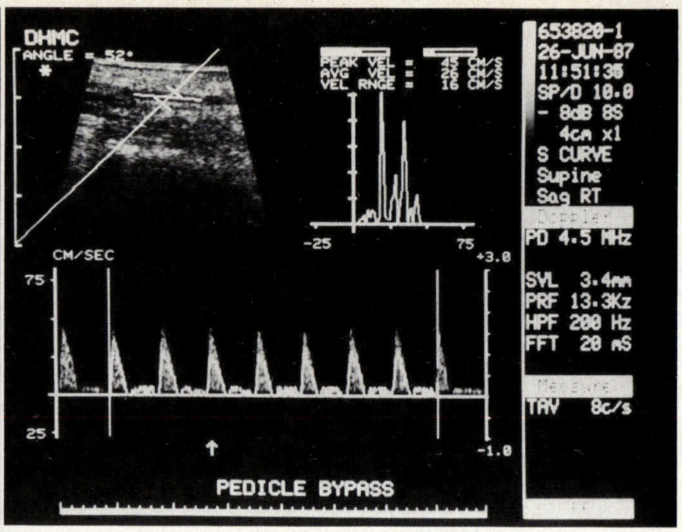

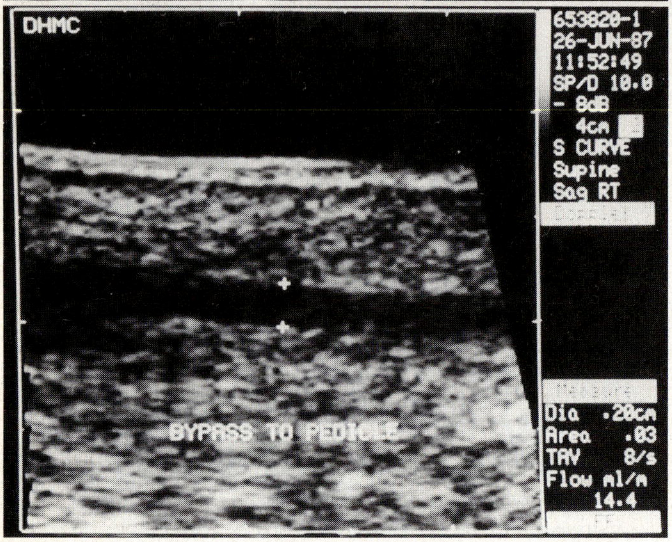

Fig 1.—Duplex ultrasound evaluation of arterial flow in free flap pedicles. Top left, Image of the microvascular anastomosis between the thoracodorsal artery of a latissimus dorsi free flap and a popliteal–posterior tibial vein graft. Top right, Velocity measurement in the thoracodorsal artery of a serratus anterior free flap with the use of a duplex imager, (Diasonic DRF 400, Diasonic Inc, Milpitas, Calif) with a 10-mHz imaging probe and a 4.5-mHz pulsed Doppler. A peak velocity of 45 cm/s was recorded. Bottom, Time-averaged volume flow of 14.4 mL/min was recorded in this 2-mm-diameter artery.

superficial femoral and popliteal stenoses followed by an ISSVG from the below-knee popliteal artery to the posterior tibial artery at the malleolar level. The ankle ulcer was débrided, including the tendons of peroneus longus and brevis, extensor digitorum communis, and osteomyelitis in the distal fibula, lateral tibia, and talus (Fig 2, top right). One week later, a latissimus dorsi free flap was transferred to obtain wound coverage, and an STSG was applied. The thoracodorsal artery was anastomosed end to side to the previously placed ISSVG. Although an uncomplicated myocardial infarction occurred postoperatively, weight bearing ambulation was achieved with assistance after 4 weeks and independent ambulation within 2 months of flap placement. The patient remained ambulatory with a healed free flap after 29 months of follow-up (Fig 2, bottom).

The location, size, tendon necrosis, and underlying osteomyelitis would normally have prevented primary healing of this wound despite adequate revascularization. Arterial reconstruction combined with adequate débridement allowed early free flap coverage and prompt rehabilitation. Although the myocardial infarction was uncomplicated, it emphasizes the need for aggressive cardiac evaluation and management in these elderly diabetic patients.

Case 12.—A 72-year-old diabetic man required a right below-knee amputation for severe distal ischemia that was not reconstructible. While convalescing from that procedure, he developed a pressure-induced neurotrophic ulcer on the posterior aspect of his left heel that gradually enlarged to a 4×4-cm ulcer that exposed the calcaneus. Arteriography revealed diffuse atherosclerotic disease in the superficial femoral and popliteal arteries, occlusion of the tibial and peroneal arteries, and reconstitution of only the distal medial branch of the peroneal artery. Although the distal arterial outflow was poor, the remainder of the foot was viable, and an attempt at conserving his remaining foot was made. The patient underwent right femorodistal peroneal bypass with an ISSVG. The distal end of the vein bifurcated, enabling anastomosis of one limb to the medial branch of the peroneal artery, with end-to-end anastomosis of the other limb to a serratus anterior muscle flap during the same procedure. An STSG was applied. Postoperatively, the femoroperoneal graft flow measured by duplex ultrasound decreased from 42 mL/min to 6 mL/min on the third postoperative day, when the vein graft branch to the peroneal artery occluded. The vein graft remained patent, however, with a palpable pulse and flow of 4 to 6 mL/min to the free flap itself. During the subsequent 2 months the foot became progressively more ischemic, and, despite viability of the free flap, the incision did not heal. Progressive ischemia of the foot led to below-knee amputation 2 months after the initial procedure. At the time of amputation, the femoral–free flap bypass was patent and the free flap completely viable.

Very low graft blood flow, achieved only from outflow into a muscular free flap, maintained distal ISSVG patency for at least 2 months in this patient. However, the inability to revascularize successfully the remainder of the foot precluded a successful outcome. The presence of a viable free flap did not allow healing of the flap-foot suture line and did not transfer any additional vascularity to the

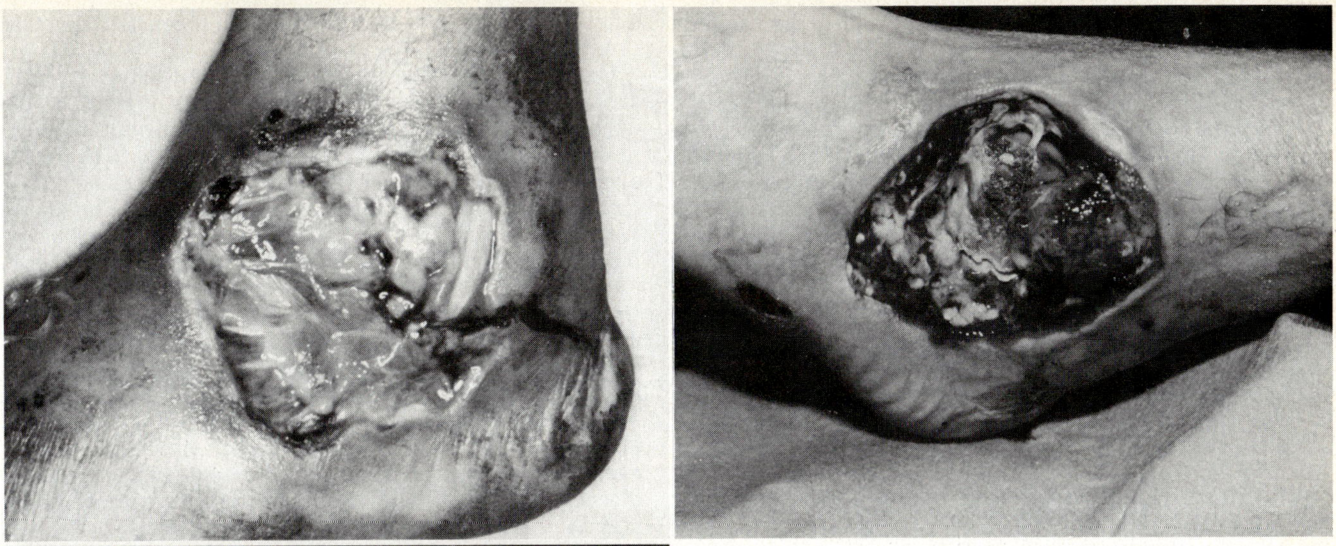

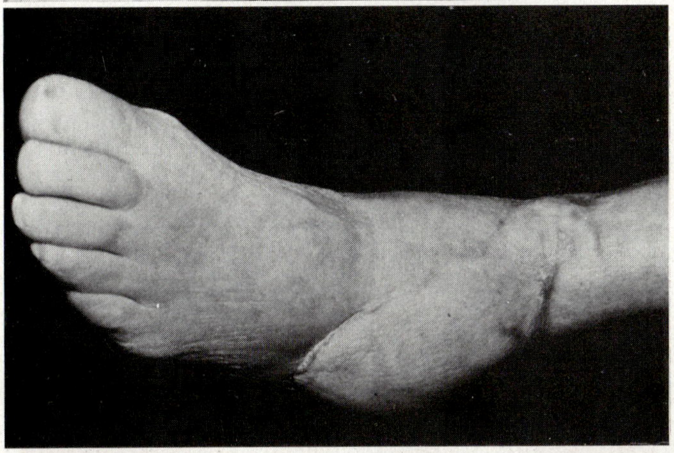

Fig 2.—Top left, Traumatic ankle ulcer in a 72-year-old diabetic woman with popliteal-tibial occlusive disease (patient 7). Tendons were exposed and osteomyelitis was present. Top right, Operative débridement of wound edges, tendons, and infected fibula, lateral tibia, and talus was performed after popliteal–posterior tibial bypass. Bottom, A latissimus dorsi free flap and skin graft were used to cover this defect. Complete healing was achieved, shown here 2 months postoperatively.

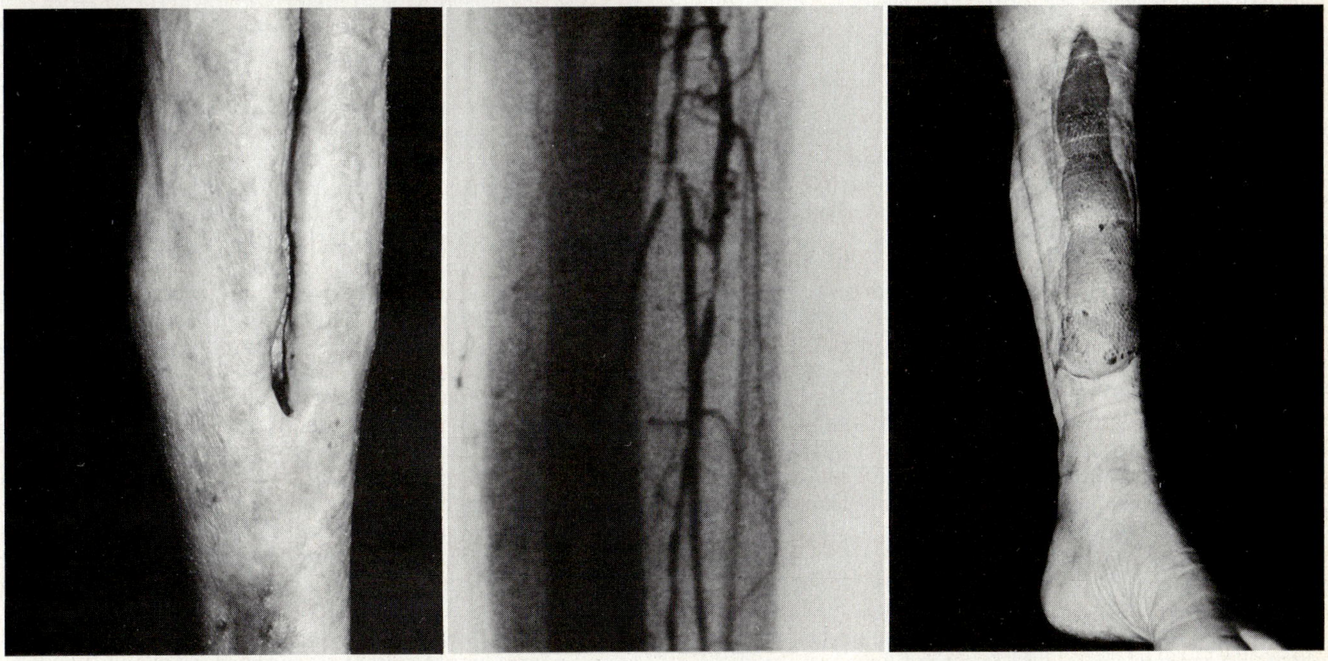

Fig 3.—Left, Chronic lower-leg ulcer associated with tibial osteomyelitis that had been present for 58 years and resisted multiple previous attempts to achieve local healing in a 65-year-old diabetic man (patient 13). Center, Tibial-peroneal occlusive disease shown in this distal subtraction arteriogram prevented free flap transfer without revascularization. Therefore, a femoral–distal posterior tibial in situ saphenous vein bypass was performed. Right, During the same procedure a rectus abdominis free flap, shown here postoperatively, was transferred with anastomosis directly to the vein bypass graft. Complete healing resulted without evidence of further infection.

ischemic foot during this interval. Since this is the single failure in our series to date, we must conclude that successful revascularization of the remaining extremity is essential. When this is in doubt, we would now advocate delaying the free flap placement until adequate revascularization has been proved. In this particular case, the arterial outflow was judged so tenuous that the procedures were purposely combined at the same operation to improve graft flow by providing the free flap anastomosis. Although the free flap maintained ISSVG patency, it did not improve foot ischemia, which led to amputation.

CASE 13.—A 65-year-old ambulatory diabetic man presented with purulent drainage from a 7 × 25-cm pretibial wound associated with chronic tibial osteomyelitis that had resulted from a childhood injury. This wound had been present for 58 years despite multiple previous surgical débridements and attempted closures (Fig 3, left). The patient had no symptoms of claudication, rest pain, or more distal tissue loss, but he had intermittent cellulitis and chronic drainage. Arteriography demonstrated diffuse superficial femoral artery occlusive disease and severe tibial-peroneal stenoses with reconstitution of the distal posterior tibial artery (Fig 3, center). After operative débridement of the chronic tibial osteomyelitis, the patient underwent a femoral–distal posterior tibial bypass with the use of vein segments from both legs. During the same operation, a rectus abdominis muscle flap based on the inferior epigastric vessels was anastomosed directly to the vein graft. An STSG was applied (Fig 3, right). Primary healing occurred and allowed independent ambulation within 2 weeks. This ulcer remained healed without evidence of recurrent drainage or cellulitis 11 months after free flap coverage.

This patient did not meet the conventional indications for arterial reconstruction. Although lower-extremity ischemia may have contributed to poor healing, it did not directly jeopardize the patient's more distal extremity. However, the popliteal, tibial, and peroneal arteries were sufficiently diseased that they would not allow satisfactory free flap arterial anastomosis. The saphenous vein bypass was constructed to allow direct arterial anastomosis of the free flap pedicle necessary for reconstruction of this chronic wound.

COMMENT

Lower-extremity revascularization combined with free tissue transfer is appropriate only for a small subgroup of patients with threatened limb loss. These patients are usually diabetic, with large, deep ulcers on the hindfoot or ankle that have developed in association with peripheral neuropathy. Many similar patients develop forefoot ulcers that are best treated with local plastic procedures or distal amputations and do not require free tissue transfer after revascularization.[7] Similarly, ulcers in many patients with less extensive tissue loss heal primarily after revascularization or after STSG application. Diabetic patients with neurotrophic ulcers and adequate arterial circulation are candidates for free tissue transfer without revascularization.[5] These subgroups must be clearly differentiated from patients in whom combined revascularization and free tissue transfer is required.

When initially evaluating patients with extensive lower-leg tissue loss, it is important to assess their need for arterial revascularization before contemplating free tissue transfer. We have performed initial revascularization when the ankle-brachial index was less than 0.70 and the distal ankle Doppler waveforms less than good biphasic quality. Because of this approach, we have not rigorously defined whether less adequate arterial inflow could sustain long-term flap healing. However, using these criteria, we have not yet experienced free flap failure due to inadequate arterial inflow, whether or not arterial reconstruction was required.[8]

Contemporary reports of infrapopliteal arterial reconstruction demonstrate limb salvage rates of 80% to 92% during 2 to 3 years of follow-up.[9-13] These include patients in whom distal anastomoses must be extended to the ankle or foot level. Despite this success rate, extensive tissue loss may preclude healing. Such wounds in the distal extremity are difficult to manage because little skin and muscle are available for local flap procedures.[4,6] Since muscles in the midcalf that are potentially available for transfer are supplied by proximal arteries, their distal rotation is limited. Conversely, free tissue transfer provides several significant benefits in the distal part of the leg. Since muscular, fascial, or fasciocutaneous flaps can be selected according to the size of a specific defect, it is possible to débride chronic granulation tissue adequately, even though this requires enlargement of the primary ulcer. Coverage of weight-bearing defects with the substantial bulk of a muscular flap has usually prevented subsequent ulceration even with insensate flaps, while previous STSGs failed despite early healing.[2-4] Application of a well-vascularized free flap also promotes healing in the presence of local infection.[4,6] Finally, free tissue transfer provides additional arterial outflow, which may enhance vascular graft patency and aid healing of immediately surrounding tissue if neovascularization from the free flap occurs.

Flap selection in our patients was dictated by the specific requirements of each ulcer. Patients with osteomyelitis underwent free muscle transfer (and STSG) since this technique has proved effective in the definitive treatment of bone infection.[14] Ulcers without osteomyelitis were covered with fascial or muscle flaps (plus STSG) or fasciocutaneous flaps, as dictated by the required length of the vascular pedicle and the size and location of the defect. Donor flaps were harvested above the waist when possible to avoid atherosclerosis in donor pedicle arteries from the thigh. No attempt was made to use sensate flaps due to the severe diabetic peripheral neuropathy present in most patients.

Free tissue transfer is now a standard technique for closing soft-tissue defects. In wounds associated with trauma or chronic infection, 93% of all free flaps, and 81% to 82% of lower-extremity free flaps, achieve successful healing when adequate arterial inflow is present.[2-4] We are aware of only one previous report describing the successful treatment of four patients by means of combined distal arterial reconstruction and free tissue transfer.[15] However, the high success rates of distal arterial reconstruction and lower-extremity free tissue transfer done separately support the results obtained in our series.

A legitimate concern in these patients is whether primary amputation with subsequent prosthetic rehabilitation would be more appropriate than revascularization plus free tissue transfer. In some patients, revascularization is necessary even to achieve amputation healing. Although 100% rehabilitation has been reported in selected amputation centers,[16] rehabilitation rates of 64% to 67% are more commonly achieved after below-knee amputation.[17,18] Furthermore, in patients with bilateral below-knee amputation, rehabilitation is only half as successful.[18] Subsequent contralateral amputation is required in approximately 50% of surviving patients within 2 years of an initial major amputation.[19] The percentage of diabetic patients requiring subsequent amputation is even higher, as is the development of serious contralateral foot infection, which approaches 50% within 2 years of initial diabetic foot infection.[20] In our series, 29% of patients had already undergone contralateral amputation, and 10% required this during follow-up. Thus, we believe that an aggressive limb salvage effort was appropriate in our patients and is supported by the 93% successful rehabilitation that was achieved. Close collaboration of vascular and plastic surgeons is essential to achieve this success in patients previously considered only for amputation. We believe that this is a valuable approach for a selected subgroup of patients with severe lower-extremity ischemic tissue loss.

References

1. Daniel RK, Talor GI. Distant transfer of an island flap by microvascular anastomosis. *Plast Reconstr Surg.* 1973;52:111-117.
2. Shaw WW. Microvascular free flaps: the first decade. *Clin Plast Surg.* 1983;10:3-19.
3. Swartz WM, Mears DC. The role of free-tissue transfers in lower extremity reconstruction. *Plast Reconstr Surg.* 1985;76:364-373.
4. Zubowicz VN, Coleman JJ III. Treatment of severe leg wounds with muscle and musculocutaneous flaps. *Arch Surg.* 1984;119:921-925.
5. Dabb RW, Davis RM. Latissimus dorsi free flaps in the elderly: an alternative to below-knee amputation. *Plast Reconstr Surg.* 1984;73:633-640.
6. May JW Jr, Gallico GG III, Lukash FN. Microvascular transfer of free tissue for closure of bone wounds of the distal lower extremity. *N Engl J Med.* 1982;306:253-257.
7. Morain WD, Dellon AL, MacKinnon SE, Colen LB. Current concepts in plastic surgery for the diabetic. *Adv Plast Reconstr Surg.* 1987;4:1-36.
8. Colen LB. Limb salvage in the patient with severe peripheral vascular disease: the role of microsurgical free-tissue transfer. *Plast Reconstr Surg.* 1987;79:389-395.
9. Karmody AM, Leather RP, Shah DM, Corson JD, Naraynsingh V. Peroneal artery bypass: a reappraisal of its value in limb salvage. *J Vasc Surg.* 1984;1:809-816.
10. Taylor LM Jr, Phinney ES, Porter JM. Present status of reversed vein bypass for lower extremity revascularization. *J Vasc Surg.* 1986;3:288-297.
11. Maini BS, Mannick JA. Effect of arterial reconstruction on limb salvage: a 10-year appraisal. *Arch Surg.* 1978;113:1297-1304.
12. Andros G, Harris RW, Salles-Cunha SX, Dulawa LB, Oblath RW, Apyan RL. Bypass grafts to the ankle and foot. *J Vasc Surg.* 1988;7:785-794.
13. Buchbinder D, Pasch AR, Rollins DL, et al. Results of arterial reconstruction of the foot. *Arch Surg.* 1986;121:673-677.
14. Mathes SJ, Alpert BS, Chang N. Use of the muscle flap in chronic osteomyelitis: experimental and clinical correlation. *Plast Reconstr Surg.* 1982;69:815-829.
15. Briggs SE, Banis JC, Kaebnick H, Silverberg B, Acland RD. Distal revascularization and microvascular free tissue transfer: an alternative to amputation in ischemic lesions of the lower extremity. *J Vasc Surg.* 1985;2:806-811.
16. Malone JM, Moore W, Leal JM, Childers SJ. Rehabilitation for lower extremity amputation. *Arch Surg.* 1981;116:93-98.
17. Hobson RW II, Lynch TG, Jamil Z, et al. Results of revascularization and amputation in severe lower extremity ischemia: a five-year experience. *J Vasc Surg.* 1985;2:174-185.
18. Couch NP, David JK, Tilney NL, Crane C. Natural history of the leg amputee. *Am J Surg.* 1977;133:469-473.
19. Bodily KC, Burgess EM. Contralateral limb and patient survival after leg amputation. *Am J Surg.* 1983;146:280-282.
20. Kucan JO, Robson MC. Diabetic foot infections: fate of the contralateral foot. *Plast Reconstr Surg.* 1986;77:439-441.

Discussion

Bruce S. Cutler, MD, Worcester, Mass: Dr Cronenwett and his group are to be congratulated for having successfully combined two recently developed surgical techniques: the in situ saphenous vein bypass graft and the free musculocutaneous tissue graft, to produce a powerful new method for salvaging extremities with large tissue defects. We have also had some experience with combined arterial reconstruction and free tissue transfer at the University of Massachusetts over the past 4 years. Our series includes seven lower and two upper extremities. Healed, stable, nonpainful wounds have been achieved in seven of the nine patients.

One of our patients was a 48-year-old man with Buerger's disease who had amputation of portions of the second through fifth fingers of both hands. He developed ischemic rest pain of the left hand and an ulceration of the thumb. An arteriogram showed occlusion of the radial and ulnar arteries just above the wrist. He underwent a combined revascularization and free tissue transfer procedure. The plastic surgery team raised a vascularized serratus muscle flap, while we performed an orthograde devalved saphenous vein graft from the brachial artery to the arterial pedicle of the free graft at the wrist with the use of an end-to-end anastomosis. It was then covered with a meshed split-thickness graft. A year later, his entire hand, not just the free graft, was pink and warm with prompt capillary blood flow. Cutaneous fluorescein quantitative blood flow studies of the palm of the hand now exceeded a reference point in the axilla. Remember that the anastomosis of the free graft to the saphenous vein was end to end, so that the only way that there could be improved blood flow to the ischemic portion of the hand was through linking of capillaries between the free graft and the palm of the hand. An arteriogram obtained 1 year postoperatively showed "corkscrew" arterioles, which we believe represent new vessels growing in from the tissue graft to the ischemic hand.

My question for Dr Cronenwett is this: Have you made any similar observations regarding neovascularization of ischemic tissue from free tissue grafts?

Frank W. LoGerfo, MD, Boston, Mass: We recently presented our results with lower-extremity arterial reconstruction in diabetic patients, showing that we can obtain excellent long-term results with a vein graft patency rate of 89% at 4 years. I think we really have solved the problem of distal arterial reconstruction in the diabetic patient, with many of these grafts extending to the distal tibial or pedal arteries. But the remaining problems are those of tissue necrosis and wound coverage. We have had a similar experience at the New England Deaconess Hospital, Boston, with local flaps rather than free grafts in the diabetic foot, and these flaps have been very successful in areas that are non–weight bearing. However, we have had some difficulty in maintaining healing in flaps that are placed on the weight-bearing surface. I wonder if the authors could comment on that.

The other area where I see this coming along as an improved modality of treatment is the area of trauma. I wonder if they have had any experience in using these techniques in the trauma patient.

Dr. Cronenwett: Although I agree with Dr Cutler that free flap transfer can improve blood flow in adjacent tissue by neovascularization, this effect will not be immediate. On the basis of our single failure, we have concluded that free flap healing will not occur without sufficient vascularity in the tissue adjacent to the flap. We have recently obtained an arteriogram in a patient 1 year after distal bypass and free flap placement and have seen evidence of late neovascularization of the foot adjacent to the free flap.

We have not staged the revascularization and tissue transfer in all of our patients. In fact, we did not stage our one case that ultimately failed, since we hoped that early neovascularization might improve limb salvage. However, staging does have the benefit of allowing you to ensure patency of the arterial bypass before you subject the patient to a long and difficult free flap procedure. In addition, staging allows you to débride and better care for the revascularized ulcer before placing the flap. Because of these factors, we try to make that decision on an individual basis.

We also prefer the latissimus dorsi flap, but we use the serratus anterior flap when a longer pedicle is required. Both of these flaps are harvested with the thoracodorsal pedicle, but the serratus flap provides a longer pedicle that is useful if you have done a femoropopliteal graft and have to use a proximal tibial artery rather than a distal vein graft as the recipient artery for a heel or ankle flap.

We have not had difficulty with weight-bearing areas except in one patient; after a successful flap was applied to the heel, this patient had ulceration of the flap 22 months later and required a second flap. This was obviously a neurotrophic situation. We have, however, insisted on a relatively strict 3-week period of nonambulation in patients with flaps applied to weight-bearing surfaces to try to ensure initial healing. We have used free flap techniques in trauma patients, but this series reviewed only those free flaps combined with revascularization.

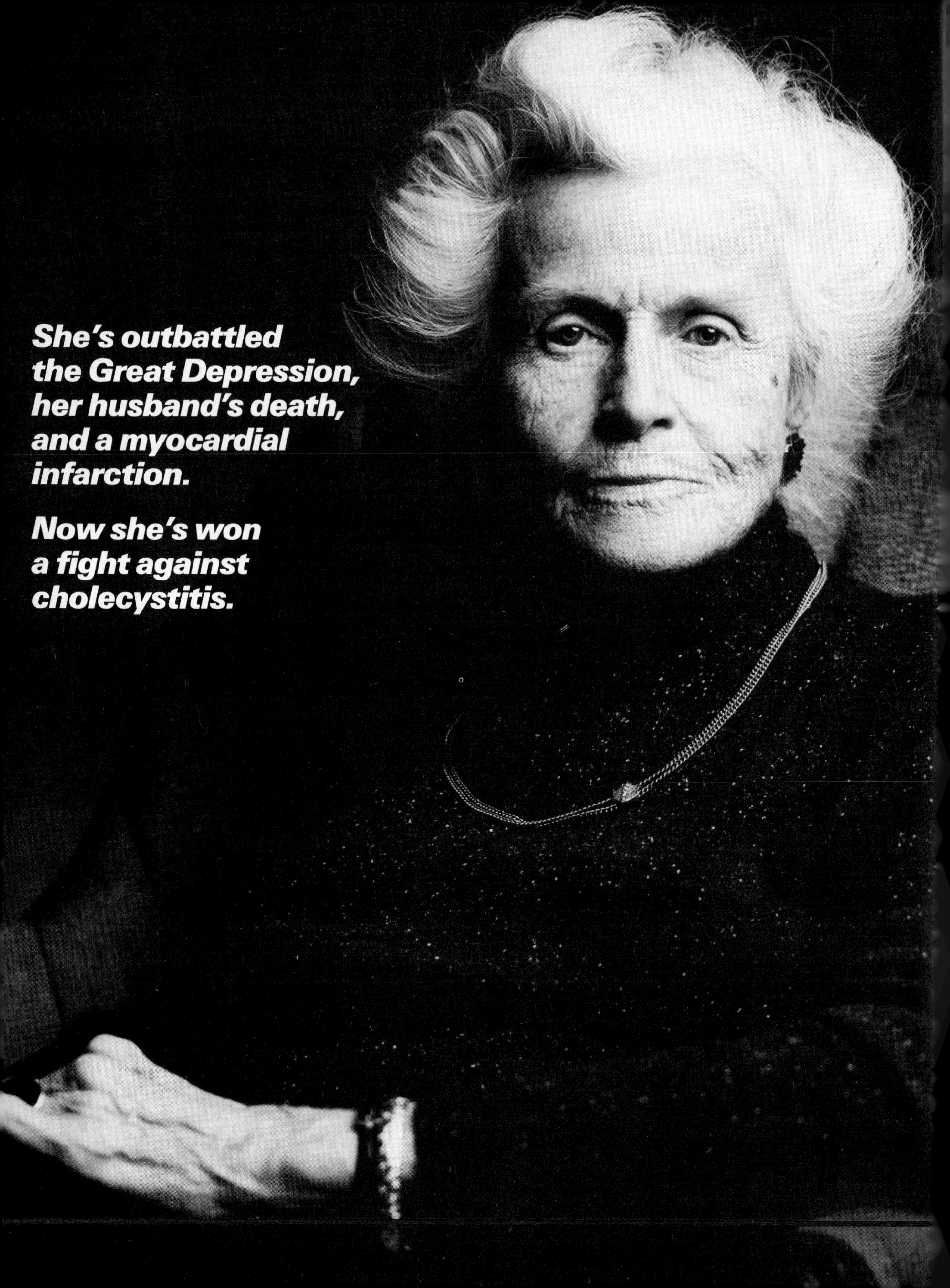
She's outbattled the Great Depression, her husband's death, and a myocardial infarction.
Now she's won a fight against cholecystitis.

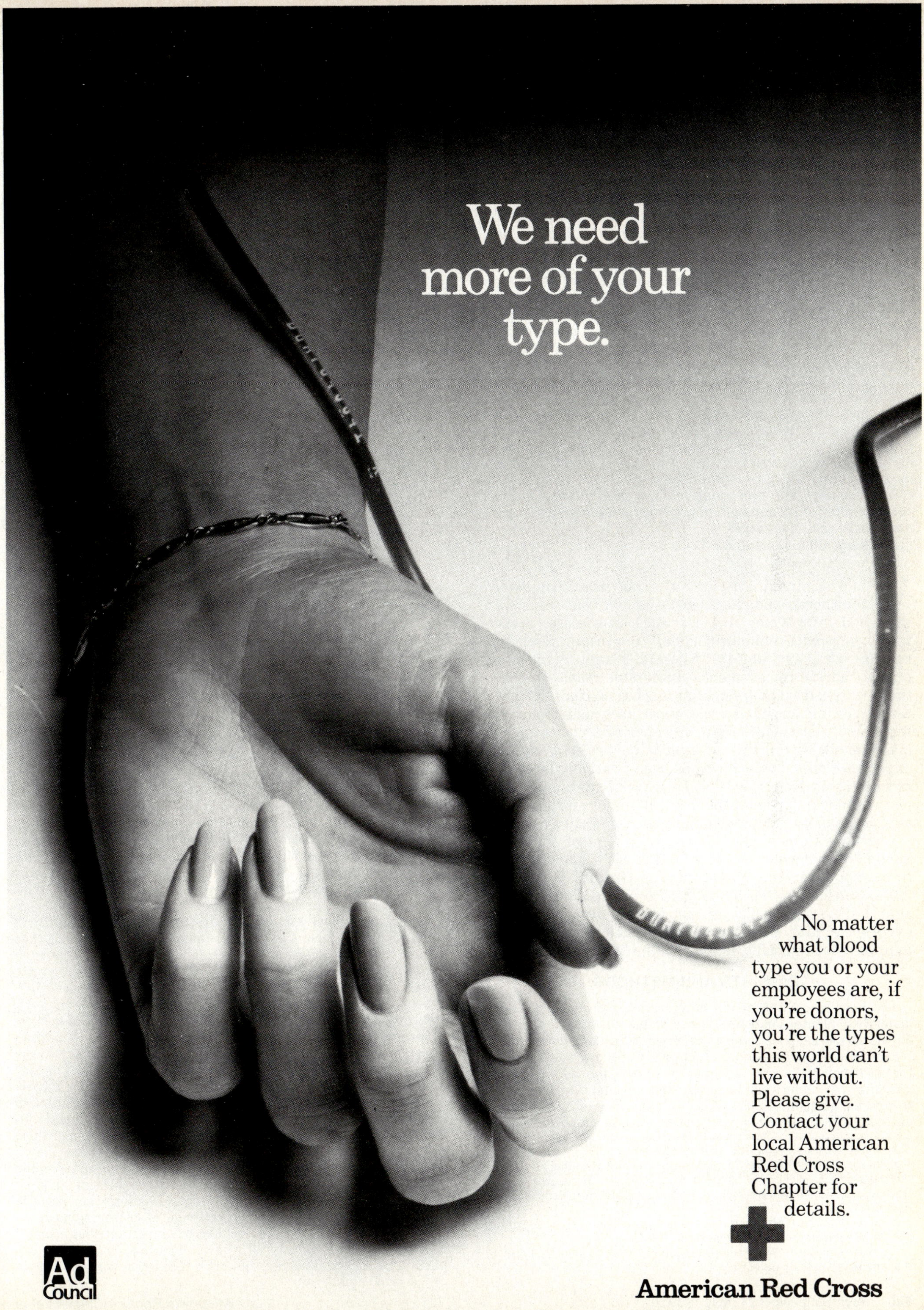
We need more of your type.
No matter what blood type you or your employees are, if you're donors, you're the types this world can't live without. Please give. Contact your local American Red Cross Chapter for details.
American Red Cross
Ad Council

Recent Experience With Thoracoabdominal Aneurysm Repair

Richard P. Cambria, MD; David C. Brewster, MD; Ashby C. Moncure, MD;
Bengt Ivarsson, MD; R. Clement Darling, MD; J. Kenneth Davison, MD; William M. Abbott, MD

• Thoracoabdominal aneurysm repair was carried out in 55 patients during the period from January 1978 to June 1988. Considering the volume of experience and application of a routine for preoperative and intraoperative management, the experience was divided as follows: group 1 1978 to 1985 (26 patients) and group 2 1985 to 1988 (29 patients). Clinical features of the two groups differed only in the incidence of emergency operations (group 1 [6/18, 30%] vs group 2 [2/29, 8%]). Operative mortality in elective operations improved substantially in recent experience (group 1 [50%] vs group 2 [7.4%]). Significant reductions in total operative time, operative blood loss, and total aortic cross-clamping times paralleled and, in part, explained the improvement in overall surgical results seen in group 2 patients. Spinal cord injury occurred in 7.2% of the entire cohort. Nonfatal but major complications occurred in 25% of group 2 patients, with the most common being prolonged ventilatory assistance (12%). Current results with thoracoabdominal aneurysm repair both establish its safety and help to provide guidelines in selecting patients for elective repair.
(*Arch Surg.* 1989;124:620-624)

While relatively uncommon, aneurysms that involve the thoracoabdominal aorta, and/or that segment of the aorta from which the visceral vessels arise, present the surgeon with a unique challenge to prevent death from rupture while avoiding the potential complications of extensive aortic replacement. Successful management of these extensive aneurysms on a routine basis is now a reality, owing largely to the experience and techniques reported by Crawford.[1] Yet, correction of a thoracoabdominal aneurysm remains a formidable undertaking, and experience outside Houston has been relatively limited. A recent report from the Mayo Clinic while detailing excellent results, emphasized the frequent major morbidity that may accompany thoracoabdominal aortic replacement.[2]

Crawford's techniques for the treatment of thoracoabdominal aneurysms were reported in 1974, and they were first applied at the Massachusetts General Hospital in 1978. Considering both the numbers of patients treated and the overall results of surgical therapy, our recent experience with thoracoabdominal aneurysm repair has improved substantially, and forms the basis of this report.

PATIENTS AND METHODS

The hospital and surgeon's office records of all patients who underwent thoracoabdominal aortic replacement for aneurysm during the period from January 1978 (when the Crawford inclusion technique was first utilized) to June 1988 were reviewed. However, the inclusion technique was not routinely applied until 1985. Patients who underwent reconstruction for stenotic disease due to aortitis, acute aortic dissection, or bypassing of infection were excluded. Patients with a pararenal or suprarenal aneurysm, not extending to the diaphragm but approached with thoracoabdominal incisions, were also excluded. A total of 55 patients underwent operations, 45 of which were elective procedures, and 10 were performed urgently for ruptured (n=6) or acutely symptomatic (n=4) aneurysms. The volume of experience, routine adoption of the techniques popularized by Crawford,[1] and routine intraoperative management by a specialized anesthesia team permitted the convenient division of the total experience into two time intervals, hereafter referred to as group 1 (1978 to 1985) and group 2 (1986 to June 1988) (Fig 1). In group 1, there were 18 elective and 8 urgent procedures, while the respective figures for group 2 were 27 and 2. Clinical and demographic characteristics of the groups 1 and 2 patients were similar and are summarized as follows:

Characteristic	Value
Mean age/y	66
Sex ratio, M/F	36/19, 2/1
Smoking, % (No.)	84 (46/55)
Hypertension, %	73
History of coronary artery disease, %	40
Associated visceral occlusive disease, %	45
History of infrarenal aortic aneurysm repair, % (No.)	25 (14/55)

Notable among these characteristics were the frequency of associated visceral occlusive disease, prior infrarenal aneurysm repair, and an excess of female patients when compared with the known preponderance of male patients when considering infrarenal abdominal aortic aneurysms.

Most aneurysms were degenerative (atherosclerotic) in nature, with only four patients (7%) having a chronic aneurysm secondary to an old aortic dissection. Aneurysms were classified by the segments of the aorta involved according to the scheme of Crawford: type I, most of the descending thoracic and upper abdominal aorta; type II, left subclavian to aortic bifurcation; type III, distal descending thoracic aorta and varying segments of the abdominal aorta; and type IV, total abdominal aorta. The distribution of patients by aneurysm type is summarized in Fig 2. This classification is useful in discussing certain technical aspects of operation, in addition to stratifying the risk for spinal cord injury. Surgery in the 26 group 1 patients was inconsistent with respect to use of the inclusion technique (20, yes; 6, no), and intraoperative heparin was used in nine patients. A Gott shunt was used in four group 1 patients. Group 2 patients all were operated on without systemic heparin/shunts/bypasses and with the Crawford[1] inclusion technique. Current diagnostic modalities include the complementary (not competitive) use of computed tomographic scanning and complete aortography. Magnetic resonance imaging scanning has been useful in recent experience if a question of aortic dissection is raised.[3]

Anesthetic management is standardized and involves a high-dose narcotic technique as the primary anesthetic. A double-lumen endotracheal tube is mandatory for all type I and type II aneurysm repairs. Monitoring includes a right radial artery catheter and pulmonary artery thermodilution catheter. Hypertension, associated with proximal clamping, is managed with sodium nitroprusside and nitroglycerin. Sodium bicarbonate infusion is started, and further needs are met at unclamping. Blood pressure support during unclamping is augmented with phenylephrine or dopamine. Other currently employed adjunts include continuous cold (4°C) perfusion of renal arteries during clamping, liberal use of mannitol, use of albumin-impregnated vascular grafts, and intrathecal catheter drainage of cerebrospinal fluid (last 15 patients) for whatever spinal cord protection it may confer. Reimplantation of intercostal arteries has been irregularly applied. The technical aspects of aortic reconstruction are largely

Accepted for publication December 14, 1988.
From the Surgical Service, Massachusetts General Hospital, Boston and the Departments of Surgery (Drs Cambria, Brewster, Moncure, Ivarsson, Darling, and Abbott) and Anesthesia (Dr Davison), Harvard Medical School, Boston, Mass.
Read before the 69th Annual Meeting of the New England Surgical Society, Montreal, Canada, September 18, 1988.
Reprint requests to Massachusetts General Hospital, 15 Parkman St, Boston, MA 02114 (Dr Cambria).

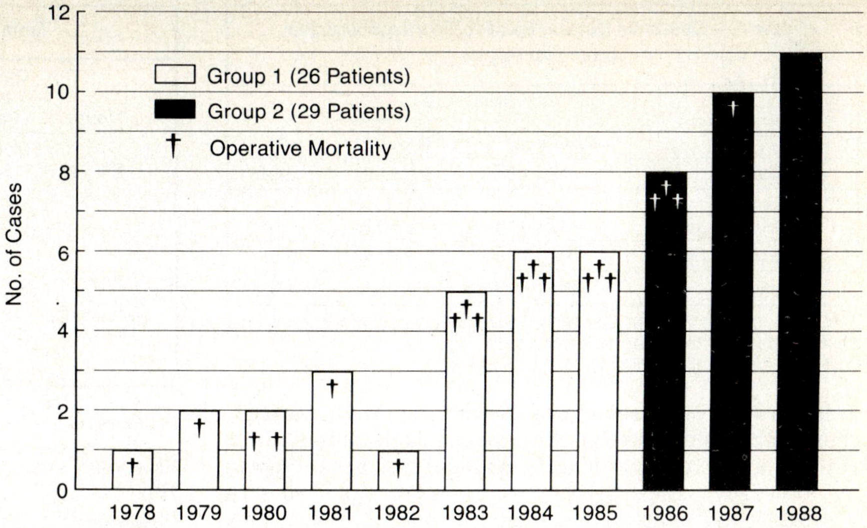

Fig 1.—Experience with thoracoabdominal aneurysm repair as function of time with attendant operative mortality.

dictated by the extent of the aneurysm and generally follow those precepts advocated by Crawford. At the end of the procedure, an oral or nasal endotracheal tube replaces the double-lumen endotracheal tube, and postoperative ventilatory support is planned. Intrathecal narcotic is injected through the cerebrospinal fluid catheter, which is then removed.

Statistical analysis was done by means of Student's unpaired *t* test and Fisher's Exact Test.

RESULTS

Operative Details

As noted above, application of the inclusion technique and avoidance of systemic heparin and shunts were routine in group 2 patients. Other details of surgery, including operative time, blood loss, and cross-clamp times for elective operations, are displayed in Table 1. All of these variables showed improvement with increasing experience in group 2 patients as compared with those in group 1.

Operative Mortality

Salvage was rare when an operation was conducted for rupture or acute expansion, and considering the entire experience, 8 of 10 such patients died. There was a distinct improvement in operative mortality when group 2 patients were compared with our earlier experience. When both elective and urgent operations were included, operative mortality in group 1 vs group 2 was 57% vs 13% ($P<.001$). Since a larger percentage of earlier operations were conducted in the presence of rupture, it is useful also to examine operative mortality in strictly elective cases. The improvement over time remains dramatic in that 9 (50%) of 18 group 1 patients died after an operation, while only 2 (7.4%) of 27 group 2 patients failed to survive surgery. This improvement in operative survival was highly significant ($P<.003$). Causes of perioperative mortality are detailed in Table 2. While hemorrhage will always be a problem in ruptured aneurysms, the early experience was notable for a 22% (4/18) mortality in elective cases due to intraoperative or perioperative hemorrhage. In group 2 patients, this had been reduced substantially to less than 4% (1/27).

Postoperative Complications

Among patients who survived an operation, major complications occurred in 4 of 11 group 1 and 5 of 25 group 2 patients. The most common complication was the requirement for prolonged (>5 days) ventilatory assistance, which was necessary in 36% of group 1 and 12% of group 2 patients. A tracheostomy was required in all of these patients, but eventual weaning from respiratory assistance was universal. In the recent experience, contributing

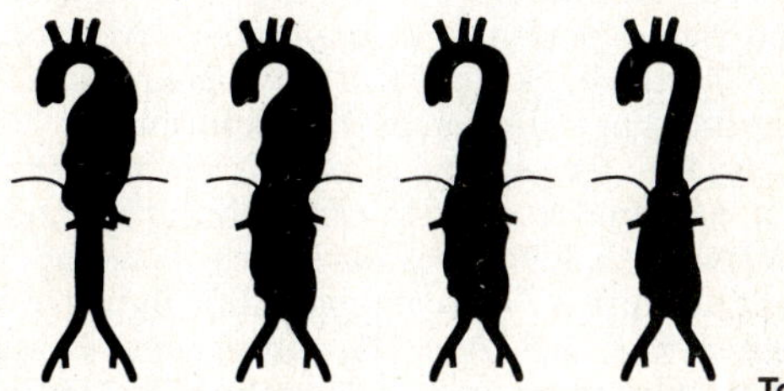

	Type I	Type II	Type III	Type IV	Total
Group 1	7	4	11	4	**26**
Group 2	5	4	9	11	**29**
Total	**12**	**8**	**20**	**15**	**55**

Fig 2.—Distribution of patients by aneurysm type.

factors to respiratory failure included one instance each of severe preoperative respiratory compromise, concomitant renal failure, and postoperative paraplegia.

Paraplegia or paraparesis occurred in four patients (7.2%) in the entire series. Two of these patients died, with the spinal cord injury contributing to postoperative respiratory compromise. The experience is too small to examine contributory factors, but two of four patients with a spinal cord injury were operated on for a ruptured aneurysm, and all four patients required resection of most of the thoracic aorta. In our last 15 cases, intrathecal catheters for cerebrospinal fluid drainage have been used, and there has been no spinal cord injury.

Significant renal failure among survivors of an operation was generally limited to a nonoliguric rise in the serum creatinine level. Many, if not most, patients experienced a rise of 88.4 μmol/L (1.0 mg/dL) or greater in the serum creatinine level over baseline values. Such transient renal dysfunction was clinically insignificant. Two patients (one each in groups 1 and 2) required dialysis, which in the most recent case was temporary.

COMMENT

No discussion of the surgical management of thoracoabdominal aneurysm can begin without an acknowledgment of the contributions of Crawford with respect to both the natural history of the disease, if untreated, and those tenets of operative management that have permitted suc-

Table 1.—Operative Details: Elective Thoracoabdominal Aneurysm Repair

	Mean ± SD		
	Group 1	Group 2	*P*
Operative time, h	7.2 ± 1.9	5.1 ± 1.9	<.005
Visceral cross-clamp time, h*	0.83 ± 0.18	0.79 ± 0.29	NS†
Total cross-clamp time, h	1.9 ± 0.79	1.5 ± 0.43	<.05
Blood loss, U	20.3 ± 14.02	13.8 ± 7.1	<.05

*Clamp time till right renal/superior mesenteric/celiac when performed after a separate proximal aortic anastomosis.
†NS indicates not significant.

Table 2.—Causes of Operative Mortality*

Group	Operation, No. of Patients	Cause, No.	No. (%)
1 (1978-1985)	Elective, 9/18	Perioperative hemorrhage, 4; perioperative MI, 4; ARDS, 1	15/26 (57)
	Urgent, 6/8	Perioperative hemorrhage, 4; empyema-sepsis, 1; renal failure, 1	
2 (1986-1988)	Elective, 2/27	Perioperative hemorrhage, 1; respiratory and renal failure, 1	4/29 (13)
	Urgent, 2/2	Perioperative hemorrhage, 2	

*MI indicates myocardial infarction; ARDS, adult respiratory distress syndrome.

cessful repair of these extensive lesions.[1,4,5] It is clear that thoracoabdominal aneurysms have the same potential for rupture as the more common infrarenal lesions, and operative therapy is appropriate if it can be accomplished with acceptable morbidity and mortality. In our institution, this is presently a reality with our current results with elective resection (operative mortality, 7.4%), comparable with those reported by Crawford et al.[5] Yet, it is also clear that the present results are the product of a "learning curve" period (group 1 patients) wherein operative mortality was in the 50% range. Several factors appear to be important in reviewing the evolution of this experience.

Clearly, the percentage of patients who were operated on for a ruptured aneurysm changed during the period of this review, with 30% of our earlier cases being done in the presence of rupture. The corresponding figure in our recent experience was less than 7%, more along the 4% figure quoted by Crawford and colleagues.[5] Certainly, a reluctance to proceed with elective resection because of prohibitive mortality was a factor in the past. This was further emphasized by the excess (25%) of our patients who had undergone prior infrarenal aortic aneurysm repair, the majority of which were performed in our institution. While these patients may have had significant progression of their more proximal aneurysmal component, it is clear that many prior infrarenal aneurysm repairs amounted to a compromise or partial repair of the largest, or certainly the most easily treated, part of more diffuse aneurysmal disease. This is best illustrated by the aortogram of a recently encountered patient with a type IV thoracoabdominal aneurysm (Fig 3) that demonstrated an apparent "neck" at the level of the superior mesenteric artery. In the past, an attempt would have been made to treat such a patient with an infrarenal graft through an anterior approach, ignoring the more proximal component of the aneurysm. Such an approach is an error in view of our current experience, as it leaves the patient with an uncorrected aneurysm. Furthermore, an attempt at infrarenal repair when the visceral vessels arise from an aneurysmal aorta is potentially more hazardous than formal thoracoabdominal repair (Fig 4), which was performed in the patient illustrated with a good result.

What other factors are responsible for the dramatic improvements in our results as a function of time? First, it must be stated that the current results should not obscure the fact that this operation remains a massive surgical undertaking for both patient and surgeon. Other recently reported series have quoted mortality for elective resection of 9.6% and 17%.[2,6] Important elements responsible for improved results can be ascertained by examining the causes of death in our earlier experience (Table 2). Clearly, intraoperative and perioperative hemorrhage was a major problem in the past but occurred only once in our recent experience with elective cases. Indeed, the scenario of a technically adequate operation and a patient dying of dilutional coagulopathy was common in past experience. Blood transfusion requirements in elective cases were decreased by one third ($P<.05$) when our group 2 patients were compared with those in group 1 (Table 1), and 50% of our current transfusion requirements are met by intraoperative autotransfusion. Crawford et al[5] have emphasized the attendant morbidity and mortality of those patients who require reexploration for hemorrhage. Avoiding hemorrhage is, therefore, an integral part of the entire operative strategy and the purview of both surgeon and anesthesiologist. The breadth of the surgical field is large, and inattention to blood loss can result in a substantial transfusion requirement before clamps are ever applied. Volume replacement must be in the form of warmed fresh-frozen plasma, in the operating room and thereafter. Those precepts promulgated by Crawford, ie, the avoidance of heparin, use of rapid autotransfusion, vigorous blood component replacement, minimal dissection, and use of impermeable prostheses, are strictly adhered to. Finally, and perhaps self-apparent, the bleeding suture line, particularly the poorly accessible inferoposterior aspect of an inclusion button, may require undesirable reclamping in a nonheparinized patient. Suture lines must be perfect—the first time.

Other technical aspects of the operation deserve emphasis as they relate to avoidance of the major complications of hemorrhage, renal and respiratory failure, and spinal cord injury. The clamp-and-sew approach is routine in our practice, as temporary shunts/or bypasses have not been helpful in decreasing complications.[7] Despite routine protection of the myocardium with pharmacologic manipulation, minimization of cross-clamp times is vitally important to avoid renal dysfunction, to minimize the lactate load from the ischemic gut, and to decrease the chance of limb ischemia in these nonheparinized patients. As displayed in Table 1, cross clamp times are currently minimal and, in our view, strongly correlated with our present results. In addition, continuous instillation of cold (4°C) renal preservation solution is used, as we believe it adds a measure of renal protection. This is likely not to be essential if visceral artery clamp times are less than 1 hour in the patient with normal renal function. Yet, most patients will demonstrate a degree of renal ischemic damage by a nonoliguric rise in the serum creatinine level, which generally is transient. The dual strategy of minimal clamp time and renal preservation solution has resulted in minimal renal-related morbidity. In recent experience, renal failure was contributory in one of two deaths, and one patient with a single kidney required temporary dialysis. Two other technical matters relate to minimizing renal (and visceral) ischemia, namely, handling of the left renal artery and the approach to the patient with a type IV aneurysm. We favor complete detachment of the left renal artery orifice and reconstruction with a previously sewn side-arm graft (Fig 4). This

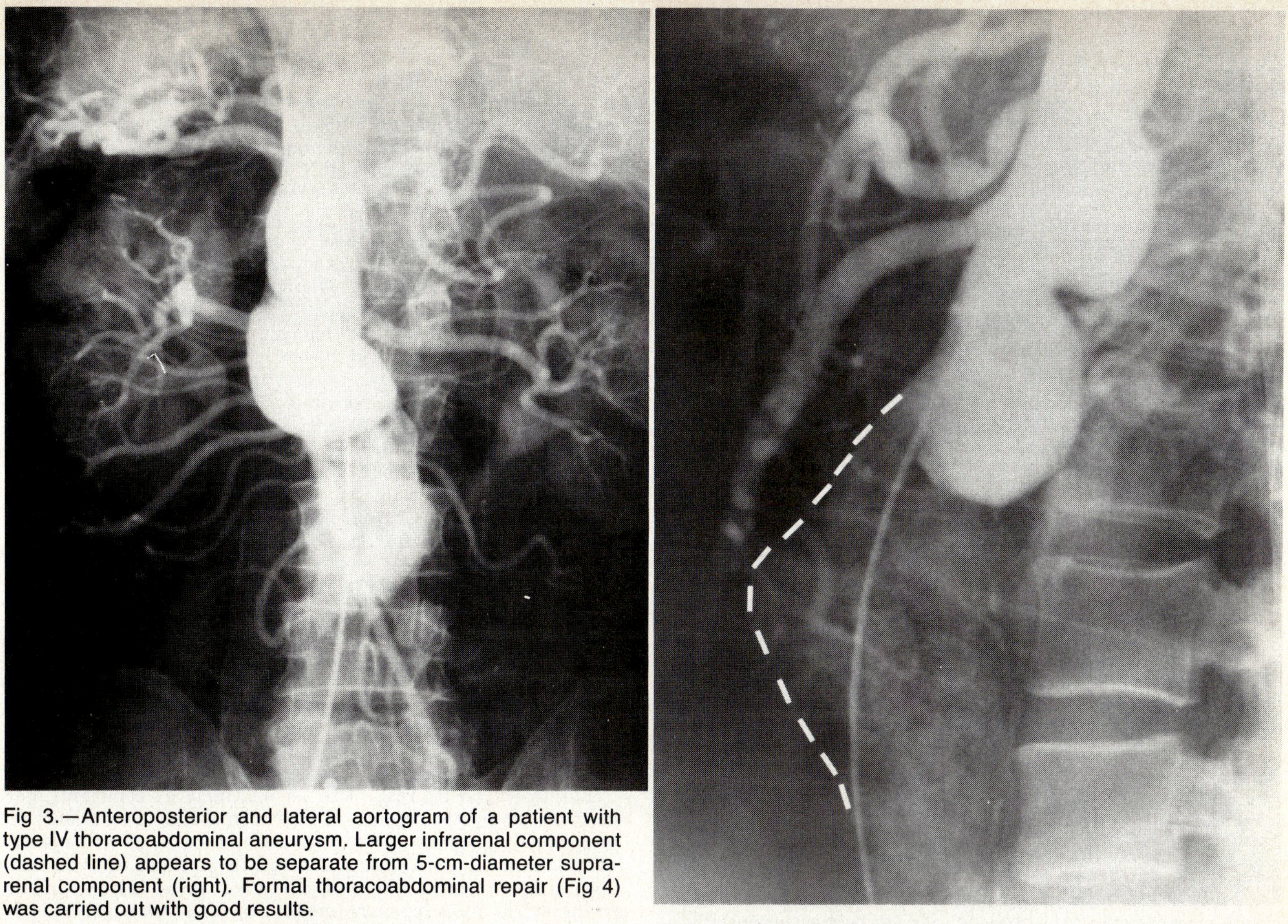

Fig 3.—Anteroposterior and lateral aortogram of a patient with type IV thoracoabdominal aneurysm. Larger infrarenal component (dashed line) appears to be separate from 5-cm-diameter suprarenal component (right). Formal thoracoabdominal repair (Fig 4) was carried out with good results.

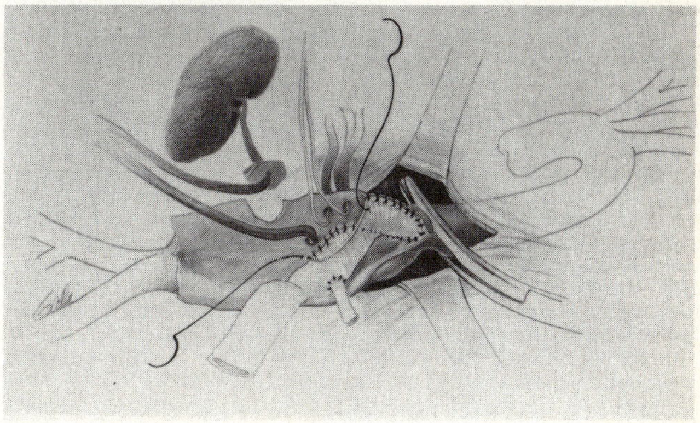

Fig 4.—Operative technique for type IV thoracoabdominal aneurysm. Diaphragm has been partially divided and retracted through thoracoabdominal incision. Proximal aortic, celiac, superior mesenteric, and right renal artery anastomoses are all accomplished with one long beveled suture line. Note renal perfusion catheters and separate side-arm graft for left renal artery.

allows for maximal exposure and precision of the left renal artery anastomosis, after careful planning as to the position of the left renal graft with respect to the inclusion button for the right renal, superior mensenteric, and celiac arteries. In patients with type IV aneurysms, it is generally possible to limit the amount of diaphragm divided and perform the proximal aortic, right renal, superior mesenteric, and celiac artery reconstruction with one long beveled anastomosis (Fig 4). A similar maneuver has been employed for the *distal* anastomosis for a type I aneurysm. Furthermore, the classification as to extent of aneurysm (Fig 2) is helpful to the surgeon in planning incisions, anticipating the need for collapsing the left lung (generally required only in types I and II aneurysms), and preparing for intercostal artery reattachment.

Spinal cord injury occurred in 7.2% of our patients. In our recent experience, this complication contributed to one death and caused flaccid paraplegia in a survivor. Crawford and associates[5] have clearly demonstrated those factors that seem to correlate with this complication, and the benefit of intercostal reattachment is unclear. Like others,[2] we have recently used cerebrospinal fluid pressure monitoring and drainage in the operating room for whatever protection it may afford and, to date, have experienced no spinal cord injury when this modality has been used.[8,9] Obviously, it is not possible to draw a cause and effect type of conclusion with respect to our experience with cerebrospinal fluid drainage, as the numbers of patients at high risk for spinal cord injury has been small.

The last consideration in reviewing our improved results relates to a *system* of preoperative evaluation and intraoperative anesthetic, or perhaps better stated, physiologic management of these patients. All patients are evaluated for coexistent coronary artery disease with dipyridamole-thallium scanning and "positive" tests further clarified with coronary angiography.[10] In the truly elective cases, we believe that the profound physiologic derangements that accompany thoracoabdominal aneurysm repair mandate prior correction of significant coronary artery disease. In the operating room, a single team of anesthesiologists cares for all of these patients and the management of blood pressure, avoidance of acidemia and hypothermia, and timely replacement of blood components are under their direction. Absolute coordination of surgical maneuvers, pharmacologic manipulations, and volume replacement are crucial to avoid wide fluctuations in blood pressure and unacceptably low or high levels of the same.

With respect to the current indications for thoracoabdominal aneurysm repair, our position is largely inferential, based on the available natural history data of thoracoabdominal aneurysms and our present overall approach to aneurysmal disease of the aorta. Clearly, the potential for rupture of a thoracoabdominal aneurysm is at least equal to the more common infrarenal aneurysm,[4,11] and it must be assumed that the risk of rupture is proportional to the size of the aneurysm. However, size criteria will likely never be well delineated for thoracoabdominal aneurysm since it is a relatively uncommon lesion. Our current approach to aneurysmal disease of the aorta is simply that the risk-benefit ratio in most patients is weighted toward elective resection. Furthermore, patients with a thoracoabdominal aneurysm are likely to present with symptoms (usually back pain) or be discovered during an evaluation for repair of an infrarenal aneurysm. Current results with elective resection justify an aggressive approach to thoracoabdominal aneurysms in appropriate surgical candidates.

References

1. Crawford ES. Thoraco-abdominal and abdominal aortic aneurysms involving renal, superior mesenteric and celiac arteries. *Ann Surg.* 1974; 179:763-772.

2. Hollier LH, Symmonds JB, Pairolero P, Cherry K, Hallett JW, Gloviczki P. Thoracoabdominal aortic aneurysm repair: analysis of postoperative morbidity. *Arch Surg.* 1988;123:871-875.

3. Cambria RP, Brewster DC, Moncure AC, Steinberg F, Abbott WM. Spontaneous aortic dissection complicating coexistent or previously repaired atherosclerotic aortic aneurysm. *Ann Surg.* 1988;208:619-624.

4. Crawford ES, DeNatale RNP. Thoracoabdominal aortic aneurysm: observations regarding the natural course of the disease. *J Vasc Surg.* 1986; 3:578-582.

5. Crawford ES, Crawford JL, Safi JH, et al. Thoracoabdominal aortic aneurysm: preoperative and intraoperative factors determining immediate and long-term results of operations in 605 patients. *J Vasc Surg.* 1986;3:389-404.

6. Vaccaro PS, Elkhammas E, Smead WL. Clinical observations and lessons learned in the treatment of patients with thoracoabdominal aortic aneurysm. *Surg Gynecol Obstet.* 1988;166:461-465.

7. Crawford ES, Walker HS, Saleh SA, et al: Graft replacement of aneurysm in the descending thoracic aorta: results without bypass or shunting. *Surgery.* 1981;89:73-85.

8. Hollier LH. Protecting the brain and spinal cord. *J Vasc Surg.* 1987; 3:524-528.

9. McCullough JL, Hollier LH, Nugent M. Paraplegia after thoracic aorta occlusion: influence of cerebrospinal fluid drainage: experimental and early clinical results. *J Vasc Surg.* 1988;7:153-160.

10. Brewster DC, Okada RD, Strauss HW, et al. Selection of patients for pre-operative coronary angiography: use of dipyridamole-stress-thallium myocardial imaging. *J Vasc Surg.* 1985;2:504-510.

11. Bickerstaff LK, Parrolero PC, Hollier LH, et al. Thoracic aortic aneurysm: a population based study. *Surgery.* 1982;92:1103-1107.

Discussion

Jeremy R. Morton, MD, Portland, Me: Our results have been very similar to those described here, and my colleagues and I are as fearful of spinal cord injury as anyone else. Dr Crawford has used no heparin, but we have found that a small amount of heparin (5000 U) makes blood salvage much easier and seems to lessen the incidence of postoperative coagulopathy. Presumably, this results from preservation of platelets by avoiding coagulation in the field before aspiration by the blood salvage system.

When the aneurysm does not involve much of the thoracic aorta, we have found it helpful to stay low with the intercostal incision by using the 10th interspace where the rib is only loosely connected to the costal arch. If one interrupts the solid portion of the costal arch, the patients seem to have much greater postoperative pain and respiratory problems.

We have used interthecal drainage on these cases and have added to that interthecal papaverine as described by Svensson in 1987 to lessen the risk of paraplegia. With thoracic aneurysms, we have recently begun employing a left-sided heart bypass without heparin by using a centrifugal pump (Biomedicus).

Anthony D. Whittemore, MD, Boston, Mass: I commend Dr Cambria on his characteristically lucid presentation and for his admirable results. This discussion reflects Dr Crawford's monumental efforts in reducing the operative mortality to the 10% level, and the incidence of its most dreaded complication, spinal cord injury, to approximately 5% overall. There exists an uncanny similarity between the authors' experience and that of our own, both of which emphasize a fairly steep learning curve. Our group of patients at the Brigham and Women's Hospital, Boston, Mass, is smaller, numbering 30 during the past 10 years, and the overall mortality was 33% for both elective and emergent indications. Dr Cambria's mortality, recalculated, is 34% for the total 10-year experience. During the past 2 years in our experience, 18 patients sustained an operative mortality of 11%, again paralleling the authors' 13%. The reasons for this improvement are multifactorial and also reflect an increase in the incidence of elective procedures. Twenty-five percent of the authors' patients had had infrarenal aneurysms that had been repaired in the past, despite many of them demonstrating a suprarenal aneurysm at the time. Today, we probably should be looking at the entire aortic pathologic condition to develop a more comprehensive plan that might avoid subsequent major procedures.

If one examines Dr Crawford's patients with type II aneurysms that involved the entire aorta, a 10% incidence of paraplegia with a 10% incidence of paraparesis is anticipated for a total incidence of spinal cord injury of 20%. Of the 55 patients in the authors' series, four demonstrated spinal cord injury did all four occur in patients in whom cerebrospinal fluid decompression was used; how many had type II aneurysms? Although no spinal cord injury occurred in the group with cerebrospinal fluid drainage, how many, were at the higher risk level for this complication? Could Dr Cambria speculate regarding the mechanism by which spinal cord decompression avoids spinal cord injury and delineate the parameters that he has found useful in monitoring this decompression?

Dr Cambria: With respect to Dr Whittemore's comments, our attitudes toward the suprarenal extension of abdominal aneurysm have indeed changed, and it is clear that in a fourth of our patients, infrarenal aneurysm repair amounted to partial treatment of a more diffuse disease. There is, of course, great interest in the cerebrospinal fluid pressure monitoring and drainage. This is based on experimental data that are not new, first being delineated by Dr Cooley in the early 1960s. One can certainly see a dramatic increase in cerebrospinal fluid pressure with the application of a very proximal thoracic aortic clamp. We do not have any magic formulas about how much cerebrospinal fluid to withdraw. We do establish a baseline of pressure, which generally runs to 10 to 15 mm Hg, and we withdraw whatever we need to keep it in that range. This has amounted in some patients with very proximal aneurysms to as much as 45 mL of cerebrospinal fluid. We do not replace it. As mentioned by Dr Morton, it seems to cost nothing. For whatever added protection it may afford, we have been enthusiastic about its use.

A word of caution with respect to your comments, about the concomitant use of papaverine. Papaverine has a tendency to crystallize in a number of intravenous solutions; we've been fearful of intrathecal crystallization and arachnoiditis, so we have not used it.

Dr Whittemore did ask me to provide more detail on our recent patients concerning the extent of aneurysm and spinal cord injury. Dr Crawford has delineated those factors that seem to correlate most with spinal cord injury. Clearly, the most important is the extent of the aneurysm and the nature of the pathologic condition, with atherosclerosis vs dissection being most important. In the last group of 15 patients, we have had two patients with the extensive type II aneurysms, and with the use of the cerebrospinal fluid catheter, there has been no spinal cord injury.

Dr Morton added a few comments about heparin, incisions, and partial left-sided heart bypass. We believe strongly in strict adherence to those measures designed specifically to prevent hemorrhage, namely, avoidance of heparin and avoidance of shunts and bypasses which have never been shown in anyone's experience to decrease complications including spinal cord injury.

A word of caution about keeping the incision too low. It has been our empiric observation that the respiratory morbidity attendant with this operation is largely a function of the destruction of the left hemidiaphragm, rather than dividing the costal margin, and we have not hesitated to use the thoracoabdominal incision for the type IV aneurysm.

Splenectomy

The Treatment of Choice for Human Immunodeficiency Virus–Related Immune Thrombocytopenia?

Thanjavur S. Ravikumar, MD; J. Davis Allen, MD;
Albert Bothe, Jr, MD; Glenn Steele, Jr, MD

• Immune thrombocytopenia is a well-recognized part of the clinical spectrum of infection with the human immunodeficiency virus. From November 1985 to February 1988, 15 patients who were human immunodeficiency virus–positive underwent splenectomy for refractory immune thrombocytopenia. Eight patients had thrombocytopenia only, and 7 others were pancytopenic prior to splenectomy. Three of the 15 patients fulfilled criteria for acquired immunodeficiency syndrome before splenectomy, and acquired immunodeficiency syndrome developed in 5 patients during the follow-up period. The median duration of thrombocytopenia prior to surgical therapy was 6 months. A bone marrow biopsy specimen showed hypercellularity with increased megakaryocytes. All patients had a therapeutic response to splenectomy. Long-term remission from thrombocytopenia/pancytopenia was achieved in 14 of the 15 patients during a follow-up period of 2 to 21 months. Splenectomy can be accomplished with an acceptable morbidity. Pneumonia developed postoperatively in 2 patients, but they did not manifest the characteristic picture of overwhelming postsplenectomy sepsis. They had received vaccinations against encapsulated organisms preoperatively. We conclude that splenectomy provides a durable and lasting response for HIV-related thrombocytopenia. Vaccination for *Streptococcus pneumonia* and *Haemophilus influenzae* should be given prior to splenectomy although its efficacy is not clear in this group.

(*Arch Surg.* 1989;124:625-628)

Infection with human immunodeficiency virus (HIV) results in a variety of clinical syndromes, the principal sequelae being acquired immunodeficiency syndrome (AIDS) and its opportunistic infections.[1] The widespread disruption of hematologic elements, most notably T- and B-lymphocyte lineage, has been the hallmark of HIV pathogenesis.[2] Pancytopenia is a common finding in patients with HIV infection; a mechanism of "pseudoautoimmunity" has been espoused by Donohue et al,[3] in which the HIV antibody reacts with a product of the virus expressed in a progenitor cell membrane, thereby suppressing proliferation. A characteristic form of autoimmune thrombocytopenia has been well documented in the population at risk for the development of AIDS. The specific pathologic mechanism of this HIV-related immune thrombocytopenia (ITP) is unclear. The condition reflects an accelerated peripheral destruction of platelets but is immunologically distinct from classic ITP purpura.[4] A heightened production of nonspecific immunoglobulins in HIV infection and deposition of immune complexes on platelets have been postulated and may result in an autoimmune process, leading to thrombocytopenia.[5] The treatment of HIV-related thrombocytopenia includes steroids, intravenous immunoglobulin, vinca alkaloids, danazol, and splenectomy. Since the natural history of the development of AIDS in patients with HIV-related thrombocytopenia has not been well defined, the role of immunosuppressive modalities like steroid therapy and splenectomy has been viewed with skepticism because such methods may enhance immune dysfunction. Herein, we report our experience with splenectomy in HIV-related thrombocytopenia.

Accepted for publication December 13, 1988.

From the Department of Surgery, New England Deaconess Hospital, Harvard Medical School, Boston, Mass.

Read before the 69th Annual Meeting of the New England Surgical Society, Montreal, Canada, September 17, 1988.

Reprint requests to Department of Surgery, New England Deaconess Hospital, Harvard Medical School, 110 Francis St, Suite 3A, Boston, MA 02215 (Dr Ravikumar).

PATIENTS AND METHODS

The medical records of 15 HIV-positive patients who underwent splenectomy from November 1985 to February 1988 were reviewed. Their ages ranged from 26 to 56 years, with a median age of 33 years. There were 12 men and 3 women. Risk factors for HIV included homosexuality (n = 10), intravenous drug abuse (n = 4), and prior transfusion of blood products (n = 2). One patient had two risk factors, namely, homosexuality and intravenous drug abuse. Eight patients had thrombocytopenia only, and 7 others were pancytopenic prior to splenectomy. The median preoperative blood counts were as follows: platelets, 13×10^9/L; white blood cells, 3.7×10^9/L; and hematocrit, 0.36. A bone marrow biopsy specimen showed hypercellularity with increased megakaryocytes in all but 1 patient. This patient had received intensive chemotherapy for leukemia in the past. Antiplatelet antibodies were detectable in 2 of 5 patients tested.

The median interval between HIV positivity and splenectomy was 16 months (range, 1 to 36 months). T-lymphocyte subset ratios (helper-suppressor ratios) were reversed in all patients (median, 0.34; range, 0.10 to 0.76). The duration of thrombocytopenia prior to surgical therapy ranged from 1 to 30 months (median, 6 months). Eleven of the 15 patients fulfilled criteria for AIDS-related complex preoperatively. Lymphadenopathy was the most common finding. Three of these 11 patients had the criteria of AIDS diagnosed prior to splenectomy (infection with cytomegalovirus or *Pneumocystis carinii*, Kaposi's sarcomas). Four of the 15 patients presented only with the hematologic abnormalities (thrombocytopenia/pancytopenia) without other AIDS-related complex findings.

Splenectomy was carried out through an upper midline or a left subcostal incision. Perioperative antibiotic prophylaxis with cephalosporin was used routinely. Suction drains in the splenic bed were not routinely used. All patients except one were vaccinated against *Streptococcus pneumoniae* and *Haemophilus influenzae* prior to splenectomy.

RESULTS

Response to Medical Therapy

A number of drugs have been used by other centers with variable results. We have used steroids, danazol, vincristine, and azathioprine (Imuran) for the treatment of HIV-related thrombocytopenia. It should be stated that the efficacy of drugs was not evaluated in a protocol setting. Rather, the treatment was individualized on the basis of the patient's comorbid problems and the physician's preferences. We did not demonstrate any response to vincristine, danazol, or azathioprine, as shown in the following tabulation:

Treatment	Response
Corticosteroid (n = 3)	1 response; 1 transient response; 1 no response
Danazol (n = 4)	No response
Vincristine (n = 3)	No response
Azathioprine (Imuran) (n = 1)	No response
Splenectomy (n = 15)	14 responses; 1 transient response

One of the three patients treated with steroids responded, and one other patient had a transient response for about 4 weeks. Seven patients in the latter part of this study were referred directly to surgery after our initial unsatisfactory experience with medical management of thrombocytopenia.

Response to Splenectomy

Splenic weight ranged from 189 to 2320 g. All patients had a therapeutic response to splenectomy. The median platelet counts at 1 week and 1 month post splenectomy were: 464×10^9/L (range, 130 to 509×10^9/L) and 222×10^9/L (range, 125 to 884×10^9/L), respectively. Long-term remission from thrombocytopenia/pancytopenia was achieved in 14 of the 15 patients during a follow-up period ranging from 2 to 21 months. The only patient who had a decreased bone marrow reserve as a result of prior chemotherapy exhibited a transient increase in platelet count lasting for up to 6 weeks following splenectomy. The magnitude of T-cell subset reversal and the size of spleen at operation did not correlate with therapeutic response to splenectomy. Additionally, the presence or absence of antiplatelet antibodies did not correlate with the magnitude or duration of response to splenectomy.

Postoperative Morbidity and Mortality

There was no postoperative mortality. The postoperative complications were as follows:

Complication	No. (%) of Patients
Postoperative fevers up to 5 days	8 (54)
Pneumonia	2 (13)
Delayed wound infection	2 (13)
Transient suction drain amylasemia	2 (13)
Clostridium difficile enterocolitis	1 (7)

Almost all patients had low-grade fever (temperature <38.3°C) postoperatively for up to 72 hours. Spiking fevers (temperature, 38.3°C) were observed in eight patients for up to 5 days, without any documentable infection despite diligent culture workup. Lobar pneumonia developed in two of these patients, *S pneumoniae* and *H influenzae* being the pathogens. Interestingly, both of these patients had presplenectomy vaccination against encapsulated organisms. Increased amylase content in the splenic bed's Jackson-Pratt suction drain was recorded in two patients; both of these patients showed no other signs of pancreatitis. Both of these drains were removed on postoperative days 4 and 8, respectively, following the normalization of fluid amylase content. One patient developed *C difficile* enterocolitis presumed to be secondary to cephalosporin administration. Delayed wound infections were observed in two patients, one of whom had a ventral hernia develop during the follow-up period.

Development of AIDS Post Splenectomy

Among the 12 patients who did not fulfill criteria for AIDS at the time of splenectomy, opportunistic infections conforming to AIDS developed in 4 (33% conversion). Despite this, the therapeutic effect of splenectomy persisted and may have improved their hematologic tolerance of antiretroviral and cytotoxic agents needed to treat these sequelae.

COMMENT

The salient findings in our study are that splenectomy provides a durable and lasting response for HIV-related ITP and that this surgery can be accomplished with acceptable morbidity. Splenectomy is an effective method to correct thrombocytopenia of diverse origins, of which ITP remains the most common indication, with an 86% sustained response.[6] The success of splenectomy in controlling HIV-related thrombocytopenia parallels that of idiopathic thrombocytopenic purpura and is stated to be in the range of 60% to 100%.[4] Like ITP, the rationale has been removal of the major source of antiplatelet antibody and to eliminate a major site of removal of "antibody-coated" platelets. Despite this similarity, immunologic studies showed differences between the homosexual patients with thrombocytopenia and patients with classic autoimmune thrombocytopenia, with respect to markedly increased platelet-bound IgG and complement levels and the presence of polyethylene glycol–precipitable immune complexes in homosexual patients.[5] Other studies, however, demonstrated the development of antiplatelet antibody in serum of homosexual men with isolated ITP, and a target platelet antigen value of 25 000 d has been postulated.[7] Five of our initial patients were tested for antiplatelet antibodies before they underwent splenectomy. Antiplatelet antibodies were detectable in two of the five patients, but there was no correlation with the presence or absence of antiplatelet antibodies and therapeutic response to splenectomy. We have since stopped using this as an indication for splenectomy.

Since splenectomy has been associated with significant immunosuppression and postsplenectomy sepsis, there has been an understandable reluctance in subjecting patients with HIV to this procedure. Several nonsurgical treatments have been tried. Intravenous gamma globulin (antithymocyte globulin) has been used in postinfectious thrombocytopenia associated with both varicella-zoster infection or HIV infection.[8] Intravenous gamma globulin is successful in the treatment of chronic ITP in children and adults, associated with a concomitant IgG Fc-receptor blockade demonstrable in vivo.[9] Unlike the experience in childhood ITP, however, there was no sustained response unless the IgG infusion was closely associated with splenectomy.[10] In HIV-related thrombocytopenia a variable response (median duration, 22 days) has been observed following single- and multiple-dose regimens; intravenous gamma globulin may be the treatment of choice in patients with acute bleeding or when an invasive procedure is needed in the thrombocytopenic.[11] Danazol increases platelet counts in some patients with ITP and HIV-related thrombocytopenia.[12,13] Danazol and vinblastine mediate their clinical effect in thrombocytopenic states by influencing the number of available Fc (IgG) receptors on phagocytic cells.[14] Their use in HIV-related thrombocytopenia thus far has been transient and anecdotal.

The suppressive effect of corticosteroid therapy on cell-mediated immunity makes its role in HIV-related thrombocytopenia problematic. Anecdotal observations of activation and regression of some AIDS-associated lesions (eg, Karposi's sarcoma) have been reported that coincided with administration of corticosteroids and withdrawal of the drug, respectively.[15] Shafer et al[16] described three HIV-positive patients in whom fulminant *Pneumocystis* pneumonia developed shortly after corticosteroid treatment. Although a majority of patients with HIV-related ITP responded initially to steroid treatment, less than 8% achieved sustained remission in long-term studies.[17]

Two major concerns in recommending a splenectomy for HIV-related thrombocytopenia are acceleration of AIDS and predisposition to overwhelming bacterial sepsis. The exact incidence of thrombocytopenia in the population with HIV and AIDS is not entirely known. Cohen et al[18] examined 50 homosexual men with AIDS for their coagulation profiles over a 2-year period. Ten patients had in vitro evidence of circulating anticoagulant; mild to moderate decreases in platelet counts were noted in 3 of the 10 patients. An incidence of 6% thrombocytopenia was thus observed in this 2-year follow-up study. The incidence of AIDS following splenectomy in HIV-positive patients was analyzed in several series. The rate of development of AIDS in patients with ITP varies from 12.5% to 37.5% and does not appear to be related to steroid use or splenectomy.[19,20] Although in a collected series AIDS developed in 25% of patients previously treated with steroids and eventually undergoing splenectomy, compared with 8% who had not had a splenectomy, the overall incidence was not dissimilar to that for HIV-positive nonthrombocytopenic patients during the same period of follow-up.[21]

Splenectomy might be expected to predispose patients with AIDS to bacterial sepsis, but this has not been reported in patients following splenectomy for HIV-related thrombocytopenia. The development of pneumonia in two of four patients despite appropriate prior vaccination calls into question the efficacy of vaccination in this group. The reasons for vaccine failure may be the absence of a particular bacterial serotype in the vaccine, poor antibody response as a result of an immunologic dysfunction, or infection by an organism other than the three common bacteria against which the patient has been vaccinated.[22] Acquired immunodeficiency syndrome is associated with an acquired T-cell as well as B-cell immunodeficiency. Ammann et al[23] demonstrated that patients with AIDS fail to respond with significant antibody levels after primary immunization with both polysaccharide (pneumococcal) and protein (KLH) antigens. B-cell abnormalities, consisting of polyclonal activation with high immunoglobulin levels (which has been invoked to explain the HIV-related thrombocytopenia) and a poor antibody response to normal antigens are common in AIDS and may be the direct consequence of HIV infection.[24] This B-cell dysfunction has been postulated to explain the frequent pyogenic infections, particularly with *S pneumoniae* and *H influenzae* in the HIV-infected population.[25] Despite the questionable efficacy of these vaccinations, we strongly recommend preoperative protection against encapsulated organisms in this group.

Appropriate timing of splenectomy is crucial in HIV-related thrombocytopenia. Patients can generally tolerate extremely low platelet counts, and we have advocated splenectomy at a median platelet count of 13×10^9/L in our population. The median duration of significant thrombocytopenia in our study has been 6 months. Walsh et al[26] observed that 18% of patients with HIV-related thrombocytopenia will have normal platelet counts develop spontaneously over a median period of 10 months and recommend avoidance of splenectomy for 6 to 12 months if possible.

Thus, splenectomy can be accomplished with acceptable morbidity in patients with HIV-related thrombocytopenia and provides durable and lasting response. Additionally, splenectomy may improve the hematologic tolerance to antiretroviral and cytotoxic drugs needed to treat other HIV-related complications.

References

1. Ho DD, Pomerantz RJ, Kaplan JC. Pathogenesis of infection with human immunodeficiency virus. *N Engl J Med.* 1987;317:278-286.

2. Lane HC, Masur H, Gelman ER, et al. Correlation between immunologic function and clinical subpopulations of patients with the acquired immunodeficiency syndrome. *Am J Med.* 1985;78:417-422.

3. Donohue RE, Johnson MM, Zon LI, Clark SC, Groopman JE. Suppression of in vitro hematopoiesis following HIV infection. *Nature.* 1987; 326:200-203.

4. Selwyn PA. AIDS: what is now known, III: clinical aspects. *Hosp Pract Off.* 1986;21:119-153.

5. Walsh CM, Nardi MA, Karpatkin S. On the mechanism of thrombocytopenic purpura in sexually active homosexual men. *N Engl J Med.* 1984;311:635-639.

6. Schwartz SI. Splenectomy for thrombocytopenia. *World J Surg.* 1985; 9:416-421.

7. Stricken RB, Abrams DI, Corash L, Shuman MA. Target platelet antigen in homosexual men with immune thrombocytopenia. *N Engl J Med.* 1985;313:1375-1380.

8. Ordi J, Vilardell M, Alijotas J, Barquinero J, Vila M. Serum thrombocytopenia and high-dose immunoglobulin treatment. *Ann Intern Med.* 1986; 104:282-283.

9. Bussel JB, Kimberly RP, Inman RD, et al. Intravenous gammaglobulin treatment of clinical ITP. *Blood.* 1983;62:480-486.

10. Newland AC, Treleaver JG, Minchinton RM, Waters AH. High-dose IV IgG in adults with autoimmune thrombocytopenia. *Lancet.* 1983;1:84-87.

11. Tertian G, Risler N, LeBras P, et al. Intravenous gammaglobulin treatment for thrombocytopenic purpura in patients with HIV infection. *Eur J Haematol.* 1987;39:180-181.

12. Fischl M, Ahn YS, Klimas N, et al. Use of danazol in autoimmune thrombocytopenia associated with AIDS. Presented at the International Conference on AIDS; April 14, 1985; Atlanta, Ga.

13. Ahn YS, Harrington WJ, Simon SR, Mylvaganam R, Pall LM, So AG. Danazol for the treatment of idiopathic thrombocytopenia purpura. *N Engl J Med.* 1983;308:1396-1399.

14. Schreiber AD, Chien P, Tomaski A, Cines DB. Effect of danazol in immune thrombocytopenic purpura. *N Engl J Med.* 1987;316:503-508.

15. Real FX, Krown SE. Spontaneous regression of Kaposi's sarcoma in patients with AIDS. *N Engl J Med.* 1985;313:1659.

16. Shafer RW, Offit K, Macrus NT, et al. Possible risk of steroid

administration in patients at risk for AIDS. *Lancet.* 1985;934-935.
17. Abrams DI, Kiprov DD, Goedert JJ, Sarngadharan MG, Gallo RC, Volberding PA. Antibodies to human T-lymphotrophic virus type III and development of the acquired immunodeficiency syndrome in homosexual men presenting with immune thrombocytopenia. *Ann Intern Med.* 1986; 104:47-50.
18. Cohen AJ, Philips TM, Kessler CM. Circulating coagulation inhibitors in the acquired immunodeficiency syndrome. *Ann Intern Med.* 1986; 104:175-180.
19. Ferguson CM. Surgical complications of human immunodeficiency virus infection. *Am Surg.* 1988;54:4-9.
20. Rosenfeld FP, Rosenblood BE, Weinstein IM. Thrombocytopenia in homosexual men. *Ann Intern Med.* 1987;106:911-913.
21. Barbui T, Cortelazzo S, Minetti B, Galli M, Buelli M. Does splenectomy enhance risk of AIDS in HIV positive patients with chronic thrombocytopenia? *Lancet.* 1987;2:342-343.
22. Dickerman JD. Splenectomy and sepsis: a warning. *Pediatrics.* 1979; 63:938-941.
23. Ammann AJ, Schiffman G, Abrams D, Volberding P, Zigler J, Conant M. B-cell immunodeficiency in acquired immune deficiency syndrome. *JAMA.* 1984;251:1447-1449.
24. Bowen DL, Lane HC, Fauci AS. Immunopathogenesis of the acquired immunodeficiency syndrome. *Ann Intern Med.* 1985;103:704-709.
25. Polsky B, Gold JWM, Whimbey E, et al. Bacterial pneumonia in patients with the acquired immunodeficiency syndrome. *Ann Intern Med.* 1986;104:38-41.
26. Walsh C, Krigel R, Lennette E, Karpatkin S: Thrombocytopenia in homosexual patients. *Ann Intern Med.* 1985;103:542-545.

Discussion

Leslie W. Ottinger, MD, Boston, Mass: The role of the abdominal surgeon in the management of patients with AIDS–related complex has previously included laparotomy for gastrointestinal complications of opportunistic infections or neoplasms and for the diagnosis of the cause of retroperitoneal lymphadenopathy. Immunodeficiency-associated thrombocytopenia occurs in otherwise asymptomatic patients with HIV infection as well as those with AIDS and the AIDS-related complex. Clinically, it resembles idiopathic thrombocytopenia purpura, and there are other similarities as well. Antiplatelet antibodies are often found in both. The underlying pathologic process in immunodeficiency-associated thrombocytopenia is, however, clearly different. The report of Ravikumar and associates provides further evidence that splenectomy can promote a sustained reversal of thrombocytopenia, with a low operative risk and without a subsequent increase in either the risk of bacterial infections or the rate of progression of the disease complex toward the final end point of standard AIDS and its complications.

Questions related to the appropriate timing for splenectomy remain. Some cases of immunodeficiency-associated thrombocytopenia have been reported to have a spontaneous return to normal platelet levels. In other cases, patients have a sustained response to corticosteroids or antithymocyte globulin and therefore have not required splenectomy. The actual risk of major bleeding complications in patients with thrombocytopenia is not known. Before the use of steroids and splenectomy for patients with ITP, the incidence was estimated to have been between 10% and 20%. Finally, some physicians believe that life expectancy in the patient with AIDS is too short to justify splenectomy.

I would like to know whether any of the patients sustained major bleeding complications resulting from thrombocytopenia and the present indications for splenectomy in these cases. Second, though I suspect many surgeons have not yet, at least knowingly, operated on patients who were HIV-positive, universal precautions, like universal health care, are commendable in concept but threadbare at bedside. Did the surgeons take specific precautions for themselves and their operating team and were any alterations in technique used to perform the splenectomy on an HIV-positive patient?

Peter J. Deckers, MD, Hartford, Conn: Patients who have hypersplenism for platelets or ITP do not have splenomegaly. I noticed in the range of splenic weights that there was an extreme up to 2000 g. I would like to know the results of the pathologic examination of those spleens over 200 g. Were they infiltrated with lymphoma or leukemia and is that the source of the sequestration of platelets in the spleen?

George A. May, Jr, MD, Newton, Mass: I want to follow up on the second question Dr Ottinger asked. During my training at a county sanatorium, precautions were taken to protect me in my enthusiasm from some of the patients with tuberculosis. Some of these precautions were quite subtle, and I never realized that I was not permitted to touch the specimen after surgery and that there were certain places in the hospital where I was not supposed to go because no one wanted me as a young surgeon to get tuberculosis.

Is splenectomy an operation that should be done by older surgical personnel and has some thought been given to keeping the medical students out of this area where there is such high exposure to a lot of blood?

Dr Ravikumar: In regard to bleeding risks and timing of surgery, bleeding complications are rare unless the platelet count is less than 30×10^9/L. The median platelet count in our study was 13×10^9/L. We safely watch patients until the platelet counts are in the range of 20×10^9/L. Spontaneous remission in one study occurred in 18% of the patients, but did not occur if the platelet count was less than 30×10^9/L.

The use of immunoglobulin in pediatric ITP has been successful. In adult classic ITP, it has been of anecdotal success. In patients with HIV-related thrombocytopenia, the immunoglobulin works temporarily (median, 22 weeks). Our indication to use immunoglobulin in these patients is as a temporizing measure when the patient has any bleeding complication or as an adjunct to upcoming surgery.

As to the specific precautions during the operation, we usually have either a senior resident or an attending surgeon as the primary surgeon and follow universal precautions. There are no formal data to prove that double-gloving helps. The glove puncture rate is about 12.5% if the operation exceeds 1 hour. From a theoretical standpoint, changing gloves every hour and double-gloving may minimize blood contamination of the surgeon's hands.

Another caveat is to use the knife only during the skin incision and then to switch to electrocautery and scissors for all subsequent dissection and cutting. The use of self-retraining retractors not only for retracting the abdominal wall but also to retract other viscera (eg, stomach) during the procedure may minimize the risk of accidental stabbing. Lastly, splenectomy is performed in a controlled fashion with ligation of the splenic artery in the lesser sac first, followed by dissection of short gastrics and mobilization of the spleen from the bed. We use nonabsorbable or long-absorbable sutures for closure. These patients can have delayed wound infections and disruption.

Original Article

Gallstone Disease

The Clinical Manifestations of Infectious Stones

Alison L. Smith, MD; Lygia Stewart, MD; Robert Fine, MD;
Carlos A. Pellegrini, MD; Lawrence W. Way, MD

• Gallstones from 82 patients were examined under a scanning electron microscope for evidence of bacteria, and the findings were compared with the clinical manifestations of the disease. Bacteria were present in 68% of pigment stones and the pigment portions of 80% of composite stones. These gallstones were referred to as infectious stones. No bacteria were found in cholesterol gallstones. Acute cholangitis was diagnosed in 52% of patients with infectious stones and in 18% of patients with noninfectious stones. Over half of the patients with noninfectious stones presented with mild symptoms. Infectious stones were more often associated with a previous common duct exploration, an urgent operation, infected bile, a common duct procedure, and complications. These data show that gallstone disease is more virulent in patients whose gallstones contain bacteria.

(*Arch Surg* 1989;124:629-633)

The severity of gallstone disease has previously been shown to be related to stone composition. In particular, septic complications are much more common in patients with pigment gallstones than in patients with cholesterol gallstones.[1-4] For example, Bernhoft et al[1] analyzed common duct stones from 96 patients and found that acute cholangitis was four times more common in patients with pigment common duct stones than in patients with cholesterol common duct stones.

In a previous study,[5] we postulated that bacteria play a primary role in the formation of many pigment gallstones. Scanning electron microscopy (SEM) of gallstones from 85 patients demonstrated evidence of bacterial microcolonies throughout the interior of 75% of pigment stones and the pigment portions of composite stones, whereas no bacteria were found in the interiors of cholesterol stones.[6] The findings supported a theory of pigment stone formation in which bacteria and glycocalyx are responsible for the precipitation and subsequent agglomeration of bilirubin pigment and other solids into macroscopic gallstones.[6]

Accepted for publication Nov 7, 1988.

From the Surgical Service, Veterans Administration Medical Center, and the Department of Surgery, University of California, San Francisco.

Read before the 59th Annual Meeting of the Pacific Coast Surgical Association, San Francisco, Feb 24, 1988.

Reprint requests to Surgical Service (112), Veterans Administration Medical Center, 4150 Clement St, San Francisco, CA 94121 (Dr Way).

In view of these observations, we studied the relationship between the presence of bacteria in gallstones and the clinical manifestations of gallstone disease.

PATIENTS AND METHODS

There were 26 new patients and 56 patients from our previous study[5] for whom detailed clinical data were available. The patients were divided into two groups. The first group comprised 57 patients treated between October 1985 and January 1988 whose gallstones and clinical data were collected prospectively. The stones from these patients were processed for SEM examination immediately on removal. The second group comprised 25 patients treated between October 1978 and October 1985. Clinical data from these patients were obtained retrospectively, and the stones, which had been air-dried, were examined by SEM weeks to months after removal. There were 27 women and 55 men ranging in age from 19 to 96 years. Their ethnic backgrounds included 51 whites, 16 Asians, nine blacks, four Hispanics, and two Middle Easterners.

Gallstone Morphologic Findings

The fresh stones were photographed and processed for SEM immediately after removal from the patient.[5] The dried stones did not require processing in fixative. All stones were dried, sputter-coated with gold or platinum to a 25- to 40-nm thickness, and examined at 10 to 20 kV with an SEM. During the examination, particular attention was paid to a search for bacteria within the interior of the stones.

The gallstones were classified according to source (gallbladder, common duct, or both) and composition. Composition was listed as pigment, cholesterol, or composite (substantial amounts of cholesterol and pigment solids in different layers) based on gross visual appearance and characteristic features when examined under an SEM. The reliability of these methods has previously been established.[7] Evidence of bacteria in the interior of the stones was documented and tabulated according to stone composition. Stones that contained bacteria were called "infectious" stones, based on evidence presented previously.[5]

Clinical Correlations

Clinical information obtained on all patients included demographic data, symptoms and physical signs, length of illness before operation, presence of other medical illnesses, history of previous biliary tract surgery, and laboratory data. The clinical diagnoses were as follows: six patients had asymptomatic gallstones and had a cholecystectomy as part of surgery for another illness (eg,

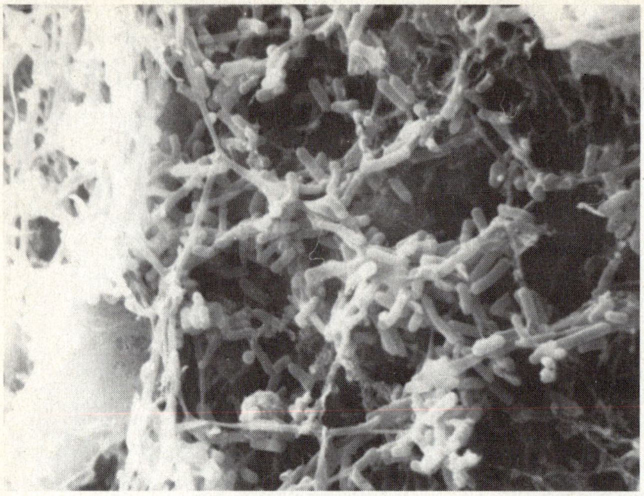

Fig 1.—Scanning electron micrograph of interior of pigment gallstone covered with bacteria (original magnification ×4170).

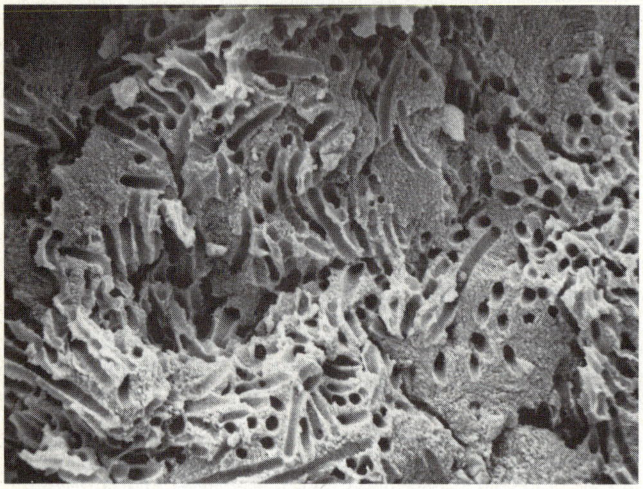

Fig 2.—Scanning electron micrograph of air-dried pigment gallstone with bacterial casts throughout interior. Casts are spaces previously occupied by bacteria (original magnification ×3530).

Fig 3.—Scanning electron micrograph of interior of cholesterol gallstone with no bacteria seen (original magnification ×2670).

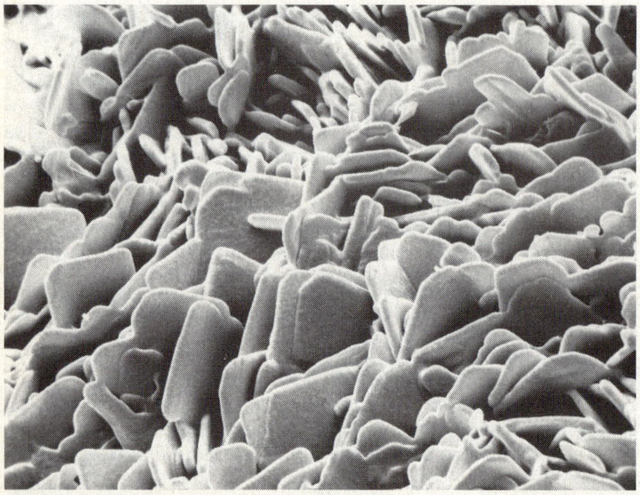

Whipple procedure); 36 patients had chronic, mild biliary tract symptoms (ie, biliary colic) but no evidence of infection; 14 patients had a clinical and pathologic diagnosis of acute cholecystitis; and 26 patients had bacterial cholangitis.

Three types of operations were performed: cholecystectomy, 35 patients; common bile duct exploration with or without cholecystectomy, 30 patients; and permanent biliary drainage procedure, such as sphincteroplasty, choledochoduodenostomy, or choledochojejunostomy, 17 patients. Although 47 common duct procedures were performed, only 42 common duct stones were actually recovered. Three duct explorations failed to reveal gallstones, and two drainage procedures in patients without common duct stones were performed for malignant biliary obstruction. The urgency of the procedure was classified as elective, urgent, or emergent based on clinical information. Pathologic findings, bile culture results, length of postoperative hospital stay, need for care in the intensive care unit, and postoperative complications were noted.

Patients with infectious stones were compared with those whose stones were free of bacteria. In addition, the ten patients with noninfectious pigment stones were compared with the 21 patients with infectious pigment stones.

Statistical analyses were performed using the χ^2 test.

RESULTS
Gallstones

Pigment Stones.—Thirty-one patients had pigment stones, 15 in the gallbladder only, four in the gallbladder and bile duct, and 12 in the common bile duct only (all of the patients in this last group had had a previous cholecystectomy). Twenty-one (68%) of the 31 patients had evidence of bacteria throughout the interior of their stones. Bacteria were identified in the fresh specimens as characteristic coccus or bacillus shapes of about 1 μm in diameter that occurred in small groups (microcolonies) (Fig 1). Previous bacterial inhabitation of air-dried pigment stones was reflected by the presence of "bacterial casts" (Fig 2), which are spaces in the pigment once occupied by bacteria.[5]

Cholesterol Stones.—Thirty-six patients had cholesterol gallstones: gallbladder, 22 patients; common duct, ten patients; and both sites, four patients. On SEM examination, only one patient had bacteria on the surface of a cholesterol common duct stone. The interior of this and all other cholesterol stones was free of bacteria (Fig 3).

Composite Stones.—Fifteen patients had composite gallstones, which were distributed as follows: three patients, gallbladder only; eight patients, common duct only; and four patients, gallbladder and common duct. The stones from 12 (80%) of these patients displayed evidence of bacteria when examined under an SEM, but only in the pigment portions. None of the cholesterol portions of these stones, whether in the center or the periphery, contained bacteria.

Infectious Stones.—The infectious stones, therefore, included 21 pigment and 12 composite stones. None of the cholesterol stones contained bacteria.

Gallbladder Stones.—The patients who had stones in their gallbladders and no stones in their bile ducts were analyzed separately: 15 had pigment stones, 22 had cholesterol stones, and three had composite stones. Twenty-three percent of these 40 stones contained bacteria (seven pigment stones and two composite stones). Thus, 45% of the 40 gallbladder stones contained pigment, and half of these stones were infectious.

Common Duct Stones.—The patients with common duct or common duct and gallbladder stones were also separately analyzed: 16 had pigment stones, 14 had cholesterol stones, and 12 had composite stones. Fifty-seven percent of these 42 stones contained bacteria (14 pigment stones and ten composite stones). Thus, 67% of the 42 common

Table 1.—Clinical Correlations in 85 Patients With Gallstones							
	Stone Composition, No. (%)			Stone Type, No. (%)		Pigment Stones, No. (%)	
Variables	Pigment (n=31)	Cholesterol (n=36)	Composite (n=15)	Infectious (n=33)	Noninfectious (n=49)	Infectious (n=21)	Noninfectious (n=10)
Clinical presentation							
Cholangitis	12 (39)	7 (19)	7 (47)	17 (52)	9 (18)*	11 (52)	1 (10)
Acute cholecystitis	4 (13)	6 (17)	4 (27)	5 (15)	9 (18)	3 (14)	1 (10)
Biliary colic	13 (42)	19 (53)	4 (27)	10 (30)	26 (53)*	6 (29)	7 (70)
Asymptomatic	2 (6)	4 (11)	0 (0)	1 (3)	5 (10)	1 (5)	1 (10)
Temperature							
Afebrile	23 (74)	31 (86)	12 (80)	22 (67)	44 (90)	13 (62)	10 (100)
>38.5°C	8 (26)	5 (14)	3 (20)	11 (33)	5 (10)*	8 (38)	0 (0)
Laboratory data†							
Hematocrit <0.37	8 (26)	9 (25)	6 (40)	14 (42)	9 (18)*	9 (100)	0 (0)
Leukocytes >10.8 × 10⁹/L	10 (32)	13 (36)	2 (13)	9 (27)	16 (33)	8 (80)	2 (20)
Total bilirubin >21 μmol/L	14 (48)	14 (39)	11 (79)	19 (59)	20 (43)	10 (71)	4 (29)
Alkaline phosphatase >125 U/L	17 (59)	16 (46)	14 (100)	25 (78)	21 (46)*	15 (88)	2 (12)
Alanine aminotransferase >35 U/L	17 (61)	19 (53)	12 (86)	22 (69)	26 (57)	13 (76)	4 (24)
Amylase >110 U/L	5 (33)	5 (26)	5 (40)	8 (40)	6 (25)	4 (80)	1 (20)

*$P<.05$.
†Not all laboratory values were obtained on all patients.

duct stones contained pigment, and 86% of these were infectious stones.

Clinical Correlations

Table 1 lists the major clinical manifestations and laboratory data in the 82 patients, divided according to stone composition (pigment, cholesterol, or composite) and stone type (infectious or noninfectious). The 31 patients with pigment stones were further analyzed (Table 1) according to whether or not the stones were infectious. Cholangitis was more common in patients with pigment and composite stones than in patients with cholesterol stones. The difference was more striking, however, when patients were divided according to stone type: cholangitis was nearly three times more frequent in patients with infectious stones. Most patients with noninfectious stones presented with chronic biliary symptoms, such as biliary colic, and no evidence of infection. Infectious stones were present in 17 (65%) of 26 patients presenting with cholangitis but in only ten (28%) of 36 patients with mild, chronic biliary symptoms ($P<.05$).

Nine (27%) of 33 patients with infectious stones had had a previous common duct procedure. This was the case in seven (14%) of 49 patients with noninfectious stones ($P<.05$). Fever was twice as common in patients with infectious stones. Other manifestations, including abdominal pain, nausea and vomiting, diarrhea, jaundice, or a positive Murphy's sign, occurred with similar frequency in both groups. Hypotension occurred in only one patient, an elderly man with infectious pigment common duct stones and toxic cholangitis.

The number of associated diseases affecting other organ systems was no different in the patients with infectious stones than in those with bacteria-free stones. However, a history of hemolysis was present in three of the ten patients with noninfectious pigment stones and in none of the other patients.

Patients with infectious stones more often had low hematocrit values and elevated alkaline phosphatase levels than did patients with noninfectious stones. The presence of leukocytosis was unrelated to bacteria in the stones. Table 2 lists the operative findings and postoperative course of these patients. The majority of patients with noninfectious stones had cholecystectomy alone, while 76% of patients with infectious stones required either a common bile duct exploration or a drainage procedure. Fifteen patients underwent permanent drainage procedures as therapy for ductal stone disease, and this was about evenly split between patients with infectious and noninfectious stones. Thirty patients had a common duct exploration without a drainage procedure, 18 of whom had infectious stones, and 12 of whom had noninfectious stones. Infectious stones were more likely to be retrieved from the common duct: 24 (73%) of 33 infectious stones were found in the common duct or both gallbladder and common duct, whereas this was the case for only 18 (37%) of 49 noninfectious stones.

Table 2.—Operation Performed and Postoperative Course Compared With Stone Type		
	Stone Type, No. (%)	
	Infectious	Noninfectious
Operation		
Cholecystectomy	8 (24)	27 (55)
Common bile duct exploration/drainage	25 (76)	22 (45)*
Status of operation		
Elective	23 (70)	39 (80)
Urgent/emergent	10 (30)	10 (20)*
Positive bile culture	28 (97)	14 (35)*
Complications		
Minor	5 (15)	7 (15)
Major	5 (15)	4 (9)

*$P<.05$.

Bile stasis due to an obstructing lesion was present in

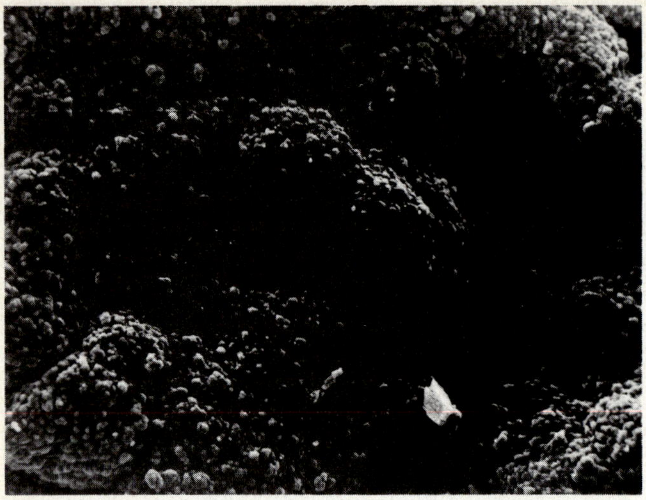

Fig 4.—Scanning electron micrograph of pigment gallstone from patient with hereditary spherocytosis, with no bacteria seen (original magnification ×1920).

seven patients. These included three patients with postoperative anastomotic biliary strictures, two patients with Oriental cholangiohepatitis, one patient with a biliary stricture due to chronic pancreatitis, and one patient with a choledochal cyst. Three of these patients had infectious stones.

Bacteria were almost always (97%) cultured from the bile of patients with infectious stones, but they were also found in 35% of patients with noninfectious stones.

Only three patients required admission to the intensive care unit: two of these patients had infectious common duct stones, and one of them died. The third patient had composite gallbladder stones that were also infectious. There was no difference in the rate of minor or major complications between the two groups.

Of the 31 patients with pigment stones, 21 (68%) had evidence of bacteria inside their stones and ten (32%) were bacteria free. Patients with infectious pigment stones were more likely to have fever (38% vs 0%), leukocytosis (48% vs 20%), a positive bile culture (89% vs 33%), and the need for an urgent or emergent operation (33% vs 20%). The two septic complications in patients with pigment stones were associated with bacteria in the stones. Seventy-six percent of patients with infectious pigment stones spent more than a week in the hospital postoperatively, compared with only 30% of patients with noninfectious pigment stones.

Four of the ten patients with noninfectious pigment stones had a hemolytic process (aortic valve prosthesis, hereditary spherocytosis) or another metabolic reason for pigment stone formation (Gilbert's disease, prolonged preoperative total parenteral nutrition). None of these risk factors was present in patients who developed infectious pigment stones.

COMMENT

Gallstones are classified according to composition into pigment and cholesterol stones. The steps in cholesterol gallstone formation are reasonably well established, but less clear is what leads to the formation of pigment stones. In some patients, pigment stones result from hemolysis[8] or other metabolic conditions,[9-11] but the factors responsible for the formation of most pigment gallstones remain obscure.

Maki et al[12-14] and other investigators[3] postulated a role for bacteria in the formation of pigment gallstones in Asia. The theory involved secretion by bacteria of the enzyme β-glucuronidase, which deconjugates bilirubin in bile. The unconjugated bilirubin precipitates with calcium to form calcium bilirubinate particles. We[5] recently reported evidence that bacteria are also involved in the formation of pigment stones in Western cultures. The most significant finding of our study was the presence of large numbers of bacteria within most pigment stones.

The present findings are consistent with our previous report: 68% of patients with pigment stones had bacteria within the interior of their stones, while no cholesterol stones contained bacteria. In addition, 80% of composite stones contained bacteria in their pigment portions.

In this study, we found that the major clinical manifestations of gallstone disease were more severe in patients whose stones contained bacteria. Over half of such patients presented with cholangitis, compared with one fifth of patients with noninfectious stones. Biliary colic was the most common manifestation in patients with noninfectious gallstones, and 10% of patients with bacteria-free stones were asymptomatic.

More patients with infectious stones had had a previous common duct operation. The kind of operation required had no relationship to the kind of stones found in the duct. Interestingly, four (33%) of 12 patients with infectious stones and previous biliary surgery had had an unsuccessful endoscopic sphincterotomy. The significance of this finding is unclear, because patients who had had a successful endoscopic sphincterotomy did not come to surgery. Nevertheless, none of the patients with noninfectious stones had had an endoscopic sphincterotomy preoperatively.

Infectious stones were more common among stones from the duct (57%) than stones from the gallbladder (25%). This helps to explain some of the correlations, because only patients with common duct stones, for example, would experience cholangitis.

Bernhoft et al[1] found that nearly one half of common duct stones in their study were composed of pigment. Sixty-seven percent of common duct stones in the present study were pigment or composite stones, but this probably overestimates the prevalence of pigment stones in general, because not every cholesterol common duct stone encountered during the period of this study was examined. Still, it is clear that pigment stones are more common in patients with common duct stones than in patients with only gallbladder stones. Possible reasons are as follows: infectious stones may be more likely to migrate from the gallbladder into the common duct and remain there; infectious stones may be likely to form primarily in the duct; or infectious stones may be more likely to cause symptoms (as shown above) and require surgery.

Considering patients with gallbladder stones alone, those with infectious stones were more likely to have suffered acute cholecystitis, while those with noninfectious stones more often presented with biliary colic. Among patients with common duct stones, those with infectious stones were more likely to present with acute cholangitis than were patients with noninfectious stones.

Because most, but not all, pigment stones are infectious stones, we compared the findings in patients with pigment stones in relation to whether or not the stones contained bacteria. Patients with infectious pigment stones more often had fever on admission, had leukocytosis, had infected bile, and required an urgent or emergent operation than those with bacteria-free pigment stones. The only two septic complications in patients with pigment stones occurred in patients with infectious stones. Thus, even in patients with pigment stones, gallstone disease was more severe in the subgroup with infectious stones.

Forty percent of the patients with bacteria-free pigment stones had specific risk factors for the development of pigment stones. For example, pigment stones that resulted from hemolysis did not contain bacteria (Fig 4). None of the patients with infectious pigment stones had these risk factors.

How bacteria enter the biliary tree and contribute to pigment stone formation is not clear. A few patients had mechanical causes of stasis (eg, biliary stricture) and two had Oriental cholangiohepatitis, which is generally assumed to have infection as an initial event. In the patients without these factors, no other cause was apparent. In this regard, it is interesting to note that a higher percentage of common duct pigment stones were infectious (86%) compared with gallbladder pigment stones (50%). Eventually, this observation will have to be incorporated into etiologic theories for infectious stones.

Although nearly half of the patients who had a drainage procedure had infectious stones, 60% of patients who had a choledocholithotomy without drainage also had infectious stones. The latter group had grossly normal ducts and no obvious reasons for biliary stasis. The finding of infectious stones in patients with normal-caliber ducts suggests that the traditional indications for a drainage procedure may need to be revised. The classical indications include (1) gross evidence of bile stasis (eg, mechanical obstruction, dilated duct) or (2) recurrent stones after an earlier common duct exploration. Both indicate that stones will recur if nothing more than a choledocholithotomy is done.[15] If bacteria colonize the duct and participate in stone formation even in the absence of anatomic changes, it seems likely that stones will recur in such cases unless something is done to interrupt the process. Consequently, the indications for a drainage procedure should probably be expanded to include the presence of infectious duct stones, even in cases where there are no signs of bile stasis. Since such a high proportion (86%) are infectious, pigment common duct stones per se should probably become an indication for a drainage procedure.

Based on these data, we propose that (1) bacteria play an important role in the formation of many pigment gallstones, whether from the gallbladder or the common duct; (2) the severity of pigment gallstone disease correlates with the presence of bacteria inside the stones; (3) if the patient has infectious common duct stones they will probably recur after choledocholithotomy alone, so a drainage procedure is indicated; and (4) the greater severity of pigment gallstone disease is probably a reflection of the bacteria that inhabit these stones.

References

1. Bernhoft RA, Pellegrini CA, Motson RW, et al: Composition and morphologic and clinical features of common duct stones. *Am J Surg* 1984; 148:77-85.
2. Lygidakis NJ: Incidence of bile infection in patients with choledocholithiasis. *Am J Gastroenterol* 1982;77:12-17.
3. Tabata M, Nakayama F: Bacteria and gallstones: Etiologic significance. *Dig Dis Sci* 1981;26:218-224.
4. Cetta FM: Bile infection documented as initial event in the pathogenesis of brown pigment biliary stones. *Hepatology* 1986;6:482-489.
5. Stewart L, Smith AL, Pellegrini CA, et al: Pigment gallstones form as a composite of bacterial microcolonies and pigment solids. *Ann Surg* 1987;206:242-250.
6. Costerton JW, Irvin RT: The bacterial glycocalyx in nature and disease. *Annu Rev Microbiol* 1981;35:299-324.
7. Trotman BW, Soloway RD: Pigment gallstone disease: Summary of the National Institutes of Health–international workshop. *Hepatology* 1982; 2:879-884.
8. Soloway RD, Trotman BW, Maddrey WC, et al: Pigment gallstone composition in patients with hemolysis or infection/stasis. *Dig Dis Sci* 1986; 31:454-460.
9. Boucher IAD: Postmortem study of the frequency of gallstones in patients with cirrhosis of the liver. *Gut* 1969;10:705-710.
10. Roslyn JJ, Pitt HA, Mann L, et al: Parenteral nutrition–induced gallbladder disease: A reason for early cholecystectomy. *Am J Surg* 1984; 148:58-63.
11. Schwesinger WH, Kurtin WE, Levine BA, et al: Cirrhosis and alcoholism as pathogenetic factors in pigment gallstone formation. *Ann Surg* 1984;201:319-322.
12. Maki T: Pathogenesis of calcium bilirubinate gallstone: Role of *E coli*, β-glucuronidase and coagulation by inorganic ions, polyelectrolytes and agitation. *Ann Surg* 1966;164:90-100.
13. Maki T, Matsushiro T, Suzuki N, et al: Role of sulfated glycoprotein in gallstone formation. *Surg Gynecol Obstet* 1971;132:846-854.
14. Maki T, Matsushiro T, Suzuki N: Pathogenesis of the calcium bilirubinate stone, in *Intrahepatic Calculi*. New York, Alan R Liss Inc, 1984, pp 81-90.
15. Allen B, Shapiro H, Way LW: Management of recurrent and residual common duct stones. *Am J Surg* 1981;142:41-47.

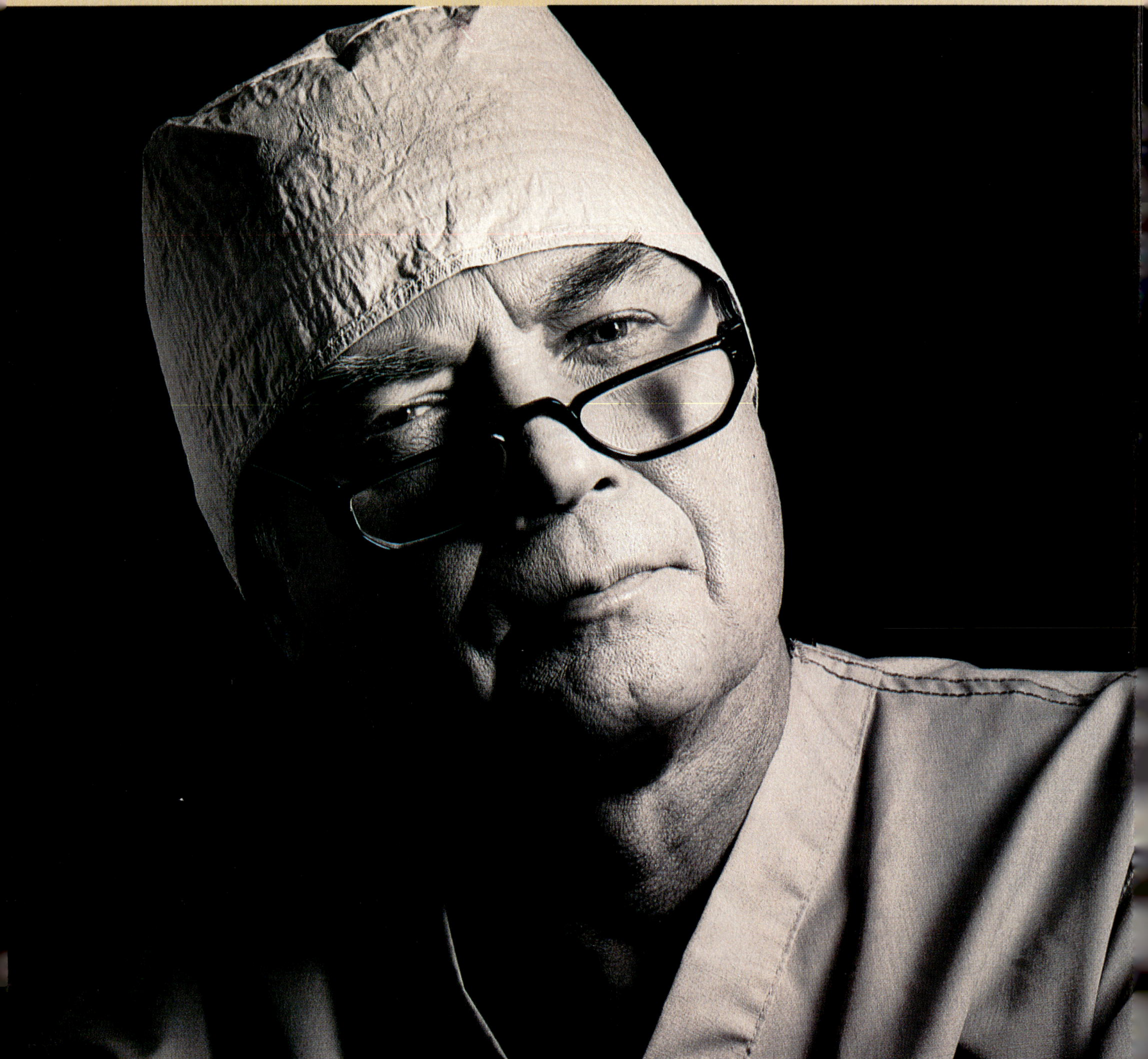

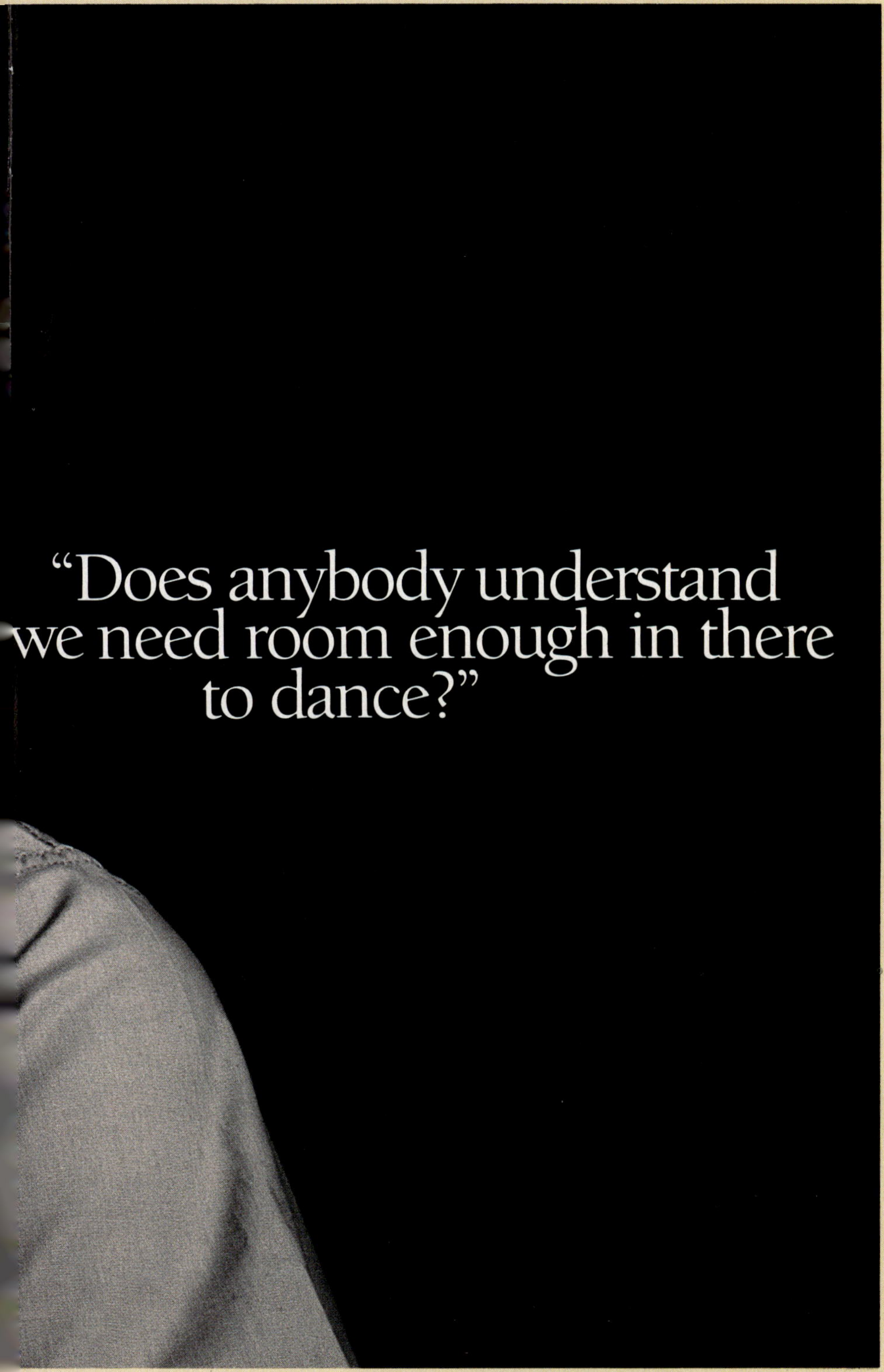
"Does anybody understand we need room enough in there to dance?"

Massive Upper-Extremity Edema Following Forearm Fistula: Cause and Treatment With Salvage of the Fistula

To the Editor.—Among the complications of arteriovenous fistulas created for hemodialysis, one of the most challenging to treat is massive arm edema. We report a case of massive arm edema with threatened gangrene following the formation of a forearm fistula in which the arm and fistula were salvaged by axillary vein–to–axillary vein bypass.

Report of a Case.—A left forearm loop fistula was created in a 68-year-old woman whose history included a previous left subclavian hemodialysis catheter. Postoperatively, the patient developed massive left arm edema, leading to pregangrenous changes in her fingers. A presumptive diagnosis of proximal venous obstruction was made. In an effort to salvage not only the arm but also the fistula, we performed left axillary vein–to–right axillary vein polytetrafluoroethylene bypass after operative venography (Figure), which demonstrated a completely thrombosed left innominate vein.

The postoperative course was extraordinarily rewarding, with overnight relief of considerable arm edema and finger cyanosis. Although mild forearm edema remains, it is not bothersome to this very appreciative patient 13 months after bypass surgery.

Comment.—Major upper-extremity venous stenosis or thrombosis combined with increased inflow (arteriovenous fistulas), such as occurs in patients undergoing dialysis, can result in serious morbidity.[1,2]

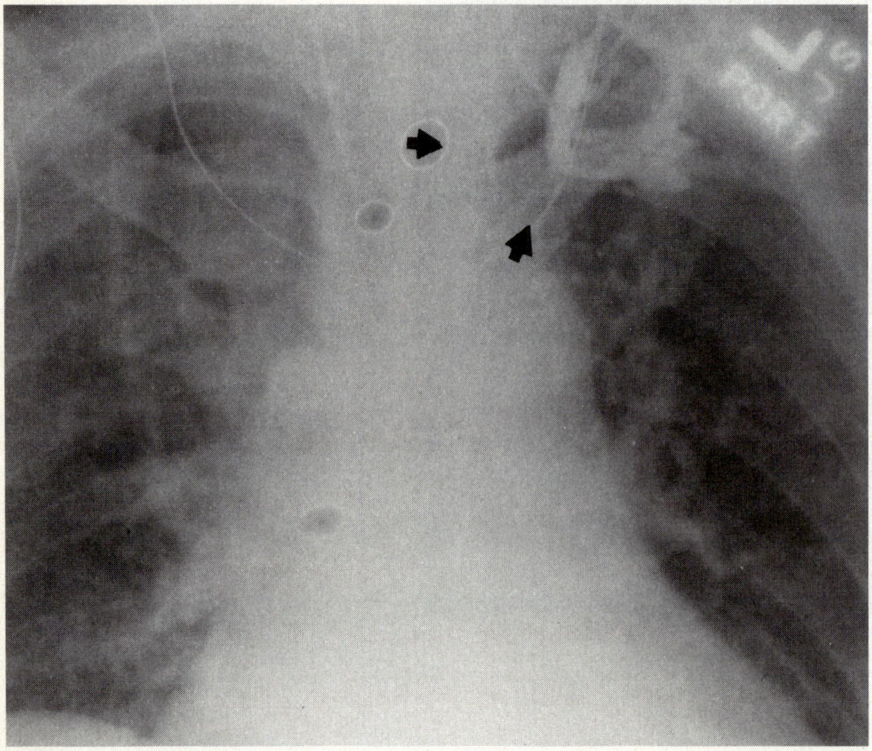

Operative venogram through left internal jugular vein demonstrates complete obstruction of left innominate vein (arrows).

Treatment of significant venous obstruction in the presence of a functioning vascular access depends on the following: (1) severity of edema; (2) degree of stenosis/occlusion; (3) duration of thrombosis; and (4) location of obstruction, ie, axillary, subclavian, or innominate stenosis/occlusion. With mild edema, arm elevation may allow progressive development of adequate collateral flow. However, with edema unresponsive to elevation, surgical intervention may be required.[2] We believe that fistula ligation should rarely be performed as preferred management. Ligation would immediately limit the patient's venous access. With inaccessible or completely occluded veins, bypass surgery may relieve the symptoms and salvage the fistula. The exact type of bypass will depend on the location of the obstructed or stenotic vein. We used axillary vein–to–contralateral axillary vein bypass, although axillary vein–to–contralateral jugular vein bypass would also be an option. Unlike other vein-to-vein grafts, it is a graft placed between an arterialized (high-flow) vein and a normal vein, which allows for high patency rates.

Proximal venous obstruction is a significant, though infrequently recognized, sequela of subclavian venous catheterization, particularly with augmented venous inflow.

Arasu Rajagoplan, MD
Robert B. Wagner, MD
Cheverly, Md

1. Glaze RC, MacDougall ML, Wiegmann TB: Thrombotic arm edema as a complication of subclavian vein catheterization and arteriovenous fistula formation for hemodialysis. *Am J Kidney Dis* 1986;7:437-441.

2. Currier CB Jr, Widder S, Ali A, et al: Surgical management of subclavian and axillary vein thrombosis in patients with a functioning arteriovenous fistula. *Surgery* 1986;100:25-28.

Sclerosing Cholangitis Associated With Hydatid Liver Disease

To the Editor.—In the October 1986 issue of the ARCHIVES, Belghiti et al[1] referred to a case commented on but unpublished. We present a description and the final outcome of this case.

Report of a Case.—A 56-year-old woman was operated on for a hydatid liver cyst in 1978. After aspiration of a small amount of bile-stained hydatid fluid, 20 mL of 40% ethanol was injected into the cyst. The entire biliary tree was found to be filled with hydatid membranes. After the bile ducts were emptied a choledochoduodenostomy was performed because of papillary stenosis. A fistulography done two weeks after the operation because of persistent biliary drainage showed multiple strictures of the intrahepatic bile ducts. The biliary fistula closed spontaneously but several bouts of cholangitis were observed over the years. An endoscopic retrograde cholangiopancreatogram showed multiple biliary strictures compatible with sclerosing cholangitis (Figure) and a liver biopsy disclosed inflammatory multicellular reaction around the portal spaces. The patient died of end-stage liver failure seven years after the operation.

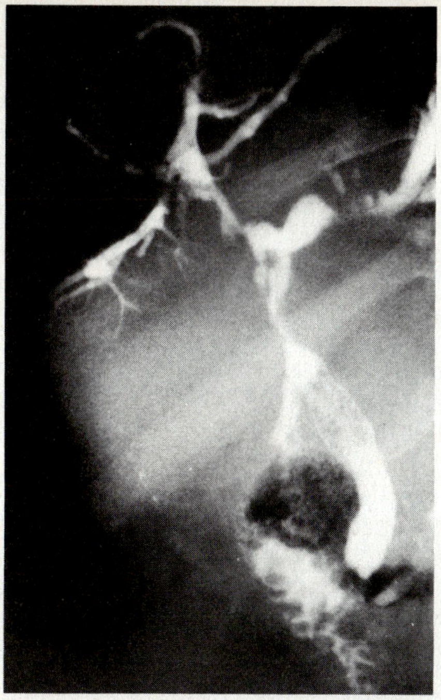

Endoscopic retrograde cholangiopancreatogram showing multiple biliary structures compatible with sclerosing cholangitis.

Comment.—As other authors have commented, it is difficult to determine a clear relationship between the intracystic use of any scolicidal solution and the occurrence of sclerosing cholangitis because of the scarcity of reported cases of this condition among thousands of hydatid cases treated with different scolicidal agents. In our patient we are dubious of alcohol's role as the causative agent because other factors, including intrabiliary hydatid disease, were involved. However, we agree with Belghiti and colleagues[1] that intracystic scolicidal solutions do not seem useful and can be dangerous.

JOSE R. POLO, MD, PHD
JOSE L. GARCIA-SABRIDO, MD, PHD
Madrid

1. Belghiti J, Benhamou J-P, Houry S, et al: Caustic sclerosing cholangitis: A complication of the surgical treatment of hydatid disease of the liver. *Arch Surg* 1986;121:1162-1165.
2. Polo-Melero J, quoted by Tères J, Gomez-Moli J, Bruguera M, et al: Sclerosing cholangitis after surgical treatment of hepatic echinococcal cysts: Report of three cases. *Am J Surg* 1984; 148:694-697.

Books

A spate of books relating to the esophagus have been published during the past six months. Such unexpected attention to what Skinner has called the "Cinderella of surgery" may simply be fortuitous, but more likely reflects the frequency of esophageal disease, the controversies that surround its management, and, perhaps, the renewed attention paid by general surgeons to the esophagus while their cardiac surgical colleagues are occupied constructing conduits from the aorta to the coronary vessels.

Management of Esophageal Disease, by D. B. Skinner and R. H. R. Belsey, 895 pp, with illus, $145, Philadelphia, Pa, WB Saunders Co, 1988.

This weighty monograph is a delightful throwback in textbook style to the first half of this century. The two confident, authoritarian, and experienced British and American surgeon-authors have produced a book in their own personal images. Not for them to rely on others in various supporting disciplines to write chapters on a subject in which they are the experts. As a result, what may be lost in scientific depth is compensated for by the authors' judgment in culling from the literature what they deem important for a fellow surgeon to know. Having thus weighed the evidence, Skinner and Belsey boldly state their conclusions based on these data.

Few readers will agree with all of the positive judgments made by these authors, but there will be no doubt where the authors stand. For example, they have but thinly veiled disdain for stapled anastomosis, transhiatal resection of the esophagus, or antireflux operations other than their own.

This encyclopedia of esophageal disease covers everything from anatomy, physiology, and diagnosis to details of operations. It is perhaps typical that most of the illustrations are of barium contrast studies or of operative techniques, not of pressure tracings or of computed tomographic scans.

Both authors are experienced teachers, which makes for a clear text. Belsey's editorial trademark of enumerating his reasons is in evidence.

Management of Esophageal Disease contains the personal comments, reflections, judgments, and opinions of two acknowledged world leaders in

(Continued on p 640.)

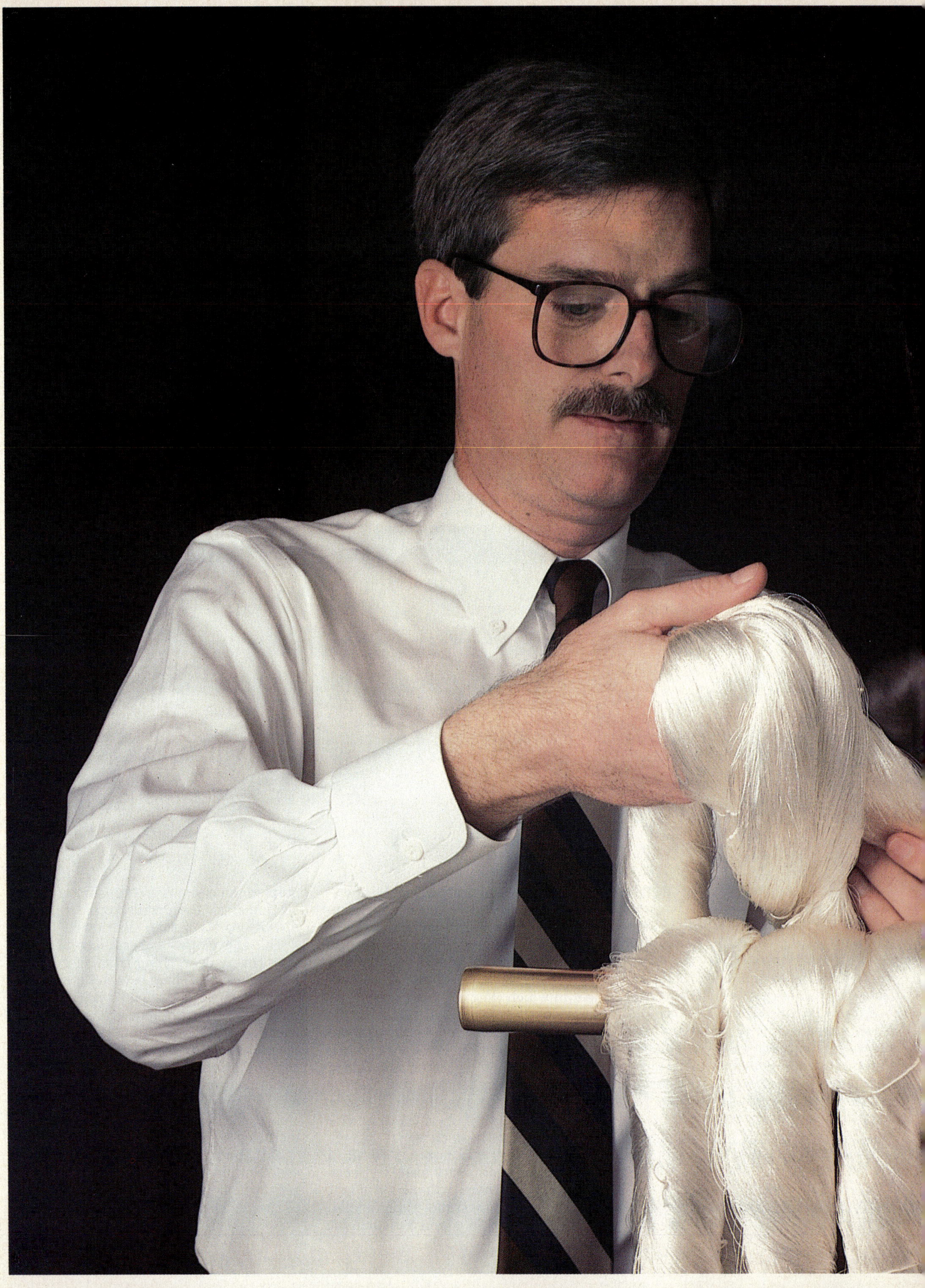

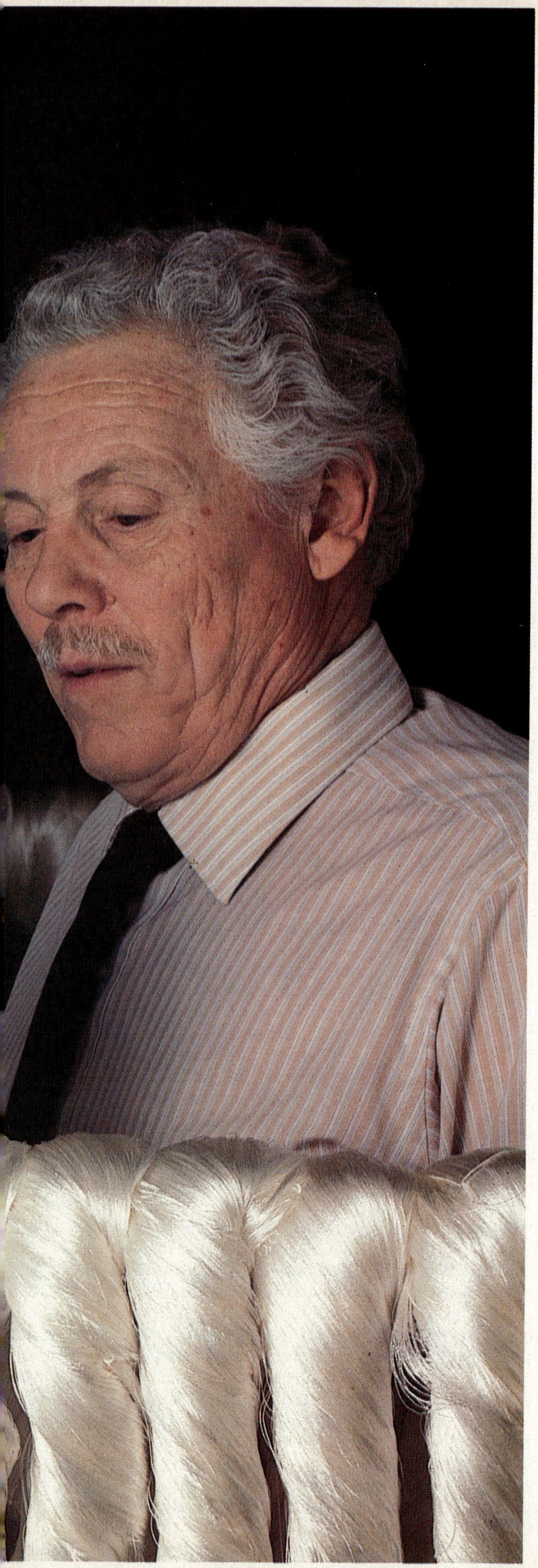

(Continued from p 637.)
esophageal surgery. Few will agree with all of their freely expressed opinions, but only a fool would not listen.

Benign Esophageal Disease, vol 3, edited by T. R. DeMeester and H. R. Mathews, 385 pp, in *International Trends in General Thoracic Surgery*, St Louis, Mo, CV Mosby Co, 1987.

At the other end of the editorial and literary spectrum lie two books sponsored by an international group of general thoracic surgeons who because of clinical interest differentiate themselves both from general surgeons, who primarily operate on the abdomen, and their thoracic surgical colleagues, who specialize in cardiac operations. The wisdom of such divisiveness among specialties may be questioned, but there can be no argument that this prestigious international group has produced two superb reviews concerning the esophagus.

Seventy-nine authors from 13 countries have written 26 chapters and almost an equal number of formal commentaries on problems of benign esophageal disease. On the face of it, this could have been a linguistic and editorial nightmare, but it is not. Thanks to excellent editorial and publishing supervision, what has emerged is a scholarly, fact-filled, well-documented current overview of a controversial clinical subject. Protagonists for competing methods of diagnosis and treatment present their subjects in forceful and critical styles. The authors are from many disciplines in addition to surgery. The resulting collection of articles is diametrically opposite to the book by Skinner and Belsey. Both sides of a controversy are presented, and it is up to the reader to choose which one to follow. Differences of opinion are expressed with verve, and no statement by the opponent in the debate is beyond challenge. Esophagologists turn out to be a feisty lot, at least in print.

With 79 authors (and an average of five pages of text per author) there inevitably is some duplication, but all needed and few extraneous data are included to support the authors' theses.

This third volume in the series sets a high intellectual and editorial standard. It is a book for the serious student of esophageal disease, but not for the beginner, who could perhaps be confused by the disagreement of experts concerning conflicting methods of patient management. This volume makes an excellent current reference source for surgeons wanting to review complex problems of benign esophageal disorders in infants and adults.

Esophageal Cancer, vol 4, edited by N. C. Delaure, E. W. Wilkins, Jr, and J. Wong, 456 pp, in *International Trends in General Thoracic Surgery*, St Louis, Mo, CV Mosby Co, 1988.

Esophageal cancer is a subject most appropriate for a multiauthored, international monograph. The international experience of the three editors guarantees a sophisticated evaluation of the differences with this tumor in various parts of the world.

The 456 pages contain chapters written by 104 authors from six continents. It is interesting that only half the articles are from countries where English is the lingua franca of medicine.

As is well known, the Japanese and Chinese experience with management of early lesions stands in stark contrast with the usually dismal results of treatment in most Western countries. The chapters describing the techniques for early detection of esophageal cancer in high-risk populations are particularly well done.

The large number of articles, some of which are only one to three pages long, makes for uneven reading. Some of the shorter chapters might have been omitted. The editors have seen to it that each contribution, however short, is fact filled and to the point.

As in other volumes within the series, emphasis is on the new and controversial. Surgeons in North America have much to learn about esophageal cancer from their colleagues in Hungary, France, South Africa, Japan, and China, where the disease is so much more frequent. Topics such as sonography, submucography, double-contrast radiography, and variants of endoscopy and brush biopsy will be of particular interest to many North American surgeons and gastroenterologists.

The Esophagus: Medical and Surgical Management, edited by L. Hill, R. Kozarek, R. McCollum, and C. D. Mercer, 327 pp, with illus, $75, Philadelphia, Pa, WB Saunders Co, 1988.

This monograph is designed to provide the physician with a practical current evaluation of competing methods of diagnosis and treatment of patients with esophageal disease. It is far less pretentious than the books reviewed above. It focuses primarily on benign disease; only 20 pages concern cancer.

The 28 contributors from seven countries represent various clinical specialties. Each author provides a 4 to 10-page review of a single method of diagnosis or management of esophageal disease. Hill supervised the surgical chapters. Though he obviously favors his own operation for benign disease, he has seen to it that competing operations have enthusiastic advocates and are given a fair hearing.

The Seattle group, of which many of these authors are members, has had experience with more than 15 000 patients with esophageal disease and with over 2000 operations. These authors' well-documented clinical experience adds authority to their presentations.

This book will be of particular value to a busy practitioner faced with the need to review the current status of a patient with benign esophageal problems. In contrast with the other volumes reviewed, this is a balanced, multidisciplined distillate that yields sensible clinical advice. What it lacks in basic scientific sophistication it makes up in the practical help it provides the clinician.

Gastroesophageal Reflux, edited by G. G. J. Amieson and A. Duranceau, 281 pp, Philadelphia, Pa, WB Saunders Co, 1988.

Two experienced esophageal surgeons, one from Montreal, Canada, and the other from Adelaide, Australia, have edited this book. As the title indicates, coverage is limited to gastroesophageal reflux (GER). It is a tidy, extensively referenced, current review of the subject in the editorial style of a classic textbook. It starts with fundamentals and manages to mention most important controversial aspects of GER in a balanced, scholarly fashion. This book will appeal to students, residents, and primary physicians who only occasionally face esophageal problems. In contrast to several of the other books reviewed, these authors and editors are almost too polite to take sides in the obvious controversies concerning GER.

One cannot but wonder why the diametrically opposed methods for the operative management of GER seem to produce good to excellent result rates of 85% in the hands of its advocates, but show far less benefit when performed by many others.

This work by Jamieson and Duranceau will be available for residents and registrars reviewing the subject of GER for fellowship and board examinations. Users will find that its scholarly balanced discussion of GER contains uncorrosive answers to examiners, whatever their bias.

Ben Eiseman, MD
Denver, Colo

Preliminary Clinical Experience With the Titanium Greenfield Vena Caval Filter

Lazar J. Greenfield, MD; Kyung J. Cho, MD; S. Osher Pais, MD; Michael Van Aman, MD

• Preliminary clinical experience in 40 patients from three institutions is reported for a new titanium model of the Greenfield vena caval filter. The titanium filter is slightly larger than the standard stainless steel filter and can be loaded into a 12 F diameter carrier system as opposed to the 24 F stainless steel filter. In patients ranging from 17 to 94 years of age, percutaneous insertions were made from the right femoral vein in 24 patients, the left femoral vein in 11 patients, and the right internal jugular in 2 patients. Operative access was obtained in 1 patient each from the right femoral, right jugular, and a lumbar vein at laparotomy. Insertion was completed in all cases but 1 and only 1 patient (3%) showed postoperative femoral vein thrombosis. Distal filter migration was seen in 3 cases (7.5%) without sequelae, and there was no proximal migration. The titanium Greenfield vena caval filter provides improved ease of insertion, and the sheath technique should prevent misplacement. Distal migration should be preventable by techniques to promote hook engagement at the time of insertion.

(*Arch Surg.* 1989;124:657-659)

Mechanical protection against pulmonary thromboembolism often is required instead of or as an adjunct to anticoagulation. Since it was introduced in 1972, the Greenfield inferior vena caval filter has established a record of safety and effectiveness with long-term patency rates in excess of 95% in the experience of several institutions.[1-3] This predictable patency is a feature of the cone-shaped design that allows emboli to be trapped without occlusion of the cava, thereby promoting subsequent spontaneous thrombolysis independent of anticoagulation. The high rate of long-term patency has allowed positioning of the filter above the level of the renal veins when indicated, usually because of thrombus propagation to that level.[4,5]

The original technique for insertion of the filter carrier system was by surgical exposure of the jugular or femoral vein. With further development of the Seldinger technique for percutaneous insertion of catheters and dilators over a guide wire, it has been possible to insert the carrier system percutaneously through a 24 F sheath.[6] However, percutaneous insertion from the femoral route has been associated with a higher incidence of postinsertion femoral vein thrombosis.[7] To reduce the size of the carrier system and to facilitate percutaneous insertions, a titanium alloy model of the Greenfield filter (TGF) has been developed and has been shown to be effective in trapping experimental emboli.[8] In addition, a modification of the technique of insertion has been made using a longer sheath through which the carrier system is passed, and additional safety features have been incorporated into the control handle. This article summarizes our preliminary clinical experience with the modified filter and insertion system.

Accepted for publication November 17, 1988.

From the Departments of Surgery (Dr Greenfield) and Radiology (Dr Cho), the University of Michigan Medical Center, Ann Arbor; the University of Maryland, Baltimore (Dr Pais); and Ohio State University, Columbus (Dr Van Aman).

Reprint requests to the University of Michigan, Department of Surgery, 2101 Taubman Center/0346, Ann Arbor, MI 48109 (Dr Greenfield).

MATERIALS AND METHODS

The TGF is fabricated from a titanium alloy that has elastic properties allowing it to be compressed into a 12 F carrier. It is slightly longer than the standard stainless steel filter (SGF), with a length of 4.7 cm as opposed to the 4.4 cm length of the SGF (Fig 1). The TGF is also broader at the base (38 mm) than the SGF (30 mm, Fig 1) and lighter in weight at 0.25 g as compared with 0.56 g for the SGF. The mechanical properties of the TGF have been tested extensively, and it shows remarkable resistance to flexion fatigue and induced corrosion.[9] It exerts a force of fixation on the wall of the vena cava that is greater than the SGF at diameters over 22 mm but less than the SGF at diameters less than 22 mm.

The technique for placement uses a guide wire inserted from either the femoral or jugular vein over which a dilator system and attached 14 F sheath can be passed. Once the sheath and dilator are in the inferior vena cava at the level of filter placement, the dilator is withdrawn, and the TGF carrier is then passed under fluoroscopic control to the level of intended insertion. Both the carrier catheter and sheath are withdrawn as a unit to release the filter. After discharge, the carrier and sheath are withdrawn and gentle pressure is applied to the insertion site.

Preliminary clinical experience was obtained in 40 patients from April to October 1988 in the hospitals of the University of Michigan, Ann Arbor (16 patients), the University of Maryland, (8 patients), and Ohio State University, Columbus (16 patients). Their ages ranged from 17 to 94 years, and the sex distribution was 23 female patients and 17 male patients. Percutaneous access for insertion was obtained from the right femoral vein in 24 patients, the left femoral vein in 11 patients, and the right internal jugular vein in 2 patients. Operative access for insertion was utilized in 3 patients, 1 each from the right femoral vein, the right internal jugular vein, and a lumbar vein as part of a resection of a retroperitoneal sarcoma. In the latter case, the lumbar vein was the final connection of the tumor mass and because fluoroscopy was not available, the carrier was palpated in the vena cava for suprarenal discharge.

The indications for filter placement included a contraindication to anticoagulation in 33 patients, a complication of anticoagulation forcing it to be discontinued in 5 patients, failure of anticoagulation to prevent pulmonary embolism in 1 patient, and for prophylaxis in the absence of embolism in 1 patient with severe pulmonary hypertension. Preoperatively, it was planned to position the filter below the renal veins in 35 patients and above the renal veins in 5 patients. Follow-up studies included duplex Doppler and B-mode ultrasound examination, computed tomographic scans, plain roentgenograms, and magnetic resonance imaging in 1 patient.

RESULTS

The percutaneous introducer system generally worked well at each of the institutions, but one us (S.O.P.) found it necessary to use balloon dilation in the tract of three patients. Most cases were managed by progressive dilation over the guidewire to 14 F, after which the carrier was passed through the sheath for filter discharge. Failure to pass the dilators occurred in 1 patient, a 56-year-old woman with terminal adenocarcinoma who had a very tight stricture of the inferior vena cava at the level of the hepatic veins. No further attempts at filter placement were made because her narrowed

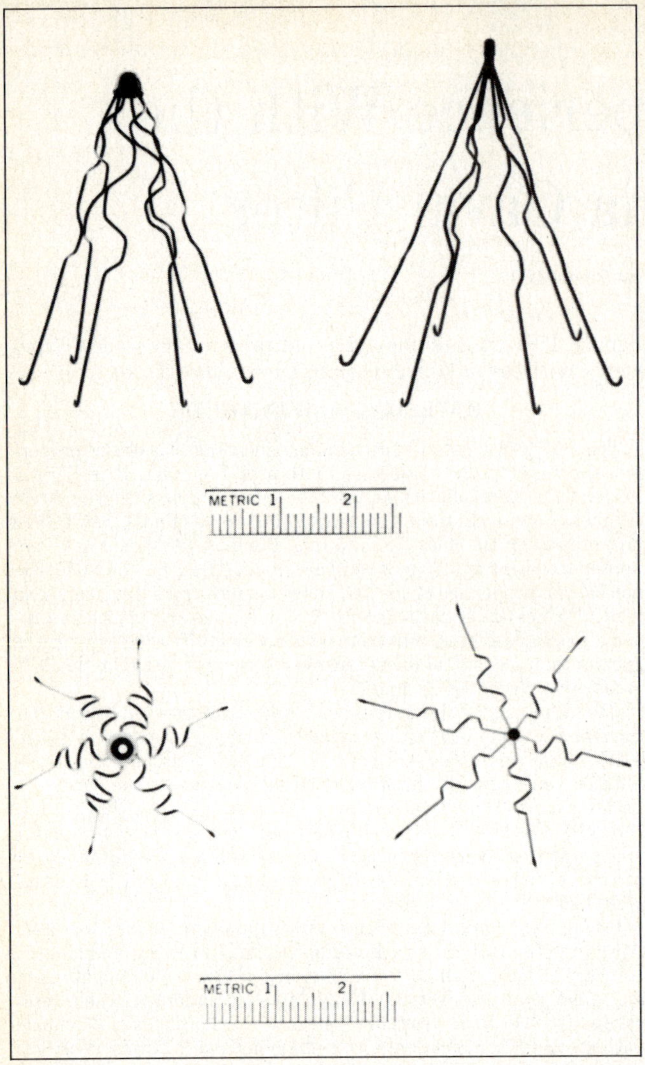

Fig 1.—Top, Side view of the stainless steel (left) and titanium (right) models of the Greenfield vena caval filter. Bottom, Axial view of the stainless steel (left) and titanium (right) models of the Greenfield filter. The titanium filter has a broader base (38 mm) than the steel filter (30 mm), allowing it to be placed in larger veins.

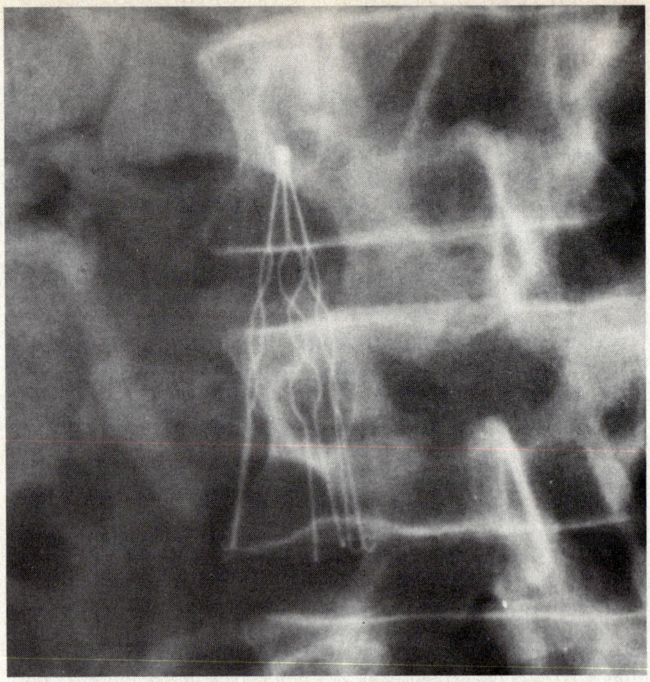

Fig 2.—The titanium Greenfield filter is shown as inserted percutaneously in an infrarenal position.

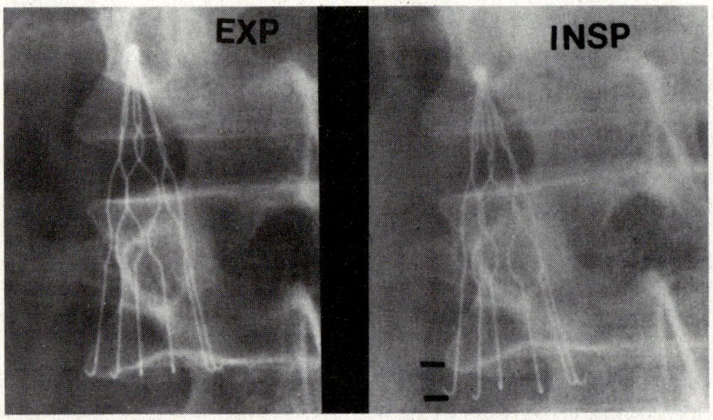

Fig 3.—Three patients were observed to have filter movement with respiration as shown. One of these patients showed a subsequent distal migration of the filter, but the other two remained stable. EXP indicates expiration; INSP, inspiration.

cava was felt to provide some protection against massive thromboembolism. She died 10 days later with no evidence of pulmonary embolism. The remainder of the insertions were uncomplicated, although the angle between the iliac vein and vena cava occasionally required simultaneous advancement of carrier and sheath to enter the vena cava. The TGF was inserted below the renal veins in 35 patients (Fig 2) and above the renal veins in 4, as intended. All of the filters were aligned well within the cava with the exception of one with a tilt of 20°.

There were no complications related to the insertion technique, but at follow-up at 1 week, one patient (3%) showed femoral vein thrombosis at the site of insertion. Filter movement of 4, 5, and 7 mm was noted with respiration in three patients who showed reversible downward displacement with inspiration (Fig 3). One of these patients showed subsequent distal migration of the filter that was also seen in two other patients (7.5%) for distances of 2 to 3 cm. Two of the filters were placed suprarenally in very large vena cavas (30 and 32 mm in diameter) and found subsequently to have slipped with angulation and entry of some of the limbs of the filter in the right renal vein. There was no proximal migration and no evidence of occlusion of any of the filters or recurrent embolism, although the period of follow-up was limited.

There were two deaths that occurred postoperatively in addition to the patient who had an unsuccessful attempt at filter placement. A 46-year-old woman with end-stage carcinoma died of sepsis, and an 82-year-old man with hypertension and bradycardia died 1 day postoperatively. Neither was felt to have sustained recurrent embolism, but autopsies were not obtained. There was one late death in a 31-year-old woman with an inherited disorder of antithrombin III who continued to have recurrent episodes of venous thrombosis despite anticoagulation therapy. Follow-up duplex and magnetic resonance imaging scans showed continued patency of her filter, but she developed subclavian vein thrombosis and progressive pulmonary hypertension. She died 4 months after filter insertion and may have sustained recurrent embolism, al-

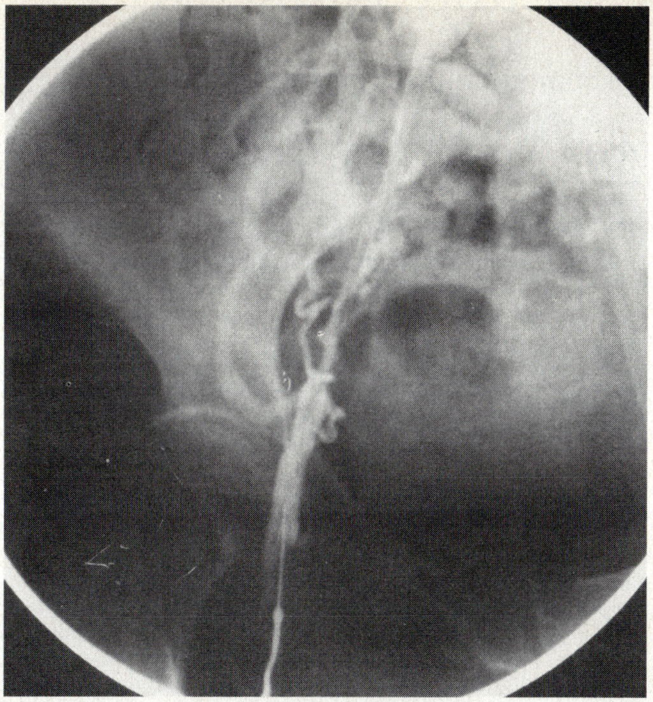

Fig 4.—A patient with thrombosis of her jugular and iliac veins had vena caval access only through the Hickman catheter shown on venogram. Balloon dilation of the catheter tract was necessary to allow passage of the 12 F carrier system for filter placement.

though repeated lung scans were unchanged before her death.

COMMENT

Although most patients with deep vein thrombosis or pulmonary embolism can be managed by anticoagulation alone, it is essential to provide timely mechanical protection from thromboembolism for those patients who have a contraindication to anticoagulation, who have a complication of anticoagulation forcing it to be discontinued, who fail anticoagulation and sustain recurrent embolism, who have a propagating tail on a thrombus in a major vein, who have required pulmonary embolectomy, or who sustain recurrent embolism after another device within or ligation of the inferior vena cava. Although most patients have adequate protection from infrarenal filter placement, the predictable high patency rate of the SGF has allowed it to be inserted above the renal veins and in the superior vena cava under special circumstances.[10] Most commonly, however, placement below the level of the renal veins is made using a guidewire that facilitates passage of the carrier system and reduces the likelihood of misplacement.[11]

The present carrier for the SGF is large enough to present mechanical problems occasionally in both introduction into the vein and passage through the eustachian valve at the atriocaval junction. Reducing the diameter of the carrier system from 24 F to 12 F has facilitated both entry and positioning from the jugular or femoral vein and completely eliminated bleeding during percutaneous filter insertion. Only one patient had sufficient stenosis of the vena cava to prohibit passage of the smaller carrier. In another patient, the first one to receive a TGF, the jugular, femoral, and iliac veins were thrombosed and the only access was through a Hickman catheter in the right femoral vein. After balloon dilatation of that tract (Fig 4), it was possible to pass the TGF carrier into position for filter placement.

The higher proportion of patients intended for suprarenal placement of the filter in this series (12.5%) reflects our increasing satisfaction with the performance of the filter at this level. In a review of the long-term experience at the Medical College of Virginia, the 10-year follow-up of suprarenal Greenfield filters showed that all of the filters remained patent in the patients who returned for yearly examination. The distal migration of two TGF suprarenal filters in our study may be due to the larger diameter of the vena cava at that level, and in each patient the cava was larger than the recommended limit for insertion of the SGF.

Although measurements of lateral force show a greater force for the TGF than the SGF at larger diameters, the lack of migration is likely due to lack of penetration of the hooks of the filter into the vena cava wall. This could be addressed by an additional tap on the filter from below at the time of discharge to engage the hooks into the wall of the cava, but further studies will be necessary to determine the optimal method of fixation. Minimal filter movement over time was reported in 27 patients in two series[12,13] and in the experience of one of us (L.J.G.) in 69 patients with measured radiographic follow-up over a period of 9 years.[14] Most importantly, proximal migration has been reported only when the filter was discharged into a markedly dilated vein[15] or when a thrombus formed within the carrier tethering the limbs of the filter and preventing fixation.

The behavior of titanium in the circulation has been studied and it shows neither additional thrombogenicity nor greater tissue reaction compared with stainless steel.[9] Experimental thrombus capture and resolution is similar to the SGF,[8] and its durability should be comparable in view of its increased corrosion resistance and tolerance to flexion stress. The addition of a sheath to the delivery system adds additional protection against premature discharge and misplacement since discharge before the intended location would be into the sheath that could easily be withdrawn.

References

1. Greenfield LJ, Michna BA. Twelve-year clinical experience with the Greenfield vena caval filter. *Surgery.* 1988;104:706-712.
2. Wingerd M, Bernhard VM, Maddison F, Towne JB. Comparison of caval filters in the management of venous thromboembolism. *Arch Surg.* 1978; 113:1264-1271.
3. Chimochowski GE, Evans RH, Zarins CK, Lu CT, DeMeester TR. Greenfield filter versus Mobin-Uddin umbrella: the continuing quest for the ideal method of vena caval interruption. *J Thorac Cardiovasc Surg.* 1980; 79:358-365.
4. Stewart JR, Peyton JWR, Crute SL, Greenfield LJ. Clinical results of suprarenal placement of the Greenfield vena cava filter. *Surgery.* 1982;92:1-4.
5. Orsini RA, Jarrell BE. Suprarenal placement of vena caval filters: indications, techniques and results. *J Vasc Surg.* 1984;1:124-135.
6. Tadavarthy SM, Castaneda-Zuniga W, Salamonowitz E, et al. Kimray-Greenfield filter: percutaneous introduction. *Radiology.* 1984;151:525-526.
7. Kantor A, Glanz S, Gordon DH, Sclafani SJA. Percutaneous insertion of the Kimray-Greenfield filter: incidence of femoral vein thrombosis. *Am J Res.* 1987;1065-1066.
8. Burke PE, Michna BA, Harvey CF, Crute SL, Sobel M, Greenfield LJ. Experimental comparison of percutaneous vena caval devices: titanium Greenfield filter versus bird's nest filter. *J Vasc Surg.* 1987;6:66-70.
9. Greenfield LJ, Savin MA. Comparison of titanium and stainless steel Greenfield vena caval filters. *Surgery.* In press.
10. Hoffman MJ, Greenfield LJ. Central venous septic thrombosis managed by superior vena cava Greenfield filter and venous thrombectomy: a case report. *J Vasc Surg.* 1986;4:606-611.
11. Greenfield LJ, Stewart JR, Crute SL. Improved technique for Greenfield vena caval filter insertion. *Surg Gynecol Obstet.* 1983;156:217-219.
12. Berland LL, Maddison FE, Bernhard VM. Radiologic follow-up on vena cava filter devices. *Am J Res.* 1980;134:1047-1052.
13. Gomez GA, Cutler BS, Wheeler HB. Transvenous interruption of the inferior vena cava. *Surgery.* 1983;93:612-619.
14. Messmer JM, Greenfield LJ. Greenfield caval filters: long term radiographic follow-up study. *Radiology.* 1985;156:613-618.
15. Castaneda F, Herrera M, Cragg AH, et al. Migration of a Kimray-Greenfield filter to the right ventricle. *Radiology.* 1983;149:690.

Arterial Mycotic Aneurysm and Rupture

A Potentially Fatal Complication of Pancreas Transplantation in Diabetes Mellitus

Andreas G. Tzakis, MD; Patricia B. Carroll, MD; Robert D. Gordon, MD;
Itsuo Yokoyama, MD; Leonard Makowka, MD, PhD; Thomas E. Starzl, MD, PhD

• Mycotic aneurysm at the site of a Carrel patch arterial anastomosis occurred in four patients who had undergone whole pancreas transplantation 2.5 to 14.5 months previously. In all patients, the graft had been removed, leaving the Carrel patch on the iliac artery. The aneurysms ruptured into the intestine or the extraperitoneal space. The ruptures were sudden and life-threatening in three of four cases. This diagnosis must be suspected in patients with a history of pancreas transplantation in the immediate or distant past if they present with unexplained hypotension, cardiac arrest, or gastrointestinal tract bleeding.

(Arch Surg. **1989;124:660-661)**

Pancreas transplantation has been performed with increasing frequency in patients with diabetes mellitus, often at the same time as renal transplantation.[1-5] Mycotic arterial aneurysms developed in four patients at the site of the Carrel patch, which was used to rearterialize the whole pancreas homograft. This life-threatening complication could be confused with cardiac arrhythmias or myocardial infarction, the most common causes of sudden death in advanced diabetes.

PATIENTS AND METHODS

The four complications occurred in 16 patients who received 17 pancreas grafts between 1983 and 1985 in a pilot study of whole pancreas transplantation at the University of Pittsburgh (Pa).[6] The 4 patients were 24 to 36 years of age and had type I diabetes mellitus and a history of ketosis for 18 years or more. All patients had neuropathy and retinopathy. All but 1 had renal failure, which was treated earlier or at the same time with cadaveric kidney transplantation.

A pancreaticoduodenal graft was used in each case. The donor celiac axis and origin of the superior mesenteric artery were included in a Carrel patch of the donor aorta, which was anastomosed to the side of the recipient common iliac artery.[6,7] The end of the graft portal vein was anastomosed to the side of the common iliac vein of the recipient. The graft exocrine secretions were directed into the recipient jejunum by anastomosing the duodenum directly into the recipient jejunum (cases 1 and 2) or through a defunctionalized Roux-en-Y limb of jejunum (cases 3 and 4), with techniques that have been described elsewhere.[6,7] Immunosuppression was achieved with cyclosporine and prednisone, supplemented with azathioprine and monoclonal antibody (OKT3, Orthoclone), as indicated.

Perioperative antibiotics administered at the time of transplantation consisted of cefazolin in patients 1 and 2, cefotaxime in patient 3, and cefotaxime and ampicillin in patient 4.

RESULTS

Clinical Presentation

Failed pancreatic grafts had been removed 5 days to 14 months before the aneurysm ruptures occurred (Table). In patients 1, 2, and 3, the ruptures occurred, fortunately, while the patients were in the hospital. Patient 1 had a peripancreatic abscess drained 1 week before pancreatectomy. No abscess was encountered in patient 2. There was no disruption of the enteric anastomosis. Both patients became pulseless at the same time that they developed swelling in the area of the graft and bleeding through the graft pancreatectomy incision. The incisions were opened at the bedside, and the bleeding was controlled as the patients were rushed to the operating room.

The graft in patient 3 had been removed 2½ months previously because of venous thrombosis, 10 days after the transplantation. The reason for his hospitalization was persistent serous wound drainage. A few hours after admission he had a cardiac arrest after suddenly developing abdominal pain and distention. The diagnosis was obvious, and the patient was resuscitated as he was brought to the operating room.

Patient 4 presented with upper gastrointestinal tract bleeding 1 year after graft pancreatectomy for pancreatitis. Upper and lower gastrointestinal tract endoscopy, technetium bleeding scanning, ultrasound examination, and arteriography of the abdominal aorta and iliac and visceral arteries did not reveal a bleeding source. She was discharged. Two months later, another episode of massive upper and lower gastrointestinal tract bleeding occurred. She was readmitted and collapsed within a few hours. At emergency operation, a rupture was found of the arterial anastomosis site into the tip of the Roux-en-Y loop previously used for enteric drainage.

Bacterial Cultures

The bacteria cultured from the rupture sites are listed in the Table. Results of cultures were negative in patient 4 but were considered to be falsely negative because there was communication with the intestine.

Surgical Treatment

All patients underwent ligation of the proximal and distal common iliac artery. In all but patient 4, crossover femoral-femoral bypass was performed immediately. In patient 4, the extremity seemed well perfused, and the limb was not revascularized. Ten months later, she developed intermittent claudication in the left leg. At the time of this writing, she is scheduled for arterial bypass.

The patients are all alive and well and are currently receiving exogenous insulin. Renal function, if it was present before, was not adversely affected by the complication (Table).

COMMENT

Since the advent of immunosuppression with cyclosporine, 1-year graft survival has improved and is currently reported to be 50% or more.[1-6] Breakdown of the constructed anastomoses for exocrine drainage has been common and has often been ascribed to the proteolytic activities of the pancreatic juices, or less often to infections.

Both factors could have contributed to the aneurysm formation and rupture in our four patients. The bacteria cultured from the rupture site in three patients were indigenous to the gastrointestinal tract, and in the patient with a negative culture, the rupture was into the intestine. Thus, we classified all of the pseudoaneurysms as mycotic.

Mycotic aneurysm and rupture may be a relatively specific complication of whole pancreas transplantation. Although Carrel patches to the iliac vessels are almost always used for kidney transplantation at the University of Pittsburgh, only one mycotic aneurysm was observed after 1375 cadaveric

Accepted for publication February 20, 1989.

From the Departments of Surgery (Drs Tzakis, Gordon, Yokoyama, Makowka, and Starzl) and Medicine (Dr Carroll), University of Pittsburgh (Pa) Health Center; and Veterans Administration, Pittsburgh (Drs Tzakis, Carroll, Gordon, Yokoyama, Makowka, and Starzl).

Reprint requests to Falk Clinic Transplantation Section, 3601 Fifth Ave, Pittsburgh, PA 15213 (Dr Tzakis).

Clinical Characteristics of Patients With Arterial Aneurysms After Pancreatic Transplantation*							
Patient/ Age, y/Sex	Time of Kidney Transplant	Time Between Pancreas Transplant and Removal	Aneurysm Rupture, Time After Pancreas Transplant Graft Removal	Findings	Arterial Site Culture Results	Repair	Current Status
1/30/M	Previous	15 mo (rejection)	5 d	Pseudoaneurysm of LCIA	*Citrobacter freundii, Bacteroides melaninogenicus, Enterobacter aerogenes, Clostridium subtermindi*	Femoral-femoral, bypass ligation of LCIA	Alive and well; functional kidney transplant
2/28/M	Previous (10 nonfunctional transplants)	2.5 mo (rejection)	1 wk	Pseudoaneurysm of LCIA	*Bacteroides fragilis, Fusobacterium nucleatum*	Femoral-femoral, bypass ligation of LCIA	Alive and well; dialysis
3/36/M	Simultaneous	10 d (venous thrombosis)	2.5 mo	Pseudoaneurysm of LCIA	*C freundii,* microaerophilic philic strept *Viridans*	Femoral-femoral, bypass ligation of LCIA	Alive and well; functional kidney transplant
4/24/F	None	3 wk (pancreatitis)	14 mo	Pseudoaneurysm of LCIA	Negative	Ligation of LCIA	Alive and well; native renal function

*LCIA indicates left common iliac artery.

renal transplantations between 1981 and 1988. In contrast, mycotic aneurysms developed after 4 of our 17 whole pancreas transplantations between 1983 and 1986. At the University of Iowa, Iowa City, aneurysm rupture was seen in 3 of 80 cases (Robert Corry, MD,oral communication, September 1988). The same incidence of 3 in 80 cases has been seen at the Karolinska Institute in Stockholm (Carl G. Groth, MD, oral communicaton, September 1988). In all 10 cases of the Pittsburgh-Iowa City-Stockholm collection, exocrine pancreatic drainage had been into the gastrointestinal tract. This complication was not seen in 3 other patients in our series who had failed grafts removed. Two of these patients' grafts were grossly infected. A fourth patient has had a failed graft left in situ for 3 years without this complication.

Intraperitoneal placement of the pancreatic allograft offers a theoretical advantage of having the arterial anastomosis exposed to the peritoneal cavity rather than the closed extraperitoneal space. Patient 4 had the only intraperitoneal pancreas graft in our series.

Whether this frightening complication will be minimized with the increasingly popular techniques of exocrine drainage into the less contaminated bladder[8,9] remains to be seen. Walstra et al[10] have reported a successfully treated mycotic aneurysm after bladder drainage, which has also been observed with a fatal outcome (D. Nghiem, MD, oral communication, June 1988)

The most important lesson from this cumulative experience is the necessity for a high index of suspicion in the event of wound complications, unexplained shock syndromes, gastrointestinal tract hemorrhage, or unexplained abnormalities with examination performed physically or by imaging techniques. Appropriate surgical care then can be planned, sometimes electively instead of under the catastrophic circumstances that existed in all of our cases. In our patient 4, in whom a wound infection with *Candida stellatoidea* and *Candida albicans* was documented at the time the pancreas was removed for pancreatitis, prophylactic ligation of the common iliac artery was seriously considered but not done. This proved to have been an error when the aneurysm ruptured into the intestine more than 1 year later.

This study was supported by the Veterans Administration, Pittsburgh, Pa; grants DK-29961 and RR0005625 from the National Institutes of Health, Bethesda, Md; and the E. Clarence Rice Fellowship of the American Diabetes Association, Washington, DC (Dr Carroll).

References

1. Sutherland DR. Pancreas transplant registry: history and analysis of cases 1966-1986. *Pancreas.* 1987;473-488.

2. Groth CG, Tyden G. Segmental pancreatic transplantation with enteric exocrine drainage. In: Groth CG, ed. *Pancreatic Transplantation.* Philadelphia, Pa: WB Saunders Co; 1988:99-112.

3. Sollinger HW, Kalayoglu M, Hoffman RM, Deierhoi MH, Belzer FO. Quadruple immunosuppressive therapy in whole pancreas transplantation. *Transplant Proc.* 1987;19:2297-2299.

4. Landgraf R, Landgraf L, Burg M, et al. Longterm follow-up of segmental pancreas transplantation in type I diabetics. *Transplant Proc.* 1986;18:1118-1124.

5. Corry RJ, Nghiem D, Schulak J, Budtel WD, Gonwa TA. Surgical treatment of diabetic nephropathy with simultaneous pancreaticoduodenal and renal transplantation. *Surg Gynecol Obstet.* 1986;162: 547-555.

6. Starzl TE, Tzakis AG. Pancreatico-duodenal transplantation with enteric exocrine drainage. In: Groth CG, ed. *Pancreatic Transplantation.* Philadelphia, Pa: WB Saunders Co; 1988:113-129.

7. Starzl TE, Iwatsuki S, Shaw BW, et al. Pancreaticoduodenal transplantation in humans. *Surg Gynecol Obstet.* 1984;159:265-272.

8. Corry RJ. Pancreatic-duodenal transplantation with urinary tract drainage. In: Groth CG, ed. *Pancreatic Transplantation.* Philadelphia, Pa: WB Saunders Co; 1988:147-153.

9. Sollinger HW, Kalayoglu M, Hoffman R, et al. Experience with pancreaticocystostomy in 24 consecutive pancreas transplants. *Transplant Proc.* 1985;17(suppl 2):141-143.

10. Walstra BJ, Jorning PG, Kootstra G, van Hoof JP, Janevski BK. Pancreas transplantation complicated by a mycotic false aneurysm: diagnostic features. *J Med Imaging.* 1988;2:133-136.

Editorial Comment

This concise article describes a devastating complication (mycotic aneurysm at the arterial suture line) that has occurred with surprisingly high frequency in patients with pancreatic transplantation at the University of Pittsburgh. There have also been a significant number of identical complications reported by the Iowa City and Stockholm groups. The common denominator in all of these cases has been drainage of the pancreatic secretions into the gastrointestinal tract. There is little general recognition even in the transplant community as to the prevalence of this complication, even though the danger of gastrointestinal tract contamination in the immunosuppressed patients is well known. The authors' recommendation for a high index of suspicion of this complication and for its aggressive treatment by ligation of the iliac artery and extra-anatomic bypass is well taken, as is their suggestion that ligation of the artery should even be considered prophalactically in instances where contamination of the suture line is recognized.

CLYDE F. BARKER, MD
Philadelphia, Pa

Results of Operative Treatment of Gastrointestinal Tract Tumors in Patients Over 80 Years of Age

Ph. Morel, MD; R. A. Egeli, MD; S. Wachtl, MD; A. Rohner, MD

• Between 1981 and 1986, 140 patients over 80 years of age were operated on for a gastrointestinal tract tumor in our service. There were 24 gastric, one small-bowel, 91 colonic, and 24 rectal cancers. Only 40% of the patients were preoperatively free of any systemic disorder other than tumor. We performed surgical procedures with a curative intent for 90 (64%) of them. Our mean overall postoperative mortality was 17%, but this rate could be decreased by performing elective operations on well-prepared patients. Over 80% of the deaths were related to systemic organ failures. Eighty-three percent of the survivors (96 patients) returned to their homes; 82% (94 patients) had normal activities for their age. The actuarial survival curve showed a 50% survival rate at three years, all tumoral stages included. These results support the view that surgery is a safe, valid option in the face of gastrointestinal tract tumors in the elderly.

(*Arch Surg* 1989;124:662-664)

Various factors, including preventive medicine, medical progress, and improved social conditions, have increased life expectancy in our societies, and the elderly population continues to expand. Between 1900 and 1970, the general population worldwide multiplied by 2.5, whereas during the same period the geriatric population increased sevenfold. At present, the geriatric population comprises 11% of the general population. This proportion will increase in the coming decades.[1]

Among the causes of death in the geriatric population, cancer represents 15%, being the second leading cause after heart diseases (45%). In the group with cancer, colorectal cancers rank first for women and third for men after lung cancer and prostate cancer. Gastric tumors occur less frequently, and their incidence will decrease over time.[2]

In accordance with these figures, we often face the problem of treating a gastrointestinal tract tumor occurring in an older patient. Since surgery is the main therapeutic option for gastrointestional cancers, we must consider this option for geriatric patients. The surgical approach is dependent on the incurred risk, the tumor's extension and probable evolution, and the agreement of the patient. Other factors should also be taken into consideration, such as life expectancy and quality of survival.

The aim of this study, conducted in a university hospital with surgeons in training, was to assess the morbidity and mortality related to surgical treatment of gastrointestinal tumors in patients older than 80 years and to establish the quality and length of their survival.

Accepted for publication May 16, 1988.

From the Department of Surgery, University Hospital, Geneva.

Reprint requests to Department of Surgery, Digestive Surgery, University Hospital, 1200 Geneva, Switzerland (Prof Rohner).

MATERIAL AND METHODS

From January 1981 to December 1986, we prospectively studied 140 patients older than 80 years operated on for gastrointestinal tract tumors in the Service of Digestive Surgery, Geneva University Hospital. The criteria for inclusion in the study were as follows: patient aged 80 years or more at the time of operation; histological proof of a malignant tumor originating from the digestive tract from stomach to rectum; performance of a laparotomy with or without tumor resection; and no previous digestive tract tumor.

We surveyed 56 men and 84 women. The mean age at operating was 85 years (range, 80 to 94 years). Ninety-eight patients (70%) were between 80 and 84 years, 35 (25%) were between 85 and 89 years, and seven (5%) were over 90 years of age. Sex division among these age groups was similar.

We observed 24 gastric, one small-bowel, 91 colonic, and 24 rectal cancers.

According to the International TNM classification, the gastric cancers were divided as follows: two at stage I; six at stage II; seven at stage III; eight at stage IV; and one not classified. Following Dukes' classification for the colonic cancers, we had two Dukes' class A, 52 Dukes' class B, 25 Dukes' class C, and nine Dukes' class D; three patients could not be classified properly. For rectal cancers, we had two Dukes' class A, nine Dukes' class B, four Dukes' class C, five Dukes' class D, and four not classified.

The number of patients operated on every year does not vary significantly, and ranges from 20 to 29 per year.

The preoperative evaluation of the surgical risk was assessed by using the classification of the American Society of Anesthesiology (ASA), dividing the patients into five groups[3] as follows: 56 patients (40%) in class II; 64 (45%) in class III; and 11 (8%) in classes IV and V. Nine patients could not be classified because some data were not available preoperatively.

Our surgical intent based on a previous retrospective study[4] was to perform operations with a curative view every time that it was technically possible. We tried at least to resect the tumor itself, even if not carcinologically. We performed an operation with a curative view for 90 patients (64%), as 48 (34%) were submitted to an obvious palliative procedure (internal bypass, proximal stomy, or incomplete resection of a macroscopically disseminated disease). Figure 1 summarizes the operative procedures performed.

All survivors were assessed by contacting either them or their families, as well as their physicians. We were mainly interested in the quality of their survival. This appraisal was based on both their social postoperative environment after leaving the hospital and on their possible activities. For this last criterion, we used the activity index proposed by the Swiss Group for Clinical Cancer Research (SAKK).[5] It divides patients into five groups as follows: 0, normal activity; 1, normal activity with symptoms; 2, marked decrease of autonomy (<50% of the day in bed); 3, important decrease of autonomy (>50% of the day in bed); and 4, bedridden. The length of survival was also established.

RESULTS

Our overall postoperative *mortality,* defined as death occurring during the hospital stay, was 17% (25 patients)

(Table). Cardiac (12 cases) and pulmonary (ten cases) insufficiencies accounted for most deaths. We observed one brain stroke. Two patients died following septic complications related to intra-abdominal collections, one due to an anastomotic leakage. (We rarely used the facilities of the intensive care unit due to unsuitable local conditions.)

We observed a good correlation between preoperative evaluation with the ASA score and our postoperative mortality. The 56 patients in class II had a 10% mortality (six cases), the 64 in class III had an 18% mortality (12 cases), and the 11 in classes IV and V had a 36% mortality (four cases). Emergency operations, performed mainly for occlusive colonic cancers, induced a higher mortality (Table).

Postoperative morbidity applied to 21 patients (18%). Most of the complications (14 cases) were related to systemic disorders (pulmonary, cardiac, and neurologic). Seven were due to local problems (two small colonic anastomotic leakages and five septic wound problems).

The mean hospital stay was 17 days (range, six to 44 days), with a median of 15 days. After leaving the hospital, most of the patients immediately returned home (43 cases). The others convalesced either in a specialized home (39 cases) or in a medical recovery center (33 cases). Later, 83% (96 cases) of all patients had returned to their homes without any change in their social environments. A few (14 cases) had to be moved to a specialized institution or to a nursing home, since some (five cases) required nursing assistance at home or went to the family's home.

We compared the preoperative index activity with the postoperative index activity. Fifty-six (49%) of our patients belonged to class 0 preoperatively, 45 (39%) were in class I, ten (9%) were in class II, and four (3%) were in class III. Postoperatively, 94 patients (82%) were in class 0, 16 (14%) were in class I, four (3%) were in class II, and one (1%) was in class III. Thirty-eight patients shifted from classes I and II toward class 0 after removal of the tumor.

We can confirm that most of these elderly patients became independent following surgery and that they enjoyed their survival time.

The length of survival appears to be an important criterion in this age group, and we were pleased to note that the actuarial survival curve (Fig 2) shows a survival rate of 48% at three years (55 patients) and a rate of 32% at five years (37 cases), all stages of tumor development and all localizations included. At the time this report was written, 48 (42%) patients were alive with no evidence of disease, seven were alive with a documented recurrence, 39 (34%) were dead of disease, and 21 were dead of other causes. The mean survival time was three years two months (range, six months to five years eight months). The survival time correlated satisfactorily with the carcinologic stage of the disease. For colonic cancers, the survival rates for patients with Dukes' class B and Dukes' class C tumors were 65% and 26%, respectively, at three years. For patients with gastric cancers, we had an overall 31% survival rate at three years. In this group, the prognosis is slightly better for localized tumors.

COMMENT

Surgery on elderly patients is a continuous challenge. Operations performed for cancer on patients over 80 years of age can seem excessive, and the discovery of a gastrointestinal tract tumor at this age always raises the question of whether to perform a surgical resection. The challenge is to allow the patients to survive the operation and then to offer them a decent quality and length of survival.

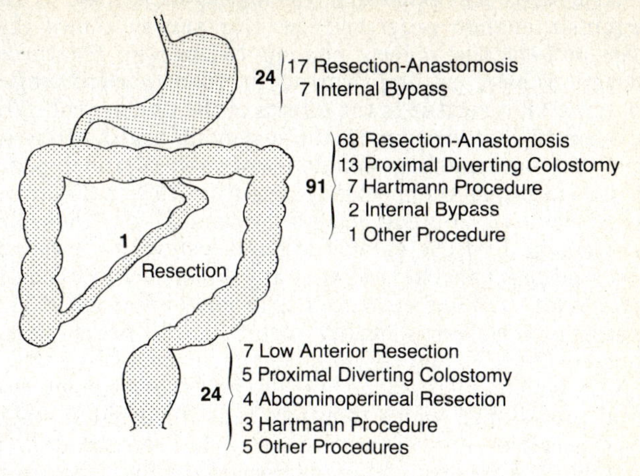

Fig 1.—Localization of tumors and operative procedures performed.

Postoperative Mortality

Procedure	Stomach Cancer (n=24)	Small-Bowel Cancer (n=1)	Colon Cancer (n=91)	Rectum Cancer (n=24)	Total (n=140)
Emergency operation					
No.	1	1	20	2	**24**
Deaths, No.	0	0	5	1	**6**
Mortality, %	0	0	25	50	**26**
Elective operation					
No.	23	0	71	22	**116**
Deaths, No.	2	...	15	2	**19**
Mortality, %	9	...	21	9	**16**
Overall mortality, %	8	...	21	12	**17**

Fig 2.—Actuarial survival curves for our patients. DOC indicates dead of other cause.

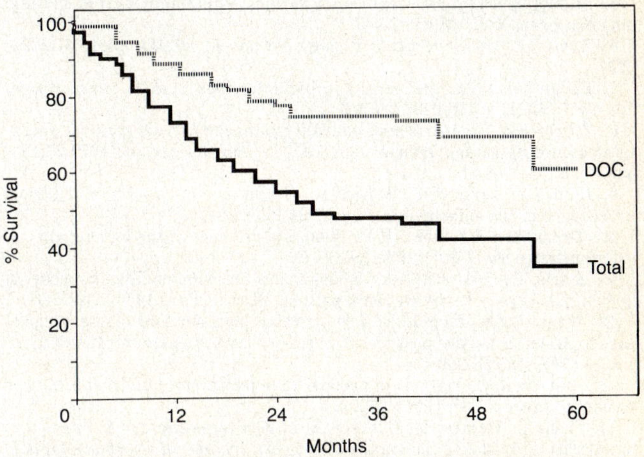

With age, the general physiological capacities of the organism change progressively.[6] Our survey shows that over 50% of the elderly coming to surgery for tumor resection have an impairment in their various organ systems[7,8] not related to the effects of the tumor itself. The relationship between preoperative general health and postoperative outcome has been demonstrated[7,9-11] and appears in our survey, as the mortality rose from 10% to 36% from ASA class II to ASA classes IV and V. We therefore recommend that the various organic systems be carefully assessed preoperatively so that any deficiency or disorder can be detected and corrected or at least improved.[10] This assessment concerns mainly metabolic disorders, nutritional defects,[12,13] and cardiopulmonary abnormalities.[14]

This management cannot be applied to emergency surgical procedures, which therefore must be avoided whenever possible. A preoperative delay for resuscitation is required.[11] This preparation decreased the mortality from 26% to 16% in our survey when the results of emergency procedures were compared with the results of elective operations.[15-17] This relationship between the timing of an operation and the postoperative outcome is also encountered in the younger population.[9]

In the elderly, the immediate postoperative course is of great importance[10,15] and prompt detection of any organic failure is required. The use of an intensive care unit for at least 48 hours is recommended.[17]

Our overall 17% mortality is within the reported range of 6% to 20% for elderly patients.[7,17-20] Systemic disorders accounted for 88% (22 cases) of those fatalities, with the number of local intra-abdominal fatal complications being low.[15] We must point out that, in this age group, the risk factors for surgery for gastrointestinal tract tumors is the same as for other major surgical procedures, such as thigh amputation or hip-joint operations.[9,21]

The postoperative morbidity is also mainly related to systemic disorders (75%). Local anastomotic leakage or septic complications have the same low incidence as for younger people.[18]

Our option to attempt a curative resection whenever possible was successful in as many as 64% of our patients. From our previous study,[4] we estimated that it would prolong the length of survival and improve its quality. Even in the elderly, it is recommended that some operative time be spent to achieve this goal, as the length of the operation is not related to the postoperative outcome,[20] although some controversy remains about this attitude.[21] If a curative resection cannot be achieved, we always favor at least a tumor resection, even palliative, rather than a proximal diverting stoma. At this age, patients have difficulties in managing a stoma bag properly,[18] and the bag does affect their psychological well-being. A one-stage procedure with immediate anastomosis is the best option, and it can be achieved even in occlusive colonic tumors by using "on-table" cleansing of the colon.

The elderly can still enjoy life. Surgical treatment of gastrointestinal tract tumor will prolong their survival, as illustrated by our 50% survival rate at three years. This result correlates with other data[18,22] and illustrates the fact that the long-term prognosis for patients with resected gastrointestinal tract tumors is similar in all age groups.[23,24]

The quality of survival is of major importance in this age group: it would be unjustifiable to recommend an aggressive surgical approach in the elderly if the results were to dramatically alter the course of life. Our survey tends to prove the opposite. The hospital stay is short (mean, 17 days). The index of activity demonstrates that 82% of our patients spent an active normal life and could carry on their previous physical and social activities following surgery. Unexcised growing tumors would have resulted in major discomfort in terms of pain, complications, and debility. Moreover, 83% of the patients returned to their homes, though several spent some convalescent time elsewhere before returning. This issue is important, since the elderly feel secure if they can return to their preoperative environment.

Aggressive surgical treatment of gastrointestinal tract tumors in the elderly will, of course, lead to fairly high health care costs, and it is a matter of health policy to decide whether this cost is worthwhile.[25] Schelling[26] pointed out that the quality of survival should be taken into account at any age when establishing the cost-value relationship in health care. From our encouraging results, we learn that the elderly can well tolerate the attempt of a surgical resection of their gastrointestinal tract tumors. For most of them, it will prolong a worthwhile survival.

References

1. Stromborg M: Early detection of cancer in the elderly: Problems and solutions. *Int J Nurs Stud* 1982;19:139-156.
2. Silverberg E: Cancer statistics, 1985. *CA* 1985;35:19-35.
3. Owens WD, Felts JA, Spitznagel EL: ASA physical status classifications: A study of consistency of ratings. *Anesthesiology* 1978;49:239-243.
4. Morel Ph, Egeli RA, Rohner A: La chirurgie dans le cancer chez les patients de plus de 80 ans. *Schweiz Med Wochenschr* 1981;111:1309-1313.
5. Stanley K: Prognostic factors for survival in patients with inoperable lung cancers. *JNCI* 1980;56:25-32.
6. Kohn RR: Cause of death in very old people. *JAMA* 1982;247:2793-2797.
7. Bader TF: Colorectal cancer in patients older than 75 years of age. *Dis Colon Rectum* 1986;29:728-732.
8. Ziffren SE: Comparison of mortality rates for various surgical operations according to age groups, 1951-1977. *J Am Geriatr Soc* 1979;27:433-438.
9. Linn BS, Linn MW, Wallen N: Evaluation of results of surgical procedures in the elderly. *Ann Surg* 1982;195:90-96.
10. Greenburg AG, Saik RP, Pridham D: Influence of age on mortality of colon surgery. *Am J Surg* 1985;150:65-70.
11. Reiss R, Deutsch AA, Eliashiv A: Decision-making process in abdominal surgery in the geriatric patient. *World J Surg* 1983;7:522-526.
12. Meguid MM, Meguid V: Preoperative identification of the surgical cancer patient in need of postoperative supportive total parenteral nutrition. *Cancer* 1985;55:258-262.
13. Silberman H: The role of preoperative parenteral nutrition in cancer patients. *Cancer* 1985;55:254-257.
14. Reiss R, Haddad M, Deutsch A, et al: Prognostic index: Prediction of operative mortality in geriatric patients by use of stepwise logistic regression analysis. *World J Surg* 1987;11:248-251.
15. Greenburg AG, Saik RP, Coyle JJ, et al: Mortality and gastrointestinal surgery in the aged. *Arch Surg* 1981;116:788-791.
16. Waldron RP, Donovan IA, Drumm J, et al: Emergency presentation and mortality from colorectal cancer in the elderly. *Br J Surg* 1986;73:214-216.
17. Greenburg AG, Saik RP, Farris JM, et al: Operative mortality in general surgery. *Am J Surg* 1982;144:22-28.
18. Payne JE, Chapuis PH, Pheils MT: Surgery for large bowel cancer in people aged 75 years and older. *Dis Colon Rectum* 1986;29:733-737.
19. Mohr DN: Estimation of surgical risk in the elderly: A correlative review. *J Am Geriatr Soc* 1983;31:99-102.
20. Djokovic JL, Hedley-Whyte J: Prediction of outcome of surgery and anesthesia in patients over 80. *JAMA* 1979;242:2301-2306.
21. Palmberg S, Hirsjärvi E: Mortality in geriatric surgery. *Gerontology* 1979;25:103-112.
22. Hobler KE: Colon surgery for cancer in the very elderly. *Ann Surg* 1986;203:129-131.
23. Wied U, Nillson T, Knudson JB, et al: Postoperative survival of patients with potentially curable cancer of the colon. *Dis Colon Rectum* 1985;28:333-335.
24. Umpleby HC, Bristol JB, Rainey JB, et al: Survival of 727 patients with single carcinomas of the large bowel. *Dis Colon Rectum* 1984;27:803-810.
25. Avorn J: Benefit and cost analysis in geriatric care. *N Engl J Med* 1984;310:1294-1301.
26. Schelling TC: The life you save may be your own, in Chase S (ed): *Problems in Public Expenditure Analysis*. Washington, DC, Brookings Institution, 1968, pp 127-176.

Surgical Manipulation and the Tensile Strength of Polypropylene Sutures

Philip B. Dobrin, MD, PhD

• Laboratory studies were performed on 509 size 6-0 polypropylene sutures to examine the effects of surgical manipulation on suture tensile strength. Results showed that dragging sutures over the torn edge of the foil package, permanently kinking sutures, or axially twisting them up to four times did not decrease tensile strength. Similarly, the tug exerted by operating room nurses on polypropylene sutures did not decrease their tensile strength. Two manipulations, however, did decrease breaking strength. The presence of a stray knot reduced suture strength 17%, and grasping sutures with DeBakey forceps decreased suture strength in a dose-dependent fashion. When experienced surgeons grasped sutures with forceps out of direct vision, their grasping forces were well below that which alters tensile strength. Nevertheless, these results demonstrate that sutures that have acquired a stray knot should be discarded and that sutures should not be grasped with mechanical devices such as forceps.

(*Arch Surg* 1989;124:665-668)

The adequacy of a suture depends on the strength of the filament relative to the load placed on it. For most surgical applications, sutures have sufficient strength to sustain the load applied to them with an adequate margin of safety.[1,2] This is especially true of polypropylene, which shows virtually no decrease in tensile strength following prolonged exposure to load and to tissue fluids.[3] Occasionally, however, sutures break,[4-11] raising the possibility that they may have been damaged during surgery.[10,11] Intraoperative manipulation of sutures can alter them structurally,[12,13] and it is presumed that this also weakens them mechanically. This is especially of concern in the case of monofilament sutures, where all the mechanical strength resides in a single strand.

The purpose of this investigation was to examine the extent to which surgical manipulation alters the breaking strength of 6-0 polypropylene sutures. This is of particular interest since recent evidence suggests that most of the strength of polypropylene sutures may lie in their outer "skin" rather than in the "core" of the filament.[14]

Accepted for publication April 14, 1988.

From the Department of Surgery, Loyola University Medical Center, Maywood, Ill, and Hines (Ill) Veterans Administration Hospital.

Reprints not available.

MATERIALS AND METHODS

Short segments of new 6-0 polypropylene sutures were prepared by placing 1-cm-long chains of square knots near both ends of the segments. A 4- to 5-cm-long region was maintained without knots between the chains at the two ends. The knotted chains were placed in clamps with soft plastic jaws to hold the suture segments firmly. One clamp was rigidly connected to a calibrated force transducer, and the other clamp was mounted on a nonrotating blade micrometer (Fig 1). The micrometer was manipulated to extend the suture in 0.25-mm increments and was held at each length for 10 s. This stepwise lengthening process was repeated until the suture broke. In all cases, the sutures broke where the straight portion of the filament entered the knot or where they were deliberately injured. In no case did the sutures break where they were held by the clamps. All experiments were performed in air at room temperature after it was demonstrated that there was no measurable difference in acute breaking strength for sutures studied dry at room temperature as compared with those studied in buffered physiologic salt solution at 37°C, pH 7.4.

Foil Abrasion

When sutures are removed from their foil package, the filaments may be dragged across the torn edge of the foil, which may damage the suture. To evaluate this, 28 polypropylene sutures were carefully removed from their foil packages. Fourteen sutures were dragged forcefully over the torn edge of the foil. Fourteen others were not subjected to contact with the foil to serve as controls. Chains of knots were placed at each end of the suture segments. Each segment was mounted in the soft-jawed clamps (Fig 1) and was extended in 0.25-mm steps until it broke.

Kinks and Knots

When sutures are removed from their package, the filaments may be inadvertently kinked or knotted. To examine the effect of kinks and knots, 54 polypropylene sutures were prepared for study by placing chains of knots at both ends of each segment. Eighteen segments were designated as control sutures. Eighteen others were folded and then rolled firmly between the thumb and forefinger to produce a visible, permanent kink in the knot-free region of the suture. Eighteen others were prepared by placing a single-throw knot in the usually knot-free region between the chains of knots. This was done to simulate the occasional stray knot, which may be formed as the suture is removed from the package. Each suture then was tested for tensile strength.

Nurses' Tugs

Some operating room nurses tug briefly on polypropylene sutures to remove their accordionlike folds. These folds are

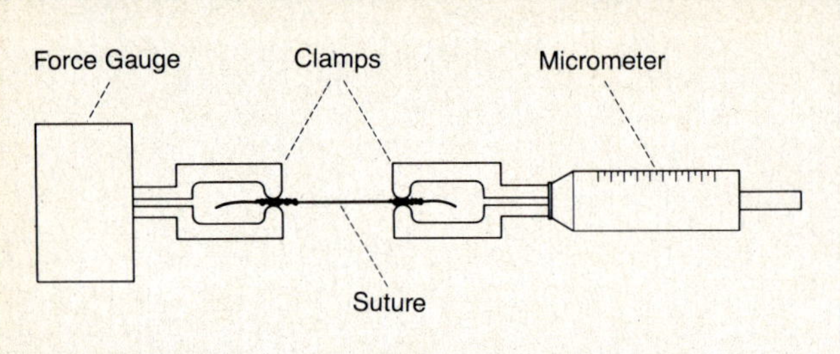

Fig 1.—Apparatus used to extend sutures in steps to breakage (from Dobrin[2]).

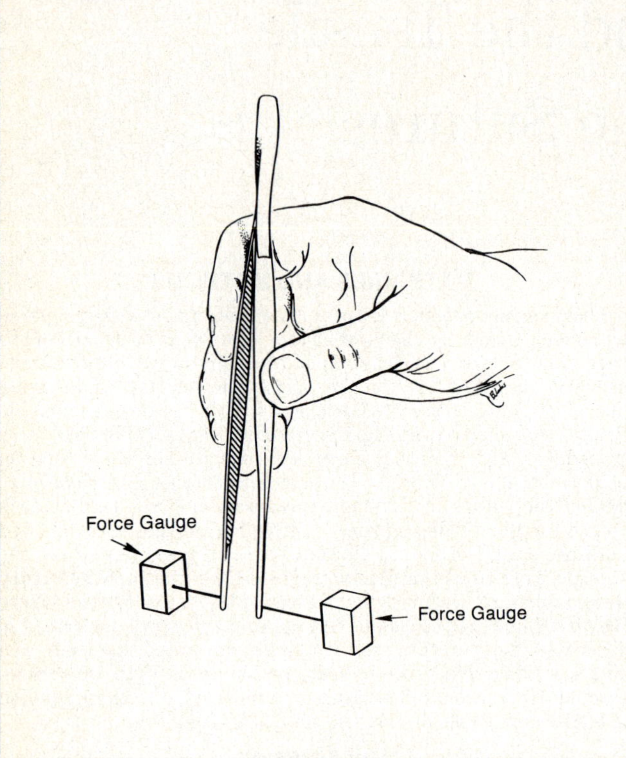

Fig 2.—Method used to measure grasping force exerted by surgeons.

acquired by the suture from having been wrapped for a prolonged period around the cardboard package insert. Experiments were performed to evaluate the force exerted by the nurses' tugs. Eight experienced scrub nurses were studied in the laboratory. Polypropylene sutures were tied to force transducers. The nurses were instructed to tug on the suture just as they would in the operating room. Forces were recorded out of direct vision of the nurses. The mean (±SEM) tug force recorded was 89±8 g. The mean rate of tug exerted by the nurses was recorded to be 130 g/s, with durations of 1 to 4 s.

Experiments then were performed to determine whether the nurse's tug weakens the suture. One hundred sixty polypropylene sutures were prepared with chains of knots at both ends. One hundred forty-four suture segments were subjected to single tugs exerted at 129 g/s. Forces up to 450 g were applied. Sixteen other sutures were studied as controls. The sutures were then mounted in the test apparatus and extended in steps until they broke.

Axial Twist

During construction of an anastomosis, the needle may be grasped and regrasped with the wrist oriented in different ways, and this may axially twist the suture. Studies were performed on 100 polypropylene suture segments to examine the effect of axial twist. Twenty 4-cm segments were not twisted. Twenty others were axially twisted once (360°), twice (720°), three times (1080°), or four times (1440°). Each suture was mounted in the clamps while twisted and was extended in steps until it broke.

Table 1.—Effects of Surgical Manipulation on Suture Strength

	Control Segments	Kinked Segments	Knotted Segments
No.	18	18	18
Breaking force, g (mean ± SEM)	339.3 ± 12.3	323.9 ± 11.6	280.7 ± 10.2*

*Significantly different from control ($P<.05$).

Forceps Injuries

Grasping sutures with forceps may injure and weaken them. To examine this insult, 167 polypropylene suture segments were prepared for study with chains of knots at both ends. Four DeBakey forceps (three V Mueller forceps and one Pilling forceps) were mounted in a horizontal position, and polypropylene suture segments were draped between the jaws of the forceps 1 to 2 mm from their tips. A "pinching" force was applied for 3 s at the tips directly over the suture. Pinching forces were applied by hanging weights from the upper arm of the horizontally mounted forceps. Pinching forces used ranged from 0 g (control) to 5000 g. After these pinches, the sutures were removed from the forceps and were mounted in the test apparatus to measure their tensile strength.

After all these data were obtained, the forceps were mounted vertically. Stainless steel wires were wrapped around each arm of the forceps 1 mm from their tips. These wires were attached to force gauges (Fig 2). The wires were connected with enough slack to permit the arms of the forceps to be grasped and brought within 2 mm of closure. The subjective sensation to the surgeon was that of closing the forceps about a grasped object. Five experienced surgeons then were asked to close the forceps out of direct vision and were directed to "grasp subcutaneous fat." They did so without knowing that the forceps were not grasping tissue but actually were attached to force gauges. These experiments provided data on the force exerted by surgeons when forceps are grasped to produce a subjectively satisfactory force.

RESULTS

Foil Abrasion

Fourteen sutures that had been dragged over the cut edge of the foil package broke at 332.8±9.3 g (mean±SEM). This was compared with 14 control sutures that broke at 334.1±10.9 g. These data were not significantly different as tested by a noncorrelated *t* test.

Kinks and Knots

Table 1 compares the breaking stresses recorded for 54 polypropylene suture segments subjected to no manipulation (control), kinking, or the placement of a single stray knot in the center of the filament. Deliberately kinking sutures did not alter their breaking strength (*P*, not significant). However, placing a single knot in the middle of the usually unknotted region reduced the breaking force 17%. This decrease was statistically significant ($P<.05$), as tested by analysis of variance and Scheffé's test.

Nurses' Tugs

Eight experienced operating room nurses were studied in the laboratory as they tugged on 6-0 polypropylene sutures. Forces recorded were 89±8 g (mean±SEM), well below the usual breaking force (about 315 to 330 g).

Table 2 summarizes the effect of applying a brief, controlled tug in the laboratory to remove the accordionlike

Table 2.—Effect of Tugs on Strength of 160 6-0 Polypropylene Sutures		
No.	**Tug Force, g**	**Breaking Force, g***
16	0 (control)	328.6±13.6
16	50	321.3±13.3
16	100	305.3±12.7
16	150	311.9±7.5
16	200	313.9±12.1
16	250	305.8±14.7
16	300	288.8±9.7
16	350	303.1±11.2
16	400	284.2±11.7
16	450	296.9±10.1

*Breaking force given as mean±SEM.

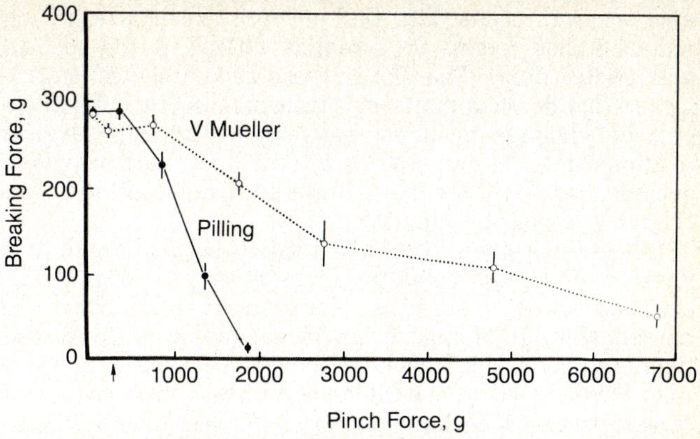

Fig 3.—Tensile strength of 167 6-0 polypropylene sutures following exposure to pinching forces with surgical forceps. Arrow is mean grasping force exerted by five surgeons.

Table 3.—Effects of Axial Twist on Suture Strength

	Control Segments, 0°	**1 Twist, 360°**	**2 Twists, 720°**	**3 Twists, 1080°**	**4 Twists, 1440°**
No.	20	20	20	20	20
Breaking force, g (mean±SEM)	333.1±9.1	318.7±12.4	312.6±12.1	319.4±14.0	315.4±0.5

folds from the suture. The rate of loading was 129 g/s. Table 2 shows that single, brief tugs did not greatly alter the tensile strength of sutures. In fact, because of the brevity of the tugs, it was possible to apply loads up to 450 g without breaking the sutures. This is about 150 g greater than usual breaking forces. The values shown in Table 2 were not significantly different from each other as tested by analysis of variance.

Axial Twist

Table 3 presents the results of axially twisting 100 polypropylene sutures 0, 1, 2, 3, or 4 times. Because this axial twist was imposed on a suture about 4 cm long, four twists are comparable to those that might occur if a suture were twisted with each passage of a needle across an anastomosis. The data shown in Table 3 demonstrate that there was no reduction in breaking force due to this manipulation even after four axial twists. These data were not significantly different from each other as tested by analysis of variance. Therefore, moderate axial twisting does not seem to decrease suture strength.

Forceps Damage

Figure 3 presents suture tensile strength plotted as a function of forceps pinching force for 167 polypropylene sutures. Means and SEs are shown. These data demonstrate that low pinching forces had little or no effect. However, after a threshold was encountered, there was a graded decrease in breaking force in a dose-dependent fashion. It also is evident that the Pilling forceps produced a greater decrease in tensile strength than did the V Mueller forceps. For the V Mueller forceps, all pinching forces greater than 1770 g produced a statistically significant decrease in breaking strength as compared with the unpinched control sutures ($P<.05$). The force required to just bring the arms of the V Mueller forceps together without exerting any measurable pinch was 278 g. For the Pilling forceps, pinching forces greater than 1000 g produced a statistically significant decrease in tensile strength as compared with unpinched control sutures ($P<.05$). The force required to bring the arms of the Pilling forceps together without exerting any measurable pinch was 125 g. Thus, for both the V Mueller and Pilling forceps, the critical pinching force was about six times that required to just bring the tips together. Although it was not the purpose of this study to compare forceps, it is evident that the injury potential varies with different forceps designs. Interestingly, the gripping surfaces of the two forceps could not be differentiated when they were palpated out of direct vision.

The mean force exerted by five surgeons when closing either brand of forceps was 269±29 g. This is shown as the vertical arrow placed on the x-axis of Fig 3. Thus, the pinching force exerted by the participating surgeons was only about 20% of that necessary to decrease the strength of 6-0 polypropylene sutures. Although these findings do not encourage surgeons to grasp polypropylene sutures with forceps, it does suggest that gentle grasping of the suture may not decrease the strength of the filament.

Of all the surgical manipulations examined, only the presence of a stray knot and the grasping of sutures with instruments decreased the tensile strength of the sutures.

COMMENT

During the 1950s and 1960s, silk and polyethylene sutures were used for vascular anastomoses. However, when these sutures were loaded and exposed to tissue fluids for prolonged periods, they degraded and lost their tensile strength.[11] As a result, suture failure resulted in an alarming number of anastomotic disruptions.[15-19] Starr and coworkers[19] reported that 39 false aneurysms developed in 1330 peripheral vascular operations. Of these 39 aneurysms, 16 were associated with the fracture of silk, polyethylene, or Dacron sutures.

Currently, polypropylene has replaced silk and polyethylene sutures in vascular surgery, which has dramatically decreased the incidence of anastomotic aneurysms. In a review of 4214 patients who had undergone arterial reconstruction, Szilagyi and coworkers[20] found 205 cases of anastomotic aneurysms but concluded that suture failure was responsible for only 3.4% of disruptions. Similarly, Gaspar and coworkers[21] reviewed 2400 anastomoses or arteriotomy closures. Ten anastomotic false aneurysms developed after these procedures, but only one could be attributed to the failure of a polypropylene suture. It is evident from these data that polypropylene is a strong material that retains its strength when exposed to load and tissue fluid. Therefore, those few cases of suture failure that do occur may result from manufacturing defects or from damage incurred inadvertently during surgical manipulation. In our studies of over 1000 polypropylene sutures, we have never encountered a defective one, although it is possible that they exist.

In the laboratory, stretched sutures usually break at a knot,[2,14] for at this point the filament crosses over itself, creasing its outer surfaces. However, when a filament is passed through living tissue in a running fashion, the filament may break anywhere along the continuous suture line. It will break at the region of highest concentration of stress, provided the local load exceeds the tensile strength of the filament. Polypropylene slides easily through tissue as it is being inserted. After a continuous suture line has been constructed, however, the filament is bound by friction at each loop. Because of this segmenting effect, the load can be distributed unevenly along the suture line. Evidence for this segmenting effect is the fact that pulling the end of the suture after completion of a continuous suture line usually will not tighten a distant loose loop. As a suture line is being constructed, the filament may break if it is pulled too forcefully in an attempt to snug a given loop. Similarly, if pulling the suture to snug the loop results in a force that is just less than the breaking force, it may fracture when subsequently subjected to pressure and tissue tension. If the suture is defective or is damaged by surgical manipulation, it may break at a lower than normal force.

The present experiments show that the presence of a stray knot or the application of a strong grasping force weakens 6-0 polypropylene sutures. These findings are consistent with the observation that the stiffness and tensile strength of polypropylene sutures correlate with the circumferential skin of the filament rather than with its core.[14] Published data demonstrate that surgical manipulation can result in gouges, shards, and creases in the suture surface,[11,12] and it generally is assumed that these morphologic changes are associated with significant changes in tensile strength. It is remarkable, therefore, that the present data showed little loss of tensile strength with usual surgical manipulations. Application of large compressive loads by pinching with DeBakey forceps does decrease the strength of the suture, but the forces required to do so are greater than that exerted by most surgeons. In any case, the present findings demonstrate that damage can result to sutures from careless handling. Specifically, they indicate that sutures that have acquired a stray knot should be discarded and that sutures should not be grasped with mechanical devices such as forceps.

New polypropylene (Prolene) suture samples were provided by Ethicon Inc, Somerville, NJ. No other support, direct or indirect, was provided by the manufacturer.

References

1. Landymore RW, Marble AE, Cameron CA: Effect of force on anastomotic suture line disruption after carotid arteriotomy. *Am J Surg* 1987;154:309-312.
2. Dobrin PB: Polypropylene suture stresses following closure of longitudinal arteriotomy. *J Vasc Surg* 1988;7:423-428.
3. Nilsson T: Mechanical properties of Prolene[R] and Ethilon[R] sutures after three weeks in vivo. *Scand J Reconstr Surg* 1982;16:11-15.
4. Cornel G: Fracture of polypropylene suture. *Ann Thorac Surg* 1982; 33:641.
5. Myre OA: Breakage of Prolene suture. *Ann Thorac Surg* 1983;36:121.
6. Szarnicki RJ: Polypropylene suture fracture. *Ann Thorac Surg* 1983; 35:333.
7. Dhasmana JP, Blackstone EH, Kirklin JW, et al: Factors associated with periprosthetic leakage following primary mitral valve replacement with special considerations of the suture technique. *Ann Thorac Surg* 1983; 35:170-178.
8. Aldrete V: Polypropylene suture fracture. *Ann Thorac Surg* 1984;37: 264.
9. Alajmo F, Vicari M: Polypropylene suture fracture. *Ann Thorac Surg* 1985;39:400.
10. Calhour TR, Kitten CM: Polypropylene suture—is it safe? *J Vasc Surg* 1986;4:98-100.
11. Reul GJ Jr: The role of sutures in complications in vascular surgery and their relationship to pseudoaneurysm formation, in Bernhard VM, Towne JB (eds): *Complications in Vascular Surgery.* New York, Grune & Stratton, 1981, pp 615-637.
12. Roy J, Guidoin R, Carlou A, et al: Cardiovascular sutures as assessed by scanning electron microscopy. *Scan Electron Microsc* 1980;3:203-210.
13. Allen MV, Jones E, Snow R, et al: Long-term study of iris sutures in rabbits. *Ophthalmic Surg* 1982;13:733-736.
14. Dobrin PB: Some mechanical properties of polypropylene sutures: Relationship to the use of polypropylene in vascular surgery. *J Surg Res* 1988;45:568-573.
15. Stoney RJ, Albo RJ, Wylie EJ: False aneurysms occurring after arterial grafting operations. *Am J Surg* 1965;110:153-161.
16. Moore WS, Hall AD: Late suture failure in the pathogenesis of anastomotic false aneurysms. *Ann Surg* 1970;172:1064-1068.
17. Richardson JV, McDowell HA Jr: Anastomotic aneurysms following arterial grafting: A 10-year experience. *Ann Surg* 1976;184:179-182.
18. Knox WG: Peripheral vascular anastomotic aneurysms: A 15-year experience. *Ann Surg* 1976;183:120-123.
19. Starr DS, Weatherford SC, Laurie GM, et al: Suture material as a factor in the occurrence of anastomotic false aneurysms. *Ann Surg* 1970; 172:1064-1068.
20. Szilagyi DE, Smith RF, Elliott JP, et al: Anastomotic aneurysms after vascular reconstruction: Problems of incidence, etiology and treatment. *Surgery* 1975;78:800-816.
21. Gaspar MR, Movius HJ, Rosental JJ, et al: Prolene sutures are not a significant factor in anastomotic false aneurysms. *Am J Surg* 1983;146:216-219.

Thromboxane A_2-Receptor Blockade and Prostacyclin in Porcine *Escherichia coli* Shock

Erik Svartholm, MD, PhD; David Bergqvist, MD; Ulla Hedner, MD, PhD; June Ljungberg; Ulf Haglund, MD, PhD

• Septic shock was induced by intravenous infusion of live *Escherichia coli* in pigs to investigate the influences on central hemodynamic, coagulation, and fibrinolytic reactions by a thromboxane A_2 (TxA_2)–receptor blocker (BM 13.177; n=6) and a prostacyclin analogue (iloprost or ZK 36374; n=7). The early pulmonary vasoconstriction following *E coli* infusion was attenuated, but not abolished, by BM 13.177. Only minor effects were seen after pretreatment with iloprost. Neither drug had any major effect on the coagulation and fibrinolytic activation. These results confirm that TxA_2 is an important, but not the only, mediator of early pulmonary vascular response in porcine septicemia and that neither TxA_2 nor prostacyclin is of major importance for the hemostatic reactions in this shock model.

(*Arch Surg* 1989;124:669-672)

Cyclo-oxygenase products of arachidonic acid cascade metabolism are involved in the circulatory changes in septic shock,[1-5] which include pulmonary hypertension, increased pulmonary vascular resistance (PVR), systemic hypotension, and decreased cardiac output (CO). Mean pulmonary arterial blood pressure (MPAP) and PVR increase early, coincident with the generation of thromboxane A_2 (TxA_2), detectable as the increased concentration of the stable metabolite thromboxane B_2 (TxB_2).[1,5,6] These pulmonary circulatory changes have been reported to be attenuated, but not abolished, with different TxA_2 synthetase inhibitors.[2,5-7] The pathophysiologic role of TxA_2 is still under debate. Prostacyclin (prostaglandin [PG] I_2) is also generated in septicemia, but according to some studies to a lesser extent and in a later period than TxA_2. Prostaglandin I_2 counteracts the platelet aggregation and vascular constriction induced by TxA_2.[1,8-11] The circulatory reactions in septicemia could be caused by an imbalance of the prostacyclin-TxA_2 ratio.[3,11,12] Such an imbalance could be one explanation for the inability of TxA_2 synthetase inhibitors to normalize the circulatory impairment in septic shock. Furthermore, the precise role of TxA_2 in the pathophysiology of sepsis-induced circulatory and hemostatic reactions is difficult to evaluate from synthetase inhibition studies alone, because in this situation other metabolites with a TxA_2-like action could be generated when this pathway is blocked,[2,13,14] and even small concentrations of TxA_2 could be enough to cause substantial effects.[13]

The aim of this porcine study of septic shock was to investigate if a TxA_2-receptor blocker (BM 13.177) could achieve a more complete inhibition of the vascular response in a standardized experimental septic model than the earlier used TxA_2 synthetase inhibitors. Our aim was to study if and how modulation of the TxA_2/PGI_2 balance by infusion of a prostacyclin analogue (iloprost or ZK 36374) influenced this vascular response. As earlier studies in our laboratory have not shown any major effect by pretreatment with a TxA_2 synthetase inhibitor on the substantial activation of the coagulation and fibrinolytic systems in septic pigs,[15] we also wanted to investigate if these reactions could be modified by the TxA_2-receptor blocker, by the prostacyclin analogue, or by both.

Accepted for publication July 15, 1988.

From the Departments of Surgery (Drs Svartholm, Bergqvist, and Haglund) and Experimental Research (Drs Svartholm, Bergqvist, Hedner, and Haglund, and Ms Ljungberg), Lund University, Malmö (Sweden) General Hospital; and Research Department, Novo Industri, A/S, Bagsvaerd, Denmark (Dr Hedner).

Reprint requests to Department of Surgery, University Hospital, S-751 85 Uppsala, Sweden (Dr Haglund).

MATERIALS AND METHODS

This experimental porcine septic shock model was described in detail earlier.[7,15]

Pigs of either sex weighing 18 to 25 kg were used. The animals were anesthetized with thiopental sodium (25 mg/kg of body weight intravenously [IV] for induction and supplemental IV infusion as needed to ensure anesthesia). The preparation included orotracheal intubation (Mallinckrodt cuffed tube, size 7) and mechanical ventilation with mixed room air and oxygen (Engström respirator, ER 300). Arterial and venous lines were established for recordings of central hemodynamic parameters, blood sampling, and infusions, respectively (Figs 1 and 2, Tables 1 through 3). Tracheal pressures were recorded through a catheter in the cuffed tube. Pulmonary vascular resistance (mm Hg × minutes × l^{-1}) was calculated from the following ratio:

$$\frac{\text{MPAP} - \text{Pulmonary Wedge Pressure}}{\text{CO}}$$

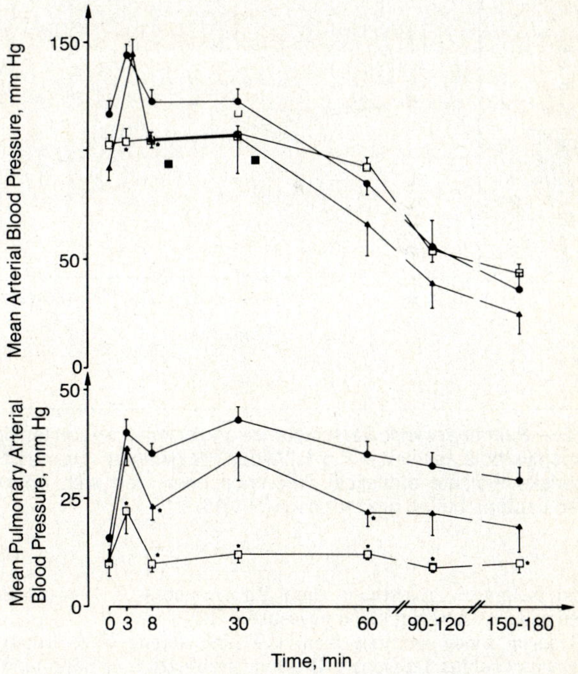

Fig 1.—Mean arterial blood pressure and mean pulmonary arterial blood pressure before and after bacterial infusion in untreated animals (n=7, circles) and in animals pretreated with either BM 13.177 (n=6, squares) or iloprost (ZK 36374) (n=7, triangles). Values are given as means±SE. Asterisks indicate statistical difference compared with animals given bacteria but no pretreatment ($P<.05$).

Table 1.—Platelets and Polymorphonuclear Leukocyte Values*

Group	Before Bacterial Infusion	Minutes 8	60	90-120	150-180
Platelets, $\times 10^9 \times 1^{-1}$					
Sham controls (n=8)	319±78	336±87	315±69	271±62†	272±75†
Bacteria (n=6)	268±34	202±12	179±23	120±12	79±18
BM 13.177 (n=6)	343±10	345±33†	277±29†	217±17†	142±20
Iloprost (n=7)	333±25	311±28†	258±32	240±26†	191±14
Polymorphonuclear leukocytes, $\times 10^9 \times 1^{-1}$					
Sham controls (n=8)	11.1±1.8	10.2±1.1	10.5±1.9†	12.4±2.4†	13.2±1.1†
Bacteria (n=6)	13.4±2.0	11.0±1.0	2.0±0.3	0.4±0.1	0.5±0.1
BM 13.177 (n=6)	9.7±1.3	7.9±0.5†	1.4±0.2	0.4±0.1	0.6±0.1
Iloprost (n=7)	9.2±1.4	6.5±0.9	1.5±0.3	0.2±0.1	0.3±0.1

*Before bacterial infusion and minutes after infusion in untreated animals and in animals pretreated with either BM 13.177 or iloprost (ZK 36374). Sham control group was untreated and infused with Ringer's solution instead of bacteria. Values are given in means ± SE.
†Statistical significance compared with animals given bacteria but no pretreatment ($P<.05$).

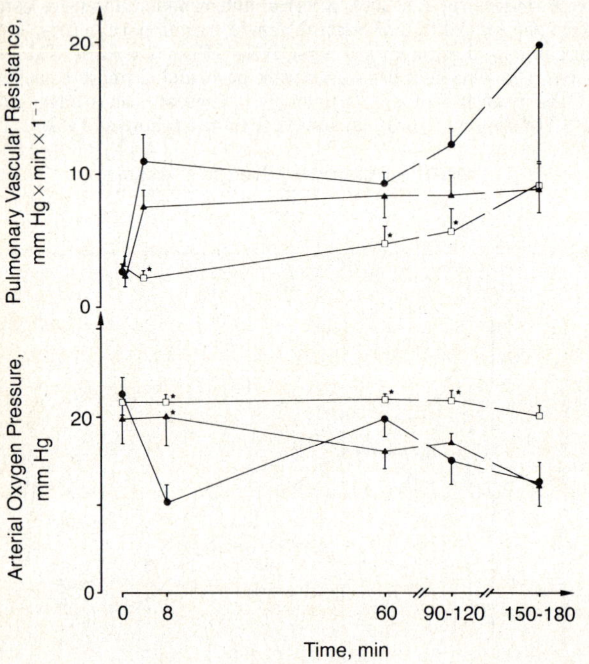

Fig 2.—Pulmonary vascular resistance and arterial oxygen tension. Same symbols as used in Fig 1. Values are given as means ± SE. Asterisks indicate statistical difference compared with animals given bacteria but no pretreatment ($P<.05$).

Table 2.—Activity (Percent) of Antithrombin III, α_2-Macroglobulin, α_2-Antiplasmin, and Prothrombin Complex (Simplastin A) Values*

Group	Minutes 60	90-120	150-180
Antithrombin III			
Sham controls (n=6)	97±11	104±10†	103±4†
Bacteria (n=6)	94±4	84±4	71±7
BM 13.177 (n=6)	105±3	89±4	73±5
Iloprost (n=6)	97±3	76±3	57±19
α_2-Antiplasmin			
Sham controls (n=6)	108±6†	106±5†	107±3†
Bacteria (n=6)	93±4	82±7	62±11
BM 13.177 (n=6)	115±11†	93±4	80±5
Iloprost (n=7)	96±4	81±10	69±5
α_2-Macroglobulin			
Sham controls (n=7)	99±3	100±2†	98±3†
Bacteria (n=6)	99±2	87±5	82±7
BM 13.177 (n=6)	101±3	94±2	92±3
Iloprost (n=7)	101±3	99±5†	99±5†
Prothrombin complex			
Sham controls (n=6)	109±4	111±6†	109±4†
Bacteria (n=6)	98±6	87±5	70±4
BM 13.177 (n=6)	88±9	80±5	79±10
Iloprost (n=7)	105±10	93±5	83±5

*Minutes after bacterial infusion in untreated animals and in animals pretreated with either BM 13.177 or iloprost (ZK 36374). Baseline, prebacteremic activity was 100%. Sham control group was untreated and infused with Ringer's solution instead of bacteria. Values are given in means ± SE.
†Statistical difference compared with animals given bacteria but no pretreatment ($P<.05$).

Total peripheral resistance (mm Hg × minutes × 1^{-1}) was calculated as mean arterial blood pressure × CO^{-1}.

Arterial blood samples from the iliac artery were taken at intervals (Tables 1 through 3) for determination of polymorphonuclear leukocytes, platelets, hematocrit, blood gases, and for preparing plasma samples for detection of changes in the coagulation and fibrinolytic systems. The diagnostic methods of these analyses have been described in detail earlier.[15] The blood losses from the sampling procedure were compensated for with Ringer's solution approximately twice the volume of the aspirated blood. To study the concentration of TxA_2 and PGI_2 during the course of the experiments, blood samples were taken in some pigs chosen at random for assessment of the arterial concentration of the stable metabolites TxB_2 and 6-keto-$PGF_{1\alpha}$, respectively, before the induction of septicemia and 120 minutes afterward. The analyses were performed using a modified radioimmunoassay for TxB_2 as reported by Fitzpatrick et al[16] and a radioimmunoassay utilizing a nuclear kit for 6-keto-$PGF_{1\alpha}$ (New England Nuclear Corp, North Billerica, Mass). The limit of sensitivity was 0.5 pg per tube for TxB_2 and 3.8 pg per tube for 6-keto-$PGF_{1\alpha}$, and the specificity (% cross-reactivity) was 0.025% to 0.9%.

The dose of the TxA_2-receptor blocker and the PGI_2 analogue used in this study has previously been used and validated by others.[8,17-19] The effect of the TxA_2-receptor blockade was further investigated by analyzing, according to the method of Born and Cross,[20] the antiaggregating effect of the TxA_2-receptor blocker on pig platelets activated in vitro by collagen or adenosine diphosphate. The incubation concentrations of the TxA_2-receptor

Table 3.—Fibrinolytic Activity on Fibrin Plates, Alcohol Gelation Test, and Fibrinogen Concentration*

Group	Before Bacterial Infusion	Minutes 60	90-120	150-180
Fibrinolytic activity, mm^2				
Sham controls (n=6)	0	0†	0†	0†
Bacteria (n=6)	0	236±56	162±85	22±22
BM 13.177 (n=6)	7±6	223±23	239±39	34±13
Iloprost (n=7)	7±7	241±66	224±43	0
Alcohol gelation test				
Sham controls (n=6)	–	–	–	–
Bacteria (n=6)	–	(+)	+	+
BM 13.177 (n=6)	–	(+)	(+)	+
Iloprost (n=7)	–	–	(+)	+
Fibrinogen concentration, $g \times 1^{-1}$				
Sham controls (n=6)	3.2±0.1	3.3±0.2	3.2±0.1	3.4±0.1†
Bacteria (n=6)	3.8±0.4	4.2±0.5	3.4±0.5	2.9±0.6
BM 13.177 (n=6)	3.4±0.3	3.3±0.2	2.9±0.4	2.2±0.3
Iloprost (n=7)	3.0±0.1	2.9±0.1	2.7±0.2	2.2±0.2

*Before bacterial infusion and minutes after infusion in untreated animals and in animals pretreated with either BM 13.177 or iloprost (ZK 36374). Sham control group was untreated and infused with Ringer's solution instead of bacteria. Values are given in means±SE. Pluses indicate all animals are positive; minuses, all animals are negative; and pluses in parentheses, more positive than negative animals.

†Statistical difference compared with animals given bacteria but no pretreatment ($P<.05$).

blocker were equivalent to the relevant range of plasma concentrations obtained by the IV doses used in the present experiments (1 to 2.5 mg/mL) and an incubation time of six to 12 minutes.

Experimental Procedure

Septic shock was induced by an IV infusion of live *Escherichia coli* (10^9/mL; 1 mL/kg/min for two minutes and thereafter 1 mL/kg/h continuously) suspended in Ringer's solution.[7,15]

Eight pigs were used as sham controls. Twenty pigs given *E coli* were divided into three groups. One group (n=6) was pretreated with the TxA_2-receptor blocker BM 13.177 (10 mg/kg of body weight during three minutes (concentration, 25 mg/mL), starting 15 minutes before bacterial challenge, followed by an infusion of 0.3 mg/kg/min. Another group (n=7) was given the prostacyclin analogue iloprost (100 ng/kg/min, starting 15 minutes before the bacterial infusion) suspended in 12 mL of Ringer's solution per hour and infused at a rate of 0.2 mL/min. The third group (n=7) was given bacteria but no pretreatment (untreated sepsis). The control group (n=8) was infused IV with the same amount of Ringer's solution as bacteria received by the other animals. The sham control animals were observed for three hours without further treatment. Some of the results of the untreated sepsis and sham control groups have been published previously.[7,15]

Statistical Analyses

Data are expressed as means±SE. For the overall statistical comparison between the different series, the Kruskal-Wallis (H-test) was used. The Mann-Whitney U test was employed for intergroup analyses, and the Wilcoxon matched-pairs signed-rank test was used for comparison within each series. P values less than .05 were considered significant.

RESULTS

Control animals were stable with respect to all cardiopulmonary hemodynamics recorded. After an initial increase in mean arterial blood pressure, all animals infused with bacteria developed severe hypotension that started about 30 minutes following the *E coli* infusion (Fig 1). Cardiac output was approximately 3.5 $L \times minutes^{-1}$ in all series. In the untreated sepsis series, CO declined to a terminal level of 21% of the prebacteremic control values, and treatment did not significantly influence this pattern. The MPAP increased abruptly during the first three minutes after *E coli* infusion (250%±19% of preinfusion control values) in the untreated sepsis series and remained increased throughout. This reaction was attenuated and only transient in the animals pretreated with the TxA_2-receptor blocker, but it was not abolished completely (Fig 1). The animals pretreated with the prostacyclin analogue had the initial MPAP increase as the untreated animals infused with bacteria but attenuated pulmonary hypertension at eight and 60 minutes (Fig 1). The calculated PVR was significantly lower early in septic shock in animals pretreated with the TxA_2-receptor blocker ($P<.05$). Later, the PVR increased in all the animals infused with bacteria (Fig 2). Total peripheral resistance increased transiently the first 30 minutes in all the animals infused with bacteria ($P<.05$). The end inspiratory to expiratory airway pressure difference increased slightly following bacterial infusion but did not differ significantly between the bacterial groups. In the two pretreated groups, arterial oxygen pressure declined following the infusion of bacteria but later and to a lesser degree (Fig 2).

Hematocrit values remained stable in all series (range, 0.23 to 0.44). A pronounced reduction of the arterial concentration of polymorphonuclear leukocytes and platelets was demonstrated after bacterial infusion ($P<.05$, Table 1). There was no difference between the bacterial groups concerning the polymorphonuclear leukocytes, but the early decrease in platelets was less pronounced in the two pretreated groups (Table 1). The TxA_2-receptor blocker showed an antiaggregatory effect on pig platelets in vitro when added in the same concentration as was calculated from the IV doses given in the animals receiving the receptor blocker (aggregation calculated from the optical transmission was 45%±3% compared with 65%±3% in normal plasma, and the maximum slope on the aggregometric curve was 23±2 vs 42±3 mm/min, respectively; $P<.05$).

The hemostatic reactions are summarized in Tables 2 and 3. Decreased levels of antithrombin III, α_2-macroglobulin, prothrombin complex (Simplastin A), and α_2-antiplasmin were found in all pigs with septic shock (Table 2). Fibrinolytic activity on fibrin plates (Table 3) could be demonstrated in all three bacterial groups. This was a transient phenomenon in all animals infused with bacteria, with maximal activity between one and two hours. Fibrin monomers, formed by thrombin action on fibrinogen, appeared earlier in the untreated septic pigs compared with the pretreated bacterial groups (Table 3). Alterations of fibrinogen concentration were moderate (Table 3). The 6-keto-$PGF_{1\alpha}$ levels were not increased 120 minutes after bacterial infusion except in the group pretreated with the prostacyclin analogue (698%±249% of the preinfusion value).

No hemodynamic or hemostatic influences by the TxA_2-receptor blocker or prostacyclin analogue were seen before the bacterial infusion. The TxB_2 level increased following bacterial infusion (2000±671 and 6040±776 pg/mL at baseline and 120 minutes after *E coli* infusion, respectively; $P<.05$) irrespective of pretreatment.

All eight animals in the sham control group survived the three-hour experiment. In the untreated bacterial group, two of seven animals died before three hours, and the remaining five animals died at the end of this bacteremic period. All six animals pretreated with the TxA_2-receptor blocker survived the experimental period. In the group pretreated with the prostacyclin analogue, three pigs died abruptly at 30, 60, and 100 minutes, respectively, while the other four survived the three-hour period and were killed.

COMMENT

This porcine septic model induces hemodynamic changes qualitatively equal to those of previous studies in both pigs and other species using endotoxins or live bacteria.[2,21-23] Inhibition of TxA_2 synthesis is known to attenuate these hemodynamic changes in septic shock.[2,5,6] Such results are also reported from the present model.[7] A complete normalization of circulation, however, has not been reported after TxA_2 synthesis inhibition in septic shock. This only partial circulatory restitution could be explained either by effects of small residual concentrations of TxA_2 or a metabolic "shunting" phenomenon, resulting in increased synthesis of other vasoactive PGs, endoperoxides, or both acting at the same receptor as TxA_2 but not being influenced by TxA_2 synthesis inhibition.[2,5,9,13,14] Because of the shunting after TxA_2 synthesis inhibition, prostacyclin is reported to be synthesized in increasing amounts,[2,13,14,24] which to some extent may explain the results from studies using TxA_2 synthetase inhibitors in septic shock.[5,14]

With the TxA_2-receptor blocker, we obtained an attenuating effect on MPAP and PVR in early sepsis, as was found in series using a TxA_2 synthetase inhibitor.[2,7] Earlier investigations have shown the specificity and site of action of this TxA_2-receptor blocker and validated the dosage used in this series as relevant for a complete blocking effect.[17-19] Studies with cyclo-oxygenase inhibitors, eg, indomethacin, have shown unaltered MPAP and PVR in early sepsis, indicating that prostanoids other than TxA_2 are involved.[25,26] Present results support that early pulmonary hypertension is mediated by arachidonic acid metabolites not acting on the TxA_2 receptor. After TxA_2-receptor blockade, the PVR increased slowly and was not significantly different from the values registered in the untreated bacterial group in the later septic phase, in accordance with studies using indomethacin or specific TxA_2 synthetase inhibitors, indicating that this later phase of disturbed pulmonary circulation is due to substances other than cyclo-oxygenase products of arachidonic acid.[2,7,25,26] Using this septic model, we have earlier shown that a protease inhibitor, aprotinin, has an attenuating effect on this later phase, indicating sepsis-induced protease activation as the mediating factor.[25] This was also confirmed in a small series with this model, in which a combined indomethacin-aprotinin pretreatment prevented early and late deteriorated pulmonary circulation (E.S., U.H., U.H., unpublished data, 1988).

Previously, increased and decreased plasma levels of 6-keto-$PGF_{1\alpha}$ following septicemia have been reported.[1,3] One explanation for these variations is suggested by Yellin et al,[11] who found differences in 6-keto-$PGF_{1\alpha}$ levels between periods of sepsis and septic shock. They demonstrated that the 6-keto-$PGF_{1\alpha}$ concentrations were unchanged from control values during sepsis in swine but increased significantly when the septicemia was aggravated into a shock state.[11] Our results, increased TxB_2 levels but unchanged 6-keto-$PGF_{1\alpha}$ levels, were obtained from plasma determinations performed at 120 minutes, when the animals were in a state of sepsis but before a severe shock state was established. Furthermore, Yellin et al reported the most pronounced disturbance of the TxB_2/6-keto-$PGF_{1\alpha}$ ratio in the sepsis period, with a more than twofold increase and normalized ratio in the shock phase.[11] A similarly increased ratio in the septic period was also seen in untreated sepsis in this study. Infusion of the prostacyclin analogue normalized the TxB_2/6-keto-$PGF_{1\alpha}$ ratio in the septic phase. However, this was not followed by significant differences in pulmonary vascular response (Figs 1 and 2). Thus, a disturbed TxA_2-prostacyclin ratio seems to be of minor importance for the recorded impairments of pulmonary hemodynamics.

This work was aided by grants 4502, 759, and 05477-088 from the Swedish Medical Research Council, Stockholm, the Medical Faculty of Lund (Sweden) University, Malmö (Sweden) General Hospital, Syskonen Svensson's Foundation, Malmö, and the Trygg-Hansa 80-Years Foundation, Stockholm.

The BM 13.177 was supplied by Boehringer-Mannheim Ltd, and the iloprost (ZK 36374) was supplied by Schering AG. The bacteria were provided by the Department of Clinical Bacteriology, Institute of Medical Microbiology, Lund University, Malmö General Hospital.

The thromboxane B_2 and 6-keto-$PGF_{1\alpha}$ determinations were done by the Ligand Laboratory, University Hospital of Michigan, Ann Arbor.

References

1. Parratt JR, Sharma N, Zeitlin IJ: Prostaglandins and pulmonary hypertension following *E coli* endotoxin infusion in sheep. *Br J Pharmacol* 1984;82:281-288.

2. Ball HA, Parratt JR, Zeitlin IJ: Effect of dazoxiben, a specific inhibitor of thromboxane synthetase, on acute pulmonary responses to *E coli* endotoxin in anaesthetized cats. *Br J Clin Pharmacol* 1983;15:127S-131S.

3. Carmona RH, Tsao TC, Trunkey DD: The role of prostacyclin and thromboxane in sepsis and septic shock. *Arch Surg* 1984;119:189-192.

4. Slotman GJ, Quinn JV, Burchard KW, et al: Thromboxane interaction with cardiopulmonary dysfunction in graded bacterial sepsis. *J Trauma* 1984;24:803-810.

5. Watkins WD, Hüttemeier PC, Kong D, et al: Thromboxane and pulmonary hypertension following *E coli* endotoxin infusion in sheep: Effect of an imidazole derivative. *Prostaglandins* 1982;23:273-285.

6. Brigham KL: Metabolites of arachidonic acid in experimental lung vascular injury. *FASEB J* 1985;44:43-45.

7. Svartholm E, Bergqvist D, Lindblad B, et al: Pulmonary vascular response to live *E coli:* The influences of different antiplatelet substances. *Circ Shock* 1987;22:173-183.

8. Casals-Stenzel J, Buse M, Losert W: Comparison of the vasodepressor action of ZK 36374, a stable prostacyclin derivative, PGI_2 and PGE_1 with their effect on platelet aggregation and bleeding time in rats. *Prostaglandin Leukotrienes Med* 1983;10:197-212.

9. Lefer AM: Role of prostaglandins and thromboxanes in shock states, in Altura BM, Lefer AM, Schumer W (eds): *Handbook of Shock and Trauma*. New York, Raven Press, 1983, pp 355-376.

10. Utsunomiya T, Krausz MM, Shepro D, et al: Prostaglandin control of plasma and platelet 5-hydroxytryptamine in normal and embolized animals. *Am J Physiol* 1981;241:H766-H771.

11. Yellin SA, Nguyen D, Quinn JV, et al: Prostacyclin and thromboxane A_2 in septic shock: Species differences. *Circ Shock* 1986;20:291-297.

12. Moncada S, Vane JR: Pharmacology and endogenous roles of prostaglandin endoperoxides, thromboxane A_2 and prostacyclin. *Pharmacol Rev* 1979;30:293-325.

13. Hornby EJ, Skidmore IF: Evidence that prostaglandin endoperoxides can induce platelet aggregation in the absence of thromboxane A_2 production. *Biochem Pharmacol* 1982;31:1158-1160.

14. Gresele P, Van Houtte E, Arnout J, et al: Thromboxane synthase inhibition combined with thromboxane receptor blockade: A step forward in antithrombotic strategy? *Thromb Haemost* 1984;52:364.

15. Svartholm E, Bergqvist D, Haglund U, et al: Coagulation and fibrinolytic reactions in experimental porcine septic shock: Pretreatment with different antiplatelet factors. *Circ Shock* 1987;22:291-301.

16. Fitzpatrick FA, Gorman RR, McGuire JC, et al: A radioimmunoassay for thromboxane B_2. *Anal Biochem* 1977;82:1-7.

17. Stegmeier K, Pill J, Müller-Beckman B, et al: The pharmacological profile of the thromboxane A_2 antagonist BM 13.177: A new anti-platelet and anti-thrombotic drug. *Thromb Res* 1984;35:379-395.

18. Hüttemeier P, Eliasen K, Mogensen T, et al: Effects of a thromboxane antagonist (BM 13.177) during endotoxin induced pulmonary vasoconstriction in the sheep. *Clin Physiol* 1986;6:415-422.

19. Van der Giessen WJ, Zijlstra FJ: The thromboxane antagonist BM 13177, inhibits experimentally induced coronary thrombosis, unlike aspirin, abstracted. Read before the Cardiovascular Pharmacotherapy International Symposium, Geneva, April 22-25, 1985, No. 140.

20. Born GVR, Cross MJ: Effects of inorganic ions and of plasma proteins on the aggregation of blood platelets by adenosine diphosphate. *J Physiol* 1964;170:397-414.

21. Falk A, Kaijser B, Myrvold HE, et al: Intestinal vascular and central hemodynamic responses in the cat following i.v. infusion of live *E coli* bacteria. *Circ Shock* 1980;7:239-250.

22. Myrvold HE, Lewis DH: Platelets, fibrinogen and pulmonary haemodynamics in early experimental septic shock. *Circ Shock* 1977;4:201-209.

23. Bredenberg CE, Taylor GA, Webb WR: The effect of thrombocytopenia on the pulmonary and systemic hemodynamics of canine endotoxin shock. *Surgery* 1980;87:59-68.

24. Parry MJ, Randall MJ, Hawkeswood E, et al: Enhanced production of prostacyclin in blood after treatment with selective thromboxane synthetase inhibitor, UK-38,485. *Br J Pharmacol* 1982;77:547P.

25. Svartholm E, Haglund U, Ljungberg J, et al: The influences of aprotinin, a protease inhibitor, in porcine *E coli* shock: Effects on coagulation, fibrinolytic and hemodynamic responses. *Acta Chir Scand*, in press.

26. Parratt JR, Sturgess RM: The effect of indomethacin on the cardiovascular and metabolic responses to *E coli* endotoxin in cat. *Br J Pharmacol* 1974;50:177-183.

Inflammatory Aneurysms of the Abdominal Aorta

Hans H. Moosa, MD; Andrew B. Peitzman, MD; David L. Steed, MD; Thomas B. Julian, MD; Fredric Jarrett, MD; Marshall W. Webster, MD

• Inflammatory aneurysms of the abdominal aorta (IAAAs) have distinctive clinical and physical characteristics that separate them from typical atherosclerotic aneurysms. They were identified in 19 (7.2%) of 265 patients undergoing abdominal aortic aneurysm repair. Symptoms were present in 12 (63%) of 19, with one patient presenting with rupture, and multiple symptoms were present in six (32%). Intraoperatively, all aneurysms exhibited dense periaortic inflammation. Adjacent structures most frequently involved were the duodenum in 15 (79%) of 19 patients, the left renal vein in six (32%) of 19, and the ureter in five (26%) of 19. Seventeen (94%) of the 18 patients who underwent elective aneurysm resection survived. The involvement of retroperitoneal structures varied in number and severity, demonstrating that a wide spectrum of inflammation is present in IAAAs, making diagnosis and definition difficult.

(*Arch Surg* 1989;124:673-675)

The term *inflammatory aneurysm* was first coined by Walker et al[1] in 1972 to describe a group of 19 patients whose abdominal aortic aneurysm showed excessive mural thickening and adherence of structures adjacent to the aneurysm. The association between perianeurysmal fibrosis and ureteral obstruction has been described in a series of reports[2-12] originating with James' description in 1935.[2] Although several vascular surgeons have emphasized the unique clinical features of inflammatory aneurysms and the necessity for modifications in the surgical approach, the number of retroperitoneal structures involved and the extent of inflammation required to categorize an aneurysm as "inflammatory" have not been defined.[13-17]

Inflammatory aneurysms of the abdominal aorta (IAAAs) are variants of atherosclerotic aneurysms that have distinctive clinical and physical characteristics. Despite the gradual accumulation of experience in treating patients with IAAAs, this variant continues to present a diagnostic and therapeutic challenge to the vascular surgeon. The purpose of this study was to review the experience at the University of Pittsburgh to characterize further the clinical presentation, the severity of the inflammatory process, and the operative management of IAAA.

Accepted for publication Oct 14, 1988.
From the Department of Surgery, University of Pittsburgh School of Medicine.
Read before a meeting of the Eastern Vascular Society, Washington, DC, May 9, 1987.
Reprint requests to Department of Surgery, University of Pittsburgh, Montefiore Hospital, Pittsburgh, PA 15213 (Dr Moosa).

METHODS

The records of 265 patients who underwent repair of abdominal aortic aneurysm from 1970 to 1987 were reviewed. Inflammatory abdominal aortic aneurysms were identified in 19 patients (7.2%). Criteria for the diagnosis of IAAA were the intraoperative presence of perianeurysmal fibrosis, marked thickening of the aneurysm wall, and adherence of adjacent structures to the aneurysm. Follow-up data were obtained in all cases through outpatient evaluation and telephone conversations.

RESULTS

Nineteen (7.2%) of 265 patients with abdominal aortic aneurysms had inflammatory aneurysms. None were identified prior to 1979. There were 17 men and two women ranging in age from 53 to 81 years (mean, 65 years). Twelve patients (63%) presented with symptoms as follows:

Symptom	No. of Patients
Abdominal pain	7
Back pain	3
Flank pain	1
Obstructive uropathy	2
Tenderness	1
Rupture	1

Multiple symptoms were present in six patients (32%).

All patients were heavy smokers (mean, 44 pack-years). Hypertension was the most common associated finding, occurring in ten patients (53%). Additional associated diseases included coronary artery disease in three, diabetes mellitus in two, stroke in one, and cirrhosis in one. Preoperative diagnostic studies included angiography in 15 patients, sonography in ten patients, and computed tomographic (CT) scanning in five patients.

Intraoperatively, all 19 patients had perianeurysmal inflammation, with thick, dense, glistening fibrous tissue that often involved adjacent structures, as noted in the following tabulation:

Structure	No. of Patients
Duodenum	15
Left renal vein	6
Ureter	5
Inferior vena cava	2
Small intestine	1
Sigmoid colon	1
Inferior mesenteric vein	1

Control of the aorta was obtained below the renal arteries in all patients, except the single patient with a ruptured aneurysm. The left renal vein was divided in three patients. No involved bowel was dissected. Ureterolysis was performed on four patients, three of whom presented with obstructive uropathy while one had renal insufficiency. One patient had ureteral entrapment without elevation of serum urea nitrogen or creatinine levels and did not undergo ureterolysis. Cultures of the aneurysm obtained at operation were negative in all but one case in which group D streptococcus grew. No postoperative infections were seen. All aneurysms were resected, and the aorta was reconstructed with a prosthetic graft. Aortoiliac grafts were placed in 16 patients (84%), while tube grafts were used in the remainder.

The single patient with a ruptured aneurysm died of sepsis two months postoperatively. Seventeen (94%) of the 18 patients undergoing elective aneurysm resection survived. The single postoperative death was due to anaphylaxis from iodine contrast from an intravenous pyelogram two weeks postoperatively. Fifteen patients (79%) were alive six months to seven years after aneurysm repair (mean, 3.2 years). Deaths at one year and two years were due to myocardial infarction and lung cancer, respectively. In one patient, abdominal exploration for small-bowel obstruction four months after aneurysm repair showed resolution of the perianeurysmal inflammation.

COMMENT

Inflammatory abdominal aortic aneurysms have clinical characteristics distinct from ordinary atherosclerotic aneurysms, although the correlation with clinical symptoms is imprecise and makes preoperative diagnosis difficult. The inflammatory variant is more likely to produce symptoms of abdominal, flank, or back pain.[1,13-18] Eleven (58%) of our patients had pain as a primary complaint. Erythrocyte sedimentation rates (ESRs) were not measured in our series but may be elevated in some patients.[1,14,16,18] The triad of chronic abdominal pain, weight loss, and an elevated ESR has been described as highly suggestive of the inflammatory nature of an abdominal aortic aneurysm.[16]

Angiography does not demonstrate the presence of inflammation.[16] The most reliable preoperative investigation appears to be a contrast-enhanced CT scan.[15-22] In one series, CT scanning suggested the diagnosis in 50% of the patients, while ultrasonography identified it in only 13.5%.[16] Computed tomographic scanning may show a dense, thick, anterolateral mass of periaortic tissue lying outside the calcified media, with sparing of the posterior wall.[22] Of the five CT scans obtained in our series, four demonstrated the characteristic findings, although the diagnosis was not made preoperatively (Figure). One patient had a large retroperitoneal hematoma consistent with rupture. The inflammatory component is composed of hypervascular tissue and usually displays delayed enhancement following intravenous contrast treatment, while the thick fibrous adventitia does not enhance[22] (Figure). However, exaggerated contrast enhancement of the periaortic mass may occur and may have the same appearance as

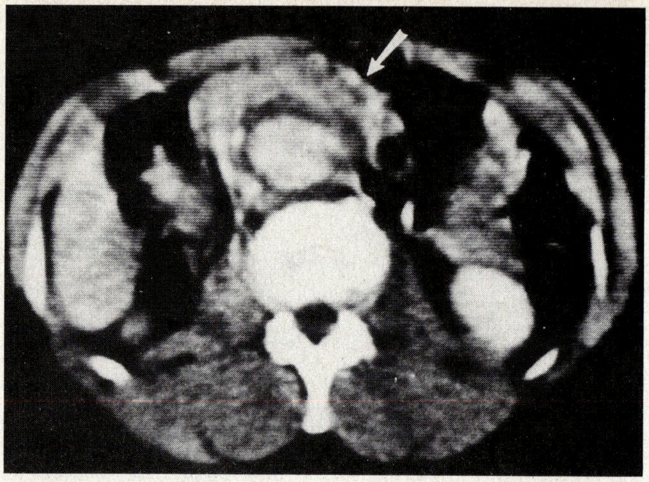

Computed tomographic scan of inflammatory aneurysms of abdominal aorta showing enhancement of thick inflammatory tissue involving arterolateral aortic wall (arrow). Note sparing of posterior wall.

blood in the aortic lumen, leading to a mistaken diagnosis of rupture or aortic dissection.[20,23]

Sonographically, an echo-free halo may be present around the aorta, corresponding to the fibrous tissue located anterolateral to the aorta. The aortic wall is not obliterated by the sonolucent rim of tissue that distinguishes aortic inflammation from other retroperitoneal structures, such as enlarged lymph nodes.[24] These sonographic findings have not been consistent in patients with IAAA.[16] Of the ten aortic sonograms performed in this series, no characteristics specific for IAAA were demonstrable, suggesting that thickening of the aortic adventitia may be subtle and may vary in severity, making preoperative detection by sonogram difficult.

Perianeurysmal fibrosis may cause ureteral entrapment and obstruction. The ureters are drawn toward the midline by the inflammation, unlike the lateral displacement seen with large atherosclerotic aneurysms. Disagreement exists about the need to perform ureterolysis on patients with ureteral obstruction.[11,12,15] We performed ureterolysis on patients who had ureteral entrapment associated with obstructive uropathy or renal insufficiency. Crawford et al[15] reported resolution of ureteral obstruction following aneurysm repair, suggesting that ureterolysis may not be necessary.

The diagnosis of IAAA is usually made at the time of operation.[13-17] Extension of the retroperitoneal process to involve adjacent structures is likely. Sixteen patients (84%) in this series had involvement of one to three adjacent structures, while only three patients had perianeurysmal inflammation alone. The posterior wall is often spared from involvement in the fibrotic process, making it the most likely point for rupture to occur.[17] One of our patients presented with a contained retroperitoneal rupture that occurred posteriorly. This was also the only patient in the series in whom aortic control was obtained at the diaphragm. Control may normally be obtained below the renal arteries, although occasionally division of the left renal vein may be required. Three of our patients required division of the left renal vein to allow exposure to the aneurysm neck, and none suffered postoperative renal complications. Dissection of the adherent duodenum or intestine is technically difficult, can lead to entry into the gastrointestinal tract, and should be avoided.[13] The repair can then proceed by suturing the replacement graft from within the aneurysm.

The etiology of IAAA is unknown.[7] Rose and Dent[25] described a pathologic spectrum of inflammatory changes present in patients with IAAA. They suggested that these aneurysms are variants of the usual atherosclerotic aneurysm in which the chronic inflammation and fibrosis seen in response to atherosclerosis is accentuated.[25] Mitchinson[26] stated that the inflammation may be due to hypersensitivity antigens in the atheromatous plaque. Removal of the presumed stimulus for the exaggerated inflammatory reaction (the atherosclerotic plaque) should lead to resolution of the inflammation. Follow-up CT scans after aneurysm resection and after steroid administration have demonstrated resolution of retroperitoneal fibrosis.[12,15,27] Repeated CT scans in other studies have shown no improvement after aneurysm repair.[17] One patient in our series had no gross evidence of inflammation at subsequent laparotomy, suggesting that regression of retroperitoneal inflammation can occur after aneurysm repair. The etiology of IAAA and the response to operative intervention remain to be elucidated.

The variable extent of periaortic fibrosis seen clinically in this study suggests that a clinical as well as a pathologic spectrum of inflammation is present. Abdominal atherosclerotic aneurysms can be associated with an inflammatory fibrotic process that may involve up to several retroperitoneal structures or just the aortic wall itself. Inflammation associated with atherosclerosis and aneurysm formation may progress to a point where distinct physical features become evident. Aneurysms exhibiting any characteristic fibrotic process may be described as inflammatory, making definition and diagnosis of IAAA difficult.

The diagnosis of IAAA can be made preoperatively by the presence of symptoms and an elevated ESR in a patient with an abdominal aortic aneurysm. A CT scan with contrast exhibiting periaortic inflammation or involvement of adjacent structures is the most reliable diagnostic test. Modifications in the operative approach are dictated by the severity of the retroperitoneal inflammation and the adjacent organs involved. Resection of the aneurysm with prosthetic graft replacement is recommended and can be performed with excellent results.

References

1. Walker DI, Bloor K, Williams G, et al: Inflammatory aneurysms of the abdominal aorta. *Br J Surg* 1972;59:609-614.
2. James TGI: Uremia due to aneurysm of the abdominal aorta. *Br J Urol* 1935;7:157.
3. DeWeerd JH, Ringer MG Jr, Pool TL, et al: Aortic aneurysm causing bilateral ureteral obstruction: Report of case. *J Urol* 1955;74:78-81.
4. Crane JF: Ureteral involvement by aortic aneurysm. *J Urol* 1958;79: 403-409.
5. Pearlman K, Mackey JF: Anuria resulting from abdominal aneurysm. *J Urol* 1960;83:184-187.
6. Labordini MM, Ratliff RK: The abdominal aortic aneurysm and the ureter. *J Urol* 1967;98:590-596.
7. Albers DD, Bettaglio A: Ureteral obstruction from an unsuspected aortic aneurysm: Case report. *J Urol* 1961;85:249-250.
8. Abercrombie GF, Hendry WF: Ureteric obstruction due to perianeurysmal fibrosis. *Br J Urol* 1971;43:170-173.
9. Wagenknecht LV, Madsen PO: Bilateral ureteral obstruction secondary to aortic aneurysm. *J Urol* 1970;103:732-736.
10. Abbott DL, Skinner DG, Yalowitz PA, et al: Retroperitoneal fibrosis associated with abdominal aortic aneurysms: An approach to management. *J Urol* 1973;109:987-989.
11. Darke SG, Glass RE, Eadre DGA: Abdominal aortic aneurysm: Perianeurysmal fibrosis and ureteric obstruction and deviation. *Br J Surg* 1977;64:649-652.
12. Sethia B, Darke SG: Abdominal aortic aneurysm with retroperitoneal fibrosis and ureteric entrapment. *Br J Surg* 1983;70:434-436.
13. Goldstone J, Malone JM, Moore WS: Inflammatory aneurysms of the abdominal aorta. *Surgery* 1973;83:425-430.
14. Baskerville PA, Blakeney CG, Young AE, et al: The diagnosis and treatment of peri-aortic fibrosis (inflammatory aneurysm). *Br J Surg* 1983; 70:381-385.
15. Crawford JL, Stowe CL, Safi HJ, et al: Inflammatory aneurysms of the aorta. *J Vasc Surg* 1985;2:113-124.
16. Pennell RC, Hollier LH, Lie JT, et al: Inflammatory abdominal aortic aneurysms: A 30 year review. *J Vasc Surg* 1985;2:859-869.
17. Savarese RP, Rosenfeld JC, DeLaurentis DA: Inflammatory abdominal aortic aneurysm. *Surg Gynecol Obstet* 1986;162:405-410.
18. Bainbridge ET, Woodward DA: Inflammatory aneurysms of the abdominal aorta with associated ureteric obstruction or medial deviation. *J Cardiovasc Surg* 1982;23:365-370.
19. Pahira JJ, Wein AJ, Barker CF, et al: Bilateral complete ureteral obstruction secondary to an abdominal aortic aneurysm with perianeurysmal fibrosis: Diagnosis by computed tomography. *J Urol* 1979;121:103-106.
20. Vint VC, Usselman JA, Warmath MA, et al: Aortic perianeurysmal fibrosis: CT density enhancement and ureteral obstruction. *AJR* 1980;134: 577-579.
21. Ramirez AA, Riles TS, Imparato AM, et al: CAT scans of inflammatory aneurysms: A new technique for preoperative diagnosis. *Surgery* 1982; 91:390-393.
22. Cullerward MJ, Scanlan KA, Pozzniak MA, et al: Inflammatory aortic aneurysm (periaortic fibrosis): Radiologic imaging. *Radiology* 1986;159:75-82.
23. Aiello MR, Cohen WN: Inflammatory aneurysm of the abdominal aorta. *J Comput Assist Tomogr* 1980;4:265-267.
24. Henry LG, Doust B, Korns ME, et al: Abdominal aortic aneurysm and retroperitoneal fibrosis: Ultrasonic diagnosis and treatment. *Arch Surg* 1978;113:1456-1460.
25. Rose AG, Dent DM: Inflammatory variant of abdominal atherosclerotic aneurysm. *Arch Pathol Lab Med* 1981;105:409-413.
26. Mitchinson MJ: Chronic periaortitis and periarteritis. *Histopathology* 1984;8:589-600.
27. Clyne CAC, Abercrombie GF: Perianeurysmal retroperitoneal fibrosis: Two cases responding to steroids. *Br J Urol* 1977;49:463-467.

Strategy in Reoperative Surgery for Hyperparathyroidism

Polly S. Y. Cheung, MBBS, FRCS; Anders Borgstrom, MD; Norman W. Thompson, MD

• Eighty-three patients undergoing reoperations for hyperparathyroidism were studied. Preoperative diagnosis was reviewed, and localization was employed in selected patients. Cervical reexploration was carried out in a systematic manner, and mediastinotomy was required in 11 patients. Sixty patients had had previous parathyroid exploration. Missed adenomas were found in 34, of which 28 were single and 6 were double adenomas. Fourteen single adenomas were in normal locations and 14 were in ectopic locations. Seventeen patients had hyperplasia; 6 were wrongly diagnosed as adenoma, 3 had inadequate excision, 2 had supernumerary glands, and 6 had remnant hypertrophy. Three patients had recurrent carcinoma. Two had wrong diagnoses and 4 had uncertain diagnoses. Reoperation eliminated hypercalcemia in 71 patients (85.5%). Eight patients developed permanent hypoparathyroidism, and 1 had a permanent recurrent nerve palsy. Reoperative parathyroid surgery can be minimized with thorough initial cervical exploration, correct pathologic interpretation, and adequate parathyroid resection.

(*Arch Surg.* 1989;124:676-680)

Primary cervical exploration for hyperparathyroidism by experienced surgeons is associated with a success rate of over 95% and is better than any localization procedures.[1-3] However, good results depend entirely on the experience of the surgeon and his or her knowledge of anatomy, embryology, and pathology of the parathyroid glands. Though many primary operations appear easy when the tumor is identified, failure in the initial operation poses a great problem for the reoperating surgeon. Because of scarring, tissue planes are often obliterated and the anatomy is distorted. Structures such as the recurrent laryngeal nerves are difficult to define. Both normal and abnormal parathyroid glands are obscured, and the blood supply to normal parathyroid glands may be jeopardized. Reoperative parathyroid explorations are therefore associated with increased chance of failure and a much greater risk of complications.

Accepted for publication November 29, 1988.

From the Division of Endocrine Surgery, University of Michigan Medical Center, Ann Arbor. Dr Cheung is now with the Department of Surgery, University of Hong Kong, Queen Mary Hospital.

Reprint requests to Department of Surgery, University of Hong Kong, Queen Mary Hospital, Hong Kong (Dr Cheung).

To identify the factors leading to failure at primary operation and to establish guidelines for managing reoperative parathyroid problems, we reviewed our experience with reoperations for hyperparathyroidism.

PATIENTS AND METHODS

Between 1970 and 1985, 754 patients who were operated on for primary or secondary hyperparathyroidism were evaluated. Eighty-three patients had had previous neck explorations for either thyroid or parathyroid disease. Twenty-three had had previous thyroid operations, 42 had persistent hypercalcemia after a primary operation, and 18 had recurrent hyperparathyroidism as determined by hypercalcemia recurring more than 6 months after the initial exploration.[4] There were 21 men and 62 women. Their ages ranged from 21 to 83 years, with a mean age of 54 years. Seventy-seven patients had primary and 6 had secondary hyperparathyroidism. In 3 patients, hyperparathyroidism was associated with multiple endocrine neoplasia type I or II syndrome.

Evaluation Before Reexploration

The diagnosis of hyperparathyroidism was reviewed in every patient, and the clinical symptoms were assessed. Inquiries were made about a family history of hypercalcemia or multiple endocrine neoplasia syndromes. Serum calcium, phosphorus, and parathyroid hormone concentrations were measured to redetermine the diagnosis. Urinary calcium levels were also determined to rule out the possibility of familial hypocalciuric hypercalcemia.

The operative notes and pathology reports of the previous operations were studied, taking note in particular of the following points: number of parathyroid glands visualized and subjected to biopsy; location and pathologic features of the resected parathyroid glands; and status of the thyroid gland, ie, any resection in search of missing parathyroids. The locations of the parathyroid glands identified or removed were scrutinized in relation to the thyroid lobe surfaces, recurrent laryngeal nerve, and inferior thyroid artery to determine whether they were superior or inferior glands. Adequacy of exploration and technique of removing tumor were assessed, taking note in particular of any breach in the capsule of the tumor. Histologic slides of the previous resected specimen were reexamined. The side of the neck bearing the missing gland, its embryologic origin, and its possible location were determined.

Patients who were determined to have had an adequate initial cervical exploration underwent localization studies before reoperation. Selective arteriography and venous samplings were employed in the early part of the series. Computed tomography, ultrasonography, and thallium-technetium isotopic scanning were used when they became available. Subsequently, only noninvasive studies were done if the result of localization was positive.

Operative Approach

Cervical exploration was chosen when the diseased gland was suspected to be in the neck. The side of the neck to be explored first was determined from the analysis of operative notes and localization studies. The previous neck incision was used in all cases, after which the standard skin–platysmal muscle flaps were developed. For exploration of missing superior glands, an incision was made along the anterior border of the sternocleidomastoid muscle, lateral to the strap muscles (lateral approach). The lateral and posterior aspects of the thyroid gland were mobilized and the space between the pharyngoesophagus and the prevertebral fascia was explored from the carotid bifurcation down to the posterosuperior mediastinum. When the inferior gland was missing, the lower portion of the strap muscles were split in the midline (medial approach), and dissection was followed from the lower pole of the thyroid gland along the thyrothymic tract to the thymic tongue into the anterior mediastinum. When no abnormal glands were identified after a thorough exploration, cervical thymectomy was performed.

When localization studies suggested a mediastinal lesion, a cervical approach was attempted for lesions above the aortic arch. If neck exploration failed to uncover the abnormal parathyroid or the lesion was localized too low in the mediastinum, further exploration was performed through a median sternotomy or thoracotomy.

The reexploration was terminated when the abnormal gland was identified and removed. Any remaining normal parathyroids were not sought, so that their blood supply would not be jeopardized by further mobilization through the scar tissue.

RESULTS

A total of 92 reoperations were performed on 83 patients. Seventy-seven patients were operated on once and four twice; one had three and another had four reoperations. Of those with multiple reoperations, three were cured but three were not, two because of recurrent carcinoma and one due to recurrent hyperplasia. An operative approach by the cervical route was chosen in most cases. Sternotomy was required when localization studies indicated a mediastinal lesion. The operative approaches were as follows.

Approach	No.
Cervical	81
Lateral	49
Medial	25
Lateral + medial	5
Strap muscles excision	2
Cervical + sternotomy	9
Sternotomy	1
Anterior thoracotomy	1
Total	**92**

Localization procedures were attempted in 36 patients and were helpful in 14 patients. Among the various modalities, thallium-technetium scintiscanning was the most accurate (Table 1).

The final diagnoses reached after reoperation are shown in Table 2. In the group with persistent hyperparathyroidism, 32 patients had missed adenomas. Sixteen were superior and 16 were inferior gland adenomas. Of the missed superior gland adenomas, 9 were in normal locations and 6 were in aberrant locations (including 1 retropharyngeal, 3 retroesophageal, and 2 in the tracheoesophageal groove). Only one was truly ectopic, buried in the esophageal wall above the level of the inferior thyroid artery (Fig 1). Of the missed inferior gland adenomas, 1 was in the thyrothymic tract, 2 were intrathyroidal, 4 were in the thymic tongue, 4 were in the mediastinal thymus, 4 were in the mediastinum at the root of the great vessels, and 1 was lying within the pericardium at the root of the superior vena cava (Fig 2). The median size of the missed glands was 2 cm, with a range of 0.5 to 7 cm in the longest diameter. Among these 32 missed adenomas, 2 were fifth-gland adenomas, found after 4 normal glands had been identified during the first exploration. Four were second ("double") adenomas, 2 in normal sites for superior glands, 1 in the esophageal wall, and the other in the thymus. Two were missed because thyroid neoplasms were misinterpreted as intrathyroidal parathyroid adenomas on frozen section and the remaining parathyroid glands were not explored.

Five patients had persistent hyperparathyroidism due to hyperplasia. Three cases were caused by inadequate excision (two with asymmetric hyperplasia were incorrectly diagnosed as adenoma, and one had a missing inferior gland despite reoperation, probably in an ectopic site). One patient had an apparently adequate initial excision of 3½ parathyroid glands, but the presence of an overlooked supernumerary gland led to persistent hyperparathyroidism. One patient developed hypertrophy of the remnant, which grew to 1 cm in 6 months.

In the group with recurrent hyperparathyroidism, two patients developed a second adenoma. One occurred 2 years later, and the tumor was found in the thyrothymic tract. The other occurred 22 years later, and the tumor was located in the posterosuperior mediastinum. Both patients had undergone incomplete exploration at the initial operation. Twelve patients had recurrence due to hyperplasia: 4 had asymmetric hyperplasia incorrectly diagnosed as adenoma, 2 had inadequate excision due to unidentified glands (1 was found in the paraesophageal area, and the other was not found despite reexploration), 1 had a 1-cm supernumerary gland in the carotid sheath, and 5 had remnant hypertrophy (one of whom also had multiple endocrine neoplasia type I syndrome).

Three patients had recurrent parathyroid carcinomas, all incorrectly diagnosed as adenomas at the initial exploration. One had residual tumor invading the strap muscles and esophageal wall requiring local excision, subtotal thyroidectomy, and modified neck dissection. Another had seeding of tumor in the pharyngeal wall as a result of rupture of the tumor capsule during previous removal. The third patient had recurrent tumor along the tracheoesophageal groove in the posterosuperior mediastinum below the level of the original tumor.

Two patients were diagnosed as having other disease after reexploration. One had hypercalcemia suppressible by steroid therapy, and the other had repeated renal stone formation and hypercalcemia despite normal serum calcium and parathyroid hormone concentration. Four patients had doubtful diagnoses: two were found to have four normal glands, and the other two had one adenoma plus two normal glands at reoperation.

Hypercalcemia was eliminated in 71 patients (85.5%), and complications occurred in 31 patients (37.3%) (Table 3). One patient who had undergone four reoperations for recurrent carcinoma had permanent recurrent laryngeal nerve palsy and Horner's syndrome on one side and transient recurrent laryngeal nerve palsy on the other side. Another patient who developed a transient esophageal fistula had excision of recurrent carcinoma in the neck. The three pulmonary complications occurred in patients who had median sternotomies. Congestive heart failure occurred in one patient after dialysis for chronic renal failure. One patient had cardiac and renal failure secondary to hypercalcemic crisis. There was one operative

Table 1.—Result of Preoperative Localizing Procedures

Procedure	Result, No. Correct	False Positive	Negative	Total	Accuracy, %
Selective arteriography	2	1	6	**9**	22.2
Selective venous samplings	9	6	8	**23**	39.1
Computed tomography	4	3	8	**15**	26.6
Ultrasonography	4	1	12	**17**	23.5
Thallium-technetium scan	5	1	3	**9**	55.5

Table 2.—Final Diagnoses at Reoperation and Causes of Failure at Initial Parathyroid Operation

Final Diagnosis	Total No. of Patients	No. With Previous Thyroid Operation	Cause of Failure at Initial Operation	No. With Persistent HPT*	No. With Recurrent HPT*
Adenoma	**56**	22	**Total**	**32**	**2**
			Insufficient anatomic knowledge	8	0
			Aberrant location	5	0
			Ectopic location	11	0
			5th-gland adenoma	2	0
			Double adenoma	4	2
			Wrong pathologic diagnosis	2	0
Hyperplasia	**18**	1	**Total**	**5**	**12**
			Inadequate excision		
			Due to wrong diagnosis	2	4
			Due to unidentified glands	1	2
			Supernumerary gland	1	1
			Remnant hyperplasia	1	5
Carcinoma	**3**	0	Recurrence	0	3
Wrong diagnosis	**2**	0	...	1	1
Doubtful diagnosis	**4**	0	...	4	0
Total	**83**	**23**	...	**42**	**18**

*HPT indicates hyperparathyroidism.

death; the patient died of pulmonary embolism 5 days after reexploration.

COMMENT

Missed adenomas are the cause of persistent hyperparathyroidism in 50% to 80% of cases.[5-7] A sound knowledge of the anatomic location of normal and ectopic parathyroid glands together with a systematic neck exploration would have uncovered most of the abnormal glands in the first operation. Often, a superior gland adenoma is missed when it is located under the dorsal surface of the thyroid gland. We have found that incising the fascia connecting the lateral border of the thyroid lobe to the carotid sheath (exposing the prevertebral fascia) allows adequate mobilization of the thyroid gland.[8] Its posterior aspect can then be completely visualized without the need for dividing the superior thyroid vessels. Six of the missed superior gland adenomas were quickly identified and excised after this maneuver. When the superior gland is not readily seen, incising the thyroid sheath may reveal a hidden parathyroid gland. This occurred in the remaining three patients with normally located superior gland adenomas missed by the first surgeon. Superior gland adenomas may be located aberrantly in the retropharyngeal and retroesophageal space, the tracheoesophageal groove, and down in the posterosuperior mediastinum.[9,10] Digital exploration of the prevertebral space behind the pharynx and esophagus may locate a parathyroid adenoma, which is usually felt as a soft, pliable, freely mobile mass in this location and can be easily removed by dividing the vascular pedicle from the inferior thyroid artery.

The positions of the inferior glands are more variable.[10,11] It is therefore important to explore systematically from the lower pole of the thyroid lobe, along the principal inferior thyroid vein or the thyrothymic tract to the cervical part of the thymus. Eight of the 11 missed inferior gland adenomas referred from other hospitals could have been found by following this approach. If an inferior parathyroid gland is still not found, a thyroidotomy in the lower pole of the ipsilateral thyroid lobe or excision of the lower pole is advised. One intrathyroidal parathyroid adenoma in our series was discovered in this way.

Apart from knowledge of normal, aberrant, and ectopic locations of the parathyroids, a complete exploration of all four parathyroid glands is important because of the possibility of double adenomas, asymmetric hyperplasia, or supernumerary glands.[12-17] In the four cases of double adenomas in our series, the second tumor was on the contralateral side of the neck. These were missed because only one side of the neck was explored. Two cases of asymmetric hyperplasia were also misdiagnosed as adenoma when only a unilateral exploration was carried out.

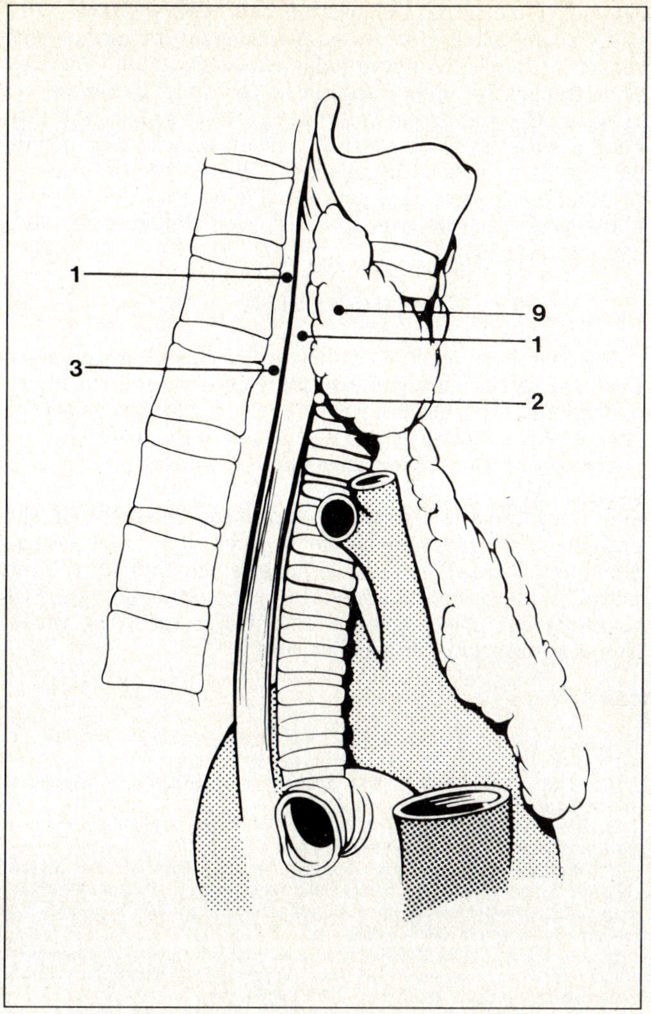

Fig 1.—Locations of 16 missed superior gland adenomas.

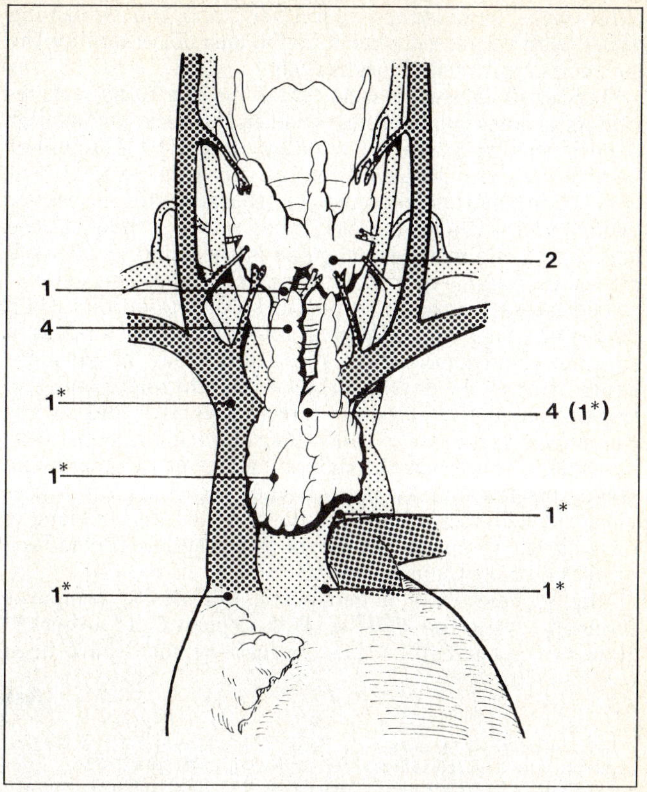

Fig 2.—Locations of 16 missed inferior gland adenomas (those requiring mediastinotomy are marked with asterisks).

Table 3.—Complications of Reoperation

Complication*	No. of Patients
Transient hypocalcemia	10
Permanent hypocalcemia	8
Transient RLN palsy + transient hypocalcemia	1
Transient RLN palsy	1
Permanent RLN palsy + Horner's syndrome + transient RLN palsy	1
Esophageal fistula	1
Wound seroma	1
Laryngeal edema	1
Lung atelectasis	1
Pleural effusion	1
Pleural effusion + wound infection	1
Acute tubular necrosis	1
Halothane hepatitis	1
Congestive heart failure	1
Cardiac + renal failure	1
Total	**31**

*RLN indicates recurrent laryngeal nerve.

Differences in glandular cellularity and intracytoplasmic fat staining, or the presence of a rim of normal parathyroid tissue around an adenoma, have been used to distinguish between adenoma and hyperplasia.[18] However, this is not totally reliable because in asymmetric hyperplasia, the parathyroid glands can exhibit great variation in glandular size and cellularity. Furthermore, the presence of a rim of normal parathyroid tissue around an adenoma is not a constant feature. Therefore, the final diagnosis relies greatly on the surgeon's judgment of the gross morphologic finding of all parathyroid glands at operation, together with the difference in the degree of glandular hypercellularity and amount of intracytoplasmic fat stain in the parathyroid glands. Complete neck exploration is thus important.

While removing an apparent adenoma, it is important to avoid breaching the capsule so that the chance of seeding hyperplastic parathyroid cells is minimized. It is especially important when the diagnosis of carcinoma is in doubt because spilling of malignant cells may lead to local recurrence, as illustrated by our two cases of recurrent parathyroid carcinoma.

Remnant hypertrophy is a major cause of recurrence in patients with hyperplasia, in our experience. This represents the natural course of primary or secondary hyperplasia. Block et al[19] reported a 14% persistence or recurrence rate after subtotal parathyroidectomy for multiglandular disease. Total parathyroidectomy with autotransplantation may be an alternative measure to avoid this recurrence.

Localization procedures before reoperation are particularly valuable when the previous cervical exploration is deemed complete. They can be especially useful in localizing mediastinal and intrathyroidal lesions and determining the side of the neck to be reexplored. However, the reported success rates of computed tomography, ultrasound, arteriogram, selective venous samplings, and thallium-technetium scan have varied widely from 36% to 85%.[20-23] These cannot replace an experienced surgeon with a systematic operative approach.[24] In fact, of the six mediastinal lesions removed via a median sternotomy or thoracotomy, only three were localized preoperatively, and the remaining three were recovered after a meticulous dissection by the surgeon despite failed localization.

Our result showed that 64 (91.4%) of the 70 hyperfunctioning glands could be removed from the neck, and similar experiences have been reported by others.[2-6,25] Most upper mediastinal lesions can be retrieved from a cervical incision.[7,24] Median sternotomy or thoracotomy is rarely needed unless the mediastinal lesion is located beneath the aortic arch or the abnormal gland is not found in the neck after a thorough exploration by an experienced surgeon.

The lateral approach in cervical exploration described by Feind[24] has an advantage in reoperative cases where a superior gland adenoma is suspected. It allows for adequate exploration of the dorsal surface of the thyroid gland, the tracheoesophageal groove, retropharyngeal and retroesophageal space, and posterosuperior mediastinum, without having to dissect through the adhesions between the strap muscles and the thyroid lobe, especially when previous thyroidectomy has been done. If an inferior gland is missing, the strap muscles can be either split in the midline or divided near their insertion.

Our success rate of reoperation of 85.5% compares favorably with the 78% to 90% reported by others.[2-7] However, about half of these operations could have been avoided if the initial exploration had been adequate. Despite reoperation, the rate of transient or permanent recurrent laryngeal nerve palsy was acceptable. The risk of postoperative hypocalcemia is certainly increased by previous thyroid or parathyroid operations. It could have been avoided in most cases if normal parathyroid glands had not been excised injudiciously during the first operation and might have been prevented in others by autotransplantation of parathyroid tissues, even though they were hyperplastic tissue.[26]

CONCLUSION

Reoperative parathyroid surgery carries a higher failure rate and increased complications compared with primary operations. Its success relies on a careful preoperative review of the diagnosis and evaluation of the anatomic and pathologic status of the excised and remaining parathyroid glands. With the selective use of localization procedures and a systematic operative approach, recovery of the pathologic parathyroid tissue is assured in most cases. However, the need for reoperations can be minimized if the initial exploration is adequate, the pathologic type is correctly identified, and the extent of parathyroid resection is appropriate for the disease.

References

1. Satava RM Jr, Beahrs OH, Scholz DA. Success rate of cervical exploration for hyperparathyroidism. *Arch Surg.* 1975;110:625-628.
2. Granberg PO, Johansson G, Lindvall N, et al: Reoperation for primary hyperparathyroidism. *Am J Surg.* 1982;143:296-300.
3. Roslyn JJ, Mulder DG, Gordon HE. Persistent and recurrent hyperparathyroidism. *Am J Surg.* 1981;142:21-25.
4. Muller H. True recurrence of hyperparathyroidism: proposed criteria of recurrence. *Br J Surg.* 1975;62:556-559.
5. Brennan MF, Norton JA. Reoperation for persistent and recurrent hyperparathyroidism. *Ann Surg.* 1985;201:40-44.
6. Billings PJ, Milroy EJG. Reoperative parathyroid surgery. *Br J Surg.* 1983;70:542-546.
7. Van Vroonhoven TJ, Muller H. Causes of failure in the surgical treatment of primary hyperparathyroidism: lessons from 51 successful reoperations. *Br J Surg.* 1978;65:297-300.
8. Thompson NW. The techniques of initial parathyroid exploration and reoperative parathyroidectomy. In: Thompson NW, Vinik AI, eds. *Endocrine Surgery Update 1983.* New York, NY: Grune & Stratton; 1983:365-384.
9. Thompson NW, Eckhauser FE, Harness JK. The anatomy of primary hyperparathyroidism. *Surgery.* 1982;92:814-821.
10. Wang CA. The anatomic basis of parathyroid surgery. *Ann Surg.* 1976;183:271-275.
11. Gilmour JR. The gross anatomy of the parathyroid glands. *J Pathol Bacteriol.* 1938;46:133-149.
12. Harness JK, Ramsburg SR, Nishiyama RH, Thompson NW. Multiple adenomas of the parathyroids: do they exist? *Arch Surg.* 1979;114:468-474.
13. Verdonk CA, Edis AJ. Parathyroid 'double adenomas': fact or fiction? *Surgery.* 1981;90:523-526.
14. Ljungberg O, Tibblin S. Perioperative fat staining of frozen sections in primary hyperparathyroidism. *Am J Pathol.* 1979;95:633-642.
15. Wang CA, Mahaffey JE, Axelrod L, Perlman JA. Hyperfunctioning supernumerary parathyroid glands. *Surg Gynecol Obstet.* 1979;148:711-714.
16. Liechty RD, Weil R. The anatomy of parathyroid hyperplasia. *Surgery.* 1984;96:1099-1102.
17. Akerstrom G, Malmaeus J, Bergstrom R. Surgical anatomy of human parathyroid glands. *Surgery.* 1984;95:14-21.
18. Monchik JM, Farrugia R, Teplitz C, Teplitz J, Brown S. Parathyroid surgery: the role of chief cell intracellular fat staining with osmium carmine in the intraoperative management of patients with primary hyperparathyroidism. *Surgery.* 1983;94:877-886.
19. Block MA, Frame B, Kleerekoper M, Rao DS. Surgical management of persistence or recurrence after subtotal parathyroidectomy for primary hyperparathyroidism. *Am J Surg.* 1979;138:561-566.
20. Brennan MF, Doppman JL, Kurdy AG, Marx SJ, Spiegel AM, Aurbach GD. Assessment of techniques for preoperative parathyroid gland localization in patients undergoing reoperation for hyperparathyroidism. *Surgery.* 1982;91:6-11.
21. Grant CS, Van Heerden JA, Charboneau JW, James EM, Reading CC. Clinical management of persistent and/or recurrent primary hyperparathyroidism. *World J Surg.* 1986;10:555-565.
22. Clark OH, Okerlund MD, Moss AA, et al. Localization studies in patients with persistent or recurrent hyperparathyroidism. *Surgery.* 1985;98:1083-1094.
23. Thompson NW. Localization studies in patients with primary hyperparathyroidism. *Br J Surg.* 1988;75:97-98.
24. Feind CR. Re-exploration for parathyroid adenoma. *Am J Surg.* 1964;108:543-546.
25. Wang CA. Parathyroid reexploration: a clinical and pathological study of 112 cases. *Ann Surg.* 1977;186:140-145.
26. Brennan MF, Brown EM, Spiegel AM, et al. Autotransplantation of cryopreserved parathyroid tissue in man. *Ann Surg.* 1979;189:139-142.

How Accurate Is Fine-Needle Biopsy in Malignant Neoplasia of the Pancreas?

Livingston Parsons, Jr, MD, Charles H. Palmer, MD

• The accuracy of fine-needle aspiration biopsy of the pancreas in 77 patients was studied, in 47 by the percutaneous route and in 30 under direct vision at the time of operation. Seventeen (49%) of 35 pancreatic malignant neoplasms were detected percutaneously and 13 (65%) of 20 at surgery. The predictive value of a positive test was 100% in both situations. The sensitivity of the percutaneous test was 57%; the sensitivity of the test done at operation rose to 72%. No complications were encountered. The test, when positive, can be relied on in surgical decision making but is of limited value when negative. Our findings are essentially similar to those of others who have reported their experience in the literature.

(*Arch Surg* 1989;124:681-683)

Percutaneous fine-needle biopsy is a technique that has become useful in the diagnosis of pancreatic malignant neoplasia. It can enable the surgeon to obtain a positive diagnosis of malignant neoplasm before laparotomy, enabling her or him to better plan her or his operative procedure and often to shorten her or his operating time. It can also help to avoid laparotomy in those patients who are not good candidates for surgery because of their age or poor health, and in those who have unresectable disease but do not have either biliary tract or gastrointestinal obstruction and are candidates for nonsurgical palliation.

In addition, fine-needle biopsy has been utilized at the time of laparotomy to biopsy pancreatic masses under direct vision to obtain an immediate diagnosis on the basis of microscopic tissue examination. It is believed to be safer and less likely to result in complications when compared with shave, wedge, or large-bore needle biopsies. This study was undertaken to determine the accuracy of this technique and its sensitivity and specificity when done both percutaneously in the radiology suite and under direct vision in the operating room.

MATERIALS AND METHODS

From 1978 to 1987 inclusive, percutaneous fine-needle biopsies of the pancreas were performed on 87 patients in Presbyterian and St Joseph Hospitals, Albuquerque. Fifty-five of these were done in the radiology departments and 32 were done at laparotomy in the operating room.

Smears prepared from tissue aspirated in gauge 20-22 needles at the time of the procedure were immediately fixed in 95% alcohol. For rapid diagnosis of aspirations performed during surgery, representative smears were stained with hematoxylin-eosin with standard procedure used for staining frozen section slides. The remaining smears were stained with the Papanicolaou stain. In addition, following smear preparation, the aspiration needle and syringe were washed out with 95% alcohol; a cell block was prepared from the tissue fragments in the alcohol. Step sections of the cell block were prepared and stained with hematoxylin-eosin. Percutaneous needle biopsies were done with the aid of computed tomography on GE 8800 and GE 8900 scanners.

The accuracy of cytological diagnoses from fine-needle aspirations was determined whenever possible by examination of patients' medical records to see the results of subsequent microscopic tissue examination at surgical procedures or postmortem examinations. Where this was not available, a clinical course that was progressively downhill and resulted in death within two years was considered a presumptive confirmation of positive cytology. Of patients in this latter category, only one survived longer than 18 months. A course of continuing good health or symptoms compatible with chronic pancreatitis were considered confirmation of cytological examination negative for malignant neoplasm. Patients who had negative cytological examinations and who did not have surgery done, but had a course compatible with benign disease, were all followed up for at least 18 months. None of the patients who had percutaneous aspiration biopsies had aspiration biopsies subsequently at operation, although 14 of these had wedge or shave biopsies.

Sensitivity is defined as true-positives minus (true-positives plus false-negatives) and specificity as true-negatives minus (true-negatives plus false-positives). Predictive value (accuracy) for a positive test is defined as true-positives minus (true-positives plus false-positives) and for a negative test, true-negatives minus (true-negatives plus false-negatives).

RESULTS

Of the 55 percutaneous fine-needle biopsies performed in the radiology suite, 47 had an adequate follow-up. This forms our determinate group. Of these 47 patients (Table), biopsies of 17 were unequivocally positive for carcinoma, five were reported as showing "suspicious" or "atypical cells," and 25 were negative for carcinoma. Of the 17 patients who had unequivocally positive aspirations (Ta-

Accepted for publication Aug 26, 1988.

From the Department of Surgery, St Joseph Hospital, and the Departments of Surgery (Dr Parsons) and Pathology (Dr Palmer), Presbyterian Hospital, Albuquerque.

Reprint requests to 4208 Aspen NE, Albuquerque, NM 87110 (Dr Parsons).

Results of Percutaneous and Intraoperative Aspirations of the Pancreas					
Cytology	No.	Tissue Confirmation	Confirmation by Course	False-positive	False-negative
		Percutaneous			
Positive (unequivocal)	17	3	14	0	. . .
"Suspicious" or "atypical" cells	5	2	3	0	. . .
Negative (unequivocal)	19	5	5	. . .	9
Pancreatitis	1	. . .	. . .	. . .	1
Fat necrosis	1	. . .	1	. . .	. . .
"Unsatisfactory"	1	. . .	1	. . .	. . .
Atypical mucous epithelium	1	. . .	. . .	. . .	1
Liver cells	2	. . .	. . .	. . .	2
Total	**47**	**10**	**24**	**0**	**13**
		Intraoperative			
Positive (unequivocal)	13	3	10	0	. . .
"Suspicious" or "atypical" cells	3	1*	2	0	. . .
Negative (unequivocal)	9	3	2	. . .	4
"Inflammation"	3	. . .	3	. . .	. . .
Acinar cells	1	. . .	. . .	. . .	1
Biliary mucosa	1	. . .	1	. . .	. . .
Total	**30**	**7**	**18**	**0**	**5**

*Immunoblastic sarcoma.

ble), three had tissue confirmation by surgical specimens removed at operative procedures and 14 had a course compatible with pancreatic carcinoma. Of the five patients who had suspicious or atypical cells, two were confirmed at subsequent surgical procedures as having pancreatic carcinoma, and three died within six months following aspiration with a course compatible with pancreatic carcinoma. There were no false-positives. There were 13 patients with negative cytological examinations for carcinoma who were subsequently found to have pancreatic carcinoma on the basis of tissue removed at surgery or at autopsy, or on the basis of their clinical course. The predictive value of a positive test was 100% in the 17 patients with unequivocally positive biopsy.

Of the 47 patients with adequate follow-up, 19 patients had biopsies that showed normal pancreatic tissue (unequivocally negative); two biopsies were reported as showing "liver cells," one as "pancreatitis," one as "fat necrosis," one as "unsatisfactory," and one as "atypical mucinous epithelial cells that do not appear to be pancreas" (Table). Twelve patients were confirmed as not having pancreatic carcinoma by either subsequent operations or a benign course of more than 18 months. There were 13 false-negative aspirations; nine patients were found at operation or autopsy to have histologically documented pancreatic carcinoma, and four had a course compatible with pancreatic carcinoma, dying in less than 18 months. The patient reported as having pancreatitis was one of those subsequently found to have pancreatic carcinoma at surgery, and three of the patients who had cells other than pancreas aspirated had a course compatible with pancreatic carcinoma. The predictive value of a negative test was 48%. Considering only unequivocal tests as positive, the sensitivity of the percutaneous biopsy was 57%. The specificity was 100%.

Thirty-two fine-needle aspirations were done under direct vision in the operating room, of which 30 had an adequate follow-up (Table). Thirteen of these were reported as unequivocally positive, three as suspicious or atypical cells, and 14 as negative. In the unequivocally positive group, three were confirmed by histological examination of the surgical specimen removed at operation, and ten patients died in less than 18 months with a course compatible with pancreatic carcinoma (Table). In the patients with suspicious and atypical cells, two had a course compatible with pancreatic carcinoma ending in death, and one was found to have immunoblastic sarcoma on the basis of a surgical specimen consisting of a bowel segment and fatty tissue. There were no false-positives, so in this setting the predictive value of a positive test was also 100%.

Nine of the 14 fine-needle biopsies negative for carcinoma were confirmed as true-negatives; three were confirmed by histological examination of resected surgical specimens, and six patients had a benign course and are alive and well after 18 months or more (Table). There were five false-negative aspirations. Two of the false-negatives were confirmed as adenocarcinomas of the pancreas by Whipple procedures, one by positive cytological examination that was rendered the day following surgery (therefore not available to the surgeon at the time of the initial operation), one at a second operation, and one by a course compatible with pancreatic malignant neoplasm. Considering only those tests where pancreatic tissue was obtained and was negative for carcinoma, the predictive value of a negative test was 62%. The sensitivity of the operating room biopsy was 72%; specificity was 100%.

Of all the 47 patients in the percutaneous aspiration group, 35 had pancreatic carcinoma; 17 (49%) of these were diagnosed by the procedure, and 18 (51%) were not. Of the latter 18, five were in the group with suspicious or atypical cells, and all five were subsequently determined to have pancreatic carcinoma. In 13 the diagnosis was not made, presumably because of failure to get the needle in the tumor or obtaining an inadequate or poorly prepared specimen. In the group of 30 patients with open biopsies performed at surgery with adequate follow-up, 20 had pancreatic carcinoma; 13 (65%) of these were identified by needle aspiration and seven (35%) were not. Of the seven patients who were not correctly diagnosed, two were reported equivocally as having suspicious or atypical cells, and five were false-negatives. As anticipated, there was increased accuracy at the operating table (65% vs 49%)

due to a decrease in false-negative aspirations; for these values, $P = .32$, which is not significant and is related to the small size of the sample.

COMMENT

We believe that fine-needle aspiration biopsy of the pancreas is a helpful modality in diagnosing pancreatic carcinoma. When positive, it can be relied on when the cytological examination is done by an experienced pathologist.

Pathologists do not give a positive diagnosis of pancreatic malignant neoplasm on fine-needle aspiration cytology unless they are very sure. False-negative cytology reports and reports of suspicious cells will continue to be presented to surgeons due to failure of the needle to hit the tumor mass or due to hitting areas of necrotic tissue or surrounding pancreatitis. In addition, the presence of well-differentiated carcinoma, where individual tumor cells show little or no cellular atypia, will always be a problem. Some improvement may be expected as additional skill in doing and interpreting this procedure is gained, but this improvement will be small, since our findings are essentially the same as the findings of those who have had the opportunity to look at a large amount of clinical material.

Holm et al[1] reported a 9.8% predictive accuracy on percutaneous fine-needle aspiration of malignant pancreatic lesions. Their two false-positives were due to initial cytological misinterpretations, which were later revised. For nonmalignant lesions, their predictive accuracy was 70%. Dickey et al[2] reported an overall accuracy of 97.3% with one false-negative and no false-positive results; their sensitivity was 71.9%. Others have reported a specificity of 100%.[3-6] No complications were reported in our series in either the percutaneous or open biopsies. There was no evidence in any of the percutaneous studies of seeding of the tumor, although this has been reported,[7] as has pancreatitis[8] following percutaneous pancreatic aspiration.

We are grateful to Julia Lujan, CTR, Presbyterian Hospital Tumor Registrar, and Dolores Moya, St Joseph Hospital Tumor Registrar, for their assistance in this study.

References

1. Holm HH, Torp-Pederson S, Larsen T, et al: Percutaneous fine needle biopsy. *Clin Gastroenterol* 1985;14:423-448.
2. Dickey JE, Haaga JR, Stellato TA, et al: Evaluation of computed tomography guided percutaneous biopsy of the pancreas. *Surg Gynecol Obstet* 1986;163:497-503.
3. Forsgren L, Orell S: Aspiration cytology in carcinoma of the pancreas. *Surgery* 1973;73:38-42.
4. Soreide O, Skoarland E, Pederson OM, et al: Fine-needle biopsy of the pancreas: Results of 204 routinely performed biopsies in 190 patients. *World J Surg* 1985;9:960-965.
5. Evander A, Ishe I, Sunderquist A, et al: Percutaneous cytodiagnosis of carcinoma of the pancreas and bile duct. *Ann Surg* 1987;188:90-92.
6. Yamamoto LT, Tatsuto M, Noguchi S, et al: Histological diagnosis of pancreatic cancer by percutaneous aspiration biopsy under ultrasonic guidance. *Am J Clin Pathol* 1985;83:409-414.
7. Ferrucci JT, Wittenberg J, Margolies MN, et al: Malignant seeding of the trait after thin needle aspiration biopsy. *Radiology* 1979;130:345-346.
8. Beazley RM: Needle biopsy diagnosis of pancreatic cancer. *Cancer* 1981;47:1685-1687.

In Other AMA Journals

ARCHIVES OF INTERNAL MEDICINE

Serum Cholesterol and 25-Year Incidence of and Mortality From Myocardial Infarction and Cancer: The Zutphen Study

Daan Kromhout, PhD, MPH; Edward B. Bosschieter, MD; Marjon Drijver, MD, RD; Cor de Lezenne Coulander, MSc

In the Zutphen Study, cholesterol determinations were carried out in 1960 in serum of 829 middle-aged men. Between 1960 and 1985, detailed information was collected on morbidity and mortality in these men. During 25 years of follow-up, 179 men developed myocardial infarctions and 203 developed cancer. During this period, 110 men died of myocardial infarction, 144 of cancer, and 410 of all causes. Survival analysis showed that the serum cholesterol level in 1960 was independently related to the 25-year incidence of myocardial infarction. This long-term relation was mainly due to the strong association between serum cholesterol level and 15-year incidence of myocardial infarction. Similar but less pronounced relations were found between serum cholesterol level and 15- and 25-year mortality from myocardial infarction. Serum cholesterol level was related neither to long-term incidence of and mortality from cancer nor to mortality from all causes (*Arch Intern Med* 1988;148:1051-1055).

Reprint requests to Institute of Social Medicine, University of Leiden, PO Box 9605, 2300 RC Leiden, the Netherlands (Dr Kromhout).

Colorectal Neodymium-YAG Photoablative Therapy

Comparing Applications and Complications on Both Sides of the Peritoneal Reflection

Donald E. Low, MD; Richard A. Kozarek, MD; Terrence J. Ball, MD; David J. Patterson, MD; Lucius D. Hill, MD

• Laser photoablative therapy has seen wide application in the esophagus, stomach, and rectum. Its use in the suprapetoneal colon has been less extensive because of fear of complications. One hundred fifteen patients who presented during a four-year period and underwent neodymium-YAG laser treatment on both sides of the peritoneal reflection (rectum, 47 patients; colon, 68 patients) were reviewed. The various lesions treated with laser therapy included 32 malignant tumors that presented with bleeding or obstruction, 44 large broad-based villous adenomas, six carcinoid tumors, and 33 patients with arteriovenous malformations or radiation proctitis who presented with acute hemorrhage or chronic blood loss. Overall treatment efficiency was 83% in the rectal group vs 87% in the colonic group. There was no significant difference in complication frequency or severity between the two groups, even though 45% of the colonic lesions were located in the thin-walled cecum. There was no laser-related mortality in this series. Laser photoablative therapy is safe and effective treatment for a wide variety of colorectal lesions. In experienced hands, it can be used on either side of the peritoneal reflection with equal efficiency and no increased risk of complications.

(*Arch Surg* 1989;124:684-688)

Laser photoablative therapy has seen increasing utilization throughout the gastrointestinal tract within the last decade. Its application in treating malignant and benign neoplasms of the esophagus,[1-3] stomach,[4] and colorectum,[5-9] as well as various forms of intestinal hemorrhage,[10-12] has been well documented. Despite the increasing level of experience, there continues to be a general reticence to treat colonic lesions above the peritoneal reflection because of concern regarding severity and frequency of potential complications.

The intraperitoneal colon and especially the cecum do not allow the margin for error that exists when treating rectal lesions. Intestinal perforation can result in general abdominal contamination and peritonitis with an expected high mortality rate. This is especially true, considering that many of the patients who are thought to be best suited for laser treatment are older individuals; often, they have concomitant medical problems. Although an increased risk is generally accepted, we are not aware of any reports that have examined whether this risk translates into actual increased morbidity and mortality. This study analyzes and compares a large experience with laser treatment both above and below the peritoneal reflection.

Accepted for publication Sept 30, 1988.

From the Departments of Surgery (Drs Low and Hill) and Gastroenterology (Drs Kozarek, Ball, and Patterson) Virginia Mason Clinic, Seattle.

Reprint requests to Department of Gastroenterology, Virginia Mason Clinic, C3-S, 1100 Ninth Ave, Seattle, WA 98111 (Dr Kozarek).

PATIENTS AND METHODS

All patients referred to the Virginia Mason Medical Center, Seattle, for laser photoablative therapy of colorectal lesions were reviewed. Patients who were not obstructed or who were not hemorrhaging acutely underwent a full bowel preparation with magnesium citrate, bisacodyl (Dulcolax) tablets, and phosphosoda (Fleet) enemas. Intravenous meperidine hydrochloride or diazepam sedation was individualized for each patient, and whenever possible, a total colonoscopic examination was carried out to rule out the presence of synchronous colonic lesions. General anesthesia was never required, and cases were done as outpatient procedures whenever possible. Prophylactic intravenous antibiotics were used in all patients with indwelling prostheses or a history of bacterial endocarditis.

Endoscopic examination was carried out with either a colonoscope (Olympus CF-1T-10L) or a flexible sigmoidoscope (CFP-105). We used a neodymium (Nd)-YAG high-powered laser (Cooper model 8000) with an energy delivery capability between 1 and 100 W. A flexible quartz laser fiber was introduced through the biopsy port of the endoscope, and treatment was aided by a visible aiming light that parallels the size and position of the laser treatment beam. We have used a bare fiber without coaxial air or carbon dioxide infusion and varied the power setting according to the lesion being treated and whether a hemostatic or photoablative effect was desired.

Treatment of Neoplasms

Treatment of villous adenomas, malignant tumors, and carcinoids was initiated with a patient in the left lateral decubitus position although other positions were frequently used to improve access in lesions that were difficult to visualize initially. Lesions that included a major intraluminal component were initially débrided by utilizing either a piecemeal snare resection or the "artificial sapphire" contact tip laser probe. The crystal contact tips provide a selection of various dissecting probes that are connected to the tip of the laser fiber and deliver energy to tissues through actual contact. This delivery system can work at lower power settings and does not produce the same depth of tissue damage as the external-beam laser. The shape and configuration of these crystals can be changed, depending on whether a hemostatic, vaporization, or dissection effect is required.

Piecemeal snare débridement was used whenever possible before laser therapy to decrease the intraluminal mass of tissue that required treatment. Villous adenomas can usually be resected down to the level of the broad-based stalk, while malignant tumors can be débrided to enlarge the residual colonic lumen to facilitate examination and treatment of the entire lesion. Snare débridement can also produce large volumes of tissue for histologic analysis; this is particularly important in the treatment of large villous adenomas. The discovery of an invasive malignant neoplasm within a colonic adenoma should always result in surgical excision and proper staging. Tissue samples of villous adenomas are obtained for pathologic analysis at the time of initial treatment, before repeated treatments, and during additional treatments carried out on recurrent lesions. However, treatment is not delayed to obtain the pathologic findings, because laser therapy does not interfere with subsequent surgical resection should it be required. In this series, all patients with malignant polyps were sent for surgical resection, with the exception of two patients who were not considered candidates for surgery because of coexistent medical disabilities.

Villous adenomas and carcinoids were treated in a circumferential fashion, beginning at their outside border and progressing inward. Malignant tumors were treated from the proximal to distal extent following snare débridement; this may have involved identifying the lumen with a flexible wire before passing the pediatric colonoscope or beginning snare resection. Neoplastic lesions were treated with energy settings of 50 to 80 W with a pulse duration of 0.5 to 1 s. Following initial treatment sessions, patients with large villous adenomas or malignant tumors were re-treated at two to four days, then every three to four weeks until complete photoablation or adequate palliation had been achieved. For benign lesions, additional follow-up was done every six months for one year, then annually. Patients who presented with extensive obstructing tumors were treated according to the rapidity of their symptom recurrence.

The laser treatment effect resulted from thermal damage, and the length of individual treatments in each patient was modified according to the visualized tissue effect. We utilized a constant-suctioning apparatus that continually evacuated smoke through the biopsy port during treatment. Clear visibility was essential to ensure that excessive cavitation did not result in perforation. Cavitation occurs when tissue is vaporized deeply into the lesion and potentially into the bowel wall. Smoke evacuation is especially important when treating lesions in the thin-walled cecum where the potential for perforation is increased.

Treatment of Arteriovenous Malformations (AVMs) and Radiation Proctitis

Patients who were selected for laser therapy for AVMs had a history of acute gastrointestinal hemorrhage or chronic blood loss. Those patients with AVMs all had their vascular lesions previously documented, either endoscopically or with arteriography. They also had upper tract endoscopy to rule out the presence of additional AVMs proximal to the ligament of Treitz.

These lesions were treated in a circumferential fashion with pulses of 0.1 to 0.5 s at an energy setting of 30 to 50 W. Treatments were not routinely repeated unless there was persistent evidence of ongoing blood loss. Radiation proctitis was treated at similar energy settings, but treatment was usually required over a larger area for treating multiple individual telangiectasias.

Treatment was deemed to be successful in the various groups when, after a minimum of two months of follow-up, (1) patients with malignant tumors had no problems with hemorrhage or obstruction and required no surgical intervention, (2) patients with villous adenomas or carcinoids demonstrated complete photoablation, and (3) patients with AVMs and radiation proctitis demonstrated no evidence of persistent or recurrent hemorrhage.

RESULTS

The charts of 115 patients who underwent colorectal Nd-YAG laser therapy in the four-year period between October 1983 and October 1987 were reviewed. This group included 53 males and 62 females, with a mean age of 70.1 years (age range, 25 to 90 years).

Laser was considered to be definitive therapy in approximately half of the patients, whereas in the other half, it was utilized because of poor operative risk, surgery refusal, or disease extent (Table 1). The type of lesions treated and their relative location to the peritoneal reflection are shown

Table 1.—Pretreatment Status of Patients Undergoing Nd-YAG Photoablative Therapy*

	No. of Patients		
	Rectum	Colon	Total No. (%) of Patients
Not eligible for surgery	17	24	**41** (36)
Refused surgery	4	2	**6** (5)
Extent of disease	10	2	**12** (10)
Definitive treatment	16	40	**56** (49)

*Nd indicates neodymium.

Table 2.—Malignant and Benign Lesions Treated With Nd-YAG Laser*

	Location and Presentation, No.	
	Rectum	Colon
Malignant Lesions		
Hemorrhage	7	0
Obstruction	10	2
Combined hemorrhage/obstruction	7	4
Photoablation	1 villous adenoma	1 villous adenoma
Total	**25**	**7**
Benign Lesions		
Hemorrhage	3 (radiation proctitis, 2; AVM†, 1)	33 (villous adenoma, 3; AVM, 30)
Obstruction	1 villous adenoma	2 villous adenomas
Photoablation	18 (villous adenoma, 12; carcinoid, 6)	26 villous adenomas
Total	**22**	**61**

*AVM indicates arteriovenous malformation; Nd, neodymium.
†Previous ileorectal anastomosis.

Table 3.—Type, Location, and Presentation of Benign Lesions Treated With Nd-YAG Laser Therapy*

	No.	
	Rectum	Colon
Hemorrhage	3 (radiation proctitis, 2; AVM, 1)	33 (AVM, 30; villous adenoma, 3)
Obstruction	Villous adenoma, 1	Villous adenoma, 2
Photoablation treatment	(18 villous adenoma, 12; carcinoid, 6)	Villous adenoma, 26

*AVM indicates arteriovenous malformation; Nd, neodymium.

Table 4.—Relationship of Treatment Frequency and Energy Delivery in Individual Lesions

	Rectum	Colon
Mean No. of treatments	2.4	1.8
Mean joules/treatment	4783	2415
Mean joules/total treatment	11 500	4225

Table 5.—Treatment Results

	Rectum*		Colon*	
	No. (%) Successful	Mean Follow-up (Range), mo	No. (%) Successful	Mean Follow-up (Range), mo
Malignant Lesions				
Hemorrhage	6/7 (86)	7 (2-28)		
Obstruction	7/10 (70)	10 (2-36)	2/2 (100)	8 (2-16)
Both	5/7 (72)	11 (2-28)	3/4 (75)	19 (4-37)
Photoablation	1/1 (100)	14	1/1 (100)	21
Total	... (76)		... (86)	
Benign Lesions				
Hemorrhage	2/3 (66)	14 (7-24)	27/33 (82)	18 (3-40)
Obstruction	1/1 (100)	6	2/2 (100)	29 (21-37)
Photoablation	17/18 (95)	13 (2-36)	24/26 (89)	11 (2-32)
Total	... (91)		... (87)	

*The entries without parenthetic values indicate no range of follow-up in single patients.

in Tables 2 and 3. Forty-seven patients had lesions located in the rectum, while 68 patients had a colonic pathologic condition. Lesions were considered to be in the "extraperitoneal rectum" if they were located within 15 cm of the anal verge. Reasons for laser therapy included hemorrhage from AVMs (n = 31), radiation proctitis (n = 2), and various types of neoplasms, ie, villous adenomas (n = 44), carcinoids (n = 6), and malignant tumors (n = 32). Presentation was variable, with some patients demonstrating rectal hemorrhage (n = 43), colonic obstruction (n = 15), or both (n = 11). Forty-six patients presented for nonsurgical definitive treatment of colorectal neoplasms. Villous adenomas were treated if they were broad based and removal with snare cautery alone would be unsafe or incomplete. Polyp size ranged from 1 to 6 cm, with 75% being larger than 3 cm^2. Patients with bleeding or obstructing neoplasms were treated only when surgery was refused or contraindicated. Patients with acute or chronic gastrointestinal hemorrhage and documented colorectal AVMs were treated after upper gastrointestinal tract endoscopy had been done to rule out coexistent AVMs proximal to the ligament of Treitz.

Abdominal pain was the most common presenting complaint (n = 14), followed by nausea (n = 7), diarrhea (n = 7), vomiting (n = 2), and mucous discharge (n = 2). Thirty-seven patients (13 rectum and 24 colon conditions) presented with bleeding that required intermittent transfusions, and 11 patients had undergone previous colonic resections (six with cancer, two with AVMs, two with familial polyposis, and one with chronic ulcerative colitis). A total of seven patients (one rectum and six colon conditions) had coagulation abnormalities, including either chronic anticoagulation (n = 5), von Willebrand's disease (n = 1), or idiopathic thrombocytopenic purpura (n = 1).

The treatment frequency and energy delivery to lesions in the colon and rectum are compared in Table 4, and the treatment results for malignant and benign lesions are reported in Table 5. The overall treatment success rate was 83% in rectal lesions (mean follow-up, 11 months) vs 87% in colonic lesions (mean follow-up, 15 months).

Neoplasms

In lesions that were treated for complete photoablation (44 villous adenomas and six rectal carcinoids), 43 had a complete response, with two additional patients with villous adenomas undergoing continued treatment and one patient unavailable for follow-up (Table 6). Recurrence following photoablation of villous adenomas occurred in four patients (10%) during follow-up; however, in every instance, the recurrence was controlled with one additional laser treatment. Ongoing treatment has continued in three patients with bleeding and obstructing cancers (one colon and two rectum conditions) and in one patient with an obstructing colonic cancer. These patients were at very high surgical risk, but they have been successfully palliated with laser treatment for 15, 15, 24, and 28 months, respectively. Treatment failures were seen in seven patients with cancer (rectal [n = 6] and colonic [n = 1]) who ultimately required either a colostomy or resection (n = 5) or who had ongoing low-grade blood loss despite treatment (n = 2).

Table 6.—Overall Treatment Success Related to Type of Lesion Undergoing Nd-YAG Laser Treatment*

	Total No.	Mean Follow-up, mo	Treatment Success No. (%)	Definition
Cancer	32	10.3	25 (78)	Effective palliation of bleeding and obstruction or photoablation of malignant polyps (n = 2)
AVMs	31	16.5	26 (81)	No further evidence of hemorrhage or chronic blood loss
Radiation proctitis	2	8.5	1 (50)	No further evidence of hemorrhage or chronic blood loss
Villous adenomas	44	23.4	37 (84)	Complete photoablation
Carcinoids	6	13	6 (100)	Complete photoablation
Total	**115**	...	...	...

*AVMs indicates arteriovenous malformations; Nd, neodymium.

AVMs and Radiation Proctitis

Failures also occurred in six patients with colonic AVMs who required resection or had persistent evidence of chronic blood loss and in one patient with radiation proctitis who had persistent blood loss and required a colostomy for incontinence. Overall results of colorectal lesions treated with laser therapy, stratified according to the type of lesion under treatment, is shown in Table 6.

Complications

A total of 233 laser treatments were carried out with 178 (80%) done on an outpatient basis. There was no laser-

Table 7.—Complications Following Laser Therapy

	Rectum	Colon
Hemorrhage, No.	3	3
Requiring transfusion	1	0
Pain, No.	2	4
Stenosis, No.	2	1
Requiring dilation	0	0
Persistent ulceration, No.	3	0
Perforation, No.	0	1
Laser-related mortality, No.	0	0
Other, type	Respiratory arrest	Postprocedure dizziness, hypotension, and delayed colocutaneous fistula

related mortality, and overall complications in rectal and colonic lesions are compared in Table 7. Delayed hemorrhage was the most common complication, occurring in three patients in both groups. Stenosis occurred in three patients (rectum [n=2] and colon [n=1]) but was never clinically significant. The perforation in the colonic group occurred in a patient who was being treated for chronic bleeding secondary to a right colonic AVM. The perforation actually occurred in the ileum when it was examined during colonoscopy and an additional AVM was treated at that time. A colocutaneous fistula occurred in one patient who was transferred to our institution after having three previous colorectal resections for malignant neoplasms during the previous 16 years; she had a completely obstructing tumor of her residual transverse colon, a significant component of which was secondary to extrinsic compression. She was a borderline candidate for surgical treatment due to severe cardiorespiratory disease and was therefore given six laser treatments via her colostomy during the following two years to maintain a patent colonic lumen. She developed a colocutaneous fistula two months after her last laser treatment and ultimately required a defunctioning ileostomy.

COMMENT

The Nd-YAG laser is an effective treatment modality in a variety of bleeding and neoplastic conditions within the gastrointestinal tract. The majority of reports on lower intestinal tract applications have examined predominantly rectal lesions.[5,13-16] The Nd-YAG laser utilizes a near-infrared wavelength of 1.06 μm with a potential penetration depth of 4 mm. The laser energy is only partially absorbed by water and hemoglobin, and it can therefore penetrate deeply into tissue to vaporize tissue or coagulate actively bleeding vessels. The penetrating power of the Nd-YAG laser is four times greater than the argon laser and 40 times greater than the carbon dioxide laser. It is this increased power delivery that not only makes it an effective therapeutic tool but increases the chance of perforation in inexperienced hands. The current applications of Nd-YAG laser technology in the colorectum include treatment of sites of colonic hemorrhage and benign neoplasms and nonsurgical palliation of malignant tumors.

Neoplasms

Fully 7% of all rectal and distal sigmoid tumors are not suitable for surgical resection on the basis of medical disabilities or extent of disease.[17] In addition, mortality rates of up to 22% have been reported in operations on obstructed rectal tumors before decompression.[18] Laser treatment provides excellent palliation in nonresectable

Table 8.—Location of Colonic Lesions*

	No.		
	Cancer	Villous Adenomas	AVM†
Cecum	0	11	22
R colon	0	6	1
Transverse colon	2	7	4
L colon/sigmoid	3	9	8

*AVM indicates arteriovenous malformation.
†Five patients with AVMs had lesions in more than one region of the colon.

rectal tumors[14,15,19] and improves morbidity and mortality figures by avoiding two- and three-stage procedures in patients who present with obstructing malignant lesions of the rectosigmoid.[7,20]

Historical management of these tumors has included electrocoagulation, cryotherapy, and external radiation. We believe that laser therapy provides significant advantages over all these treatments. Electrocoagulation usually requires a general anesthetic, cannot be applied proximal to the peritoneal reflection, and has been associated with high complication rates.[21] Cryotherapy is effective, but it is associated with weeks of posttreatment rectal discharge and has a significant propensity for delayed hemorrhage.[22,23] External radiation is effective on smaller lesions but less so with extensive rectal tumors[24,25] and is associated with an increased incidence of side effects and complications.[26]

Broad-based villous adenomas have traditionally been managed surgically, either via a colotomy or with a transanal or segmental surgical resection. There is, as yet, no good evidence that malignant polyps should be treated with any modality other than surgical resection. Virtually all patients with villous adenomas at our institution undergo extensive snare débridement before laser treatment, which provides significant volumes of neoplastic tissue for histologic analysis. This is an important step that will help rule out the presence of malignancy in these large polyps and ultimately decrease the number of treatments necessary for complete photoablation. The chance of finding an invasive malignant focus is greater as the polyp size increases,[27-29] and the incidence of missing a malignant neoplasm with visual inspection alone is approximately 10%[30]

AVMs

The treatment of colonic AVMs with laser therapy is more controversial, although reports have shown that effective treatment can be achieved in up to 82% of patients with 24 months of follow-up.[12] These are good results when compared with recurrence rates as high as 10% in patients with AVMs who undergo surgical resection.[31] Although the treatment of individual AVMs requires fewer treatments and less overall energy delivery, the risk of perforation when treating these lesions is actually higher than in neoplastic lesions. The AVMs occur in the submucosa and can involve the mucosa or muscularis of an otherwise normal, unaltered colonic wall. Endoscopic management, whether laser, heater probe, sclerotherapy, or monopolar biopsy forceps involves treatment without the increased safety associated with chronic inflammation or neoplastic growth. Therefore, when carrying out a single treatment of an isolated AVM by applying 200 to 600 J, it would seem safer in relative terms when compared with delivering many thousands of joules in multiple treatments to a rectal malignant neoplasm. However, in actual fact, it is quite the contrary.

Energy delivery, as reported in all laser studies, can be very misleading. The actual tissue effect produced by laser treatment is as much an expression of the operator's skill and technique as it is the actual laser power settings. Bursts of laser energy delivered at greater than 1.5 cm from the lesion will have relatively little tissue effect regardless of the power setting. The absence of a correlation among the total energy level, duration of treatment, and complication rates has been noted previously.[32] Treatment duration and timing must be gauged on the basis of visualized tissue effect alone. Laser endoscopists can vary power settings to enhance a hemostatic or vaporizing effect, but most importantly, they must be able to recognize and avoid excessive cavitation.

Initial examination of Table 4 would indicate that a lower energy delivery in fewer treatment sessions might explain the absence of more serious colonic complications. However, the lesions treated within the colon were more likely to be AVMs (48%), and lesions were most often treated in the thin-walled cecum (45%) (Table 8). As a result, the lower energy delivery is a simple expression of adapting treatment to the individual lesion and its location. This is particularly true when overall treatment efficiency is virtually identical (rectum, 83%; colon, 87%).

Even though 33 individual lesions were treated in the cecum, no serious complications occurred in this high-risk area. Overall, there was no statistically significant difference between treatment success or incidence of major complications between the rectal and colonic groups. Major complications, ie, delayed hemorrhage, stenosis, and perforation, occurred in five rectal patients and six colonic patients.

The colocutaneous fistula and two treatment failures in patients with rectal cancers occurred in situations that included significant extrinsic compression at initial presentation. We believe that patients with obstruction due to extrinsic compression respond poorly to laser treatment and may be more vulnerable to laser-induced complications. The incidence of delayed hemorrhage was the same in rectal (n=3) and colonic (n=3) lesions although the colonic group contained a higher percentage of patients with major coagulation abnormalities, such as chronic anticoagulation, von Willebrand's, or idiopathic thrombocytopenic purpura. A bleeding abnormality likely contributed to one treatment failure in a patient with a right colonic AVM, but this was not a factor in any patient with delayed hemorrhage. Taken as a total group, the incidence of major complications was 10%, which compares favorably with other large laser series.[33]

CONCLUSION

In this group of 115 patients, 47 of whom had a rectal lesions and 68 of whom had a colonic lesion, we could find no significant difference in overall treatment efficiency or incidence of major complications between the two groups. We would emphasize, however, that there was a significant learning curve in utilizing the Nd-YAG laser endoscopically. It is important therefore that all potential laser endoscopists learn the visual cues associated with laser effect and cavitation before applying this modality to lesions above the peritoneal reflection.

This work was supported in part by the Ryan Hill Research Foundation, Seattle.

The authors acknowledge the contributions of Bette Glass and George Maupin in the preparation of this manuscript.

References

1. Fleischer D, Kessler F, Haye O: Endoscopic Nd:YAG laser therapy for carcinoma of the esophagus: A new palliative approach. *Am J Surg* 1982; 143:280-283.

2. Pietrafitta JJ, Dwyer RM: Endoscopic laser therapy of malignant esophageal obstruction. *Arch Surg* 1986;121:395-400.

3. Murray FE, Bowers GJ, Birkett DH, et al: Palliative laser therapy of advanced esophageal carcinoma: An alternative perspective. *Am J Gastroenterol* 1988;83:816-819.

4. Fleischer D, Sivak MV: Endoscopic Nd:YAG laser therapy as palliative treatment for advanced adenocarcinoma of the gastric cardia. *Gastroenterology* 1984;87:815-820.

5. Souquet JC, Sabben G, Chavaillon A, et al: Traitement laser des tumeurs villeuses rectales. *Ann Gastroenterol Hepatol* 1987;23:311-314.

6. Lambert R, Sabben G, Guyot P, et al: Villous adenoma in the rectum: Follow-up after laser therapy. *Gastrointest Endosc* 1985;31:147.

7. Kiefhaber P, Kiefhaber K, Huber F: Preoperative neodymium-YAG laser treatment of obstructive colon cancer. *Endoscopy* 1986;18:44-46.

8. Mathus-Vliegen EMH, Tytgat GNJ: Laser ablation and palliation in colorectal malignancy: Results of a multicenter inquiry. *Gastrointest Endosc* 1986;32:393-396.

9. Russin DJ, Kaplan SR, Goldberg RI, et al: Neodymium-YAG laser: A new palliative tool in the treatment of colorectal cancer. *Arch Surg* 1986;121:1399-1403.

10. Rutgeerts P, Vantrappen G, Broeckaert L, et al: Controlled trial of YAG laser treatment of upper digestive hemorrhage. *Gastroenterology* 1982;83:410-416.

11. Bown SG, Swain CP, Storey DW, et al: Endoscopic laser treatment of vascular anomalies of the upper gastrointestinal tract. *Gut* 1985;26:1338-1348.

12. Rutgeerts P, Van Gompel F, Geboes K, et al: Long term results of treatment of vascular malformations of the gastrointestinal tract by neodymium YAG laser photocoagulation. *Gut* 1985;26:586-593.

13. Brunetaud JM, Mosquet L, Houcke M, et al: Villous adenomas of the rectum: Results of endoscopic treatment with argon and Nd:YAG lasers. *Gastroenterology* 1985;89:832-837.

14. Brunetaud JM, Maunoury V, Ducrotte P, et al: Palliative treatment of rectosigmoid carcinoma by laser endoscopic photoablation. *Gastroenterology* 1987;92:663-668.

15. Escourrou J, Delvaux M, Frexinos J, et al: Treatment of rectal cancer with the neodymium-YAG laser. *Gastroenterol Clin Biol* 1986;10:152-157.

16. Kuvshinov IP, Poddubnyi BK, Veselov VV, et al: Immediate results of the treatment of cancer patients. *Vopr Onkol* 1986;32:58-60.

17. Goligher J: *Surgery of the Anus, Rectum, and Colon*, ed 5. London, Bailliere Tindall, 1984, pp 741-743.

18. Phillips RKS, Hittinger R, Fry JS, et al: Malignant large bowel obstruction. *Br J Surg* 1985;72:296-302.

19. Naveau S, Roulot D, Zourabichvili O, et al: Tratement palliatif des adenocarcinomes du rectum par le laser YAG neodyme: Resultats immediats et a long terme: Etude des facteurs lies a la destruction tumorale initiale. *Gastroenterol Clin Biol* 1986;10:651-655.

20. Bown SG, Barr H, Matthewson K, et al: Endoscopic treatment of inoperable colorectal cancers with the Nd YAG laser. *Br J Surg* 1986;73:949-952.

21. Madden JL, Kandalaft SI: Electrocoagulation as a primary curative method in the treatment of carcinoma of the rectum. *Surg Gynecol Obstet* 1983;157:164-179.

22. Mlasowsky B, Duben W, Jung D: Cryosurgery for palliation of rectal tumours. *J Exp Clin Cancer Res* 1985;4:81-83.

23. Osborne DR, Higgins AF, Hobbs KEF: Cryosurgery in the management of rectal tumours. *Br J Surg* 1978;65:859-861.

24. Papilon J: New prospects in the conservative treatment of rectal cancer. *Dis Colon Rectum* 1984;27:695-700.

25. Sischy B: The place of radiotherapy in the management of rectal adenocarcinoma. *Cancer* 1982;50:2631-2637.

26. Puthawala AA, Syded AMN, Gates TC, et al: Definitive treatment of extensive anorectal carcinoma by external and interstitial irradiation. *Cancer* 1982;50:1746-1750.

27. Kellokumpu I, Husa A: Colorectal adenomas: Morphologic features and the risk of developing metachronous adenomas and carcinomas in the colorectum. *Scand J Gastroenterol* 1987;22:833-841.

28. Christenson CE, Nemer FD, Schottler JL, et al: Villous adenomas of the rectum: The accuracy of clinical assessment. *Acta Med Scand* 1981;210:187-192.

29. Stulc JP, Petrelli NJ, Herrera L, et al: Colorectal villous and tubulovillous adenomas equal to or greater than four centimeters. *Ann Surg* 1987;207:65-71.

30. Nivatvongs S, Nicholson JD, Rothenberger DA, et al: Villous adenomas of the rectum: The accuracy of clinical assessment. *Surgery* 1980;87:549-551.

31. Boley SJ, Sammartano R, Brandt LJ, et al: Vascular ectasias of the colon. *Surg Gynecol Obstet* 1979;149:353-359.

32. Mathus-Vliegen EM, Tytgat GN: ND:YAG laser photocoagulation in colorectal adenoma: Evaluation of its safety, usefulness, and efficacy. *Gastroenterology* 1986;90:1865-1873.

33. Mathus-Vliegen EMH: Complications and pitfalls of laser therapy. *Endoscopy* 1986;18:69-72.

Small-Bowel Perforation Complicating the Open Treatment of Generalized Peritonitis

Walter J. B. Mastboom, MD; Han H. C. Kuypers, MD, PhD; Frans J. Schoots, MD; Theo Wobbes, MD, PhD

• Fourteen patients were found to have developed 53 small-bowel perforations in the absence of pathogenic factors during "open abdominal treatment" for generalized peritonitis. They occurred after three to 17 laparotomies, on average at the eighth postoperative day (one to 120 days). Forty-nine lesions were located superficially. A relation with organ system failure, routine blood tests, type of nutrition, or microorganisms could not be demonstrated. The etiology of the lesions remains uncertain, but the open abdominal treatment must play some important role in its pathophysiology. Five patients survived. The therapy of choice appears to be mobilization of the bowel with resection of the affected part and primary anastomosis.

(*Arch Surg* 1989;124:689-692)

The occurrence of nontraumatic small-bowel perforations is rare. Several pathophysiological factors are known, such as vascular disorders, infectious diseases such as tuberculosis and typhus, Crohn's disease, disseminated malignant disease, medication with potassium tablets or corticosteroids, and radiotherapy.[1-6] In some cases the cause is unknown or uncertain, and such cases are classified as "spontaneous."

We have noticed the occurrence of small-bowel perforations during "open treatment" of patients with intra-abdominal sepsis when factors predisposing to intestinal perforations were absent. This group of patients has been studied in an attempt to establish under which circumstances these perforations occurred, what the cause might have been, and how they should be treated.

PATIENTS AND METHODS

Open Treatment of Intra-abdominal Sepsis

In patients who remain septic during the treatment of generalized peritonitis, we perform relaparotomy when extra-abdominal causes for sepsis have been excluded.[7] During this operation, the whole bowel is mobilized to detect and drain all abscesses. Frequently, persisting sepsis necessitates multiple laparotomies. Sometimes primary closure of the abdominal wall is impossible without extreme tension on the fascial sutures. To avoid complications caused by fascial disruption, the abdominal wall is then left open and a nylon mesh is sutured to the wound edges to prevent intestinal eventration.[8] Occasionally the bowel is so stiff, due to fibrosis and edema, that protrusion through the abdominal wound is unlikely to occur and application of a mesh is omitted.

When reexploration is indicated within a few days, the mesh can easily be removed since it is not attached yet to the underlying bowel loops. However, with time, exploration of the abdominal cavity becomes more difficult. Progressive formation of fibrous granulation tissue overgrowing the abdominal wound complicates removal of the mesh, and complete mobilization of the bowel loops is hindered by diffuse adhesions. Consequently, extensive exploration of the peritoneal cavity performed in these patients might be complicated by iatrogenic bowel perforations. Usually, these lesions are detected during the surgical procedure. So as not to miss undetected lesions, the whole bowel is always checked before terminating the operation. Serosal lesions occur frequently under these circumstances. Extensive serosal avulsions, sometimes including more than half the bowel circumference, are closed in one layer as much as possible, whereas small lesions are considered unimportant and left undisturbed. As a result of the complicated course of their intra-abdominal sepsis, most patients with an "open abdomen" need intensive care unit (ICU) treatment.

Gauzes drenched in isotonic saline solution (0.9% sodium chloride) are applied and changed at least twice a day to prevent both sticking to the wound and dehydration. Thus, leakage from a bowel perforation is detected within hours. Superficial intestinal lesions can be seen as mucosal blowouts producing bowel fluids; deeper lesions are only detected during surgery. Bowel perforations detected within 24 hours after laparotomy were considered to occur from unnoticed iatrogenic lesions.

When reexploration is no longer necessary, the granulating layer becomes thicker and contracts. Epithelialization from the wound edges occurs, and mesh grafts may be applied.

Between July 1977 and July 1987, 394 patients were treated for generalized peritonitis in the Department of General Surgery at University Hospital Nijmegen, Nijmegen, the Netherlands. During the course of the disease, the abdominal wall was left open in 135 patients, and a mesh was applied for some period in all. Twenty-seven patients developed perforations in the jejunum or ileum. After exclusion of factors predisposing to small-bowel perforations, as already mentioned, 14 patients remained for analysis. The records were reviewed only when perforations had appeared more than 24 hours after laparotomy and no suture material was found at or near the site of the lesion.

To detect factors that might have contributed to the occurrence of small-bowel perforations, several factors were examined. Multiple perforations diagnosed at the same time were considered as one event for further analysis. Medical history, primary cause of the intra-abdominal sepsis, and duration of ICU treatment were examined for each patient.

Several variables were analyzed at the time of each perforation, including individual functions of seven organ systems, which were scored according to the Multiple Organ Failure (MOF) Scale modified by Goris et al[9] (Table 1), the presence of a mesh, type of nutrition, and cultures taken from intra-abdominal foci during laparotomy. Other variables were only studied when they were determined within 24 hours before occurrence of the lesions, such as hemoglobin concentration, serum albumin and protein concentrations, and blood cultures.

RESULTS

Small-bowel perforations occurred in five women and nine men during open treatment for intra-abdominal sepsis (Table 2). Their mean age was 51 years (ranging from 19 to 79 years). Primary causes of the generalized peritonitis were necrotizing hemorrhagic pancreatitis (six patients), anastomotic dehiscence (three), septic aortoiliac graft (two), septic cholangitis (one), diverticulitis (one), and colonic perforation (one).

All underwent several laparotomies, varying from four to 20 times. Overall, 20 iatrogenic perforations occurred during these procedures.

Altogether, 53 noniatrogenic perforations were found. Several perforations were diagnosed simultaneously on ten occasions; six times there were two and twice there were three lesions. Thus, the diagnosis of small-bowel perfora-

Accepted for publication Nov 16, 1988.

From the Department of Surgery, St Radboud University Hospital, Nijmegen, the Netherlands.

Reprint requests to Department of Surgery, University Hospital Nijmegen, PO Box 9101, 6500 HB Nijmegen, the Netherlands (Dr Mastboom).

tion of unknown origin was made 43 times, varying from one to 13 times per patient. The perforations occurred after the third to 17th laparotomy, varying from the first to the 120th postoperative day (mean, day 8; Figure). In ten patients, the diagnosis was made several times. The intervening periods varied from one to 88 days. Forty-nine lesions were located superficially, whereas four deep lesions were found at laparotomy. Nine perforations (17%) were observed while a mesh was absent. All 14 patients needed ICU treatment for their intraabdominal sepsis; admittance to the ICU varied from one to six times. Total length of stay ranged from three to 275 days (mean, 74 days). Twenty-two times (51%) the diagnosis of small-bowel perforation was made on this ward.

Table 3 shows that respiratory insufficiency was present during diagnosis of 37% of the perforations. Concerning the digestive tract, hepatic failure was present ten times (23%) and stress ulcer was present on one occasion. Forty-four percent of the small-bowel perforations were diagnosed in the absence of serious insufficiency of the organs checked, according to Table 1, but eight times the MOF score was 4 or more, indicating serious disturbances of several organ systems.

MOF Score	No. (%) of Perforations
0	19 (44)
1	3 (7)
2	4 (9)
3	9 (21)
4	4 (9)
5	3 (7)
6	0 (0)
7	0 (0)
8	1 (2)

Five times (12%) perforations were detected while the patient was anemic (hemoglobin level, <95 g/L; normal, 120 to 180 g/L).

Hemoglobin Level, g/L	No. of Perforations
<80	2
80-95	3
95-110	15
≥110	17
Not measured	6

Hypoalbuminemia and hypoproteinemia were often present; severe deficiencies were present, respectively, in 18% (serum albumin concentration, ≤20 g/L; normal, 35 to 50 g/L) and 9% (serum total protein concentration, ≤44 g/L; normal, 65 to 80 g/L) of the times measured.

Level, g/L	No. of Perforations
Albumin	
≤20	6
21-27	15
28-34	7
≥35	6
Not measured	9
Protein	
≤44	3
45-54	11
55-64	9
≥65	12
Not measured	8

Most lesions were diagnosed when patients were parenterally fed. Sixteen times they received enteral nutrition, seven times in combination with parenteral support.

Type of Nourishment	No. of Perforations
Probe feeding or normal diet	9
Parenteral nutrition	25
Combination	7
No feeding	2

Table 1.—Scoring of Multiple Organ Failure*

Organ System	Score	Variable
Respiratory	0	No mechanical ventilation
	1	PEEP ≤10 cm H_2O and F_{IO_2} ≤0.4
	2	PEEP >10 cm H_2O and/or F_{IO_2} >0.4
Cardiovascular	0	Normal blood pressure without vasoactive substances
	1	Blood pressure >100 mm Hg by volume loading; dopamine hydrochloride ≤10 μg/kg/min or nitroglycerin ≤20 μg/kg/min
	2	Blood pressure ≤100 mm Hg and/or dopamine hydrochloride >10 μg/kg/min and/or nitroglycerin >20 μg/kg/min
Renal	0	Serum creatinine <177 μmol/L
	1	Serum creatinine ≥177 μmol/L
	2	Hemodialysis or peritoneal dialysis necessary
Hepatic	0	AST <25 U/L and total bilirubin <30 μmol/L
	1	Total bilirubin 30-89 μmol/L or AST 25-49 U/L
	2	Total bilirubin ≥90 μmol/L or AST ≥50 U/L
Hematological	0	Normal counts of thrombocytes and leukocytes
	1	Thrombocytopenia <50 × 10^9/L and/or leukocytes 0.03-0.059 × 10^9/L
	2	Hemorrhagic diathesis or leukocytes <0.0025 × 10^9/L or leukocytes ≥0.06 × 10^9/L
Gastrointestinal	0	. . .
	1	Acalculous cholecystitis or stress ulcer
	2	Bleeding from stress ulcer necessitating >2 U/24 h blood, necrotizing enterocolitis and/or pancreatitis, and/or spontaneous perforation of gallbladder
Neurological	0	Normal functioning
	1	Clearly diminished responsiveness
	2	Severely disturbed responsiveness and/or diffuse neuropathy

*PEEP indicates positive end-expiratory pressure; F_{IO_2}, fraction of inspired oxygen; and AST, aspartate aminotransferase.

Microorganisms cultured from blood samples and abdominal foci are detailed in Table 4. A wide variety of microorganisms was cultured showing no relation with the occurrence of the intestinal perforations.

Forty-six of the 53 perforations were treated surgically. Twenty-nine laparotomies were performed for 41 lesions. Twenty-two perforations were closed in layers, with a secondary dehiscense in four. Thirteen resections were performed for 19 lesions. A stoma was constructed in seven cases, whereas continuity was restored in six. Dehiscence was not observed. Five superficial lesions were directly closed in one layer without performing adhesiolysis or laparotomy. Dehiscence occurred in two.

Surgical treatment was rejected in four patients. They had already been treated previously for spontaneous small-bowel perforations, and new lesions occurred during the terminal stage of the intra-abdominal sepsis. Altogether, nine patients (64%) died, all due to the underlying diseases.

Four patients also developed colonic perforations without demonstrable cause. All these lesions were located superficially in the wound. Two of them occurred together with small-bowel perforations, the others on unrelated occasions. These colonic lesions were not analyzed in this study.

Table 2.—Clinical Data of 14 Patients With Small-Bowel Perforations*

Patient No./ Sex/Age, y	Medical History	No. of Laparotomies	No. of Perforations	No. of Events	Occurrence After Laparotomy No.†	Corresponding Postoperative Days	Course
1/F/63	Perforated sigmoid diverticulitis, 3-staged operation	19	15	13	10-19	2-88	Died, MI‡
2/M/58	MI, infected ruptured aortoiliac graft with sigmoid necrosis	9	4	2	7-8	3-4	Died, aspergillosis septicemia
3/M/72	Polycythemia, resection of infected aortoiliac graft, axillobifemoral bypass	5	2	2	3-4	1-10	Recovered
4/M/39	Cholelithiasis, alcohol abuse, acute hemorrhagic pancreatitis	20	3	2	17	28-33	Died, sepsis‡
5/M/53	Septic cholangitis	9	3	2	7-9	5-8	Died, sepsis‡
6/M/31	Acute hemorrhagic pancreatitis	15	3	3	5-14	1-5	Recovered
7/M/79	Pacemaker, MI, COPD, incarcerated inguinal hernia with colon perforation	4	1	1	3	32	Died, respiratory insufficiency; pneumonia
8/M/57	MI (myopathy), cholecystitis, pancreatitis	14	4	4	13-15	4-8	Died, cardiac insufficiency
9/F/19	Cholecystectomy, pancreatitis	17	1	1	1	10	Recovered
10/F/70	Acute hemorrhagic pancreatitis	8	4	2	6-8	2-17	Died, sepsis‡
11/F/29	Ovarian thecal cell carcinoma, uterus-adnexa extirpation and partial colon resection, dehiscence of anastomosis	10	5	5	5-10	2-19	Died, uremia‡
12/M/35	Pancreas pseudocyst, dehiscence of gastrocystostomy	6	1	1	5	120	Recovered
13/F/51	Diabetes mellitus, cholecystectomy, acute necrotizing pancreatitis	18	5	4	10-16	2-8	Recovered
14/M/58	Gastric ulcer, BII gastrectomy, leakage of duodenal stump	8	1	1	6	3	Died, sepsis, pulmonary abscess
Total	...	**164**	**53**	**43**	...	...	...

*MI indicates myocardial infarction; COPD, chronic obstructive pulmonary disease; and BII, Billroth II.
†First and last laparotomy after which perforations were diagnosed.
‡Persistent intra-abdominal sepsis when death occurred.

Frequency distribution of occurrence of 53 small-bowel perforations of unknown origin and corresponding postoperative days.

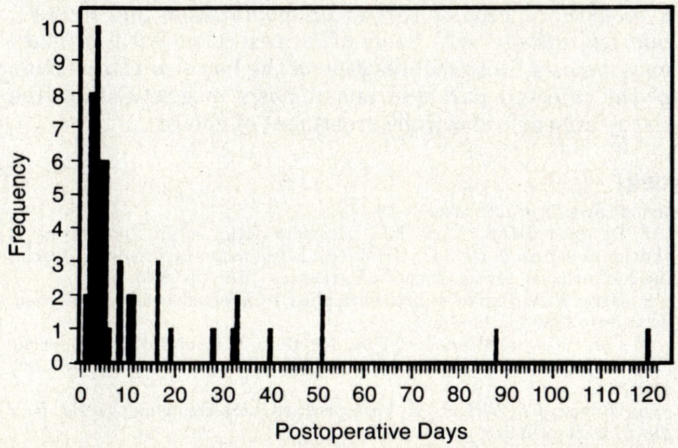

Table 3.—Scoring According to MOF Score of Individual Organ Failure During 43 Times Perforations Were Diagnosed*

	Score		
Organ System	0	1	2
Respiratory	27 (63)	8 (18.5)	8 (18.5)
Cardiovascular	33 (77)	4 (9)	6 (14)
Renal	38 (88)	3 (7)	2 (5)
Hepatic	33 (77)	5 (12)	5 (12)
Hematological	38 (88)	5 (12)	0 (0)
Gastrointestinal	42 (98)	1 (2)	0 (0)
Neurological	38 (88)	1 (2)	4 (9)

*MOF indicates Multiple Organ Failure Scale (Table 1). Values are number (percent).

Table 4.—Frequency of Microorganisms Cultured in Blood Samples and From Intra-abdominal Contaminated Pockets*

Microorganism	Blood Culture Positive	Positive Culture of Intra-abdominal Focus
Staphylococcus albus	7	5
Staphylococcus aureus	3	2
Bacteroides fragilis	...	1
Citrobacter	...	3
Enterobacter cloacae	...	3
Escherichia coli	...	5
Klebsiella pneumoniae	...	4
Morganelli	...	2
Pseudomonas aeruginosa	1	5
Proteus mirabilis	...	5
Serratia marcescens	...	1
Streptococcus faecalis	...	7
Candida albicans	1	3
Aspergillus fumigatus	1	...

*Blood samples taken within 24 hours before the occurrence of perforations (43 events); intra-abdominal contaminated pockets found during surgical treatment of the perforations. In blood samples, only solitary specimens of microorganisms were cultured. Once a single kind of microorganism was cultured from intra-abdominal foci (*S albus*); 13 times a mixture of two or more different microorganisms was cultured.

COMMENT

To our knowledge, the occurrence of intestinal perforations during open treatment for generalized peritonitis has not been described so far. We are aware that in our series some iatrogenic or mechanical factor cannot be denied. All perforations occurred after at least three preceding laparotomies for intra-abdominal sepsis, in which surgery is known to be technically difficult,[10] and only when the abdominal cavity had been left open. Thus, iatrogenic perforations and serosal lesions will inevitably occur. Since iatrogenic perforations are easily recognized during surgery, it is unlikely that they have been missed and have caused symptoms after a few days. Moreover, most perforations definitely would have been detected immediately postoperatively or during the first changing of the wound dressings, since 92.5% of the lesions were located in the exposed bowel surface, which was clearly visible at inspection.

Small serosal lesions, made during operation, were considered to be unimportant and not sutured. When, for some reason, relaparotomy was necessary after a few days, the mucosa on the spot was noted to bulge out and to be tense. It may be imagined that perforation would only be a matter of days, but it is our experience that this hardly ever happens. We believe this is due to the extrinsic counterpressure of the surrounding loops covering the lesions.

Even if serosal lacerations would be predisposing sites for perforations, this would only account for the early perforations, since the bowel loops in which late lesions occurred were covered with a thick, granulating, fibrotic plate. A mechanical factor as the only cause of the late perforations, ie, changing of a wound dressing sticking to the underlying layer, is rejected for the same reason. The nylon mesh applied to the wound edges seems to be a less important mechanical factor since 17% of the lesions had been diagnosed while a mesh was absent. All patients had been suffering from intra-abdominal sepsis and had been treated in the ICU for support of several organ systems; however, only 51% of the perforations were diagnosed on this ward. Nineteen (44%) of the 43 times, the patient was in a reasonable condition, as organ system failure was present in only 56%.

Although serious anemia, hypoalbuminemia, and hypoproteinemia did occur on some occasions, they were not clearly related to the lesions, as in most patients these deficiencies were absent or only moderate. It might be expected that ileus and parenteral feeding were predisposing factors, but 16 times the lesions occurred while the patient was enterally fed. No predisposing microorganisms have been cultured. Since no common causative factor could be found, we can only hypothesize about the pathophysiology of the perforations. In a few cases, we were able closely to follow the development of a superficial perforation several weeks after surgery. When the wound gauzes were changed, a small blisterlike elevation could be observed in the diffusely granulating surface. On palpation these felt like weak spots in a stiff, fibrotic plate. Within a few days they burst open. At first, small mucosal blowouts were seen, but within a few hours, while awaiting surgery, they became rather large defects, sometimes even mimicking a loop enterostomy. This demonstrates that traction forces are prevalent in the granulating wound. The abdominal wall, when left open, retracts sideways, enlarging the wound dehiscence, while the granulation tissue contracts in an effort to reduce it. Weak spots in the fibrotic plate may give way to these counteracting forces and cause bulging and rupture of the underlying bowel, which is stuck to it. The high recurrence rate (40%) of the lesions directly sutured without laparotomy supports this theory.

The occurrence of a spontaneous small-bowel perforation should not be considered as an indication that the patient is in the terminal phase of intra-abdominal sepsis. After all, 35% of the patients survived. Surgery, as difficult as it may be, should therefore not be rejected.

Mobilization of the bowel appears to be a sheer necessity. The granulating area is detached from the wound edges and split up, so that the prevalent traction forces are neutralized. When laparotomy was performed, there was a recurrence rate of 18% after mobilization and closure, but no leakage was seen after resection with primary anastomosis. Both mobilization of the bowel with resection of the affected part and anastomosis in granulation-free tissue appear to form the treatment of choice.

References

1. Leijonmarck CE, Fenyo G, Raf L: Nontraumatic perforation of the small intestine. *Acta Chir Scand* 1984;150:405-411.
2. Nadkarni KM, Shetty SD, Kagzi RS, et al: Small-bowel perforations. *Arch Surg* 1981;116:53-57.
3. Orringer RD, Coller JA, Veidenheimer MC: Spontaneous free perforation of the small intestine. *Dis Colon Rectum* 1983;26:323-326.
4. Schmitt EH III, Symmonds RE: Surgical treatment radiation induced injuries of the intestine. *Surg Gynecol Obstet* 1981;153:896-900.
5. Chaikof EL: Nontraumatic perforation of the small bowel. *Am J Surg* 1987;153:355-358.
6. ReMine SG, McIlrath DC: Bowel perforation in steroid-treated patients. *Ann Surg* 1980;192:581-586.
7. De Boer HHM, Goris RJA, Cremers JEL, et al: Reoperation in abdominal sepsis, in De Boer HHM (ed): *Intra-abdominal Sepsis.* Utrecht, the Netherlands, Bunge Scientific Publishers, 1979, pp 59-67.
8. Goris RJA: Ogilvie's method applied to infected wound disruption. *Arch Surg* 1980;115:1103-1106.
9. Goris RJA, te Boekhorst TPA, Nuytinck JKS, et al: Multiple-organ failure: Generalized autodestructive inflammation? *Arch Surg* 1985;120:1109-1115.
10. Rogers PN, Wright IH: Postoperative intra-abdominal sepsis. *Br J Surg* 1987;74:973-975.

Angiotropin Treatment Prevents Flap Necrosis and Enhances Dermal Regeneration in Rabbits

Michael Höckel, MD, PhD, John F. Burke, MD

• **Angiotropin is a potent angiogenesis factor isolated from the serum-free media of cultured, lectin-activated peripheral monocytes. In vitro, the purified substance stimulates migration, phenotypic differentiation, and tube formation, but not proliferation of capillary endothelial cells. When injected intradermally, angiotropin induces, in dose-dependent fashion, angiogenesis associated with skin hyperplasia. We have developed a flap model with insufficient blood supply and a model for contraction-free defect healing in rabbit skin. We show that (1) local pretreatment with angiotropin can prevent flap necrosis and (2) dermal regeneration after wounding can be augmented by angiotropin. From these results, we conclude that angiotropin might be of use as an adjuvant to healing in surgery.**

(Arch Surg **1989;124:693-698)**

Tissue ischemia due to impaired or reduced local blood flow is involved in the pathogenesis of a variety of diseases. It may also cause surgical complications, such as delayed wound healing, anastomotic insufficiency, or acute graft necrosis. Radiation-associated ulcer and fistula formation as well as major wound healing problems in burn patients are also consequences of insufficient microcirculation.

Since the discovery and isolation of biomolecules capable of inducing the neomorphogenesis of blood vessels ("angiogenesis factors"), a potential clinical use of these substances for the prevention or treatment of at least some of these pathological conditions has been suggested.[1] Moreover, biomolecules mediating angiogenesis and other cellular reactions involved in tissue regeneration and repair might also be applied to speed up normal wound healing processes.[2]

Angiotropin has recently been discovered as an angiogenesis factor acting on capillary endothelial cells in vitro by stimulating migration and differentiation into tube-forming cell phenotypes.[3] It has been isolated and highly purified from conditioned serum-free media of large-scale cultures of porcine peripheral monocytes activated with concanavalin A by Wissler et al.[4] Chemically, angiotropin was found to be a metallopolyribonucleopolypeptide complex consisting of one copper ion per 38 amino acids and 43 ribonucleotides as a least-common unit of all components. Selective enzymatic splitting indicated that the polypeptide as well as the polyribonucleotide portions are essential for the angiogenic activity.[4]

Intradermal injection of angiotropin into the skin of rabbit ear lobes in the concentration range of 1 to 20 ng/mL induces "controlled angiogenesis" in terms of defined time-dependent dynamics and dose-dependent vascular changes. These are characterized by an extension of the vascular bed and subsequent increase of blood perfusion, which is initially caused by dilation of the microvessels into large sinusoidal blood channels and later by local capillary growth.[5]

Angiotropin did not exhibit mitogenic activity on endothelial cells and fibroblasts in vitro when injected intradermally into rabbit skin.[3] Autoradiographic studies with tritiated thymidine demonstrated a strong increase of labeled endothelial cells, pericytes, and perivascular cells as well as stromal and epidermal cells. Within the site of angiotropin injection, resting hair follicles were activated to grow.[5,6]

The effects observed in the skin after intradermal injection of angiotropin prompted us to test the possibility that ischemic necrosis might be prevented and that the proliferative reaction in tissue regeneration/repair could be accelerated by use of angiotropin. We therefore studied the effects of angiotropin treatment in a miniflap model with inadequate vascular supply and in a model for contraction-free dermal regeneration.

MATERIALS AND METHODS

Animals

In our study we used adult long-eared New Zealand white rabbits of both sexes that weighed 2.5 to 3.5 kg and were kept in accordance with institutional guidelines. For the injections and operations, the animals were anesthetized by intramuscular application of 40 mg/kg of ketamine sodium (Ketanest, Parke Davies Co, Munich, West Germany) and 5 mg/kg of xylazine (Rompun, Bayer, Leverkusen, West Germany).

Intradermal Injections

After removing the hair with a depilatory (PILCA, Olivin Co, Hamburg, West Germany) and disinfection with povidone-iodine

Accepted for publication July 6, 1988.

From the Universitätsfrauenklinik Mainz, West Germany (Dr Höckel), and the Department of Surgery, Harvard Medical School, Massachusetts General Hospital, Boston (Dr Burke).

Reprint requests to Trauma Services, Bigelow 12, Massachusetts General Hospital, Boston, MA 02114 (Dr Burke).

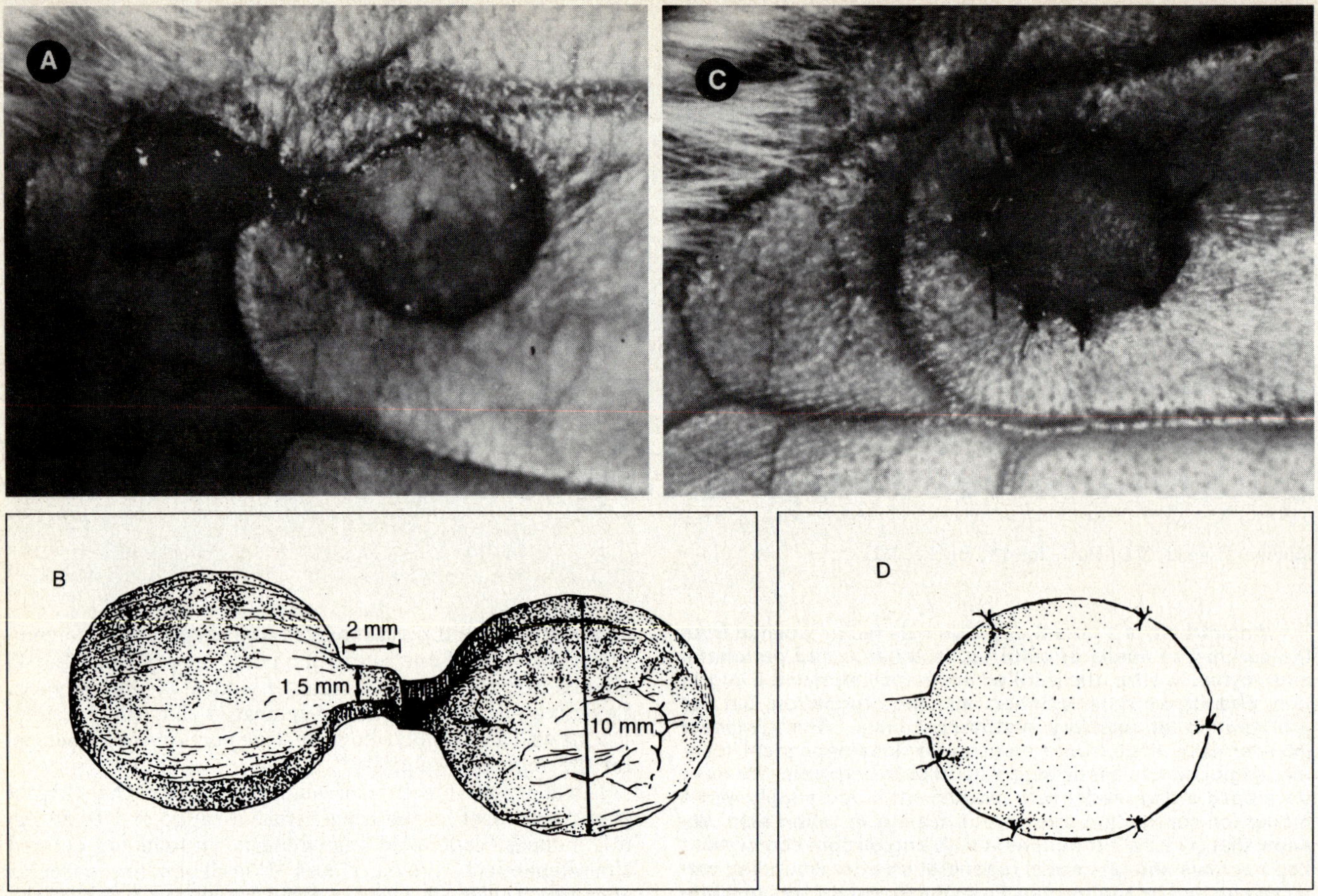

Fig 1.—Design of flap model in ear lobe of rabbit. Racket-shaped whole-skin perichondrial tissue flap is raised from cartilage (A and B) and resutured in its former bed (C and D).

solution, intradermal injections were made in the skin of the dorsal aspect of the ear lobes. The injections were placed approximately at the junction of the middle and distal third of the ear and located to avoid visible blood vessels. The injections were done under direct vision.

A sterile 50-mL glass syringe (Hamilton, Bonaduz Co, Switzerland) was equipped with a 31-gauge needle. A shorter, 26-gauge needle was inserted into the epidermis at a low angle to serve as trocar, and the 31-gauge needle was directed through the trocar and pushed forward into the dermis for about 2 mm. The standard 50-mL aliquot injection produced a transient papule of about 1 cm in diameter.

Angiotropin

The preparation of angiotropin used in this study was shown to migrate as a single band in sodiumdodecyl sulfate polyacrylamide gel electrophoresis (SDS PAGE) gel[3] and to possess no endotoxin-like activity in the rabbit fever test. It was stored as frozen stock solution at a concentration of 50 ng/mL and dissolved in 1 mmol/L of L-cysteine and 3.65 mmol/L of pyrogen-free porcine serum albumin[3] as carrier protein. Thawed aliquots of stock solution were diluted with sterile pyrogen-free phosphate-buffered saline solution (GIBCO Inc, Grand Island, NY) prior to intradermal injections for the flap experiments. For the neodermis experiments, aliquots of the undiluted stock solution were used.

Flap Model

Dorsal aspects of both ear lobes were depilated and disinfected and racket-shaped full-thickness skin flaps, including the perichondrial tissue, were dissected from the cartilage (Fig 1, A and B). The diameter of the circular part of the flap was 10 mm; pedicle length, 2 mm; and pedicle width, 1.5 mm. Via a template flap, size and design were kept constant for all experiments. After hemostasis by gentle pressure with a gauze swab for three minutes, the flaps were reattached to their former beds with 6-0 monophilic single sutures (Fig 1, C and D). Wound dressings were not applied.

Inadequate perfusion of the transplants was achieved in the control experiments under the following conditions: The flaps were placed in the upper third of the dorsal aspect of the ear lobes of adult animals medially or laterally to the central ear artery. The skin at the transplantation site contained only hair follicles in the resting state. The location of the pedicle was chosen so that no macroscopically detectable vessel leading through it entered the circular part of the flap.

The rabbit ears were pretreated in the area of the future flap as follows: After the intended location of the transplant was drawn on the skin (Fig 2, D), two intradermal injections of 50 mL of phosphate-buffered saline solution containing 5 ng/mL of angiotropin and 25 mg/mL of porcine serum albumin were made in the prospective pedicle area and the center of the circular area. The angiotropin injections were repeated at the same sites 48 hours later. The flap experiments were performed 48 hours after the second injections of angiotropin. For the control experiments in the homologous sites of the contralateral ears, analogous injections were made with the carrier solution (phosphate-buffered saline and 25 mg/mL of porcine serum albumin) alone. All injected solutions were sterile and pyrogen free. The base of all flaps was placed at the distal margin of the ear.

Flaps were clinically judged each day for a ten-day period; the sutures and all necrotic tissue were then removed. Flap survival was judged by two investigators who did not know the mode of treatment.

Neodermis Model

In the depilated and disinfected dorsal skin of the rabbit ear lobe, an 8-mm circular defect was made that included the peri-

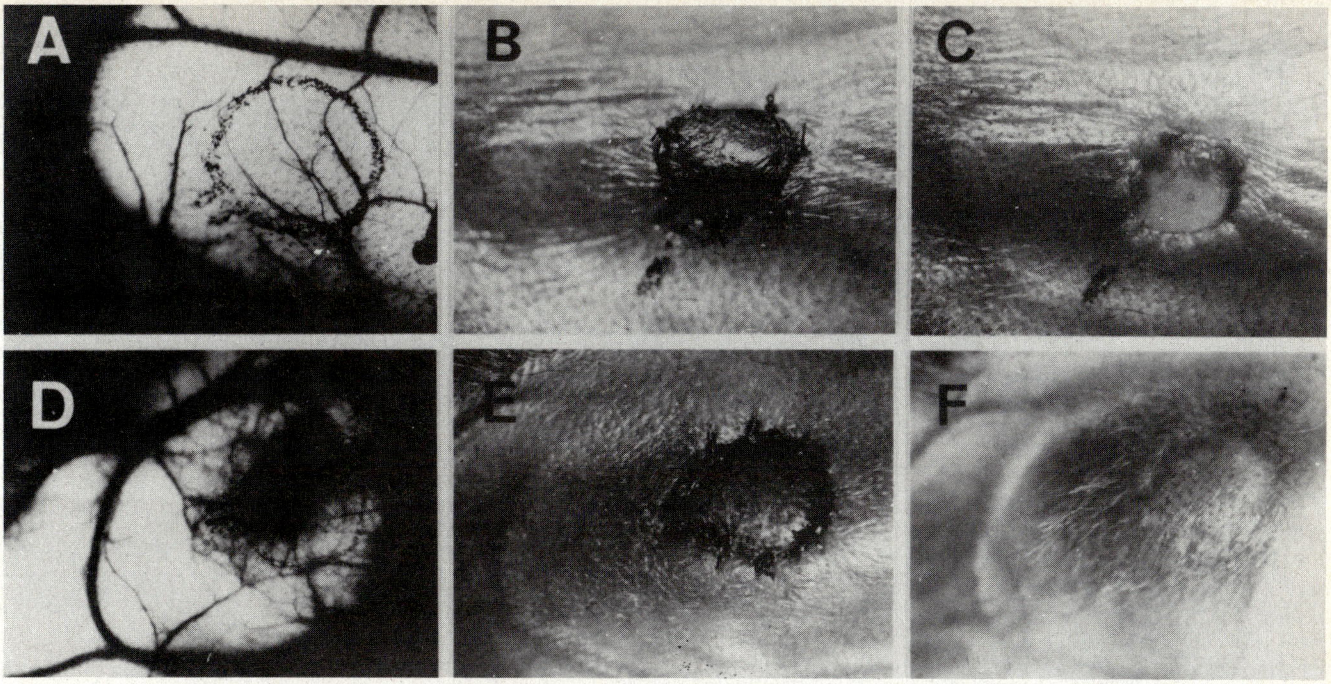

Fig 2.—Prevention of total flap necrosis by angiotropin in flap model. A, B, and C, Control ear. D, E, and F, Treated ear. See text for details.

chondrial tissue and denuded the cartilage (Fig 3, A and B). The defect was then covered by an equally sized graft of "artificial skin" fixed by 6-0 monophilic single sutures (Fig 3, C and D).

The operations were performed under strictly aseptic conditions on homologous sites of both ear lobes, each rabbit serving as its own control. One ear of each animal received an artificial skin graft that contained either 0.25 ng or 0.5 ng of angiotropin to test for a dose-related response. Only the carrier solution was added to the artificial skin graft of the control ear. No dressings were used to cover the artificial skin grafts.

On days 7 to 10, when loosening of the sutures was evident, the animals were killed for histologic examination by an overdose of pentobarbital sodium (Nembutal, Ceva Co, Paris). Fibrovascular ingrowth into the artificial skin matrix was determined morphometrically by measuring the area covered by "neodermal" tissue continuous to the primary wound margins with a computer-aided MOP videoplan (Kontron Co, Zurich). Morphometry was performed in Masson trichrome–stained paraffin sections of the whole ear, which were cut in the midline planes perpendicular to the long ear axis. The evaluation was done by two investigators who did not know the mode of treatment.

RESULTS

Flap Model

In all eight control experiments, no change of the vascular pattern could be observed preoperatively (Fig 2, A). Within 24 hours, all skin flaps became gangrenous (Fig 2, B), and after removing the sutures on the tenth postoperative day, the black and dry skin flaps stripped off, leaving a circular defect to the cartilage (Fig 2, C). The wound margins were covered by small rims of epithelialized granulation tissue. In only one case a narrow tongue of granulation tissue, extending from the edge, reached the center of the defect.

Corresponding flap experiments were performed at homologous sites of the contralateral ears. The sites, however, were pretreated with intradermal injections of a total of 1 ng of angiotropin, which resulted in marked engorgement of the microvascular bed within the skin sites where the flaps were raised (Fig 2, D).

After 24 hours, the flaps usually were somewhat edematous (Fig 2, E). Small focal demarcation areas were found in four treated transplants at that time. When the sutures were removed on the tenth postoperative day, four of eight skin flaps had healed completely, with intact epidermis and hair follicles (Fig 2, F). The remaining four flaps showed only epithelial defects of less than half of each transplant's area. However, the sites with impaired epidermis were covered by viable (bleeding) tissue. The tissue was continous to the wound edge corresponding to intact deeper layers of the dermis and/or granulation tissue. No overall skin defect denuding the cartilage was seen, as was the case in all untreated control flaps. The blindly evaluated results demonstrate a highly significant ($P=.0002$, Fisher's exact test) reduction of skin-flap necrosis following pretreatment with angiotropin.

Neodermis Model

Of the 14 experiments performed with this model, two cases had to be excluded because of local infection. A third case was also discarded because the animal damaged the artificial skin grafts by scraping. The results with the remaining 11 animals were evaluated in Masson trichrome–stained histological sections of the whole-ear specimens containing the artificial skin grafts in midplane transverse sections. The histological slides of a typical experiment are shown in Fig 4.

The fibrovascular tissue expanding into the artificial skin matrix (neodermis) could clearly be distinguished from the wound margins at the periphery and from the "empty" parts of the artificial skin matrix in the center (Fig 4, A and B). As a rule, the neodermis originated from the adjacent dermal and perichondrial wound margins. Occasionally, in the area of denuded cartilage, there was a small blood vessel perforating from the volar site of the ear through the cartilage. In a few cases, a small amount of fibrovascular tissue grew through these small holes in the cartilage, as seen in Fig 4, A (arrowhead). However, the

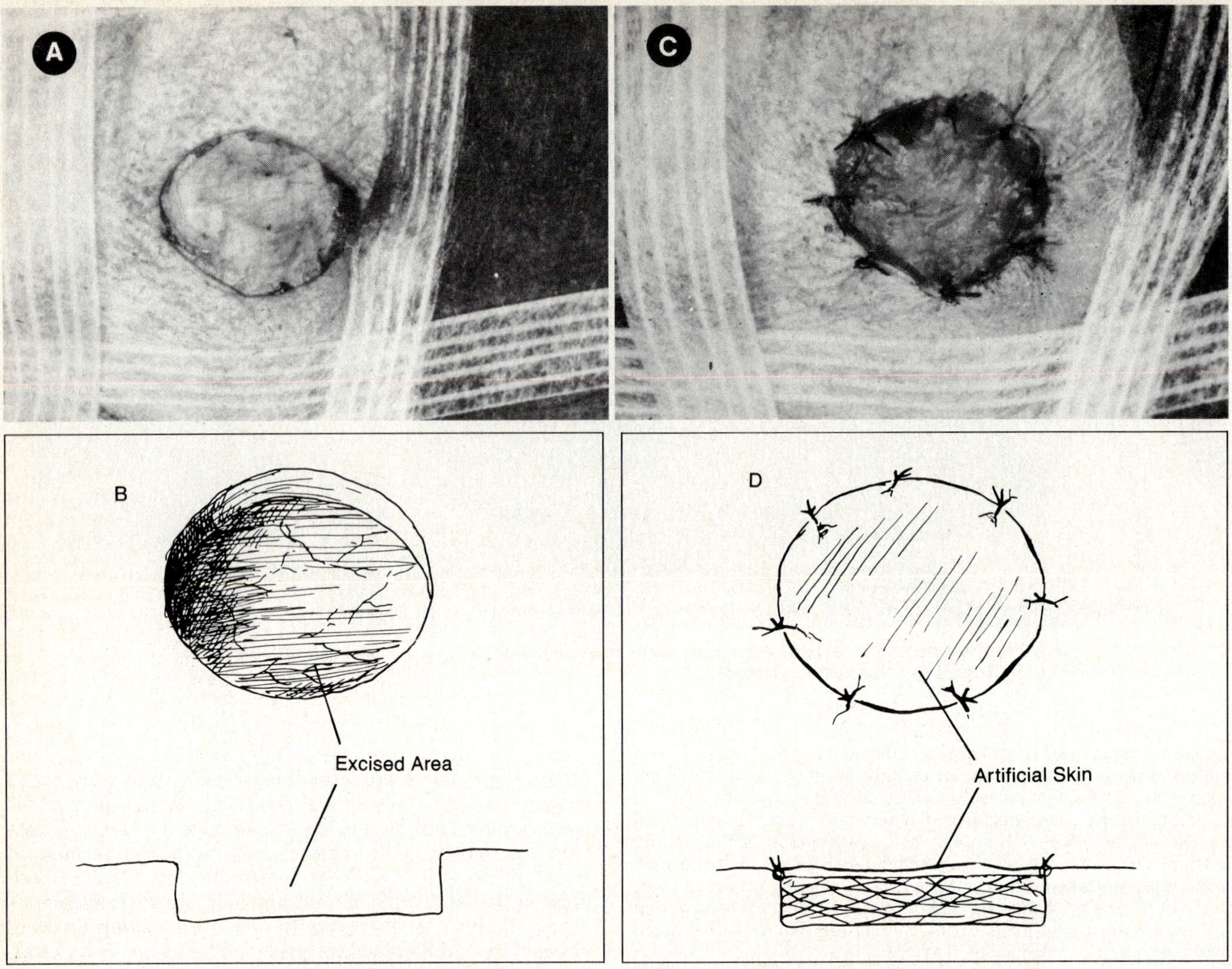

Fig 3.—Design of neodermis model in ear lobe of rabbit. Whole-skin perichondrial tissue defect denuding cartilage is made (A and B) and covered by equally sized artificial skin graft (C and D).

contribution of the tissue that grew through these small holes in the cartilage to the overall formation of the fibrous tissue ingrowth was not important.

In the majority of the control experiments, the wound margins were covered by a downward-growing, irregular epidermal layer that even reached the cartilage in some cases (Fig 4, A). Only small areas of the artificial skin matrix were filled with fibroblastic cells. Blood vessels were rarely found in the artificial skin grafts that contained only the carrier solution.

In the artificial skin grafts soaked with 0.5 ng of angiotropin, most of the matrix was filled by neodermal tissue (Fig 4, B). At the periphery, the original collagen fibers of the matrix were replaced by a loose network of newly synthesized fine collagen fibrils. Many fibroblasts and dilated neocapillaries were seen herein (Fig 4, C). Fibroblastic cells admixed with mononuclear cells filled the pores of the artificial skin matrix toward the center (Fig 4, D).

The fibrovascular ingrowth from the margins of the primary defects into the artificial skin matrix was determined morphometrically. The results obtained by two investigators who did not know the mode of treatment are shown in the Table. Neodermis formation was significantly ($P=.0039$, signed rank test) increased in the grafts containing angiotropin. The relative increase of the neodermis formation (mean ± SD) compared with the controls was 235% ± 39% when the artificial skin grafts were treated with 0.5 ng of angiotropin and 73% ± 37% when 0.25 ng of angiotropin was used, demonstrating the dose dependence of the angiotropin effects ($P=.047$, rank sum test).

COMMENT

Based on the in vivo actions of purified monocytic angiotropin—angiogenesis associated with tissue proliferation—we designed a pedicle flap and a skin graft model in rabbits with respect to a potential clinical relevance of this bioactive substance in surgery. With the flap model, we could demonstrate that ischemic necrosis due to the reduction of the microvasculature flow via surgical procedure was prevented by local pretreatment with angiotropin. In this model, the microvessels of both the graft and its bed were expanded by angiotropin treatment prior to the operation. The survival of the flaps pretreated with angiotropin compared with that of the controls might therefore be explained by (1) the enlarged vascular flow in the pedicle, providing increased perfusion of the flap with blood immediately after the operation, and (2) the presence of "activated" blood vessels or capillary sprouts at the time of surgery, leading to an earlier fusion of the blood vessels

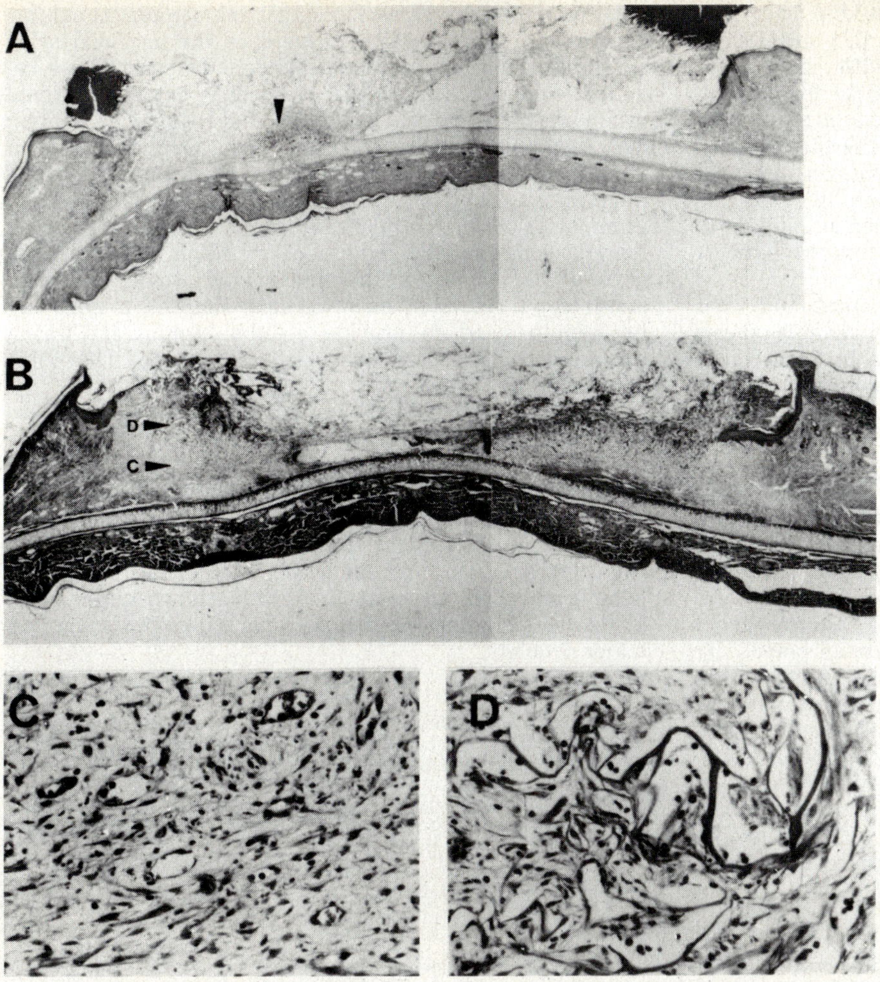

Fig 4.—Stimulation of fibrovascular ingrowth by angiotropin in neodermis model. A, Control experiment. Arrowhead indicates small area of tissue vascularized through hole in cartilage connecting dorsal with ventral side of ear. No other vascularized tissue is present in grafted defect (Masson trichrome, original magnification ×30). B, C, and D, Defect covered by artificial skin matrix that received 0.5 ng of angiotropin, showing presence of extensively vascularized neodermis. Masson trichrome–stained transverse sections of rabbit's ear lobes on day 10 (B, original magnification ×30; C and D, original magnification ×300).

Stimulation of Fibrovascular Ingrowth Into Artificial Skin Grafts Treated With Angiotropin Compared With Control (Carrier Alone) Artificial Skin Grafts*

Animal No.	Angiotropin, ng	Fibrovascular Tissue in Control and (Angiotropin-Treated) Artificial Skin Grafts, mm^2	Relative Increase Compared With Control, %
1	0.25	0.78 (2.10)	170
2	0.25	0.80 (1.56)	93
3	0.25	2.02 (2.22)	13
4	0.25	1.86 (2.18)	17
5	0.5	2.26 (5.64)	150
6	0.5	1.38 (3.02)	119
7	0.5	1.26 (5.78)	356
8	0.5	0.64 (3.14)	385
9	0.5	1.36 (4.82)	252
10	0.5	1.30 (3.26)	152
11	0.5	0.98 (3.26)	230
1-4	0.25	1.37 ± 0.33 (2.02 ± 0.15)	73 ± 37
5-11	0.5	1.31 ± 0.19 (4.13 ± 0.47)	235 ± 39

*The total areas of neodermal tissue in midplane histologic sections are given for each experiment. Mean ± SEM values were calculated for animals 1 through 4 and 5 through 11 to show dose dependency.

of the flap with those of the surrounding wound margins.

The effects of angiotropin treatment in this model show remarkable morphological similarities with the "delay" phenomenon.[7,8] The mechanisms responsible for the improved survival of delayed whole-skin flaps are not fully understood at present. Although α-adrenergic vascular effects, as well as many others, are reported to be involved, a role for angiotropin or related substances in mediating the vascular effects of the delay phenomenon appears to be possible as well. Further studies must test this hypothesis.

This is, to the best of our knowledge, the first study that demonstrates the successful use of a purified angiogenesis factor to prevent tissue necrosis caused by insufficient microvascular supply. "Therapeutic" angiogenesis with physiological angiogenesis factors, such as pharmacological agents, appears to be a promising new approach as an adjuvant means in surgery.

The neodermis model was designed to demonstrate effects of angiotropin treatment on stromal tissue regeneration. It provided this information through quantitative determination of the ingrowing fibrovascular tissue by morphometry. Since the defects in the rabbit skin were extended below the perichondrium down to the cartilage, their geometry was anatomically defined in all planes. By use of the artificial skin matrix, wound contracture that otherwise might have interfered with the morphometrical evaluation could be avoided. In animal and human series, it was shown that artificial skin, a collagen chondroitin-6-sulfate matrix developed by other investigators,[9-13] leads to "regenerationlike" repair without skin contracture. Moreover, by soaking the artificial skin matrix with angiotropin solution, a homogeneous local application to the wound margins was achieved.

By use of the model, we found that angiotropin stimulates the growth of connective tissue into the artificial skin, resembling dermis, in dose-dependent fashion. These results also show that the tissue defect is not the maximal stimulus for regeneration or repair and that wound healing can be accelerated by chemical mediators used as local pharmacological agents. Considering the cellular effects of angiotropin in vitro[3] and in vivo,[5] we suggest that the stimulation of fibrovascular ingrowth into the artificial skin matrix is due to the increased activation of endothelial cells of capillaries in the undamaged wound margins. Angiotropin-activated microvascular endothelial cells can be hypothesized to provide cellular signals for tissue proliferation via several proposed mechanisms.[5] This point remains to be tested.

The successful use of (angiogenic) growth factors to accelerate dermal and epidermal wound healing has been reported recently.[14-22] However, these growth factors had to be applied in greater than 1000-fold–higher doses to produce a stimulation of wound healing comparable with that of angiotropin treatment. Angiotropin is therefore regarded as a very potent accelerator of dermal wound healing and should be tested in further studies with respect to its use for clinical situations where wound healing is a major problem.

Angiotropin and artificial skin were provided by J. J. Wissler, Bochum, West Germany, and Marion Laboratories, Kansas City, Mo, respectively.

Dr Höckel thanks V. Friedberg, MD, Mainz, West Germany, for generous support of this work.

The authors thank D. Costa and G. Kind for excellent technical assistance and R. Lippold, Institut für Statistik und Medizinische Dokumentation, Mainz, for his help with the statistical evaluation of the data.

We acknowledge the critical reading of the manuscript by P. Vaupel, PhD, Harvard Medical School, Boston.

References

1. Folkman J, Klagsbrun M: Angiogenic factors. *Science* 1987;235:442-447.

2. Hunt TK: Can repair processes be stimulated by modulators (cell growth factors, angiogenic factors, etc.) without adversely affecting normal processes? *J Trauma* 1984;24(suppl 9):S39-S47.

3. Höckel M, Sasse J, Wissler JH: Purified monocyte-derived angiogenic substance (angiotropin) stimulates migration, phenotypic changes and 'tube formation' but not proliferation of capillary endothelial cells in vitro. *J Cell Physiol* 1987;133:1-13.

4. Wissler JH, Logemann E, Meyer HE, et al: Structure and function of a monocytic blood vessel morphogen (angiotropin) for angiogenesis in vivo and in vitro: A copper-containing metallo-polyribonucleo-polypeptide as a novel and unique type of monokine. *Protides Biol Fluids* 1986;34:525-536.

5. Höckel M, Jung W, Vaupel P, et al: Purified monocyte-derived angiogenic substance (angiotropin) induces controlled angiogenesis associated with regulated tissue proliferation in rabbit skin. *J Clin Invest*, in press.

6. Höckel M, Beck T, Wissler JH: Neomorphogenesis of blood vessels in rabbit skin induced by a highly purified monocyte-derived polypeptide (monocyto-angiotropin) and associated tissue reactions. *Int J Tissue React* 1984;6:323-331.

7. Myers MB, Cherry G: Augmentation of tissue survival by delay: An experimental study in rabbits. *Plast Reconstr Surg* 1967;39:397.

8. Pearl RM: A unifying theory of the delay phenomenon: Recovery from the hyperadrenergic state. *Ann Plast Surg* 1981;7:102-108.

9. Yannas IV, Burke JF: Design of an artificial skin: I. Basic design principles. *J Biomed Mater Res* 1980;14:65-81.

10. Yannas IV, Burke JF, Gordon PL, et al: Design of an artificial skin: II. Control of chemical composition. *J Biomed Mater Res* 1980;14:107-131.

11. Dagalakis N, Flink J, Stasikelis P, et al: Design of an artificial skin: III. Control of pore structure. *J Biomed Mater Res* 1980;14:511-528.

12. Burke JF, Yannas IV, Quinby WC, et al: Successful use of a physiologically acceptable artificial skin in the treatment of extensive burn injury. *Ann Surg* 1981;194:413-428.

13. Yannas IV, Burke JF, Orgill DP, et al: Wound tissue can utilize a polymeric template to synthesize a functional extension of skin. *Science* 1982;215:174-176.

14. Sporn MB, Roberts AB, Shull JH, et al: Polypeptide transforming growth factors isolated from bovine sources and used for wound healing in vivo. *Science* 1983;219:1329-1331.

15. Buckley A, Davidson JM, Kamerath CD, et al: Sustained release of epidermal growth factor accelerates wound repair. *Proc Natl Acad Sci USA* 1985;82:7340-7344.

16. Davidson JM, Klagsbrun M, Hill KE, et al: Accelerated wound repair, cell proliferation, and collagen accumulation are produced by a cartilage-derived growth factor. *J Cell Biol* 1985;100:1219-1227.

17. Brown GL, Curtsinger L, Brightwell JR, et al: Enhancement of epidermal regeneration by biosynthetic epidermal growth factor. *J Exp Med* 1986;163:1319-1324.

18. Knighton DR, Ciresi KF, Fiegel VD, et al: Classification and treatment of chronic nonhealing wounds. *Ann Surg* 1986;204:322-330.

19. Laato M, Niinikoski J, Lebel L, et al: Stimulation of wound healing by epidermal growth factor. *Ann Surg* 1986;203:379-381.

20. Lawrence WT, Norton JA, Sporn MB, et al: The reversal of an Adriamycin induced healing impairment with chemoattractants and growth factors. *Ann Surg* 1986;203:142-147.

21. Mustoe TA, Pierce GF, Thomason A, et al: Accelerated healing of incisional wounds in rats induced by transforming growth factor-β. *Science* 1987;237:1333-1336.

22. Schultz GS, White M, Mitchell R, et al: Epithelial wound healing enhanced by transforming growth factor-α and vaccinia growth factor. *Science* 1987;235:350-352.

Simple Intestinal Obstruction Causes Bacterial Translocation in Man

Edwin A. Deitch, MD

• Indirect clinical evidence has accumulated indicating that the gut may be a reservoir for microorganisms causing systemic infection in man. Our experimental results, in a variety of animal models, demonstrate that bacteria can translocate across the mucosal barrier and cause systemic infections. To determine directly whether bacterial translocation occurs in man, we cultured mesenteric lymph nodes (MLNs) obtained at laparotomy from 42 patients, none of whom were clinically infected. Ten (59%) of 17 patients with intestinal obstruction (none of whom had necrotic bowel) had bacteria in their MLNs, in contrast to one (4%) of 25 patients operated on for other reasons. The most common bacteria cultured from the MLNs was *Escherichia coli*. Thus, it appeared that simple intestinal obstruction of the colon or small bowel in the absence of necrotic bowel was associated with bacterial translocation.

(*Arch Surg* 1989;124:699-701)

Under normal circumstances, the gut performs many functions, including the complex processes of digestion, selective absorption, and secretion. However, the gut contains bacteria and bacterial products that must be excluded as well as nutrients that must be absorbed. Therefore, the gut has developed a complex immune system that works in synchrony with local antibacterial barrier systems to prevent the escape of luminal contents. Although it is well recognized that intestinal motility, absorption, and secretion may be altered, it has only recently been recognized that the gut's immunologic and barrier functions may also fail.[1,2]

We have demonstrated experimentally that indigenous bacteria colonizing the gastrointestinal tract can cross the epithelial mucosa to infect the mesenteric lymph nodes (MLNs) and systemic organs, a process termed *bacterial translocation*.[3,4] Factors that promote the translocation of bacteria from the gastrointestinal tract in animal models include disruption of the ecologic balance of the normal indigenous microflora, resulting in bacterial overgrowth,[4,5] impaired host immune defenses,[6] physical disruption of the gut mucosal barrier,[7] trauma,[8] endotoxemia,[9] intra-abdominal abscesses,[10] and hemorrhagic shock.[11,12] Furthermore, systemic sepsis occurred in endotoxin-challenged, protein-malnourished, or immunocompromised mice, since the spread of bacteria from the gut could not be controlled and the translocating bacteria could not be cleared.[1,2] Thus, in some experimental circumstances, bacteria translocating from the gut caused septicemia and death. In addition, indirect clinical evidence has accumulated indicating that the gut may be a reservoir for microorganisms causing systemic infections in man.[2,13,14] To determine whether bacterial translocation occurs in man, we quantitatively cultured MLNs from 42 noninfected patients undergoing laparotomy. The results of this study indicate that intestinal obstruction is associated with bacterial translocation to the MLN in the absence of intra-abdominal infection.

Accepted for publication Aug 26, 1988.

From the Department of Surgery, Louisiana State University (LSU) Medical Center, Shreveport.

Reprint requests to Department of Surgery, LSU Medical Center, 1501 Kings Hwy, PO Box 33932, Shreveport, LA 71130-3932 (Dr Deitch).

PATIENTS AND METHODS

At laparotomy, the MLNs of 42 patients operated on between April and November 1987 for a variety of conditions underwent biopsy. Patients with an intra-abdominal infection, necrotic bowel, or a perforated viscus were excluded from study. All patients received perioperative antibiotics. At the time of laparotomy, prior to performance of any further operative manipulations, a lymph node from the mesentery of the small or large intestine was excised and sent for culture. Cultures of peritoneal fluid when present were obtained in patients operated on for intestinal obstruction.

The excised lymph node was immediately taken to the laboratory, where it was weighed and then placed into grinding tubes containing sterile tryptic soy broth and processed as previously described.[3,4] Briefly, the MLN was homogenized with glass-reinforced Teflon grinders, and aliquots (0.3 mL) of the MLN homogenate were plated on selective MacConkey agar to culture gram-negative, enteric bacilli, on blood agar to culture gram-positive cocci, and on selective agar to culture lactobacilli. The plates were incubated at 37°C for 24 hours. Three milliliters of tryptic soy broth was added to the remaining 0.1 mL of MLN homogenate and incubated overnight at 37°C. Any growth was gram-stained and subcultured on MacConkey agar. The gram-negative, enteric bacteria were identified with an enteric (API 20E) identification system and gram-positive cocci and lactobacilli were identified by standard procedures. Strict anaerobic bacteria were not measured, since obligate anaerobic bacteria rarely translocate from the gut.[15] The translocation levels of the various bacteria were calculated per gram of MLN. Comparisons between groups were performed by χ^2 analysis.

RESULTS

The 42 patients were divided into two groups according to whether or not intestinal obstruction was present. Only one of the 25 patients, who did not have intestinal obstruction, had viable bacteria in her MLN (Table 1). This patient had previously received radiation therapy and chemotherapy for an ovarian carcinoma and the current procedure was an elective cholecystectomy for symptomatic cholelithiasis. Thus, with the exception of the patient who had received intestinal radiation therapy, the MLNs of patients without intestinal obstruction were sterile.

Of the 17 patients operated on for intestinal obstruction, the small bowel was the most common site of obstruction (71%) (Table 2). None of the patients with small-bowel obstructions had necrotic bowel or required intestinal resections. The incidence of bacterial translocation to the MLNs of the patients with intestinal obstruction (59%) was significantly higher than in the patients without intestinal obstruction (4%) ($P<.001$). The presence of bacteria in the MLN was not due to surface contamination with intraperitoneal bacteria, since peritoneal fluid cultures were sterile in nine of the ten patients with small-bowel obstruction who had peritoneal fluid cultures performed. The MLN was sterile in the patient who had a positive peritoneal fluid culture. In fact, this peritoneal fluid specimen contained *Staphylococcus aureus*, an organism that was not cultured from any of the MLNs. The most common bacterium cultured from the MLNs of these patients was *Escherichia coli*, which was present in eight of the MLNs (72%) containing viable bacteria (Table 3).

There was no apparent clinical difference between the six patients with small-bowel obstructions who had sterile MLNs and the six patients whose MLNs contained bacteria. The mean ($\pm$SD) age of the patients with sterile MLNs was similar (59 ± 15 years) to that of the patients (55 ± 21 years) with bacteriologically positive MLNs, as were their clinical histories and preoperative findings. None of the patients from either group developed postoperative intra-abdominal infections.

COMMENT

The results of this study indicate that the MLNs draining the small and large intestine generally do not contain viable bacteria. However, intestinal obstruction will promote the translocation of bacteria from the intestine to the MLNs, since 59% of the patients with simple intestinal obstruction had viable bacteria cultured from their lymph nodes. The presence of bacteria within the lymph nodes was not due to contamination by intraperitoneal bacteria, since the peritoneal cavities of all but one of these patients were sterile. In fact, the incidence of bacteria translocation may have been underestimated for two reasons. First, all of these patients received perioperative antibiotics and second, only one lymph node was cultured per patient. Thus, if antibiotics were not used and/or more lymph nodes had had biopsy specimens taken from them, the incidence of bacterial translocation may have been higher.

The results of the present study are similar to those reported by Ambrose et al,[16] who sampled ileal serosa and MLNs from patients with or without Crohn's disease. They found that only 5% of the patients without Crohn's disease had viable bacteria in their MLNs, in contrast to the patients with Crohn's disease, in whom 33% of the MLNs contained bacteria. These authors concluded that leakage of bacteria from the gut lumen may be responsible for the high incidence of intra-abdominal infections in this group of patients. Unfortunately, information is not available on the indications for surgery in those patients with Crohn's disease. Therefore, the possible role of intestinal obstruction in the escape of bacteria from the gut in these patients cannot be determined. Nevertheless, there is no evidence from two studies indicating that, under certain circumstances, bacteria can translocate from the gut to the MLN in man.

To our knowledge, the mechanism(s) responsible for the translocation of bacteria from the gut to the MLN in patients with intestinal obstruction is not known. Based on our previous animal studies,[2,4,7,9,11] however, it is likely that intestinal obstruction induces bacterial translocation by promoting bacterial overgrowth, increasing intestinal permeability, or physically disrupting the mucosal barrier. Which of these mechanisms are operative will require further study both in animals and in man.

Table 1.—Incidence of Bacterial Translocation ot MLNs* in 25 Patients Undergoing Elective Surgery

Organ System	*n*	Incidence of Translocation
Biliary tract	10	1
Pancreas†	6	0
Stomach	3	0
Colon	3	0
Aorto-iliac	3	0

*MLNs indicate mesenteric lymph nodes.

†Three patients had cancer and obstructive jaundice; two patients had pancreatic pseudocysts; and one patient had pancreatitis.

Table 2.—Incidence and Magnitude of Bacterial Translocation to MLNs* in 17 Patients Operated on for Intestinal Obstruction

Intestinal Segment	*n*	Incidence of Translocation	CFUs per Gram of MLN†
Stomach	1	1	110
Small intestine	12	6	128 ± 118
Colon‡	4	3	1382 ± 1571

*MLNs indicate mesenteric lymph nodes.

†Data are expressed as mean±SD colony-forming units (CFUs) of bacteria per MLN.

‡Three patients had obstructing colon cancers and one patient had sigmoid volvulus.

Table 3.—Microbiologic Findings of 11 Patients With Positive MLNs*

Bacteria	*n*	Abnormality
Escherichia coli	4	Gastric, colon, SBO†
Klebsiella pneumoniae and *E coli*	1	SBO
Proteus mirabilis and *E coli*	1	Biliary tract
Enterococcus and *E coli*	1	SBO
Bacillus species and *E coli*	1	SBO
Bacillus species	2	Sigmoid volvulus, SBO
Enterobacter aerogenes and *Citrobacter freundii*	1	SBO

*MLNs indicate mesenteric lymph nodes.

†One patient had gastric outlet obstruction; two patients had obstructing colon cancers; and one patient had small-bowel obstruction (SBO).

In the 1960s Caridis et al[17] and Woodruff et al[18] proposed that bacteria and endotoxin could leak from the intestines into the systemic circulation in certain disease states. Since the early anecdotal studies of these authors, several epidemiologic studies have been reported documenting that bacteria colonizing the gut can cause systemic infections in bone marrow recipients and in patients with cancer.[13,14] Life-threatening infections with gut-associated bacteria are not limited to bone marrow recipients and patients with cancer. Patients who have undergone surgery also frequently develop bacteremias for which a source of infection is never found even at autopsy. These high-risk patients include patients who have sustained burns,[19,20] victims of trauma,[21] and patients developing multiple organ failure.[22,23] The patient populations at increased risk of developing bacteremias from clinically occult foci tend to share certain common predisposing factors, including an immunocompromised state, altered intestinal function, and previous exposure to therapeutic regimens that may have altered the ecology of the indigenous gut flora. Thus, indirect clinical evidence has accumulated indicating that the gut may be a reservoir for microorganisms causing systemic infections in man.

The current study presents direct evidence that bacteria can translocate across the intestinal barrier and spread to the MLNs in patients with simple intestinal obstruction in the absence of necrotic bowel or bacteriologically positive peritoneal cultures. These findings add further support to the hypothesis that systemic infections may be caused by microorganisms translocating across the intact gut.

This investigation was supported by grant GM36376 from the National Institutes of Health, Bethesda, Md.

References

1. Deitch EA, Winterton J, Li M, et al: The gut as a portal of entry for bacteremia: Role of protein malnutrition. *Ann Surg* 1987;205:681-692.
2. Deitch EA, Berg R: Bacterial translocation from the gut: A mechanism of infection. *J Burn Care Rehabil* 1987;8:475-482.
3. Berg RD, Garlington AW: Translocation of certain indigenous bacteria from the gastrointestinal tract to the mesenteric lymph nodes and other organs in a gnotobiotic mouse model. *Infect Immun* 1979;23:403-411.
4. Deitch EA, Maejima K, Berg R: Effect of oral antibotics and bacterial overgrowth on the translocation of the gastrointestinal tract microflora in burned rats. *J Trauma* 1985;25:385-392.
5. Berg RD: Inhibition of *Escherichia coli* translocation from the gastrointestinal tract by normal cecal flora in gnotobiotic or antibiotic-decontaminated mice. *Infect Immun* 1980;29:1073-1081.
6. Deitch EA, Winterton J, Berg R: Deficiency of T-cell mediated immunity promotes bacterial translocation from the gastrointestinal tract after thermal injury. *Arch Surg* 1986;121:97-101.
7. Morehouse J, Specian R, Stewart J, et al: Promotion of the translocation of indigenous bacteria of mice from the gastrointestinal tract by oral ricinoleic acid. *Gastroenterology* 1986;91:673-682.
8. Deitch EA, Bridges RM: Effect of stress and trauma on bacterial translocation from the gut. *J Surg Res* 1987;42:536-542.
9. Deitch EA, Berg R, Specian R: Endotoxin promotes the translocation of bacteria from the gut. *Arch Surg* 1987;122:185-190.
10. Wells CL, Rotstein OD, Pruett TL, et al: Intestinal bacteria translocate into experimental intra-abdominal abscesses. *Arch Surg* 1986; 121:102-107.
11. Baker JW, Deitch EA, Li M, et al: Hemorrhagic shock induces bacterial translocation from the gut. *J Trauma* 1988;28:896-906.
12. Rush BF Jr, Sori AT, Murphy TF, et al: Endotoxemia and bacteremia during hemorrhagic shock: The link between trauma and sepsis? *Ann Surg* 1988;207:549-554.
13. Wells CL, Podzorski RP, Peterson PK, et al: Incidence of trimethoprim-sulfamethoxazole-resistant Enterobacteriaceae among transplant recipients. *J Infect Dis* 1984;150:699-706.
14. Bodey GP: Antibiotic prophylaxis in cancer patients: Regimens of oral, nonabsorbable antibiotics for prevention during induction of remission. *Rev Infect Dis* 1981;3(suppl):259-268.
15. Steffen EK, Berg RD, Deitch EA: Comparison of translocation rates of various indigenous bacteria from the gastrointestinal tract to the mesenteric lymph node. *J Infect Dis* 1988;175:1032-1038.
16. Ambrose NS, Johnson M, Burdon DW, et al: Incidence of pathogenic bacteria from mesenteric lymph nodes and ileal serosa during Crohn's disease surgery. *Br J Surg* 1984;71:623-625.
17. Caridis DT, Reinhold RB, Woodruff PW, et al: Endotoxemia in man. *Lancet* 1972;2:1381-1386.
18. Woodruff PW, O'Carroll DE, Koizumi S, et al: Role of the intestinal flora in major trauma. *J Infect Dis* 1973;128(suppl):S290-S294.
19. Jarrett F, Balish L, Moylan JA, et al: Clinical experience with prophylactic antibiotic bowel suppression in burn patients. *Surgery* 1978;83:523-527.
20. Chitkara YK, Feierabend TC: Endogenous and exogenous infections with *Pseudomonas aeruginosa* in a burn unit. *Int Surg* 1981;66:237-240.
21. Garrison RN, Fry DE, Berborich S, et al: Enterococcal bacteremia: Clinical implications and determinants of death. *Ann Surg* 1982;196:43-47.
22. Fry DE, Garrison RN, Polk HC Jr: Clinical implicatios in *Bacteroides* bacteremia. *Surg Gynecol Obstet* 1979;149:189-192.
23. Border JR: Trauma and sepsis, in Worth MH (ed): *Principles and Practice of Trauma Care.* Baltimore, Williams & Wilkins, 1982, pp 330-387.

In Other AMA Journals

ARCHIVES OF INTERNAL MEDICINE

Cancer of the Nongastric Hollow Organs of the Gastrointestinal Tract After Gastric Surgery

Ravi Thiruvengadam, MD; Victoria Hench, MS; L. Joseph Melton III, MD; Eugene P. DiMagno, MD

To estimate the risk of esophageal, gallbladder, small-bowel, and colon cancers after gastric surgery for benign disease, all 337 residents of Olmsted County, Minnesota, who had surgical treatment of benign peptic ulcer disease during the years 1935 through 1959, were followed up. Patients were followed up for 6552 person-years of observation. No esophageal cancers developed (0.8 were expected). Members of the cohort developed one small-bowel malignant neoplasm (0.2 were expected), two gallbladder cancers (1.1 was expected), and four colon cancers (11.2 were expected), but these figures do not reflect a significant increase in the risk of these malignant neoplasms. In particular, the relative risk of developing colon cancer was only 0.4 when this analysis had 88% power to detect a relative risk of two or more. When the present investigation and two previous studies of this cohort were taken together, there was no strong evidence for an increased risk of any gastrointestinal cancer following gastric surgery (*Arch Intern Med* 1988;148:405-407).

Reprint requests to Gastrointestinal Diagnostic Unit, Mayo Clinic, Rochester, MN 55905 (Dr DiMagno).

Management of Severe Incisional Abscesses Following Laparotomy

Early Reclosure Under Cover of Metronidazole and Ampicillin

Finn Gottrup, MD, PhD; P. Gjøde, MD; F. Lundhus, MD; H. Andrup, MD; C. N. Holm, MD; S. Terpling, MD

• Patients developing severe incisional abscesses following laparotomy were treated with incision and drainage followed by early reclosure under antibiotic cover with metronidazole and ampicillin anhydricum. Patients with subcutaneous abscesses were randomized into two groups that were treated with antibiotics for one day (n = 23) or four days (n = 27). These patients all underwent reclosure four days later. In a third group of patients (n = 14) abscesses had developed down to, but not through, the peritoneum. These patients received antibiotic treatment for four days and underwent reclosure a mean of 5½ days later (range, four to eight days). No abscesses reappeared in any group and all wounds healed by first intention. Five patients healed totally, with minor defects, but there was no need for surgical intervention. We conclude that the early reclosure technique is a safe procedure under antibiotic cover with metronidazole and ampicillin. One day and four days of antibiotic treatment are equally safe in patients with subcutaneous abscesses.

(*Arch Surg* 1989;124:702-704)

Early reclosure of incisional abscesses, before granulation tissues become visible, is biologically comparable to delayed primary closure of wounds. This surgical procedure increases the resistance of the wound against infection and improves healing of the wound. The resulting appearance of the wound is comparable to that of an uncomplicated, primarily healed wound.[1] Early reclosure of contaminated wounds four days after drainage of severe incisional abscesses down to the fascia following laparotomy has recently been described in retrospective studies.[2,3] In those studies, clindamycin phosphate was administered for four days. However, this drug is bacteriostatic, and severe side effects have been described.[4] To our knowledge, no prospective studies on early reclosure of subcutaneous abscesses breaking through the fascia have been published.

In this randomized, prospective, double-blind study, early reclosure under antibiotic cover with metronidazole and ampicillin anhydricum for one or four days was performed on incisional wounds extending to the fascia. In all cases where the abscess broke through the fascia, but the peritoneum was intact, the antibiotic was administered for four days.

PATIENTS AND METHODS

This study was carried out over a period of 20 months from 1985 to 1987. Seventy-three consecutive patients with severe incisional abscesses following laparotomy were randomized into groups 1 and 2, with abscesses to the fascia, and group 3, where the abscess went through the fascia but the peritoneum remained intact. Severe incisional abscess was defined as an accumulation of pus necessitating surgical opening of the wound. All wounds were drained of pus and cleaned daily. After four days in groups 1 and 2 and four to eight days in group 3, patients underwent the excision of necrotic tissue. The wounds were closed using interrupted polypropylene (Prolene) sutures. In groups 1 and 2 a large needle was passed through the skin and subcutaneous layer at a distance of 2.5 cm to 3 cm from the wound margins and underneath the fascia (Figure). In cases where the fascia was broken (group 3), it was reclosed by interrupted polyglycolic (O-Dexon) sutures. These surgical procedures allowed complete occlusion of the wound cavity with few or no sutures in the cavity itself.

The antibiotic cover consisted of 500 mg of metronidazole and 1 g of ampicillin anhydricum, both administered three times daily. Five hundred milligrams of metronidazole and 1 g of ampicillin were administered half an hour preoperatively and every eight hours thereafter. The antimicrobial agents were administered intravenously on the day of resuturing. On postoperative days 1, 2, and 3, metronidazole and ampicillin were administered as suppositories and capsules in group 2, while in group 1, placebo suppositories and capsules were administered. In group 3, all patients were treated with antibiotics for four days.

While the patients were hospitalized, daily postoperative observations of the wounds were performed. Sutures were removed on the tenth day and the patients were seen in the hospital eight weeks after reclosure to discover any delayed septic complications. During each observation, the wounds were observed for tissue reaction (swelling, erythema, or tenderness), pus accumulation, and defects of the incision line.

The investigation was conducted according to the Declaration of Helsinki II. The protocols and methods were accepted by the Danish National Health Service and the local committee concerning ethics in science.

The statistical evaluation included the χ^2 test applied with Yates' correction.

RESULTS

Of 71 patients meeting the criteria, four were excluded due to error of the surgical procedure and three were excluded due to error of the medical procedure, leaving 64 patients for study.

The groups were well matched in regard to age, sex, and primary operations (Table 1). Group 1 had a relatively higher percentage of women than groups 2 and 3. The results of the study are shown in Table 2. Forty-four patients (69%) had no tissue reaction, such as swelling, erythema, or tenderness, after ten days of healing, when the sutures were removed. No abscesses reappeared within 60 days, but five patients healed with minor defects, which were defined as defects less than one third the total wound length. Minor defects were found in three patients (21%) in group 3 and one each (4%) in groups 1 and 2. In no

Accepted for publication Nov 16, 1988.
From the Department of Surgical Gastroenterology A, Aalborg Hospital (Drs Gjøde and Andrup), and the Departments of Surgery, Randers Hospital (Drs Gottrup, Lundhus, and Terpling) and Viborg Hospital (Dr Holm), Denmark.

Reprint requests to V Kyhnsalle 4, DK-8270 Højbjerg, Denmark (Dr Gottrup).

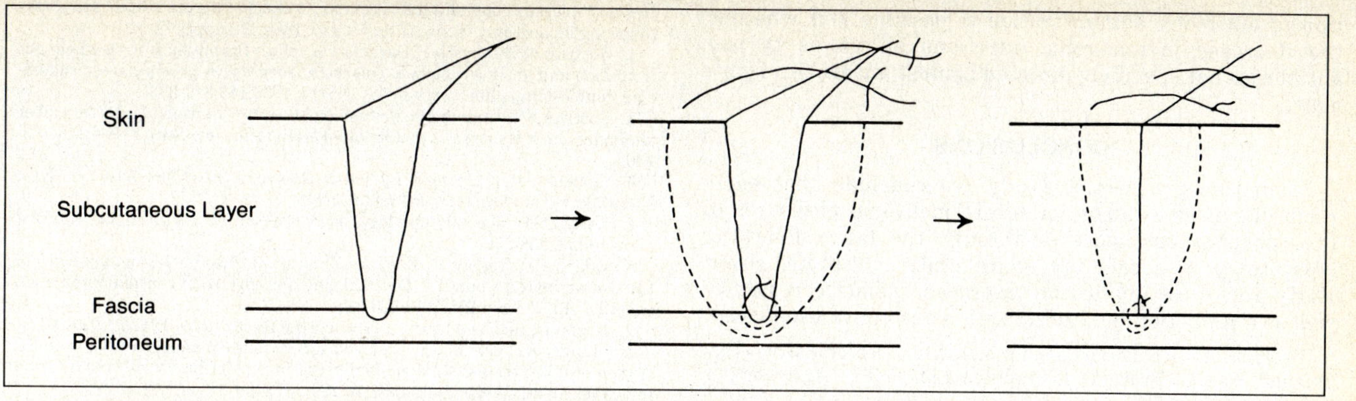

Closure of wounds after incisional abscesses extending to peritoneum (group 3). Monofil sutures are placed 2.5 cm to 3 cm from edge of wound. Defect of fascia is closed by absorbable sutures. If fascia is intact (groups 1 and 2), monofil sutures are placed as shown.

Table 1.—Patients' Age, Sex, and Primary Operation

	Group		
Variable	1 (n=23)	2 (n=27)	3 (n=14)
Median age, y (range)	61 (16-79)	53 (14-83)	61 (19-83)
F/M ratio	18/5	13/14	6/8
Primary operations			
Gastric	4	1	1
Biliary	6	7	1
Intestinal	13	17	10
Urologic	0	0	1
Gynecologic	0	2	1
Median No. of days from drainage to resuture (range)	4 (4-4)	4 (4-4)	5.5 (4-8)

Table 2.—Results of Early Reclosure

	Group		
Variable	1 (n=23)	2 (n=27)	3 (n=14)
No tissue reaction after 10 d	16	19	9
Healed by first intention	23	27	14
Healed with minor defects (<⅓ length of incision)	1	1	3
Wound sepsis within 60 d	0	0	0

patients with minor defects of the healing wound was further surgical intervention needed. No fistula formation or other surgical complications were encountered during the observation period. Bacteriological findings of the primary infected wounds were similar to earlier reported bacteriological findings from our hospital departments.[4,5]

No significant differences were found between the three groups in regard to primary healing, recurring abscesses, or healing with minor defects.

COMMENT

In this study, early reclosure of incisional wounds down to and through the fascia has been shown to be a safe procedure under antibiotic cover with metronidazole and ampicillin. The results are similar to those of an earlier retrospective study using clindamycin as an antibiotic cover.[3] Compared with clindamycin, the metronidazole/ampicillin regimen is bactericidal, has few side effects, has a broad antibacterial spectrum covering almost all bacterias involved, and is inexpensive. Clindamycin is a bacteriostatic drug with a spectrum that includes anaerobic organisms and *Staphylococcus aureus*.[6] Our employment of ampicillin was based on our knowledge of the sensitivity of the predominant organisms isolated after colorectal surgery in our hospitals. *Escherichia coli* was isolated from most postoperative wound infections and the incidence of ampicillin resistance was about 15% for several years. This sensitivity of *E coli* to ampicillin is higher than that reported in England and the United States.[6,7] For this reason, selection of antibiotics always has to be based on the present sensitivity of the dominant organisms isolated from infections. Ampicillin has been shown to be effective against enterococci, but some strains of *S aureus* were resistant.[4]

The decision to close a contaminated wound is based on a few important factors: timing, technique of wound closure, and antibiotics.[1] The use of specific antibiotics is probably of minor importance compared with timing and closure technique. The wounds were resutured on the fourth day after they were opened and drained. This is in accordance with the principle of delayed primary closure, which is defined as closure that is delayed a few days but accomplished before granulation tissue becomes visible, usually eight to ten days after wounding.[1] Secondary closure refers to either spontaneous closure or closure by operation after granulation tissue has developed and the wound macroscopically looks "clean." This has been found 12 days after drainage of the wound abscesses.[3]

The ideal time for closure of contaminated wounds has experimentally,[8] as well as clinically,[9,10] been found to be on or shortly after the third or fourth day. Earlier closure will not allow the wound to be prepared for enhanced healing or resistance to infection.[11] In later closures (secondary closure), the wound edges will become increasingly difficult to approximate because the granulation tissue induces an increasing collagen content in the wound.

The closure technique used in this study is based on known surgical principles, such as débridement with removal of foreign bodies and devitalized tissue. Furthermore, the suture technique, without sutures in the wound itself, results in a complete occlusion of the wound cavity, thus inhibiting formation of hemorrhage or fluid collection. This has been shown to decrease the risk of infection in contaminated wounds.[12,13]

Future investigation will show whether a shorter duration of antibiotic administration is possible and whether the decrease in anaerobic infections allows us to use antibiotics not specificly directed against anaerobic organisms.

CONCLUSIONS

From this prospective study, we conclude that early reclosure after drainage of severe incisional abscesses of the subcutaneous space or through the fascia following laparotomy is a safe procedure under antibiotic cover. Early reclosure implies an improved cosmetic result as well as a reduction in hospitalization and convalescence.

We thank A/s Rhône-Poulenc for supplying metronidazole (Flagyl) and A/s Gist-Brocades for supplying ampicillin (Anhypen).

References

1. Gottrup F: Delayed primary closure of wounds. *Infect Surg* 1985;4: 171-178.
2. Moesgaard F, Larsen PN, Nielsen ML, et al: New approach to treatment of severe incisional abscesses following laparotomy. *Dis Colon Rectum* 1983;26:701-702.
3. Lykkegaard-Nielsen M, Moesgaard F, Nørgaard Larsen P, et al: Early reclosure versus conventional secondary suture of severe wound abscesses following laparotomy. *Scand J Infect Dis* 1984;43(suppl):67-70.
4. Gottrup F, Diederich P, Sørensen K, et al: Prophylaxis with whole gut irrigation and antimicrobials in colorectal surgery: A prospective, randomized double-blind clinical trial. *Am J Surg* 1985;149:317-322.
5. Gottrup F: Prophylactic metronidazole in prevention of infection after appendectomy: Report of a double blind trial. *Acta Chir Scand* 1980;146:133-136.
6. Simmons RL, Howard RJ (eds): *Surgical Infections Disease.* East Norwalk, Conn, Appleton & Lange, 1982.
7. Eykyn SJ: The microbiology of postoperative bacteriemia. *World J Surg* 1982;6:268-272.
8. Edlich RF, Rogers W, Kaspers G, et al: Studies in the management of the contaminated wound: I. Optimal time for closure of contaminated open wounds. *Am J Surg* 1969;117:323-329.
9. Rosfeld L: Delayed suture of war wounds. *Surgery* 1947;21:200-207.
10. Lowry KF, Curtis GM: Delayed suture in the management of wounds: Analysis of 721 traumatic wounds illustrating the influence of time interval in wound repair. *Am J Surg* 1950;80:280-287.
11. Gottrup F, Fogdestam I, Hunt TK: Delayed primary closure: An experimental and clinical review. *J Clin Surg* 1982;1:113-124.
12. Edlich RF, Rodeheaver G, Thacher JG, et al: Technical factors in wound management, in Hunt TK, Dunphy JE (eds): *Fundamentals of Wound Management.* East Norwalk, Conn, Appleton & Lange, 1979, pp 364-455.
13. Alexander JW, Kaplan JZ, Altemeier WA: Role of suture material in development of wound infection. *Ann Surg* 1967;165:192-199.

In Other AMA Journals

ARCHIVES OF INTERNAL MEDICINE

Is Mammography Painful? A Multicenter Patient Survey

Paul C. Stomper, MD; Daniel B. Kopans, MD; Norman L. Sadowsky, MD; Marian R. Sonnenfeld, MD; Cynthia A. Swann, MD; Rebecca S. Gelman, PhD; Jack E. Meyer, MD; Maxine S. Jochelson, MD; Myla S. Hunt, MA; Paul D. Allen, MD, PhD

Anecdotal reports of pain experienced during mammography have been a source of anxiety and concern for some women considering screening. To determine what asymptomatic women actually experience during mammography, a survey of 1847 women was performed at seven breast-imaging centers. Women recorded their experience on a six-point scale ranging from no discomfort to severe pain. Eighty-eight percent of the women experienced no discomfort (49%) or mild discomfort (39%). Only 9% experienced moderate discomfort; 1%, severe discomfort; and 1%, moderate pain. No woman had pain so severe that it would make her reconsider having a mammogram again. The degree of discomfort was slightly greater in women who complained of breast tenderness within three days prior to the mammogram but was not strongly related to age, menstrual status, or week of the menstrual cycle. We conclude that in a vast majority of women mammography causes no or mild physical discomfort and that actual pain is an uncommon occurrence (*Arch Intern Med* 1988;148:521-524).

Reprint requests to Department of Radiology, Dana-Farber Cancer Institute, 44 Binney St, Boston, MA 02115 (Dr Stomper).

Oral Prophylaxis With Neomycin and Erythromycin in Colorectal Surgery

More Proof for Efficacy Than Failure

Per-Arne Kling, MD, Sven Dahlgren, MD

• In an open, prospective, and randomized investigation on the prophylactic efficacy of peroral neomycin sulfate–erythromycin base vs intravenous ceftriaxone-metronidazole preparation in colorectal surgery, no significantly diverging results between regimens were recorded (1/27 [3.7%] and 2/27 [7.4%] wound infections, respectively). Commentary is made about the diverging results from earlier studies on antimicrobial prophylaxis and on the multifactorial causality of surgical infection. We believe that variables such as physical condition of the patients, virulence and local resistance patterns of bacteria, and technical skill of the surgeons are far more important in regard to the postoperative outcome concerning septic complications than is the choice of proper antibiotics. Thus, to determine the efficacy of antimicrobial prophylaxis, we call for larger investigations in the future, preferably double-blind, where it is possible to better control and diminish the influence of determinants other than the antibiotics being compared.

(*Arch Surg* 1989;124:705-707)

Throughout the last 15 years, innumerable studies have been carried out to estimate the efficacy of different enteral and/or systemic antibiotic regimens for prophylaxis of infection in colorectal surgery. By tradition, enteral/peroral (PO) antimicrobial regimens have been, and probably still are, favored by many American surgeons, whereas systemic/intravenous (IV) prophylaxis has become more and more common in western Europe. Oral prophylaxis, which by tradition is paralleled by a thorough mechanical bowel-cleansing procedure, is theoretically aimed at lowering the bacterial counts in the colon lumen, thereby diminishing the bacterial inoculum in case of intraoperative spillage.[1] Intravenous preparation, on the other hand, does not necessarily include the same meticulous bowel-cleansing procedure, and the antimicrobial effect on the colonic bacterial flora is probably negligible, the aim instead being to achieve antibiotic concentrations in blood and tissues high enough to deal with the fecal spillage that might occur intraoperatively.

To compare the efficacy of these two main prophylactic regimens, a two-center trial was conducted in Birmingham (United Kingdom) and Umeå (Sweden) in 1985 to 1986. After identical mechanical bowel-cleansing procedures, one study group was orally prepared with three standard loading doses of erythromycin base and neomycin sulfate[2] (PO group), whereas the other group of patients was subjected to a single IV administration of metronidazole (Elyzol) and ceftriaxone (Rocephin, a rather new long-acting cephalosporin[3]; IV group). The original intention of the two-center investigation was to present a mutual study report after the entrance of about 100 patients in each group, with the reservation that for "safety reasons" a sequential analysis would be carried out and the study discontinued in case of "very high sepsis rates" in either prophylactic regimen.

As infection rates for the Birmingham PO group turned out to be unacceptably high, the study was concluded at the English center after the entrance of only 60 patients. At that time the preliminary Swedish figures were in no way alarming, and it was decided that our part of the investigation should not be discontinued until a comparable number of patients had been entered into the study. Results from the English center (41% wound infections in the PO group vs 9.6% in the IV group) were presented in 1986.[4] Since results from the Swedish study differ greatly from those obtained at the English center, we believe it is important that they be reported.

PATIENTS AND METHODS

This open, randomized study was undertaken at the Department of Surgery of Umeå University Hospital between May 1985 and December 1986. Only patients admitted for elective surgery for either colonic or rectal carcinomas were included in the study. A total of 63 patients were randomized. Nine of these patients were excluded from the final evaluation: six of them, three in each group, because their bowels were never opened at operation (exploratory laparotomy alone) and three patients, two from the PO and one from the IV group, because additional antibiotics were given within 48 hours after operation. In spite of minute inquiry, no obvious reasons for any of these additional antibiotic treatments were found. After these exclusions, the study comprised 54 evaluable patients, 27 in each group. The localization of carcinomas is given below:

	PO	IV
Cecum	4	4
Ascending colon	2	6
Transverse colon	3	0
Descending colon	2	1
Sigmoid	9	9
Rectum	7	7

Accepted for publication Oct 28, 1988.

From the Department of Surgery, Umeå University Hospital, Umeå, Sweden.

Reprint requests to Department of Surgery, University Hospital, S-901 85 Umeå, Sweden (Dr Kling).

The operative procedures performed were as follows:

	PO	IV
Right hemicolectomy	4	9
Ileotransversostomy	2	1
Transverse resection	2	0
Left hemicolectomy	3	1
Sigmoid resection	6	8
High anterior resection	3	1
Low anterior resection	3	2
Rectal amputation	3	5
Colostomy alone	1	0

Mechanical Bowel Preparation

Day	Regimen
1	Low-residue diet; bisacodyl, 5 mg orally at 6 PM
2	Continue low-residue diet; magnesium sulfate, 7 g orally at 10 AM, 2 and 6 PM; water enema in evening
3	Clear liquid diet; magnesium sulfate, in above dose, at 10 AM and 2 PM; no enemas
4	Rectal washout at 6 AM; operation

The mean age for patients in the PO group was 70 years (range, 53 to 81 years) and for the IV group, 64 years (range, 44 to 81 years). The female-male ratio was 14:13 in the IV and 11:16 in the PO group. Diabetes mellitus was the only complicating disease found among the patients: four in the IV and five in the PO group.

Before surgery all patients were subjected to mechanical bowel preparation slightly modified from that described by Nichols et al[1] in 1972 (Table). Patient discomfort, if any, as well as bowel-cleansing efficacy, was followed up throughout the entire investigation.

Patients in the PO group were given 1 g of neomycin sulfate and 1 g of erythromycin base at 1, 2, and 11 PM on the day before operation. In the IV group, single doses of metronidazole (1.5 g) and ceftriaxone (2.0 g) were administered at the induction of anesthesia.

Immediately after surgery, all surgeons were questioned about the occurrence and quantity of fecal spillage during the operation. They were also asked about other possible surgical complications such as bleeding, unintentional damage to other structures, and other technical problems. All patients who entered the investigation were meticulously followed up for any signs of postoperative infection until at least six weeks after the operation.

Postoperative infection was monitored by a specially trained and experienced nurse-epidemiologist. Wound infection was defined as the discharge of pus, either spontaneously or by débridement. It was planned that intra-abdominal abscess formation, if any, would be monitored by ultrasonographic or computer tomographic examinations and ultimately diagnosed by relaparotomy. All infections directly related to the operative field are referred to herein as surgical infections. Material from infected sites was quickly taken to the bacteriological laboratory for routine aerobic and anaerobic cultivation. The occurrence of urinary (UTI) and respiratory (RTI) tract infections, designated herein as nonsurgical infections, was also monitored. Furthermore, fecal material randomly collected from 12 of the patients who received PO prophylaxis was specially examined during the postoperative course for the possible appearance of *Clostridium difficile* enterotoxin. The 54 evaluable patients were operated on by 22 surgeons, none with less than five years of surgical experience. Only one of the surgeons operated on more than ten patients in this investigation.

RESULTS

None of the six patients, three in the PO and three in the IV group, who were excluded because their bowels were not opened at operation experienced any postoperative septic complications. Among the three patients excluded as a consequence of early postoperative administration of antibiotics, only one, randomized to the PO group, had a nonsurgical infection (RTI) during the postoperative course.

Only three surgical infections occurred among evaluable patients (3/54, 5.6%): one perineal wound infection after rectal amputation in the PO group (1/27, 3.7%) and two perineal wound infections, one of them with extension also to the abdominal wound, in the IV group (2/27, 7.4%). No cases of septicemia were documented during the course of this investigation. In the PO group, the infecting organism was *Staphylococcus aureus*, whereas the two IV group infections were caused by *Escherichia coli* plus *Klebsiella aerogenes* and *Pseudomonas aeruginosa* plus *S aureus*, respectively. Anaerobic pathogens were not obtained from any of the surgical infection sites. In the IV group, one patient was operated on for ileus 20 days after the primary operation. Although there were no signs of intra-abdominal infection at the time of this relaparotomy, for unknown reasons imipenem was instituted in the postoperative course.

In the PO group, five patients developed UTI. Three of them were given antibiotic treatment with trimethoprim-sulfamethoxazole and one received amdinocillin pivoxil. One patient with UTI recovered without antimicrobial treatment. In none of the UTI cases were antibiotics instituted before the tenth postoperative day, and none of the nonsurgical infections gave rise to any septic complications.

Clostridium difficile enterotoxin was not isolated from any of the fecal samples randomly obtained from patients in the PO group, and no patients suffered from postoperative diarrhea. On the other hand, 11 patients (11/54, 20%) experienced discomforting diarrhea from the preoperative bowel-cleansing procedure. In both the PO and the IV groups, the cleanness of the bowel was considered very good in 22 patients (44/54, 81.5%) and poor or bad in five patients from each group; all the latter had stricturating carcinomas in the rectosigmoid colon. Fecal spillage was considered insignificant in 20 patients in the IV group and 22 in the PO group. A fairly large spillage was registered in five patients in the IV group and five in the PO group, whereas in two in the IV group the spillage was considered to be massive. The latter two patients—both with rectal amputations, one of them suffering from diabetes mellitus—constituted the infected cases in the IV group. For the only surgical infection occurring in the PO group, also a rectal amputation, the intraoperative spillage was reported as insignificant.

COMMENT

Following the first presentation by Nichols et al[1] in 1972 on the subject of neomycin-erythromycin bowel preparation in colorectal surgery, the beneficial effects of this regimen on the postoperative infection rate have been confirmed by several investigators. By far the largest and most impressive tribute to the idea of "gut sterilization" was given by Condon et al,[5] who in 1983 presented results from a multicenter study comparing the efficacy of oral neomycin-erythromycin with and without the addition of IV cephalothin (5.7% and 7.8% infectious complications, respectively). The significance of these results is underlined by the fact that each study group contained more than 540 patients, an unusually large number for this kind of investigation. In a recent European investigation on the same topic, Figueras-Felip et al[6] presented results from a study with one tenth the number of patients comparing the standard neomycin-erythromycin PO preparation with IV gentamicin-metronidazole prophylaxis. They found significantly fewer wound infections in the PO than in the IV group (5% and 21%, respectively; $P<.05$).

In regard to systemic prophylaxis, the number of antibiotic combinations, investigators, and study designs has been considerable during the last ten years. It is not so far-fetched to assume that the large number of investigations containing few patients is simply a reflection of the ceaseless flow of new and potent antibiotics from manufacturers, and an eagerness to achieve rapid results to get the antibiotics registered also for prophylaxis of infection within the broad field of gastrointestinal surgery. These factors are open for discussion, since development of postoperative infection after contaminated surgery is most certainly a question of multifactorial causes, and the choice of proper antibiotics constitutes only one of these. Variables difficult to standardize, such as the physical condition of the patients, disease state, virulence and resistance patterns among fecal pathogens, and differences both in surgical conditions and in technical qualifications of the surgeons, are probably far more decisive in regard to postoperative outcome than is the choice of proper prophylactic antibiotics. This constitutes neither a lack of approval for antibiotics in contaminated surgery nor a denial of the fact that different antibiotics may be more or less effective against fecal pathogens, but merely a claim for larger studies (multicenter, double-blind studies involving centers with genuine interest in these problems) to determine the significance of the above-mentioned uncontrollable variables. In our rather small study on the efficacy of PO and IV antimicrobial prophylaxis, we were unable to detect any difference between the regimens. Our results for the PO group are in sharp contrast to those obtained by our Birmingham colleagues (one of 27 infected PO cases in Umeå vs 14 of 29 in Birmingham; $P<.001$). We have not been able to discover any plausible explanation here at the Swedish center for this large difference in results between two identical studies based on a common study protocol.

One gets the impression from many investigations that traditional PO prophylaxis is effective in significantly lowering postoperative morbidity from infectious complications in elective colorectal surgery. We also know from several studies that both single and multiple doses of IV antibiotics (such as metronidazole for anaerobes and third-generation cephalosporins for aerobes) have likewise proved effective in lowering infection rates after contaminated surgery. Furthermore, neither the PO nor the IV regimen has proved harmful to the patients or to the ecology of the fecal flora of the patients. Thus, it is somewhat surprising that the emergence of resistance to neomycin and erythromycin, which was observed and made responsible in part for the discouraging Birmingham PO figures, did not give rise to related problems in the multicenter trial performed by Condon et al.[5]

Perhaps the correct answer to the question as to whether to use the American (PO) or the European (IV) model for antibiotic prophylaxis should be to use both, ie, a thorough mechanical bowel-cleansing procedure, PO neomycin-erythromycin on the day before operation to reduce colonic bacterial counts, and single-dose systemic antibiotics administered preoperatively to achieve high enough antibiotic concentrations in blood and tissue to deal with the spillage that sometimes is difficult to avoid in a potentially contaminated operative field.

References

1. Nichols RL, Condon RE, Gorbach SL, et al: Efficacy of preoperative antimicrobial preparation of the bowel. *Ann Surg* 1972;176:227-232.
2. Nichols RL, Broido P, Condon RE, et al: Effect of preoperative neomycin-erythromycin intestinal preparation on the incidence of infectious complications following colon surgery. *Ann Surg* 1973;178:453-459.
3. Shepherd A, Roberts A, Ambrose NS, et al: Ceftriaxone (a long acting cephalosporin) with metronidazole as single dose prophylaxis in colorectal surgery. *Colo-proctology* 1986;8:90-94.
4. Weaver M, Burdon DW, Youngs DJ, et al: Oral neomycin and erythromycin compared with single-dose systemic metronidazole and ceftriaxone prophylaxis in elective colorectal surgery. *Am J Surg* 1986;151:437-442.
5. Condon RE, Bartlett JG, Greenlee H, et al: Efficacy of oral and systemic antibiotic prophylaxis in colorectal operations. *Arch Surg* 1983; 188:496-502.
6. Figueras-Felip J, BasilioBouet E, Lara-Eisman F, et al: Oral is superior to systemic antibiotic prophylaxis in operations upon the colon and rectum. *Surg Gynecol Obstet* 1984;158:359-362.

Editorial Comment

This is a report of a study of 54 patients in a randomized clinical trial comparing PO neomycin-erythromycin with IV ceftriaxone-metronidazole for antibiotic bowel preparation in patients undergoing elective resections for cancer. The study showed no significant difference in postoperative infectious complications between the two study groups. Under usual circumstances, this report would not be of great interest, primarily because of the small numbers of patients involved. However, there are special circumstances surrounding this report.

This report from Sweden gives the results from a part of a multi-institutional trial, the other part of which has previously been reported from Birmingham.[1] What makes the present article interesting, and justifies its publication, is the disparity in results between Umeå and Birmingham. The Birmingham part of the study, which was published without referring to the fact that another institution was also participating in the trial, showed an unexpectedly high postoperative infection rate following PO bowel preparation.[2] The reason for this result, which is clearly different from the experience with PO antibiotics in many other institutions around the world, was never satisfactorily explained by the Birmingham authors.[3] The explanation still remains obscure.

This report from Umeå documents a second instance in which the Birmingham group has participated in a multi-institutional trial, and reported their results unilaterally, with a disparate experience as compared with the other institution. The previous example was a report comparing IV vs PO regimens of kanamycin-metronidazole. Very different results were obtained between Birmingham[4] and Switzerland.[5]

It is important for surgeons to realize that the results from studies of infections following surgical procedures, as reported from some institutions in Britain today, are unique. The reasons for this phenomenon are not immediately apparent. Indeed, one can only speculate about the possibilities; but this is a fact. Surgeons should be aware so that they are not misled by unique British experiences of relatively high rates of surgical infectious complications, outcomes that do not characterize surgical experience in the rest of the developed world.

Robert E. Condon, MD, MS
Milwaukee

References

1. Weaver M, Burdon DW, Youngs DJ, et al: Oral neomycin and erythromycin compared with single-dose systemic metronidazole and ceftriaxone prophylaxis in elective colorectal surgery. *Am J Surg* 1986;151:437-442.
2. Condon RE, Nichols RL, Bartlett JG: Letter to the editor. *Am J Surg* 1986;152:564.
3. Keighley MRB, Burdon DW: Letter to the editor. *Am J Surg* 1986; 152:564-565.
4. Keighley MRB, Arabi Y, Alexander-Williams J, et al: Comparison between systemic and oral antimicrobial prophylaxis in colorectal surgery. *Lancet* 1979;1:894-897.
5. Fluckiger M, Berger J, Casey P, et al: Antibiotics darmvorbereitung oder peroperative parenterale Abschirmung bei Kolon Eingriffen? Eine randomsierte Studie. *Helv Chir Acta* 1980;47:659-662.

The Effect of New Monofilament Absorbable Sutures on the Healing of Musculoaponeurotic Incisions, Gastrotomies, and Colonic Anastomoses

Pamela A. Foresman; Richard F. Edlich, MD, PhD; George T. Rodeheaver, PhD

• The purpose of this study was to quantitate the effect of two new synthetic monofilament absorbable sutures, Maxon and PDS, on the healing of musculoaponeurotic incisions, gastrotomies, and colonic anastomoses. Wound healing was assessed by measuring the resistance of the closed wound to leak or burst with controlled infusion of fluid. Bursting strength measurements of these incisions were compared with those undertaken in age-weight matched controls without wounds to determine the rate of gain of wound strength. The bursting strength measurements of unwounded tissue was found to vary according to the age, weight, and specific tissue. As the animals gained weight over 42 days, the bursting strength of their colons and musculoaponeurotic tissues significantly increased. In general, the regain of prewounding bursting strength was inversely proportional to the bursting strength of the unwounded tissue. The bursting strength of abdominal musculoaponeurotic tissue was the highest, followed by the stomach and then the colon. The time intervals in which the wounded musculoaponeurotic tissues, gastrotomies, and colonic anastomoses regained the strength of the unwounded tissue was 42, 14, and 7 days, respectively. The performance of Maxon and PDS sutures in the musculoaponeurotic tissues, gastrotomies, and colonic anastomoses was similar.

(*Arch Surg* 1989;124:708-710)

Polyglycolic acid and polyglactin 910 sutures are used routinely in surgery. These braided sutures degrade in tissue by simple hydrolysis, resulting in a tissue response and absorption rate that is more predictable and reliable than gut sutures.[1,2] Because of the inherent rigidity of polyglycolic acid and polyglactin 910 polymers, monofilament sutures produced from these polymers are stiff and inflexible, precluding their use as a monofilament in sizes larger than 7-0.

An extensive research program has led to the discovery of novel polymers that can be converted into two uniquely flexible monofilament absorbable sutures of all sizes. One monofilament is prepared by polymerizing the monomer, paradioxanone, in the presence of a suitable catalyst to the polymer, polydioxanone (PDS).[3] The other is made from a copolymer of glycolide and trimethylene carbonate (Maxon).[4] Like the braided absorbable sutures, these new monofilament sutures are absorbable by simple hydrolysis with minimal tissue response. However, these monofilament sutures retain their strength for a substantially longer period of time than the braided synthetic absorbable sutures. By 21 days, the braided synthetic absorbable sutures have lost their strength, while the monofilament absorbable sutures still retain 30% to 40% of their initial strength at 42 days after implantation.[3,4]

Their retention of strength for an extended period should permit secure apposition of the divided edges of different incised tissues until the healing wounds can withstand stress without mechanical sutural support. Consequently, the purpose of this study was to determine the relative importance of these new synthetic monofilament absorbable sutures to the strength of healing wounds in various gastrointestinal tissues—musculoaponeurotic incisions, gastrotomies, and colonic anastomoses. The results of this experimental study demonstrate that these monofilament sutures maintain sufficient strength to permit secure repair of these incised tissues in healthy animals.

MATERIALS AND METHODS

Sutures

All sutures were obtained from commercial sources. The size of suture and needle available, respectively, for use on the various wounds were as follows: (1) colon—Maxon, 7-0 and TE-10; PDS, 7-0 and BV-1; (2) stomach—Maxon, 6-0 and TE-10; PDS, 6-0 and C-1; and (3) abdomen—Maxon, 5-0 and TE-1; PDS, 5-0 and RB-1.

Experimental Design

Two hundred male Sprague-Dawley rats, weighing between 225 and 255 g, were used for this study. All animals were assessed for good health during a one-week period before the study as evidenced by a gain in weight. The animals were caged individually and given free access to water and rat chow (Purina 5012). Room conditions were maintained at 23°C ± 1°C and 50% relative humidity, with a 12-hour light/dark cycle. The animals were then randomly assigned into two treatment groups. One group (160 animals) underwent a standardized surgical procedure, while the other group (40 animals) served as the controls. In the surgical group, all animals underwent a colonic anastomosis, closure of a gastrotomy, and closure of the midline abdominal incision. In each animal, the same type of synthetic monofilament absorbable suture was utilized for each surgical procedure. By random assignment, Maxon sutures were utilized in half of the animals, while PDS sutures were used in the remaining animals. Randomly selected groups of control animals and those receiving Maxon or PDS sutures were selected for wound-healing measurements at the following time intervals after surgery: immediately after surgery (0) and at 7, 14, 21, and 42 days. At each time interval, the interrupted suture loops used in wound closure remained intact during the healing measurements in half the animals, while they were cut before the healing measurements were undertaken in the remaining animals. With a dissecting microscope and microsurgical instruments, the suture loops were cut at the knot with as little disturbance of the tissue as possible and left in the tissue.

Surgical Procedure

Each animal fasted for 24 hours before surgery. Anesthesia was accomplished with an intraperitoneal injection of pentobarbital sodium (43 mg/kg). The abdominal hair was clipped with electric clippers and then depilated with a depilatory preparation. After

Accepted for publication Oct 28, 1988.
From the Department of Plastic Surgery, University of Virginia School of Medicine, Charlottesville.

Reprint requests to Department of Plastic Surgery, Box 443, University of Virginia School of Medicine, Charlottesville, VA 22908 (Dr Rodeheaver).

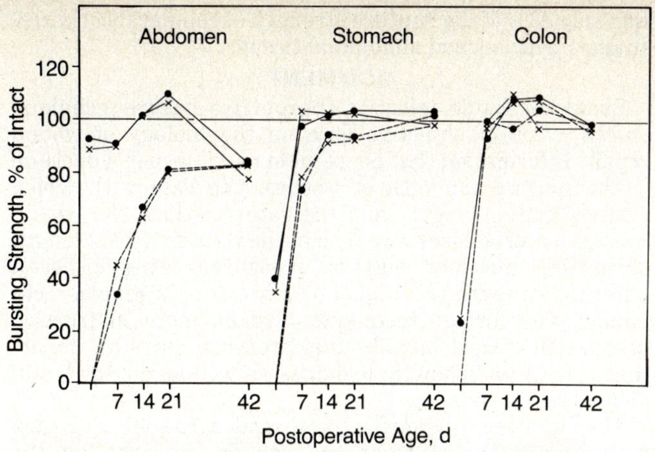

Bursting strength of wounds was determined at time of surgery (0) and at various periods over 42 days. Bursting strength was determined with sutures intact (solid lines) or sutures cut (dashed lines). Two different suture materials were evaluated—a copolymer of glycolide and trimethylene carbonate (Maxon), solid circles; and polydioxanone (PDS), pluses.

Table 1.—Animal Weights*

Group	0†	1 wk	2 wk	3 wk	6 wk
Controls	246±11	267±13	336±13	357±17	406±10
Maxon	242±11	267±13	317±20	364±20	411±30
PDS	245±11	276±12	321±16	359±20	410±23

*Data expressed in grams±SD. Maxon is a copolymer of glycolide and trimethylene carbonate; PDS, polydioxanone.
†All animals had fasted for 24 hours before anesthesia.

copious rinsing with water, the skin was prepared with an iodophor antiseptic solution and then isolated with sterile drapes for surgery. With aseptic technique, a 5.5-cm midline incision was made through the abdominal skin, beginning 0.5 cm below the xiphoid process. The linea alba and underlying peritoneum were then incised. The length of this incision through this musculoaponeurotic layer and peritoneum was identical to that of the skin.

The site for the left colon anastomosis was identified 2.5 cm above the pelvic floor. The left colon was divided transversely. The anastomosis was accomplished using one layer of interrupted 7-0 synthetic monofilament absorbable sutures spaced approximately 2 mm apart. Eight sutures were used in each anastomosis.

A gastrotomy was then performed in each animal. A 10-mm-long incision was made in the anterior gastric wall in the glandular portion of the stomach. The incision began 10 mm from the pylorus to avoid injury to the antrum and extended 5 to 7 mm from the nonglandular portion (rumen) of the stomach. The gastrotomy was approximated by one layer of interrupted 6-0 synthetic monofilament absorbable sutures spaced about 2 mm apart.

The linea alba was approximated by a one-layer closure with interrupted 5-0 synthetic monofilament absorbable sutures. The distance between the entrance and exits of each interrupted suture and the cut edges of the linea alba was 5 mm. The distance between each interrupted suture loop was also 5 mm. The divided skin edges were apposed by wound closure tapes. Each animal was bandaged with sterile gauze and wrapped in cloth tape. All animals were allowed food and water ad libitum 24 hours after surgery. No postoperative deaths occurred.

Analysis of Healing Strength

Healing strength was defined as the pressure at which leakage or rupture occurred when the tissue was inflated with a constant infusion of water provided by an infusion pump (Harvard). The pressure generated in each test sample was measured by a pressure transducer (Bentley Trantes Model 800). The signal from this transducer was amplified and connected to a calibrated strip chart recorder. At the instant of leakage or rupture, the pressure was recorded for each specimen. The site of rupture (eg, incision

Table 2.—Colonic Anastomoses: Burst or Leak Strength*

		Sutures Intact		Sutures Cut	
Days	Controls	Maxon	PDS	Maxon	PDS
0	145±3	35±4†	36±6†	0±0†	0±0†
7	141±6	132±2	142±6	141±5	139±7
14	145±6	158±9	161±4	142±2	157±3
21	152±5	167±4	149±9	160±10	162±5
42	160±7	159±6	157±7	158±11	155±3

*Data expressed in millimeters of mercury as mean±SEM where N=8 in each group. Maxon is a copolymer of glycolide and trimethylene carbonate; PDS, polydioxanone.
†$P<.001$ compared with the mean value of the controls.

Table 3.—Gastrotomies: Burst or Leak Strength*

		Sutures Intact		Sutures Cut	
Days	Controls	Maxon	PDS	Maxon	PDS
0	246±8	99±7†	85±4†	0±0†	0±0†
7	255±6	251±13	266±10	189±9	201±13†
14	249±11	255±8	257±8	236±9	230±11
21	247±12	257±7	254±8	232±12	229±10
42	239±12	248±8	237±9	246±6	237±9

*Data expressed in millimeters of mercury as mean±SEM where N=8 in each group. Maxon is a copolymer of glycolide and trimethylene carbonate; PDS, polydioxanone.
†$P<.005$ when compared with the mean value of the controls.

Table 4.—Musculoaponeurotic Tissues: Burst or Leak Strength*

		Sutures Intact		Sutures Cut	
Days	Controls	Maxon	PDS	Maxon†	PDS†
0	252±2	234±6†	226±4†	0±0	0±0
7	301±9	275±5†	272±7†	102±12	135±4
14	337±5	340±14	340±6	227±10	211±7
21	306±8	338±7†	327±10	247±15	249±15
42	325±15	316±8†	292±13†	311±7	313±11

*Data expressed in millimeters of mercury as mean±SEM where N=8 in each group. Maxon is a copolymer of glycolide and trimethylene carbonate; PDS, polydioxanone.
†$P<.025$ compared with the mean value of the controls.

or unwounded tissue) was also noted. The weight of each animal was recorded before each wound-healing measurement.

Musculoaponeurotic Tissue

The strength of the abdominal wall was determined by measuring the wound-bursting pressure. The musculoaponeurotic tissue of the abdominal wall was exposed by incising the 5.5-cm-long skin wound and reflecting back the skin. A condom was placed over the tip of a filling catheter, inserted into the peritoneal cavity through a rectal perforation, then passed along the ventral surface of the abdominal cavity until its tip was below the xiphoid. The abdominal cavity was isolated by using strong cotton cords to bind circumferentially the abdomen at the levels of the xiphoid and the pelvic crest. The condom was filled with water at a rate of 35.37 mL/min. Because the condom provided no resistance to distention, all resistance to filling was derived from the musculoaponeurotic tissues. When the abdomen burst, the site of rupture and the bursting pressure were recorded.

Stomach

The entire stomach was removed from the burst abdomen. Because the closed gastrotomy incision was located in the glandular half (corpus) of the stomach, only the glandular part of the stomach was subjected to the wound-healing measurements. The nonglandular part (rumen) was isolated from the corpus by a circumferential 4-0 silk suture. The filling catheter was inserted through the pylorus into the stomach and secured by another 4-0 silk suture. The corpus with its healing incision was then filled with water at a constant rate of 7.08 mL/min. The pressure and the site at which rupture or leakage occurred were recorded.

Colon

A 5.0-cm segment of the left colon with the anastomosis as its midpoint was excised. The distal end of the transected colon was ligated with a 4-0 silk suture, and the filling catheter was passed into the proximal end and secured by a 4-0 silk suture. The isolated colon was filled with water at a constant rate of 1.79 mL/min until leakage or rupture occurred. The pressure and site at which rupture or leakage occurred were noted.

RESULTS

The animals tolerated the surgical procedure well. They were alert and physically active within three hours of being bandaged. Food was withheld for 24 hours to allow for adequate recovery of basic functions. After being given access to solid food, the animals were excreting solid waste within 48 hours. All animals ate heartily and showed no signs of fever or discomfort.

Efforts were made to standardize the weights of the animals undergoing surgery. Thereafter, the homogeneity of their weights was used as a monitor of well-being. No animals had to be eliminated because of a malfunctioning gastrointestinal tract as determined by subsequent weight loss. All animals steadily gained weight during the study (Table 1). At the end of six weeks, the animals had almost doubled their weight since the time of surgery.

The presence of suture material in the tissue played a variable role in the tissue's ultimate security, depending on the tissue being examined and its rate of healing (Figure). The type of suture material used did not seem to influence the level of wound security or rate of healing. As expected, the security of incised wounds in the colon, stomach, and musculoaponeurotic tissues immediately after surgery was supplied by the interrupted sutures (Tables 2 through 4). When these sutures were cut, no pressure was required to burst these wounds. The rate of wound repair was different in each of the tissues examined. Within one week, the mean burst or leak strength of colonic anastomoses was comparable with that of intact colons, even when the interrupted suture loops were cut. The mean burst or leak strength of gastrotomies with sutures intact was similar to that of the control stomachs within seven days after surgery. The synthetic monofilament sutures in the gastrotomies seven days after surgery obviously contributed to the strength of these wounds as evidenced by the significantly reduced mean burst or leak strength of the gastrotomies after cutting the interrupted suture loops. By 14 days, the mean burst or leak strength of gastrotomy incisions with cut suture loops was comparable with that of the control stomachs.

Sutures played an important role in maintaining the strength of the musculoaponeurotic wounds until 42 days after surgery. At 7, 14, and 21 days after surgery, division of the interrupted suture loops was associated with a significant reduction in the mean burst strength of the musculoaponeurotic wounds. The mean burst strength of incised musculoaponeurotic tissues with intact sutures was comparable with that of the control musculoaponeurotic tissues by 14 days after surgery. Sutures did not contribute to the burst strength of musculoaponeurotic wounds 42 days after surgery as evidenced by the mean burst strength with sutures intact being similar to that of musculoaponeurotic tissues tested with sutures cut. By 42 days after surgery, it seemed that these abdominal wounds had attained their maximum level of healing strength, which was only 83% of the rupture strength of comparable control animals with normal abdominal tissue.

COMMENT

Surgeons should select an appropriate closure technique on the basis of objective data on the biology of wound repair. Information that is useful in making such a decision is the normal strength of tissues, the rate with which wounds gain strength, and the rate at which the wound closure material loses strength in the tissues. The strength of healing incisions may be measured using either a bursting strength technique[5] or a breaking strength technique.[6] The former technique may be more instructive because increased intraluminal pressure plays an important role in anastomotic leakages as well as disruption of abdominal wounds.[7]

The bursting strength of unwounded tissues will vary according to the animal's age, weight, and the specific tissue. As the rats gained weight over the 42 days of observation, the bursting strength of the colon and abdominal musculoaponeurotic tissue significantly increased. Levenson and coworkers[7] demonstrated that the breaking and tensile strength of rat skin increased with age and body weight. Because the animal's weight and age seem to be important determinants of tissue strength, the use of age-weight–matched controls is recommended for experimental studies of wound repair.

Immediately after surgery, the burst or leak strength of all the wounds was low. During this period, wound security depends primarily on the interrupted suture loop, as evidenced by the absence of bursting strength after division of the suture loops. In general, the time required for the tissues to regain maximum strength was inversely proportional to the bursting strength of the unwounded tissue. Thus, abdominal musculoaponeurotic incisions, gastrotomies, and colonic anastomoses regained their maximum strength 42, 14, and 7 days, respectively, following surgery. Once the wounded tissue attained the burst strength of unwounded tissue, the tissues frequently burst at sites other than the wound. This finding suggests that the wounds were stronger than the surrounding unwounded tissue. Although we can see no advantage in the wound being stronger than the unwounded tissue, these findings serve to emphasize that the sutures adequately restored the integrity of the divided tissue. The performance of the two synthetic monofilament sutures in the musculoaponeurotic tissues, colonic anastomoses, and gastrotomies was similar. While our studies provide considerable support for the use of these new absorbable monofilament synthetic sutures in musculoaponeurotic tissue, stomach and colon, we must reiterate that our studies were restricted to healthy animals. The use of these sutures for closure of wounds in animals with impaired healing should be the subject of additional investigations.[8]

References

1. Katz AR, Turner R: Evaluation of tensile and absorption properties of polyglycolic acid sutures. *Surg Gynecol Obstet* 1970;131:701-716.
2. Herrmann JB, Kelly RJ, Higgins GA: Polyglycolic sutures. *Arch Surg* 1970;100:486-499.
3. Ray JA, Doddi N, Regula D, et al: Polydioxanone (PDS), a novel monofilament synthetic absorbable suture. *Surg Gynecol Obstet* 1981;153:497-507.
4. Katz AR, Mukherjee DP, Kaganov AL, et al: A new synthetic monofilament absorbable suture made from polytrimethylene carbonate. *Surg Gynecol Obstet* 1985;161:213-222.
5. Scheinin TM, Viljanto J: Bursting pressure on healing gastrointestinal wounds in the rat. *Ann Med Exp Biol Fenn* 1966;44:49-51.
6. Herrmann JB, Woodward SC, Pulaski EJ: Healing of colonic anastomoses in the rat. *Surg Gynecol Obstet* 1964;119:269-275.
7. Levenson SM, Geever EF, Crowley LV, et al: The healing of rat skin wounds. *Ann Surg* 1965;161:293-308.
8. Adamsons RJ, Enquist IF: The relative importance of sutures to the strength of healing wounds under normal and abnormal conditions. *Surg Gynecol Obstet* 1963;117:396-401.

Diagnosis and Treatment of Duodenoenteric Fistulas Complicating Crohn's Disease

Kenneth K. W. Lee, MD, Wolfgang H. Schraut, MD

• **A duodenoenteric fistula is an unusual complication of Crohn's disease that requires surgical intervention and may present a difficult management problem. Eleven patients with this condition were treated with an ileocolectomy with primary anastomosis and closure of the duodenal defect after takedown of the fistula. In all patients, the duodenal tissues were free of pathologic evidence of Crohn's disease. The fistula was found to result from Crohn's disease limited to the ileocolonic segment or from anastomotic complications in some patients who had previously undergone ileocolonic resections. Satisfactory healing at the ileocolonic anastomosis and at the duodenal closure site occurred in ten patients; breakdown of the duodenal closure leading to sepsis and death occurred in one patient with an unusually large defect in the first portion of the duodenum. In most instances, these fistulas can be treated safely and adequately by resection of the diseased intestinal segment and simple direct duodenal closure. However, safe management of large duodenal defects may require the use of other methods, such as a serosal patch or creation of a duodenojejunostomy.**

(*Arch Surg* 1989;124:712-715)

Fistulous communication between the duodenum and the small or large intestine is an unusual condition that may pose challenging problems for the surgeon. Duodenoenteric fistulas most often have been associated with colonic carcinomas near the hepatic flexure, which penetrate into the underlying duodenum and pancreas. Welch and Warshaw[1] have estimated that these malignant fistulas occur in one of 900 carcinomas of the colon. Less commonly, duodenoenteric fistulas have resulted from benign conditions, such as peptic ulcer disease,[2] cholecystitis,[3] duodenal diverticulitis,[4] and appendicitis.[5]

Although internal and external fistulas commonly form in association with Crohn's disease, with some investigators reporting the incidence of fistulous disease to be as high as 60%,[6] duodenoenteric fistulas resulting from Crohn's disease are distinctly uncommon, having been reported, to our knowledge, in fewer than 40 patients.[7-18] Recently, however, we have encountered this disorder with increasing frequency. We therefore undertook a review of our experience with duodenoenteric fistulas associated with Crohn's disease to develop principles for the diagnosis and treatment of this potentially difficult problem.

PATIENTS AND METHODS

The clinical records, operative reports, and pathology reports of all patients undergoing laparotomy for Crohn's disease at The University of Chicago Hospitals and Clinics between 1970 and 1986 were reviewed. This review included 467 patients who had Crohn's ileitis, ileocolitis, or colitis. In 191 (41%) of these patients, internal or external fistulas were present. Eleven patients (2.4%) had a duodenoenteric fistula.

RESULTS

Patient Characteristics

The group of 11 patients consisted of nine men and two women. Their ages ranged from 28 to 74 years (mean, 42.2 years). The diagnosis of Crohn's disease was made five to 32 years before the development or detection of the duodenoenteric fistula. Six of the 11 patients had undergone previous ileoascending colectomies with ileotransverse anastomosis (one at our hospital and five at other institutions) between one and seven years earlier.

Clinical Data

The most common symptoms and signs encountered in evaluating these patients were chronic fatigue, weight loss, abdominal pain, anorexia, and diarrhea. Anemia, intermittent fever, and an abdominal mass were noted in seven patients. Two patients had symptoms consistent with recurrent partial small-bowel obstruction. Feculent emesis, a finding highly suggestive of a duodenocolic fistula, occurred in a single patient; this was the only patient in whom the diagnosis of a duodenoenteric fistula could be made based on the medical history and physical examination.

Diagnostic Studies

All 11 patients underwent preoperative barium contrast studies of the gastrointestinal tract, following which the duodenoenteric fistula was detected in nine of the patients. The examination of the stomach and small bowel demonstrated the fistula in five patients (Figure, left), suggested the presence of a duodenal fistula in five patients, and

Accepted for publication Dec 7, 1987.
From the Department of Surgery, University of Chicago Medical Center. Dr Schraut is now with the University of Pittsburgh.

Reprint requests to Department of Surgery, University of Pittsburgh, 497 Scaife Hall, Pittsburgh, PA 15261 (Dr Schraut).

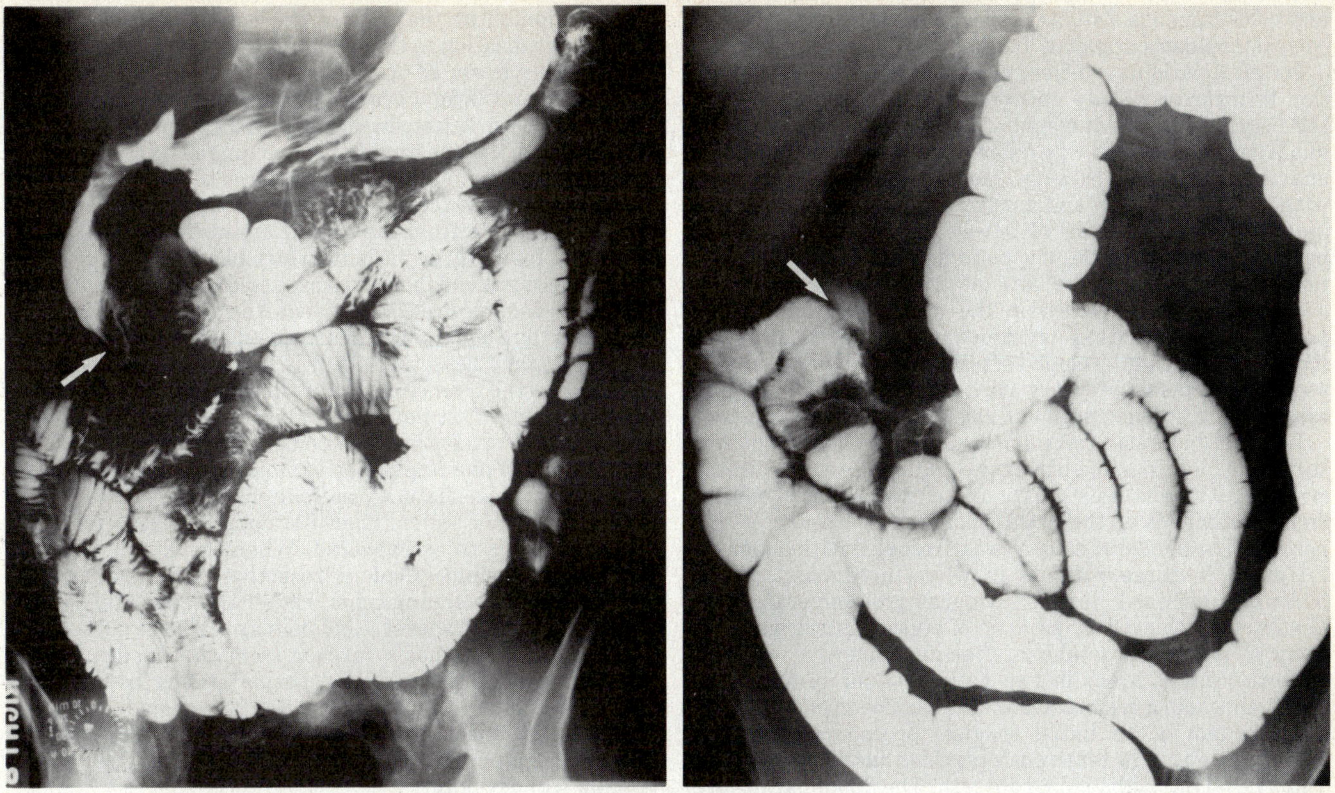

Definitive diagnosis of duodenoenteric fistula most often is made by upper or lower gastrointestinal tract contrast roentgenography. The two examinations are complementary, with one examination often yielding normal results and the other demonstrating presence of fistula. Left, Upper gastrointestinal tract roentgenogram showing fistulous tract at junction of second and third portions of duodenum (arrow). Right, Lower gastrointestinal tract roentgenogram showing fistula (arrow), which permits passage of air and contrast material into duodenum.

yielded normal findings in one patient. Barium enema examination demonstrated the fistula in six patients (Figure, right) and was nondiagnostic in the others. The fistula was also seen in the duodenum of one of three patients who underwent preoperative esophagogastroduodenoscopy.

Indications for Surgery and Preoperative Preparation

In the nine patients with roentgenographic evidence of the duodenoenteric fistula, the fistula was an indication for surgery, but in no case was it the sole indication. In all patients, several factors indicated surgery, including recurrent small-bowel obstruction; failure of medical management to halt weight loss, abolish abdominal pain, and control severe diarrhea; enterocutaneous fistulas; and septic complications, such as an abdominal mass/abscess with recurring fever. Two patients received total parenteral nutrition for six and 16 months, respectively, before surgery. Although symptoms such as feculent emesis and abdominal pain resolved, the fistula did not close in either patient. In six other patients, a short course (two to four weeks) of total parenteral nutrition similarly improved the general state of health but did not cause closure of the fistula. In the immediate preoperative period, all patients underwent thorough mechanical bowel preparation (gut lavage with oral electrolyte solution, enemas). Perioperative antibiotic therapy (parenterally administered broad-spectrum cephalosporins) was given to all patients.

Surgical Findings and Procedures

At operation, the precise pathologic anatomy of the duodenoenteric fistula was determined. In four of the six patients who had undergone previous ileocolectomy, the fistula was found to communicate between the site of anastomosis and the duodenum. In two of these four patients, active Crohn's disease was present at the site of the previous ileocolonic anastomosis; in the other two, there was no evidence of active Crohn's disease at the previous anastomotic site, and the fistulas were probably the result of anastomotic complications, such as formation of a perianastomotic abscess or leakage. In the remaining two patients who had undergone previous ileocolonic resection, the fistulous tract was found to arise from the preanastomotic area harboring recurrent Crohn's disease.

Among the five patients who had not undergone previous intestinal resections, the anatomy of the fistulous communication was more variable. In one patient, two fistulas were found between the transverse colon and the first and second portions of the duodenum. In two patients, the fistulas connected the cecum or proximal transverse colon with the first or second portion of the duodenum. In another patient, the fistulous tract extended from the transverse colon through the mesocolon into the third portion of the duodenum and the pancreas. In the fifth patient, the fistula arose in the distal transverse colon and communicated with the fourth portion of the duodenum at the ligament of Treitz. Although an active inflammatory response at the site of the duodenal fistula and in the surrounding tissues, including the pancreas, was encountered in all patients, none had evidence of Crohn's duodenitis or gastritis.

A wide range of pathologic abnormalities was found in addition to the duodenoenteric fistulas, including mesenteric abscesses and a variety of other fistulas, such as enteroenteric, enterocolonic, enterocutaneous, colocolonic, and colocutaneous fistulas, and one particularly tortuous cologastropleurocutaneous fistula.

For all 11 patients, surgery consisted of ileocolonic resection to macroscopically uninvolved margins, takedown of the fistula from the duodenum, and primary repair of the duodenal defect. This was followed by primary ileocolonic anastomosis in ten patients. Total abdominal colectomy with an end ileostomy and a mucous fistula was performed in one patient because of severe pancolitis and active perineal disease. In the six patients who had undergone previous resections, the site of the existing intestinal anastomosis was included in the new resection. In one patient, a coexisting gastropancreatopleurocutaneous fistula, which had developed after a vagotomy and antrectomy performed six years earlier, required distal pancreatectomy, splenectomy, and closure of the gastric defect.

In all 11 patients, the duodenal site of the fistula was treated by débridement of this site and simple closure of the resulting duodenal defect. A nearly circumferential end-to-end anastomosis of the duodenum was necessary in one patient. The duodenal closure was protected with an omental patch in three patients in whom a remnant of the omentum remained. Temporary decompression of the duodenum was achieved by passage of a nasogastric, gastrostomy, or jejunostomy tube into the duodenum.

Complications arose in two patients—one of these patients, in whom a mesenteric abscess had been encountered and drained in the initial surgical procedure, required reexploration on the tenth postoperative day for drainage of a subfascial intra-abdominal abscess. The duodenal closure was intact, and the patient recovered uneventfully. In the second patient in whom simple closure of a 3.5-cm defect in the anterior wall of the first portion of the duodenum was undertaken, a leak developed in this closure. After a prolonged hospital course marked by recurrent sepsis, recurrent leakage, and intra-abdominal bleeding that required two additional laparotomies, the patient died of sepsis. The ten surviving patients have now been followed up for periods ranging from one to nine years. Recurrent active Crohn's disease has been diagnosed in four patients, but in none of these has a recurrence of the duodenoenteric fistula been diagnosed, nor have any of these patients developed duodenal Crohn's disease.

COMMENT

As this article demonstrates, the unusual finding of fistulous communication between the duodenum and the small or large intestine as a complication of Crohn's disease characteristically results from enterocolonic, rather than duodenal, involvement by Crohn's disease. This was the finding in other reports of duodenoenteric fistulas associated with Crohn's disease and in reports of duodenal Crohn's disease. Although Crohn's duodenitis may coexist with Crohn's enterocolitis in patients with such fistulas, fistulas resulting from isolated duodenal disease are extremely rare. Abnormalities of the duodenum, which are detected roentgenographically or endoscopically in patients with duodenoenteric fistulas, most commonly arise secondary to the fistula itself and are nonspecific (non–Crohn's disease) inflammatory changes, that resolve following adequate treatment of the fistula (ie, resection of the primarily diseased bowel, which gives rise to the fistula).

The proximity of the second and third portions of the duodenum to the proximal transverse colon facilitates fistulous communication between these regions, particularly in the setting of Crohn's colitis. However, the first portion of the duodenum and other portions of the intestine also may be involved. The position of the fourth portion of the duodenum at the root of the small-bowel mesentery makes fistulization to this area less likely, but it is possible, as was seen in one of our patients.

In patients who have undergone previous ileocolonic resection with ileoascending or ileotransverse colostomy, the region of the anastomosis is a common site of origin for a duodenoenteric fistula. In this series, the duodenoenteric fistulas in four of the six patients who had undergone such resections arose from the earlier anastomosis. Wilk et al[13] similarly found three patients who had undergone previous ileal resections and ileotransverse colostomies and who had fistulous communication between the perianastomotic region and the duodenum. The ileocolonic anastomosis following ileocolonic resection often is in proximity to the duodenum. As recurrence of Crohn's disease is likely to occur in the preanastomotic ileum, the frequency of duodenoenteric fistulas that arise from the perianastomotic region is not surprising. If one implicates technical factors in the development of these fistulas, as may have been true for two patients in this series, then fistulous involvement of the anastomosis is to be expected. When the existing disease permits, more limited colonic resection with anastomosis to the proximal ascending colon, rather than to distal ascending or proximal transverse colon, may place the subsequent ileocolonic anastomosis further from the duodenum and thereby reduce the risk of a fistula arising between the duodenum and the anastomotic site. Placement of omentum between the anastomosis and the duodenum at the time of the ileocolectomy also may reduce the likelihood that such a fistula will develop.

To our knowledge, no association exists between the risk of developing a duodenoenteric fistula and either the patient's age or the length of the interval since the onset of symptoms of Crohn's disease. A duodenoenteric fistula has been found as little as one year after the onset of symptoms.[8] For reasons that are not clear, there is a marked male preponderance in this series and among other reported cases (28:10) of duodenoenteric fistulas secondary to Crohn's disease.

In the surgical management of a fistulous communication between the duodenum and the small or large bowel involved by Crohn's disease, the surgeon must be aware of the condition of the bowel at both ends of the fistula. Although duodenoenteric fistulas resulting from duodenal Crohn's disease are extremely rare, it is advisable to exclude the presence of Crohn's duodenitis in these patients when it is known preoperatively that the fistula exists. If the duodenal mucosa is normal (with the exception of local inflammatory changes at the fistula site), then the fistula can be disconnected, the diseased ileocolonic segment resected with reanastomosis, and the duodenal defect closed by simple suture after excision of the margins back to normal tissue. In three of our patients, the duodenal defect was found near the pancreatic border and required dissection of the pancreas from the duodenum to allow a secure closure of the duodenal defect. In these situations, meticulous hemostasis and diligent dissection are necessary to prevent injury to the pancreas.

Although the value of an omental or peritoneal patch to buttress the duodenal closure has not been proved scientifically, this is a simple maneuver that may protect the duodenal closure and that is incorporated easily in the repair of the duodenal defect. If the retroperitoneum is markedly inflamed and is the site of an abscess or phlegmon, then vigorous débridement is strongly recommended before the anastomotic suture line is placed in the retroperitoneal bed. Closure of the duodenal defect by a duodenojejunostomy, as advocated by Wilk et al,[13] is not necessary as a routine procedure. Furthermore, a duodenojejunostomy bypasses a portion of the small bowel; in a patient with Crohn's disease who has undergone previous small-bowel resections, the nutritional consequences of rendering a segment of the remaining small bowel nonfunctional may be substantial. However, in the presence of a large duodenal defect that cannot be closed simply, creation of a duodenojejunostomy or use of a serosal patch may be necessary. This approach might have secured the closure of the large duodenal defect and prevented its leakage in one of our patients. If Crohn's disease should arise in the small-bowel segment used for the serosal patch, however, the duodenal fistula may recur.

We have abstained from placing a drain in the area of the duodenal closure but routinely have inserted an intraluminal tube into the duodenum for decompression either by a gastrostomy or a jejunostomy. At present, we prefer the transgastric placement of such a duodenal tube. This tube is placed across the duodenal closure and allows for enteral alimentation if the duodenal closure should remain edematous and temporarily obstruct gastric emptying during the early postoperative course.

The bowel involved by Crohn's disease is treated according to established guidelines. The extent of the bowel resection and decisions for or against primary anastomosis and primary wound closure must be made on an individual basis, as dictated by the degree of intra-abdominal contamination.

References

1. Welch JP, Warshaw AL: Malignant duodenocolic fistulas. *Am J Surg* 1977;133:658-661.
2. Herrington JL Jr: Duodenocolic fistula with perforation secondary to peptic ulcer. *Am J Surg* 1967;113:285-288.
3. Neville WE: Duodenocolic fistula due to acute cholecystitis. *Am J Surg* 1954;87:300-302.
4. Dey KR, Latchmore AJ: Steatorrhea due to duodeno-colic fistula from perforation of a duodenal diverticulum with ectopic gastric epithelium. *Br J Clin Pract* 1970;24:444-445.
5. Clayton RS, Thornton WL: Benign duodenocolic fistula: Review of the literature and case report. *Radiology* 1953;60:832-836.
6. Schraut WH, Abraham VS: A comparison of complications following ileocolonic resection for Crohn's disease and for non-inflammatory bowel disease. *Colo-proctology* 1987;9:289-295.
7. Masters H: Duodenal-colic fistula as a complication of regional ileitis. *NY Mt Sinai Hosp* 1948;15:264-265.
8. Grayson MJ, O'Connell ND: Benign duodeno-colic fistulae. *Postgrad Med J* 1960;36:549-556.
9. Leichtling JJ, Garlock JH: Granulomatous colitis complicated by gastrocolic, duodenocolic, and colopulmonic fistulas. *Gastroenterology* 1962;42:152-165.
10. Greenstein AJ, Kark AE, Dreiling DA: Crohn's disease of the colon. *Am J Gastroenterol* 1974;62:419-429.
11. Thompson WM, Cockrill H Jr, Rice RP: Regional enteritis of the duodenum. *AJR* 1975;123:252-261.
12. Smith TR, Goldin RR: Radiographic and clinical sequelae of the duodenocolic anatomic relationship. *Dis Colon Rectum* 1977;20:257-262.
13. Wilk PJ, Fazio V, Turnbull RB Jr: The dilemma of Crohn's disease: Ileoduodenal fistula complicating Crohn's disease. *Dis Colon Rectum* 1977;20:387-392.
14. Korelitz BI: Colonic-duodenal fistula in Crohn's disease. *Dig Dis Sci* 1977;22:1040-1048.
15. Fitgibbons TJ, Green G, Silberman H, et al: Management of Crohn's disease involving the duodenum, including duodenal cutaneous fistula. *Arch Surg* 1980;115:1022-1028.
16. Goldwasser B, Mazor A, Wiznitzer T: Enteroduodenal fistulas in Crohn's disease. *Dis Colon Rectum* 1981;24:485-486.
17. Mosca F, Della Giovampaola C, Parra PF, et al: Enterocolite granulomatosa e fistola colo-duodenale. *Minerva Chir* 1984;39:1745-1749.
18. Glass RE, Ritchie JK, Lennard-Jones JE, et al: Internal fistulas in Crohn's disease. *Dis Colon Rectum* 1985;28:557-561.

In Other AMA Journals

AJDC

Necrotizing Enterocolitis in Full-term Infants: A Case-Control Study

LTC Thomas E. Wiswell, MC, USA; CPT Carol F. Robertson, MC, USA;
CPT Timothy A. Jones, MC, USA; Capt Deborah J. Tuttle, MC, USAF

We performed a case-control investigation of 43 full-term infants with necrotizing enterocolitis (NEC) to identify possible risk factors and unique features of the disorder in the more mature infant. Two control groups were used. The first consisted of "healthy" term infants. The second was a group of "sick" term infants who did not develop NEC. The 43 term infants with NEC represented 12.7% of all 338 neonates with NEC. The median age at onset of symptoms was 2 days, and 18 infants developed NEC on the first day of life. Two (4.7%) of the 43 affected term infants died, while 35 (11.9%) of 295 preterm infants with the disorder died. Only three of the full-term infants who subsequently developed NEC had entirely unremarkable courses prior to the onset of symptoms. Sick infants, in particular those who are small for gestational age or require exchange transfusions, are at risk for NEC. Several other features that may be associated with the subsequent development of NEC include the following: perinatal asphyxia, presence of umbilical catheters, antecedent respiratory distress, polycythemia, and maternal preeclampsia. Full-term infants with these features should be treated with cautious observation and aggressive management early in the neonatal period should they develop signs and symptoms suggestive of NEC (*AJDC* 1988;142:532-535).

Reprint requests to 7727 Iron Forge Ct, Derwood, MD 20855 (Dr Wiswell).

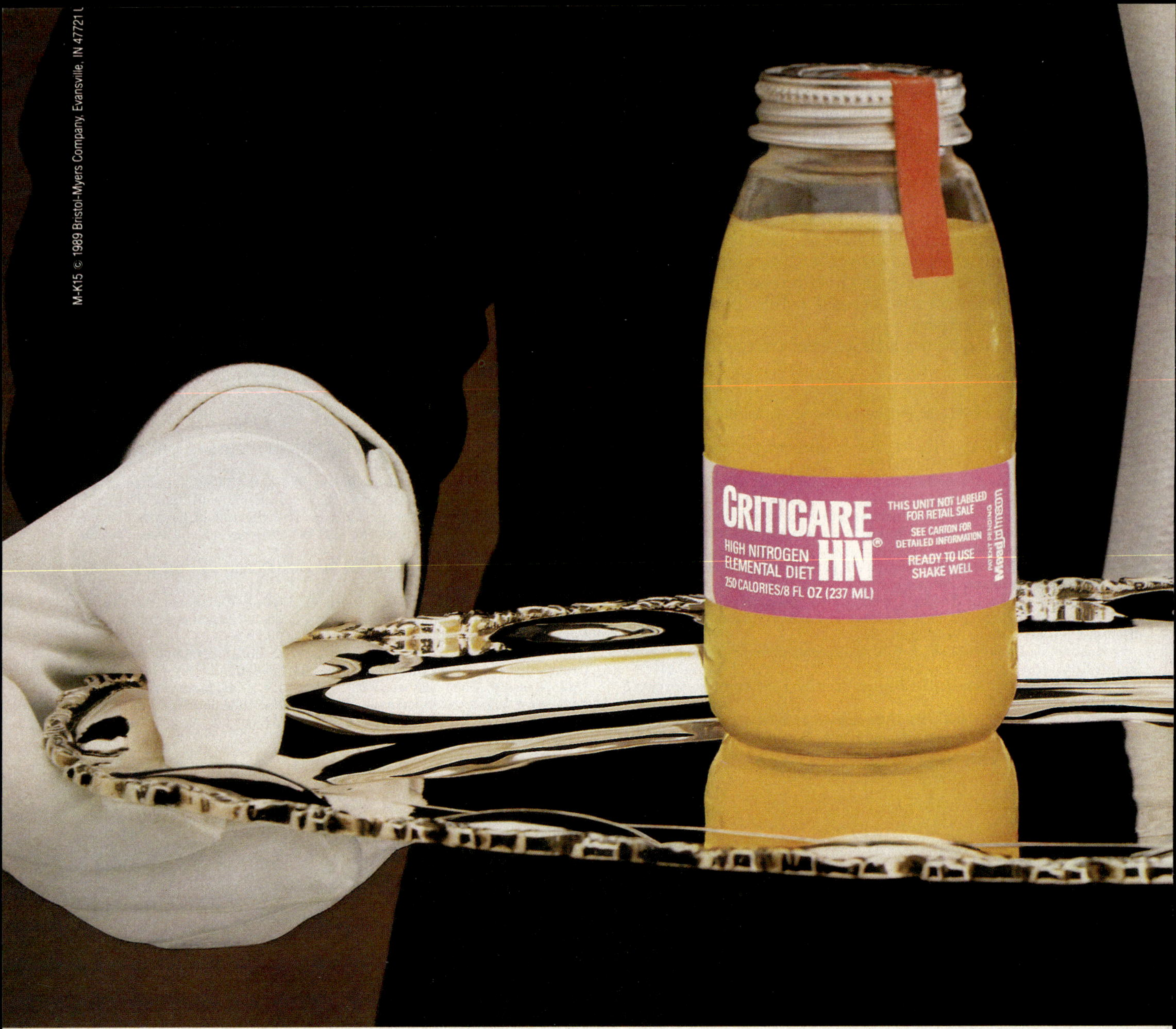

CRITICARE HN®

Because patients with impaired digestion and absorption are often those who need essential nutrients most.

The *only* complete, high-nitrogen elemental diet in a commercially sterile, ready-to-use form.

Dietitians told us that they needed a highly specific nutritional formulation in sterile, ready-to-use form to rapidly renourish their malnourished patients and a product which minimized the risks associated with prepared powdered formulas.

Criticare HN was formulated in response to that need. Developed to provide patients, even those suffering from problems of maldigestion or malabsorption, with the elemental nutrition they so critically need.

Formulated to provide generous levels of the preferred elemental protein for these patients, Criticare HN offers 50% free amino acids and 50% small peptides. Plus 100% of U.S. RDAs for vitamins and minerals in 2000 Calories.

Criticare HN. For stressed patients, it's just what the dietitian ordered.

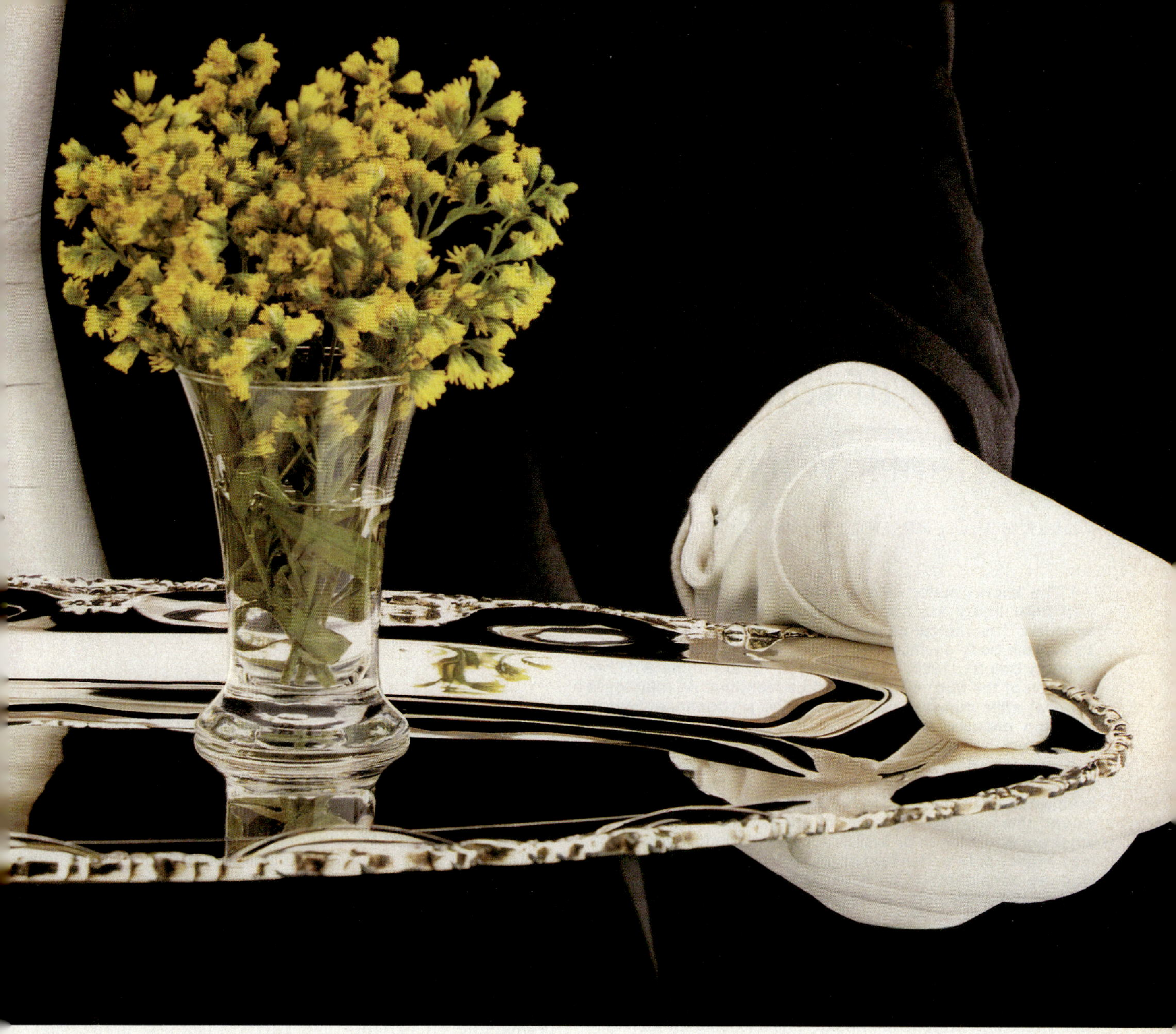

The complete line of clinically validated, xceptionally well-tolerated adult enteral nutritionals.

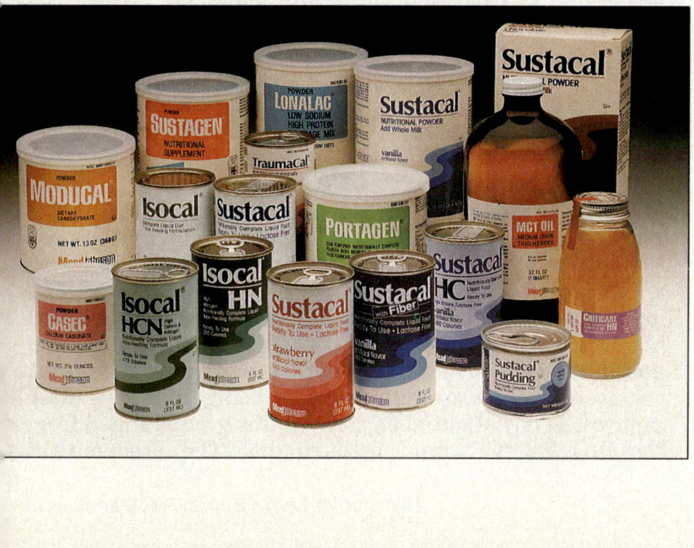

This important product is part of what we believe to be one of the broadest lines of technologically advanced, lactose-free enteral nutritionals. Each product is formulated with the precise nutrient values you demand and the exceptional patient tolerance you expect.

For more information about Mead Johnson enteral nutritionals, call toll-free: 1-800-892-9201.

Mead Johnson

ENTERAL NUTRITIONALS

Bristol-Myers Institutional Products

A Bristol-Myers Company

75 YEARS OF CATERING TO YOUR PATIENTS' NUTRITIONAL NEEDS.

Excision of the Burn Wound in Patients With Large Burns

William F. McManus, MD; Arthur D. Mason, Jr, MD; Basil A. Pruitt, Jr, MD

• The known major determinants of survival for patients with burn injury are age, burn size, inhalation injury, and infection. The clinical courses of 210 patients with burns of 30% of the body surface or greater treated from Jan 1, 1983, through Dec 31, 1985, were reviewed to determine whether excision of the burn wound could be identified as a factor in survival after massive burn injury. The predominant site of infection changed from the burn wound to the lung, with pneumonia being the most common bacterial infection in patients whose wounds were treated as described. Effective topical control of bacterial proliferation and excision of the burn wound have resulted in replacement of invasive bacterial wound infection by nonbacterial burn wound infection. The apparent advantages of excision, particularly in large burns, may reflect only patient selection, since only those patients who are considered to be physiologically stable and able to tolerate the physiologic stress of excision are considered for operation.

(*Arch Surg* 1989;124:718-720)

The known major determinants of survival for patients with burn injury are age, burn size, inhalation injury, and infection. In light of the current enthusiasm for early excision of the burn wound and reports of general improvement in outcome after burn injury, we reviewed our recent results of care of patients with massive burn injury to evaluate the applicability of excision in such patients.

PATIENTS AND METHODS

The hospital records of 571 burned patients admitted to the US Army Institute of Surgical Research, Fort Sam Houston, Tex, between Jan 1, 1983, and Dec 31, 1985, were reviewed. Of these patients, 474 were male, reflecting the preponderance of male admissions to this center. The ages of this group of patients ranged from 2 months to 97 years, and 62% were admitted to the burn center within 24 hours of injury. Two hundred ten patients (37%) were identified as having massive burn injury, which for this review was defined as involvement of 30% or more of the body surface. The clinical courses of those 210 patients were reviewed.

RESULTS

Among the 210 patients who met the arbitrary definition of massive burn injury, 186 were male and 24 were female. Age ranged from 8 months to 93 years, with a mean of 35.7 years. The mean burn size in this subset was 52.6% of the total body surface, with an average of 32.6% of the surface involved in full-thickness injury. A diagnosis of inhalation injury, established by history, physical examination, fiberoptic bronchoscopy, and xenon 133 ventilation perfusion scan, was made in 118 (56%) of these patients.

One hundred seventeen patients (55.7%) survived. The mean age of surviving patients was 27.9 years, and the mean burn size was 44.5% of the body surface, with a mean of 21.1% full-thickness injury. Inhalation injury was present in 39 surviving patients 33.3%. Excision of the burn wound was carried out in 104 of these 117 patients; the remaining 13 patients had partial-thickness injury that healed spontaneously, without any necessity for excision or autografting of their wounds. Tangential excision of the burn wound, excision to a level within subcutaneous fatty tissue, and excision to the level of the investing fascia were performed as necessary to remove nonviable tissue. The average time to initial excision in surviving patients was 13.5 days after injury (range, fourth to the 31st postinjury day). Those patients undergoing wound excision later in their burn course characteristically had extensive burns with a limited area of full-thickness injury that was excised after spontaneous reepithelialization of the large areas of partial-thickness injury.

Ninety-three (44.3%) of the 210 patients died. The average age among patients who died was 45.1 years, and their mean burn size was 61.9% of the body surface, with an average of 46.6% of the surface involved in full-thickness injury. Seventy-nine (85%) of the patients who died had inhalation injury. Excision of the burn wound was deemed possible in only 40 (43%) of the nonsurviving patients, with the average time to initial excision being 12.5 days after injury. The day of initial excision in this group ranged from the fifth to the 23rd postburn day. The predominant

Accepted for publication Sept 30, 1988.

From the US Army Institute of Surgical Research, Fort Sam Houston, Tex.

Read before the 94th Annual Session of the Western Surgical Association, Detroit, Nov 18, 1986.

The opinions or assertions contained herein are the private views of the authors and are not to be construed as official or as reflecting the views of the Department of the Army or the Department of Defense.

Reprint requests to Medical Library, US Army Institute of Surgical Research, Fort Sam Houston, TX 78234.

contraindication to excision of the burn wound in this group was pulmonary insufficiency. The complications of inhalation injury and/or pneumonia necessitating maximal ventilatory support either precluded safe transport of the patient to the operating room or reduced to an unacceptable level the assessed ability of the patient to tolerate the physiologic stress of excision. In some patients renal failure, hemodynamic instability secondary to sepsis, or serum electrolyte derangements precluded or delayed burn wound excision.

Infection was the cause of death in 71 (76.3%) of these 93 nonsurviving patients. Pneumonia was the single most common infection and was identified as a cause of death in 54 patients. Invasive burn wound infection was identified in 24 of the patients who died. Bacterial wound infection occurred in only six patients, while yeast or fungal burn wound infection was identified in 18 of the 24 patients with histologically documented invasive burn wound infection. Causes of death other than infection identified in 22 patients included severe inhalation injury in 12, acute myocardial infarction in five, and pulmonary embolism, resuscitation failure, phenol toxic reaction, aspiration due to a tracheoesophageal fistula, and cerebral edema secondary to hypoxia in one patient each.

COMMENT

Various investigators have reported the consequences of early burn wound excision.[1-3] Among these reports, only one[1] claimed that excision improved the survival of burned patients. In that study, however, there were no controls, the study spanned a period of approximately 45 years during which there was a general improvement in survival after burn injury not necessarily attributable to excision, and most of the described patients had burns of 20% of the body surface or less. Another study[2] reported the results of early excision in patients with burns of 20% to 40% of the body surface and identified no survival advantage. A third article[3] reported on a controlled study in which there was no survival advantage of early excision of burns that exceeded 15% of the body surface. When one compares reported outcomes, comparable populations must be used for such analysis, with particular attention paid to the distribution of inhalation injury and pneumonia within the populations. If excision of the burn wound is to be cited as the reason for improved survival, concurrent controls must be included to validate that conclusion, since without such controls, improvement in survival may merely reflect unintentional selection of patients without inhalation injury or life-threatening infection.

The Figure displays the plane describing the improvement in survival of patients treated at this burn center over the past three decades. The plane was generated by subtracting the calculated death rate, corrected for burn size and age, of patients treated during the years 1980 through 1984 from the similar death rate of patients treated during the period 1950 through 1963. The improvement in survival is indicated on the vertical axis in terms of percentage difference at any combination of burn size and age. The control of burn wound infection is, in part, responsible for the improvement in survival, but to what degree excision of the burn wound is related to the reduction of wound infection is difficult to document.

As previously reported from this institute,[4] inhalation injury alone is associated with a maximum added mortality of 20%, related to burn size and age. Pneumonia is associated with a maximum added mortality of 40%, and the combination of inhalation injury and pneumonia, which are significant independent and additive comorbid factors,

Table 1.—Survival by Patient Age and Burn Size

Age, y	No. of Survivors/No. of Nonsurvivors — Burn Size, % of Body Surface: 30-50	51-70	71-100
0-15	15/5	5/1	0/0
16-40	51/3	18/11	3/20
41-60	16/7	5/10	0/8
≥61	4/18	0/3	0/7

Table 2.—Characteristics of 210 Patients With Massive Burn Injury

	Survivors	Nonsurvivors
No. (%)	117 (55.7)	93 (44.3)
Average age, y	27.9	45.1
Average burn size, % of body surface	44.5	61.9
Full-thickness burn, % of burn	22.1	46.6
Inhalation injury, No. (%) of patients	39 (33)	79 (85)
Excision, No. (%) of patients	104 (89)	40 (43)
Postburn day of 1st excision		
Mean	13.5	12.5
Range	4-31	5-23

Table 3.—Reasons for Not Performing Excision in 53 Patients

Reason	No. of Patients
Pulmonary insufficiency	**43**
Inhalation injury and pneumonia	19
Inhalation injury	14
Pneumonia	6
Aspiration	2
Acute asthma	1
Pulmonary embolus	1
Nonpulmonary/hemodynamic instability	**10**
Acute myocardial infarction	4
Septic shock (not wound)	3
Resuscitation failure	2
Sepsis with disseminated intravascular coagulation	1

Difference in deaths per 100 patients (1950 to 1963 minus 1980 to 1984) by patient age and burn size.

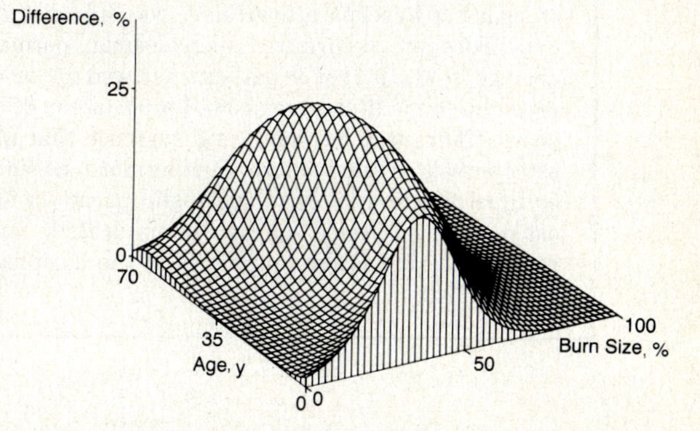

is associated with a maximum added mortality of 60%, related to burn size and age.

The effects of age and burn size on mortality are given in Table 1. As anticipated, mortality in these 210 patients increased, in general, as either age or burn size increased. The high mortality in the pediatric patients with burns of 30% to 50% of the body surface was anticipated because of the high burn-related mortality in the extremely young. The mean age of the nonsurvivors in that group was 18.8 months, and all were less than 33 months of age.

The generally accepted indications for excision of the burn wound include full-thickness burns of limited extent, deep dermal dorsal hand burns when the total burn is of limited extent, débridement and definitive treatment of high-voltage electric injury, and removal of areas of burn wound infection. The advantages of excision and closure of the burn wound include reduction in the time during which the patient is at risk of invasive burn wound infection and reduction in the magnitude and duration of burn size–related physiologic stress.

These indications and advantages must be balanced against the associated blood loss, which has been estimated to be as high as 9% of the blood volume for each 1% of the body surface excised by tangential technique,[5] the risk of hepatitis and acquired immunodeficiency syndrome after the administration of blood and blood products, and the uncertainty of graft take on subcutaneous fat. Additionally, excision at the levels below the dermis results in loss of viable skin in those areas of partial-thickness injury interspersed with areas of full-thickness injury, thus compounding the donor-recipient site disparity in a patient with extensive burn injury.

Table 2 demonstrates that in these 210 patients there was a marked difference between surviving and nonsurviving patients with massive burn injury in terms of age, total burn size, extent of full-thickness burn, and the presence of inhalation injury.

Table 3 identifies the conditions that precluded operation in the 53 nonsurviving patients whose burns were not excised. Pulmonary insufficiency prevented excision in 43 patients. Inhalation injury and/or pneumonia commonly requiring maximum ventilator settings for ventilatory support were the common causes of pulmonary insufficiency. Hemodynamic instability with or without sepsis and commonly requiring pharmacologic support was the other principal cause of deferring excision (ten patients).

CONCLUSIONS

Apparent advantages of excision, particularly in patients with massive burns, may reflect only patient selection, since complications of the injury per se or of treatment resulted in 57% of the nonsurvivors vs 11% of the survivors being considered too unstable or unable to tolerate excision. Age, burn size, inhalation injury, and infection were, as anticipated, the principal determinants of mortality in this group of patients. The preponderant site of infection, the burn wound in earlier years, is now the lung, and pneumonia is presently the most frequently occurring bacterial infection in massively burned patients. Current techniques of wound care employing topical chemotherapy and, when feasible, excision of the burn wound have reduced the occurrence of invasive burn wound infection. Associated with the decrease in invasive bacterial burn wound infection has been a relative increase in nonbacterial, predominantly fungal, burn wound infection.

References

1. Tompkins RG, Burke JF, Schoenfeld DA, et al: Prompt eschar excision: A treatment system contributing to reduced burn mortality. *Ann Surg* 1986;204:272-281.
2. Gray DT, Pine RW, Harnar TJ, et al: Early surgical excision versus conventional therapy in patients with 20 to 40 percent burns. *Am J Surg* 1982;144:76-80.
3. Sorenson B, Fisker NP, Steensen JP, et al: Acute excision or exposure treatment? *Scand J Plast Reconstr Surg* 1984;18:87-93.
4. Shirani KZ, Pruitt BA Jr, Mason AD Jr: The influence of inhalation injury and pneumonia on burn mortality. *Ann Surg* 1987;205:82-87.
5. Snelling CF, Shaw K: The effect of topical epinephrine hydrochloride in saline on blood loss following tangential excision of burn wounds. *Plast Reconstr Surg* 1983;72:830-836.

In Other AMA Journals

ARCHIVES OF INTERNAL MEDICINE

Primary Hyperparathyroidism: A Review of the Long-term Surgical and Nonsurgical Morbidities as a Basis for a Rational Approach to Treatment

Fred W. Lafferty, MD, Charles A. Hubay, MD

We studied long-term morbidity after parathyroid surgery for primary hyperparathyroidism in 100 patients and compared it with the long-term morbidity of medical follow-up from the literature. The surgical treatment of primary hyperparathyroidism was associated with negative results of neck explorations, persistent hypercalcemia, recurrent hypercalcemia, permanent hypoparathyroidism, or recurrent laryngeal nerve damage in 13 (19%) of 68 patients followed up for five years postoperatively. A review of medical follow-up as reported in the literature showed progression of disease in 8% to 22% of patients followed up for five to ten years. There was no convincing evidence that mild primary hyperparathyroidism resulted in progressive osteoporosis or renal failure. Furthermore, no significant improvement in hypertension, peptic ulcer disease, or renal function followed successful parathyroid surgery. Unless future studies demonstrate progressive osteoporosis or renal damage in untreated, mild primary hyperparathyroidism, medical follow-up is a reasonable alternative to surgery in the compliant patient over 50 years of age. (*Arch Intern Med.* 1989; 149:789-796).

Diagnostic Pneumoperitoneum in the Pediatric Patient With a Unilateral Inguinal Hernia

Gregory A. Timberlake, MD; M. Gage Ochsner, MD; Randall W. Powell, MD

• Controversy continues among surgeons over the management of pediatric patients with unilateral groin hernias. Currently, advocated treatment modalities include repair of only the clinically apparent side, exploration of the contralateral side when the ipsilateral hernia is repaired, or performance of contrast herniography before surgery. Another technique for consideration—diagnostic intraoperative pneumoperitoneum—is a simple, quick, safe, and highly accurate means of detecting a clinically inapparent contralateral inguinal hernia during the initial surgery. This technique, the results of its use, and a review of the literature are included.

(*Arch Surg* 1989;124:721-723)

Controversy continues to provoke interest among surgeons concerning management of pediatric patients with unilateral inguinal hernias. Many methods of handling the asymtomatic contralateral groin have been advocated. The treatment modalities currently recommended include (1) repair of the clinically apparent hernia only, (2) exploration of the contralateral side when the clinically apparent hernia is repaired, or (3) performance of contrast herniography before surgery, with repair of both sides if the herniogram is abnormal.

At the US Naval Hospital, San Diego, we have used intraoperative diagnostic pneumoperitoneum to evaluate the contralateral groin for hernia, which has proved to be a safe, quick, humane, economical, and logical approach to the problem. It avoids "unnecessary" surgery in the guise of asymptomatic groin explorations and permits "necessary" surgery for repair of a contralateral inguinal hernia to be performed while the patient is under the same anesthetic. Our report describes the technique used and the results of inguinal hernia repair in infants, children, and adolescents over a six-year period and compares this technique to others in the literature.

PATIENTS AND METHODS

The medical records of all 552 infants, children, and adolescents undergoing repair of an inguinal hernia or communicating hydrocele for the six-year period from Oct 1, 1978, through July 5, 1984, were examined for age, sex, presenting complaint, history of previous surgery, preoperative physical findings, findings at operation, results of diagnostic pneumoperitoneum (if performed), and operative complications. Informed consent for the operative procedure was obtained from the patients' parents. All of the operations were performed by, or under the supervision of, a pediatric surgeon (R.W.P.).

Repair of the indirect inguinal hernia or communicating hydrocele was by high ligation with excision of the sac. The four direct inguinal hernias and two femoral hernias were repaired with a standard Cooper's ligament herniorrhaphy.

All patients underwent diagnostic pneumoperitoneum except those who had previously undergone surgery on the contralateral side, those with bilateral inguinal hernias or hydroceles on presentation, or those in whom the procedure was not technically possible. Also excluded were those patients with an intra-abdominal foreign body, such as ventriculoperitoneal or peritoneovenous shunts. All operations were performed under general anesthesia with endotracheal intubation. The technique, as previously described from our institution,[1] required the isolation and opening of the hernia or hydrocele sac and introduction of a small, 10- to 14-F Robinson catheter through the neck of the sac and into the peritoneal cavity. The peritoneal cavity was insufflated with room air using a bulb syringe until moderate abdominal distention was obtained, as judged on physical examination by the presence of tympany over the liver. The contralateral groin was then palpated for pneumotosis, and in males the scrotum was also palpated. The presence of crepitus in the groin or scrotum constituted an abnormal test finding; we performed exploration of that groin after the insufflated air was evacuated from the peritoneal cavity and the ipsilateral hernia or hydrocele was repaired.

RESULTS

Over the three-year review period, 552 infants, children, and adolescents (426 boys and 126 girls) underwent repair of inguinal hernias or hydroceles. Diagnostic pneumoperitoneum was not attempted in 172 patients. Fifty-six of these 172 patients had bilateral hernias or hydroceles, 30 of 172 patients had undergone previous surgery for a contralateral hernia or hydrocele, and four patients had a ventriculoperitoneal shunt in place. In the remaining patients, diagnostic pneumoperitoneum was not attempted, either because of older age or because permission to perform the procedure was not obtained from the parents before surgery.

Diagnostic pneumoperitoneum was attempted in 380 patients (291 boys and 89 girls). In 41 of the boys, the catheter could not be passed into the peritoneal cavity because of a narrow-necked hernia or hydrocele sac. In the remaining 339 patients (250 boys and 89 girls), intraoperative diagnostic pneumoperitoneum was performed satisfactorily. The data (Table 1) show that in boys having a right inguinal hernia or hydrocele, an associated diagnostic pneumoperitoneum and groin exploration that gave abnormal results were present in 19% (40/210) in whom the procedure was successfully performed. Similarly, a left inguinal hernia or hydrocele was associated with abnormal contralateral findings for 26% (21/81) of the boys. In the girls (Table 1), a right inguinal hernia was associated with a pneumoperitoneum and exploration that gave abnormal results for 31%, and a left inguinal hernia was associated with a pneumoperitoneum and exploration that gave abnormal results for 30%.

Almost one third of our patients were 1 day to 6 months old, 46% of whom had bilateral inguinal hernias on either initial physical examination or diagnostic pneumoperitoneum. The incidence of bilaterality then decreased steadily with age, although our data for those children older than 6 years may be biased or distorted. Diagnostic pneumoperitoneum was not always performed on children having a larger body size because of the difficulty in performing an adequate pneumoperitoneum.

Accepted for publication Nov 3, 1987.

From the Departments of Surgery and Clinical Investigation, US Naval Hospital, San Diego. Dr Ochsner is now with the US Naval Hospital in the Republic of the Philippines, and Dr Powell is now with the University of South Alabama in Mobile.

The views expressed in this article are those of the authors and do not reflect the official policy or position of the Department of the Navy, Department of Defense, or the US government.

Reprint requests to Clinical Investigation Department, Naval Hospital, San Diego, CA 92134-5000 (Dr Timberlake).

Table 1.—Pneumoperitoneum in Pediatric Patients

Presenting Hernia	Attempted	Diagnostic Pneumoperitoneum, No. (%)		
		Abnormal Results	Normal Results	Unsuccessful
Males				
Right inguinal hernia	150	31 (21)	106 (71)	13 (8)
Right communicating hydrocele	60	9 (15)	36 (60)	15 (25)
Left inguinal hernia	59	17 (29)	36 (61)	6 (10)
Left communicating hydrocele	22	4 (18)	11 (50)	7 (32)
Total	**291**	**61** (21)	**189** (65)	**41** (14)
Females				
Right inguinal hernia	59	18 (31)	41 (69)	0
Left inguinal hernia	30	9 (30)	21 (70)	0
Total	**89**	**27** (30)	**62** (70)	**0**

Table 2.—Complications Noted in Patients With Hernias

Patient Group	No. (%)
All patients (n = 552)	
Emesis after surgery	1 (0.2)
Apnea after surgery	1 (0.2)
Shoulder pain	1 (0.2)
Injury to vas deferens	4 (0.7)
Infection	2 (0.4)
Scrotal hematoma	4 (0.7)
Patients undergoing pneumoperitoneum (n = 380)	
Shoulder pain	1 (0.3)
Injury to vas deferens	1 (0.3)
Infection	1 (0.3)
Scrotal hematoma	2 (0.5)
Technical failure (inability to pass catheter)	21 (10.8)

To date, in follow-up of one to eight years, there have been 15 (8.7%) occurrences of symptomatic contralateral inguinal hernias in the 172 patients who did not undergo diagnostic pneumoperitoneum. In those who successfully underwent diagnostic pneumoperitoneum (339 patients), there were no false-positive results found at exploration. To date, three patients (0.9%) have had a clinically apparent hernia in the contralateral groin.

For the entire study group, there was a 2.54% complication rate. None of these complications occurred in patients in whom diagnostic pneumoperitoneum was attempted. There was a technical failure rate of 10.8% in the diagnostic pneumoperitoneum group because of an inability to pass the catheter through a narrow-necked sac. The various complications encountered are shown in Table 2.

COMMENT

The question of whether to explore the contralateral asymptomatic groin when a pediatric patient has a unilateral inguinal hernia has provoked much controversy among surgeons primarily due to the high incidence of a contralateral patent processus vaginalis in pediatric patients with inguinal hernias. Snyder and Greaney,[2] quoting autopsy studies by Sachs, Campers, and Engel, reported that at birth 80% to 94% of all neonates will have an open processus, and at 1 year of age as many as 57% of these processuses will still be patent. While the presence of a patent processus vaginalis may not constitute a hernia, as noted by Holder and Ashcraft,[3] an indirect inguinal hernia will not be clinically apparent unless a patent processus is present. In this regard, Rowe et al,[4,5] in a study of 2764 patients, showed that in an infant with a unilateral groin hernia, the contralateral processus vaginalis obliterates in only 60% of the patients by 2 years of age. In the remaining 40% of the patients, the processus remains open; in half of these patients a clinical hernia will develop. Many other studies have provided data that tend to support the high incidence of asymptomatic contralateral patent processus vaginalis or inguinal hernia in children. For example, studies in which routine contralateral groin explorations were performed indicated 40% to 74% of the patients had a patent processus vaginalis or a hernia.[3-9] Other studies, in which only the symptomatic side was repaired and patients were followed up for the occurrence of a contralateral groin hernia, reported that as many as 31% of these patients would have a groin hernia in the side not operated on.[7,8,10-12]

There are three common modes for evaluating the asymptomatic contralateral groin as follows: (1) repair of the symptomatic side only with close follow-up, (2) exploration of the contralateral side in conjunction with repair of the ipsilateral side, and (3) use of preoperative contrast herniography to assess the contralateral side for the presence of a patent processus vaginalis. A fourth method has been described as transperitoneal probing of the contralateral groin with a Bakkes dilator or other instrument at the time of ipsilateral hernia repair.[13] However, because of a high false-negative rate,[11] it has never been widely accepted.

Many surgeons advocate the repair of only the symptomatic inguinal hernia, with repair of the contralateral side only if a hernia develops.[2,10-12] These surgeons believe routine bilateral exploration should not be performed because of the high number of unnecessary procedures that would be performed, exposure of the patient to increased anesthesia time, and the increased possibility of major complications (testicular atrophy or injury to the vas deferens). The disadvantage of this approach is that a number of necessary procedures are not performed at the initial operation; thus, the child is exposed to the risk of undergoing a second anesthetizing and operation.

Other surgeons advocate routine exploration of the asymptomatic contralateral groin when the clinically apparent hernia is repaired.[3-9] The advantage of this technique is that the second hernia is detected and repaired at the initial operation, thus sparing up to 30% of the patients from the risks of a second anesthetizing and surgery. The disadvantages of this technique are that in a substantial number of patients (increasing with patient age), the exploration does not disclose an abnormality; thus, the patients have had an unnecessary inguinal incision, they undergo anesthesia longer, and, in male patients, there is a risk of injury to cord structures and testicular atrophy. Bock and Sobye[10] reported the latter two complications occurred in 1% to 13% of male patients.

Because of the problems with both of these treatment modalities, many surgeons and radiologists have enthusiastically endorsed preoperative inguinal herniography.[3,14-23] In 1967, Ducharme et al[16] first reported this technique, which utilizes the intraperitoneal injection of a water-soluble contrast agent to radiographically define pathologic lesions of the inguinal canal. Since then, this technique has been used in thousands of patients, with a 95% to 99.5% accuracy rate[15,17,19-22] and a false-negative rate of 0.5% to 4.0%, if patients with unexplored contralateral groins are followed up closely.[19,20,22] Disadvantages of this technique include the discomfort of the procedure to patients, exposure to radiation, time and expense, rare false-negative results, and a complication rate of up to 11%.[14,17-19] These complications are usually reported as minor and include fever, sweating, nausea and vomiting, and abdominal pain.[14,15,17-19] Ducharme et al[24] have recently reported two serious complications of herniography—intestinal obstruction due to a bowel hematoma and cellulitis of the abdominal wall resulting in septicemia and skin slough that requires skin grafting. Because of these two cases and a similar case reported by Butsch and Kuhn,[25] Ducharme et al have critically reexamined their indications for inguinal herniography. They now state inguinal herniography should no longer be used to rule out a hernia, to detect the presence of a contralateral sac, or to confirm the presence of a communicating hydrocele because of the risks of these rare but life-threatening complications.[24]

As noted by White et al, if a method were developed that avoided asymptomatic groin explorations, "there would appear to be few if any objections to closing a contralateral peritoneal sac at the time a unilateral hernia was repaired."[22(p825)] Intraoperative diagnostic pneumoperitoneum seems to be such a method. In this series, no false-positive results have been noted to date in those patients who successfully underwent the procedure. There have been only three false-negative results (0.9%) found in our limited follow-up. Of course, the true false-negative rate cannot be ascertained from our data because routine contralateral explorations were not done. We are convinced, however, that if the contralateral groins had been explored, few hernias would have been found.

There have been no complications related to the procedure itself, including no instances of respiratory compromise or air embolism. Because of our concern that respiratory compromise could result from the distention of the peritoneal cavity by the insufflated air, we advocate performing the technique only under general anesthesia with endotracheal intubation. We do not believe that use of mask general anesthesia, local anesthesia, or regional anesthesia is appropriate when diagnostic pneumoperitoneum is performed. We also attempt to evacuate all of the insufflated air possible before removal of the Robinson catheter and repair of the ipsilateral hernia sac. Another theoretical concern, not encountered in this series, is the risk of air embolism. We believe this risk is low and have continued to use manual insufflation with room air, as described. The use of an automatic insufflator and carbon dioxide gas in an attempt to better quantitate the degree of pneumoperitoneum and reduce the risk of air embolus, however, would be reasonable. Additionally, we do not perform the test in children with intra-abdominal foreign bodies, such as ventriculoperitoneal or peritoneovenous shunts, because of the risk of air embolism through the shunt tubing.

We were concerned about the technical failure rate of 10.8% because of our inability to pass a 10- to 14-F Robinson catheter through the neck of the hernia sac. This problem occurred only in male patients and was always a result of the narrowing in the sac at the internal ring. The frequency of this problem was equal among those with hernias and communicating hydroceles. This problem could conceivably be corrected by the use of a smaller catheter.

Scant attention has been given to this procedure in the literature. In 1924, Farr[26] first described the use of pneumoperitoneum in the preoperative diagnosis of inguinal hernia. Arner and Fernstrom[27] reported the use of this procedure in the preoperative diagnosis of clinically uncertain inguinal hernias. In 1953, Shiozaki et al[28] reported the use of intraoperative diagnostic pneumoperitoneum in 49 patients with no complications and an 83.7% accuracy rate. Bulow[29] described 117 patients studied with this technique in 1974. In 14% of the patients, a contralateral hernia was demonstrated with no false-positive results and one false-negative result. The only complication noted was one case of localized subcutaneous emphysema that resolved spontaneously. Singh et al[30] performed a prospective evaluation of preoperative pneumoperitoneum with preoperative inguinal herniorrhaphy. They found that pneumoperitoneum was more reliable than inguinal herniography, having an accuracy rate of 98.4%, fewer complications, and fewer technical failures.

References

1. Powell RW: Intraoperative diagnostic pneumoperitoneum in pediatric patients with unilateral inguinal hernia: The Goldstein test. *J Pediatr Surg* 1985;20:418-421.
2. Snyder WH, Greaney EM Jr: Inguinal hernias, in Mustard UT, Kavitch MM, Snyder WH Jr, et al (eds): *Pediatric Surgery*, ed 2. Chicago, Year Book Medical Publishers Inc, 1969, pp 692-707.
3. Holder TM, Ashcraft KW: Groin hernias and hydrocoeles, in Holder TM, Ashcraft KW (eds): *Pediatric Surgery*, ed 1. Philadelphia, WB Saunders Co, 1980, pp 594-608.
4. Rowe MI, Copelson CW, Clatworthy HW: The patent processus vaginalis and the inguinal hernia. *J Pediatr Surg* 1969;4:102-107.
5. Rowe MI, Clatworthy HW Jr: The other side of the pediatric inguinal hernia. *Surg Clin North Am* 1971;51:1371-1376.
6. Bronsther B, Abrams ML, Elboim C: Inguinal hernias in children—a study of 1000 cases and a review of the literature. *JAMA* 1972;27:522-535.
7. Clausen EG, Jake RJ, Binkley FM: Contralateral inguinal exploration of unilateral hernia in infants and children. *Surgery* 1958;44:735-740.
8. Kiesewetter WB, Parenza NL: When should hernia in the infant be treated bilaterally? *JAMA* 1959;99:45-47.
9. Tepas JJ III, Stafford PW: Timing of automatic contralateral groin exploration in male infants with unilateral hernias. *Ann Surg* 1986;52:70-71.
10. Bock JE, Sobye JV: Frequency of contralateral inguinal hernia in children. *Acta Chir Scand* 1970;136:707-709.
11. Kiesewetter WB, Oh KS: Unilateral inguinal hernias in children. *Arch Surg* 1980;115:1443.
12. McGregor DB, Halverson K, McVay CB: The unilateral pediatric inguinal hernia: Should the contralateral side be explored? *J Pediatr Surg* 1980;15:313-317.
13. Brown RK: Hernia diagnosis by transperitoneal probing of the contralateral groin. *Surg Gynecol Obstet* 1964;118:123.
14. Avery JA II, Berg RA, Widmann WD: The clinical value of pediatric herniography. *AJDC* 1977;131:1255-1257.
15. Ducharme JC, Bensoussan AL, Guttman FM, et al: Herniography: Ten years and 1200 cases later. *Ann R Coll Phys Surg Can* 1976;9:78.
16. Ducharme JC, Bertrand R, Chacar R: Is it possible to diagnose inguinal hernia by x-ray? *J Can Assoc Radiol* 1967;18:448-451.
17. Gallegos F, Glass HG, Lynch RH: Inguinal herniography in cases of unilateral hernia to detect a contralateral hernia. *Int Surg* 1974;59:279-281.
18. Guttman FM, Bertrand R, Ducharme JC: Herniography and the contralateral inguinal hernia. *Surg Gynecol Obstet* 1972;135:551-555.
19. Ruiz PL, Ducharme JC, Bertrand R, et al: Inguinal herniography: Its value in the diagnosis of silent patent vaginal process. *Ann Radiol (Paris)* 1976;19:35-40.
20. Singh JP, Nagabhushanam V, Mehra S, et al: Herniography and inguinal hernia in childhood—a study of 100 cases. *Indian J Pediatr* 1972;9:710-714.
21. White JJ: Herniography—a perspective. *Surgery* 1978;83:363-364.
22. White JJ, Haller JA, Dorst JP: Congenital inguinal hernia and inguinal herniography. *Surg Clin North Am* 1970;50:823-837.
23. Iarchy J: Peritoneography, a safe method to assess the bilaterality of inguinal hernia in children with obvious unilateral hernia or cryptorchidism (100 cases). *Acta Chir Belg* 1983;83:253-260.
24. Ducharme JC, Guttman FM, Poljicak M: Hematoma of bowel and cellulitis of the abdominal wall complicating herniography. *J Pediatr Surg* 1980;15:318-319.
25. Butsch JL, Kuhn JP: Intramural hematoma of the small bowel: A possible lethal complication of herniography. *Surgery* 1978;83:121-122.
26. Farr RE: Pneumoperitoneum as an aid in diagnosis in hernia. *JAMA* 1924;82:1774-1775.
27. Arner O, Fernstrom I: The value of pneumoperitoneum in the diagnosis of hernia in the inguinal region. *Surgery* 1970;67:741-747.
28. Shiozaki A, Wada N, Tonoda S, et al: Evaluation of pneumoperitoneum as a criterion for a contralateral exploration in pediatric inguinal herniorrhaphy. *J Wakayama Med Soc* 1973;24:103-113.
29. Bulow W: Artificial pneumoperitoneum during inguinal herniotomy in children. *Acta Chir Scand* 1974;140:127-130.
30. Singh JP, Nagabhushanam V, Grover VK: Evaluation of herniography techniques in pediatric surgical cases. *Indian J Pediatr* 1974;11:705-710.

Prostaglandin E_2 in Pyloric Stenosis

Gideon Goldman, MD; Elsa Tiomny, MD; Perry J. Kahn, MD; Dalia Somjen, PhD;
Zamir Halpern, MD; Tuvia Gilat, MD; Theodor Wiznitzer, MD

• Prostaglandins are presumed to have many cytoprotective properties that play a role in the pathogenesis of duodenal ulcer and its complications where decreased levels of prostaglandin E_2 (PGE_2) impair gastric motility, oppose ionic membrane influx, and enhance obstructive changes. These are just some of the mechanisms that may cause pyloric obstruction and may result from decreased PGE_2 levels. To evaluate this hypothesis, 17 patients with duodenal ulcer complicated by pyloric stenosis were examined. Biopsy specimens were obtained from the duodenal bulb, ulcer margins, gastric antrum, fundus, and gastric secretions. Prostaglandin E_2 levels were measured and compared with those taken from the same areas during a second endoscopy in a later quiescent or exacerbated phase. During the active phase of pyloric stenosis, decreased levels of PGE_2 were found in the gastroduodenal tissues and secretions were compared with levels found during convalescence. These level differences were statistically significant. A correlation between the severity of the clinical and endoscopic findings and the PGE_2 levels was found. A further decrease in PGE_2 levels in the second endoscopy were indicative of the presence of scar tissue, representing an irreversible obstructive peptic disease.

(*Arch Surg* 1989;124:724-726)

Prostaglandin E_2 (PGE_2) and several other types of PGs have been shown to play a major role in the prevention of gastric mucosal lesions.[1] Initial studies suggested that the antiulcer effect of PGs was related to their known potent antisecretory properties. Subsequent experimental observations demonstrated that the mechanism of protection involved factors beyond simple inhibition of acid secretion. This ability of PGs to protect the cells has been termed *cytoprotection*.[2] The mechanism underlying gastric cytoprotection is not yet fully understood. Prostaglandins may enhance gastric musocal blood flow,[3] stimulate mucus and bicarbonate secretions,[4] improve synthesis of macromolecules and transport processes,[5] increase gastric mucosal cyclic adenosine monophosphate content,[6] and affect gastric motility.[7]

Clinical investigations revealed the possible beneficial effects of PG administration on the prevention and healing of gastric and duodenal lesions.[8] These observations raised the possibility that further decreases in PGE_2 levels may be present during duodenal ulcer complications and specifically during pyloric stenosis (PS). To evaluate this hypothesis, we studied the levels of PGE_2 in patients suffering from PS. A comparison was made between levels measured during active, quiescent, and exacerbated phases of the disease.

Accepted for publication Aug 29, 1988.
From the Departments of Surgery "A" (Drs Goldman, Tiomny, Kahn, and Wiznitzer) and Gastroenterology (Drs Halpern and Gilat) and the Tissue Laboratory (Dr Somjen), Ichilov Hospital, Tel-Aviv Medical Center and Sackler School of Medicine, Tel-Aviv University, Tel-Aviv, Israel.
Reprints not available.

PATIENTS AND METHODS
Study Groups

Our study group consisted of 17 patients with duodenal ulcer. All presented at the emergency ward with symptoms of PS as the initial symptom of their peptic disease. Patients having had a history of duodenal ulcer were excluded from this study. None had received anti-PG or antiulcer drugs.

Pyloric stenosis was determined in all patients by the following criteria: (1) clinical—voluminous vomiting of gastric contents devoid of bile and a residual gastric aspirate volume above 700 mL/24 h, (2) laboratory—signs of dehydration with hemoconcentration accompanied by hypokalemic alkalosis, and (3) endoscopic findings—with a stenosed pyloric canal functional with a hyperemic, edematous, and friable mucosa or organic with a scarred rigid canal.

From admission to the emergency ward until gastroscopy was performed, nasogastric suction was continued, and no antiulcer medication was initiated. Gastroscopy was performed by the same endoscopist 12 to 24 hours from admission with a gastroscope. Premedication for gastroscopy consisted of fentanyl citrate,

Table 1.—Clinical and Endoscopic Data

Presenting Symptoms	No. of Patients: First Endoscopy	Second Endoscopy
	Group A*	
Vomiting, 11	Pyloric spasm, 11	Complete healing, 9
Epigastric pain, 8	Erosive gastritis, 4	Duodenitis, 2
Weight loss, 9	Gastric ulcer, 2	...
	Group B†	
Vomiting, 6	Pyloric stenosis, 6	Pyloric stenosis, 6
Epigastric pain, 6	Erosive gastritis, 1	Gastric dilatation, 2
Weight loss, 6	Gastric ulcer, 1	Erosive gastritis, 2

*Eleven patients; mean age, 66.7 years.
†Six patients; mean age, 69.3 years.

Table 2.—Prostaglandin E_2 Levels in Various Sites*

Phase	Ulcer Margins	Antrum	Fundus	Gastric Secretions	Mean
Group A					
Pyloric spasm	61 ± 39	113 ± 72	99 ± 62	24 ± 36	69 ± 56†
Convalescence	510 ± 61	127 ± 16	169 ± 15	213 ± 35	244 ± 101
Group B					
Pyloric stenosis	108 ± 63	173 ± 33	133 ± 86	‡	138 ± 69§
Deterioration	47 ± 12	116 ± 14	109 ± 20	‡	87 ± 18

*Values given in picograms per milligram of protein; expressed as mean ± SD.
†$P = .02$.
‡Prostaglandin E_2 levels in gastric secretions were measured as well, but chronic gastric dilatation and mucosal damage in this group rendered secretion sampling meaningless.
§$P < .05$.

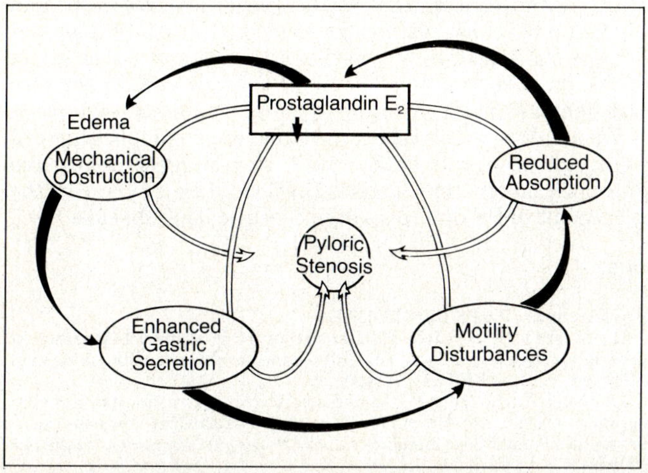

Possible role of prostaglandin E_2 in pyloric stenosis pathogenesis.

0.05 mg, atropine sulfate, 0.5 mg, and diazepam, 5 mg, all administered intravenously.

At the initial gastroscopy before any endoscopic manipulation, gastric secretions were aspirated and sampled for PGE_2 determination, following which two biopsy specimens each were obtained from the gastric antrum (3 cm from the pylorus), gastric fundus, duodenal bulb, and ulcer margins. Each biopsy specimen weighing 1 mg was assayed for PGE_2 levels separately.

A third biopsy specimen from the ulcer margin was sent for pathologic examination to ascertain that no necrotic tissue was present, and a fourth biopsy specimen was obtained from the stenosed pyloric canal for histologic typing to substantiate the endoscopic impression of the kind of stenosis, either functional, with edematous mucosa, with chronic and acute inflammatory infiltrates, or organic, with fibrotic mucosal changes.

During the initial hospitalization, after gastroscopy was performed, all 17 patients received identical treatment with nasogastric suction, nutritional maintenance of 10 500 J (2500 calories) per day through total parenteral nutrition and 1600 mg of H_2 blocker (cimetidine) per day divided into four doses. On release from the hospital, the patients were given a rigid, appropriate, identical diet.

Of the 17 patients in our study group, 11 proved to have had a functional stenosis. Biopsy specimens from the pyloric canal showed the mucosa with chronic and acute inflammatory infiltrates. These patients responded to therapy well and became asymptomatic, whereby all symptoms of nausea and vomiting ceased, and were able to ingest normal quantities of food. They received H_2-blocker treatment for five weeks and underwent endoscopy again electively eight weeks from initial admission. During the three-week interval when no H_2-blocker drugs were ingested, no symptoms of PS had recurred, and before the repeated endoscopy, gastric rest was measured by nasogastric suction. In 11 patients (group A), gastric rest did not exceed 50 mL of bile-stained aspirate. Endoscopy was repeated at the same sites (twice each) as the initial endoscopy, and gastric aspirate was sampled for determination of PGE_2 levels. These levels were compared with those found at initial endoscopy.

The remaining six patients (group B) were found to have organic PS as proved histologically by fibrotic changes in the pyloric canal. With H_2-blocker treatment, they continued to suffer intermittent obstructive symptoms, with repeated nausea and vomiting of gastric contents after food ingestion. Four patients had to be rehospitalized when their symptoms intensified, whereupon a second endoscopy was performed (five to seven weeks after the first) after initial gastric aspirate volume was measured (average, 700 mL devoid of bile). The PGE_2 levels of the biopsy specimens and gastric aspirate were again assayed and compared with those determined on the first endoscopy. Two patients underwent endoscopy electively eight weeks after the first endoscopy for PGE_2 determination (H_2-blocker treatment was ceased three weeks before the second endoscopy) but were reported to be suffering from occasional vomiting and epigastric pain during the interim between endoscopies, with a slight intensification of the symptoms during the period without H_2-blocker treatment.

The presenting symptoms and endoscopic findings of both groups are given in Table 1. The statistical significance of PGE_2 difference was analyzed by Fisher's exact test.

PGE_2 Determination

The specimens were collected in plastic tubes and frozen immediately in liquid nitrogen and kept at −18°C until analysis. The quick freezing is necessary to avoid pertrubation of the tissue and the continual production of PGE_2 as a response to trauma. Biopsy material was homogenized in 1 mL of buffered acetate (40 nmol/L; pH, 4.0). Three volumes of ethyl acetate were added and mixed well, and the organic and aqueous phases were separated. This manipulation in an acidic pH environment helps eliminate arachidonic acid. The upper organic phase containing the PGE_2 was collected, and the ethyl acetate was evaporated. The yield of PG extraction as measured by labeled tritiated PGE_2 was over 90%. The residue was dissolved in buffered 0.1% sodium azide. The aqueous phase was used for protein determination. Prostaglandin E_2 was assayed using a PGE_2 radioimmunoassay kit.[9-13] The antibodies used in this kit showed 6% cross-reactivity with PGA_2, 3% with PGA_1, about 1% with 6-keto-PGE_1 and $PGE_{2\alpha}$, and less than 1% with all other PGs. The assay is reproducible within 5% in those done at different times. Protein was assayed by the Coomassie brilliant blue dye binding method with bovine serum albumin as standard.[14] The PGE_2 levels were expressed in picograms per milligrams of protein, with each patient serving as his own control.

As gastric secretions also contain protein, PGE_2 content was calculated in the sample material per protein content.

RESULTS

Of the 17 patients studied, 11 (group A) were found to present with pyloric spasm due to an active peptic disease. Their average age was 66.7 years. The presenting symptoms, consisting of vomiting, epigastric pain, and weight loss, together with endoscopic findings, are described in Table 1.

Prostaglandin E_2 levels from various sites sampled are given in Table 2. The increase in PGE_2 levels accompanying the clinical and endoscopic findings on repeated tests two months later are also shown in Table 2. This increase in PGE_2 levels was found to be of statistical significance ($P=.02$). The PGE_2 level increase was most marked in samples from the ulcer margins and gastric secretions.

Six patients (group B), with an average age of 69.3 years, had low PGE_2 levels found at first endoscopies on admission (Table 2). Repeated tests during their clinical deterioration showed both a deterioration in the endoscopic findings and a further decrease of statistical significance ($P<.05$) in PGE_2 levels (Table 2).

COMMENT

Pyloric stenosis is a complication of peptic ulcer disease. We believe that decreased levels of PGE_2 play an important role in the pathogenesis of this complication and aggravate the condition by a positive feedback mechanism (Figure). By causing functional gastric outlet obstruction and increased histamine release, active ulcer disease leads to increased gastric secretion, reduction of mucosal absorption, and gastric motility disturbance.[15-18] These are the pathophysiologic mechanisms that presumably play an important role in the pathogenesis of PS and that may be triggered or result from a PGE_2 level decrease.

This study confirms a decrease in PGE_2 levels during the active phase of pyloric spasm and stenosis and increased levels during convalescence. Conversely, a deterioration in the clinical and endoscopic findings was associated with a continued reduction in the PGE_2 level. A correlation was observed between the severity of the clinical and endoscopic findings and the decreased levels of PGE_2 in all sites tested. The six patients with true PS that did not heal and a demonstrated decrease in PGE_2 levels required bypass operations. We believe that the inability of the tissue to produce PGs indicates the presence of fibrosis rather than normal mucosa and represents an irreversible stage of the obstructed peptic disease. Group A showed both increased PGE_2 levels concomitant with clinical improvement and needed only conservative treatment. Our study does not answer the question of whether PGs are a cause or effect of PS, but a correlation between PG levels and PS severity was demonstrated.

We emphasize the relationship between complications of peptic disease and PGE_2 levels and suggest a possible pathophysiologic mechanism that could be applied in the treatment of PS due to an active peptic ulcer disease.

References

1. Cloud WG, Ritchie WP: Evidence of cytoprotection by endogenous prostaglandins in gastric mucosa treated with bile acid. *Surg Forum* 1982;33:150-152.
2. Johansson C, Bergstrom S: Prostaglandins and protection of gastroduodenal mucosa. *Scand J Gastroenterol* 1982;77:21-46.
3. Koturek SJ, Robert A, Honchar AJ, et al: Comparison of prostacyclin and prostaglandin E_2 on gastric secretion, gastric release and mucosal blood flow in dogs. *Dig Dis Sci* 1980;25:673-679.
4. Garner A, Heylings JR: Stimulation of alkaline secretion in amphibian isolated gastric mucosa by 16.16 dimethyl PGE_2 and PGF_2. *Gastroenterology* 1979;76:491-503.
5. Dejani EZ, Callison DA, Butermann RE: Effects of prostaglandins on canine gastric potential difference. *Dig Dis Sci* 1978;23:436-442.
6. Miller TA: Protective effects of prostaglandins against gastric mucosal damage: Current knowledge and proposed mechanism. *Am J Physiol* 1983;245:G601-G603.
7. Sanders KM, Kenton M: Role of prostaglandins in regulating gastric motility. *Am J Physiol* 1984;247:G117-G126.
8. Vantrappen G, Janssens J, Papiela T, et al: Effect of 15(R)-15-methyl prostaglandin E_2 (arbaprostil) on healing of duodenal ulcer: A double blind, multicenter study. *Gastroenterology* 1982;83:357-363.
9. Jaffee B, Behrman HR, Parker CS: Radioimmunoassay measurement of prostaglandins E, A and F in human plasma. *J Clin Invest* 1973;52:398.
10. Jobke A, Peskar BA, Peskar BM: On the specificity of antisera against prostaglandins. *FEBS Lett* 1973;37:192.
11. Lingren JA, Kindahl H, Hammarstrom S: Radioimmunoassay of prostaglandins E_2 and F_2 in cell culture media utilizing antisera against PGF_2 and PGE_2. *FEBS Lett* 1974;48:22.
12. Green K, Hamberg M, Samuelsson B, et al: Extraction and chromatographic procedures for purification of prostaglandins, thromboxanes, prostacyclines and their metabolites. *Adv Prostaglandin Thromboxane Res* 1978;5:15.
13. Granstrom E, Kindahl H: Radioimmunoassay of prostaglandin and thromboxanes. *Adv Prostaglandin Thromboxane Res* 1978;5:119.
14. Bradford MM: Rapid and sensitive method for quantitation of microgram quantity of protein utilizing the principle of protein dye binding. *Anal Biochem* 1976;72:248-254.
15. Rober A: Cytoprotection of the gastrointestinal mucosa, in Stollerman GH, Harrington WJ, LaMont JT (eds): *Advances in Internal Medicine.* Chicago, Year Book Medical Publishers Inc, 1983, vol 28, pp 325-337.
16. Wilson DE: Therapeutic aspects of prostaglandins in the treatment of peptic ulcer disease. *Dig Dis Sci* 1986;31(suppl):42S.
17. Wilson DE, Kaymakalan H: Prostaglandins: Gastrointestinal effects and peptic ulcer disease. *Med Clin North Am* 1986;65:773-787.
18. Muller P, Damann HG, Simon B, et al: Prostaglandins and human gastric mucosa: Molecular aspects and protective properties, in Allen A, Flemström G, Garner A, et al (eds): *Mechanism of Mucosal Protection in the Upper Gastrointestinal Tract.* New York, Raven Press, 1984.

The Effect of Endotoxin on Glucose Metabolism in Skeletal Muscle Requires the Presence of Plasma

Joseph F. Amaral, MD; Jeffry D. Shearer, MA; Balduino Mastrofrancesco, MS;
Donald S. Gann, MD; Michael D. Caldwell, MD, PhD

• The administration of endotoxin in vivo results in an increase in glucose utilization through an as yet undetermined mechanism. This study evaluated (1) the contribution of blood to the increased glucose utilization noted following endotoxemia, (2) the direct action of endotoxin on skeletal muscle glucose uptake in an isolated hindlimb perfusion system and in incubated muscle, and (3) the possibility that the increased glucose uptake in skeletal muscle mediated by endotoxin requires the presence of plasma. Incubation of blood with 50 and 100 mg/L of endotoxin increased glucose uptake and lactate production in a dose-dependent manner. Muscle incubations and perfusions in the absence of plasma and white blood cells showed that glucose uptake and lactate production were not affected by the presence of 50 to 250 mg/L of endotoxin, while 500 mg/L of endotoxin produced a 26.2% decrease in glucose uptake. In contrast, incubation of muscle in the presence of plasma and endotoxin increased glucose uptake by 37%. These findings suggest that (1) the increased glucose utilization of endotoxemia is only partially explained by increased glucose metabolism by blood, (2) endotoxin does not have a direct effect on the glucose uptake of skeletal muscle, and (3) an interaction of endotoxin with a component of plasma is required for an endotoxin-mediated increase in glucose utilization by skeletal muscle.

(*Arch Surg* 1989;124:727-732)

Endotoxemia and septic shock are characteristically associated with transient hyperglycemia, followed by sustained hypoglycemia.[1-5] The mechanism(s) for the hypoglycemia has been the object of considerable investigation, particularly in light of the finding that the prevention of hypoglycemia by the administration of intravenous glucose prevents death in animals subjected to endotoxemia.[6]

There are at least five possible mechanisms for the development of hypoglycemia after endotoxin administration as follows: (1) a decrease in glucose production, (2) an increase in glucose utilization, (3) a decrease in glucose intake, (4) an increase in the volume of distribution for glucose, and (5) an increase in the renal loss of glucose. The last three possibilities are unlikely to contribute substantially to the development of hypoglycemia by themselves, since a concomitant inhibition of glucose production would also be necessary. Furthermore, nephrectomized animals develop hypoglycemia in the presence of endotoxemia at the same rate as nonnephrectomized dogs,[7] the blood flow to the kidneys during endotoxemia is decreased rather than increased,[8] and urinary excretion of glucose is not detectable during endotoxemia.[9]

A considerable amount of evidence supports the possibility that endotoxin mediates a decrease in hepatic glucose production. Both in vitro[10,11] and in vivo[12-14] studies have shown a decrease in hepatic gluconeogenesis during endotoxemia. A possible mechanism for the depression in hepatic gluconeogenesis following the administration of endotoxin has been described by Moore and colleagues,[15] who noted an inhibition of hepatic phosphoenolpyruvate carboxykinase by a macrophage product. However, an impairment in hepatic gluconeogenesis does not appear to be sufficient to explain the hypoglycemia that develops during endotoxemia. For example, Kelleher et al[16] and Merrill and Spitzer[17] reported an increase in hepatic glucose production during septic shock in the presence of hypoglycemia; Peyton et al[14] described the more rapid development of hypoglycemia in eviscerated, endotoxin-treated dogs than in controls; and Wolfe et al[13] described the development of hypoglycemia in endotoxemia before the development of impaired gluconeogenesis. These data suggest that an increase in peripheral glucose utilization is also necessary for the development of hypoglycemia.

An increase in the peripheral utilization of glucose following the administration of endotoxin has been well documented by in vivo studies. Wolfe et al[13] and Kelleher et al[16] noted an increase in the disappearance of glucose during endotoxic and septic shock that was associated with an increase in lactate production. The heart, lungs,[18] and central nervous system[19] do not appear to contribute to the increase in glucose utilization. However, Hinshaw and colleagues[3,20] found an increase in glucose uptake by blood and by white blood cells in the presence of endotoxin, and Holley and Spitzer[21] and Witek-Janusek and Filkins[22] noted an increase in the oxidation of glucose by adipose tissue in the presence of endotoxin. Meszaros et al[23] recently described sustained increases in glucose utilization by organs rich in mononuclear phagocytes (the liver and spleen) and found no change in glucose uptake by the brain or testis in animals exposed to endotoxin.

Skeletal muscle, which constitutes 40% to 45% of the lean body mass and accounts for 30% of the total oxygen (O_2) consumption at rest,[24] is a probable site for the increased glucose utilization in response to endotoxin. In fact, recent studies that examined the metabolism of canine hindlimbs in vivo during endotoxemia have shown an increase in glucose uptake and lactate release.[4,5] These results were variably attributed either to a direct effect[5] or to an anoxic effect[4] of endotoxin on skeletal muscle. The latter explanation is unlikely, since an increase in glucose uptake and lactate production in the hindlimb tissue was noted even in the absence of anoxia.[5] Additional studies by Meszaros et al[25] showed that glucose uptake by skeletal muscle in vivo is increased transiently following administration of endotoxin. However, these in vivo studies did not address the mechanism for this endotoxin-mediated increase in glucose utilization by skeletal muscle.

The present study evaluated (1) the contribution of blood to the increased glucose utilization noted following endo-

Accepted for publication March 15, 1988.

From the Department of Surgery, Brown University (Drs Amaral, Gann, and Caldwell, and Messrs Shearer and Mastrofrancesco) and the Surgical Metabolism Laboratory, The Rhode Island Hospital (Messrs Shearer and Mastrofrancesco and Dr Caldwell), Providence, RI.

Reprint requests to Department of Surgery, The Rhode Island Hospital, 593 Eddy St, Providence, RI 02902 (Dr Caldwell).

toxemia, (2) the direct action of endotoxin on skeletal muscle glucose uptake in an isolated hindlimb perfusion system and in incubated muscle, and (3) the possibility that the increased glucose uptake in skeletal muscle mediated by endotoxin requires the presence of plasma.

MATERIALS AND METHODS

Animals and Anesthesia

Male Sprague-Dawley rats were used in all perfusions, and male Fisher rats were used in all incubations. These animals were housed under constant environmental conditions with 12-hour light-dark cycles and maintained on rat chow (RMH 3000, Agway Inc, Syracuse, NY) with free access to water. The mean ± SEM weight of rats used was 165 ± 2.5 g in the hindlimb perfusions, 60 ± 2.5 g in muscle incubations, 125 ± 2.5 g in epididymal fat pad incubations, and 350 ± 20 g in blood incubations. Rats were anesthetized before all experiments and procedures by the intraperitoneal injection (50 mg/kg of body weight) of a commercial preparation of pentobarbital sodium (Nembutal, Abbott Laboratories, North Chicago, Ill).

Epididymal Fat Pad Incubations

Epididymal fat pads were incubated by a modification of the technique of Witek-Janusek and Filkins.[22] A portion of an epididymal fat pad that weighed approximately 100 mg was isolated with a suture, removed, and rinsed with room temperature Krebs-Ringer bicarbonate buffer (KRBB). The fat pads were then preincubated at 37°C in glass vials that contained 2 mL of a continuously oxygenated (95% oxygen [O_2]: 5% carbon dioxide [CO_2]) incubation medium composed of KRBB, 4% bovine serum albumin, and 1 mmol/L of glucose. After a 30-minute preincubation, the fat pads were removed from the vials, washed in room temperature KRBB, and blotted. They were then placed in new glass vials that contained 2 mL of fresh, preoxygenated (O_2 pressure [Po_2] approximately equal to 600 mm Hg) incubation medium with uniformly labeled (U-[^{14}C]) glucose (0.1 μCi/mmol of glucose) and either no endotoxin, 250 mg/L of endotoxin, or 1794 pmol/L of insulin. The vials were then capped with rubber stoppers that held a center well (Kontes, Vineland, NJ) containing a filter paper wick and 200 μL of Scintisorb-C (Isolabs, Inc, Akron, Ohio) and incubated for one hour in a shaking water bath at 37°C. At the end of the incubation, the fat pads were removed, blotted dry, and weighed. A 500-μL aliquot of incubate was removed from the vial and stored at −80°C until assay. The vial was then recapped, and 1.5 mL of 0.7N perchloric acid was injected into the vial to evolve the dissolved CO_2 according to the method of Rodbell.[26] At the end of an additional hour of incubation, the center wells were removed and counted in 5 mL of Scintisorb-C.

Blood Incubations

Blood was removed from the abdominal aorta with heparinized syringes, pooled, and heparinized with 0.2 mL of heparin sodium (Elkins-Sinn, Inc, Cherry Hills, NJ) per 10 mL of blood. Blood was incubated in 2-mL aliquots for one hour in a shaking water bath at 37°C, with continuous oxygenation with 95% O_2:5% CO_2 without endotoxin or in the presence of 50 or 100 mg/L of endotoxin. At the end of the incubation, 1 mL of blood was removed for determination of the hematocrit; 1 mL of blood was centrifuged to obtain plasma, and the plasma was frozen until assayed for plasma glucose and lactate.

Perfusion Experiments

Overnight-fasted animals were placed in a Vanderbilt perfusion apparatus and surgically prepared for hindlimb perfusion using a previously described technique.[27] The perfusate consisted of continuously oxygenated KRBB containing 4% bovine serum albumin, 10 mmol/L of glucose with 0.05 μCi/mL of U-[^{14}C] glucose, 2 mmol/L of lactate, 0.2 mmol/L of pyruvate, physiologic amino acid concentrations,[27] and washed, outdated human erythrocytes that were added to give a hematocrit of 0.3.

Following a five-minute flow-through period and a 15-minute recirculating preperfusion at 10 mL/min, a 5-mL bolus of either KRBB alone, B5:55 *Escherichia coli* endotoxin (Sigma Chemical Co, St Louis) dissolved in KRBB, or insulin (Humalin, Eli Lilly & Co, Indianapolis) dissolved in KRBB was added to the perfusate.

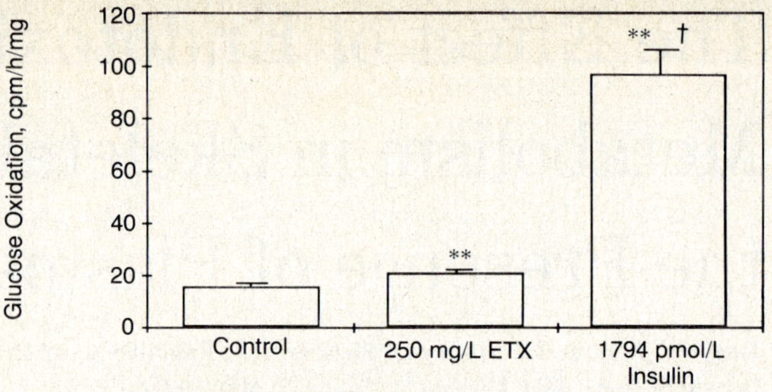

Fig 1.—Glucose oxidation by fat pads. Incubation of fat pads with 250 mg/L of endotoxin (ETX) increased glucose oxidation by 32.1%. This response was less than that seen in presence of 1.8 nmol/L (250 mU/L) of insulin in which 525% increase in glucose oxidation was noted. There was no difference in initial specific activity of glucose in this experiment. Two asterisks indicate $P<.01$ vs control; dagger, $P<.01$ vs ETX.

Fig 2.—Glucose uptake and lactate production by blood. Glucose uptake and lactate production by blood were increased by 50 and 100 mg/L of endotoxin (ETX). Data are expressed on basis of whole blood. a indicates $P<.05$ vs control; b, $P<.01$ vs 50 mg/L of ETX.

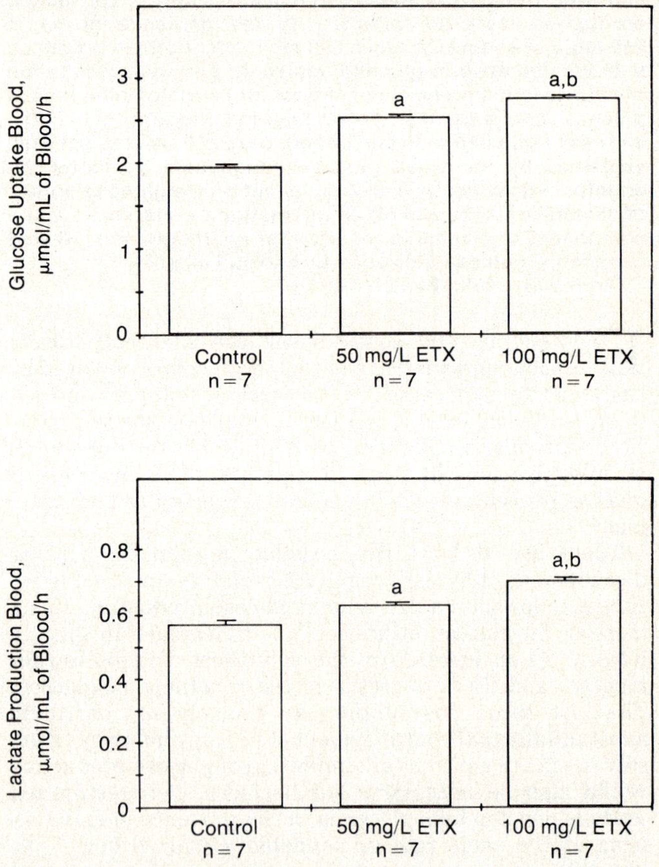

The endotoxin was added to the perfusates to achieve an initial calculated concentration of endotoxin in the perfusate of 50 or 500 mg/L. Insulin was added to the perfusates to achieve an initial calculated concentration of insulin in the perfusate of 1.8 nmol/L (250 mU/L). The hindlimbs of animals in each group were then perfused at a constant flow rate of 10 mL/min in a recirculating mode for an additional 60 minutes. Arterial and venous perfusate samples were taken at 20-minute intervals. At the end of the perfusions, approximately 1 g of muscle was rapidly frozen using tongs as described by Wollenberger and colleagues[28] and stored at −80°C. The initial pH of the perfusate in all perfusions was 7.4 to

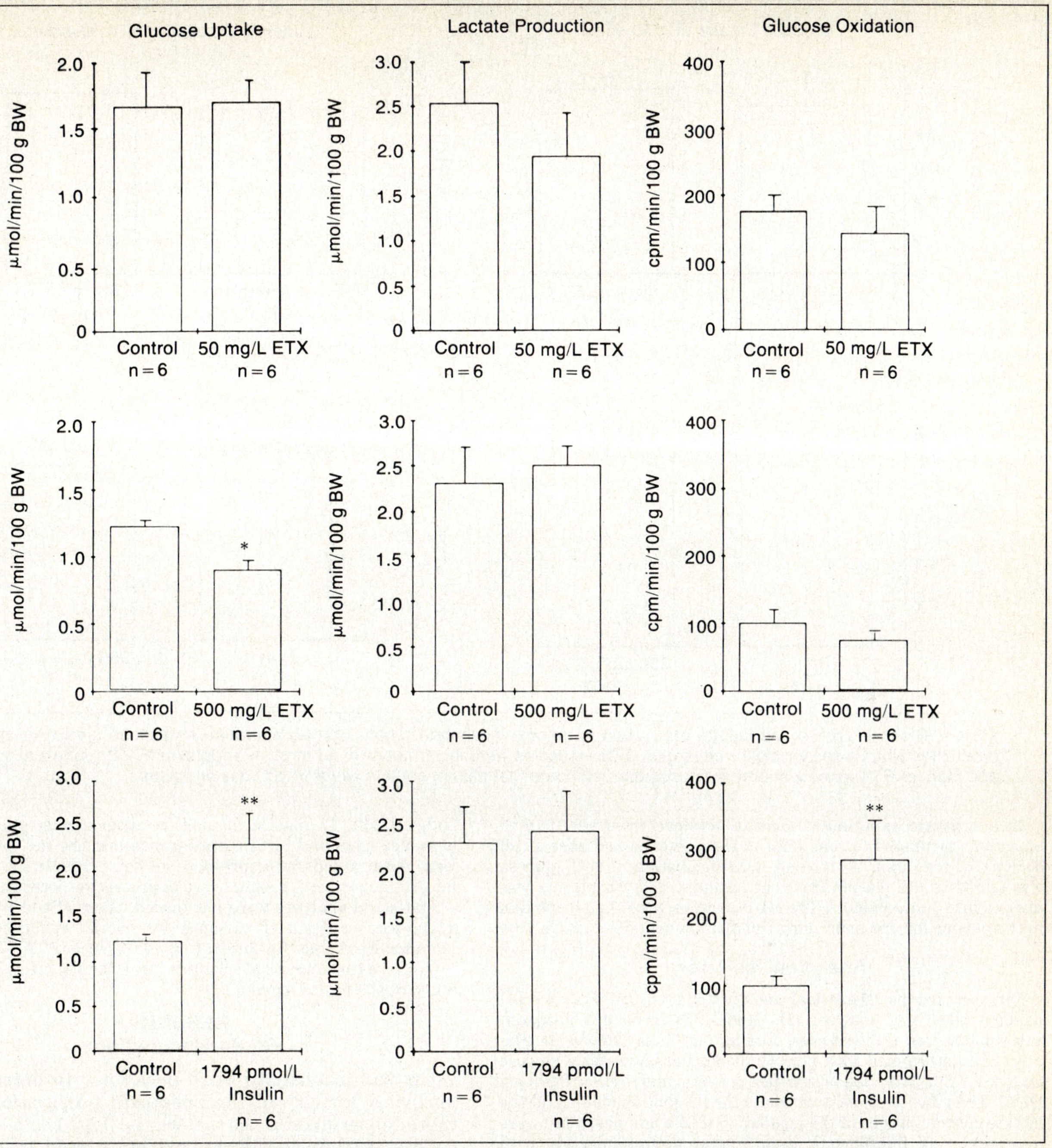

Fig 3.—Glucose metabolism in hindlimb perfusions. There was no alteration in glucose uptake, lactate production, or carbon dioxide (CO_2) production when hindlimbs were perfused with 50 mg/L of endotoxin (ETX) (panels at top). Perfusion of rat hindlimbs with 500 mg/L of endotoxin decreased glucose uptake by 26.2% with no alteration in lactate or CO_2 production (panels at center). In contrast, perfusion of hindlimb tissue with 1794 pmol/L of insulin increased glucose uptake by 90.2% and CO_2 production by 178.5% (panels at bottom). One asterisk indicates $P<.05$ vs control; two asterisks, $P<.01$ vs control; and BW, body weight.

7.5, and the initial arterial Po_2 was greater than 300 mm Hg. These values were relatively unchanged for the duration of each perfusion.

Muscle Incubation Technique

The extensor digitorum longus (EDL) muscles were incubated by a modification of the technique of Pain and Manchester.[29] The EDL muscles were rapidly removed, rinsed with room temperature KRBB, and placed on muscle holders to maintain resting length. The muscles were then preincubated at 37°C in polystyrene tubes that contained 3 mL of a continuously oxygenated (95% O_2:5% CO_2) incubation medium composed of KRBB (pH 7.4), 4% bovine serum albumin, and 1 or 5 mmol/L of glucose. After a 30-minute preincubation, the muscles were removed from the test tubes, washed in room temperature KRBB, and blotted. They were then placed in new incubation tubes that contained 3 mL of fresh incubate with U-[^{14}C] glucose (0.1 μCi/mmol of glucose) and either no endotoxin or 50 or 250 mg/L of endotoxin. The tubes were then incubated for one hour at 37°C in a shaking water bath with continuous oxygenation (95% O_2:5% CO_2). At the end of the one-hour incubation, the muscles were removed, washed in room temperature KRBB, blotted dry, rapidly frozen in liquid nitrogen, and stored at −80°C until assayed. The incubation medium was removed and stored at −80°C until assayed.

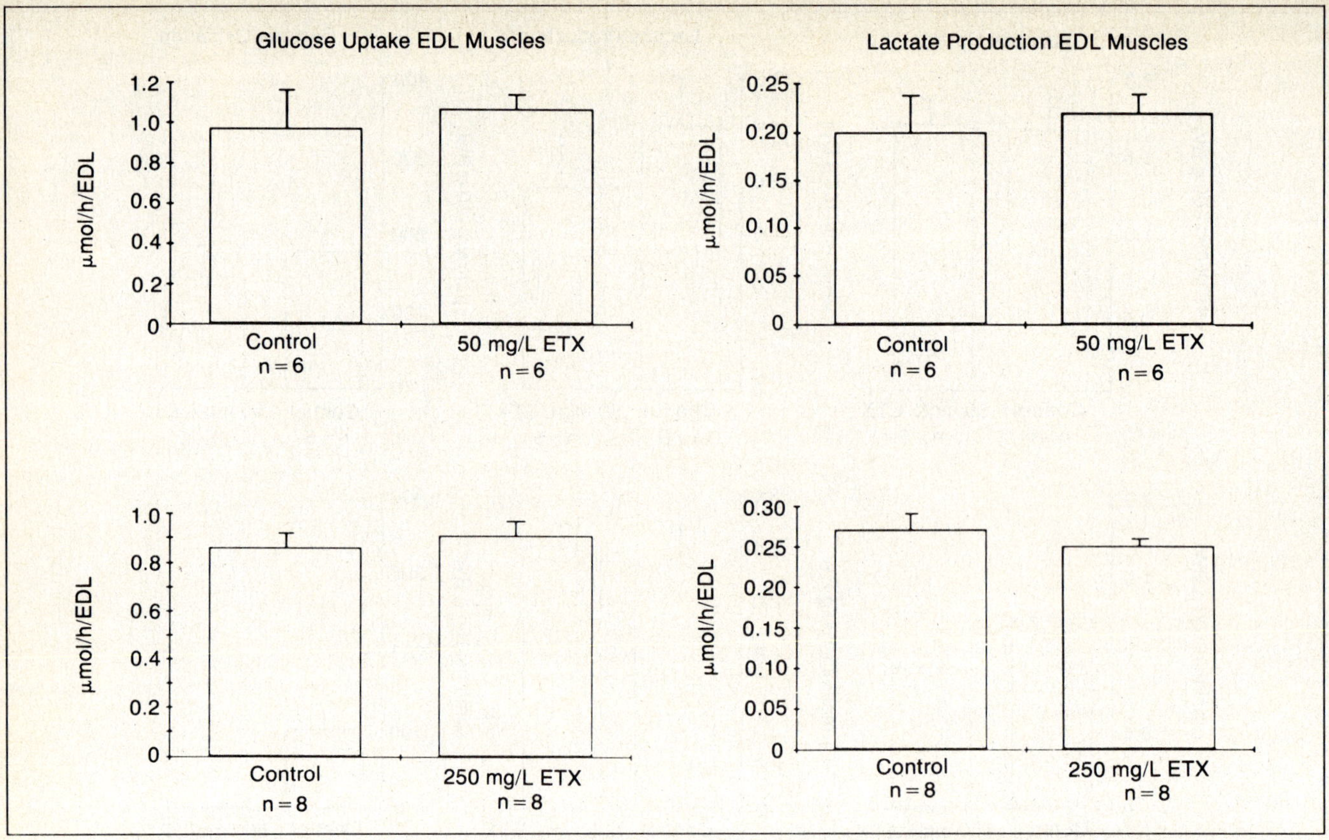

Fig 4.—Glucose uptake and lactate production in muscle incubation. There was no alteration in glucose uptake or lactate production when extensor digitorum longus (EDL) muscles were incubated with 50 mg/L of endotoxin (ETX) (panels at top) or 250 mg/L of ETX (panels at bottom) in standard incubate that did not contain white blood cells or plasma.

In a separate experiment, plasma obtained from centrifuged blood was incubated for one hour in the presence and absence of 50 mg/L of endotoxin. At the end of the incubation, U-[^{14}C] glucose was added to the plasma from both groups, and the plasma was divided into 3-mL aliquots. The EDL muscles were then incubated in the plasma for one hour using the method described above.

Analytical Methods

Perfusate samples were analyzed for CO_2 pressure, Po_2, and pH using a blood gas analyzer (IL Model 213 blood gas analyzer, Instrumentation Laboratories, Lexington, Mass). Perfusate glucose was determined by a glucose oxidase assay using a glucose analyzer (YSI-23A, Yellow Springs Instruments, Yellow Springs, Ohio). The glucose concentrations of the incubation media and the lactate concentrations of the incubation media and perfusate were determined by fluorometric assay[30] after deproteinization with 0.7N perchloric acid. Production of [^{14}C]O_2 was measured by injecting arterial and venous perfusate samples (1 mL) into the main compartment of counting vials. The counting vials contained center wells that held 0.2 mL of Scintisorb-C and filter paper wicks in gelatin capsules and 1 mL of 0.7N perchloric acid in the main compartment. After incubation of the counting vials in a shaking water bath at 37°C for one hour, the gelatin capsules in the center wells were removed and counted in 5 mL of Scintisorb-C. The specific activity of glucose and lactate in both incubate and perfusate was determined by a modification of the method of Rich et al.[31] Effluent peaks for glucose and lactate were separated by high-pressure liquid chromatography, collected, and then counted.

Calculations and Statistical Analysis of Results

The specific activity of U-[^{14}C] glucose remained constant throughout all experiments. As a result, the mean initial specific activity was used for all calculations in these experiments. In perfusion experiments, glucose uptake and lactate production were calculated on the basis of arterial concentrations at 20 and 80 minutes. All results were expressed on the basis of a 100-g body weight. In muscle incubation experiments, glucose disappearance from and lactate appearance into the incubation media were determined and expressed per total muscle. In epididymal fat pad incubations, results were expressed on a weight basis.

Statistical analyses were performed using a Student's t test or a one-way analysis of variance for overall differences with a Neuman-Keul test for intergroup differences.[32] All results are reported as mean±SEM. Sample sizes for each experiment are noted in the figure legends.

RESULTS

Fat Pad Incubations

Fat pad incubations were performed to determine the biological activity of the endotoxin preparation used in these experiments. As shown in Fig 1, 250 mg/L of endotoxin increased glucose oxidation by 32.1% (15.6±0.9 to 20.6±1.8 cpm/h/mg of fat [$P<.01$]). This response was considerably less than that seen in the presence of 1.8 nmol/L of insulin in which a 525% increase in glucose oxidation was noted (15.6±0.9 to 97.5±10.1 cpm/h/mg of fat [$P<.001$]). There was no difference in the initial specific activity of glucose in these three experiments.

Blood Incubation

The mean initial blood glucose concentration was 6.0±0.1 mmol/L of blood and that of lactate was 1.9±0.02 mmol/L of blood. As shown in Fig 2, incubation of blood with 50 mg/L of endotoxin increased glucose uptake by blood by 30% ($P<.01$). Incubation of blood with 100 mg/L of endotoxin resulted in a further increase in glucose uptake. This was equivalent to a 41% increase vs control ($P<.01$) and a 9% increase vs blood incubated with 50 mg/L of endotoxin ($P<.01$).

Lactate production paralleled glucose uptake. As shown

in Fig 2, incubation of blood with 50 mg/L of endotoxin increased lactate production by blood by 10% ($P<.01$). Incubation of blood with 100 mg/L of endotoxin resulted in a further increase in lactate production. This was equivalent to a 24% increase vs control ($P<.01$) and a 12% increase vs blood incubated with 50 mg/L of endotoxin ($P<.01$).

Hindlimb Perfusion and Muscle Incubation Studies

There was no difference in glucose uptake, lactate production, or CO_2 production when hindlimbs were perfused with or without 50 mg/L of endotoxin (Fig 3). Similarly, the incubation of the EDL muscles with endotoxin in concentrations of 50 or 250 mg/L of medium did not alter glucose uptake or lactate production over controls (Fig 4).

The perfusion of rat hindlimbs with 500 μg of endotoxin per milliliter of perfusate decreased glucose uptake by 26.2% (1.22±0.06 to 0.9±0.12 μmol/min/100 g of body weight [$P<.05$]) (Fig 3). There was no alteration in lactate or CO_2 production in the presence of 500 mg/L of endotoxin (Fig 3). In contrast, perfusion of the hindlimb tissue with 1.8 nmol/L of insulin increased glucose uptake and CO_2 production by 90.2% and 178.5%, respectively, with no alteration in lactate production (Fig 3).

Muscle Incubations in Plasma

When the EDL muscles were incubated in plasma that contained 50 mg/L of endotoxin, glucose uptake was increased by 37.6% (1.89±0.13 to 2.6±0.07 μmol/min/EDL muscle [$P<.01$]), and lactate production was increased by 26.7% (0.45±0.04 to 0.57±0.01 μmol/min/EDL muscle [$P<.05$]) (Fig 5) over EDL muscles that were incubated in plasma without endotoxin. There was no decrease in the plasma concentration of glucose when plasma was incubated for one hour with and without 50 mg/L of endotoxin.

COMMENT

The increased utilization of glucose by peripheral tissue during endotoxemia has been well documented.[3-5,13,14,16] The results of the present experiments confirm the work of Hinshaw et al[3] in that there was an increase in glucose uptake and lactate production by blood in the presence of 50 mg/L of endotoxin. Furthermore, these studies demonstrate a dose response to endotoxin since glucose uptake and lactate production were greater at 100 mg/L of endotoxin than at 50 mg/L. This is in agreement with the work of Cohn and Morse,[33] who demonstrated a nonlinear dose response for glucose uptake by polymorphonuclear leukocytes as the concentration of endotoxin was increased above 10 mg/L.

To our knowledge, the contribution of an endotoxin-stimulated increase in glucose uptake and lactate production by blood cells to the overall increase in glucose uptake demonstrated by hindlimb tissue in in vivo studies has not been previously examined. Using the data obtained in the present studies for the rat, blood exposed to 50 mg/L of endotoxin would increase its glucose uptake by 0.017 μmol/min/mL. Assuming a blood volume in the rat of 7.5% of body weight, it can be calculated that blood could increase endotoxin-stimulated total-body glucose uptake by 7.4% (from 1.72 to 1.85 μmol/min/100 g of body weight). A similar calculation can be performed for the dog by using the data of Hinshaw et al[3] for the response of blood to endotoxin and the data of Romanosky et al[5] or Raymond et al[4] for the response of hind limb tissue in vivo to endotoxin. Assuming a blood volume of 8% body weight,[34]

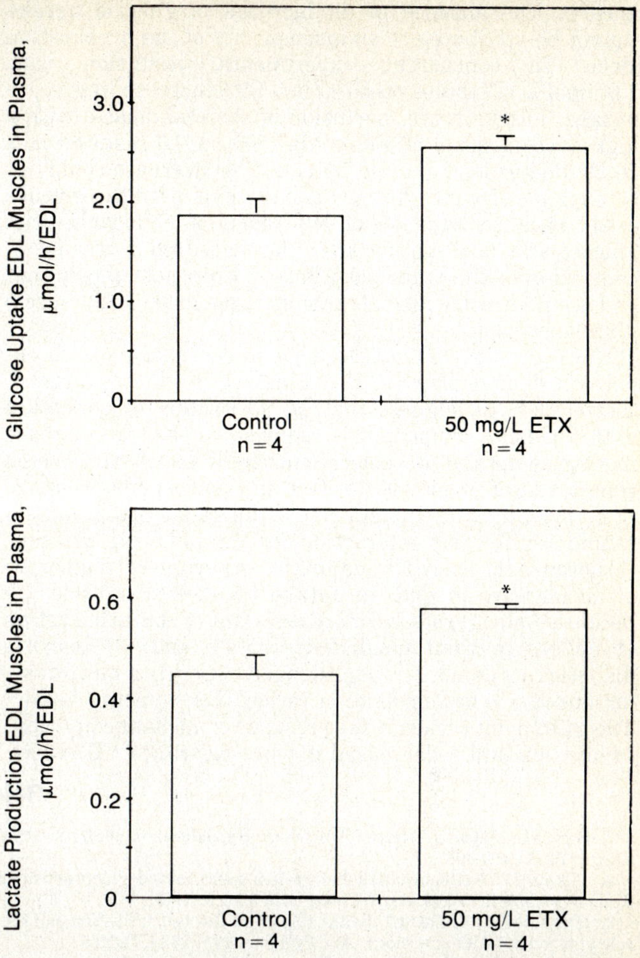

Fig 5.—Glucose uptake and lactate production by skeletal muscle incubated in plasma ± endotoxin (ETX). Glucose uptake and lactate production by extensor digitorum longus (EDL) muscles were increased when incubated in plasma with 50 mg/L of ETX. One asterisk indicates $P<.05$ vs control.

the studies of Romanosky et al[5] would predict that the response of blood to the administration of endotoxin could result in an increase in glucose uptake of 13%, and the studies of Raymond et al[4] would predict an increase of 4.5% in the whole animal. Although a leukocytosis consequent to endotoxin exposure might further increase this difference, endotoxin-induced leukocytosis does not occur until four to six hours after exposure. Thus, the increase in the metabolism of glucose by blood in the presence of endotoxin is unlikely to account for the immediate difference in glucose uptake noted in in vivo studies following endotoxin administration. The studies of Meszaros et al[23,25] evaluated the contribution of other organs to the increased glucose consumption of endotoxemic rats. The largest increase in glucose uptake per unit weight was found in the liver and spleen. However, the major contributors to the increased glucose consumption were the skin, skeletal muscle, and intestine due to the large mass of these tissues.[23,25]

An increase in glucose uptake by skeletal muscle in the presence of endotoxin may result from a direct action of endotoxin on skeletal muscle. However, the present studies suggest that endotoxin does not have a direct effect on glucose uptake in the absence of white blood cells or hormones since perfusion and incubation of skeletal muscle with up to 250 mg/L of an endotoxin preparation (shown to alter glucose oxidation in adipose tissue and glucose uptake in blood) did not alter glucose uptake by the skeletal muscle. The absence of an increase in glucose uptake cannot be attributed to an insensitivity of the preparation since, in concurrent experiments, perfusion with 1.8 nmol/L of insulin resulted in a 95% increase in glucose uptake. Furthermore, perfusion of skeletal muscle with a high concentration of endotoxin (500 mg/L) resulted in a 26.2% decrease in glucose uptake. This decrease could not be explained by interference of endotoxin with the glucose assay because addition of 500 mg/L of endotoxin to a glucose standard did not alter the measured glucose concentration of the standard. Thus, it does not appear that endotoxin directly mediates an increase in skeletal muscle glucose uptake.

However, skeletal muscle incubated in plasma with endotoxin demonstrated a 37% increase in glucose uptake. These findings suggest that an interaction of endotoxin with a plasma component is required to elicit an increase in glucose uptake by skeletal muscle by endotoxin. Which component of plasma is involved in this response remains to be investigated. Insulin or insulinlike factors are likely candidates for this interaction for the following reasons: (1) because these are the major known peripheral mediators of an increase in glucose uptake by skeletal muscle; (2) because diabetic rats are more resistant to the lethal action of endotoxin than nondiabetic rats[35]; and (3) because diabetic rats demonstrate prolonged hyperglycemia following endotoxin administration rather than hypoglycemia.[36] The third point occurs in the presence of unchanged glucose production and a decreased glucose clearance.[9] However, an increase in the plasma insulin concentration may not be necessary for an increase in glucose utilization during endotoxemia, since Romanosky et al[5] and Raymond et al[4] both noted increased glucose uptake in muscle in the absence of an increased plasma insulin concentration, and Adeleye et al[37] reported the development of hypoglycemia and elevated blood lactate concentrations in rats after the administration of endotoxin in the absence of hyperinsulinemia.

Several additional mechanisms by which endotoxin may mediate an increase in skeletal muscle glucose uptake are possible. Briefly, an increase in glucose uptake by skeletal muscle in the presence of endotoxin could also be the result of an alteration in substrate delivery to the muscle that is mediated by endotoxin. An increase in glucose uptake may result from tissue anoxia or ischemia. Finally, endotoxin may increase glucose uptake in skeletal muscle by stimulating the release of a product from white blood cells that, in turn, mediates the increase in glucose uptake.

In conclusion, endotoxin does not have a direct effect on the glucose uptake of skeletal muscle. An interaction of endotoxin with a component of plasma is required for an endotoxin-mediated increase in glucose utilization by skeletal muscle. The requirement of plasma for an endotoxin-mediated increase in glucose uptake by tissue other than skeletal muscle awaits further evaluation.

We thank Georgia Platonotis and William Henry for their excellent technical assistance.

References

1. Berk JL, Hagan JF, Beyer WH, et al: Hypoglycemia of shock. *Ann Surg* 1970;171:400-408.
2. Filkins JP: Reticuloendothelial system function and glucose-insulin dyshomeostasis in sepsis. *Am J Emerg Med* 1981;2:70-73.
3. Hinshaw LB, Archer LT, Beller BK, et al: Glucose utilization and the role of blood in endotoxin shock. *Am J Physiol* 1977;233:E71-E79.
4. Raymond RR, Harkema JM, Emerson TE: Mechanism of increased glucose uptake by skeletal muscle during *Escherichia coli* endotoxin shock in the dog. *Circ Shock* 1981;8:77-83.
5. Romanosky AJ, Bagby GJ, Bockman EL, et al: Increased muscle glucose uptake and lactate release after endotoxin administration. *Am J Physiol* 1981;239:E311-E316.
6. Hinshaw LB, Peyton MD, Archer LT, et al: Prevention of death in endotoxin shock by glucose administration. *Surg Gynecol Obstet* 1974;139:851-859.
7. Archer LT, Benjamin B, Lane MM, et al: Renal gluconeogenesis and increased glucose utilization in shock. *Am J Physiol* 1976;231:872-879.
8. Van Lambalgen AA, Bronsveld W, Van Den Bos GC, et al: Distribution of cardiac output, oxygen consumption and lactate production in canine endotoxin shock. *Cardiovasc Res* 1984;18:195-205.
9. Kellehee DL, Bagby GI, Spitzer JJ: Glucose metabolism following endotoxin administration in diabetic rats. *Horm Metab Res* 1980;12:595-601.
10. Filkins JP, Buchanan BJ, Cornell RP: Hepatic carbohydrate metabolism alterations during endotoxin and traumatic shock. *Circ Shock* 1975;2:129-135.
11. Filkins JP, Cornell RP: Depression of hepatic gluconeogenesis and the hypoglycemia of endotoxin shock. *Am J Physiol* 1974;227:778-781.
12. Groves AC, Woolf LI, O'Regan PJ, et al: Impaired gluconeogenesis in dogs with *Escherichia coli* bacteremia. *Surgery* 1974;76:533-541.
13. Wolfe RR, Elahi D, Spitzer JJ: Glucose and lactate kinetics after endotoxin administration in dogs. *Am J Physiol* 1977;232:E180-E185.
14. Peyton MD, Hinshaw LB, Greenfield LJ, et al: Hypoglycemic effects of endotoxin in eviscerated dogs. *Surg Gynecol Obstet* 1975;141:727-730.
15. Moore RN, Goodrum KO, Berry LJ: Mediation of an endotoxic effect by macrophages. *J Reticuloendothelial Soc* 1976;17:187-197.
16. Kelleher DL, Puinno PA, Fong BC, et al: Glucose and lactate kinetics in septic rats. *Metabolism* 1982;31:252-257.
17. Merrill GF, Spitzer JJ: Glucose and lactate kinetics in guinea pigs following *Escherichia coli* administration. *Circ Shock* 1978;5:11-21.
18. Hinshaw LB, Benjamin B, Coalson JJ, et al: Hypoglycemia in lethal septic shock in subhuman primates. *Circ Shock* 1975;2:197-208.
19. Raymond RM, Emerson TE Jr: Cerebral metabolism during endotoxin shock in the dog. *Circ Shock* 1978;5:407-414.
20. Hinshaw LB, Beller BK, Archer LT, et al: Hypoglycemic response of blood to live *Escherichia coli* organisms and endotoxin. *J Surg Res* 1976;21:141-150.
21. Holley DC, Spitzer JA: Insulin action and binding in adipocytes exposed to endotoxin in vitro and in vivo. *Circ Shock* 1980;7:3-12.
22. Witek-Janusek L, Filkins JP: Insulin-like action of endotoxin: Antagonism by steroidal and non-steroidal anti-inflammatory agents. *Circ Shock* 1981;8:573-583.
23. Meszaros K, Lang CH, Bagby GJ, et al: Contribution of different organs to increased glucose consumption after endotoxin administration. *J Biol Chem* 1987;262:10965-10970.
24. Havel R: *Utilization of Body Fuels by Muscle in Energy Metabolism and Body Fuel Utilization.* Cambridge, Mass, Harvard University Press, 1966, p 20.
25. Meszaros K, Bagby GJ, Lang CH, et al: Increased uptake and phosphorylation of 2-deoxyglucose by skeletal muscles in endotoxin-treated rats. *Am J Physiol* 1987;253:E33-E39.
26. Rodbell M: Metabolism of isolated fat cells: I. Effects of hormones on glucose metabolism and lipolysis. *J Biol Chem* 1964;239:375-380.
27. Caldwell MD, Lacy WW, Exton JH: Effects of adrenalectomy on the amino acid and glucose metabolism of perfused rat hindlimbs. *J Biol Chem* 1978;253:6837-6844.
28. Wollenberger A, Ristau O, Schoffa G: Ein einfarche Technik der extrem schellen Abkuhlung groberer Gewebestucke. *Pflugers Arch* 1970;270:399-412.
29. Pain VM, Manchester KL: The effect of electrical stimulation in vitro on protein synthesis and other metabolic parameters of the rat extensor digitorum longus muscle. *Biochem J* 1970;118:209-220.
30. Lowry OH, Passonneau JV: *Flexible System of Enzymatic Analysis.* Orlando, Fla, Academic Press Inc, 1972.
31. Rich W, Johnson E, Lois L, et al: Determination of organic acids in body fluids by ion chromatography: Plasma lactate and pyruvate and urinary vanillylmandelic acid. *Clin Chem* 1980;26:1492-1498.
32. Winer BJ: *Statistical Principles in Experimental Design.* New York, McGraw-Hill International Book Co, 1971.
33. Cohn ZA, Morse SI: Functional and metabolic properties of polymorphonuclear leucocytes: II. The influence of a lipopolysaccharide endotoxin. *J Exp Med* 1960;111:689-703.
34. Reeve EB, Gregerson MI, Allen TH, et al: Validity of cell and blood volume measurements in the splenectomized dog. *Am J Physiol* 1953;175:211-217.
35. Pieroni RE, Levine L: Enhancing effect of insulin on endotoxin lethality. *Experientia* 1969;25:507-508.
36. Kelleher DL, Fong BC, Bagby GJ, et al: Metabolic and hormonal changes following endotoxin administration to diabetic rats. *Am J Physiol* 1982;243:R77-R81.
37. Adeleye GA, Al-Jibouri LM, Furman BL, et al: Endotoxin-induced metabolic changes in the conscious rat: Hypoglycemia and elevated blood lactate concentrations without hyperinsulinemia. *Circ Shock* 1981;8:543-555.

Hypertonic Saline Resuscitation in a Porcine Model of Severe Hemorrhagic Shock

Gregory G. Stanford, MD; C. Richard Patterson, MD; Lynda Payne, RN; Timothy C. Fabian, MD

• The purpose of this study was to investigate the effect of 7.5% hypertonic saline solution (HTS) as the initial solution in resuscitation of a pig in shock. Twenty-two animals were bled 50% of their blood volume over 30 minutes and maintained in shock for 60 minutes. The 14 survivors were divided into two groups. The first group was given 20 mL/kg of lactated Ringer's solution (LR) over a ten-minute period, while the second group was given 10 mL/kg of HTS. Both groups were then given LR at 2 mL/kg/min until the mean arterial pressure reached 80 mm Hg. The HTS group achieved a more rapid rise in mean arterial pressure over the first ten minutes of resuscitation. During this period, the cardiac index increased significantly more in the HTS group when compared with the LR group. All animals in the HTS group developed an adequate urine output. Only two animals in the LR group developed an adequate urine output. Hypertonic saline solution markedly improved survival, and there were significant improvements in hemodynamics. This was accomplished with smaller volumes of resuscitation fluid and may prove useful under conditions where intravascular access is limited.

(*Arch Surg* 1989;124:733-736)

The rapid infusion of crystalloid solutions remains the cornerstone of early therapy for trauma victims in severe hemorrhagic shock. An alternative to conventional crystalloids for early fluid resuscitation is a crystalloid solution that may be effective in smaller volumes, permitting more rapid resuscitation. Hypertonic saline solution (HTS) and hyperosmotic solution used in small volumes have been beneficial in animal shock models[1-5] and human burns.[6-8] These studies have consistently shown marked hemodynamic improvement with the use of HTS to treat hemorrhagic shock; however, in most studies, these improvements have been transient. It appears that HTS is very effective in the treatment of hemorrhagic shock for a short period. On the other hand, in the early resuscitation of patients in hemorrhagic shock, when time is all important and the rate of infusion is limited, HTS may improve their circulatory status while more conventional methods of resuscitation are begun.

The purpose of this study was to compare a resuscitation regimen that incorporates an initial infusion of HTS in a porcine hemorrhagic shock model with one that incorporates lactated Ringer's solution (LR). We attempted to test the hypothesis that an initial infusion of HTS would restore hemodynamic stability more rapidly, since less volume would be required to do so.

Accepted for publication Oct 28, 1988.

From the Department of Surgery, University of Tennessee, Memphis.

Reprint requests to University of Tennessee, 956 Court Ave, Room E228, Memphis, TN 38163 (Dr Fabian).

MATERIALS AND METHODS

Twenty-two young female pigs (8 to 12 weeks old), weighing 15 to 20 kg, were obtained from a single supplier. All experiments were monitored and approved by the Animal Care Committee of the University of Tennessee, Memphis. On the morning of the experiment, each animal was sedated intramuscularly with ketamine hydrochloride (Ketaset, Bristol Laboratories, Syracuse, NY) in a dose of 10 mg/kg. An intravenous line was then established through which an additional 5 mg/kg of ketamine hydrochloride was injected. Many of the animals exhibited random, nonpurposeful muscular activity while under the influence of ketamine and were paralyzed with 1 mg of pancuronium bromide (Pavulon, Organon Laboratories, West Orange, NJ) to facilitate placement of the intravenous catheters. During this period, the pigs underwent mechanical ventilation with room air. After insertion of all necessary catheters, pancuronium was withheld, and the animals were spontaneously allowed to breathe room air. Mechanical ventilation was then only used in the occasional animal that became apneic during the hemorrhage phase of the experiment and was discontinued as soon as the animal resumed an adequate ventilatory pattern.

Catheters were placed in each external jugular vein for measurement of central venous pressure as well as administration of fluids during the resuscitation phase of the experiment. The femoral artery was used for continuous measurement of arterial pressure and collection of shed blood during the hemorrhage phase of the experiment. The femoral vein was used to pass a 7F Swan-Ganz catheter (American Edwards Laboratories, Irvine, Calif) into the pulmonary artery for measurement of pulmonary artery pressures, pulmonary capillary wedge pressure, and thermodilution cardiac outputs. When the catheter was not being used for cardiac output determinations, it was set to give continuous readings of central venous blood temperatures. The distal port was used for collection of mixed venous blood samples. A Foley catheter was inserted through a superpubic cystostomy to continuously monitor urine output.

After each animal had been prepared in this fashion, it was allowed to lie undisturbed for a 60-minute period to minimize the effect of the preparation on the subsequent experiment. Baseline measurements were taken at the end of this period. Over the next 30 minutes, each animal was bled 50% of its estimated blood volume based on the regression equation for swine reported by von Engelhardt[9]: estimated blood volume per kilogram = 95 (body weight)$^{-0.068}$. Over the subsequent 60 minutes, each animal was kept in shock by maintaining its mean arterial pressure (MAP) between 40 and 60 mm Hg by either reinfusing shed blood or withdrawing more blood. At the end of this shock period, the surviving animals were divided into two groups. One group, the HTS group, received 10 mL/kg of 7.5% hypertonic sodium chloride solution (2400 mOsm/L) over the first ten minutes of the experiment. The other group, the LR group, received 20 mL/kg of LR

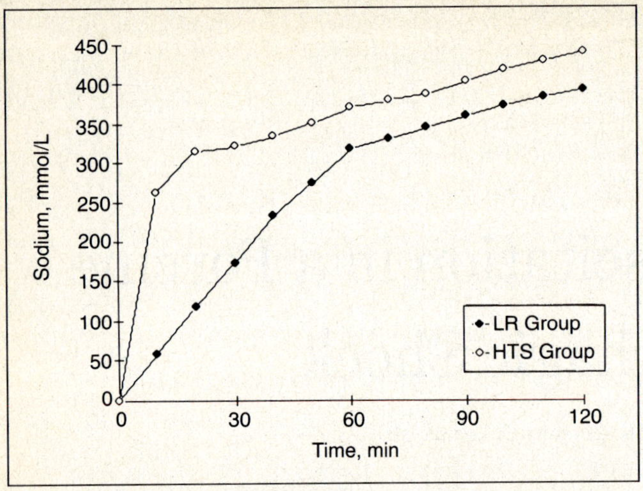

Fig 1.—Cumulative average amount of sodium per animal in hypertonic saline solution (HTS) and lactated Ringer's solution (LR) groups given during resuscitation.

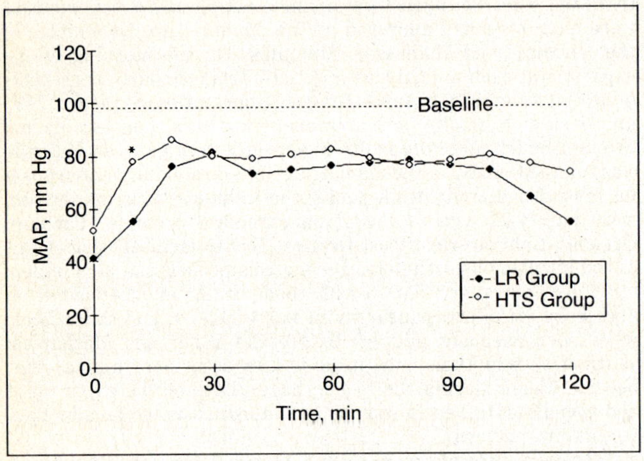

Fig 2.—Average mean arterial pressure (MAP) of hypertonic saline solution (HTS) and lactated Ringer's solution (LR) groups throughout experiment. Baseline represents MAP just prior to beginning of hemorrhage. Asterisk indicates $P<.05$.

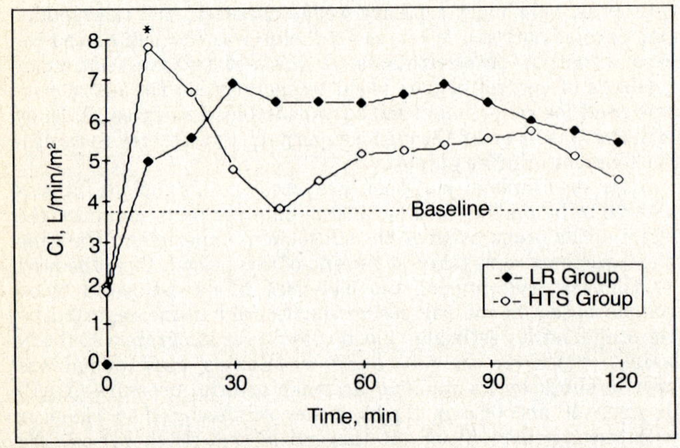

Fig 3.—Average cardiac index (CI) of hypertonic saline solution (HTS) and lactated Ringer's solution (LR) groups during study. Baseline CI represents CI just prior to beginning of hemorrhage. Asterisk indicates $P<.05$.

during the same ten-minute period. For the remainder of the experiment, both groups received LR at the rate of 2 mL/kg/min until the end point of resuscitation was reached, at which time the rate of infusion was decreased to a maintenance rate of 2 mL/kg/h. The end point of resuscitation was defined as reaching and maintaining an MAP of 80 mm Hg for two consecutive measurements taken ten minutes apart.

Measurements of temperature, respirations, heart rate, arterial pressure, central venous pressure, pulmonary artery pressure, pulmonary capillary wedge pressure, cardiac output, and urine output were recorded at baseline, every ten minutes for the first 40 minutes of resuscitation, and every 20 minutes for the remainder of the experiment.

Blood samples for levels of sodium, lactate, potassium, bicarbonate, and arterial blood gas tensions were withdrawn from the femoral artery catheter and analyzed prior to hemorrhage (baseline), prior to resuscitation, and at the end of the experiment. Mixed venous blood gas tensions taken from the pulmonary artery catheter were analyzed at the same time points.

Statistical analyses were performed using the Wilcoxon paired *t* test. Body surface area was calculated using the formula of DuBois and DuBois[10]: body surface area = $\text{height}^{0.725} \times \text{weight}^{0.425} \times 0.007184$.

RESULTS

Of the 22 pigs entered into the study, eight animals did not survive the hemorrhage, yielding a mortality rate for this model of 36%. Fourteen animals survived the shock to enter the study: seven were placed in the LR group and seven in the HTS group. Of the seven animals placed in the LR group, two did not survive the two-hour resuscitation period. Five were successfully resuscitated, and two achieved an adequate urine output (defined as 2 mL/kg/h). Of the seven pigs placed in the HTS group, there were no deaths. All animals reached or exceeded an MAP of 80 mm Hg, and all regained an adequate urine output.

The animals in the LR group required an average of 2704 mL of intravenous fluid by the end of the resuscitation period, while those in the HTS group received an average of 1234 mL (46% of the LR group average). The animals in the LR group consistently required more volume of intravenous fluid to reach and maintain a stable blood pressure when compared with the HTS group so that, by the conclusion of the experiment, the animals in the LR group required an average of almost 2.5 times the volume received by the HTS group. Even though the HTS animals received markedly more sodium in the first ten minutes of resuscitation during the HTS infusion, as seen in Fig 1 (HTS group, 260 mmol/L; LR group, 60 mmol/L), both groups received similar amounts of sodium by the conclusion of the experiment (HTS group, 420 mmol/L; LR group, 360 mmol/L).

The MAP throughout the experiment is shown graphically in Fig 2. With the onset of resuscitation, there was an initial rapid increase in the HTS group following the 7.5% HTS infusion. At the conclusion of the HTS infusion, the MAP was significantly higher in the HTS group when compared with the LR group ($P<.05$). The MAP in the LR group rose more slowly, but after 30 minutes, both groups stabilized around 80 mm Hg for the remainder of the study period, with the LR group requiring more volume to maintain this pressure.

As shown in Fig 3, the cardiac index (CI) was seen to improve dramatically in both groups at the beginning of resuscitation but was significantly higher at ten minutes ($P<.05$) in the HTS group. The means for the two groups approached significance ($P<.07$) at 30 minutes, with the LR group being greater, but there were no other statistical differences between the two groups during the study period. Following this peak at the conclusion of the HTS infusion, the CI fell in the HTS group but remained above

Table 1.—Hematocrit and Serum Chemistry Changes				
Variable	Group*	Baseline	End of Shock	End of Resuscitation
Hematocrit	LR	0.321±0.053	0.211±0.052	0.161±0.036
	HTS	0.327±0.033	0.257±0.036	0.181±0.023
Sodium, mmol/L	LR	141±3.6	141±7.0	138±6.6
	HTS	140±2.7	142±4.5	158±5.9
Potassium, mmol/L	LR	3.4±0.6	4.0±0.5	3.8±0.6
	HTS	3.5±0.6	4.0±0.7	2.6±0.9
Bicarbonate, mEq/L	LR	23.4±1.8	11.6±5.3	12.9±7.0
	HTS	23.4±3.1	9.4±3.5	11.9±2.4
Lactate, mmol/L	LR	3.9±2.0	21.7±16.3	14.9±5.7
	HTS	5.7±3.8	19.5±4.2	15.9±6.2

*LR indicates group given 20 mL/kg of lactated Ringer's solution; HTS, group given 10 mL/kg of 7.5% hypertonic saline solution.

Table 2.—Acid-Base and Oxygen Transport Changes*				
Variable	Group	Baseline	End of Shock	End of Resuscitation
pH	LR	7.50±0.10	7.30±0.18	7.22±0.14
	HTS	7.60±0.09	7.25±0.17	7.26±0.13
Base deficit, mmol/L	LR	4.9±3.2	21.0±6.6	19.9±8.1
	HTS	5.0±2.3	25.5±5.7	22.8±2.2
Arterial O_2 content, mL/dL	LR	15.3±1.8	9.6±2.0	7.4±1.7
	HTS	14.8±2.9	11.3±1.6	7.5±1.2
$AVDo_2$, mL/dL	LR	5.8±2.4	6.6±2.4	3.2±1.2
	HTS	4.6±0.8	7.6±1.3	3.4±1.9
O_2 delivery mL/min/m²	LR	628±71	165±71	392±137
	HTS	526±99	214±58	430±89
O_2 consumption, mL/min/m²	LR	235±86	108±48	157±34
	HTS	164±28	144±34	177±70
O_2 extraction ratio	LR	0.37±0.11	0.69±0.20	0.44±0.22
	HTS	0.32±0.04	0.68±0.05	0.44±0.22

*LR indicates group given 20 mL/kg of lactated Ringer's solution; HTS, group given 10 mL/kg of 7.5% hypertonic saline solution; and $AVDo_2$, arteriovenous oxygen difference.

baseline throughout the remainder of the experiment. The LR group CI peaked at 30 minutes and also remained above baseline for the remainder of the resuscitation period.

The systemic vascular resistance fell sharply in both groups during resuscitation when compared with the baseline. After reaching a minimum at ten minutes, the HTS group stabilized at a level somewhat higher than the LR group, but the differences between the groups were not significant. Values obtained for the hematocrit value and the sodium, potassium, bicarbonate, and lactate levels are shown in Table 1. The hematocrit value dropped to just over 50% of baseline in both groups. The sodium level was elevated to 158 mmol/L in the HTS group at the end of resuscitation but remained normal in the LR group. The potassium level did not change in either group. The bicarbonate level fell precipitously in both groups by the end of the shock period but had begun to recover by the end of resuscitation. The lactate level was predictably elevated by the hemorrhage but had begun to revert toward normal at the conclusion of the study in both groups.

Tissue oxygenation and acid-base data are illustrated in Table 2. The severe shock produced in this model is demonstrated by the presence of significant metabolic acidosis, elevated base deficit, and depression of both oxygen delivery and consumption, with a marked increase in the oxygen extraction ratio. At the end of resuscitation, both groups remained acidotic, but the base deficit was partially replenished. Oxygen delivery doubled from the shock level but did not reach the baseline values, which can be attributed to hemodilution and the fall in hematocrit value. The oxygen extraction ratio fell toward baseline, indicating at least a partial restoration of tissue perfusion.

COMMENT

The hemodynamic effects of HTS have been evaluated in several hemorrhagic shock models, with most studies involving canine models anesthetized with various regimens incorporating phenobarbital sodium. Few studies have reported hemorrhagic shock models involving ketamine anesthesia in the young pig. Ketamine has fewer hemodynamic side effects than barbiturates, even though it appears to stimulate the sympathoadrenal axis.[11,12] Pentobarbital sodium, on the other hand, disrupts the venous compensatory response to shock,[13,14] with a loss of venomotor tone.[15] In a study by Simon and Olsen,[16] pentobarbital alone produced greater abnormalities in relatively nutrient-rich capillary blood flow than did an acute 40% hemorrhage in the young pig. Ketamine was also chosen because it is often used clinically in hemorrhagic shock when the patient cannot tolerate more potent agents. Another benefit of this model is that the functional characteristics of the pig cardiovascular system more resemble those of humans[9,17]; studies in swine, therefore, may be more relevant to clinical applications.

The results presented herein demonstrate the rapid cardiovascular effects of HTS in hemorrhagic shock. Mean arterial pressure rose rapidly during and immediately following the infusion, and it was associated with the statistically significant early rise in the CI and the stroke index, when compared with isotonic crystalloid resuscitation, even though 60% less volume was required. The systemic vascular resistance fell below baseline values early in the resuscitation, which implied that the elevated arterial pressure and cardiac output resulted in a rapid increase in tissue blood flow and perfusion. Varying concentrations of HTS have been shown to increase the cardiac output when given to animals in both the shock and nonshock states. In normovolemic dogs, hyperosmolar solutions increased cardiac contractility[11,18] and gave ventricular work a lowered peripheral vascular resistance.[19] In mongrel dogs subjected to hemorrhage, 5.2% saline produced large initial increases in cardiac output, mesenteric flow, and oxygen consumption.[2] The cause of this inotropic effect, combined with arterial dilatation, was first thought to be a redistribution of fluid from the interstitium to the vascular system. Lopes et al[20] investigated the effect of HTS in the canine model, with and without vagotomy, and showed that vagally mediated reflex venoconstriction was triggered by the influx of HTS in the pulmonary vasculature. This mechanism may also contribute significantly to the effect of the solutions, as evidenced by the rapid improvement that follows initiation of treatment.

It is interesting to speculate that the improvements

described herein corresponded to the rapid infusion of sodium. As seen in Figs 1 and 3, the improvements seen in the first ten minutes of resuscitation were more closely related to the dose of sodium given than the volume. It is important to note that the animals in the LR group achieved hemodynamic stability only after they had received a similar amount of sodium as the HTS group at the time the latter became stable. The effect of HTS may be due to the sodium ion, but it could also be due to the chloride ion or the osmolar effect. Nonionic osmotic agents have been used in the treatment of hemorrhagic shock with similar results to those described herein[2,6,21]; however, the responses seen are more dramatic and prolonged if the resuscitative regimen incorporates sodium either as the bicarbonate or chloride salt. Sodium has profound effects at the cell membrane,[5] and it may help to restore the membrane potential damaged by the hypotensive insult and prevent the decompensation of the second phase of blood volume restitution, which is caused by the shift of fluid into the cell in severe hemorrhagic shock as described by Gann et al.[22] The increased interstitial sodium might also offset the plasma factor-mediated poisoning of the sodium pump described by Cunningham et al.[23] The extracellular fluid volume deficit described by Shires et al[24] may also be accompanied by a sodium deficit that is more rapidly corrected with HTS.

Another measure of the improved hemodynamic status in the animals receiving HTS was the rapid resumption of urine production. The rapid restoration of renal perfusion is not only indicative of increased cardiac output but may also be a secondary cause of decreased renal vascular resistance that is due to the increased osmolality and increased osmotic clearance as was shown by Gazitua et al.[25] In their study, the renal vascular resistance fell when HTS was infused into the renal artery. In a study by Yesberg et al,[26] intravenous HTS caused increases in urine flow, sodium and potassium excretion, vasopressin excretion, and free water reabsorption. Hypertonic solutions thus appear to aid renal preservation in hemorrhagic shock by triggering both the systemic effects of shortening the ischemic period and the direct effects on the renal parenchyma itself.

Although most investigators have described the effects of HTS as transient, Velasco et al[1] achieved improved survival and sustained recovery of blood pressure by restoring cardiac output and stroke volume to normal. In the present study, CI, stroke index, and left ventricular stroke work increased to levels higher than the prehemorrhage values, and then slowly declined to levels just above baseline. The animals receiving HTS had a marked hypernatremia following the conclusion of the experiment. There were no adverse effects that could be attributed to this finding. In studies done on human burns, patients reached serum sodium values as high as 170 mmol/L without any signs or symptoms of acute hypernatremia.[7,8] The serum sodium level rapidly fell after the conclusion of the infusion of HTS, as the added sodium was diluted in the extracellular water and excreted by the kidneys. These improvements continued throughout the two-hour resuscitation period; the animals required markedly less volume to maintain a stable cardiovascular status.

Although LR has been the fluid of choice for patients in shock, HTS may offer a superior alternative for the initial resuscitation of the patient in hemorrhagic shock. There are situations where LR cannot be infused as rapidly as necessary to reverse the hemodynamic derangements seen in the severely traumatized patient. A solution as effective as LR, but used in a much smaller volume, would aid in resuscitating these patients prior to their arrival at the hospital. The battlefield and other similar mass casualty situations would be other areas where HTS could be beneficial. As demonstrated in this study, HTS rapidly corrects many of the hemodynamic deficits caused by severe hemorrhage as effectively as larger volumes of LR. Hypertonic saline solution, when given either initially in the prehospital period or shortly after arrival, might improve a patient's survival by rapidly restoring tissue perfusion while conventional treatment modalities are begun.

References

1. Velasco IT, Pontieri V, Silva RE Jr, et al: Hyperosmotic NaCl and severe hemorrhagic shock. *Am J Physiol* 1980;239:664-673.
2. Baue AE, Tragus ET, Parkins WM: A comparison of isotonic and hypertonic solutions and blood on blood flow and oxygen consumption in the initial treatment of hemorrhagic shock. *J Trauma* 1967;7:743-756.
3. Prough DS, Johnson JC, Stump DA, et al: Effects of hypertonic saline versus lactated Ringer's solution on cerebral oxygen transport during resuscitation from hemorrhagic shock. *J Neurosurg* 1986;64:627-632.
4. Prough DS, Johnston JC, Poole GV Jr, et al: Effects on intracranial pressure of resuscitation from hemorrhagic shock with hypertonic saline versus lactated Ringer's solution. *Crit Care Med* 1985;13:407-411.
5. Nakayama S, Kramer GC, Carlsen RC, et al: Infusion of very hypertonic saline to bled rats: Membrane potentials and fluid shifts. *J Surg Res* 1985;38:180-186.
6. Caldwell FT, Bowser BH: Critical evaluation of hypertonic and hypotonic solutions to resuscitate severely burned children. *Ann Surg* 1979;189:546-552.
7. Monafo WW, Chuntrasakul C, Ayvazian VH: Hypertonic sodium solutions in the treatment of burn shock. *Am J Surgery* 1973;126:778-783.
8. Monafo WW: The treatment of burn shock by the intravenous and oral administration of hypertonic lactated saline solution. *J Trauma* 1970;10:575-586.
9. Von Engelhardt W: Swine cardiovascular research: A review, in Bustad LK, McClellan RO (eds): *Swine in Biomedical Research*. Richland, Wash, Pacific Northwest Laboratory and Batelle Memorial Institute, 1966, pp 307-329.
10. DuBois D, DuBois EF: A height-weight formula to estimate the surface area of man. *Arch Intern Med* 1916;17:863-871.
11. Yamanaka I, Dowdy EG: The effects of ketamine on spiralcut strips of rabbit aorta. *Anesthesiology* 1974;40:222-227.
12. Chernow B, Lake CR, Barton M, et al: Sympathetic nervous system sensitivity to hemorrhagic hypotension in the subhuman primate. *J Trauma* 1984;24:229-232.
13. Dow RW, Fry WJ: Venous compensatory mechanisms in acute hypovolemia. *Surg Gynecol Obstet* 1967;125:511-515.
14. Zweens J, Frankena H, Zijlstra WG: The effect of pentobarbital anesthesia upon the volume and ionic composition of the extracellular space in the dog. *Bibl Anat* 1977;241-244.
15. Eckstein JW, Hamilton WK, McCammond JM: The effect of thiopental on peripheral venous tone. *Anesthesiology* 1961;22:525-528.
16. Simon J, Olsen WR II: Hemorrhage in the anesthetized pig. *Arch Surg* 1969;99:634-636.
17. Douglas WR: Of pigs and men in research: A review of applications and analogies of the pig, *Sus scrota*, in human medical research. *Space Life Sci* 1972;3:226-243.
18. Wildenthal K, Mierzwiak DS, Mitchell JH: Acute effects of increased serum osmolality on left ventricular performance. *Am J Physiol* 1969;216:898-904.
19. Rowe GG, McKenn DH, Corliss RJ, et al: Hemodynamic effects of hypertonic sodium chloride. *J Appl Physiol* 1972;32:182-184.
20. Lopes OU, Pontieri V, Rocha-E-Silva M Jr, et al: Hyperosmotic NaCl and severe hemorrhagic shock: Role of the innervated lung. *Am J Physiol* 1981;241:H883.
21. Baue AE, Tragus ET, Parkins WM: Effects of sodium chloride and bicarbonate in shock with metabolic acidosis. *Am J Physiol* 1967;212:54-60.
22. Gann DS, Carlson DE, Byrnes GJ, et al: Impaired restitution of blood volume after large hemorrhage. *J Trauma* 1981;21:598-603.
23. Cunningham JN, Shires GT, Wanger Y: Changes in intracellular sodium and potassium content of red blood cells in trauma and shock. *Am J Surg* 1971;70:215-222.
24. Shires GT, Coln D, Carrico J, et al: Fluid therapy in hemorrhagic shock. *Arch Surg* 1964;88:688-692.
25. Gazitua S, Scott JB, Chou CC, et al: Effect of osmolality on canine renal vascular resistance. *Am J Physiol* 1969;217:1216-1223.
26. Yesberg NE, Henderson M, Budtz-Olsen OE: The effect of intravenous hypertonic saline infusion on renal function and vasopressin excretion in sheep. *Q J Exp Physiol* 1978;63:331-339.

Instructions for Authors

Manuscripts are to be sent by first-class mail to the Editor, Claude H. Organ, Jr, MD, Professor, Dept of Surgery, University of California–Davis, East Bay 1411 E 31st St, Oakland, CA 94602. The procedures listed must be followed carefully and all materials requested must be enclosed for prompt review and consideration for publication in the *Archives of Surgery.* Use the checklist to ensure completeness.

Manuscript Preparation.—*The original typescript and two high-quality copies* of the entire manuscript must be submitted, including copies of all illustrations, legends, tables, and references. All copy, including references, legends, and tables, must be typed double-spaced on 8½ × 11-in, heavy-duty white bond paper. Margins must be at least 1 in. If a word processor is used, do *not* use justified right margins.

Abstract.—*Submit an abstract* (135-word maximum) of the manuscript, which must include a statement of the problem, methods of study, results, and conclusions. The synopsis-abstract replaces a summary or conclusions.

Copyright.—*A copyright release* form signed by *all* authors of manuscripts, brief communications, and correspondence is required by the Copyright Revision Act of 1976. The following statement, dated and signed by all authors, may be used: **"In consideration of the American Medical Association's taking action in reviewing and editing my submission, the author(s) undersigned hereby transfers, assigns, or otherwise conveys all copyright ownership to the AMA in the event that such work is published by the AMA."**

Financial Interest.—List all affiliations with or financial involvement in any organization or entity with a direct financial interest in the subject matter or materials of the research discussed in the manuscript (eg, employment, consultancies, stock ownership). All such information will be held in confidence during the review process. Should the manuscript be accepted, the Editor will discuss with the author the extent of disclosure appropriate for publication.

References.—*References* should be listed in *consecutive numerical order* as they are cited in the text, *not alphabetically.* Once a reference is cited, all subsequent citations should be to the original number. All references must be cited in the text or tables. Unpublished data and personal communication may not be listed as references. References to journal articles should include (1) authors, (2) title, (3) journal name as abbreviated in *Index Medicus,* (4) year, (5) volume number, and (6) inclusive page numbers—in that order. References to books should include (1) authors, (2) chapter title, if any, (3) editor, if any, (4) title of book, (5) year, (6) city, and (7) publisher. Volume and edition numbers, specific pages, and name of translator should be included when appropriate. **The author is responsible for the accuracy and completeness of the references and for their correct text citation.**

Author Responsibility.—One author must be designated *corresponding author,* with his or her address and telephone number provided. All correspondence and copy editing are sent to this author. The corresponding author will receive an edited typescript rather than galley proofs for approval. The authors are responsible for all statements in their work, including changes made by the copy editor. Order reprints at the time the typescript is returned after editorial processing. Specify the address to which requests for reprints should be sent.

Titles.—*The title* must be *short,* specific, and clear. It cannot exceed 42 characters per line, including punctuation and spaces, and is limited to two lines. The title page should include the full names and academic affiliations of all authors. If the manuscript was presented at a meeting, indicate the name of the organization, the place, and the date on which it was read.

SI Units.—Use Système International (SI) measurements throughout the manuscript.

Illustrations.—Use only illustrations that clarify and augment the text. Submit illustrations in triplicate, unmounted and untrimmed. Do not send original artwork. Send high-contrast glossy prints (not photocopies). Figure number, name of senior author, and arrow indicating "top" should be typed on a gummed label and affixed to the back of each illustration. All lettering must be legible after reduction to column size. Artwork submitted for publication may be relettered to achieve uniformity of lettering style throughout the journal. Illustrations should preferably be in a proportion of 5 × 7 in. *Color illustrations* are accepted for publication if the editors believe that color will add significantly to the published manuscript. The ARCHIVES will pay only part of the expense of color reproduction and printing color illustrations. The author's share of the expense is $400 for up to six square finished illustratons that can be arranged on a one-page layout. Any additional illustrations or special effects will be billed to the author at cost. Positive color transparencies (35-mm preferred) must be submitted for an evaluation. Do not send color prints unless accompanied by original transparencies.

CHECKLIST FOR AUTHORS

Send:

- Three copies of manuscript.
- Three copies of synopsis-abstract.
- Three copies of attached photographs, legends, tables, and/or illustrations clearly marked as described in the instructions.
- A copyright release statement signed by *all* authors.
- The address and telephone number of the designated corresponding author.
- Send to Claude H. Organ, Jr, MD
Archives of Surgery
Professor, Dept. of Surgery
University of California–Davis, East Bay
1411 E 31st St
Oakland, CA 94602
- Use sufficient postage.

(Continued on p 738.)

(*Continued from p 737.*)

Legends.—*Legends* must be typed double-spaced, beginning on a separate sheet of paper. Length is limited to a maximum of 40 words.

Tables.—Each table must be typed double-spaced, including all headings, on a separate sheet of 8½×11-in paper. Do not use larger-size paper. If a table must be continued, use a second sheet and repeat all heads and stubs. Each table must have a title.

Manuscript Acceptance.—Manuscripts are received with the understanding that they *are not* under simultaneous consideration by another publication. Accepted manuscripts become the permanent property of the ARCHIVES and may not be published elsewhere without permission from the publisher (AMA).

OTHER INFORMATION

Brief Clinical Notes.—The ARCHIVES welcomes the submission of Brief Clinical Notes for review. These are generally reports of cases that provide a new or unique contribution and are to consist of no more than 400 words, two references, and one illustration. The synopsis-abstract may not exceed 80 words.

Correspondence and Brief Communications.—The Editor is pleased to receive letters that pertain to material published in the ARCHIVES as well as brief communications concerning other matters of interest to our readers. An interesting case may be published as a brief communication. Such contributions should be 250 words or less, typewritten, double-spaced without an abstract, and clearly marked "for publication." No more than two references are permitted and illustrations or tables are acceptable only when essential to the message.

News and Announcements.—Brief notices may be submitted of meetings, seminars, or symposiums that are of interest to surgeons.

Acknowledgments.—Illustrations from other publications must be acknowledged. Include the following when applicable: authors, title of article, title of journal or book, volume number, pages, month and year. The publisher's permission to reprint must be submitted to the ARCHIVES when the manuscript has been formally accepted.

Statistical Review.—Manuscripts containing statistical evaluation should include the name and affiliation of the statistical reviewer.

Informed Consent.—Manuscripts reporting the results of experimental investigations on human subjects must include a statement to the effect that informed consent was obtained after the nature of the procedure(s) had been fully explained.

Reference to Patients.—Patients should be referred to by number or, in anecdotal reports, by fictitious given names. Real names or initials must not be used in the text, tables, or illustrations.

Photographic Consents.—A letter of consent must accompany all photographs of patients in which a possibility of identification exists. It is *not* sufficient to simply cover the eyes to mask identity.

AMA Manual of Style.—This 1988 edition, formerly the *Manual for Authors & Editors*, is available from Williams & Wilkins, 428 E Preston St, Baltimore, MD 21202. Single copy price: $24.95. A shipping charge is added on all orders not prepaid. If additional ordering information is needed, or to order by telephone, call 1-800-638-0672.

Percutaneous Nephrostomy in the Management of Renal Candidiasis

Orlando Ortiz, MD, Won J. Lee, MD

• **A case of *Candida* infection of the kidney was successfully managed by percutaneous means. This case demonstrates that percutaneous nephrostomy is a simple, effective technique not only for drainage, extraction of fungus balls, and irrigation with amphotericin B, but also for examining the renal collecting system and obtaining urine samples for diagnostic culture verification. Because of the toxicity of antifungal drugs, the incorporation of this percutaneous technique into standard management will benefit the patient with a life-threatening renal fungal infection.**

(*Arch Surg* 1989;124:739-740)

Fungal infections of the urinary tract are uncommon but seem to be increasing in frequency partly due to an increase in opportunistic infection from the common complication of modern therapeutics and debilitating disease.[1,2] As one indicator, the medical literature has seen an almost 400% increase in the reporting of genitourinary fungal infections.[3] Such infections are predominantly candidal and have become increasingly prevalent because of the alteration of host resistance caused by aggressive use of broad-spectrum antibiotics, corticosteroids, and immunosuppressive agents. Most fungal infections of the upper urinary tract involve the drainage structures rather than the renal parenchyma and produce fungal pyonephrosis.[4] We report a case of renal candidiasis in an adult in which percutaneous nephrostomy was used to counteract this pathophysiologic condition via extraction of the fungus ball, drainage, and antifungal irrigation of the renal collecting system.

REPORT OF A CASE

A 59-year-old man with a history of diet-controlled diabetes mellitus, hypertension, chronic renal failure, and multiple urinary tract infections complained of left flank pain and fever. His medical history included left-sided nephrolithiasis that had required pyelolithotomy six years prior to the current admission. Four years after this initial episode, the patient underwent ureteral surgery for left ureteral stricture. The patient subsequently underwent multiple urologic procedures for left-sided obstructive uropathy complicated by *Candida* sepsis. In addition, a nonfunctioning right kidney had been identified two years prior to admission. Physical examination at the time of admission revealed left costovertebral angle tenderness.

Significant laboratory findings were a serum urea nitrogen level of 50 mmol/L of urea, a serum creatinine level of 1360 μmol/L, and a white blood cell count of 20.2×10^9/L. Urine Gram's stain did not demonstrate any yeast forms but did show gram-positive cocci that were later identified as enterococci. A left percutaneous nephrostomy was performed on the third hospital day; nephrostogram showed marked hydronephrosis, with small, irregular filling defects in the renal collecting system representing fungus ball and debris, which were evacuated via nephrostomy tube (Figure). Blood and urine cultures revealed *C albicans*. Systemic and local amphotericin B were added to the antibiotics being given. Noncontrast computed tomography immediately after percutaneous nephrostomy revealed a nephrostomy-induced perinephric hematoma, which required no additional management.

His condition improved, and prior to discharge an arteriovenous fistula was placed for long-term hemodialysis. His serum urea nitrogen and serum creatinine levels steadily improved for three months while the percutaneous nephrostomy tube was in place. Other than a clogged arteriovenous graft, which required emergency thrombectomy, the patient remained asymptomatic for 12 months following the nephrostomy tube removal.

COMMENT

Renal candidiasis with fungus ball formation remains an uncommon entity, though its frequency has increased over the past few decades. Nonetheless, the significant morbidity and potential mortality associated with this condition make it imperative that a diagnosis be arrived at as expeditiously as possible. The afflicted patient already may have impaired health status. In addition, since the involved therapies are not without inherent risks, it is extremely important that the correct diagnosis be made.

Renal candidiasis is an uncommon presentation of an organism that, under normal circumstances, is commonly found within the human host. When host resistance is altered, the organism may assume pathogenic properties. Possible predisposing factors include the following: (1) states of compromised health (diabetes mellitus, acquired immunodeficiency syndrome, premature birth, or chronic debilitating illness); (2) pregnancy; (3) disturbance of urine flow (congenital genitourinary anomalies, neurogenic bladder, ureteropelvic junction obstruction, nephrolithiasis, genitourinary tuberculosis, ileal conduit, or other genitourinary surgery); (4) drugs (antibiotics, steroids, chemotherapy, or drug abuse); (5) radiation therapy; (6) major surgery or renal transplant; (7) trauma; and (8) indwelling catheter devices.[5] Under these circumstances, the patient may remain asymptomatic or may develop fever, flank pain, hematuria, dysuria, anuria, or renal failure.[6] The clinical presentation, therefore, will identify pertinent risk factors and symptoms that may herald a renal fungal process.

Laboratory findings demonstrate that less than 5% of clean-voided urine specimens should be expected to yield yeast in culture and that candiduria, in many instances, reflects improper collection, sampling, and processing of urine specimens.[7] Nevertheless, the presence of yeast in the urine warrants serious attention in the compromised host. It has been reported that a candidal colony count of 10 000 to 15 000 per milliliter in the absence of an indwelling Foley catheter represents a useful index of separation between colonization and infection.[8] It is also important to stress that though *Candida* is the most common cause of fungus balls in the genitourinary tract, *Penicillium*, Phycomycetes, and *Aspergillus* fungus balls can also occur. Renal fungus balls can also result from systemic fungal disease, as the kidney is involved in over 85% of cases of systemic candidiasis.[9]

Despite a wide selection of imaging modalities, a definitive diagnosis of fungus ball often remains elusive. This phenomenon can partly be explained by the composition

Accepted for publication March 10, 1988.

From the Department of Radiology, Long Island Jewish Medical Center, New Hyde Park, NY, and the State University of New York Health Sciences Center at Stony Brook.

Reprint requests to Long Island Jewish Medical Center, New Hyde Park, NY 11042 (Dr Lee).

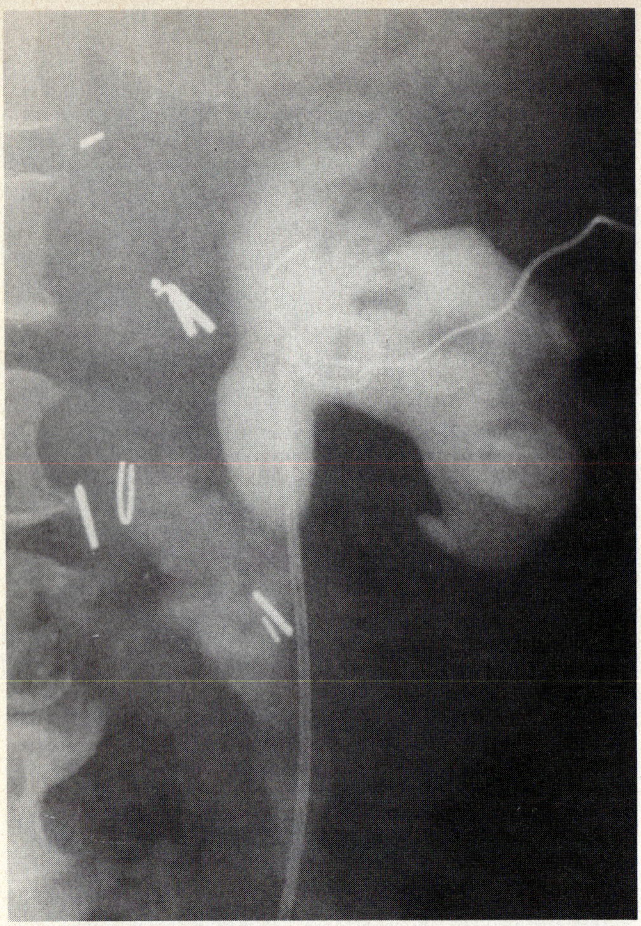

Nephrostogram showing hydronephrosis and irregular filling defects simulating blood clots, stones, or debris. Double pigtail ureteral stent is noted in place.

and location of the fungus ball. The fungus ball represents a conglomerate of hyphal elements and exudative debris resulting from inflamed, necrotic tissue within the renal collecting system.

The findings on plain-film roentgenography are highly nonspecific. Excretory urography may yield a smooth, mobile filling defect within the renal pelvis or an elongated, castlike ureteral filling defect.[2] Other, less specific features include a nonvisualized kidney, a delayed nephrogram, calyceal blunting or widening, hydronephrosis, hydroureter, or nodular ureteral filling defects. The diagnosis is confounded by the fact that many of these abnormalities are associated with tumor, calculus, blood clot, or papillary necrosis.

Noncontrast computed tomography will identify a nonradiopaque calculus due to the increased density resulting from the crystal structure of the calculus, and then one must differentiate between blood clot, sloughed papilla, tumor, and fungus ball.[4] Ultrasonometry readily detects hydronephrosis and can potentially detect an echogenic, nonshadowing mass in the renal pelvis.[10] As with excretory urography, retrograde pyelography may reveal a filling defect in the renal collecting system. From a nonimaging standpoint, ureterorenoscopy may also assist in evaluating the renal collecting system, as well as in extracting a fungal mass. Obviously, though beneficial, these tests do not always provide the clinician with the exact diagnosis.

Percutaneous nephrostomy is a versatile approach combining diagnostic and therapeutic modalities. Indications for percutaneous nephrostomy are relief of obstruction, confirmation of the diagnosis, and aggressive administration of fungicides. Percutaneous nephrostomy is performed under local anesthesia with an aseptic technique. In skilled hands, this procedure exposes the patient to minimal morbidity.[1] Not only can antegrade pyelography be performed, but aspirates from the renal pelvis can also be studied to determine the presence of fungi. The presence of a mobile filling defect in the collecting system with a positive aspirate virtually confirms the diagnosis of a fungus ball. An attempt is made to extract and thereby debulk the fungal mass. The usefulness of this maneuver is twofold: it reduces the possibility of distal ureteral obstruction by fungal debris and shortens the interval of irrigation required for sterilization of the renal pelvis.[11]

Local irrigation with an antifungal agent is performed via the nephrostomy tube. We consider 50 mg of amphotericin B prepared in 1 L of water to be a safe nephrostomy tube dose, and administration can be discontinued after five days if the blood cultures are sterile. The therapeutic goal is to relieve obstructive uropathy and completely eradicate all fungal organisms from the renal collecting system. Concurrent systemic antifungal therapy may also be administered. The most effective and only parenteral agent, amphotericin B, has serious side effects, such as hepatic dysfunction, nephrotoxic changes, gastrointestinal disturbances, hypotension, electrolyte derangements, and anaphylactoid reactions.

Large perirenal hematoma was demonstrated on computed tomographic scan. In one of the first reviews of the percutaneous nephrostomy, which encompassed 1207 patients, Stables[12] found significant bleeding in 1.3%. We found perirenal hematomas not requiring treatment in three of the 20 patients we studied by computed tomography following percutaneous nephrolithotomy.[13] To minimize the frequency of blood loss after percutaneous nephrostomy, any clotting abnormalities should be corrected before the procedure, and the operator should choose the puncture site carefully through Brodel's avascular line.

Percutaneous nephrostomy has proved to be extremely useful in the management of fungus ball and renal drainage. It supplements the previously described diagnostic modalities and affords a relatively less invasive means of treatment, thus obviating the need for surgery in these characteristically high-risk patients.

Peter G. Herman, MD, reviewed the manuscript and provided editorial guidance. Patricia Petersen assisted in preparing the manuscript.

References

1. Dembner AG, Pfister RC: Fungal infection of the urinary tract: Demonstration by an antegrade pyelography and drainage by percutaneous nephrostomy. *AJR* 1977;129:415-418.
2. Mindell HJ, Pollack HM: Fungal disease of the ureter. *Radiology* 1983;146:46.
3. Tacker JR: Fungal infections in the genitourinary system. *Monogr Urol* 1986;7:11-17.
4. Mazer MJ, Bartone FF: Percutaneous antegrade diagnosis and management of candidiasis of the upper urinary tract. *Urol Clin North Am* 1982;9:157-164.
5. Hamory BH, Wenzel RP: Hospital associated candiduria: Predisposing factors and review of the literature. *J Urol* 1978;120:444-445.
6. Sales JL, Mundy HB: Renal candidiasis: Diagnosis and management. *Can J Surg* 1973;16:139-143.
7. Fisher JF, William HC: Urinary tract infections due to *Candida albicans*. *Rev Infect Dis* 1982;4:1107-1117.
8. Kozinn PJ, Taschdjian CL, Goldberg PK, et al: Advances in the diagnosis of renal candidiasis. *J Urol* 1978;119:184-187.
9. Gerle RD: Roentgenographic features of primary renal candidiasis: Fungus ball of the renal pelvis and ureter. *AJR* 1973;119:731-738.
10. Aragona F, Glazel GP: Upper urinary tract obstruction in children caused by *Candida* fungus balls. *Eur Urol* 1985;11:188-191.
11. Abramowitz J, Fowler JE, Tarwrik: Percutaneous identification and removal of fungus ball from renal pelvis. *J Urol* 1986;135:1232-1233.
12. Stables DP: Percutaneous nephrostomy: Technique, indications and results. *Urol Clin North Am* 1982;9:15-29.
13. Lee WJ, Smith AD, Cubelli V, et al: Complications of percutaneous nephrolithotomy. *AJR* 1987;148:177-180.

Echinococcal Disease in an Extended Family and Review of the Literature

CPT Franco Musio, MC, USA, Dimitrios Linos, MD

• Echinococcal disease occurred in an extended family from Athens, Greece. Seven of the 11 family members were noted to be infected with *Echinococcus granulosus*, and five members have undergone surgical treatment. The potential sources of infection are discussed, although localization was impossible. There is no genetic basis for this disease and no apparent pattern of family member interrelationship or visceral involvement. Although echinococcal infection is frequently diagnosed in large urban centers, its transmission within a family is rare. Review of the literature and the current diagnostic and therapeutic measures are presented.

(*Arch Surg* 1989;124:741-744)

Echinococcal disease has plagued mankind from the time of Hippocrates, who most likely was referring to this condition in his description of patients with "livers full of water." The words *Echinococcus* and *hydatid* are derived from the ancient Greek language meaning "hedgehog berry" and "a drop of water," respectively. Infection by the parasite most commonly involves the liver, followed by the lungs, with the spleen,[1] central nervous system,[2] muscles,[3] kidneys,[4] adrenal glands,[5] heart,[6] bones,[7] retroperitoneum,[8] and other organs being affected with much less frequency. According to Fossati,[9] the "familial" form of echinococcosis was first mentioned by Thorstensen in 1840 and later described by Krabbe in 1866 as a "chronic disease which in the opinion of those in Ireland is hereditary." Deve,[10] in 1907, was the first to conduct an in-depth study of a number of family members afflicted with the echinococcal cysts in regard to the clinical features and pulmonary and hepatic locations. In 1946, Ferro[11] examined 29 affected families with a total of 66 cases, 59% of which were found between siblings. Since then, there have been scattered reports in the literature of the parasite affecting nuclear and extended families. There is no genetic basis for the disease, because human echinococcal infection is transmitted from the definite host to humans via the fecal-oral route.

Although relatively rare in the United States, echinococcal disease may still be diagnosed in large urban centers and also transmitted within a family. Such a case of echinococcosis occurred in seven of 11 members of an extended family from Athens, Greece, who were infected with *Echinococcus granulosus*, five of whom have undergone surgical treatment (Fig 1). These patients are described, with a review of the current diagnostic and therapeutic methods applied in the management of this disease.

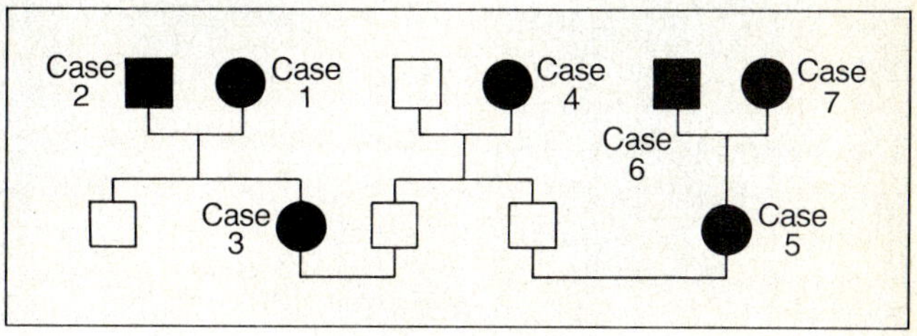

Fig 1.—Pedigree of case reports.

REPORT OF CASES

CASE 1.—A 52-year-old woman had previously been in good health. The patient discovered a mass directly beneath the right costal margin in May 1985. Abdominal roentgenograms were normal. In September 1985, the patient presented with dyspnea and shortness of breath. Chest roentgenograms demonstrated multiple lesions on both lungs (Fig 2), and an abdominal ultrasound study revealed multiple echogenic lucencies in both hepatic lobes. Chest and abdominal computed tomographic scans demonstrated multiple, round, low-density lesions in both lung fields (Fig 3) and in both hepatic lobes, respectively. Although the initial clinical impression was that of malignancy, subsequent measurement of serum antiechinococcal antibodies by radioimmunoassay was positive.

A laporotomy was performed in late September 1985, in which multiple hepatic cysts were found. Evacuation and sterilization of each cyst was done using hypertonic saline solution. Deep O-chromic sutures on a liver needle were used to approximate the uncalcified walls of each cavity. Two drains were left in the subhepatic space. Histologic analysis was consistent with a diagnosis of *E granulosus*. The postoperative course was uneventful, and no further symptoms were noted until February 1986, when the patient presented with dyspnea and shortness of breath. Chest roentgenograms demonstrated transformation of a previously seen left inferior, round, radiodense pulmonary lesion to a well-circumscribed air-fluid level. Intravenous antibiosis was commenced, with rapid improvement of symptoms.

The patient most recently presented in April 1987 with fever, anorexia, and right-sided chest pains. Chest roentgenograms demonstrated a similar progression of a previously seen right inferior, round, radiodense pulmonary lesion to a well-circumscribed air-fluid level. In May 1987, a right thoracotomy was performed, with removal of all cysts. The patient's symptoms have subsided during the postoperative course, and she is awaiting surgical treatment of the left pulmonary lesions.

CASE 2.—A 70-year-old man, the husband of patient 1, had previously been in good health. Routine chest roentgenograms obtained two years before his presentation showed no abnormalities, although radioimmunoassay studies of serum samples were positive for antiechinococcal antibodies. A subsequent abdominal computed tomographic scan demonstrated a right hepatic cyst measuring 10 cm in diameter as well as a right renal cyst. The patient refused to undergo surgery.

CASE 3.—A 25-year-old woman, the daughter of patients 1 and 2, had previously been in good health and had been married for the last two years. A routine chest roentgenogram obtained on January 1986 demonstrated a left inferior pulmonary lesion. Chest and abdominal computed tomographic scans were abnormal for one pulmonary and multiple hepatic cysts, respectively (Fig 4). The patient underwent a left thoracotomy in October 1986, with the removal of the pulmonary cyst, and laparotomy in March 1986, with evacuation of all hepatic cysts and obliteration of the cavities by approximating their uncalcified walls. Histologic analysis of all

Accepted for publication Feb 18, 1988.

From Hellenikon Air Force Base Hospital, Athens, Greece (Dr Musio), and the Department of Surgery, University of Athens (Greece) (Dr Linos). Dr Musio is now with the Department of Surgery, General Surgery Service, Brooke Army Medical Center, Fort Sam Houston, Tex.

Reprint requests to the Department of Surgery, General Surgery Service, Brooke Army Medical Center, Fort Sam Houston, TX 78234-6200 (Dr Musio).

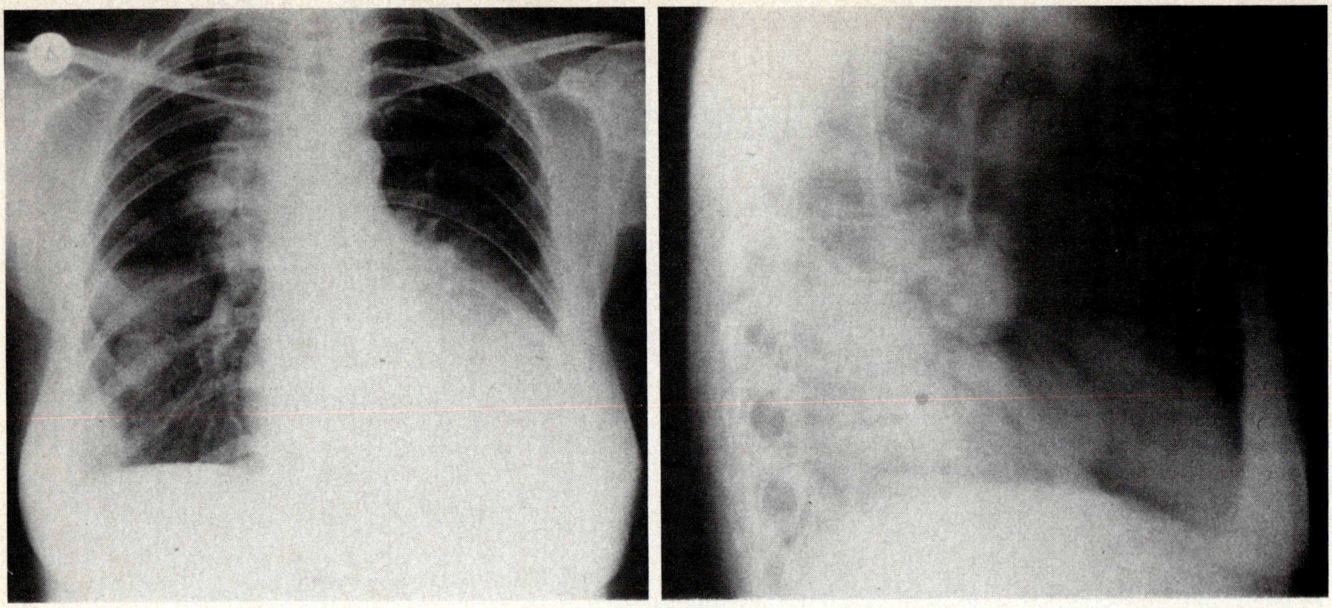

Fig 2.—Posteroanterior (left) and lateral (right) chest roentgenograms demonstrating multiple pulmonary lesions (case 1).

Fig 3.—Chest computed tomographic scan demonstrating multiple pulmonary lesions (case 1).

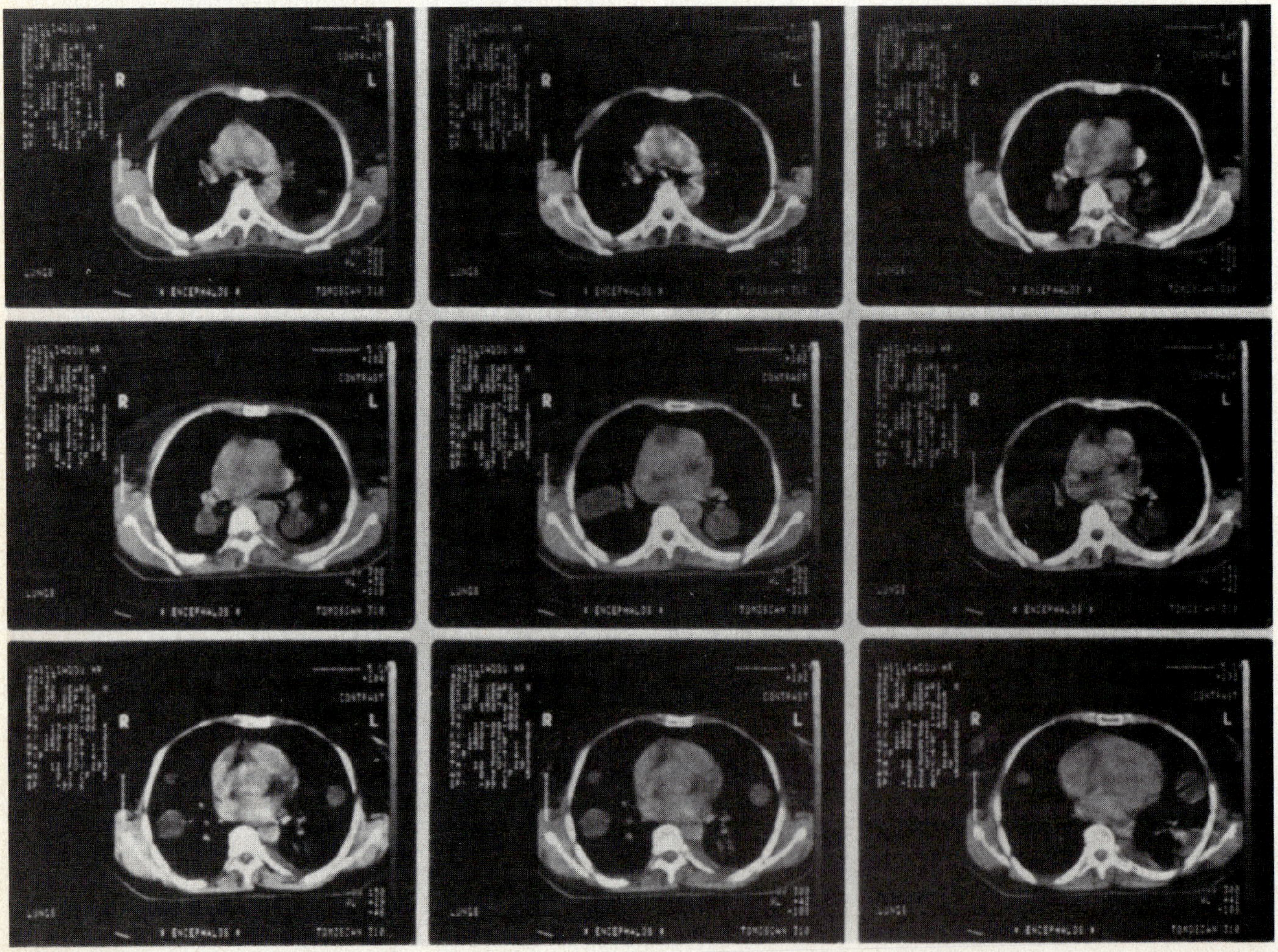

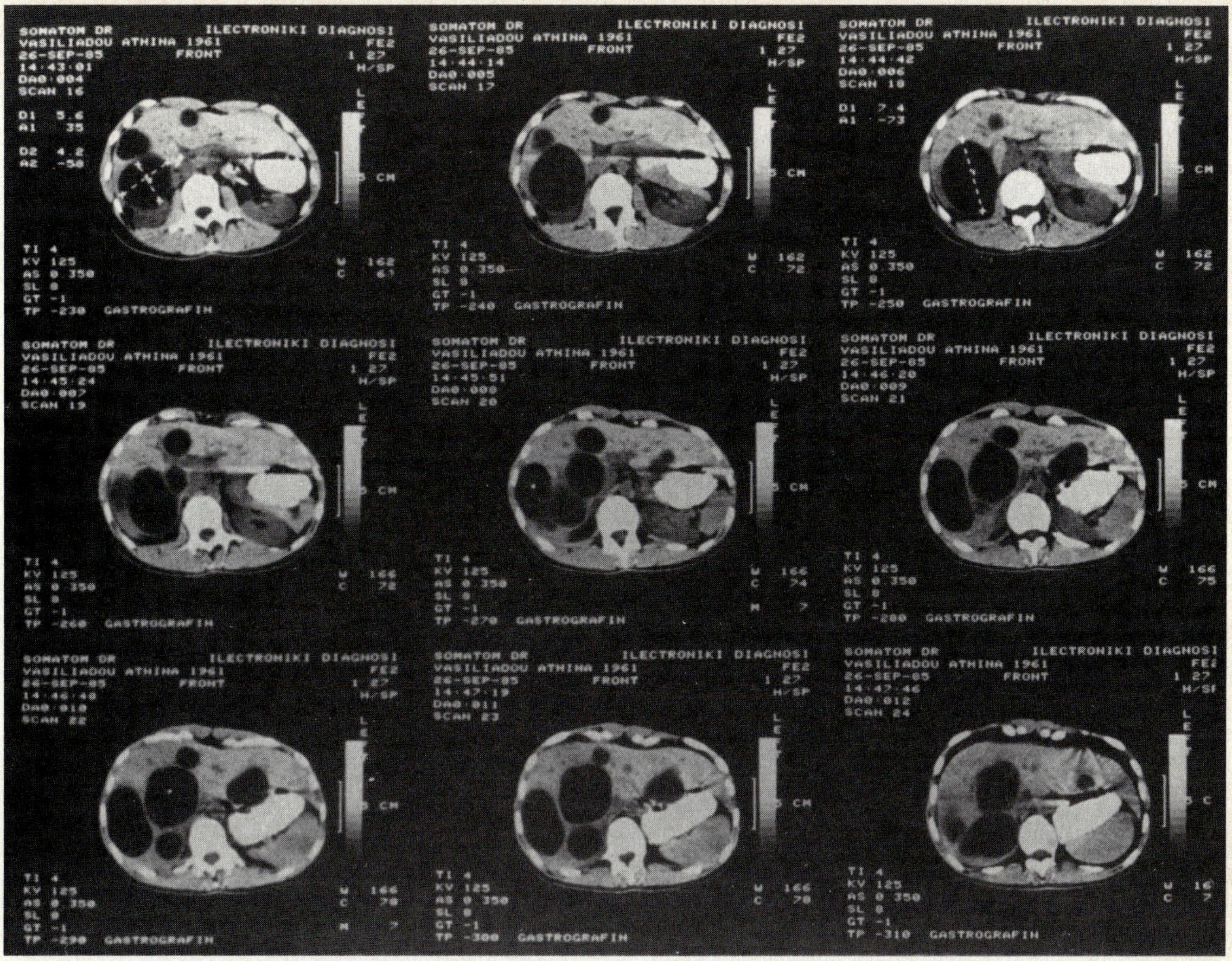

Fig 4.—Abdominal computed tomographic scan demonstrating multiple hepatic lesions (case 3).

cysts was consistent with a diagnosis of *E granulosus*. The postoperative course has been normal.

CASE 4.—A 64-year-old woman, the mother-in-law of patient 3, was previously in good health until January 1986, when she presented with right upper quadrant pains. Workup revealed cholelithiasis, and an abdominal computed tomographic scan showed four hepatic cysts. The serum sample was positive by radioimmunoassay for antiecchinococcal antibodies. The patient underwent cholecystectomy in January 1986, with synchronous treatment of the hepatic cysts. In this case, the large cavity was closed by omentoplasty, and the remaining ones were obliterated by approximation of their uncalcified walls. Histologic analysis was consistent with a diagnosis of *E granulosus*. The postoperative course was normal.

CASE 5.—A 29-year-old woman, the daughter-in-law of patient 4, had previously been in good health. Routine chest roentgenograms in March 1986 demonstrated a right inferior, round, radiodense pulmonary lesion. A thoracotomy revealed a cyst, which was removed and proved to be *E granulosus* by histologic study. The postoperative course was normal.

CASE 6.—A 64-year-old man, the father of patient 5, had undergone two separate thoracotomies, with the removal of pulmonary echinococcal cysts, and two laparotomies, with evacuation of hepatic echinococcal cysts. All procedures were performed at another institution.

CASE 7.—A 58-year-old woman, the mother of patient 5, had chest roentgenograms and abdominal computed tomographic scans that were normal. Serum antiechinococcal antibody tests by radioimmunoassay were positive. She is being followed up.

The remaining members of the extended family have been tested serologically and are negative for antiechinococcal antibodies.

COMMENT

Echinococcosis in humans results from infection by *E granulosus* or *Echinococcus alveolaris* (multilocularis). The latter infection is rare and only forms 2% to 3% of all known cases of the disease.[12] The involvement of humans in the life cycle commences with ingestion of the ova, which is released in the stool of the definite host. The infection is usually due to eating unboiled vegetables contaminated by the feces of dogs as well as cats, wolves, and foxes. The eggs may also be carried directly from the dog or cat to the mouth of the child or adult. Contamination of well water by such infected carnivores may also serve as a potential source of infection. Once the egg is swallowed, it develops into the six-hooklet embryo that penetrates the intestinal mucosa and is carried to the liver by the portal vein, where the primary filtering and trapping occurs. Occasionally, the embryo can escape from the liver and travel to the lungs, with rare progression beyond this second filter to the central circulation and other organs.[1-8] Rarely, the embryo may enter the lymphatic circulation from the intestinal mucosa and be carried directly to the lungs via the thoracic and mediastinal lymph vessels. The embryo grows into a cyst consisting of an external cuticle and an inner germinal epithelium. *Echinococcus granulosus* develops into a unilocular cyst that grows slowly over many years and does not penetrate tissue. The hydatid cyst of *E alveolaris* is always multilocular, with active invasion of the host tissue by germinal layer extensions. The life cycle of the parasite is complete as dogs and other carnivores eat the flesh or liver of previously infected intermediate hosts such as sheep, cattle, and pigs. This is a logical explanation for the prevalence of the disease in locations such as Greece, Australia, Central Europe, the Middle East, South America, southwestern Canada, and Alaska, where sheep and cattle breeding are important activities and there is close contact between animals and humans. The cyst develops into the adult worm in the jejunum of the definite host that measures 4 to 6 mm and resides for up to 20 months before releasing its eggs.

There seems to be no definitive pattern of family member interrelationship or visceral involvement in this "familial" form of echinococcal disease. The world literature in the last 20 years contains several accounts of identical organ infection within families to include only lung,[13] liver,[14] or muscle.[3] Fossati[9] described 24 sheep-herding families, 11 of which harbored solely pulmonary infection and five of which had solely hepatic infection among the members. Also, families such as the one we described are reported to have combinations of lung, liver, and other organ involvement.[15-18] Both types of *Echinococcus* were found in one couple from the French Jura, the wife diagnosed as having a large splenic *E granulosus* cyst and the husband having hepatic cysts of *E alveolaris*.[19] In offering a cause, a family dog was reported in only three cases,[3,15,17] and close animal association was noted in one study involving a community with constant contact between family members and dogs and sheep.[9] In our study, a pet dog was kept by the principal family of patients 1 through 3, although the other infected individuals had no contact with this animal. This dog was examined by a local veterinarian and found not to carry the parasite. All the family members lived in middle-class neighborhoods of Athens proper and had no association with apparent sources of infection, such as animals, farms, well water, other individuals harboring the organism. All the women of the family were housewives. All the men of the family, with the exception of the brother and husband of patient 3, were co-owners and clerks in a small retail store of wool products. The brother of patient 3 was a high school student. The husband of patient 3 was a butcher. Although no signs or symptoms of infection were noted in this individual, his mother, sister-in-law, and her parents had visceral involvement, antiechinococcal antibodies, or both demonstrated by radioimmunoassay. Notwithstanding the exposure of the butcher to animal viscera (in particular, lamb), his consideration as a source of infection is unlikely.

The affliction of an extended family with this disease is rare. Nevertheless, it is necessary to examine all members of the family of the afflicted patient. Computed tomographic and ultrasound scans as well as the modern serologic tests (indirect hemagglutination, complement fixation, enzyme-linked immunosorbent assay, and specific hydatid IgE tests)[20] are highly sensitive and specific and have facilitated the diagnosis of echinococcal disease. The surgical treatment of the liver echinococcosis consists of removal of the hydatid cyst, with careful protection of the abdomen from spillage of the hydatid fluid and obliteration of the remaining cavity using the many different described techniques—primary suturing,[21] omentoplasty,[22] capitonage,[23] and capsulorraphy. Before removal of the cyst, evacuation of the hydatic fluid followed by injection of hypertonic saline or silver nitrate solution is indicated to sterilize the contents. The surgical treatment of an uncomplicated hydatid cyst of the lung is much easier in that a simple incision of the surrounding pleura in conjunction with increased intrapulmonary pressure provided by the anesthesiologist will "pop out" the intact cyst. A simple suturing of the site of the delivered cyst suffices.

Medical treatment of hydatid disease has centered on the broad-spectrum antihelminthic agent mebendazole. After its initial introduction by Bekhti et al[24] in 1977, clinical studies have demonstrated the ability of mebendazole to sterilize hydatid cyst cavities.[25,26] A recently completed ten-year clinical trial of continuous therapy demonstrated increased life expectancy, subjective improvement, substantial radiologic decrease in the size of hepatic lesions, and lack of progression of distant metastases.[27] Mebendazole has therefore been recommended by many groups as a preoperative agent in inactivating the cyst and preventing possible scoliceal dissemination during surgery or for use in inoperable conditions.

References

1. Desai MB, Kamdar MS, Bapat RD, et al: Splenic cysts. *J Postgrad Med* 1981;27:251-252.
2. Bia FJ, Barry M: Parasitic infections of the central nervous system. *Neurol Clin* 1968;117-206.
3. Schmrigk K, Emser W: Parasitic myositis by *Echinococcal alveolaris*—report of a family with myotonia congenita. *Eur Neurol* 1978;17:1-7.
4. Cohen MS: Granulomatous nephritis. *Urol Clin North Am* 1986;39: 647-659.
5. Deliviotis A, Stenos J, Kyrillopoulou M: Adrenal cysts: Report of a case and review of the literature. *Acta Urol Belg* 1971;39:353-360.
6. Calamai G, Perna M, Venturini A: Hydatid disease of the heart—report of five cases and review of the literature. *Thorax* 1974;29:451-458.
7. Porat S, Joseph KN: Hydatid disease of bone: Case report and review of the literature. *Isr J Med Sci* 1978;14:223-227.
8. Sekar N, Madhavan KK, Yadav VS, et al: Primary retroperitoneal hydatid cyst. *J Postgrad Med* 1982;28:112-114.
9. Fossati C: Sull'idatidosi famigliare in Cirenaica. *Clin Pediatr* 1965;47: 280-287.
10. Deve F: L'echinococcose familiar. *Arch Gen Med* 1907;6:160-164.
11. Ferro A: Hidatidosis familiar. *Arch Int Hidatidosis* 1946;6:135.
12. Hashemian H: Hydatid disease of the liver and other viscera, in Maingot R (ed): *Abdominal Operations.* East Norwalk, Conn, Appleton-Century-Crofts, 1980.
13. Sadeghi A, Maghtader J, Navaie F: Familial multiple pulmonary hydatidosis. *J Indian Med Assoc* 1978;71:181-182.
14. Dimitrov D, Marinova L, Markov I: Suchetana ekinokozoza u drama chlera na edno semsistvo. *Khirurgila (Sophia)* 1980;33:409-415.
15. Schwabe CW: Epidemiology of echinococcosis. *Bull WHO* 1968;39: 131-137.
16. Ben-Ami M, Koren A, Goshen J: Case reports—familial echinococcal disease. *Harefuah* 1984;107:124-126.
17. Romanoff H, Krausz M: Surgical aspects of pulmonary hydatid disease and report of a familial hydatidosis. *Int Surg* 1975;60:361-364.
18. Muras DO: Hidatidosis multiple pulmonary hepatica. *Thorax* 1970; 19:144.
19. Hofstetter J: Un kyste hydatique de la rate et une echinococcose alveolaire du foie dans une meme famille de Jura Francaise. *Lyon Chir* 1968;64:113-117.
20. Kagan IG: A review of serological tests for the diagnosis of hydatid disease. *Bull WHO* 1968;39:25-37.
21. Langer J, Rose D, Keystone J, et al: Diagnosis and management of hydatid disease of the liver. *Ann Surg* 1984;199:412-417.
22. Sayek I, Yalin R, Sanas Y: Surgical treatment of hydatid disease of the liver. *Arch Surg* 1980;115:847-850.
23. Romero-Torez R, Campbell JR: An interpretive review of the surgical treatment of hydatid disease. *Surg Gynecol Obstet* 1965;121:851-864.
24. Bekhti A, Schaaps JP, Caprion M, et al: Treatment of hepatic hydatid disease with mebendazole—preliminary results in four cases. *Br Med J* 1977;2:1047-1051.
25. Smego DR, Smego RA Jr: Hydatid cyst—preoperative sterilization with mebendazole. *South Med J* 1986;79:900-901.
26. Ronconi P, Boraone A, Alquati P, et al: Preoperative treatment of hydatid cysts with mebendazole. *Int Surg* 1982;67:405-406.
27. Rausch RL, Wilson JF, McMahon BJ, et al: Consequences of continuous mebendazole therapy in alveolar hydatid disease—with a summary of a ten year clinical trial. *Ann Trop Med Parasitol* 1986;80:403-419.

Emergent Endoscopic Retrograde Cholangiopancreatography

A Highly Specific Test for Acute Pancreatic Trauma

Sharon R. Hayward, MD; Charles E. Lucas, MD; Choichi Sugawa, MD; Anna M. Ledgerwood, MD

• Emergent endoscopic retrograde cholangiopancreatography (ERCP) was assessed as the definitive diagnostic test for acute pancreatic injury in a 23-year-old male automobile driver who sustained blunt abdominal trauma. Despite the patient's quiet, tender abdomen, rising serum amylase level, and an abdominal computed tomographic scan demonstrating probable pancreatic transection, a nonoperative approach was successful when an emergency ERCP demonstrated normal ductal anatomy. This approach is advocated when the presence of a possible pancreatic injury is the only reason for a planned exploratory laparotomy.

(*Arch Surg* 1989;124:745-746)

Endoscopic retrograde cholangiopancreatography (ERCP), a valuable diagnostic test for pancreatic disease, is now being advocated for acute pancreatic trauma.[1] This report highlights a situation where early ERCP permitted successful nonoperative therapy despite abdominal tenderness and computed tomographic (CT) findings indicating transection of the distal pancreas.

REPORT OF A CASE

A 23-year-old man driving his car had a collision with a truck, during which the lower portion of his chest and upper portion of his abdomen bent the steering wheel. He was momentarily unconscious, and findings when he arrived for treatment elsewhere included stable vital signs, multiple facial abrasions, a closed right femur fracture, hypoactive bowel sounds, and diffuse abdominal tenderness greatest in the epigastrium and left upper quadrant (LUQ). Amylase levels at admission were 50 U/L and rose to 240 U/L in two hours. His hemoglobin level was 150 g/L. Chest, abdomen, cervical spine, skull, and pelvis roentgenograms were normal. A peritoneal lavage yielded normal findings (red blood cell count, 4.0×10^{12}/L; no bilirubin; no amylase). A CT scan revealed a probable transverse fracture of the distal pancreas (Fig 1). On transfer to Detroit Receiving Hospital for abdominal exploration, vital signs and hemoglobin level remained stable. Epigastric and LUQ tenderness persisted. His amylase level had risen to 478 U/L. Twelve hours after injury and two hours after arrival to Detroit Receiving Hospital, an emergency ERCP demonstrated a completely normal pancreatic duct without any extravasation (Fig 2). The patient was then treated nonoperatively with nasogastric suction until pain ceased on day 8 when a

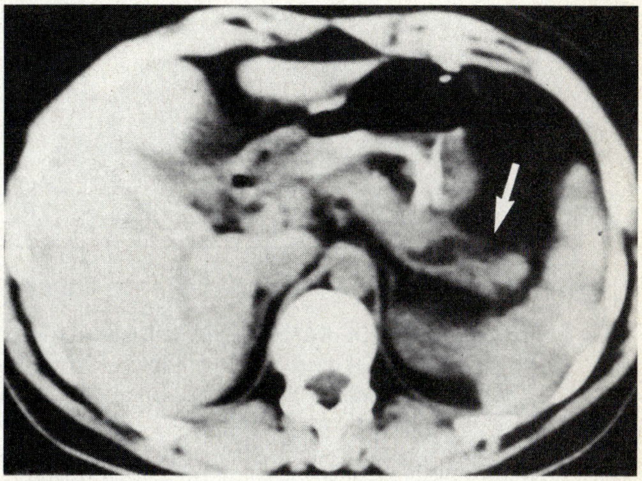

Fig 1.—Abdominal computed tomographic scan demonstrating probable transverse fracture of distal pancreas (arrow).

Fig 2.—Endoscopic retrograde pancreatography with pancreatogram demonstrating an intact ductal system without extravasation of dye.

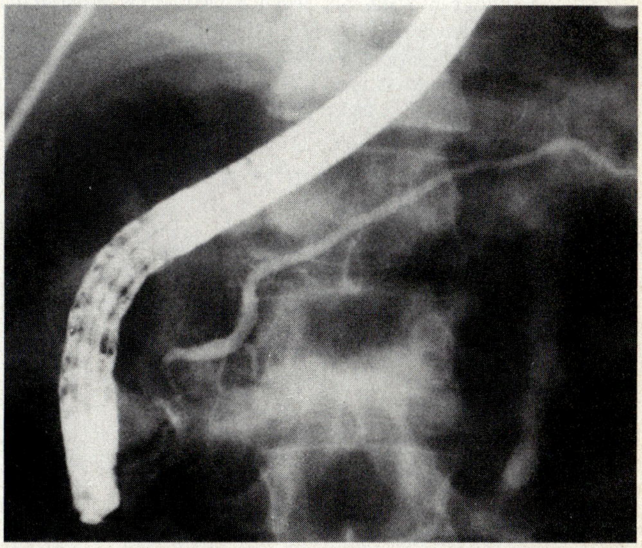

Accepted for publication June 15, 1988.
From the Department of Surgery, Wayne State University, Detroit.
Reprint requests to Department of Surgery, 6-C University Health Center, 4201 Saint Antoine, Detroit, MI 48201 (Dr Lucas).

progressive diet was started. Amylase level peaked on day 2 at 490 U/L and then decreased to 160 U/L by day 6. After operative fixation of the femur fracture on day 8, he was discharged home on day 14. Follow-up abdominal CT scan and serum amylase level at six weeks were normal.

COMMENT

Blunt pancreatic trauma must be suspected after all severe injuries. When associated intraperitoneal injuries are absent, the decision to explore for suspected pancreatic injury is based on abdominal tenderness and a rising serum amylase level as the earliest clues.[2] Both were present in this patient who, in the past, would have undergone laparotomy. Emergency ERCP in the face of abdominal tenderness, a quiet abdomen, a rising serum amylase level, and a CT scan showing probable pancreatic transection was done to define the extent and site of ductal injury. Identification of an intact ductal system permitted successful nonoperative therapy.

Thus, an emergency ERCP is proposed as the definitive test for pancreatic injury in patients in stable condition who do not require laparotomy for other reasons. Emergency ERCP is best done within 12 hours of injury since early treatment of confirmed pancreatic injuries reduces morbidity and mortality.[2] When laparotomy is performed for other injuries, intraoperative ERCP would define ductal anatomy without resorting to duodenotomy for ductography. Emergency preoperative ERCP or intraoperative ERCP is advocated in patients in stable condition with suspected pancreatic trauma.

This study was supported by the Interstitial Fluid Fund, Detroit, Account No. 444966.

References

1. Barkin JS, Ferstenberg RM, Panullo W, et al: Endoscopic retrograde cholangiopancreatography in pancreatic trauma. *Gastrointest Endosc* 1988;34:102-105.

2. Lucas CE: Diagnosis and treatment of pancreatic and duodenal injury. *Surg Clin North Am* 1977;57:49-65.

In Other AMA Journals

ARCHIVES OF PATHOLOGY & LABORATORY MEDICINE

Expression of Pan-Neuroendocrine Proteins in 53 Neuroblastic Tumors: An Immunohistochemical Study With Neuron-Specific Enolase, Chromogranin, and Synaptophysin

Yoichi Hachitanda, MD; Masazumi Tsuneyoshi, MD; Munetomo Enjoji, MD

The presence and distribution of pan-neuroendocrine markers such as neuron-specific enolase (NSE), chromogranin (CG), and synaptophysin (SYP) were investigated by immunohistochemistry in 53 cases of neuroblastic tumors, including three cases of ganglioneuromas, 17 ganglioneuroblastomas, and 33 neuroblastomas. In ganglioneuromas, all three markers were observed both in ganglion cells and in neurofibrils. All cases of ganglioneuroblastoma were positive for these markers, however, some variability of staining intensity was noted. Of the 33 cases of neuroblastomas, all were positive for NSE, 23 (70%) for CG, and 31 (94%) for SYP. Neuron-specific enolase was detected not only in the majority of the neuroblasts showing signs of differentiation, but also in some undifferentiated neuroblasts. Chromogranin was found mainly in differentiated neuroblasts with enlarged cytoplasm and nuclei, but was scarcely found in undifferentiated cells. Synaptophysin was detected in some undifferentiated neuroblasts, as well as in differentiated neuroblasts. Two cases without SYP-positive cells were also negative for CG. Our observations conclude that antibodies against NSE and SYP are helpful as a diagnostic aid for neuroblastic tumors. (*Arch Pathol Lab Med.* 1989; 113:381-384).

Percutaneous Transhepatic Ultrasonic Cholelithotripsy

Anurag K. Das, MD; John L. Weinerth, MD; Steven C. Rose, MD; R. Randal Bollinger, MD, PhD

• **In a patient with acute cholecystitis whose body habitus precluded cholecystectomy, we used percutaneous transhepatic ultrasonic cholelithotripsy. We compare it with other modalities applicable in such cases. Although not commonly used, these alternatives may be the most appropriate therapy in certain unusual circumstances.**
(*Arch Surg* 1989;124:747-748)

In addition to the usual open surgical techniques, the treatment of renal calculi now includes various types of lithotripsy: extracorporeal shock wave, electrohydraulic, ultrasonic, and laser. These modalities can also be adapted to the treatment of gallstones, although most of the reported cases in the literature depict their use in the treatment of retained cystic duct and common bile duct stones. However, there has been limited experience in the fragmentation of gallstones by extracorporeal shock wave lithotripsy[1,2] and rapid dissolution of stones by instillation of methyl tert-butyl ether.[3] We present the use of percutaneous transhepatic ultrasonic cholelithotripsy in a patient whose body habitus precluded cholecystectomy or extracorporeal shock wave lithotripsy, and where stone calcium content did not allow dissolution.

REPORT OF A CASE

A 69-year-old man presented with an eight-day history of worsening epigastric and right-sided abdominal pain, fever, nausea, and vomiting. Medical history was remarkable for a coal-mining accident with "crush" injury to the spine resulting in disability due to severe kyphoscoliosis and hip angulation. Physical examination revealed an elderly man in moderate distress. The patient had a blood pressure of 110/70 mm Hg, respiratory rate of 24 breaths per minute, pulse of 100 beats per minute and regular, and temperature of 38.9° C. Abdominal examination revealed bilateral compression of the rib cage on the pelvis with almost no room between the right subcostal margin and the iliac crest. There was right-sided tenderness to palpation but no signs of peritoneal irritation. Laboratory studies revealed a white blood cell count of 11.6×10^9/L (normal, 4.5 to 10.5×10^9/L) with a left shift, normal hemoglobin level, normal serum chemistry results, aspartate aminotransferase level of 118 U/L (normal, 5 to 35 U/L), alanine aminotransferase level of 68 U/L (normal, 5 to 35 U/L), total bilirubin level of 22 μmol/L (normal, 3 to 21 μmol/L), and normal amylase level. An intravenous urogram was normal, and abdominal ultrasound revealed a 2-cm gallstone impacted at the cystic duct.

The patient was given intravenous antibiotics and transferred to our facility for further care. At our institution, abdominal computed tomography (Fig 1) revealed a thick-walled, dilated gallbladder, two gallstones with lamellated calcification (one impacted in the neck of the gallbladder and a second in the fundus), and pericholecystic fluid, all consistent with acute cholecystitis.

Since the patient's body habitus precluded a cholecystectomy, a percutaneous transhepatic 7.0F pigtail catheter was placed in the body of the gallbladder and 150 mL of purulent, sludge-laden bile was aspirated. A tube cholecystocholangiogram demonstrated two gallstones (2.5 and 1.0 cm in diameter). With the cholecystostomy tube left on external drainage, the patient was discharged for two weeks, then readmitted; he underwent dilation of the cholecystostomy tract with serial dilators with sheaths (Amplatz dilators) to 26F. A 24F Foley catheter and a 5F Kumpe catheter were then placed in the gallbladder through the Amplatz sheath. In addition, an 11.5-mm deflated venous occlusion balloon catheter was negotiated into the cystic duct (Fig 2).

Two days later the patient was taken to the operating room. Using general anesthesia, the Foley and Kumpe catheters were exchanged over heavy guide wires for a 26F Amplatz sheath. The cystic duct venous occlusion balloon catheter was inflated, and a

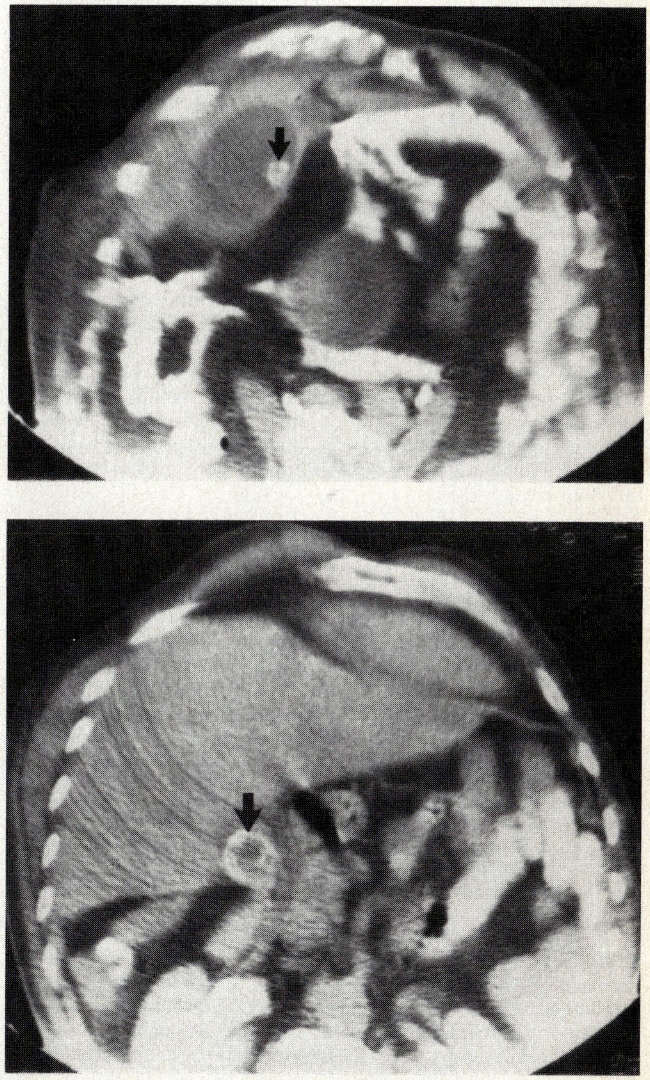

Fig 1.—Abdominal computed tomographic scan. Top, Near gallbladder fundus, at approximate level of subsequent percutaneous cholecystostomy; 1-cm lamellated calculus and thickened gallbladder wall (arrow). Bottom, Gallbladder neck with impacted 2.5-cm calcified calculus (arrow). Pericholecystic fluid present on sections between top and bottom.

Accepted for publication Aug 29, 1988.
From the Divisions of Urology (Drs Das and Weinerth) and General Surgery (Dr Bollinger) and the Department of Radiology (Dr Rose), Duke University Medical Center, Durham, NC.
Reprint requests to Box 3343, Duke University Medical Center, Durham, NC 27710 (Dr Weinerth).

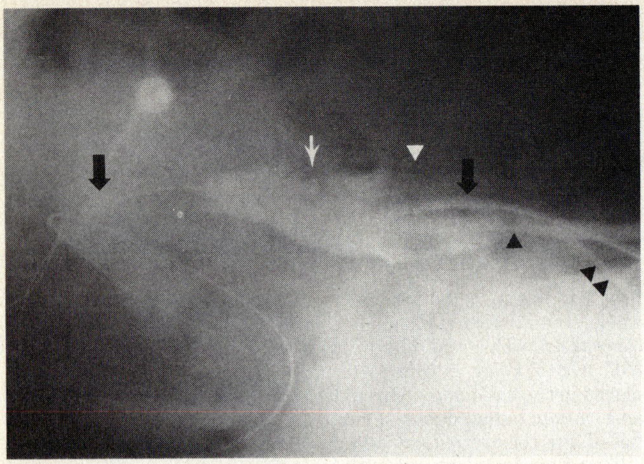

Fig 2.—Lateral view cholecystogram before gallstone lithotripsy; patient's head to left. During catheter manipulations, calculus positions reversed such that 2.5-cm stone (white arrowhead) lies in gallbladder fundus and 1.0-cm stone (white arrow) resides near gallbladder neck; 24F Foley catheter (black arrowhead) and 5F Kumpe catheter (double black arrowhead) reside in gallbladder; venous occlusion balloon catheter (black arrows) is inflated with tip in cystic duct and guide wire into common bile duct and duodenum. Incidental electrocardiographic lead superiorly.

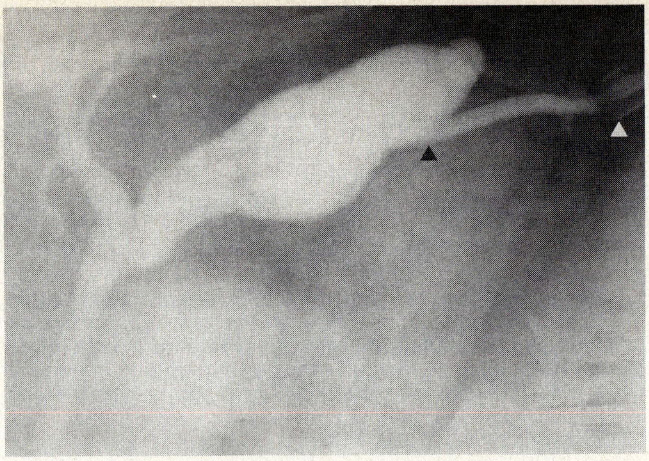

Fig 3.—True lateral view, cholecystogram following gallstone lithotripsy; 24F Foley catheter (black arrowhead) is inflated within gallbladder. Back-loaded 26F Amplatz sheath (white arrowhead) lies outside patient. No evidence of residual gallstones; free flow into common bile duct. No apparent biliary debris. Incidental film processor artifact (dark horizontal stripes).

24.5F Wolf nephroscope was placed in the gallbladder over a heavy guide wire. A 3.5-mm ultrasonic probe was then used to fragment the gallstones under direct vision, and the fragments were aspirated through the suction port. The procedure was uncomplicated. A 24F Foley catheter was left in the gallbladder for drainage. A tube cholecystocholangiogram on the second postoperative day (Fig 3) showed no retained fragments and free flow of contrast through the cystic and common bile ducts into the duodenum.

Before discharge on the fourth postoperative day, the 24F Foley catheter was exchanged for an 11F nephrostomy-type self-retaining catheter. One week later, a repeated tube cholecystocholangiogram was normal, and the cholecystostomy tube was removed. The patient remains asymptomatic and has a normal bilirubin level.

COMMENT

Cholecystectomy remains the accepted treatment of symptomatic cholelithiasis and cholecystitis. Percutaneous transhepatic electrohydraulic lithotripsy,[4] endoscopic mechanical and electrohydraulic lithotripsy,[5] and extracorporeal shock wave lithotripsy[6,7] have all been utilized in the treatment of retained cystic duct and common bile duct stones. In addition, Gacetta et al[8] reported two cases of ultrasonic lithotripsy of noncalcified gallstones after surgical cholecystostomy. These cases were done in a manner similar to ours except that the cystic duct was not occluded during the procedure.

Our patient's anatomy made it impossible to perform a cholecystectomy, and since the patient had percutaneous access, it was much easier to perform a percutaneous lithotripsy rather than to attempt a retrograde endoscopic procedure. The patient's anatomy also precluded extracorporeal shock wave lithotripsy on the Dornier HM-3 machine, and although the second-generation machines such as the Wolf Piezolith 2200 may not have been limited by the patient's anatomy, they are not used to treat calcified gallstones. Ultrasonic fragmentation of stones was chosen because the 3.5-mm hollow ultrasound probe allows suctioning capability, reducing the chance for small fragments to accumulate and possibly obstruct the cystic duct or the common bile duct ("steinstrasse" phenomenon, from the German word for street of stone).

References

1. Sauerbruch T, Delius M, Paumgartner G, et al: Fragmentation of gallstones by extracorporeal shock waves. *N Engl J Med* 1986;314:818-822.
2. Brown B, Loening S, Johlin F, et al: Fragmentation of biliary tract stones by lithotripsy using local anesthesia. *Arch Surg* 1988;123:91-93.
3. Allen M, Borody T, Bugliosi T, et al: Rapid dissolution of gallstones by methyl tert-butyl ether. *N Engl J Med* 1985;312:217-220.
4. Lear J, Ring E, Macoviak J, et al: Percutaneous transhepatic electrohydraulic lithotripsy. *Radiology* 1984;150:589-590.
5. Riemann J, Demling L: Lithotripsy of bile duct stones. *Endoscopy* 1983;15:191-196.
6. Becker C, Fache J, Gibney R, et al: Treatment of retained cystic duct stones using extracorporeal shockwave lithotripsy. *AJR* 1987;148:1121-1122.
7. Gelfand D, McCullough D, Myers R, et al: Choledocholithiasis: Successful treatment with extracorporeal lithotripsy. *AJR* 1986;148:1114-1116.
8. Gacetta D, Cohen M, Crummy A, et al: Ultrasonic lithotripsy of gallstones after cholecystostomy. *AJR* 1984;143:1088-1089.

Editorial Comment

This article is representative of a spate of reports that describe alternatives to cholecystectomy. In this instance, the patient's body habitus precluded cholecystectomy. The acute infection was treated by percutaneous cholecystostomy, which is being used experimentally in critically ill patients who develop acute cholecystitis after surgery or trauma or during another illness. The stones were fragmented by ultrasonic lithotripsy and removed by manual extraction. The authors discuss the currently available techniques for breaking up stones and removing them from the gallbladder. Although the treatment was effective in this unique circumstance, the report raises broader issues of importance to those who care for patients with biliary tract disease. Will one or a combination of high-technology procedures replace cholecystectomy for acute cholecystitis? Which procedure is safest and least troublesome for the patient? Changes in the management of biliary tract disease are inevitable because of the availability of these new techniques. Carefully designed, prospective studies must be done to determine the safest and most effective procedures. As surgeons, our skepticism is healthy, but we must not close our minds to the likelihood of change, and we must be at the forefront in conducting the necessary studies.

David L. Nahrwold, MD
Chicago

Argon Laser Treatment of Radiation Proctitis

John J. O'Connor, MD

• **Radiation therapy for malignant gynecologic disease and prostatic cancer has resulted in increased survival and cure rates. This modality has unfortunately produced debilitating radiation proctitis. Recently, five patients were seen with continuous rectal bleeding secondary to radiation disease of the rectum. Four of these patients were women who were being treated for cervical carcinoma and one was a man with prostatic cancer. These patients were refractory to steroid retention enemas, iron therapy, and benproperine enema therapy. Treatment was accomplished using the argon laser with a 300-μm fiber passed via flexible fiberoptic sigmoidoscope. The most proximal areas were treated first. One and a half watts at 0.5 pulses was used. Up to 50 pulses were delivered per therapy session. The fiber was placed in contact with the lesion and circumferentially for 0.5 cm surrounding each suspected area. Bleeding stopped in the four women after two sessions and in the man after four sessions.**

(*Arch Surg* 1989;124:749)

Radiation therapy for malignant gynecologic disease and prostatic cancer has resulted in increased survival and cure rates. This modality has unfortunately produced debilitating radiation proctitis. The bleeding that results from the proctitis can and does produce severe anemia that often requires replacement blood therapy. Recently, five patients were seen with continuous rectal bleeding secondary to radiation disease of the rectum. Four of these patients were women who were being treated for cervical carcinoma, and one was a man with prostatic cancer. These patients were refractory to steroid retention enemas, iron therapy, and benproperine enema therapy.

Three patients underwent endoscopy to ascertain the linear extent of the proctitis. Disease in all three patients was confined to the distal 30 cm of the colorectum. Treatment was accomplished using the argon laser with a 300-μm fiber passed via a flexible fiberoptic sigmoidoscope. The most proximal areas were treated first. One and a half watts at 0.5-s pulses was used. Up to 50 pulses were delivered per therapy session. The fiber was placed in contact with the lesion and circumferentially for 0.5 cm surrounding each suspected area.

Bleeding stopped in the four women after two sessions and in the man after four sessions. They were treated as outpatients, and did not require analgesic therapy. The patients have remained free of bleeding for five months without the use of medication.

The argon laser is well suited for the type of procedure performed on these patients. The vessels are superficial, requiring a 1- to 3-mm depth of coagulation and are usually small. Using telangiectasia as a model where the argon laser therapy is most effective, radiation proctitis should have a similar result.[1] These five cases seem to add proof to this hypothesis, at least in short-term follow-up. It seems that this method of coagulation could be used in the management of an ever-increasing group of patients.

Accepted for publication May 24, 1988.

From the Section of Colorectal Surgery, Suburban Hospital, Bethesda, Md.

Reprint requests to 4801 Massachusetts Ave NW, Suite 205, Washington, DC 20016 (Dr O'Connor).

Reference

1. Apfelberg DB, Smith T, Maser M, et al: The argon laser for cutaneous lesions. *JAMA* 1981;245:2073-2075.

YOU CAN'T WASH YOUR HANDS OF DRUG ABUSE.

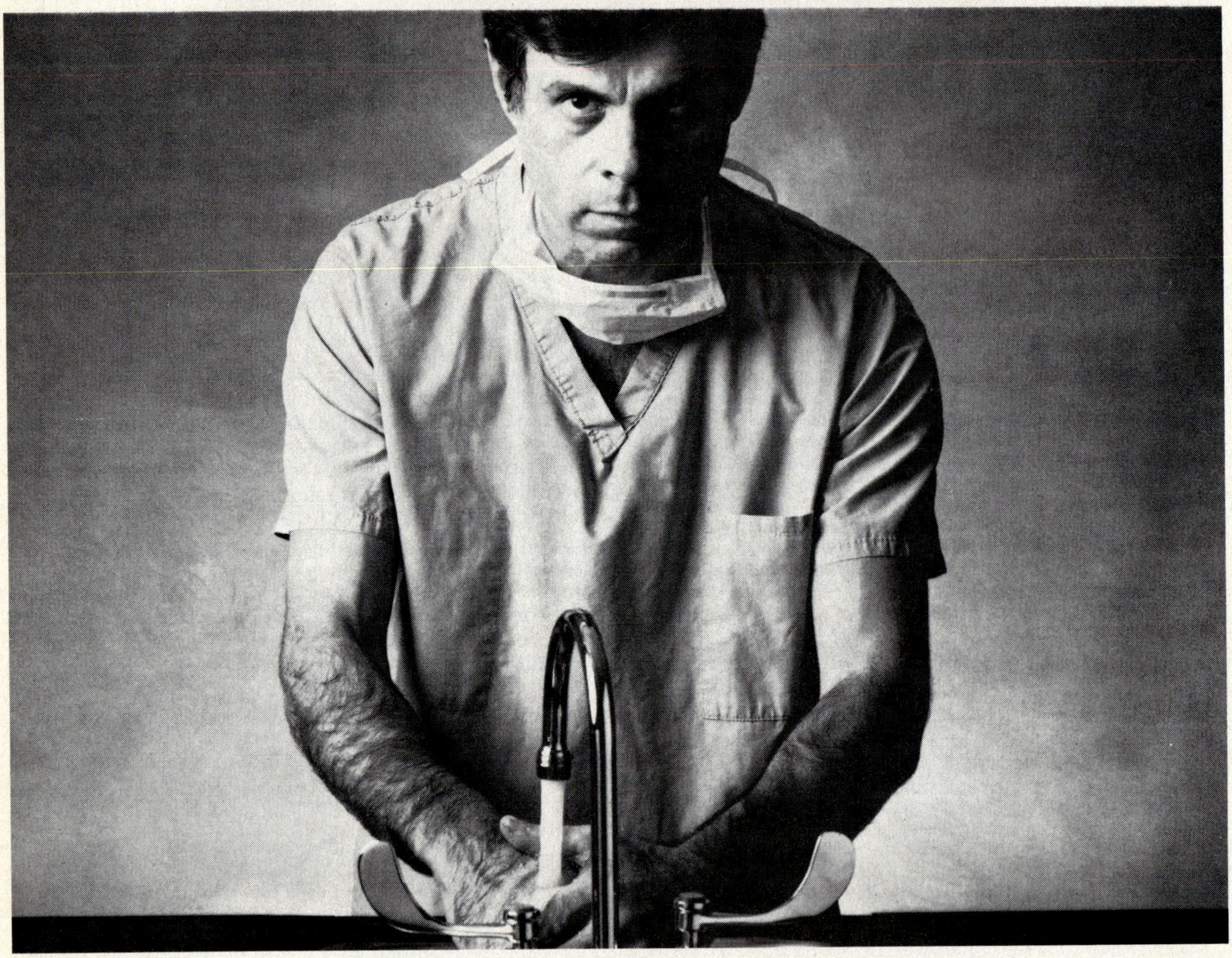

Your skill can save a life; your involvement can make life more worth living.

Surgeons prolong life. But, if your patients use illegal drugs, your hard work could be wasted. As a healer, your responsibility to your patients extends beyond the operating room. Make the most of your unique physician-patient relationship. Ask patients about their use of illegal drugs. Do it routinely. Remember, they trust you with their lives.

HELP FIGHT ILLEGAL DRUG USE. IT'S YOUR RESPONSIBILITY.

Partnership for a Drug-Free America

Pain on Coughing and Numbness in Sciatica: What Exactly Do These Symptoms Mean?

To the Editor.—In sciatica, pain on coughing and segmental numbness are generally known symptoms. They are often mentioned in the literature, but their nature and clinical meaning have never been exactly defined. The new approach to the study of clinical findings in relation to disk changes, by lumbar diskography in our material,[1,2] has not been generally noticed and understood, and it is significant that 22 book reviews on the monograph,[2] in various journals, comment on the morphologic diagnosis but not on the analysis of the clinical findings.

Pain on coughing is found in disk rupture, the gelatinous contents of the nucleus pulposus being squeezed out of the disk to spread around the nerve root where they cause aseptic inflammation; it appears about one week after onset of the complaints. Numbness, however, is found in nerve compression, when a nonruptured disk exerts pressure to the root (these patients have no pain on coughing), or when particles of fibrous tissue dislocated through a disk rupture compress the root (with both numbness and pain on coughing present). This suggests that the clinical picture of sciatica is composed of two elements—the syndrome of nerve irritation (radiculitis) and the syndrome of nerve compression—or that there is a combination of both. The other symptoms and signs are nonspecific, but, in various forms of disk lesions, differ in intensity and persistence in the decourse of a case.

Pain on coughing can thus be defined as a symptom of radiculitis caused by disk rupture; treatment is conservative. Numbness is a symptom of nerve root compression in various forms of disk lesions, some of which may require surgical intervention. This knowledge, gained with the aid of diskography, contributes to a systematic evaluation of sciatica, without the need for diskography itself to be performed in the clinical routine. It seems justified to bring this to the attention of the clinic, as new detailed studies of the clinical picture in diskographic material are unlikely to appear, the attention of the clinic at present being turned to computerized tomography and nuclear magnetic resonance.

L. Walk, MD
Solna, Sweden

1. Walk L: Diagnostic lumbar disk puncture: Clinical review and analysis of 67 cases. *Arch Surg* 1953;66:232-243.
2. Walk L. *Lumbar Diskography and Its Clinical Evaluation.* Springfield, Ill: Charles C. Thomas Publishers; 1962.

Away With Leniency Toward Gastric Pseudolymphoma

To the Editor.—Since its description in 1958, approximately 200 cases of gastric pseudolymphoma (GPL) have been reported. Gastric pseudolymphoma is regarded basically as a benign condition, although various authors have speculated on its potential for malignant transformation. Over the years, several reports associating GPL with malignant lymphoma have been published, thus implying that GPL may be a premalignant condition.[1-6] Nevertheless, to date, guidelines for treatment of GPL remain lenient.

Report of a Case.—We recently performed a subtotal gastrectomy on a 37-year-old woman who we had been observing for 20 years and in whom the diagnosis of GPL had been made, supported by repeated gastroscopic biopsy specimens. After many years of refusal, the patient finally agreed to undergo surgery, hoping to achieve the symptomatic relief that the numerous conservative treatments she had undergone had failed. At laparotomy, the gastric antrum was grossly thickened, and regional lymphadenopathy was noted. Histologic examination of the resected stomach revealed typical GPL (Figs 1 and 2), within which microscopic foci of malignant lymphoma (diffuse small cleaved cell type, poorly differentiated lymphocytic lymphoma) were detected (Figs 3 and 4). The regional lymph nodes showed reactive changes only.

Comment.—This is the 11th reported case, to our knowledge, associating GPL and malignant lymphoma. It is unique in that the histologic findings demonstrate the emergence of microscopic foci of malignant lymphoma within the bulky GPL, thus indicating malignant transformation in long-standing GPL.

Having recognized the premalignant potential of GPL, we believe that a change in our attitude toward this lesion and in the recommendations for its management is mandatory, and we suggest the following:

1. The data presented herein, together with those accumulated in the literature, strongly point to the affirmative resolution of the debate regarding the possibility of malignant transformation in GPL.
2. The true incidence of this malignant change remains unknown; data collected from the literature imply an incidence of roughly 5.5% (11/200 cases).
3. According to the data from the various cases, the lead time from the onset of symptoms to the occurrence of this malignant change differs within wide margins, but it may be as short as three months.
4. Contrary to the general concept in the literature, we believe that GPL may be diagnosed with near certainty by gastroscopic biopsy, provided that multiple deep biopsy specimens that include the submucosa are taken and cryostat immunoperoxidase studies are utilized.[7]
5. On the other hand, we presently have no absolutely reliable means for histologically monitoring GPL for the occurrence of malignant transformation, since the latter occurs in microscopic foci that are situated deep within the bulky GPL and give no corresponding changes on the mucosal surface that could help direct our bi-

Fig 1.—Transmural photomicrograph of gastric wall showing typical pseudolymphoma. Note numerous germinal centers (hematoxylin-eosin, original magnification ×40).

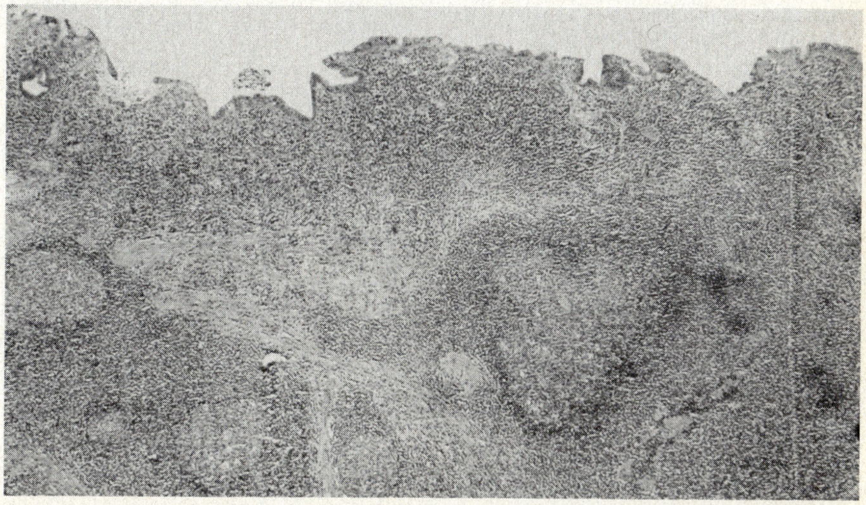

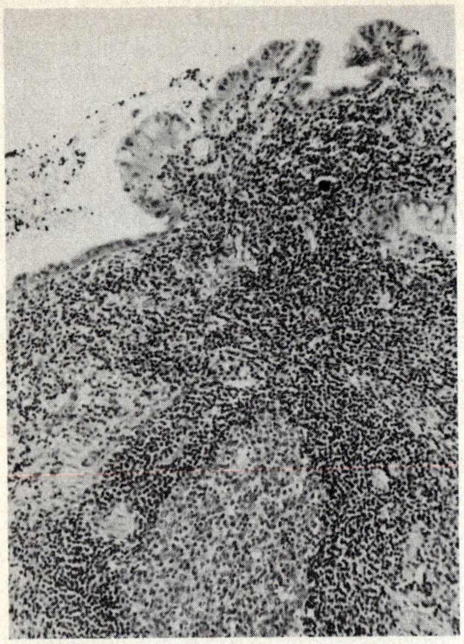

Fig 2.—Photomicrograph of lymphoid follicle with germinal center in lamina propria (hematoxylin-eosin, original magnification ×200).

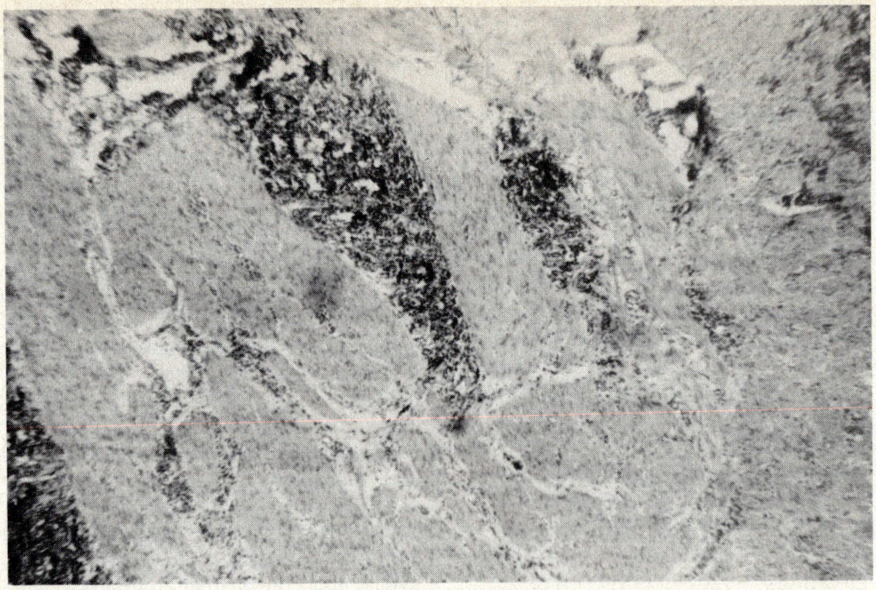

Fig 3.—Photomicrograph of gastric wall implying transformation to focal gastric lymphoma. Note muscle-fiber destruction by lymphocytic infiltrate (hematoxylin-eosin, original magnification ×200).

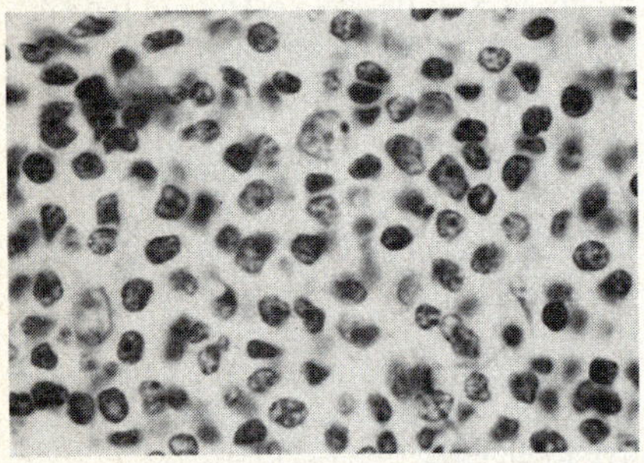

Fig 4.—Photomicrograph of focus of malignant lymphoma within gastric pseudolymphoma. Note atypical lymphocytes with prominent nucleoli and pleomorphism (hematoxylin-eosin, original magnification ×1000).

opsy. Thus, although the lesion is readily accessible to repeated gastroscopic biopsies, these would be truly random biopsies and of doubtful credibility when the results are negative.

6. We believe that in the face of a less-than-optimal ability to monitor a premalignant lesion for occurrence of malignant transformation, there is a place for consideration of prophylactic resective surgery. In fact, in case of future malignant transformation with an unfavorable outcome, not having given the patient a clear presentation of the facts and an opportunity to consider the option of early surgery might even be regarded as negligent.

7. Accordingly, we believe that the traditionally lenient attitude toward GPL should be abandoned, and a more aggressive approach adopted. The above-mentioned facts should be clearly presented to patients, and the option for early gastric resection should be discussed. Ideally, the resection should be radical to the extent of removing all diseased tissue, but the surgical procedure should be tailored to the individual case (eg, to avoid the potential complications associated with an esophageal anastomosis in cases of GPL that involve the proximal stomach). Keeping in mind the possibility of lymphoma, preoperative and intraoperative staging measures are appropriate (eg, computed tomographic scans, bone marrow studies, and regional lymph node sampling/dissection).

Ahud Sternberg, MD
Arnon Koren, MD
Uri Kadish, MD
Judith Sandbank, MD
Raphael Reiss, MD
Petah Tiqva, Israel

1. Faris TD, Saltzstein SL: Gastric lymphoid hyperplasia: A lesion confused with lymphosarcoma. *Cancer* 1964;17:207-212.
2. Case reports of the Massachusetts General Hospital: Case 39–1975. *N Engl J Med* 1975;293:712-717.
3. Vanden Heule B, Van Kerkem C, Heimann R: Benign and malignant lymphoid lesions of the stomach: A histological reappraisal in the light of the Kiel classification for non-Hodgkin's lymphomas. *Histopathology* 1979;3:309-320.
4. Wolf JA Jr, Spjut HJ: Focal lymphoid hyperplasia of the stomach preceding gastric lymphoma: Case report and review of the literature. *Cancer* 1981;48:2518-2523.
5. Brooks JJ, Enterline HT: Gastric pseudolymphoma: Its three subtypes and relation to lymphoma. *Cancer* 1983;51:476-486.
6. Orr RK, Lininger JR, Lawrence W: Gastric pseudolymphoma: A challenging clinical problem. *Ann Surg* 1984;200:185-194.
7. Sternberg A: Diagnosing gastric pseudolymphoma by gastroscopic biopsy. *Gastrointest Endosc* 1987;33:397.

Staple Line Healing in Gastric Surgery

To the Editor.—Dr Ravitch's reply to my communication[1,2] requires clarification.

I certainly do not feel that patients' behavior is to blame for leaks and perforations following bariatric surgery. However, their noncompliance may well be a factor in early, and possibly even late, staple line disruption after gastric partitioning. This is an entirely different situation. Leaks and perforations are life-threatening but staple line disruptions usually are not. A small disruption may only be apparent on upper gastrointestinal tract endoscopy or barium studies, but if the disruption is large, then gastric restriction will be lost. After a small disruption, the whole staple line could "unzip." If restriction is lost, the operation usually fails, particularly if this occurs in the early postoperative stage.

We know little about staple line healing in the morbidly obese human's stomach. If gastric restriction is going to be successful, even in carefully selected cases, knowledge of the time taken and the technique necessary to produce the strongest staple line possible is vitally important knowledge both for the bariatric surgeon and patient.

Eoghan R. T. C. Owen, FRCS
Harrow, Middlesex, England

1. Owen ERTC: Experimental evaluation of staple lines in gastric surgery. *Arch Surg* 1988;123:912.
2. Ravitch MM: Experimental evaluation of staple lines in gastric surgery. *Arch Surg* 1988;123:912.